WOMEN'S GYNECOLOGIC HEALTH

THIRD EDITION

KERRI DURNELL SCHUILING, PhD, NP-BC, CNM, FACNM, FAAN
Provost and Vice President of Academic Affairs
Northern Michigan University
Marquette, Michigan
Co-Editor-in-Chief
International Journal of Childbirth

FRANCES E. LIKIS, DrPH, NP-BC, CNM, FACNM, FAAN
Editor-in-Chief
Journal of Midwifery & Women's Health
Adjunct Assistant Professor of Nursing
Vanderbilt University
Nashville, Tennessee

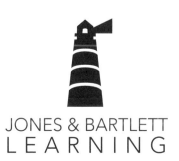

JONES & BARTLETT
LEARNING

World Headquarters
Jones & Bartlett Learning
5 Wall Street
Burlington, MA 01803
978-443-5000
info@jblearning.com
www.jblearning.com

Jones & Bartlett Learning books and products are available through most bookstores and online booksellers. To contact Jones & Bartlett Learning directly, call 800-832-0034, fax 978-443-8000, or visit our website, www.jblearning.com.

07891-6

Production Credits

VP, Executive Publisher: David D. Cella
Executive Editor: Amanda Martin
Acquisitions Editor: Teresa Reilly
Editorial Assistant: Danielle Bessette
Production Editor: Vanessa Richards
Marketing Communications Manager: Katie Hennessy
Product Fulfillment Manager: Wendy Kilborn
Composition: S4Carlisle Publishing Services
Cover Design: Kristin E. Parker
Director of Rights and Media: Joanna Lundeen
Rights & Media Specialist: Wes DeShano

Media Development Editor: Troy Liston
Printing and Binding: Edwards Brothers Malloy
Cover Printing: Edwards Brothers Malloy
Cover Image: Symbol: The symbol on the cover is adapted from *The Changer* by K Robins and is used with the permission of K Robins Designs. The editors are very grateful to K Robins for allowing us to adapt her design for our cover, and we encourage readers to visit www.krobinsdesigns.com where *The Changer* and other symbols are available as pendants. Background: © Evgenii Iaroshevskii/Shutterstock.

Library of Congress Cataloging-in-Publication Data
Names: Schuiling, Kerri Durnell, editor. | Likis, Frances E., editor.
Title: Women's gynecologic health / [edited by] Kerri Durnell Schuiling, Frances E. Likis.
Description: Third edition. | Burlington, Massachusetts : Jones & Bartlett Learning, [2017] | Includes bibliographical references and index.
Identifiers: LCCN 2016005174 | ISBN 9781284076028 (hardcover)
Subjects: | MESH: Genital Diseases, Female | Women's Health | Reproductive Physiological Processes
Classification: LCC RG101 | NLM WP 140 | DDC 618.1--dc23
LC record available at http://lccn.loc.gov/2016005174

6048

Printed in the United States of America
20 19 18 17 16   10 9 8 7 6 5 4 3 2 1

Dedication

To:

The indomitable Kitty Ernst, thank you for encouraging us to always look for ways to improve women's health care;

Our students and the women for whom we have provided care, thank you for being our best teachers;

The readers who have told us what you appreciate about our book, thank you for inspiring us as we worked on this edition; and

Our colleagues, friends, and family members who have been encouraging and patient throughout the labor of this edition. There are too many to mention each of you by name, but you know that we know who you are. We truly appreciate the support you provided.

—Kerri and Francie

To:

The memory of my dear friend Judy Pennington Adams, her granddaughter Tiffany and great-grandson Kyson, and their good friend Charlene Lewis, who were all taken from us far too soon;

Rachael Stade, MS, PA-C, for providing me with outstanding woman-centered health care;

Joani and Lisa, whose friendship supports me in ways too many to mention;

Donovan, for his unconditional love and friendship;

Judd, for his companionship and humor;

My parents, Marie and Don Hall, whose belief that I can do anything makes me believe that I can; and

My children and sons-in-law, Mary, Mike, Sean, Sarah, and Galen, who bring me life's greatest joys.

—Kerri

To:

My husband Zan, you are the one I love more with each passing day, and we make a formidable team;

My nieces Katherine and Elizabeth, my sister Mary, and my mother Katey, you are my favorite girls in the whole wide world;

My grandmother Frances, you are such an important part of who I am, and your determination and perseverance never cease to amaze me;

Ali, you are my trusted confidante and keep me hopeful about the future of midwifery;

Christy, you are a wonderful companion for adventures and an endless source of kindness;

The community of St. Augustine's Episcopal Chapel, especially our leaders Becca and Lissa, you embody love, mercy, and radical hospitality, and you help me find my way home.

—Francie

CONTENTS

PREFACE

Historically, women's health was framed within a biomedical model by clinicians. Textbooks typically used a biomedical framework to present women's health content. Although this approach can be useful on many levels, it also has limitations that can have significant negative effects on women's health, particularly gynecologic health. A biomedical model is disease oriented and focuses on curing illness—an approach that risks pathologizing normal aspects of female physiology. When a biomedical lens is used to assess women's health, there is a risk of essentializing women and reducing them to their biologic parts. As an example of this proclivity, *women's health* is frequently used to mean reproductive health, regardless of whether the woman plans to bear children. This reductionism transfers to practice when a woman's parts become the focus of diagnosis and treatment. The meaning of the diagnosis to the woman, as well as the impact that the diagnosis has on her, her significant others, and the work she does, is not addressed in this approach.

Feminist theories about women's growth and development provide a different perspective from earlier male-oriented models because they include women's lived experiences and the importance of relationships to women. Recognizing each woman as an expert knower supports women's agency. The focus with this approach is holistic, with health being assessed within the context of each woman's life.

It is important for our readers to know that we, as the editors of this book, are experienced women's health clinicians whose practice philosophy is grounded in caring for the whole woman within her lived experience. As teachers, we were repeatedly frustrated by our inability to locate a gynecologic textbook that we felt was suitable for our course. Many of the books that were available were written primarily from a biomedical perspective and, in our opinion, did not provide sufficient content about the normalcy of women's reproductive physiology. Books such as those authored by the Boston Women's Health Book Collective were extremely helpful with ideas about health and holism, but lacked the necessary content to educate student clinicians. Other books did not provide the health-oriented perspective that is vital to the philosophy of care espoused by nursing and midwifery, in which we both strongly believe. Additional books provided elements of both biomedical and health-oriented views and had very useful decision trees or categorization of concerns or problems. However, we felt that these books would not encourage students and practicing clinicians to think critically and to appreciate the importance of making decisions based on the most recent evidence.

For these myriad reasons, we embarked on producing a book that presents women's gynecologic health from a woman-centered and holistic viewpoint. Our goal was to create a book that emphasizes the importance of respecting the normalcy of female physiology, and provides clinical content appropriate for assessment, diagnosis, and treatment of pathology. We believe this book embodies these perspectives and underlines the importance of collaboration among clinicians.

Some aspects of this feminist approach will be obvious to our readers, whereas others may be more subtle. For example, we used illustrations of whole women, rather than pictures of only breasts or genitalia, when possible. We refer to a woman who has a specific condition rather than referring to the woman by her condition. For example, we speak of the woman who has HIV, as opposed to the HIV-positive woman. We use the term *birth* as opposed to *delivery* because it situates the power to give birth within the woman versus transferring it to the clinician. We purposefully use *women's* rather than *gynecologic* as the first word of this book's title. Our intention in making these deliberate choices was to encourage readers to keep first in their mind that they are treating a whole woman, not her body parts, and not just a condition. We hope that this approach emphasizes the importance of treating women holistically within their lived experiences.

We were fortunate to have many excellent contributors to this book. Some are nationally known; others might be new to many readers. The common thread among all of our contributors is their expertise in their respective areas and their recognition of the importance of evidence-based practice. Our contributors are expert clinicians, educators, and scientists. Frequently co-authored chapters represent a clinician and researcher team, whose collaboration provides readers with a real-world view that is grounded in evidence.

This book encompasses both health promotion and management of gynecologic conditions that women experience. All of the content is evidence based. The first section introduces the feminist framework that permeates the book and provides readers with a context for evaluating evidence and determining best practice. The second section provides a foundation for assessment and promotion of women's gynecologic health. The third section addresses the evaluation and management of clinical conditions frequently encountered in gynecologic health care. The fourth section provides an introduction to prenatal and postpartum care.

We are gratified by how well the first two editions of this book were received by clinicians, students, and faculty, and it was an honor to receive the Book of the Year Award from the American College of Nurse-Midwives for both previous editions. In this third edition of *Women's Gynecologic Health,* we have updated, and in many cases extensively revised, all of the chapters from the second edition to ensure comprehensive content that reflects current standards of care. For example, the chapter on health care for individuals who are lesbian, bisexual, queer, or transgender has been extensively updated, as have the chapters on intimate partner violence and sexual assault. In response to requests from a significant number of educators and readers, we have added four new chapters that provide an introduction to pregnancy and postpartum care.

We believe this edition builds upon the precedents set in the previous editions and hope it contributes to women receiving evidence-based, holistic, gynecologic care within their lived experiences. As before, we welcome feedback from our readers that will help us in future editions.

Kerri Durnell Schuiling, PhD, NP-BC, CNM, FACNM, FAAN

Frances E. Likis, DrPH, NP-BC, CNM, FACNM, FAAN

CONTRIBUTORS

Ellise D. Adams, PhD, CNM
Associate Professor
Director, Nursing Honors
College of Nursing
The University of Alabama in Huntsville
Huntsville, Alabama

Ivy M. Alexander, PhD, APRN, ANP-BC, FAANP, FAAN
Clinical Professor and Director of Advanced
    Practice Programs
School of Nursing
University of Connecticut
Storrs, Connecticut

Linda C. Andrist, PhD, RN, WHNP-BC
Assistant Dean, Graduate Programs
MGH Institute of Health Professions
Boston, Massachusetts

Kathryn P. Atkin, DNP, WHNP-BC, ANP-BC
Nurse Practitioner
Beth Israel Deaconess Obstetrics, Gynecology, and
    Midwifery
Plymouth, Massachusetts
Assistant Professor
MGH Institute of Health Professions
Boston, Massachusetts

Evelyn Angel Aztlan-James, PhD, RN, CNM, WHNP
Postdoctoral Research Associate
College of Nursing
University of Illinois at Chicago
Chicago, Illinois

Joanne Motino Bailey, CNM, PhD
Director, Nurse-Midwifery
University of Michigan Health System
Lecturer II
Department of Women's Studies
University of Michigan
Ann Arbor, Michigan

Cynthia Belew, CNM, WHNP-C, MS
Associate Clinical Professor
School of Nursing
University of California, San Francisco
San Francisco, California

Kelly A. Berishaj, DNP, RN, ACNS-BC, CFN, SANE-A
Special Instructor
Forensic Nursing Program Coordinator
School of Nursing
Oakland University
Rochester, Michigan

Sharon M. Bond, PhD, CNM, FACNM
Nurse-Midwife
Department of Obstetrics and Gynecology
Medical University of South Carolina
Charleston, South Carolina

Katherine Camacho Carr, PhD, CNM, FACNM, FAAN
Professor and DNP Internship Coordinator
College of Nursing
Seattle University
Seattle, Washington

Phyllis Patricia Cason, MS, FNP-BC
Assistant Clinical Professor
School of Nursing
University of California, Los Angeles
Los Angeles, California

Nicole R. Clark, DNP, RN, FNP-BC
Adjunct Faculty
School of Nursing
Nurse Practitioner
Graham Health Center
Oakland University
Rochester, Michigan

Simon Adriane Ellis, MSN, RN, CNM
Nurse-Midwife
Group Health
Seattle, Washington

Heidi Collins Fantasia, PhD, RN, WHNP-BC
Assistant Professor
College of Health Sciences, School of Nursing
University of Massachusetts Lowell
Lowell, Massachusetts

Brooke Faught, MSN, WHNP-BC, IF
Clinical Director
Women's Institute for Sexual Health
Division of Urology Associates
Nashville, Tennessee

Nanci Gasiewicz, DNP, RN, CNE
Associate Dean and Director
School of Nursing
Northern Michigan University
Marquette, Michigan

Mickey Gillmor-Kahn, MN, CNM
Course Faculty
Frontier Nursing University
Hyden, Kentucky

Margaret M. Glembocki, DNP, RN, ACNP-BC, CSC, SANE-A, FAANP
Assistant Professor
School of Nursing
Oakland University
Rochester, Michigan
Acute Care Nurse Practitioner
Henry Ford Health System
Clinton Township, Michigan
Sexual Assault Nurse Examiner
HAVEN
Royal Oak, Michigan

Deana Hays, DNP, RN, FNP-BC
Interim Associate Dean
School of Nursing
Oakland University
Rochester, Michigan
Nurse Practitioner
Beaumont Health
Troy, Michigan

Caroline M. Hewitt, DNS, RN, WHNP-BC, ANP-BC
Assistant Professor and DNP Program Coordinator
School of Nursing
Hunter College of the City University of New York
New York, New York

Deborah Karsnitz, DNP, CNM, FACNM
Associate Professor
Frontier Nursing University
Hyden, Kentucky

Leslye Stewart Kemp, MSN, ANP-BC, WHNP-BC
Nurse Practitioner
Tennessee Oncology
Nashville, Tennessee

Holly Powell Kennedy, PhD, CNM, FACNM, FAAN
Executive Deputy Dean and Helen Varney
    Professor of Midwifery
Yale University School of Nursing
West Haven, Connecticut

Lucy Koroma, MSN, CRNP
Nurse Practitioner, Division of Gynecology
    Specialties
School of Medicine
Department of Gynecology and Obstetrics
Johns Hopkins Medical Institute
Baltimore, Maryland

Lisa Kane Low, PhD, CNM, FACNM, FAAN
Associate Dean, Practice and Professional
    Graduate Programs
Co-Lead, Nurse-Midwifery Program
Associate Professor, School of Nursing
    and Women's Studies Program
Lecturer, Department of Obstetrics
    and Gynecology
University of Michigan
Ann Arbor, Michigan
President-Elect
American College of Nurse-Midwives
Washington, DC

Sandra Lynne, CNM, MSN, DNP
Nurse-Midwife
Bronson Women's Service
Kalamazoo, Michigan

Nancy Maas, MSN, FNP-BC, CNE
Associate Professor
School of Nursing
Northern Michigan University
Marquette, Michigan

Janis M. Miller, PhD, APRN, FAAN
Associate Professor
School of Nursing
Associate Research Professor
School of Medicine
Department of Obstetrics and Gynecology
University of Michigan
Ann Arbor, Michigan

Patricia Aikins Murphy, CNM, DrPH, FACNM, FAAN
Professor and Annette Poulson Cumming
    Presidential Endowed Chair in
    Women's and Reproductive Health
University of Utah College of Nursing
Salt Lake City, Utah

Katharine K. O'Dell, PhD, WHNP-BC, CNM (ret.)
Associate Professor
University of Massachusetts
    Medical School
Worcester, Massachusetts

Kathryn Osborne, PhD, CNM, FACNM
Associate Professor
Department of Women, Children,
    and Family Nursing
College of Nursing
Rush University
Chicago, Illinois

Julia C. Phillippi, PhD, CNM, FACNM
Assistant Professor
School of Nursing
Vanderbilt University
Nashville, Tennessee

Amy Pondo, MSN, FNP-BC
Nurse Practitioner
St. John Providence Weight Loss
Madison Heights, Michigan

Kristi Adair Robinia, PhD, RN
Professor
School of Nursing
Northern Michigan University
Marquette, Michigan

Melissa Romero, PhD, FNP-BC
Associate Professor and Graduate Program
    Coordinator
School of Nursing
Northern Michigan University
Marquette, Michigan

Ying Sheng, RN, BSN, MSN
PhD Student
School of Nursing
University of Michigan
Ann Arbor, Michigan

Katherine Simmonds, MS, MPH, WHNP-BC
Assistant Professor
MGH Institute of Health Professions
Boston, Massachusetts

Stephanie Tillman, CNM, MSN
Nurse-Midwife
University of Illinois
Chicago, Illinois

Kathryn J. Trotter, DNP, CNM, FNP-C, FAANP
Senior Nurse Practitioner, Duke Breast Program
Assistant Professor and Lead Faculty, Women's
    Health Nurse Practitioner Specialty
School of Nursing
Duke University
Durham, North Carolina

Tanya Vaughn, MS, APRN, CNM, FNP-BC, EFM-C
Nurse-Midwife and Nurse Practitioner
Partridge Creek Obstetrics and Gynecology
Macomb, Michigan

Ruth Zielinski, PhD, CNM, FACNM
Clinical Associate Professor
Midwifery Program Lead
University of Michigan
School of Nursing
Ann Arbor, Michigan

REVIEWERS

Amy Alspaugh, MSN, CNM
Nurse-Midwife
Durham Country Department
  of Public Health
Durham, North Carolina

Tia Andrighetti, DNP, CNM
Assistant Professor
Frontier Nursing University
Hyden, Kentucky

**Laura Kim Baraona, DNP,
  APRN, CNM**
Assistant Professor
Frontier Nursing University
Hyden, Kentucky

Margaret Beal, PhD, CNM
Professor
MGH Institute of Health Professions
Boston, Massachusetts

Lynne C. Browning, CNM, MSN
Certified Nurse-Midwife and
  Nurse Manager
Women and Infants, Center for Reproduction
  and Infertility
Providence, Rhode Island

Patricia W. Caudle, DNSc, CNM, FNP-BC
Associate Professor
Frontier Nursing University
Hyden, Kentucky

**Anne Z. Cockerham, PhD, CNM, WHNP-BC,
  CNE**
Associate Professor and Associate Dean
  for Academic Affairs
Frontier Nursing University
Hyden, Kentucky

Angela Deneris, PhD, CNM, FACNM
Professor Clinical
Nurse-Midwifery and Women's Health Nurse
  Practitioner Programs
University of Utah
Salt Lake City, Utah

**Renae M. Diegel, RN, BBL, SANE-A, CFN,
  CMI-III, CFC, DABFE,
  DABFN, FACFEI**
Administrator of Clinical Forensic Nursing Services
Turning Point's Clinical Forensic Nursing Program
Clinton Township, Michigan

Dawn Durain, CNM, MPH, FACNM
Faculty
School of Nursing
University of Pennsylvania
Philadelphia, Pennsylvania

Mary Ellen Egger, APN, WHNP-BC, CBPN-IC
Women's Health Nurse Practitioner
Vanderbilt University Breast Center
Nashville, Tennessee

Gina Eichenbaum-Pikser, LM, CNM
Nurse-Midwife
Community Gyn Care
Brooklyn, New York

Ami L. Goldstein, MSN, CNM, FNP
Assistant Clinical Professor
University of North Carolina
    at Chapel Hill
Chapel Hill, North Carolina

**Robin L. Hills, DNP, WHNP-BC,
    C-MC, CNE**
Assistant Professor
Vanderbilt University School of Nursing
Nashville, Tennessee

**Aimee Chism Holland, DNP, WHNP-BC,
    FNP-C, RD**
Assistant Professor
University of Alabama at Birmingham
    School of Nursing
Birmingham, Alabama

Amy Hull, MS, WHNP-BC
Assistant Professor
Division of Midwifery and Advanced
    Practice Nursing
Department of Obstetrics and Gynecology
Vanderbilt University Medical Center
Nashville, Tennessee

Lisa Kane Low, PhD, CNM, FACNM, FAAN
Associate Dean, Practice and Professional
    Graduate Programs
Co-Lead, Nurse-Midwifery Program
Associate Professor, School of Nursing and
    Women's Studies Program
Lecturer, Department of Obstetrics
    and Gynecology
University of Michigan
Ann Arbor, Michigan
President-Elect
American College of Nurse-Midwives
Washington, District of Columbia

Hayley D. Mark, PhD, RN, FAAN
Associate Professor
Johns Hopkins University
Baltimore, Maryland

Alison O. Marshall, RN, MSN, FNP-BC
Clinical Instructor
Connell School of Nursing
Boston College
Chestnut Hill, Massachusetts

Monica R. McLemore, PhD, MPH, RN
Assistant Professor
University of California, San Francisco
San Francisco, California

Tonya Nicholson, DNP, CNM, WHNP-BC, CNE
Associate Dean of Midwifery and Women's Health
Associate Professor
Frontier Nursing University
Hyden, Kentucky

**Katharine K. O'Dell, PhD, WHNP-BC,
    CNM (ret.)**
Associate Professor
University of Massachusetts Medical School
Worcester, Massachusetts

Susan Jo Roberts, DNSc, ANP, FAAN
Adult Nurse Practitioner and Professor
School of Nursing
Northeastern University
Boston, Massachusetts

**Maureen Shannon, CNM, FNP, PhD,
    FACNM, FAAN**
Associate Professor and Frances A. Matsuda
    Endowed Chair in Women's Health
School of Nursing and Dental Hygiene
University of Hawai'i at Mānoa
Honolulu, Hawaii

Penny Wortman, DNP, CNM
Instructor
Frontier Nursing University
Hyden, Kentucky

ABOUT THE EDITORS

Kerri Durnell Schuiling, PhD, NP-BC, CNM, FACNM, FAAN, earned her master's degree in advanced maternity nursing from Wayne State University and a PhD in nursing and graduate certificate in women's studies from the University of Michigan. She received her nurse practitioner education from Planned Parenthood Association of Milwaukee, Wisconsin, and her nurse-midwifery education from Frontier Nursing University. She is dually certified as a women's health care nurse practitioner and nurse-midwife, and has been an advanced practice registered nurse and educator for more than 35 years. She has presented numerous times to national and international audiences on topics that focus on women's health, and twice was invited to provide formal presentations to maternal child health committees of the Institute of Medicine. As a member of the American College of Nurse-Midwives (ACNM) Clinical Practice Committee, Kerri assisted in the development of ACNM clinical bulletins related to abnormal uterine bleeding and has been an item writer for the National Certification Examination for women's health care nurse practitioners. Kerri has authored several articles and book chapters that focus on women's health. She has received numerous awards for her work, including a Clinical Merit Award from the University of Michigan for outstanding clinical practice; the Kitty Ernst award from the ACNM in recognition of innovative, creative endeavors in midwifery and women's health care; the Esteemed Women of Michigan award from the Burnstein Clinic for her significant contributions to women's health; and, most recently, the inaugural Distinguished Service to Society Award from Frontier Nursing University. She is a Fellow of the ACNM and the American Academy of Nursing. Currently she is Provost and Vice President of Academic Affairs at Northern Michigan University and Co-Editor-in-Chief of the *International Journal of Childbirth*, the official journal of the International Confederation of Midwives.

Frances E. Likis, DrPH, NP-BC, CNM, FACNM, FAAN, earned her bachelor's and master's degrees from Vanderbilt University and her doctorate in public health from the University of North Carolina at Chapel Hill. She received her nurse-midwifery and women's health care nurse practitioner education from Frontier Nursing University, and she earned a certificate in medical writing and editing from the University of Chicago. Francie is a women's health care nurse practitioner, family nurse practitioner, and certified nurse-midwife, and she has been an advanced practice registered nurse for more than 20 years. Her clinical experience includes family practice in community health and urgent care centers, performing sexual assault examinations, and midwifery practice in a freestanding birth center and a large obstetrics and gynecology group practice. Francie has authored numerous journal articles, systematic reviews, and book chapters related to women's health, and she frequently gives presentations at national meetings and invited lectures. Her awards and honors include the Student Choice Award for Teaching Excellence at Frontier Nursing University; selection as a Vanderbilt University School of Nursing Top 100 Leader, one of 100 distinguished alumni and faculty honored in commemoration of the School's Centennial; the Kitty Ernst Award from the American College of Nurse-Midwives (ACNM); the Vanderbilt University Alumni Award for Excellence in Nursing; and induction as a Fellow of the ACNM and the American Academy of Nursing. Currently she is the Editor-in-Chief of the *Journal of Midwifery & Women's Health*, the official journal of the ACNM, and an Adjunct Assistant Professor of Nursing at Vanderbilt University.

Introduction to Women's Gynecologic Health

CHAPTER 1

Women's Health from a Feminist Perspective

Lisa Kane Low

Joanne Motino Bailey

The editors acknowledge Kerri Durnell Schuiling, who was a coauthor of the previous edition of the chapter.

WOMEN'S HEALTH CARE AND GYNECOLOGIC HEALTH

The state of women's health care today is a direct reflection of women's status and position in society. Many healthcare advances have been made in women's health, yet comprehensive, compassionate healthcare services that address the complexity and diversity of how women live their lives and experience health and disease are still lagging.

This text is based on a feminist framework in an effort to advance the quality of health care provided to women in today's society. The authors attempt to acknowledge the complexity of women's health by paying particular attention to women's status in society and their unequal access to opportunity and power, while focusing on women's gynecologic health and well-being. The purpose of this chapter is to provide an overview of women's health using a feminist perspective and gender considerations as a lens for exploring women's health in general and gynecologic health in particular. The glossary in **Box 1-1** offers definitions of key terms that are used throughout the chapter and are linked to feminist critical analysis of gender and health.

WHAT IS FEMINISM?

The author bell hooks (2000) offers a definition of feminism that is well suited for addressing the context in which women experience health and wellness: Feminism is a perspective that acknowledges the oppression of women within a patriarchal society, and struggles toward the elimination of sexist oppression and domination for all human beings. Acknowledging the oppression of women is increasingly difficult because affluence and increased opportunities within some sectors of employment and education are construed as equal access or equity in opportunity for all women. Hooks, however, defines oppression as "not having a choice." With this definition, many more individuals are able to recognize constraints in their personal experiences. Examples of such practices include unjust labor practices, lower wages for equal work, lack of maternity leave policies, limited access to a range of contraceptive options, and inability to access desired healthcare providers. These examples indicate the breadth of experiences within the context of a patriarchal society that denies women equal access to power, resources, and opportunities.

Characteristics of a feminist perspective include the use of critical analysis to question assumptions about societal expectations and the value of various roles on both sociopolitical and individual levels. The process of critical analysis is accomplished by rejecting conceptualizations of women as homogeneous. It acknowledges power imbalances, and uses the influence of gender as the foremost consideration in the analysis. Using a gender lens that is informed by feminism permits areas

---

BOX 1-1 Glossary of Key Terms

Cis-sex/gender: An individual whose gender identity coincides with that individual's birth-assigned sex/gender (e.g., a cis-man is often referred to as simply "man," a cis-woman is often referred to as simply "woman")

Classism: Discrimination or prejudice on the basis of social class

Discrimination: The prejudicial treatment of an individual based on that person's actual or perceived membership in a certain group or category (e.g., race, ethnicity, sexual orientation, national origin)

Feminism: A movement to end sexism, sexist exploitation, and oppression (hooks, 2000)

Gender: A socially constructed category addressing how people identify and act based on sex (e.g., men and women)

Homophobia: Prejudice against individuals with same-sex attraction

Intersectionality: The unique combination of multiple identities based on race, class, gender, and other characteristics, and the compounded experience of oppression based on these identities

Medicalization: Defining or treating a physiologic process or behavior as a medical condition or disease

Oppression: Exercise of authority or power in an unjust manner; according to bell hooks, "not having a choice"

Patriarchy: A social system of institutions that privileges men, resulting in male domination over access to power, roles, and positions within society

Power: The ability to do something, act in a particular way, or direct/influence others' behavior or a course of events

Race/ethnicity: Socially constructed categorization of individuals and communities based on a combination of physical attributes and cultural heritage

Racism: Individual and structural practices that create and reinforce oppressive systems of race relations

Sex: Biological classification as female or male based on chromosomes, genitalia, and reproductive organs

Sex/gender: Combined term of sex and gender acknowledging that the discreet meanings of these terms are not easily separated in research and practice

Sexism: Individual and institutional practices that privilege men over women

Social construction: The process by which societal expectations of behavior become interpreted as innate, biologically determined characteristics

Socioeconomic status (SES): An indicator that encompasses income, education, and occupation

Trans*: Represents multiple identities in transgender communities; read as "trans star" (Erickson-Schroth, 2014)

Transgender or trans: An individual whose gender identity does not coincide with that individual's assigned gender at birth

---

of disparity to be identified both between groups, based on gender, and within groups, based on the recognition of heterogeneity among women.

Feminist women's health explores the context of how women live their lives both collectively and individually within a patriarchal society. The various social, environmental, and economic aspects become integral to understanding the context in which women are able to achieve health and well-being. Furthermore, feminism requires

---

BOX **1-2** **Components of a Feminist Perspective in Women's Health**

- Works *with* women as opposed to *for* women
- Uses heterogeneity as an assumption, not homogeneity
- Minimizes or exposes power imbalances
- Rejects androcentric models as normative
- Challenges the medicalization and pathologizing of normal physiologic processes
- Seeks social and political change to address women's health issues

---

consideration of health, as influenced by the intersection of sexism, racism, class, nation, and gender, within a framework that acknowledges the role of oppression as it affects women and their health as individuals and as a group. **Box 1-2** summarizes the components of a feminist perspective when considering women's health issues or models of care, which can help to reframe one's view of women's health in a feminist perspective.

GENDER

What does gender have to do with women's health? Although women's health is focused on the female sex (as determined by chromosomes, genitalia, and sexual organs), its priorities are shaped by what are considered socially important attributes of being a woman (such as reproductive capacity and feminine appearance). Gender is defined as a person's self-representation as man or woman and the way in which social institutions respond to that person based on the individual's gender presentation. Gender is often congruent with sex (a person with female genitalia identifies as being a woman "cis-woman"), but can also be incongruent (a person with female chromosomes may identify as being a man "trans-man"). Sex and gender are ultimately "irreducibly entangled" from both the research and the practice perspectives, however, and are better referred to by the combined term

"sex/gender"—a term that acknowledges the combined contribution of both the biologic and socially constructed aspects (Springer, Stellman, & Jordan-Young, 2012).

Sex/gender is a socially constructed attribute that is shaped by biology, environment, and experience and is expressed through appearance and behavior (Fausto-Sterling, 2012). Social construction is the process by which societal expectations of behavior become interpreted as innate characteristics that are biologically determined. Thus, behaviors associated with femininity become confused with innately determined behaviors rather than being recognized as socially constructed behaviors. As a result, health risks, treatments, and approaches to care are not necessarily biologically based aspects of women's health, but rather are determined by social expectations rooted in assumptions about sex/gender differences. In addition, diagnoses can be influenced by sex/gendered assumptions regarding behavior or what is socially constructed as feminine behavior. A significant body of literature has documented such influences on the manner of diagnosis and treatment in mental health (Neitzke, 2016) and obesity (Wray, 2008), as well as in the misdiagnosis of women's cardiovascular risks (Worrall-Carter, Ski, Scruth, Campbell, & Page, 2011).

Three primary aspects must be considered when examining the impact of sex/gender on women's health. The first is the priorities assigned to research, treatment, and outcomes in women's health as compared to men's health. The second is the context of sex/gender, including how it affects the process of providing healthcare services, which encompasses an acknowledgment of power differentials. The third aspect is the social construction of sex/gender, including how it affects women's health. Each aspect has implications for the manner in which women access, receive, and respond to health care. Collectively, these three aspects provide opportunities for us to better understand women's healthcare experiences and assist in the identification of underlying factors that influence the healthcare disparities experienced by women.

Sex/gender-based social role expectations can create undue burdens for women and may subsequently lead to increased health risks. For example, limited access to all contraceptive options may create reproductive health risks for some women.

Extensive cultural preoccupation with dieting and thinness may lead to unsafe dieting practices and precipitate eating disorders. Anorexia and bulimia are more prevalent among women despite the lack of a clear biologic explanation for this predominance.

Another example of a gender-based health risk is the disproportionate amount of violence that women experience (Modi, Palmer, & Armstrong, 2014). Gender-based violence includes any act that results in physical, sexual, or psychological harm or suffering (United Nations General Assembly, 1993). The multiple health consequences of violence reveal the long-lasting layers of health consequences associated with a gender-based health risk. Refer to Chapters 13 and 14 for further discussion of this topic.

INTERSECTIONALITY

Sex/gender interacts with many other identities that affect healthcare delivery and outcomes. Intersectionality is the unique combination of multiple identities based on race/ethnicity, socioeconomic status (SES), gender, nation status, ability, and other factors and the experience of oppression based on these identities. Disparities in health outcomes are often better explained by considering the intersections of multiple forms of oppression based on identity (Etherington, 2015; Warner & Brown, 2011). For example, poor women of color often obtain fewer or receive different health services and have worse health outcomes compared to more affluent white women. Although low socioeconomic status is the single most powerful contributor to illness and premature death (Mehta, Wei, & Wenger, 2015), numerous examples of poorer health based on race/ethnicity can be cited even after controlling for SES (Williams, 2008).

"Race" as a category has been critiqued as creating a false perception of biological difference, despite gene-level similarities across defined races. Thus the term *race/ethnicity* is used to describe a socially constructed combination of physical attributes and cultural commonality (Williams, 2008). Although disparities in health outcomes across race/ethnicities are often assumed to be genetic or biologic, in reality they are significantly impacted by social forces of discrimination. Discrimination is unjust treatment that is based on appearance or identity and is often described primarily as an interpersonal construct (e.g., a person expressing racist opinions). Even more damaging than interpersonal discrimination is systemic or structural discrimination—such injustice perpetuates large-scale, often invisible processes, policies, systems, or structures (e.g., underfunded school systems in poor districts, locations of subsidized housing) that are much harder to dismantle than individual opinions. Structural discrimination impacts the social, political, geographic, and economic influences on health, yet it is very difficult to quantify and often is misidentified (Krieger, 2014).

The structural components of where we live, learn, work, and play impact health across the life span. "Where we live" encompasses factors such as access to living space with good air quality, access to safe drinking water, access to green space, a safe environment for spending time outdoors, local grocery stores with high-quality fresh food, neighborhood and community support, and even the distance needed to get to a place of employment, which dictates the ability to walk to work versus having a lengthy car commute. "Where we learn" incorporates factors such as access to well-equipped, safe schools with challenging and engaging curricula, and skill acquisition to prepare for high-quality employment and future life skills. "Where we work" reflects access to living wages, safe working conditions, healthcare benefits, and a sense of meaningful work. "Where we play" includes types of recreation that promote physical activity, community connection, and long-term healthy behaviors such as exercise. Feminist considerations in relation to health disparities in these areas include factors such as gender bias in hiring, access to resources, availability of healthcare providers, and contraceptive options. Policies or practices that impose undue stress or limit access based on gender contribute to health disparities and are a form of structural bias.

The social embeddedness of women's health must attend to all of these factors—such as types of medical care, geographic location, migration, acculturation, racism, exposure to stress, and access to resources—when exploring disparities in women's health. Only by incorporating these factors into the discussion can we fully and accurately appreciate the health disparities women experience, including factors of sexism.

A MODEL OF CARE BASED ON A FEMINIST PERSPECTIVE

A model of care that is based on a feminist perspective contrasts sharply with a biomedical model, particularly in the areas of power and control and, in the definition of what is health compared to pathology. A feminist model supports egalitarian relationships and identifies the woman as the expert on her own body. The woman is at the center of this healthcare model. The following key points provide further insights into a feminist-based model of care:

1. The model of care must focus on *being with* women, not *doing for* women. This frames the model of care as a partnership with women as opposed to a model of care in which treatment decisions are directed by others and then dictated to women.

2. Heterogeneity, rather than homogeneity, is assumed. Using broad generalizations like "all women," with their inherent gender-based assumptions, essentializes women rather than acknowledging the diversity within individual women and across populations of women's experience. An assumption of heterogeneity considers women on an individual basis, tailoring health care and services to each woman's unique needs, rather than treating all women as a group with the assumption of similarity across all considerations of health.

3. The feminist model of care seeks to minimize or expose power imbalances that are inherent in most current healthcare models, especially those based on a biomedical model. Power should be distributed equally within the healthcare interaction, and the interaction should be based on a belief in a woman's right to self-determination as well as her self-knowledge of her body. Therefore, the role of the clinician focuses on providing support, information, education and skillful knowledge, as opposed to asserting authority over the decision-making ability of the individual.

4. A feminist framework rejects androcentric models of health and disease as normative. The pervasiveness of male-based models being extrapolated and applied to women assumes that women are merely a biologic variant of men. This misapplication of androcentric models to women's health also serves to medicalize or pathologize normal physiologic processes of women, such as menstruation, childbirth, and menopause (Lorber & Moore, 2011). In contrast, the feminist model acknowledges as normal those physiologic changes that occur over a woman's life span, such as menarche and menopause.

5. A feminist perspective challenges the process of medicalization and pathologization by identifying and exploring women's unique health experiences and normalizing them. Medicalization is the process of labeling conditions as "diseases" or "disorders" as a basis for providing medical treatment. The medicalization of women's biologic functions, such as menstruation, pregnancy, and menopause, is frequently cited as an illustration of both the social construction of disease and the general expansion of medical control into everyday life (Conrad, 1992; Zola, 1972). In addition, characterizing behaviors that are not gender normative as potential pathology instead of appreciating the social context in which they occur serves as a form of pathologizing, such as defining sexual desire using androcentric models and then developing treatments for it without considering the potential for coercion or prior history of sexual trauma.

6. A feminist framework acknowledges the broader context in which women live their lives and the subsequent challenges to their health as a result of living within a patriarchal society. It argues for a process of social and political change that would eliminate gender bias and sexism. This includes consideration of how the personal health decisions and healthcare interactions a woman experiences are influenced by the larger structural and political context in which women live their lives, including access to services and resources.

SOCIAL MODELS VERSUS BIOMEDICAL MODELS OF HEALTH

As the discussion of the social construction of sex/gender and its relationship to health unfolds, it becomes evident that a broader model of health must be employed to address the health consequences of gender bias and sexism and their implications for the overall health and well-being of women. The first step in broadening the model of health requires redefining health itself. *Health* is biomedically defined as the absence of disease—a narrow definition that does not address the context in which the absence of disease may occur. Considering only the absence of disease fails to address quality of life or the opportunity to reach the individual's potential. To gain a fuller appreciation of the scope of health, the dominance of the medical model as the rubric that defines health must be challenged in an effort to broaden the lens of what is health and to expand its definition. Without a broader definition, opportunities to understand the social realities and complexities within the healthcare system and the experiences of health for an individual and the collective community will remain limited. Without a broader perspective, which aspects of health are understood or studied will also be limited to individual characteristics or behaviors devoid of the context in which those behaviors and/or experiences are occurring. The biomedical model, as a conceptualization of health, generally does not address health beyond an individual perspective.

An alternative to the biomedical definition of health is offered by the World Health Organization (WHO). WHO defines health as "a state of complete physical, mental, and social well-being and not merely the absence of disease or infirmity." This broader definition is based on assumptions of what must be present to secure health for individuals and the community in which they live. It addresses the social context in which individuals live their lives, including the communities where they live, work, and play. According to WHO, the following prerequisites must be in place before health can occur:

- Freedom from the fear of war
- Equal opportunity for all
- Satisfaction of basic needs for food, water and sanitation, education, and decent housing
- Secure work
- Useful role in society
- Political will
- Public support

Germane to this definition is the commitment to address social injustice, equity, economic development and opportunity, and accessibility of healthcare services as a basic human right for all individuals in any society. WHO's definition of health requires that the community and environment in which women live their lives must also be considered in the same context as a new medical procedure. The constraints of an individualistic, disease-only–focused biomedical model of health become readily apparent when WHO's broader context and definition of health are considered. Through the use of this definition of health, the social aspects of health and the contributors to health are acknowledged, broadening the lens of factors that must be addressed to support individual as well as collective health.

A social model of health is more congruent with a feminist perspective compared to the biomedical model. The social model of health expands the contributors to health beyond just the individual body, extending them to the family, community, and society. This broader perspective enhances the understanding of health disparities that are rooted in the social and cultural forces that affect how women live their lives.

The interconnectedness of working and living conditions, environmental conditions, and access to community-based healthcare services becomes a focus when health and well-being are framed within a social context. Questions about health and well-being for an individual hone in on these factors as well as lifestyle decisions and health habits. The prevention of health problems becomes both a social burden and an individual responsibility. This wider emphasis, in turn, forces greater consideration of the various social factors that can either support or degrade an individual's health.

A social model of health also requires asking questions about the health effects of socially situated factors such as racism, sexism, and other forms of oppression. Consideration of women as central to the health model, rather than marginal to it, is a requirement of the feminist social model of health care. The broader social models do not ignore biologic or genetic components of health, nor is the significance of individual lifestyle health habits denied. However, the broader social model frames these issues as important to health, but no more so than women's experiences within everyday life, their access to healthcare services, their socioeconomic status, their racial/ethnic identity, and their membership within a community (Schiebinger, 2003).

The health risks associated with the social construction of sex/gender and the inequities associated with gender-based assumptions are essential components of the feminist social model of health. As links are forged between human rights, social models of health, women's health disparities, and opportunities to address those disparities, a feminist perspective offers new strategies and ways of thinking or asking questions that can promote expanded approaches to women's health issues.

FEMINIST STRATEGIES FOR THE ANALYSIS OF WOMEN'S HEALTH

Several aspects of analysis are important when considering women's health from a feminist perspective. The following strategies for analyzing women's health using a feminist framework are adapted from Franz and Stewart's (1994) strategies for conducting feminist research. Each of the strategies listed in **Table 1-1** can be used to form a question one can ask about women's health issues. Taken together, they constitute a feminist lens that

TABLE 1-1	Strategies for Analysis of Women's Health from a Feminist Perspective

Strategies	Questions
Look for what has been left out or what we do not know.	• What do we know, how do we know it, and who knows it? • Why don't we know? What do we want to know and why? • Who determines what is left out or who has access to what we want to know?
Analyze your own role or relationship to the issue or topic.	• Is it personal? What is the meaning of this issue for you as an individual? • Is it political? What is the meaning of this issue for you as a woman or as a member of an identified group? • Depending on your relationship to the issue, can you be objective in its analysis or are you engaged personally and subjective? • Are you invested in the outcome or topic or not? • Why do you care about the issue?
Identify women's agency in the midst of social constraints and the biomedical paradigm.	• Are woman really victims, or are they acting with agency? • Are individuals making choices despite positions of powerlessness? • Are the choices allowing individuals to remain in control, or do they allow individuals to have some form of power in the context of the situation? • By identifying women's agency in a particular context, can we learn new ways of understanding or approach the health implications?
Consider the social construction of gender and how its assumptions may be used to define what health is, limit options, or presume which behaviors and/or choices can made within the context of health.	• Explore gendered assumptions about the value of anatomy such as breasts or facial appearance. • Would this health issue be defined or explored in the same manner if it primarily affected one sex or another? • Do socially prescribed gender norms influence how this health condition is understood or defined (e.g., mental health)?

(continues)

TABLE 1-1	Strategies for Analysis of Women's Health from a Feminist Perspective (*continued*)

Strategies	Questions	
Explore the precise ways in which gender defines or affects power relationships and the implications of those power dynamics in terms of health.	• Physician/nurse • Clinician/patient • Parent/adolescent • Husband/wife	• Parent/child • Father/daughter • Partnered or not partnered woman • Heterosexual/transgender
Identify other significant aspects of an individual's or group's social position, and explore the implications of that position as it relates to health issues.	• Consider examples such as an adolescent who is seeking reproductive healthcare services or a same-sex couple seeking fertility services. • Ask who has access to various forms of healthcare services and resources and who does not. • Consider the intersections of race, class, gender, sexuality, and socioeconomic status. • Who has a choice, what constitutes a choice, and who is able to exercise the right to make choices within the context of health?	
Consider the risks and benefits of generalizations and speaking in terms of groups versus individuals.	• Who are "all women"? Are "all women" the same? • Consider who benefits from generalizations or assumptions of homogeneity versus heterogeneity. • Is value placed on having a coherent understanding of a health issue compared to acknowledging diversity or complexity in how the issue is experienced? • Which reflects reality most accurately—a coherent story or an appreciation for diversity in the understanding of the health issue? • When "grouping" occurs, who is missing from the group or who might not be reflected in the group process?	

Data from Franz, C., & Stewart, A. (Eds.). (1994). *Women creating lives: Identities, resilience, and resistance.* Boulder, CO: Westview Press.

allows for new considerations to arise as health issues are reframed. The following discussion highlights the manner in which some of the strategies can be applied.

Look for What Has Been Left Out or What We Do Not Know

This strategy is particularly applicable to investigations into the scientific basis of women's health.

Much of what we know about women's health needs, outside of reproductive health, is historically based on androcentric models of men's health considerations. For many years, almost all medical research that was not related to gynecology was conducted using male participants (human and animal), with the findings then being generalized to women. Large-scale investigations focusing on health promotion have been based primarily on study populations composed of only men. This practice persisted prominently until the 1990s, but continues to be an issue (Pinnow, Herz, Loyo-Berrios, & Tarver, 2014; Schiebinger, 1999).

According to feminist scientist Londa Schiebinger's analysis, many common health promotion measures have been assumed to be true for both men and women, despite the fact that the evidence supporting the measures came from research in which the study populations included only men. Examples of such studies include the Physicians' Heart Study, in which the findings led to recommendations on the use of aspirin to prevent heart disease, and the Multiple Risk Factor Intervention Trial, which evaluated correlations among blood pressure, smoking, cholesterol, and heart disease. In fact, one of the first studies to investigate the use of estrogen for heart disease was conducted on a study population consisting of only men (Schiebinger, 2003)!

The lack of representation of women in research trials reflected a prioritization of men's health issues and was also rooted in gendered assumptions about the potential impact of research on women's reproductive capacity. Additional considerations focused on women's hormonal variations throughout the menstrual cycle as potentially challenging issues in studies of medications. These as well as other biases related to women's participation as research participants extended through 1988, when clinical trials of new drugs were routinely conducted predominately on men—even though women consume approximately 80% of the pharmaceuticals in the United States (Schiebinger, 2003). In employing one of the feminist strategies, the question of "What has been left out?" can be asked and answered: considerations of women's biologic variations in processing drugs! The significance of potential hormonal variations was not considered in exploring the impact of particular treatments on women or was not factored into study designs. For example, acetaminophen is eliminated in women at 60% of the rate at which it is eliminated in men. This finding obviously has sex/gender-related implications for prescribing dosage regimens. Alternatively, it should not be assumed that all medications will have variations or that variations in dosing regimens are the same for all women because women post menopause may be more similar to men at that point than they are to women who are menstruating.

Examples abound of the problematic manner in which the scientific base for women's health, beyond reproductive health, was initially developed. Even when positive study examples are cited, limitations were often present in the design of the studies. Many key women's health studies, such as the Framingham Heart Study and the Nurses' Health Study I and II, were either observational or epidemiologic investigations instead of randomized clinical trials, even though the latter design has long been considered the gold standard for investigative research (Schiebinger, 2003). Examples such as these suggest women were being left out of the scientific quest to understand many health issues that directly affected them.

Consumer health advocates, women's health activists, and members of the scientific community have been instrumental in coming together to address the many limitations concerning women's health care and scientific investigations of women's health issues. In 1993, the National Institutes of Health's (NIH) Revitalization Act was considered a milestone in this regard. The Revitalization Act required that women and minorities, and their subpopulations, be included in all NIH-supported biomedical and behavioral research, including phase 3 clinical trials, in numbers adequate to ensure valid analysis of differences in intervention effects; that the cost not be the basis for exclusion from clinical trials; and that outreach programs to recruit these individuals for clinical trials are adequately supported. As a result of this policy change, important progress has been documented in terms of significantly greater inclusion of women and minorities in research investigations. In this case, asking "what had been left out" or "what was missing" provided an opportunity to alter what had been left out of women's health research.

There is an ongoing need to employ this strategy to expose blind spots in what is being presented under the rubric of women's health. An example can be found in the current focus on heart disease in women. Heart disease is now the number one killer of women in the United States. Every step in the healthcare process related to cardiovascular disease—from identification of symptoms to diagnosis, treatment, and referral—demonstrates sex/gender-related differences. The need to explore this disease process in women becomes even clearer when the question of "what has been left out of prior studies" is asked. The answer has helped frame new ways to address this health condition. Rather than accepting the inappropriate misapplication of findings to women when the research was conducted only in men, researchers are being charged with exploring new avenues of research and new ways of asking the research question.

Analyze Your Own Role or Relationship to the Issue or Topic

Traditionally, the focus of women's health has been relegated to those systems "between the breasts and the knees." Pregnancy and childbirth were long the focus when it came to health care of women, because the value of women was based on their role in procreation and continuation of the citizenry. Historically, this focus on reproductive health created opportunities to promote maternal and child health reforms in the public health arena. In such cases, women typically took advantage of the focus on reproductive health to advance an agenda that addressed both maternal and child health. At the same time, the practice of addressing only reproductive health carried risks, as it enabled normal physiological reproductive processes to be medicalized within a biomedical context.

In response to the practice of medicalizing aspects of women's health and traditional models of women's health care, consumer activism by women has been directed at reframing women's health and calling for reforms at even the most basic levels. The strategy of "analyzing your own role or relationship to the issue" may help reveal the role women play in relation to the process of rejecting medicalization of many of the normal healthy physiologic processes they experience.

Over the past 50 years, aspects of women's health have been topics of public debate and of organized social action. Two notable waves have occurred in the women's health movement. One wave coincided with social action movements such as the civil rights and women's rights movements. A key feature of this wave was its grassroots orientation, with a key focus on access to information and expanded knowledge regarding health. One outgrowth of this movement was the creation of the Boston Women's Health Book Collective (BWHBC)

and its publication of *Our Bodies, Ourselves* for consumers in 1974. During this period, primary access to health-related information was available only through medical textbooks. In contrast to this historical practice in which women's health information and knowledge was framed as reserved for the domain of medical professionals, particularly physicians, the BWHBC promoted open access to health information for women as consumers. Members of the BWHBC were consumers who sought out information, prior to the advent of the Internet and readily available online access. Arguably, they were the forerunners to the wealth of accessible online health information sources now available today. The BWHBC's membership included women who were healthcare consumers; they developed a consumer-oriented women's health book through a process of conducting individual research related to women's health. The framework that the BWHBC used was one of reclaiming health for themselves, using the feminist perspective of reducing power differentials as access to information. Knowledge about health empowered women to seek out services, redefine what health was, and consider a wider range of treatments or choices they might not have otherwise been exposed to or offered.

With this wave of health activism came a strong rejection of the medicalization of physiologic processes, with women reclaiming control of their health by offering new definitions. A key aspect of this ongoing process has been the demystification of health conditions and processes so as to promote women's agency and autonomy and empower them to engage effectively with clinicians. This change supported women in taking control of their health away from medical professionals and assuming responsibility for their healthcare decision making, rather than simply adhering to the older biomedical model, which placed authority for decision making firmly under the control of the clinician. The BWHBC was an initial pioneer in this movement, as was the Women's Health Network.

While this phase of the women's health consumer movement in the 1970s and 1980s was pivotal in many ways in defining a women's health agenda, it also lacked an appreciation of intersectionality and diversity. Essentially, this wave of the women's health movement could be critiqued as assuming homogeneity of women's health issues rather than heterogeneity. In response, the National Black Women's Health Project was launched in 1983 by Byllye Avery, with the goal of understanding black women's health issues in the broader social context. This project, which was eventually renamed the Black Women's Health Imperative, remains the only national organization dedicated to the improving the health and wellness of black women (Black Women's Health Imperative, 2015). Importantly, this organization defines its goal as addressing health and wellness through a framework that includes physical, emotional, and financial aspects, thereby incorporating social considerations as well as the biological elements of health. According to some scholars, the launch of this project was not intended as a rejection of the importance of other women's health organizations, but rather highlighted the need for independent organizations to frame questions or areas of emphasis that were unique to them while also opening opportunities for collaboration in collective areas of interest (Hart, 2012). From a practical standpoint, this meant that instead of everyone working within one organization on what may be presumed to be all issues of women's health, individual organizations, representing various groups, defined by those groups, could organize to address their specific health concerns. However, the various organizations could build alliances and coalitions with one another when issues of common interest were identified (Hart, 2012).

The ongoing efforts directed toward close examination of how the intersections of racism and sexism affect health disparities are essential to disentangling the social determinants of health and how they impact overall health outcomes for women of color in particular. Asking the question of how a health issue relates to you personally or politically is an important first step in considering that issue's significance, but it is also important to consider how individual factors can or cannot be extended in making assumptions for a larger population of women.

Consider the Risks and Benefits of Speaking in Terms of Groups Versus Individuals

Reclaiming control of their health care from clinicians and focusing on women's role and authority over their own health was initially promoted by well-educated white, straight, cis-women from middle- and higher-income groups. This limited view within the women's health movement revealed the problematic underpinnings of presumed homogeneity across all women.

The strategy of "considering the risks and benefits of speaking in terms of groups versus individuals" acknowledges this problematic aspect of the women's health movement. Today, women's health activists demonstrate greater diversity and focus on a wider range of issues that affect the health of women and their families.

Consider the Social Construction of Gender and How Its Assumptions May Limit Options or Presume Choices That Are Made Within the Context of Health

Earlier discussions regarding the social construction of sex/gender highlighted the implications of this strategy. An additional aspect to consider is the manner in which women's health issues are described—that is, the terminology used. The language used for many women's health concerns has been described by anthropologist Emily Martin (2001) as reflecting an androcentric bias—for example, the image of menstruation in medical texts is that of "failed reproduction" (p. 92).

Another example is the practice of referring to a woman who has experienced sexual assault as a victim rather than as a survivor of the process, implying inherent weakness rather than strength. Descriptions of childbirth usually invoke the term *delivery*—that is, a woman being *delivered* rather than *giving birth*. The *delivery* terms focus on the actions of the clinician and place the woman in a passive position, rather than appreciating her as the central figure: the one giving birth.

Explore the Precise Ways in Which Gender Defines Power Relationships and the Implications of Those Power Dynamics on Health

Creating health care from a feminist perspective requires the acknowledgment of power differentials between individuals who are consuming health care and those who provide it (clinicians). It also mandates attempts to minimize power differentials by developing a partnership model of care provision. In this model, rather than invoking a level of authority by virtue of being a clinician, the clinician acknowledges the life experiences and knowledge that the woman brings to the interaction. What makes a practice "feminist" is not who provides the health care, but rather how that care is provided, how the clinician thinks about his or her work, and which populations with whom the clinician works.

While hierarchical relationships and structures are typically elements of the traditional healthcare delivery system, feminist practice requires an active process of action to decrease asymmetrical relationships. Simple actions, such as not having a woman undress prior to meeting her clinician, allow the woman to greet the clinician as an equal rather than from a vulnerable position (naked and wrapped in an ill-fitting paper gown). Having a woman check her own weight, as opposed to having someone else do this for her, places some accountability for health on her shoulders. It sends the message that she can control aspects of her health. Although these simple changes can be readily made in the healthcare office setting, each demonstrates power sharing rather than placing the woman in a dependent position in relation to aspects of her health care that she should rightly control.

Additional ways for clinicians to address gender dynamics and power relationships include supporting a feminist model of care that focuses on the ways in which the healthcare interaction is addressed. Key features of this model deal with how one listens and trusts what the woman brings to the interaction. These steps include removing assumptions from consideration and not ascribing meaning without confirming it with the woman directly. Checking power imbalances and addressing them, even simply by means of introduction and the manner in which the clinician sits in relationship to the woman, can give the woman greater power in the relationship. Careful use of language and terminology, as previously noted, must occur in all discussions and information that is provided. Seeking consent before touching and assuring the woman has control over what is or is not done during an examination are required. For additional considerations of promoting a feminist approach to healthcare interactions, see the blog series, Feminist Midwife (Tillman, 2016).

Each of the strategies discussed in this chapter provides an opportunity to consider the details as well as the global aspects of women's health care and women's health issues. These strategies can be applied both individually and collectively. They are not meant to be an exhaustive checklist to determine whether something is being considered from a feminist perspective, but rather are meant to serve as guidelines and considerations that allow for the identification of blind spots in how we are able to think about women's health issues when we are potentially constrained by the limitations of the biomedical model. Through the use of these strategies, clinicians, policy makers, and women themselves are able to reframe expectations, approaches, and the focus of women's health research, healthcare delivery, and receipt of healthcare services.

WHY A TEXT ON GYNECOLOGY?

Taking the same feminist strategies we use for analyzing women's health and applying them to this text on gynecologic aspects of women's health creates opportunities as well. Why, when a feminist perspective is being presented, along with the limitations of considering women's health as being equivalent to reproductive health, would a text purportedly using a feminist framework focus primarily on the gynecologic aspects of women's health? The reason is that gynecologic health is still important. Focusing on gynecology for clinicians is important because reframing and expanding considerations of gynecologic health from a feminist perspective may more accurately reflect the experience for women in their everyday lives. By offering a feminist perspective throughout the chapters in this text, we seek to dispel myths that pathologize normal gynecologic functioning, and we seek to support normality as opposed to medicalizing it. We also offer a framework for providing gynecologic health care that considers the social, emotional, and intimate and physical nature of this aspect of women's health care. Rather than ignoring gynecologic health and allowing it to remain within the biomedical domain, this text seeks to reframe aspects of gynecologic health issues within a feminist framework. This perspective expands the opportunities for understanding gynecologic health within a wellness-oriented, women-centered framework that considers the social elements as well as biologic and encourages providers to look beyond the medical model and to *support* normalcy instead of *manage* it.

References

Black Women's Health Imperative. (2015). Story. Washington DC: Author. Retrieved from http://www.bwhi.org/feature-blurbs /story

Boston Women's Health Book Collective. (1974). *Our bodies, ourselves*. New York, NY: Simon & Schuster.

Conrad, P. (1992). Medicalization and social control. *Annual Review of Sociology, 18*, 209–232.

Erickson-Schroth, L. (2014). *Trans bodies, trans selves: A resource for the transgender community*. New York, NY: Oxford.

Etherington, N. (2015). Race, gender, and the resources that matter: An investigation of intersectionality and health. *Women and Health 55*(7), 754–777.

Fausto-Sterling, A. (2012). *Sex/gender: Biology in a social world*. New York, NY: Routledge.

Franz, C., & Stewart, A. (Eds.). (1994). *Women creating lives: Identities, resilience, and resistance*. Boulder, CO: Westview Press.

Hart, E. (2012). *Building a more inclusive women's health movement: Byllye Avery and the development of the National Black Women's Health Project, 1981–1990* [Dissertation]. Retrieved from https://etd.ohiolink.edu

hooks, b. (2000). *Feminism is for everybody*. Cambridge, MA: South End Press.

Krieger, N. (2014). Discrimination and health inequities. *International Journal of Health Services, 44*(4), 643–710.

Lorber, J., & Moore, L. J. (2011). *Gendered bodies*. New York, NY: Oxford University Press.

Martin, E. (2001). *The woman in the body: A cultural analysis of reproduction*. Boston, MA: Beacon Press.

Mehta, P. K., Wei, J., & Wenger, N. K. (2015). Ischemic heart disease in women: A focus on risk factors. *Trends in Cardiovascular Medicine, 25*(2), 140–151.

Modi, M. N., Palmer, S. & Armstrong, A. (2014). The role of Violence Against Women Act in addressing intimate partner violence: A public health issue. *Journal of Women's Health, 23*(3), 253–259.

Neitzke, A. B. (2016). An illness of power: gender and the social causes of depression. *Culture, Medicine, and Psychiatry, 40*, 59–73. doi:10.1007/s11013-015-9466-3

Pinnow, E., Herz, N., Loyo-Berrios, N., & Tarver, M. (2014). Enrollment and monitoring of women in post-approval studies for medical devices mandated by the Food and Drug. *Journal of Women's Health, 23*(3), 218–223.

Schiebinger, L. (1999). *Has feminism changed science?* Cambridge, MA: Harvard University Press.

Schiebinger, L. (2003). Women's health and clinical trials. *Journal of Clinical Investigation, 112*(7), 973–977.

Springer, K. W., Stellman, J. M., & Jordan-Young, R. M. (2012). Beyond a catalogue of differences: A theoretical frame and good practice guidelines for researching sex/gender in human health. *Social Science Medicine, 74*(11), 1817–1824.

Tillman, S. (2016). Feminist Midwife. Retrieved from http://www .feministmidwife.com

United Nations General Assembly. (1993). Declaration of the elimination of violence against women A/RES/48/104. New York, NY: United Nations. Retrieved from http://www.un.org /documents/ga/res/48/a48r104.htm

Warner, D. F., & Brown, T. H. (2011). Understanding how race/ethnicity and gender define age-trajectories of disability: An intersectionality approach. *Social Science Medicine, 72*(8), 1236–1248.

Williams, D. R. (2008). Racial/ethnic variations in women's health: The social embeddedness of health. *American Journal of Public Health, 98*(9), S38–S47.

Worrall-Carter, L., Ski, C., Scruth, E., Campbell, M., & Page, K. (2011). Systematic review of cardiovascular disease in women: Assessing the risk. *Nursing and Health Sciences, 13*(4), 529–535.

Wray, S. (2008). The medicalization of body size and women's healthcare. *Health Care for Women International, 29*(3), 227–243.

Zola, I. (1972). Medicine as an institution of social control. *Sociological Review, 20*, 487–504.

CHAPTER 2

Women's Growth and Development Across the Life Span

Kerri Durnell Schuiling

Lisa Kane Low

A discussion of women's growth and development provides a frame for this text's discussion of variations from what many consider normative. Although this approach may *seem* comprehensive, the problem is that often a biomedical context is used for descriptions of women's growth and development. This representation deconstructs women's bodies into biologic parts and physiologic processes. While such an approach enables quantification of growth, it does not speak to the qualitative aspects of women's lives that also influence their growth and development.

The biomedical model of health is individualist and disease oriented. In contrast, a feminist and social model of health acknowledges the influence of the culture in which women live, their economic status, the social interactions they experience, and the context in which they access and receive health care. A feminist model acknowledges the many other facets of life beyond the physiologic functioning of women and the genetic inheritance that affects their growth and development. Feminism provides a framework to explore sex/gender differences with women as central while simultaneously challenging patriarchy and sexism and addressing power imbalances (Backus & Mahalik, 2011). As a result, even the manner in which we understand and explain what normative growth and development include changes in the expanded framework of a feminist perspective, thereby allowing for a clearer understanding of the complexity inherent in women's growth and development.

As a first step in considering women's development (cognitive, psychosocial, and functional behaviors), it is important to acknowledge that the traditional models that are used were developed from research about men. For example, psychoanalyst Erik Erikson (1950) expanded developmental theory beyond the years of adolescence to offer a grand theory of human development (**Table 2-1**). The expansion of this theory was viewed as transformational at the time because no one else had pushed the boundaries of psychosocial theory quite so far (Sokol, 2009). Erikson identified eight general stages of development, each of which is the sequential focus of psychological energy (Mitchell, 2014). Erikson describes psychological life of adulthood as centrally organized by four of these themes (**Table 2-1**) (Mitchell, 2014). The eight virtues that are the goals of the stages are trust, autonomy, initiative, industry, identity, intimacy, generativity, and integrity.

By explicating a process of resolving eight developmental crises that are sequentially confronted, Erikson's theory offers a comprehensive account of individual development throughout the life span that until recently was applied to both males and females. However, a critical distinction that should be noted is that Erikson's stages of psychosocial development are based on studies of

TABLE 2-1 Erikson's Epigenetic Model

Age Period for Crisis	Stages							
	1	2	3	4	5	6	7	8
Infancy	Trust vs. mistrust							
Early childhood		Autonomy vs. shame and doubt						
Play age			Initiative vs. guilt					
School age				Industry vs. inferiority				
Adolescence					Identity vs. identity diffusion			
Young adult						Intimacy vs. isolation		
Adulthood							Generativity vs. self-absorption	
Mature age								Integrity vs. despair

Used with permission from Low, L. K. (2001). *Adolescents' experiences of childbirth: Nothing is simple.* Unpublished doctoral dissertation, University of Michigan, Ann Arbor, MI.

white, middle-class males; in fact, his initial work on identity was conducted with returning war veterans in the 1950s (Erikson, 1968; Gilligan, 1986). Nevertheless, his model has been universally applied to women with some gendered assumptions. The underlying gendered assumptions within Erikson's grand theory of development are important because his theory assumes homogeneity of all individuals, with minimal attention being paid to gender, socioeconomic, or ethnic variability (Gilligan, 1982; Taylor, 1994). These assumptions include a normative linear pattern of identity, followed by marriage (intimacy), and then childbearing (generativity) in adulthood. Erikson's theory assumes the need for a female to first develop an intimate relationship with another before she can complete her sense of self as an individual. Interestingly, males (according to his theory) do not have the same requirement. Thus, while the larger context of the theory assumes the desirability of autonomy and distancing oneself from the family of origin, for females autonomy is defined as being dependent on another within the context of a relationship, with a primary focus on caretaking by females.

Other examples of grand theories that are misapplied to women include those developed by Kohlberg (1981) and Perry (1968). Kohlberg's levels of moral development are based on interviews with only men, and Perry actually discarded interviews he had with women, using only data from interviews with men to formulate his model of intellectual development. The difficulty that arises when these scales are applied to assess a woman's developmental level is that they assume universality in development and treat all women as a monolith, not acknowledging the multiple variables that can affect progress through the stages (Belenky, Clinchy, Goldberger, & Tarule, 1986; Low, 2001). As Tavris (1992) observes, "[B]ecause of the (mis)measures we use, women fail to measure up to having the right body and fail to measure up to having the right life" (p. 36). The use of these androcentric models constrains the manner in which women's development is framed, such that women's development is presented as an aberration in comparison to white male development, which is held up as the standard.

This chapter discusses growth and development by contrasting traditional male-biased theoretical constructs with newer feminist theories that challenge some of the basic assumptions about women's growth and development. Alternative theories of female development that focus on relationship and connection have been offered by feminist theorists, psychologists, and researchers (particularly those connected with the Stone Center, Wellesley College) since the 1970s (Deanow, 2011; Miller & Scholnick, 2015; Taylor, 1994). Although there is substantial variation in the emphasis of feminist scholars, a primary focus is the self in relation to others or in connection with others (family and peers) as a means of further development. Feminist theories of development emphasize the quality and nature of individual women's experiences. As a consequence, women's development is construed as broader than the traditional process of individualization and includes the value of maintaining connection and continuity within relationships; the relationships are viewed as primary sources for support and identity development (Deanow, 2011; Gilchrist, 1997; Tummala-Narra, 2013).

The definition of relationships within this model incorporates not just the self in relation to others, but also inner constructions of relationships that form the sense of self and identity development of the female (Kaplan, Gleason, & Klein, 1991; Tummala-Narra, 2013). These relationships contain progressively more conflict, and it is through resolution of this conflict that the relationships become more complex, requiring flexibility that allows connections and relationships to be maintained (Baker Miller, 1991). This view stands in opposition to traditional theories of development, which emphasize conflict resolution as entailing greater disconnection and the development of distinct boundaries around identity formation, characterized as the process of "becoming one's own man" (Baker Miller, 1991).

It is noteworthy that these relational development models were not placed into a chronological framework to compare or contrast them with the age-related stages of other theories (Deanow, 2011). Additionally, the relational development models focus on relational processes between adults and do not address what occurs relationally in childhood, or adolescence; there has been no overall developmental framework (Deanow, 2011).

A newer relational model of development (see **Appendix 2-A**) identifies two poles, normative relational growth at one end and age-relational disconnection within age-related stages at the other end, thereby incorporating a chronological relational model of development into a theoretical base that can assist clinicians' understanding of their clients. Although this model can be applied to both males and females, it is especially beneficial in assisting clinicians to better understand their female clients (Deanow, 2011). Therefore, this model has the potential to enable a better understanding and assessment of women, which in turn will enable the development of more accurate therapeutic goals.

Feminist theories are primarily offered in contrast to Erikson's theory of psychosocial development. Gilligan (1982) and other feminist scholars have critiqued his work as not only descriptive of male development in general, but also descriptive of primarily white, privileged male development. Black feminist scholarship has furthered this critique beyond that of the traditional male-based model to include limitations in contrasting models offered by early feminist theorists. A key limitation of early feminist models is that they were developed by white middle-class Euro-American women who interpret relationships and connection as being similar across all women, regardless of ethnic identity or the influence of racism (Collins, 2000). Owing to this perspective, much of early feminist scholarship was limited by a lack of understanding of the role of ethnic identity and socioeconomic level on development. The history of enslavement and current ongoing struggles with racism and gender-based oppression emphasize the importance, particularly for African American women, of race and gender in identity formation as well as the development of mature love relationships (Tyson, 2012).

Subscription to a model that delineates gender differences versus a model that identifies gender similarities and provides an explanation for differences based on gender is a key philosophical dilemma for developmental theorists. The emphasis on difference, rather than similarity, evokes a debate about the risk of essentializing women's development. The controversy arises because the gender differences described by these theories are ascribed to biologic or innate characteristics rather than considering the social and cultural context that can create these differences. The differences described within the theories are wrongly assumed to be biologic in origin, instead of reflecting social constructs of femininity (Gilligan, 1982; Martin, 1992). While lauding the work of Gilligan and other early feminist theorists who argue that women have a "different voice" through which they develop and speak, several feminist psychologists and theorists offer the critique that in later developmental theories, what feminist theorists have described as being uniquely female is instead likely to be based in the social construction of gender roles and has been inadequately explored (Deanow, 2011; Hare-Mustin & Marecek, 1998; Riger, 1998).

This perspective, which results in differing expectations at different times based on gender, is consistent with the model proposed by Erikson (1950). He argues that the particular developmental crisis is not necessarily chronologically driven, but rather is driven by social expectations for behavior. Thus expectations for caregiving and consideration by females of themselves in relation to others may have more to do with socially prescribed gender roles of femininity than with biologically differing pathways for development. More similarities than differences between males and females may become evident when gender boundaries are broken down and males have a greater level of participation in caretaking for others rather than primarily for themselves. While transformations in gender roles and caretaking are in process, contrasting developmental models with an emphasis on differences that are primarily socially constructed have generally prevailed and, therefore, will inform the perspectives presented in this chapter.

Important content added in this third edition explores the foundations of gender identity development and challenges faced by transgender youth in particular. While the research on this topic is generally sparse, it is critically important to include what is currently understood about gender identity development, social reactions to what is currently termed nonconforming gender behavior, and ways to support transgender youth as they confront cultural expectations of gender expression and strive for balance, learn to cope, and eventually become comfortable with their own gender identity and sexual orientation (Stieglitz, 2010). Being comfortable in one's *own skin* is critically important for everyone and is particularly important for healthy growth and development. For information beyond growth and development for LBQT youth, see Chapter 9.

The intention of the newer feminist models is not to replace male generalist models of development with feminist generalist models of development, but rather to offer alternatives to the constrained models that were previously misapplied to all women. This chapter provides an overview of growth and development within the linear stages of adolescence through older age using a feminist perspective. Emphasis is placed on contrasting models of development outside the traditional biomedical focus.

ADOLESCENCE

The adolescent years are generally described as the time of transition from childhood to young adulthood and are biologically defined as beginning with the onset of puberty and lasting until young adulthood (American Academy of Child and Adolescent Psychiatry [AACAP], 2015a, 2015b). In a chronological sense, this encompasses the ages of 10 to 19 years, although some clinicians prefer to define adolescence in alignment with the teenage years (12–19 years), with ages 9 to 12 years labeled the "tween" years (*Psychology Today*, 2015; World Health Organization [WHO], 2015). The stages of adolescence are commonly identified as early adolescence (ages 11–14 years), mid-adolescence (ages 15–17 years), and late adolescence (ages 18–21 years) (AACAP, 2015a, 2015b; Healthychildren.org, 2015).

Visible physical changes occur during adolescence, such as breast development and menarche, but many additional developmental processes occur during this period that are not outwardly visible but are nonetheless critically important for a healthy transition to adulthood. For example, the brains of adolescents are continuing to develop, which results in increased cognitive skills that enhance their ability to reason and think abstractly. The changes that occur in the adolescent brain are both structural and functional and support cerebral maturation (Segalowitz, Santesso, & Jetha, 2010). Although the changes that occur during this period are discussed here in the contexts of biology and physiology, there are also qualitative aspects of adolescence that must be considered from a healthcare standpoint. Indeed, the context of the adolescent's lived experience is important to appreciate to fully understand the adolescent for whom you are providing health care. Her family, neighborhood, workplace, and community are factors that are just as important as her gender, race, sexual orientation, disability or chronic disease, and religious beliefs (American Psychological Association [APA], 2002).

The Biology and Physiology of Female Adolescent Growth and Development

The onset of puberty depends on a changing body accumulation of adipose tissue. As a consequence, this event marks the beginning of a tension between biologic development and the social context in which it occurs. Our culture today demands perfection, which causes many young women to suffer great anxiety about their bodies. The challenges faced by young women vary based on ethnicity, self-esteem, the social environment, and the contrast between the individual adolescent's sense of herself and society's perceived standard for beauty. In addition, many of the changes of puberty are framed within the social context of sexual development. As their physical sexual characteristics develop, many young women are challenged by a potential mismatch between their socially perceived sexual development and their interpersonal level of maturity and development. Clinicians can be an important source of support and information during what is often framed culturally as a tumultuous phase of development.

Significant physical changes occur as an adolescent reaches puberty. Adult height and weight are usually attained during this time. Probably most significant to many young girls, however, are the physical changes associated with puberty, especially the development of secondary sex characteristics. Female pubertal events are initiated by the production of low amounts of estrogen, which stimulate long bone growth (American College of Obstetricians and Gynecologists, 2011). As the amount of estrogen increases, breast buds are developed, long bone growth slows, and epiphyseal closure occurs, signaling that peak height has been attained. It is believed that women acquire the majority of their bone mass during early adolescence; thus this critical period lays the groundwork for prevention of osteoporosis in later years of life.

The events of puberty during a young woman's adolescence trigger the onset of menses, which occurs when a positive feedback of estrogen on the pituitary and hypothalamus stimulates a surge of luteinizing hormone at midcycle, which is critical to ovulation (Fritz & Speroff, 2011). The changes that occur during puberty usually happen in an ordered sequence, beginning with thelarche (breast development) at around age 10 or 11, followed by adrenarche (growth of pubic hair due to androgen stimulation), peak height velocity, and finally menarche (the onset of menses), which usually occurs around age 12 or 13 (American College of Obstetricians and Gynecologists, 2011; Fritz & Speroff, 2011). Peak height usually occurs about 2 years after breast budding and about 1 year prior to menarche (Fritz & Speroff, 2011).

The timing of the growth spurt or peak height velocity in young girls occurs approximately 2 years earlier in puberty than it does for boys (American College of Obstetricians and Gynecologists, 2011). Thelarche normally occurs between the ages of 8 and 13 years; it is stimulated by hormones, but is also affected by race and ethnicity. Approximately 48% of African American girls will begin breast development between 8 and 9 years of age, whereas only 15% of white girls this age will experience thelarche (American College of Obstetricians and Gynecologists, 2011). Adrenarche generally begins within 6 months of the advent of thelarche; thus it generally begins between ages 11 and 12. In some girls, pubic hair may be evident prior to thelarche; this development is particularly noted in young African American girls (American College of Obstetricians and Gynecologists, 2011). Nevertheless, it is important to carefully assess whether the advent of adrenarche prior to thelarche is a normal variation or whether it is due to androgen excess or estrogen deficiency. The general time frame from thelarche to menarche is 2 to 3 years. The first several menstrual cycles usually

do not result in ovulation, and often a girl's first-year experience of menstruating is characterized by irregular anovulatory cycles, along with heavy bleeding (Fritz & Speroff, 2011).

Although the U.S. National Health and Nutrition Examination Surveys have found no change in the median age of menarche over the last 30 years, other research suggests that non-Hispanic black girls start menarche approximately 6 months earlier than they did 30 years ago (American College of Obstetricians and Gynecologists, 2011; Forbes & Dahl, 2010; Krieger et al., 2015). The median age for the onset of menstruation has remained stable despite variations worldwide and with the U.S. population—12.8 years, with a range of ages 9 to 17—in well-nourished populations in developed countries (American College of Obstetricians and Gynecologists, 2015; Fritz & Speroff, 2011). On an international scope, however, the reported age at menarche varies, especially when comparing highly resourced to less resourced countries: Menarche tends to occur later in girls from lower-resource countries (Thomas, Renaud, Benefice, de Meeus, & Guegan, 2001). It is important to remind young girls that there is a range as to when puberty begins and that the timing varies from one young girl to another. Adolescent girls often worry about "being on time" for the advent of puberty and need to be reassured of the variations of normal in timing of breast development and menarche.

Female adolescents who have not reached puberty by the age of 13 or who have not had menarche by the age of 15 should be evaluated by a clinician to assess for the pubertal delay. Even though such a delay may be due to heredity, it is important to rule out other factors that may be impacting the young woman's health, such as poor nutrition or eating disorders, involvement in sports/athletics, or genetic and medical conditions (American College of Obstetricians and Gynecologists, 2011). While participation in sports has been linked to later onset of menarche, this link has not been found to be causal—that is, many other confounding factors contribute to this relationship (Clapp & Little, 1995).

Menarche for most young girls is a pivotal milestone event with implications for a girl's sense of self. It is probably also the most anticipated, feared, and socially misconstrued aspect of female adolescent development. Menarche is often viewed as a significant life event that carries physical, social, and emotional consequences that are important for clinicians to understand so that they can promote adolescent health (Chang, Hayter, & Wu, 2010).

Menarche has many layers of social meaning for girls and women. It is an event that establishes reproduction and sexual potential (Jackson & Falmagne, 2013). Thus menarche is important both as a physiologic marker of transitioning to adulthood, albeit framed by biomedical metaphors of scientific knowledge, and as one of the social and cultural junctures at which gender identity and gender relations may be shaped (Lee, 2008). In many societies, menarche is celebrated as an important entrance into womanhood. In Western societies, however, it is often denied any significance and instead is treated as a taboo subject and an embarrassing hygienic issue (Jackson & Falmagne, 2013).

Daughters have long relied upon their mothers to help them negotiate menarche, its meaning, and ways to "manage" it. Contemporary U.S. society continues to view menstruation as a taboo subject and the dominant discourses remain highly negative, suggesting that menstruation and menarche should be kept a secret and are a source of shame and secrecy (Jackson & Falmagne, 2013). Unfortunately, the continued systemic perpetuation of the negative discourses around menstruation, womanhood, and the female body have the potential to set girls on a highly problematic trajectory that will influence their affective and behavioral experiences across the life span (Jackson & Falmagne, 2013). It is important for clinicians caring for adolescent girls to carefully explore the young adolescent's sense of self, body image, and feelings about her transition to young adulthood.

Clinicians can educate young girls and their parents (or guardians) about what to expect with the experience of puberty and menarche. Experts suggest that girls who have been educated about what to expect about puberty and menarche will be much more comfortable with its onset than girls who are not educated about what to expect. The American College of Obstetricians and Gynecologists (2015) identifies the menstrual cycle as a vital sign and as such makes the following recommendations:

- Educate young girls and their parents (or guardians) about what to expect of a first menses.
- Educate young girls and their parents or guardians about the variations of normal as well as what might signal a problem and require a clinical visit.
- Ask about the menses at each clinical visit, and identify abnormal problems and treat them early to offset potential health concerns that may arise during adulthood.
- For all clinicians providing care to women, have an understanding of the patterns of menstrual patterns of adolescents and be able to differentiate between normal and abnormal, and have the skill to accurately assess and evaluate the adolescent girl patient.

A significant body of evidence shows that early or late pubertal onset appears to put girls at risk for a number of health problems, including depression, conduct problems, and, later in life, a higher risk of substance abuse (APA, 2002).

A commonly used scale for assessing sexual maturity and pubertal development is the Tanner scale, which, for girls, relies on development of the breasts and growth of pubic hair. It divides sexual physical maturity into five stages that extend from preadolescence to the adult (**Figure 2-1**). The Tanner model is widely accepted for staging sexual maturity, but is not appropriate to use for determining chronological age (Rosenbloom & Tanner, 1998). Additionally, Rosenbloom and Tanner note that because of the variability in timing of stages and of pubic hair growth, both of which are important elements of Tanner staging, the scale should not be used as originally developed for staging individuals of Asian ethnicity.

Adolescence can be particularly challenging because growth in one area may not match growth in another and both may be mismatched with chronological age (American College of Obstetricians and Gynecologists, 2011). An adolescent's entire body, mind, and relationships are shifting during puberty (Silber, 2012). These changes can be particularly difficult for young girls to navigate,

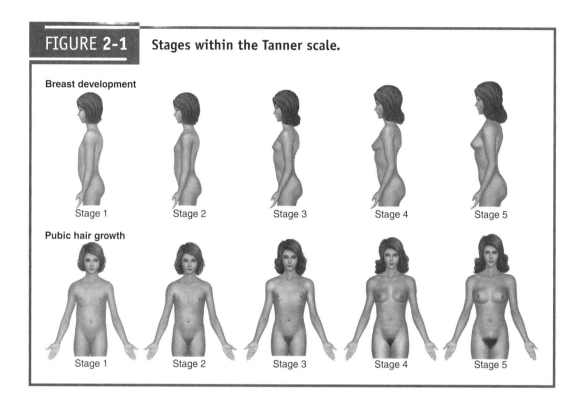

FIGURE 2-1 Stages within the Tanner scale.

Breast development

Stage 1   Stage 2   Stage 3   Stage 4   Stage 5

Pubic hair growth

Stage 1   Stage 2   Stage 3   Stage 4   Stage 5

as they are striving to conform and not appear different from their peers. Significant amounts of time are spent on appearance and fitting in with group norms. It is important for parents of adolescents to listen when their child expresses dissatisfaction or concerns related to her body or pubertal changes. She needs support to reassure her that the changes are normal, and she needs adult help in keeping her concerns in perspective.

Neurodevelopment

During the preteen years, significant proliferation of the neurons and synapses occurs, which is followed by shaping of the synaptic connections during the next 5 to 10 years (American College of Obstetricians and Gynecologists, 2011). Myelinization of neural connections from the caudal to frontal cortex is ongoing at the same time. This process begins 1 to 2 years earlier in girls than in boys (American College of Obstetricians and Gynecologists, 2011). The cerebral maturation or neurodevelopment and reorganization is both

structural and functional in nature (Segalowitz et al., 2010). Genetic disposition, hormonal influence, and experience affect which neural pathways are developed and retained; clearly, epigenetics plays an important role in the maturation of the adolescent brain (American College of Obstetricians and Gynecologists, 2011; Segalowitz et al., 2010).

As the adolescent grows older, education, experience, and role models continue to impact brain development. By late adolescence, the prefrontal cortex is more developed, which enables the adolescent to have better abilities at planning, strategizing, and thinking before acting. Thus the older adolescent has a better ability to control her impulses (American College of Obstetricians and Gynecologists, 2011).

The enhanced understanding and recognition of the development of the brain that occurs during adolescence has pushed clinicians to pay more attention to how adolescents act and react and why earlier in adolescence it is more difficult for the individual to make sound judgments. This is particularly important as clinicians teach adolescents about preventive health measures such as wearing helmets during activities where there is a risk of a blow to the head (e.g., skiing or snowboarding).

Psychosocial and Cognitive Development

The traditional developmental task of adolescence is to develop a sense of identity and autonomy before progressing toward adulthood. The role of peers tends to increase in importance, and it is normal to observe a distancing from parents and other adults as the adolescent tries to find her own identity, separate from that of her parents during this time. The interaction between an adolescent's behavior and role performance may either promote or confuse her sense of identity, depending on the social context in which it occurs. Through a process of trial and experimentation, individuals develop their own set of values and beliefs as well as a sense of themselves as they formalize or commit to their own identity. Initiation of sexual activity, pregnancy, childbearing, and parenting are all gendered roles and experiences that differ in their effects on any one individual adolescent based on the social, cultural, and historical definition that is associated with these behaviors and roles, as well as peers' and family's perceptions of these events.

In contrast, a feminist perspective of female adolescent development emphasizes the young girl's relationship with others instead of distancing from others in the process of individuation as described by Erikson (1950). Theorists argue that the hallmark of healthy identity development is development of a sense of connection to others, with a primary task being the ability to participate in mutual relationships in which the individual feels active and effective, and is not "lost within" the relationship (Kaplan et al., 1991). The self-in-relation model of adolescent development proposed by Baker Miller (1991) and her colleagues at the Wellesley College Stone Center defines a woman's sense of self as emerging out of experience with a relational process that begins in infancy. From initial interactions with caregivers through the process of becoming a caretaker, the self-in-relation theory argues that women are socialized to care more and more about the development of relationships.

Beginning with the earliest mother–daughter interactions, this relational sense of self develops out of women's involvement in progressively complex relationships, characterized by mutual identifications, attention to interplay between each other's emotions, and caring about the process and activity of relationship. (Kaplan et al., 1991, p. 123)

Laurel Silber (2012), along with other feminist scholars such as Carol Gilligan, posits that girls risk *losing their voice* during adolescence and that to stay connected and further develop an authentic sense of self, they need to gain the ability to resist cultural norms. This is a monumental task for an adolescent girl because it requires that she identify her sense of self and be comfortable enough with it that at the same time she can identify her agency, construct her own boundaries, and speak up. Few, if indeed any, cultures support this developmental challenge of female adolescents (Silber, 2012). As much as the adolescent wants and works toward individuation, she also wants and needs to feel connected. Herein lies the struggle, which further underscores "the importance of working within the intergenerational relational context in which adolescent girls' struggles are embedded" (p. 132). Girls usually interact closely with their mothers, a relationship that means girls, as compared to boys, are more apt to learn and appreciate the importance of empathy.

Reasoning changes as a child grows to adolescence. As a girl goes through adolescence, her cognitive development expands from being a very concrete thinker to gaining the ability to think abstractly, reason more effectively, problem solve, and involve herself in planning for her future (APA, 2002). By comparison, cognitive competence develops more slowly over time. As a consequence, adolescents still require guidance in some of their decision making: They are prone to jumping to conclusions and making poor decisions, which can lead to risky behavior (Jones, 2010). For example, older adolescent girls are usually able to connect intercourse with the potential for pregnancy, but younger adolescents might not be able to appreciate the logical sequencing of these events. Adolescents are particularly influenced by their peers, so it is important for adults to understand the importance of peer pressure and provide the support the adolescent needs to make healthy decisions about risky behaviors such as consuming alcohol, having unprotected intercourse, and driving too fast. Additionally, using her newly developed hypothetical and deductive reasoning skills to make decisions can be especially difficult when the adolescent is confronting her peers (American College of Obstetricians and Gynecologists, 2011). Maturation in thinking behavior is supported by understanding family members, an emotionally stable environment, parental discipline, and positive life experiences. The cognitive development of adolescents helps to lay the groundwork for their development of moral reasoning, honesty, and willingness to help and care for others (APA, 2002). Role modeling by caring adults is important as it reinforces positive behaviors.

Identity Development Among Adolescents Who Identify as Lesbian, Gay, Bisexual, or Transgender Individuals

Few would argue that adolescents face many demanding challenges as they transition to adulthood. Exploring identity is a normal process for all adolescents. In fact, Erikson (1968) suggests that forming an individual identity is one of the most pressing tasks of adolescents. Youths who do not identify within the traditional binary of sexual identities of male or female and heterosexuality experience the additional challenges of navigating a gender and sexual identity in a society that still tends to discriminate against homosexuals and a youth culture that remains largely homophobic (APA, 2002; Glover, Galliher, & Lamere, 2009). Generally an awareness of feeling "different" or being attracted to someone who is the same sex is what brings the adolescent to recognize that she may have a sexual or gender identity that is different from many of her peers. This realization can be frightening and complex, such that the adolescent may at first try to deny these feelings. While navigation of this complexity is aided by a supportive environment at home and in her peer relationships, clinicians can also aid in this process of accepting the adolescent's sexual and gender orientation (APA, 2002). Parents, friends, and significant others of the adolescent need to clearly appreciate that sexual orientation is not a mental disorder

and that sexual orientation is not a choice (AACAP, 2013). Without support, youths who identify as lesbian, gay, bisexual, or transgender (LGBT) can become socially isolated and withdraw from friends and family members. (See Chapters 1, 9 and 10 for in-depth discussion of gender.) Because such social isolation increases the risk for depression and thoughts of suicide, it is critical that parents and significant others in the adolescent's life provide support and be aware of any signs of distress (AACAP, 2013).

Early work on models for sexual identity development emerged in the United States during the 1970s (Bilodeau & Renn, 2005). The Cass Identity Model was one of the first theoretical models about lesbian and gay identity development (Cass, 1979). Although this model encompasses six sequential stages of identity development, a person may go back and forth among stages as she navigates identity development. The Cass model was based on gays and lesbians, and more men than women participated in the research undergirding its development. As more models began to emerge, it became apparent that using only one model to understand the development of sexual orientation identity was probably inadequate (Bilodeau & Renn, 2005). Later criticisms by Kaufman and Johnson (2004) argued that the Cass model is probably less valid today because (1) it did not take sociocultural factors that impact identity into account, (2) there have been many changes in the social stigma associated with lesbian and gay identity and its management since the model was first developed, and (3) the linear nature of the model suggests that if a person does not go through all of the stages, then that person could not become a well-adjusted homosexual (Kaufman & Johnson, 2004). Another, perhaps more obvious concern with the Cass model is that it does not address transgender individuals.

Very few models have been proposed that focus on the developmental issues faced by LBGT adolescents. Additionally, there is an increased awareness of the importance of race, ethnicity, nationality, spirituality, and culture as factors affecting LGBT identity development (Bildodeau & Renn, 2005). The identity processes of non-heterosexual women have often been presented as parallel with men's identity processes, even though research suggests that women tend to come out later than men (Bildodeau & Renn, 2005). And, yet again, research on men has been used to describe outcomes in women. Additionally, bisexual and transgender individuals emphasize identities that are outside the binary constructs of gender and sexuality (Bildodeau & Renn, 2005). For all these reasons, expanded models are needed to appreciate sexual identity development inclusive of LGBT identity development.

Multidimensional models of development appear to enable a more comprehensive understanding of identity and sexual orientation development. These models take into consideration the multiple influences that impact the development of a person's identity and sexual orientation. Using a multidimensional model, Glover, Galliher, and Lamere (2009) examined identity development of adolescents who identified as sexual minorities. Although the study population was small (n = 82), this investigation represents one of the very few studies that have focused on identity development of adolescents, particularly adolescents who identify as LGBT. Its findings support the use of social constructionist theories and multidimensional models of identity development. The study underscored the complexity of the ranges of adolescent sexual identity development and emphasized the need for more research in this area that will help us move away from stigmatizing youth who identify as LGBT as different from their peers, and provide a framework of normal development for this population (Glover et al., 2009).

Clinical Application

Almost from birth, females are socialized to be highly oriented to others, so it is not surprising that risky behaviors and conditions, such as depression or early sexual activity, are more likely to be influenced by the nature of an adolescent female's relational experiences with significant others, family, and peers (Baker Miller, 1991). In fact, the major health problems of adolescents relate to their risk-taking behaviors. In contrast to males, these behaviors in females are more often influenced by a desire to maintain important relationships than a desire to "take on" adult behaviors. Female adolescent morbidity is most likely to include pregnancy,

sexually transmitted infections, running away, and suicide (American College of Obstetricians and Gynecologists, 2011). Risk taking can also be a result of the young girl's environment, or it may be an expression of symptoms of depression.

The developmental self-in-relation model offered by feminist scholars can be extended into the healthcare visit for adolescents. Trust is a key component of any therapeutic relationship—a fact that cannot be emphasized enough for providers caring for adolescents. Additional time is often needed to establish a trusting relationship with an adolescent.

A relational approach can be very helpful when providing adolescent females' healthcare services because it takes into consideration the human relations that influence how adolescent females define their health. For example, "Tell me about your friends or who you hang out with" and "How would you describe yourself in relation to your friends?" are the types of questions that can be asked of an adolescent during a healthcare visit to assess who influences the adolescent and how she sees herself in relationship to others. The relational assets approach merges developmental assets frameworks and the voice-centered relational work of feminist psychologists (Sadowski, Chow, & Scanlon, 2009). This model works well with adolescents who are in a sexual minority.

The goal is not to isolate the behavior from the relational context in which it occurs, but rather to acknowledge the health implications of behaviors. This enables a more effective approach to risk reduction because the behavior is addressed along with the context in which it occurs. This relational model can be extended as a woman progresses in her healthcare needs across the life span.

EARLY ADULTHOOD

Young adulthood is generally accepted as spanning the time from late adolescence (age 18) to the beginning of the perimenopausal years (ages 35–50). This period is often referred to as the *reproductive years*, reflecting a societal valuing of women primarily for their reproductive capacities (Olshansky, 1996). Health care during the young adulthood years traditionally focuses on health promotion and maintenance, with a primary emphasis on reproductive capacity rather than a broader, comprehensive focus on health promotion throughout the life span.

Biology and Physiology

The years between ages 18 and 35 are biomedically considered optimal for reproduction. Generally, most women experience regular menstrual cycles that are ovulatory, providing opportunity for pregnancy if unprotected intercourse occurs. The biologic changes that accompany a pregnancy and that affect motherhood and aging also have a psychological impact in our youth-oriented culture (Blakenship, 2003). Contraception is an important health consideration for heterosexual couples during these years.

Physical health in young adulthood is promoted by consumption of an adequate diet, exercise, and monitoring of overall well-being. These needs for health promotion and maintenance are best met when a woman lives within a social context that is conducive to health (Olshansky, 1996). Optimal health is more readily achievable when a woman does not have to confront racism, sexism, or classism, but instead has access to quality health care, economic stability, and other resources (Olshansky, 1996). In reality, however, most women have lives that incorporate multiple and competing demands related to work, economics, childbearing, and childrearing.

Women's changing roles—specifically, the transition from traditional homemaker to working outside the home—have come at a cost to their health, probably because women working outside the home continue to have significant responsibilities within the home. Balancing these competing demands increases the stress level of many women (Condon, 2004). As stress increases, many women have coped by developing unhealthy behaviors such as smoking, lack of exercise, and poor nutrition. As a result, women's health risks for some diseases are now similar to those of men. For example, cardiac disease is now the number one killer of women in the United States (Centers for Disease Control and Prevention [CDC], 2015), whereas 2 decades ago the primary cause of illness and health risk for women was related to reproduction. Health problems that frequently occur during this stage of life include cardiac disease, arthritis, occupational injury and related illnesses, cancer, infections (sexually transmitted and otherwise),

and reproductive disorders (Olshansky, 1996). Chapters 4 and 7 discuss health promotion and health maintenance in more specific detail.

Psychosocial Development

Erikson's (1968) model identifies two crises that occur during early adulthood. The first is the development of intimacy versus isolation: the process of entering into a life partnership with another individual. It is during this developmental phase that gender assumptions about behavior become more typically defined. As previously noted, women are assumed to require intimacy as a prerequisite for the completion of their identity development, whereas males may progress into this phase without any prior development related to their ability to participate in relationships.

It is this contrast of what is described as normative for both males and females that challenged Franz and White (1985) to offer an expansion of Erikson's theory of development. Using a feminist lens, Franz and White discourage the use of a single pathway of development that primarily focuses on individuation, and instead encourage the consideration of a two-pathway process that includes both individuation and a process of attachment. They argue that Erikson does not conceptualize being female as somehow inferior or lacking in purpose, nor simply as a vehicle for childbearing and caretaking. Instead, they describe his work as not attending to the process by which attachment occurs through intimacy and relationships with others. Franz and White posit that Erikson does not provide adequate opportunity in his traditional framework for male development of the capacity for intimacy and attachment.

The expanded model that Franz and White (1985) propose includes two processes of development: individuation combined with an attachment pathway in a double-helix model. The double-helix model allows for these two separate strands to be interconnected, depicting the relationship between psychological individuation and attachment as ascending in a spiral that represents the human life span. The strand representing individuation is essentially the same as it is in Erikson's model, but the attachment strand addresses the neglected relational dimension of human development. **Table 2-2** represents the individuation and

TABLE 2-2 Franz and White's Adaptation of Erikson's Theory of Development to a Two-Path Model

Pathway	Infancy	Early Childhood	Play Age	School Age	Adolescence	Young Adulthood	Adulthood	Old Age
Individuation pathway	Trust vs. mistrust	Autonomy vs. shame and doubt	Initiative vs. guilt	Industry vs. inferiority	Identity vs. identity diffusion	Career, lifestyle exploration vs. drifting	Lifestyle consolidation vs. emptiness	Integrity vs. despair
Attachment pathway	Trust vs. mistrust	Object and self-constancy vs. loneliness and helplessness	Playfulness vs. passivity or aggression	Empathy and collaboration vs. excessive caution or power	Mutuality interdependence vs. alienation	Intimacy vs. isolation	Generativity vs. self-absorption	Integrity vs. despair

Used with permission from Low, L. K. (2001). *Adolescents' experiences of childbirth: Nothing is simple.* Unpublished doctoral dissertation, University of Michigan, Ann Arbor, MI.

attachment "strands" as described by Franz and White. The authors argue:

> With changing times and mores, [if] attachment processes were to undergo fuller development in men and individuation processes were to undergo fuller development in women, sex differences might become more elusive than ever, but individuation and attachment would retain their power as psychological variables associated with psychological value in important nomological nets. (Franz & White, 1985, p. 254)

The second crisis of early adulthood is acquiring the ability to become generative versus stagnation. Here *generative* is defined as acting on one's concern for the welfare of the next generation. Reproduction and parenting may accomplish this goal, as can service to others. Stagnation occurs when the person is unable to step outside of herself or himself and be generative.

As stated earlier, Erikson's work is based on men and may not be an accurate model for assessing women's development. Newer models of women's development emphasize the relational aspects of women's lives. Understanding women's lives within their individual social context provides a women-oriented perspective for conceptualizing the degree to which a woman reaches a particular level of psychosocial development (Olshansky, 1996).

During the young adulthood years, women's psychosocial development may involve a variety of factors, such as accepting responsibilities (parenting, caring for others), creating a career, forming enduring relationships, caring for elderly parents, and deciding whether to become a parent. Although all of these factors influence a woman's psychosocial development, they cannot be understood as generalities that are applied to all women, nor should each be assessed in isolation. Instead, each woman's relation to these factors—to herself and others, to the social context of her life, and to her lived experience—provides insight into her level of psychosocial development.

Clinical Application

A woman goes through many transitional periods from age 18 to 35. For women at risk of pregnancy,

contraceptive decisions are of paramount importance, and it is critical to have access to and receive information and education about contraceptive options. Decisions related to childbearing (or not) are also prominent and frame much of the healthcare services that women traditionally receive during this phase of their lives. Many lifestyle-related health problems may become apparent during this time. Substance abuse, intimate partner violence, and stress related to her life or those she cares for can all negatively affect a woman's health during early adulthood. Psychiatric illnesses that may become apparent during these years include bipolar disorder, schizophrenia, and psychosis, which may or may not be related to childbearing.

Although young adult women are primarily healthy, it is evident there are many opportunities for life events to negatively affect their health. Health promotion and maintenance during this period are critical to ensure optimal health in the later years of life.

MIDLIFE

Midlife for women encompasses the perimenopausal years (ages 35–50) to menopause (ages 50–65) (American College of Obstetricians and Gynecologists, 2014a). Midlife is actually a transition more than a phase of the human life cycle, and during this time many women experience a recognition that their lives are changing irrevocably. Some women will pursue goals and dreams they may have deferred while dealing with the greater life demands they faced in younger adulthood. If they were parenting during their earlier adulthood, then transitions into other aspects of their lives may be prompted by their children leaving home. Still others may be in the active phases of parenting as more women delay childbearing decisions until later into the early phases of midlife. During this phase of the life span, Erikson (1950) would continue to identify the phases of generativity versus stagnation as a continuing process.

Biology and Physiology

Perimenopause and menopause are biologic markers of the transition from young adult to midlife. Neither is a syndrome or a disease, but instead both demonstrate a natural maturing of the reproductive system. Social constructions of perimenopause and menopause abound. Martin (1992) encourages us to reframe perimenopause and menopause so that our ideas of a "single purpose" for the menstrual cycle can be reconstructed into images of healthy transitions.

During the perimenopausal years, women may experience physical changes associated with decreasing estrogen levels, such as the vasomotor symptoms of hot flashes and flushes. Other changes associated with aging include a decrease in the size of genitalia, changes in breast structure, and decreased skin elasticity. These changes are more fully described in Chapter 12.

Although for many years it was believed a preponderance of midlife women suffered mood changes caused by a deficiency of estrogen during this time of life, more recent studies suggest that psychosocial factors have a much greater effect on a midlife woman's mood than do the physiologic transitions of menopause.

Psychosocial Development

Midlife is a dynamic period of ongoing transition. Women during this time often experience increased feelings of physical and emotional well-being and greater control over their lives (American College of Obstetricians and Gynecologists, 2014b). They may pursue new interests, acquire new skills, and enjoy more time with friends and family (Boston Women's Health Book Collective, 2011). A qualitative study of midlife women born between the years 1955 and 1964 found that most of the participants had an overall positive outlook on life (Hilber, 2011). Conversely, Gilligan (1982) suggests that midlife may be a time of risk for women precisely because of their embeddedness in relationships, orientation to interdependence, ability to subordinate achievement to care, and conflicts over competitive success. However, the findings of the Hilber (2011) study suggest that important relationships lead to more positive perceptions during this time and that relational changes are consistent with personal growth through acceptance and positivity.

What is often missing from descriptions of psychosocial development of women in midlife is the social context of their lives and their own perspective (Dare, 2011). In Dare's research, women participated in a qualitative study of their perceptions of midlife transition. The findings revealed that menopause was more irritating than unmanageable or representative of a major emotional upheaval, with most women reporting that they coped well with the changes associated with this transition. Some of the participants indicated that the relief of no longer having to deal with menses overshadowed any discomfort. Women whose children had grown and left home expressed that this was a natural stage in their children's independence; while some were ambivalent about what it might mean in the way of change, just as many felt a new sense of freedom and welcomed this time in their lives. In fact, a sense of pride was expressed about having their children grown and on their own. The study participants also looked forward to an evolving relationship with their children in which they would be on more "equal" footing. One of the biggest stressors identified by the participants was divorce—particularly, its impact on their financial status and on their networks of social support. Another issue identified by the group was caring for aging parents. Overall, however, this group of women in midlife suggested that they were navigating the transitions quite well (Dare, 2011).

Clinical Application

A common myth is that women lose their interest in sex when they reach middle age and that sexual activity is still defined within the context of heterosexuality only. Aging does decrease vaginal lubrication, and therefore the use of vaginal lubricants can facilitate comfortable intercourse. A study of 286 women who were in their midlife years identified a significant decrease in sexual desire during the late menopausal transition stage. However, women who were using hormone therapy and who had a better health perception reported higher desire (Woods, Mitchell, & Smith-Di, 2010). It is important for clinicians who provide care for women who are in midlife to promote healthy sexual functioning and assess their patients' changing biology as well as life challenges that may negatively impact desire. Also, women who engage in sexual intercourse with men and who are perimenopausal should be provided with information about contraception if they want to avoid pregnancy.

Ageism and bias based on age are common in Western society. For the clinician, it is important to provide supportive care throughout a woman's life span and not assume a woman's health concerns are entirely related to her age.

OLDER WOMEN

The term *older women* refers to women who have completed menopause. Older women outnumber older men, although overall there is a continuing increase in the number of people in the United States who are 65 years or older (U.S. Census Bureau, 2014). This aging of the population is due to the "baby boomers," who began to turn 65 in 2011 (American College of Obstetricians and Gynecologists, 2014b). Many older women are living on limited and fixed incomes, and Medicare reimbursement is either poor or nonexistent for many of the healthcare services needed by this population (American College of Obstetricians and Gynecologists, 2014a). The aging process is frequently associated with a number of problematic issues, including chronic medical conditions as well as challenges related to autonomy and independence (American College of Obstetricians and Gynecologists, 2014a). Providing supportive and age-appropriate health care is critical to maintaining the health and quality of life for this population.

Biology and Physiology

Theories abound about the cause of aging and the biologic and physiologic impacts of aging, but more research is needed to produce definitive findings. What is known about aging is that "normal" aging can be distinguished from disease. As bodies age and change due to aging, and in some instances decline due to age, the changes do not inevitably lead to chronic diseases such as diabetes, hypertension, and dementia (National Institute on Aging [NIA]/National Institutes of Health [NIH], 2008, reprinted 2010). Additionally there is no chronological timetable for human aging (NIA/NIH, 2008).

People age differently, and factors such as genetics, lifestyle, and disease processes all affect the aging process. Nevertheless, research has identified some factors that support healthy aging:

- Exercise and physical activity, especially when it is done regularly
- Maintaining a healthy weight
- Maintaining good nutrition (NIA/NIH, 2008)

Overall, many more studies on aging are needed.

Psychosocial Development

Research suggests that older women are often caregivers for ailing male spouses or partners, and many end up living alone (because they outlive their male partners), but they continue to maintain a connectedness to other family members. There is a dearth of research examining the caregiver issue when the partners or spouses are both female, or the specific concerns of LGBT older adults and their families, because sexual orientation as a research variable is typically missing in the major studies of gerontology (Orel & Fruhauf, 2015). Although transgender and gender-nonconforming people (TGNC) face many of the same aging challenges as heterosexual people, they also have some unique ways of experiencing the aging process (Ippolito & Witten, 2014). It is important, therefore, that studies focusing on psychosocial development and the aging process include LGBT people as participants.

There is also a specific gap in the knowledge about gender-related distinctions and aging. The economic and social conditions in which people live are known as the social determinants of health; they have a significant impact on an individual's health and well-being. In addition to social determinants, the capacity of women to actively be part of the decision-making process and their access to the resources needed to maintain health and well-being can have a critical impact on their likelihood of healthy aging (Davidson, DiGiacomo, & McGrath, 2011). Theories suggest that as we age, we begin to disengage from society, and that we make adjustments based on our lifelong patterns, likes, and dislikes. As yet, however, relatively few studies have addressed hypotheses.

Clinical Application

The health issues of older women are substantial. For many women, older age brings social isolation and, in many cases, economic adversity (Davidson et al., 2011). Ageism—that is, stereotyping and discrimination of a person based on age—is even more common at this stage of life. Elderly women must contend not only with ageism, but also with sexism. Youth and beauty are highly valued in the United States. While older men may be viewed as attractive, often an older woman is pressured to take steps to ward off looking her age.

As the aging of the global population is recognized, what is not being acknowledged is the "feminization of aging" (Davidson et al., 2011). While more women are living longer than men and thus overcoming many of the negative impacts of communicable and chronic conditions, that trend means that more older women may be impacted by social isolation and economic adversity; living longer does not necessarily mean living healthfully (Davidson et al., 2011). The impact of this pattern on the aging population and on the well-being of women is in need of further study.

In a recent qualitative gender analysis of aging and resilience among very old men and women, it was found that even if an elderly person scores low in resilience, he or she can still experience well-being. Resilience, in this study, was defined as an enduring positive view of life despite aging and difficult circumstances. However, when elderly men and women were compared, it was clear that elderly women who had low resilience were more vulnerable than men. Moreover, it was important to strengthen their social and relational possibilities, as this in turn increased their resilience and well-being (Alex & Lundman, 2011).

Pohl and Boyd (1993) suggest that a key area in which clinicians might begin to link feminist theory with aging women is in health policies and the inequities inherent in them. To promote health and wellness in women who are older, clinicians must provide them with adequate information about their health status, risks, and ways of improving health through diet and exercise commensurate with their age and capabilities.

CONCLUSION

Other chapters within this text present more detailed discussions of the clinical assessment and management of women's gynecologic health. Through the continued use of a feminist framework, an expanded model of gynecologic health is presented that includes great opportunity to both affect change and improve health outcomes for women.

References

Alex, L., & Lundman, B. (2011). Lack of resilience among very old men and women: A qualitative gender analysis. *Research & Theory for Nursing Practice, 25*(4), 302–316.

American Academy of Child and Adolescent Psychiatry (AACAP). (2013). Gay, lesbian and bisexual adolescents. No. 63. Retrieved from http://www.aacap.org/AACAP/Families_and_Youth/Facts_for_Families/FFF-Guide/Gay-Lesbian-and-Bisexual-Adolescents-063.aspx

American Academy of Child and Adolescent Psychiatry (AACAP). (2015a). Normal adolescent development Part I. No. 57. Retrieved from http://www.aacap.org/AACAP/AACAP/Families_and_Youth/Facts_for_Families/FFF-Guide/Normal-Adolescent-Development-Part-I-057.aspx

American Academy of Child and Adolescent Psychiatry (AACAP). (2015b). Normal adolescent development Part II. No. 58. Retrieved from http://www.aacap.org/AACAP/AACAP/Families_and_Youth/Facts_for_Families/FFF-Guide/Normal-Adolescent-Development-Part-II-058.aspx

American College of Obstetricians and Gynecologists. (2011). Guidelines for adolescent health care. Retrieved from http://www.acog.org/About-ACOG/ACOG-Departments/Adolescent-Health-Care/Guidelines

American College of Obstetricians and Gynecologists. (2014a). *Guidelines for women's health care: A resource manual* (4th ed.). Washington, DC: Author.

American College of Obstetricians and Gynecologists. (2014b). Midlife transitions: Perimenopause to menopause. Retrieved from http://www.acog.org

American College of Obstetricians and Gynecologists. (2015). Menstruation in girls and adolescents: Using the menstrual cycle as a vital sign. Committee Opinion No. 651. *Obstetrics & Gynecology, 126,* e143–e146.

American Psychological Association (APA). (2002). Developing adolescents: A reference for professionals. Retrieved from http://www.apa.org/pubs/info/brochures/develop.aspx

Backus, F. R., & Mahalik, J. R. (2011). The masculinity of Mr. Right: Feminist identity and heterosexual women's idea partner. *Psychology of Women Quarterly, 35*(2), 318–326.

Baker Miller, J. (1991). The development of women's sense of self. In J. Jordan, A. Kaplan, J. Miller, I. Stiver, & J. Surrey (Eds.), *Women's growth in connection: Writings from the Stone Center* (pp. 11–34). New York, NY: Guilford Press.

Belenky, M., Clinchy, B., Goldberger, N., & Tarule, J. (1986). *Women's ways of knowing.* New York, NY: Harper Collins.

Bilodeau, B. L., & Renn, K. A. (2005). Analysis of LGBT identity development models and implications for practice, *New Directions for Student Services, 111*, 25–39.

Blakenship, V. (2003). Psychosocial development of women. In E. Breslin & V. Lucas (Eds.), *Women's health nursing: Toward evidence-based practice* (pp. 133–169). St. Louis, MO: Saunders.

Boston Women's Health Book Collective. (2011). *Our bodies, ourselves for the new century.* New York, NY: Simon & Schuster.

Cass, V. (1979). Homosexual identity formation: A theoretical model. *Journal of Homosexuality, 4,* 219–235.

Centers for Disease Control and Prevention (CDC). (2015). Women and heart disease fact sheet. Retrieved from http://www.cdc.gov/dhdsp/data_statistics/fact_sheets/docs/fs_women_heart.pdf

Chang, Y., Hayter, M., & Wu, S. (2010). A systemic review and meta-ethnography of the qualitative literature: Experiences of the menarche. *Journal of Clinical Nursing, 19*(3/4), 447–460.

Clapp, J. F., & Little, K. D. (1995). The interaction between regular exercise and selected aspects of women's health. *American Journal of Obstetrics & Gynecology, 173*(1), 2–9.

Collins, P. (2000). *Black feminist thought: Knowledge, consciousness, and the politics of empowerment.* London, UK: Harper Collins.

Condon M. C. (2004). *Women's health: Body, mind, and spirit: An integrated approach to wellness and illness.* Prentice Hall, NJ: Prentice Hall.

Dare, J. S. (2011). Transitions in midlife women's lives: Contemporary experiences. *Health Care for Women International, 32,* 111–133.

Davidson, P. M., DiGiacomo, M., & McGrath, S. J. (2011). The feminization of aging: How will this impact on health outcomes and services? *Health Care for Women International, 32,* 1031–1045.

Deanow, C. G. (2011). Relational development through the life cycle: Capacities, opportunities, challenges, and obstacles. *Journal of Women and Social Work, 26*(2), 125–138.

Erikson, E. H. (1950). *Childhood and society.* New York, NY: W. W. Norton.

Erikson, E. H. (1968). *Identity: Youth and crisis.* New York, NY: W. W. Norton.

Forbes, E. E., & Dahl, R. E. (2010). Pubertal development and behavior: Hormonal activation of social and motivational tendencies. *Brain and Cognition, 72,* 66–72.

Franz, C., & White, K. (1985). Individuation and attachment in personality development: Extending Erikson's theory. *Journal of Personality, 53*(2), 224–256.

Fritz, M., & Speroff, L. (2011). *Clinical gynecologic endocrinology and infertility* (8th ed.). Baltimore, MD: Williams & Wilkins.

Gilchrist, V. (1997). Psychosocial development of girls and women. In J. Rosenfeld (Ed.), *Women's health in primary care* (pp. 21–28). Baltimore, MD: Williams & Wilkins.

Gilligan, C. (1982). *In a different voice: Psychological theory and women's development.* Cambridge, MA: Harvard University Press.

Gilligan, C. (1986). Reply by Carol Gilligan. *Signs, 11*(2), 324–333. Retrieved from http://www.jstor.org/stable/3174055

Glover, J. A., Galliher, R. V., & Lamere, T. D. (2009). Identity development and exploration among sexual minority adolescents: Examination of a multidimensional model. *Journal of Homosexuality, 56*(1), 77–101.

Hare-Mustin, R. T., & Marecek, J. (1998). The meaning of difference: Gender theory, postmodernism and psychology. In B. McVicker Clinchy & J. K. Norem (Eds.), *The gender and psychology reader* (pp. 125–143). New York, NY: New York University Press.

Healthychildren.org. (2015). Stages of adolescence. Retrieved from https://www.healthychildren.org/English/ages-stages/teen/Pages

Hilber, T. L. (2011). A qualitative study of midlife in women born within 1955–1964: The trailing edge group of the baby boomer cohort. *ProQuest: Dissertation Abstracts International.* Retrieved from http://proquest.com

Ippolito, J., & Witten, T. M. (2014). Aging. In L. Erickson-Schroth (Ed.), *Trans bodies, trans selves: A resource for the transgender community* (pp. 476–497). New York, NY: Oxford University Press.

Jackson, T. E., & Falmagne, R. J. (2013). Women wearing white: Discourses of menstruation and the experience of menarche. *Feminism & Psychology, 23*(3), 379–398.

Jones, T. C. K. (2010). "It drives us to do it": Pregnant adolescents identify drives for sexual risk-taking. *Issues in Comprehensive Pediatric Nursing, 33*(2), 82–100.

Kaplan, A., Gleason, N., & Klein, R. (1991). Women's self-development in late adolescence. In J. Jordan, A. Kaplan, J. Miller, I. Stiver, & J. Surrey (Eds.), *Women's growth in connection: Writings from the Stone Center* (pp. 122–140). New York, NY: Guilford Press.

Kaufman, J., & Johnson, C. (2004). Stigmatized individuals and the process of identity. *Sociological Quarterly, 45*(4), 807–833.

Kohlberg, L. (1981). *The philosophy of moral development.* San Francisco, CA: Harper & Row.

Krieger, N., Klang, M. V., Kosheleva, A., Waterman, P. D., Chen, J. T., & Beckfield, J. (2015). Age at menarche: 50-year socioeconomic trends among US-born black and white women. *American Journal of Public Health, 105*(2), 388–397.

Lee, J. (2008). "A Kotex and a smile": Mothers and daughters at menarche. *Journal of Family Issues, 29*(10), 1325–1347.

Low, L. K. (2001). *Adolescents' experiences of childbirth: Nothing is simple.* Unpublished doctoral dissertation, University of Michigan, Ann Arbor, MI.

Martin, E. (1992). *The woman in the body.* Boston, MA: Beacon Press.

Miller, P. M., & Scholnick, E. K. (2015). Feminist theory and contemporary developmental psychology: The case of children's executive function. *Feminism & Psychology, 25*(3), 266–283.

Mitchell, V. (2014). The lifespan as a feminist context: Making developmental concepts come alive in therapy. *Women & Therapy, 37*(1–2), 135–140.

National Institute on Aging (NIA), & National Institutes of Health (NIH). (2008, reprinted 2010). Healthy aging: Lessons from the Baltimore Longitudinal Study of Aging. Publication No. 08-6440. Retrieved from https://d2cauhfh6h4x0p.cloudfront.net/s3fs-public/healthy_aging_lessons_from_the_baltimore_longitudinal_study_of_aging.pdf

Olshansky, E. (1996). The reproductive years. In J. Lewis & J. Bernstein (Eds.), *Women's health* (pp. 105–143). Sudbury, MA: Jones and Bartlett.

Orel, N. A., & Fruhauf, C. A. (Eds.). (2015). *The lives of LGBT older adults: Understanding challenges and resilience.* Washington DC: American Psychological Association.

Perry, W. (1968). *Forms of intellectual and ethical development in the college years.* New York, NY: Holt, Rinehart & Winston.

Pohl, J., & Boyd, C. (1993). Ageism within feminism. *Image, 25,* 200–203.

Psychology Today. (2015). Adolescence. Retrieved from https://www.psychologytoday.com/basics/adolescence

Riger, S. (1998). Epistemological debates, feminist voices: Science, social values, and the study of women. In B. McVicker Clinchy & J. K. Norem (Eds.), *The gender and psychology reader* (pp. 34–53). New York, NY: New York University Press.

Rosenbloom, A., & Tanner, M. (1998). Misuse of Tanner scale [Letter to the editor]. *Pediatrics, 102,* 1494.

Sadowski, M., Chow, S., & Scanlon, C.P. (2009). Meeting the needs of LGBTQ youth. *Journal of LGBT Youth, 6*(2–3), 174–198.

Segalowitz, S. J., Santesso, D. L., & Jetha, M. K. (2010). Electrophysiological changes during adolescence: A review. *Brain and Cognition, 72*(1), 86–100.

Silber, L. M. (2012). Adolescent girls and the transgenerational relational catch. *Journal of Infant, Child, and Adolescent Psychotherapy, 11,* 121–132.

Sokol, J. T. (2009). Identity development throughout the lifetime: An examination of Eriksonian theory. *Graduate Journal of Counseling Psychology, 1*(2), 1–11.

Stieglitz, K. A. (2010). Development, risk, and resilience of transgender youth. *Journal of the Association of Nurses in AIDS Care, 21*(3), 192–206.

Tavris, C. (1992). *Mismeasure of women.* New York, NY: Simon & Schuster.

Taylor, C. (1994). Gender equity in research. *Journal of Women's Health, 3,* 143–153.

Thomas, F., Renaud, F., Benefice, E., de Meeus, T., & Guegan, F. F. (2001). International variability of ages at menarche and menopause: Patterns and main determinants. *Human Biology, 73,* 271–290.

Tummala-Narra, P. (2013). Growing at the hyphen: Female friendships and social context. *Women & Therapy, 36,* 35–50.

Tyson, S.Y. (2012). Developmental and ethnic issues experienced by emerging adult African American women related to developing a mature love relationship. *Issues in Mental Health Nursing, 33,* 39–51.

U.S. Census Bureau. (2014). *65+ in the United States 2010.* Washington, DC: U.S. Government Printing Office.

Woods, N. F., Mitchell, E. S., & Smith-Di, J. K. (2010). Sexual desire during the menopausal transition and early postmenopause: Observations from the Seattle midlife women's health study. *Journal of Women's Health, 19*(2), 209–218.

World Health Organization (WHO). (2015). Maternal, newborn, child and adolescent health: Adolescent development. Retrieved from http://www.who.int/maternal_child_adolescent/topics/adolescence/dev/en

Deanow's Model of Development Highlighting Relational Tasks and Obstacles Throughout the Life Span

Age Clusters	Roles	Capacities/ Opportunities	Obstacles/ Challenges[a]
Infancy: 0–18 months[b]	Primary empathy/ nonresponsive	Learns primary empathy Bonds with caregivers A two-person dynamic Girls may be more encouraged to develop primary empathy, although boys are permitted to learn empathy and satisfaction of relationships	Nonresponsiveness to caregivers Disconnection to caregivers Could be due to biology (autism spectrum) or to neglect and abuse by a caregiver
Toddler: 18 months to 2–3 years[c]	Relational differentiation/ unworthiness	Little girls learning who they are, what they think and feel More attuned to feelings of others Relational differentiation occurs: differentiated from others but more connected in other ways	Develops sense of unworthiness Learns that self is not acceptable Learns not to expect satisfaction in relationships
Preschool: 3–6 years[d]	Caretaking/ diminishment	Begin to engage in authentic mutual relationships with other children Little girls are socialized to become caretakers and to take care of the relationship itself (most of the toys for girls at this age emphasize this)	Danger is that girls may begin to learn to keep aspects of themselves out of relationships if they fear it will negatively impact the relationship Girls may learn that caring about themselves first is selfish Girls may learn the father has more power than the mother This period is complex for little boys, as they begin to become involved in "boy culture," which is evidenced by distancing from their mothers and disengaging from feelings except for anger

Age Clusters	Roles	Capacities/ Opportunities	Obstacles/ Challenges[a]
			Little boys may be shamed for crying or other activities viewed as feminine
School age: 7–12 years	Chumship/hurt	Continue to develop relationships at home but also invest a lot of energy into investing relational development with same-sex peers	Learn that disconnections and conflicts in relationships always cause hurt May develop bullying behaviors; especially noted in boys, as the boy culture emphasizes winning at all costs If unsuccessful in developing positive relationships with peers, the social support for positive relational conflict and engagement is hurt
Adolescence: 12–25 years	Authenticity/ voicelessness	Bringing the evolving sense of self into relationships with parents, other adults, friends, and romantic partners Parents remain important but child begins to redefine the relationship	Very difficult for adolescent girls to bring full self to relationships, which creates a relational paradox—without authenticity, there is no real relationship; in essence, the girl "loses her voice" Growing awareness of sexuality and viewing self as a sexual being For boys, the boy culture continues to have a tight hold, often resulting in a locker-room mentality; physical and sexual dominance develop, and may include violence and risk-taking behaviors
Early adulthood and may be repeated throughout adulthood	Mutuality/ subordination or domination	Physical and societal push to "find a mate" Relationships become a major focus; goal is to achieve a true relational mutuality	Regardless of whether the relationship is same or different sexes, if one partner is male, the relational work is often distorted by the man's inability or lack of desire to be involved wholly in the relationship Dilemma is that while women usually want something to happen in the relationship, men fear it will

(continues)

Age Clusters	Roles	Capacities/ Opportunities	Obstacles/ Challenges[a]
			The difference in relational skill development between men and women is very evident and creates major challenges
			If male domination is extreme, domestic violence may result
Throughout adulthood (ongoing)	Dexterity/ imbalance	Greater opportunities for mutually enhancing relationships (e.g., spouse, partner, children, friends, colleagues)	Real challenge for women is finding time to engage in all the relationships and still have a balance in their lives
		Men at this stage tend to have left the boy culture and are now more into family relationships	Danger for men at this stage is to adhere to the belief that they need to be the breadwinner and invest in work at the expense of family and friends
		Relationships at work are especially important for women at this stage	Men at this age often have few adult male friendships and may be jealous of the friendships their female partners have
Aging/elders	Sustainment/ abandonment or withdrawal	Opportunities for sustaining relationships are strong	Diminished capacities and energies along with inevitable disconnections or loss of some friends challenge the relational lives of seniors
		Relational growth at this age may involve asking for and accepting help due to their decreasing abilities to care for themselves	Some may not want to start new relationships due to fear of loss

[a] Occur when things to not go well for the child/person.
[b] In this age cluster, there is the least difference in the expected relational behavior between boys and girls.
[c] Gender identity is thought to begin at this stage; this should not be confused with gender socialization, which occurs throughout the life cycle.
[d] Relational work takes place at home and in a variety of preschool settings.

CHAPTER 3

Using Evidence to Support Clinical Practice

Holly Powell Kennedy

Katherine Camacho Carr

WHAT IS EVIDENCE-BASED PRACTICE?

The elements of evidence-based practice (EBP) or medicine were initially defined by Sackett, Strauss, Richardson, Rosenberg, and Haynes (2000) as "the integration of the best research evidence with clinical expertise and patient values" (p. 1). EBP demands a high level of scientific evidence at all decision-making points in a woman's care, making every clinician a researcher on some level to ensure that women receive the best possible care. Since Sackett's original work, the influence of EBP has become increasingly evident in identifying best clinical practices, in the education of clinicians, in the development of health policy, and in organizational management and quality improvement (Badgett & Fernandez, 2013; Gillam & Siriwardina, 2014; Ilic & Maloney, 2014; Levin & Chang, 2014; Maggio & Kung, 2014; Melnyk, Gallagher-Ford, Long, & Fineout-Overholt, 2014; Miller & Skinner, 2012; Sackett, Haynes, Guyatt, & Tugwell, 2000; Schaffer, Sandau, & Diedrick, 2013).

EBP begins with a clinical question or query about best practice, and then proceeds to identify and evaluate the best research available to find the answer. To comprehensively and accurately answer the question, clinical experience and patient preferences must be integrated with the research evidence. Evidence generated by other researchers, which has been preappraised and synthesized by agencies or organizations, such as the National Guideline Clearinghouse of the Agency for Healthcare Research and Quality or the Cochrane Database of Systematic Reviews (CDSR), is often used as sources of evidence. The synthesis of evidence can provide guidelines for practice, diagnostic testing, and changes in procedures, treatment plans, or policies. Evidence-based pathways of care eliminate wide variations in care that may not be efficacious or safe, or that are superfluous or unnecessarily costly. Examination of the evidence can also assist with the development of clinical benchmarking and process- or outcome-based performance measures as well as provide a rationale for the elimination of unnecessary processes or procedures. The use of evidence complements the clinician's expertise and the woman's personal desires in her health care.

At times we clinicians conduct our own research to generate an answer to a clinical question by sorting and evaluating research findings to identify the most effective therapies or the best way of controlling costs. For some clinicians, conducting research may entail a small study to develop a clinical protocol. For others, it may involve supervising a clinical trial. Regardless of the scope of the research, the underlying principles are the same. This chapter reviews research principles, methods, and critique techniques to assist clinicians in developing skills in practice-based research so they can provide care that is truly evidence-based.

A FEMINIST PERSPECTIVE ON RESEARCH

This book is founded on a feminist framework that recognizes hierarchies are an oppressive reality in health care. These hierarchies are implicated in women's health disparities, as well as in the historical lack of research devoted to women's health issues (Doyal, 1995). Feminist theories provide a platform to expose gender inequities, ensure social understanding of women's perspectives, and offer "critiques of the assumptions, biases, and consequences of androcentric philosophies and practices" (Brisolara, 2014, p. 4). Most feminists would agree that science is not acontextual or ahistorical—rather, it must understand the woman's history and the context of her life.

Brisolara (2014) outlines eight evaluation principles critical to the conduct of feminist research (pp. 23–31):

1. Knowledge is culturally, socially, and temporally contingent.
2. Knowledge is a powerful resource that serves an explicit or implicit purpose.
3. Evaluation is a political activity; evaluators' [researchers'] personal experiences, perspectives, and characteristics come from and lead to a particular political stance.
4. Research methods, institutions, and practices are social constructs.
5. There are multiple ways of knowing.
6. Gender inequities are one manifestation of social injustice. Discrimination cuts across race, class, and culture and is inextricably linked to all three.
7. Discrimination based on gender is systemic and structural.
8. Action and advocacy are considered to be morally and ethically appropriate responses of an engaged feminist evaluator.

These principles provide a lens from which to examine the construction, design, and outcomes of women's health research.

THE HISTORY OF EVIDENCE-BASED PRACTICE

Nursing science has a rich heritage of applying evidence to practice. Florence Nightingale (1859/1957) outlined the basic principles of nursing science in her best-known work, *Notes on Nursing*. The Nightingale method of nursing included rigorous monitoring of all treatments for their effectiveness, which was an early version of EBP. Authority for Nightingale's work in public health and hygiene was based on trial and error, intuition, clinical experience, careful observation, and discussion with patients (McDonald, 2004). As a pioneer, Nightingale used statistical data to improve health, sanitation, administration of health services, and nursing education. Nightingale was not a romantic Victorian gentlewoman, but rather a bright, organized feminist and mathematician. She applied statistics to the study of public health and mortality data, exposing vast social injustices, and influenced health policy on multiple levels (Hegge, 2013). Her work and that of other nurse theorists, researchers, and clinicians provided the foundation for a long tradition in nursing that combines careful scientific observation, sensitivity to the individual's needs, and recognition of the influence of the contextual environment of health and illness.

The initiation of the modern EBP movement in health care is attributed to British epidemiologist, Dr. Archie Cochrane, who was concerned that clinicians often failed to evaluate the effectiveness of their own care and did not have widespread access to the scientific literature (Smith & Rennie, 2014). His initial work in the 1970s led to the review of all randomized controlled trials in perinatal medicine and ultimately to the establishment of the Cochrane Collaboration in 1992, which currently has a much wider scope covering reviews in many fields of health care. The Cochrane Database of Systematic Reviews (2014), an electronic database that is part of the Cochrane Library, remains one of the largest, most comprehensive reviews of evidence available.

The EBP movement is often described as a paradigm change in health care, moving from reliance on expert opinion and experience to reliance on scientific evidence as the basis for practice (Eisenberg, 2001; Kuhn, 1970). The present paradigm shift to evidence-based care has focused on the identification of the best drugs, clinical practices, and surgical procedures through rigorous study, with randomized clinical trials (RCTs), meta-analyses, and systematic reviews of the scientific literature forming the primary evidence base for patient care (Straus, Richardson, Glasziou, & Haynes, 2010). In response to this shift away from expert opinion, there has been a proliferation of articles, books, and websites instructing clinicians how to conduct, evaluate, interpret, and apply the medical literature over the last decade (Carlson, 2014; Guyatt, Rennie, Meade, & Cook, 2014). Marckmann, Schmidt, Sofaer, and Strech (2015) present a useful framework for application of evidence using a public health perspective (**Box 3-1**).

An examination of the state of the EBP movement, the philosophy of science, and the state of nursing science suggests that the use of evidence is not a new or revolutionary paradigm shift, and may explain only part of the science upon which the change is based (Sehon & Stanley, 2003). Quine (1952), another philosopher of science, describes the scientific worldview as a web of beliefs, like a spider web with an exterior edge or frame secured to an existing structure, and possessing an interconnecting interior of radii and connecting points. Using this metaphor, the web of scientific beliefs can be seen as encompassing sensory information and new untested theories that now exist on the developing edge of the web. Foundational theories such as the laws of nature, logic, or mathematics form the center of the web. The interconnections

between the center and the periphery are composed of well-proven hypotheses about health and clinical practice. According to Quine's metaphor, we use a vast network or web of healthcare beliefs with logical and evidential relationships to determine best practices, including the findings of experimental research, primarily RCTs, intuition, and experience (Quine, 1952).

The sciences of medicine and nursing are composed of a vast network of beliefs, scientific observations, practices, hypothetical relationships, and theories. For example, in practice we encounter observations (blood pressure), hypotheses (how the blood pressure may need to be repeated before we accept that it is an accurate measurement), and theories (the psychophysiology of blood pressure regulation). Quine (1952) also suggests that scientific observations must be contextually examined as part of a whole, rather than being viewed in isolation from the rest of scientific knowledge. The concept of a web of knowledge, along with interconnected relationships between practices and underlying theories, supports a multiple-method approach to examining phenomena.

A more recent development in health care is the recognition that management of facilities and practices should also be evidence-based—an approach termed *evidence-based management.* Managers of healthcare settings are beginning to realize that clinicians are not the only ones who should consider the importance of evidence in the provision of quality care and innovative workforce redesign in terms of both quality and cost (Palazzo, 2015). Specifically, management has a key role in preventing the overuse of interventions shown to be ineffective, the underuse of those interventions that are effective, and misuse when the evidence is unclear (Kohn, Corrigan, & Donaldson, 1999). Managers must work in concert with clinicians and patients to provide evidence-based programs and an environment of care that is highly conducive to quality outcomes, as well as both efficient and cost effective. Decisions about which evidence and outcomes are most important should not be made in a vacuum. Indeed, studies have found that the clinical settings most effective in EBP implementation have a culture that emphasizes adapting to change and encouraging strong nursing and obstetric leadership (Graham, Logan, Davies, & Nimrod, 2004).

BOX 3-1 Evidence-Based Practice from a Public Health Lens

- What are the expected health benefits of the intervention for the target population?
- What are the potential burdens and harms of the intervention?
- How does the intervention affect the autonomy of the individuals in the target population?
- Impact on equity: How are benefits and burden distributed?
- Expected efficiency: What are the costs and opportunity costs of the intervention?

Data from Marckmann, G., Schmidt, H., Sofaer, N., & Strech, D. (2015). Putting public health ethics into practice: A systematic framework. *Frontiers in Public Health, 3,* 1–7.

The California Pregnancy-Associated Mortality Review (CA-PAMR) is an excellent example of a multidisciplinary group that assisted the state in analyzing causes of maternal mortality and translating those findings into improved care (Mitchell, Lawton, Morton, McCain, & Main, 2014). Buse (2008) specifically calls for prospective policy analysis using research and best information relevant to stakeholders in care to provide effective and efficient healthcare systems.

Much of our existing science in medicine and nursing comes from a variety of sources, not all of which are evidence-based. There is not always *one best way* to obtain scientific information about clinical practice. For this reason, we must remain open to and creative about research methods that will give us the best answer or help us better define the interconnected web of knowledge related to the phenomena of interest. Korhonen, Hakulinen-Viitanen, Jylhä, and Holopainen (2013) have described the systematic review of qualitative studies, using meta-synthesis or meta-aggregation, following the principles of scientific rigor, as a means to add these findings to the evidence base and complete the web of knowledge on phenomena.

RESEARCH AND CLINICAL DECISION MAKING

The dimensions of EBP are multifaceted and often influenced by the discipline in which EBP is employed. Despite this inconsistency, EBP remains a major influence on healthcare decisions (Gillam & Siriwardina, 2014). The educational preparation of clinicians usually includes core content on the research process, which can range from actual participation in research studies to general discussions about how to apply research findings to practice. Unfortunately, the word *research* can engender anxiety in many clinicians who are years removed from their educational experience. Research, like any skill, must be used on a regular basis to be effective. Today, however, as a result of their increasing access to computerized information, guidance, and sometimes regulation, clinicians are increasingly being called upon to access, appraise, apply, and evaluate the evidence and the expected patient outcomes (Gillam & Siriwardina, 2014).

One basic premise that helps clinicians shed their tentativeness in either considering conducting research or applying research to clinical practice is the need to reformulate how they think about the entire subject. Research follows the exact same principles that any good clinician follows in everyday clinical management. These principles are ongoing and often circular in nature. One step usually leads to another, but can also raise new questions that take the clinician either back to the beginning or in a new direction. **Table 3-1** compares the steps in the clinical management and research processes.

TYPES OF RESEARCH EVIDENCE

Research evidence comes in many forms. We prefer to call them *types* of evidence, rather than *levels*, to dispel the notion that one form is necessarily better than another, or to suggest linearity. As previously mentioned, clinical experience and patient preferences are two parts of the triad of clinical decision-making criteria. To complete the triad, they are combined with an evaluation of current clinical research.

The RCT is often held up as the gold standard in Western medicine, but not all clinical problems lend themselves to this kind of research. Whatever research method is used must serve the research question being asked, and the results should be evaluated in terms of the quality of the study and the potential benefit or harm to the patient. In the United States, the U.S. Preventive Services Task Force takes the lead on setting guidelines for evaluating healthcare research evidence (USPSTF, 2015). **Table 3-2** summarizes this approach.

RESEARCH METHODS TO INFORM CLINICAL PRACTICE

The historically defined parameters of science, particularly in the Western tradition, can create tension among researchers and clinicians as to what truly qualifies as scientific evidence. Both quantitative and qualitative research approaches employ a variety of methods and techniques, and both aim to expand knowledge about a specific phenomenon. Attempting to pinpoint a defining difference

TABLE 3-1	Alignment of Clinical and Research Processes

The Clinical Management Process	The Research Process
Gathering the Data	
• Focused toward individual clinical scenario. • Historical, physical, and laboratory data may be gathered.	• Focused on a broader perspective of a health issue. • Historical data, review of literature, and pilot study may be involved.
Identifying the Problem	
• Assessment is made of the individual's clinical problem.	• A research question and/or hypothesis is generated.
Development of the Plan	
• An evidence-based clinical management plan is used to meet the patient's needs.	• A research design is constructed that will best answer the research question.
Implementation	
• The management plan is implemented.	• The research study is conducted.
Evaluation of the Results	
• Clinical follow-up is conducted to assess the effectiveness of the treatment plan.	• Data are analyzed to provide answers to the research questions.

TABLE 3-2	Recommendations for Using Research Evidence in Clinical Practice[a]

Level of Certainty[b]	Description
High	The available evidence usually includes consistent results from well-designed, well-conducted studies in representative primary care populations. These studies assess the effects of the preventive service on health outcomes. This conclusion is therefore unlikely to be strongly affected by the results of future studies.
Moderate	The available evidence is sufficient to determine the effects of the preventive service on health outcomes, but confidence in the estimate is constrained by such factors as: • The number, size, or quality of individual studies • Inconsistency of findings across individual studies • Limited generalizability of findings to routine primary care practice • Lack of coherence in the chain of evidence • As more information becomes available, the magnitude or direction of the observed effect could change, and this change may be large enough to alter the conclusion

(continues)

TABLE 3-2	Recommendations for Using Research Evidence in Clinical Practice[a] (*continued*)

Low	The available evidence is insufficient to assess effects on health outcomes. Evidence is insufficient because of: • The limited number or size of studies • Important flaws in study design or methods • Inconsistency of findings across individual studies • Gaps in the chain of evidence • Findings not generalizable to routine primary care practice • Lack of information on important health outcomes • More information may allow estimation of effects on health outcomes

Grade	Definition	Suggestions for Practice
A	The USPSTF recommends the service. There is high certainty that the net benefit is substantial.	Offer or provide this service.
B	The USPSTF recommends the service. There is high certainty that the net benefit is moderate or there is moderate certainty that the net benefit is moderate to substantial.	Offer or provide this service.
C	The USPSTF recommends selectively offering or providing this service to individual patients based on professional judgment and patient preferences. There is at least moderate certainty that the net benefit is small.	Offer or provide this service for selected patients depending on individual circumstances.
D	The USPSTF recommends against the service. There is moderate or high certainty that the service has no net benefit or that the harms outweigh the benefits.	Discourage the use of this service.
I Statement	The USPSTF concludes that the current evidence is insufficient to assess the balance of benefits and harms of the service. Evidence is lacking, of poor quality, or conflicting, and the balance of benefits and harms cannot be determined.	Read the clinical considerations section of USPSTF Recommendation Statement. If the service is offered, patients should understand the uncertainty about the balance of benefits and harms.

Reproduced from U.S. Preventive Services Task Force (USPSTF). (2015). United States Preventive Services Task Force methods and processes. Retrieved from http://www.uspreventiveservicestaskforce.org/Page/Name/grade-definitions.

Hierarchy of Research Designs

I	Evidence obtained from at least one properly conducted, randomized controlled trial.
II-1	Evidence obtained from well-designed controlled trials without randomization.
II-2	Evidence obtained from well-designed cohort or case-control analytic studies, preferably from more than one center or research group.
II-3	Evidence obtained from multiple time series with or without the intervention. Dramatic results in uncontrolled experiments (such as the introduction of penicillin treatment in the 1940s) could be regarded as this type of evidence.
III	Opinions of respected authorities, based on clinical experience, descriptive studies and case reports, or reports of expert committees.

[a] The U.S. Preventive Services Task Force grades its recommendations about specific health services or treatments according to one of five classifications, which reflect the strength of evidence and magnitude of net benefit (benefits minus harms).
[b] The USPSTF defines certainty as "likelihood that the USPSTF assessment of the net benefit of a preventive service is correct." The net benefit is defined as benefit minus harm of the preventive service as implemented in a general, primary care population. The USPSTF assigns a certainty level based on the nature of the overall evidence available to assess the net benefit of a preventive service.

Reproduced from Agency for Healthcare Research and Quality. (n.d.). Agency for Healthcare Research and Quality Archive. Retrieved from http://archive.ahrq.gov/clinic/ajpmsuppl/harris2.htm.

between the two creates the possibility of oversimplifying the complexity of each. Our goal is to help you understand the differences, understand what is credible from both perspectives, and decide what is applicable to your practice and research. We do not seek to debate whether one approach is better than another, because such a judgment assumes one approach has more truth-value than the other. In reality, both approaches help us fill in the web of knowledge where open spaces exist, as Quine (1952) suggests.

Research often begins with a clinical problem or question that needs an answer. This problem or question usually arises from a broad topical area, so the first task of the researcher is to clearly define the problem. Research questions can be inspired by everyday practice or they can emerge from other research studies, especially where discrepancies, inconsistencies, or remaining questions about patient care practices, interventions, or products used exist. Social or policy issues, such as access to care, models of care, effects of racism, gender bias or other forms of discrimination on health, health disparities, poverty, and violence can also give rise to research questions.

The question is then translated into research aims about what the study proposes to do to meet the gap in our current knowledge and to be significant (National Institutes of Health, 2001). This means your exploration of the literature must reveal a lack of prior research in this area that could specifically address your questions. It also means that the results of the study could make a difference in the healthcare delivery or outcomes for the population being studied.

Quantitative Research

Quasi-experimental design is similar to experimental design but does not include random assignment of participants to an experimental or control group for practical, ethical, or other reasons. This weakness prohibits causal inference, because it can no longer be assumed that the two groups are equal. That is, the findings might be explained by differences between the groups or some other factor. Most researchers try to establish some control over these extraneous variables by matching groups or by establishing group equivalency with a variety of quasi-experimental designs and statistical

analyses (Polit & Beck, 2012). The strength of the quasi-experimental design lies in its practicality and feasibility in the real world of health care and informed choice, where subjects often cannot be randomly assigned to groups.

Nonexperimental research answers questions that do not lend themselves to manipulation of a variable. For example, if we want to study the effects of the death of a child on the mother, the independent variable (the death of a child) is clearly not something that can be manipulated or controlled. Nevertheless, control and experimental groups could be identified, consisting of those mothers who did not experience the death of a child and those who did (as the death naturally occurs), respectively. Psychological and physical well-being could still be described and measured and compared in both groups, but cause and effect cannot be determined. In this kind of study, a vast array of human factors cannot be manipulated and, therefore, cannot be studied experimentally (Polit & Beck, 2012). These factors can, however, be described and interrelationships can be examined with nonexperimental research.

Meta-analyses and systematic reviews are considered to be highly reliable forms of evidence. Meta-analysis uses the single study as the unit of analysis and statistically combines the findings of several similarly designed studies on the same topic. This method provides a standardized way to compare findings across studies, adding together larger numbers to observe patterns and relationships that might not have otherwise been observed in a single study (Polit & Beck, 2012). A well-conducted meta-analysis allows for a more objective assessment of the evidence obtained in RCTs, especially where findings from multiple studies have produced disagreement or uncertainty. This consideration might be important when testing a new drug, procedure, or intervention that may have different effects in subgroups or varying results in different studies.

Systematic review is the method used to analyze a general body of scientific data using clearly defined criteria. Systematic reviews can include meta-analyses, appraisals of single trials, and other sources of evidence. Great care is taken to find all relevant published and unpublished studies, assess each study, synthesize the findings, present a balanced and unbiased summary of the findings, and consider any flaws that may be present in the evidence. Many high-quality systematic reviews are available in journals and online, most notably the Cochrane Library. The need for rigor in systematic reviews has led to a formal process for their conduct. Although meta-analysis always uses a quantitative statistical analysis of the findings, systematic review may include a quantitative meta-analytic combination of study results, or a more qualitative summary of the aggregated data (Korhonen et al., 2013).

Rigor in Quantitative Research

Just like clinical practice, quality research depends on adherence to standards to ensure that it is conducted accurately and ethically. The description of the research design must be clear so that the reader can fully assess what took place and replicate the study if desired. Errors in any step of the process will invalidate the results. This possibility can be minimized through careful attention to the accuracy of the instruments used for measurement, appropriate sample selection, and understanding of how to apply the findings in the acceptance or rejection of the research hypotheses.

Variables must be well defined—you must be sure you understand what is being tested and measured. Validity indicates how well the measurement actually measures the variable. For example, a sphygmomanometer must accurately reflect a blood pressure measurement. The reliability of the measure indicates how consistently it performs. For machines operated by humans, reliability includes how well the operator conducts the measurement (e.g., using the correct size cuff and positioning each time a measurement is obtained).

A research sample must reflect the population it is meant to represent. Error is minimized by use of appropriate sampling techniques and random assignment to study groups. For example, if you were measuring the reporting of menopausal symptoms, you might find a difference in prevalence if you obtained your sample from a women's clinic (where women might be seeking therapy) versus among shoppers at a local supermarket (where there might be a more representative population). In addition, where the supermarket is located might affect the outcome because of socioeconomic or cultural differences that may bias the results. These issues can potentially affect the generalizability of the study findings—that is, the ability to apply the results to populations other than the sample group studied. The size of the sample reflects its power and also affects the research findings. A sample that is too small will not have enough power to detect a significant difference between study groups. Likewise, a too-large sample may provide significant results related to size only, rather than producing meaningful findings (Kellar & Kelvin, 2013).

There are two commonly cited types of errors in research—Type I and Type II (Polit & Beck, 2012). A Type I error is made when the researcher concludes that a relationship exists—Drug A is effective in treating Disease X—when it actually does not (a "false positive" in clinical terms). The differences observed between the groups in such cases are often due to a sampling error such as self-selection bias. Random assignment to groups controls for sampling error and associated Type I error. The level of significance, referred to as *alpha* (α) and reported as a p value, will also influence a Type I error. The most frequently used levels of significance (i.e., alpha levels) are .05 and .01. With a .05 alpha, the researcher accepts the probability that out of 100 samples, a true hypothesis will be falsely rejected only 5 times, and in 95 out of 100 samples a true hypothesis will be correctly accepted. With a .01 alpha, there is only 1 chance out of 100 that the true hypothesis will be falsely rejected, so this level of significance makes the incidence of Type I error lower. Usually, the minimal acceptable level of significance in quantitative research is .05.

A Type II error, also called *beta* (β), is made when the researcher concludes that no relationship exists when it actually does (a "false negative" in clinical terms). As the risk of a Type I error decreases, the risk of a Type II error increases.

Researchers try to avoid both Type I and Type II errors. To do so, they frequently conduct a power analysis of a sample size, while taking into account the desired level of significance (alpha value) and the probability of Type II error (beta value). Random sampling, random assignment to groups to avoid selection bias, and adequate sample size are all steps that can help researchers avoid these kinds of errors.

Confidence intervals provide more information than p values because they give a range of values and allow inference of the true association of a parameter with a population (Kellar & Kelvin, 2013). The range specifies where the parameter (e.g., the mean) is most likely to lie (Polit & Beck, 2012). Most confidence ranges are set at 95%; they provide a statement of the level of confidence the researcher has about the findings.

Qualitative Research

Qualitative research methods use different techniques and answer different questions than do quantitative research methods. Guba and Lincoln (1998) proposed that how we perceive reality provides the backdrop for how we conduct science. This sets the stage for understanding the nature between the knower (researcher) and what can be known, commonly called epistemology. Together they form the question asked about method: How does one choose a way to learn about the world?

A person's view of the world shapes the answer to this question and influences his or her entire approach to science. Creswell (2012) notes that our philosophical assumptions about how we create knowledge, for what purpose that knowledge is used, and how we integrate our own values in this process shape our fundamental approach to research and science. There are many ways to tell and hear a story—to gain knowledge about people and their health. The richness and details of the individual story provide the data we need to extend our knowledge of the world. The individual's point of view within the constraints of everyday life can be known only from the specifics of each case and cannot be controlled. Scientists using qualitative methods believe that the researcher cannot be fully removed from the participants. For this reason, they sometimes call this type of research "naturalistic," referring to the fact that the testing usually takes place in a setting that is not controlled.

These perspectives differ in fundamental ways from the more objectivist stance of traditional Western science, in which quantitative methods—and particularly the RCT—are highly valued. Ultimately, however, the key features are the different language used and the different perspective assumed. Each has its place and role; each can inform the other. One induces *why* something

happens, and the other deduces *how* it happens. A simple example is the development of a hypothesis from clinical observations and discussions with women that a specific method of contraception causes weight gain (qualitative findings). To support this hypothesis, a study using quantitative methods can be designed to examine whether this effect actually does occur.

The research questions most appropriate for investigation via qualitative methods are often exploratory in nature: Why do things happen? What does it feel like? What does it mean? How should I interpret this result? All of these questions are excellent candidates for the use of qualitative methods. Such questions can arise from either clinical problems or specific gaps in clinical evidence.

A variety of lenses serve as the underlying basis for the traditions of qualitative research. The term *bricoleur* is often applied to the scientist who can navigate these traditions and lenses to answer the original research question and those questions that emerge as the study progresses. A bricoleur is characterized by his or her ability to "put together a complex array of data, derived from a variety of sources, and using a variety of methods" (Polit & Beck, 2012, p. 487). Skills required to accomplish this feat include astute observation, reflection, interpretation, and introspection.

Qualitative Research Design and Methods

Qualitative research explores a problem by induction and often moves toward hypothesis or theory development. Data are derived from multiple sources, such as interviews, fieldwork, observations, videotapes, art, media, and other documents, but are usually textual in composition rather than numerical. The researcher is considered to be the "instrument," and his or her role is closely tied to the collection and interpretation of the data. Sometimes the researcher is also a participant, such as in fieldwork where observations of specific clinical practices are being conducted. The researcher's assumption of this role can lead to an increased level of trust between the participants being observed and the researcher.

Qualitative studies are descriptive from the perspective of those who have experienced a particular phenomenon; therefore, samples are not random, but are "purposive" (Polit & Beck, 2012). In other words, specific research participants are sought who can shed the most light on the research question. For example, if you wanted to learn about the experience of postpartum depression, it would be fruitless to interview people who had never been exposed to this phenomenon.

To refine ideas based on emerging findings in the data analysis, the researcher may "theoretically sample" populations to answer specific questions (Charmaz, 2000). Sample size is usually not predetermined in such a case, and the power of the samples used in qualitative studies reflects the robust richness of the textual data. Data collection usually continues until the researcher observes saturation or redundancy, or until nothing new is coming to light or being observed. Data analysis is conducted in a variety of ways, but usually produces findings that are richly descriptive in textual or thematic language.

Choosing from among the many qualitative methods available requires that the researcher have an understanding of his or her disciplinary focus. Each area has its own complexity and methodology (a topic that goes beyond the scope of this chapter). For an easier understanding of some of the basic methods, the various qualitative research approaches have been organized here using general categories adapted from Polit and Beck (2012) to reflect the area of knowledge they explore.

Understanding the Experiences and Processes of Health and Illness Many research questions in the healthcare realm address what it is like to go through a certain health event, for the purpose of helping us find ways to improve life for others who have similar experiences. These approaches focus on understanding the basic experiences and processes of how a person moves through the event. The methods used in such investigations come from the traditions of philosophy and sociology.

Phenomenology is derived from a philosophical tradition that provides a "textual reflection on the lived experiences and practical actions of everyday life with the intent to increase one's thoughtfulness and practical resourcefulness or tact" (van Manen, 1990, p. 4). The focus is on understanding what it is like for this person to be in this experience within the context of his or her life. Such work is interpretative or hermeneutical, and its findings are

often presented as paradigm cases or exemplars, creating "a dialogue between practical concerns and lived experience through engaged reasoning and imaginative dwelling in the immediacy of the participant's worlds" (Benner, 1994, p. 99). The results provide a vivid description that can help us better understand the social, political, or historical context of the individual's experience (Polit & Beck, 2012).

Asking questions from the tradition of sociology assists us in understanding how social structures and human interactions affect people's experience of health and illness (Polit & Beck, 2012; Speziale & Carpenter, 2003). These approaches range from understanding how people make sense of their social interactions (symbolic interaction) to discovering how social processes are structured and developed (grounded theory). Charon (1992) describes four central foci of symbolic interactionism:

- The nature of the social interaction
- Human action that both causes and results from social interaction
- Present rather than past focus
- Actions of the person who is unpredictable and active in his or her world

Grounded theory was developed by Glaser and Strauss in the 1960s as a research method that addresses both the chief concern or problem for people and the basic processes available to address that concern (Glaser, 1978, 1992; Strauss & Corbin, 1998). The goal of this approach is to develop theory in a substantive area that is grounded directly in the data. Grounded theories "are likely to offer insight, enhance understanding, and provide a meaningful guide to action" (Strauss & Corbin, 1998, p. 12). One example is Cooper and colleagues' (2015) study of African American women's experiences with partner incarceration.

Understanding Human Behavior The tradition of psychology focuses specifically on how and why people act; its aim is to describe behavior. Studying human behavior can help us understand how behaviors are related to health and illness. Ethology examines the evolution of human behavior in its natural context (Polit & Beck, 2012); with this methodology, observations of human behavior are used to expose structures essential to life. This observational approach can also be used from an environmental perspective, as in ecological psychology. Ecological models examine the relationship of environmental influences with specific human attributes (Humpel et al., 2004). For example, studying the ecology of girls' bullying behaviors can expose characteristics and patterns within schools, which in turn can facilitate the development of preventive strategies (Jamal, Bonell, Harden, & Lorenc, 2015).

Learning how people communicate is another approach to learning about human behavior. Human communication has many processes and forms. To explore the construction of meaning in the nuances of these processes, researchers use methods derived from both sociology and linguistics. Sociolinguistics is the examination of the forms and rules of conversation through discourse analysis (Polit & Beck, 2012). Mishler (1984) proposes that by examining the dialogue between clinicians and patients, we can encourage the development of noncoercive discourse and humane clinical practice.

Understanding Cultural Traditions and Influences One of the oldest qualitative traditions comes from the field of anthropology, where scientists strive to understand cultural variations among the many peoples of the world. Although several approaches are used in this disciplinary area, ethnography is the most commonly employed. An ethnographer's goal is to carefully describe a specific culture. Historically, grand ethnographies often explored indigenous peoples. In health-related research, however, smaller specific subsets are often the focus of study and enable us to understand the intimate nature of women's lives. For example, Carney (2015) used ethnography to examine barriers that undocumented migrant Mexican and Central American women face in feeding their families and accessing formal health care, and their intersection with private food assistance programs.

Synthesizing Qualitative Research Findings Meta-synthesis is another qualitative method. This research method analyzes, synthesizes, and interprets a specified body of research and holds the potential to provide valuable insight and knowledge about the distinctive aspects of a phenomenon (Kennedy, Rousseau, & Kane Low, 2003). It shares some commonalties with the type of meta-analysis conducted in quantitative research, but is distinguished by some important differences. Meta-synthesis provides an organized, yet interpretive approach to a specific group of qualitative studies (Korhonen et al., 2013). Sandelowski and her colleagues (1997) note that it is essential to systematically examine qualitative findings about a specific phenomenon to keep from repeating ourselves if we are to change practice and policy making. The meta-synthesis method involves identifying similar qualitative studies about a particular phenomenon, determining how they are related, and synthesizing their findings. This analysis entails more than a systematic review; it becomes an interpretative study itself.

Rigor in Qualitative Research

Just as in quantitative research, a clearly articulated study design is essential to understanding the purpose and results of any qualitative project. Because qualitative research uses textual rather than numerical data, relative terms such as *trustworthiness* and *dependability* are used to describe results, whereas *error* is used as the corresponding term with quantitative study results (Speziale & Carpenter, 2003). Understanding the specific terminology associated with qualitative research can help you assess whether the results of such studies are valid and reliable.

Credibility reflects how much confidence you have in the study results (Polit & Beck, 2012). It is enhanced by complete descriptions of the sample and setting, data collection, analytic procedures, the way in which decisions were made, and the researcher's role in the study. Preparation and experience with the methods and acknowledgment of preconceived ideas, sometimes called bracketing, are helpful in understanding the researcher's perspective and influence on the study. This practice is similar to evaluating whether a specific statistical test is appropriate in a quantitative study.

A qualitative study should provide enough documentation for the results to be confirmed—a characteristic sometimes called *confirmability* (Polit & Beck, 2012). Confirmability helps to ensure that later researchers can follow the analysis and understand how decisions were made. The findings are enhanced when evidence is presented that a team of researchers was involved with peer debriefing and searches for negative cases. These procedures allow the research team to reflect on their analysis and to check for bias and interpretative errors. Another approach, called *member checking*, has study participants read and react to the researchers' analytic decisions to see if their findings reflect their personal experience with the phenomenon under investigation.

All research findings should make conceptual sense. The investigators should provide enough thick, rich description to prove that the results clearly fit with the data presented. *Transferability* refers to how well the findings can be applied to another setting and is similar to the concept of *generalizability* in quantitative research (Polit & Beck, 2012). A study should provide enough descriptive evidence to help you assess whether the findings could apply to your setting.

Mixed Research Methods

Sometimes the research questions beg for a mixed methods approach—that is, a combination of quantitative and qualitative methods. There are multiple ways to combine methods. Perhaps one method is more widely used than the other, or perhaps research is conducted sequentially using the various methods (Tashakkori & Teddlie, 1998). A helpful way to think about this issue is to consider how different lenses help you see different things. You might design a study that examines how a specific intervention affects women's perinatal outcomes and health behaviors (quantitative measures). Yet, within the same study, you could also interview women (qualitative methods) about their experience of the intervention—that is, how it affected their lives.

Another term appropriate to this discussion is *triangulation*, which refers to the use of multiple referents to capture a more complete and contextualized picture of the phenomenon under investigation (Polit & Beck, 2012). This approach may involve the use of multiple sources of data, time collection points, sites, and samples, as they all provide different perspectives on the same research question.

MOVING FROM BEST EVIDENCE TO BEST PRACTICE

Research can improve practice by providing answers to clinical questions; evaluating the safety, effectiveness, or cost of therapeutics; refining practice guidelines; or testing theories relevant to practice (Lanuzza, 1999). Research evidence that has been reviewed, compiled, and analyzed by a variety of credible resources enhances our ability to obtain and apply research findings; organizations that fill this role include the Cochrane Collaboration, professional organizations, and government agencies. This information has also been published on the Internet, so it is readily available to the busy clinician. Despite this access to best evidence, many clinicians continue to struggle with the issue how to apply the results of research to practice: How do you actually make it happen?

As clinicians, we must be able to use the computer and must be familiar with the EBP resources in all fields of health. We must also be cognizant of the criticisms and limitations of EBP, including overreliance on RCT-derived results and systematic reviews, an emphasis on the routinization of practice, and the daunting effort required to stay current, as today's best evidence may be tomorrow's inappropriate practice.

Clinicians must be able to critically appraise individual studies to determine how much faith they should put into their findings. The strengths and weaknesses of each study must be readily identifiable. Evidence hierarchies rank studies according to the strength of the evidence they provide (Polit & Beck, 2012). Most such hierarchies put meta-analyses of RCTs at the top and opinions of experts at the bottom. As a consequence, such hierarchies inevitably emphasize a scientific and rational focus and assume causation (the design of the tightly woven web structure) can be identified only by rigorous quantitative study. This approach fails to recognize the gaps in the web of knowledge and discounts qualitative research or naturalistic observations that focus on the understanding of the human experience. EBP attempts to escape this reductionist approach by integrating information from a variety of well-designed studies, clinical experience, existing resources, and the woman's preference. When developing clinical practice guidelines, protocols, or clinical pathways, all of these elements should be included (Camacho Carr, 2000). Put simply, no single study or group of studies can provide an infallible answer to a clinical question.

The Stetler (2001) model of research utilization was designed to help individual clinicians, as well as organizations, move the best evidence into the practice setting. Individual clinicians or organizations can use this model to critically analyze the research evidence and apply the findings to real-world practice (**Figure 3-1**). The current model includes five sequential phases:

1. The preparation phase includes the identification of the purpose of the project and the searching, sorting, and selection of the research evidence.
2. The validation phase involves a critique of the evidence.
3. If the evidence is found to be sound, then the process continues to the comparative evaluation and decision-making stage. The evidence is synthesized, and four criteria—fit of the setting, feasibility, current practice, and substantiating evidence—are used to assess the applicability of the evidence. Fit with the setting examines the similarity of the study's environment with the one in which the findings will be applied and compares the characteristics of the study population with the client population where the evidence will be applied. Feasibility implies that potential benefits outweigh any risk to patients, resources for implementation are available, and the involved persons are ready for change. Congruency with current practice philosophy and values must also be considered.
4. In the translation application phase, a dissemination plan is developed and strategies that need to be changed are revised.
5. In the evaluation phase, the level of successful integration of the evidence into practice must be assessed.

Using a model such as the one proposed by Stetler (2001) can make EBP more focused and acceptable to those clinicians who, when faced with a proposed

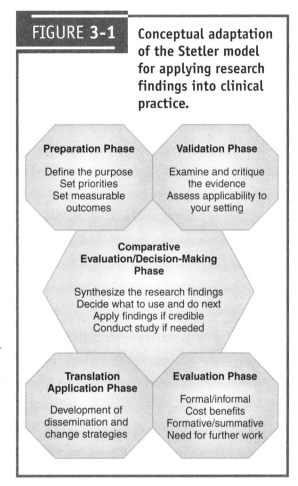

FIGURE 3-1 Conceptual adaptation of the Stetler model for applying research findings into clinical practice.

Preparation Phase

Define the purpose
Set priorities
Set measurable outcomes

Validation Phase

Examine and critique the evidence
Assess applicability to your setting

Comparative Evaluation/Decision-Making Phase

Synthesize the research findings
Decide what to use and do next
Apply findings if credible
Conduct study if needed

Translation Application Phase

Development of dissemination and change strategies

Evaluation Phase

Formal/informal
Cost benefits
Formative/summative
Need for further work

change, assert, "This is the way we've always done it." Integrating a methodical approach to applying evidence to practice can be effective in overcoming this all too frequently encountered mantra.

BARRIERS TO USING RESEARCH EVIDENCE IN CLINICAL PRACTICE

The two factors that clinicians and students most commonly cite for their failure to apply the latest research evidence are (1) lack of confidence in critiquing research studies and (2) lack of time to find the studies. We empathize with both concerns, and offer some practical strategies to overcome them in this section.

Critiquing Research Studies

Critiquing research studies takes practice and some basic knowledge about how research is conducted. We suggest that all clinicians have a basic research text on their bookshelf to look up unfamiliar terms and statistics. We have used Polit and Beck's (2012) *Nursing Research: Generating and Assessing Evidence for Nursing Practice* to provide some structure for this chapter and find it easy to read and practically written; however, many other good basic texts are available, such as *Users' Guide to the Medical Literature: A Manual for Evidence-Based Practice* (Guyatt et al., 2014).

To assess the applicability of any research findings to patient care, clinicians must evaluate the validity of the research; determine the practicality of implementing the findings; weigh any associated risks and benefits to the patient; and consider the ethical issues, available resources, and cost (Melnyk et al., 2014; Owens et al., 2010). Clinicians applying EBP guidelines must be able to recognize the limitations of the available databases as well as the limitations of scientific evidence. They must also know how to integrate clinical expertise, ethical considerations, patient individuality, and choice into the decision-making process. Additional objectives of EBP may include cost reduction, a desire to reduce wide variations in healthcare practices, and the desire to include clients as partners in their own care. None of these ideas is novel to clinicians.

Box 3-2 provides a brief summary of important points to consider when evaluating the quality of a research study and determining whether you shoud apply the findings to your practice.

BOX 3-2 Practical Points in Critiquing Research Studies

Title

Does the title of the article accurately describe the study? Is the language that is used in the title understandable and informative?

Abstract

Does the abstract accurately present the study? It should summarize the purpose of the study, the problems that were investigated, the research question or hypotheses, the study design and the methodology used, the sample, the instruments used, other data collection procedures, and the results or findings.

Research Questions and Purpose of the Study

What are the research questions? Are these questions researchable in the sense that they can be carried out by the investigators? What is the significance of the study in terms of practice, adding to the body of scientific knowledge, or other areas? Are the research questions stated in a concise and precise manner?

Research Variables

If it is a quantitative study, can you delineate the independent and dependent variables? If it is a qualitative study, is the phenomenon of study clear?

Review of the Literature and Conceptual Frameworks/Model

Is the literature review relevant to the study? Does it include timely as well as classic articles that pertain to the study? Does the review provide adequate background information? Do the authors state how this review provides support for their study (i.e., give background information for the identified research problem/question)?

Sample and Setting

Is there a description of how the sample was selected and the location of the study? What are the sources of bias, if any, that are associated with the sample selection process? Were power and effect size calculated for this study? In qualitative studies, was the sample purposive, and when was sampling stopped?

Ethical Considerations

Do the authors address protection of human study participants? Did they obtain permission to conduct this study in the setting?

Method: The Design

Is the design appropriate for the research questions? Is it described? Which extraneous variables are associated with the design, if any? Are they identified? Is the description adequate enough to allow replication of the entire study?

Instrumentation and Data Collection Procedures

How are issues of scientific rigor addressed? Are validity and reliability of the instruments described? Was collection of data conducted in a standardized manner? In qualitative research, is the "researcher as instrument" described?

Data Analysis

Are the analytic techniques supportive and appropriate for the research design? Does the article include supportive graphs, tables, or charts? Do these components help to describe the results? Are they easily understood?

Results

Do the results follow logically from the design and method? Do the authors describe the results in a way that is understandable and clear? Do the results answer the research question(s) or hypotheses?

Summary and Conclusions

What is your overall impression of the study? Does the author convince you about the conclusions that are drawn? Do the conclusions seem logical in light of the method, procedures, and other factors?

Data from Fullerton, F. (2002). Lectures and presentations at the American College of Nurse-Midwives Annual Meeting, Atlanta, GA.

Finding the Relevant Research

Today's information-rich world places the most recent research virtually at your fingertips. It is important to realize, however, that published findings are inevitably outdated the minute they are published. Journal articles can take 1 to 2 years from first submission to reach the printed page, and textbooks take even longer to be published. The advent of the Internet, however, has substantially improved our ability to keep up with the most recently published research.

Several excellent sources provide the best evidence in a succinct format for the busy clinician:

- The Cochrane Collaboration makes up-to-date, accurate information about the effects of health care readily available worldwide, including via the Cochrane Database of Systematic Reviews. The Cochrane Collaboration produces and disseminates systematic reviews of healthcare interventions and promotes the search for evidence in the form of clinical trials and other well-controlled studies (Cochrane Database of Systematic Reviews, 2014).

- PubMed provides free access to millions of citations in peer-reviewed biomedical journals, and is another excellent source for research findings, although the reader must evaluate most of the studies to determine their scientific merit and clinical applicability.
- The Agency for Healthcare Research and Quality (2012, 2014) provides evidence reports and technology assessments, consisting of technical reviews and guidelines on many clinical topics.
- The Database of Abstracts of Reviews of Effects (2013) is another healthcare-related database, produced at the University of York in England; it provides quality-assessed evidence reviews on interventions and health services organizations.

Many other agencies and organizations prepare evidence-based guidelines and protocols, which can usually be accessed conveniently on the Internet. Additional resources for EBP are listed in **Appendix 3-A**.

CONCLUSION

As a clinician, when considering the issue of research, it is helpful to look at what using evidence in practice actually means. Examples of applying evidence to clinical practice abound—from the choice of pharmaceutical treatments versus alternative therapies for vaginitis, to whether women need continuous electronic fetal monitoring during labor. Every clinical scenario needs to be addressed from the perspective of your personal experience, the woman's desires, and the best evidence to support your recommendations. Your first challenge is to blend these considerations artfully in everyday practice. Your second challenge is to work within the healthcare system to influence management and policy makers to use the best information and evidence possible to provide the highest quality of care.

If you walk away with anything from this chapter, it should be the following lesson: Question everything. The questions need not immobilize you, but rather should set the stage for thinking critically about the causes of clinical problems and ways to search for the best evidence available. The women for whom you provide health care will be your partners on this path of discovery, as they access the Internet and come to you with questions about different strategies in their health care.

For example, a recent paper published by Dahlen and colleagues (2013) proposed that the puerperium is a window of time in which clinicians and women can potentially support health (or illness) in both the short and long terms. Which kind of care and care practices influence these outcomes? The researchers' analysis of the evidence on epigenetic remodeling processes during labor and birth suggests the use of synthetic oxytocin, antibiotics, and cesarean birth may have subsequent impact on the health of both mother and child. Much of this exploration has been with animal models, and its extension requires future examination with human models. Regardless, as clinicians and researchers, we should never be caught wondering, "Why didn't I ask the question about the potential of our actions over time?" We owe it to women and to ourselves to search for the best evidence to support our healthcare practices.

References

Agency for Healthcare Research and Quality. (n.d.). Agency for Healthcare Research and Quality Archive. Retrieved from http://archive.ahrq.gov/clinic/ajpmsuppl/harris2.htm

Agency for Healthcare Research and Quality. (2012). National Guideline Clearinghouse fact sheet: Clinical practice guidelines. Retrieved from http://www.ahrq.gov/research/findings/fact sheets/errors-safety/ngc/national-guideline-clearinghouse.html

Agency for Healthcare Research and Quality. (2014). Evidence reports and technology assessments. Retrieved from http://archive.ahrq.gov/downloads/pub/evidence/pdf/literacy/literacy.pdf

Badgett, R., & Fernandez, J. (2013). Are proposals by politicians for health care reform based on evidence? *Journal of the Medical Library Association, 101*(3), 218–220.

Benner, P. (1994). The tradition and skill of interpretive phenomenology in studying health, illness, and caring practices. In P. Benner (Ed.), *Interpretive phenomenology: Embodiment, caring, and ethics in health and illness* (pp. 99–127). Thousand Oaks, CA: Sage.

Brisolara, S. (2014). Feminist theory: Its domains and applications. In S. Brisolara, D. Seigart, & S. SenGupta. (Eds.), *Feminist evaluation and research: Theory and practice* (pp. 3–41). New York, NY: Guilford Press.

Buse, K. (2008). Addressing the theoretical, practical, and ethical challenges inherent in prospective health policy analysis. *Health Policy and Planning, 23*(5), 351–360.

Camacho Carr, K. (2000). Developing an evidence-based practice protocol: Implications for midwifery practice. *Journal of Midwifery & Women's Health, 45*(6), 544–551.

Carlson, N. S. (2014). Current resources for evidence-based practice. *Journal of Midwifery & Women's Health, 59*(6), 660–665.

Carney, M. (2015). Eating and feeding at the margins of the state: Barriers to health care for undocumented migrant women and the "clinical" aspects of food assistance. *Medical Anthropology Quarterly, 29*(2), 196–215. doi:10.1111/maq.12151

Charmaz, K. (2000). Grounded theory: Objectivist and constructivist methods. In N. K. Denzin & Y. S. Lincoln (Eds.), *Handbook of qualitative research* (2nd ed., pp. 509–535). Thousand Oaks, CA: Sage.

Charon, J. M. (1992). *Symbolic interactionism: An introduction, an interpretation, an integration* (4th ed.). Englewood Cliffs, NJ: Prentice Hall.

Cochrane Database of Systematic Reviews. (2014). The Cochrane Collaboration. Retrieved from http://community.cochrane.org/editorial-and-publishing-policy-resource/cochrane-database-systematic-reviews-cdsr

Cooper, H. L. F., Caruso, B., Barham, T., Embry, V., Dauria, E., Clark, C. D., & Comfort, M. L. (2015, February). Partner incarceration and African-American women's sexual relationships and risk: A longitudinal qualitative study. *Journal of Urban Health: Bulletin of the New York Academy of Medicine, 92*(3), 527–547. doi:10.1007/s11524-015-9941-8

Creswell, J. W. (2012). *Qualitative inquiry and research design: Choosing among five approaches*. Thousand Oaks, CA: Sage.

Dahlen, H. G., Kennedy, H. P., Anderson, C. M., Bell, A. F., Clark, A., Fourer, M., . . . Downe, S. (2013). The EPIIC hypothesis: Intrapartum effects on the neonatal epigenome and consequent health outcomes. *Medical Hypotheses, 80*, 656–662.

Database of Abstracts of Reviews of Effectiveness. (2013). Retrieved from http://community.cochrane.org/editorial-and-publishing-policy-resource/database-abstracts-reviews-effects-dare

Doyal, L. (1995). *What makes women sick? Gender and political economy of health*. New Brunswick, NJ: Rutgers University Press.

Eisenberg, J. M. (2001). *Evidence-based medicine: Expert voices*. Washington, DC: Agency for Healthcare Research and Quality.

Fullerton, F. (2002). Lectures and presentations at the American College of Nurse-Midwives Annual Meeting, Atlanta, GA.

Gillam, S., & Siriwardena, A. N. (2014). Evidence-based health care and quality improvement. *Quality in Primary Care, 22*, 125–132.

Glaser, B. G. (1978). *Theoretical sensitivity*. Mill Valley, CA: Sociology Press.

Glaser, B. G. (1992). *Basics of grounded theory analysis*. Mill Valley, CA: Sociology Press.

Graham, I. D., Logan, J., Davies, B., & Nimrod, C. (2004). Changing the use of electronic fetal monitoring and labor support: A case study of barriers and facilitators. *Birth, 31*(4), 293–301.

Guba, E. G., & Lincoln, N. K. (1998). Competing paradigms in qualitative research. In N. K. Denzin & Y. S. Lincoln (Eds.), *The landscape of qualitative research: Theories and issues* (pp. 195–220). Thousand Oaks, CA: Sage.

Guyatt, G., Rennie, D., Meade, M. O., & Cook, D. J. (Eds.). (2014). *Users' guide to the medical literature: A manual for evidence-based practice* (3rd ed.). Columbus, OH: McGraw-Hill Education.

Hegge, M. (2013). Nightingale's environmental theory. *Nursing Science Quarterly, 3*(26), 211–219.

Humpel, N., Owen, N., Leslie, E., Marshall, A. L., Bauman, A. E., & Sallis, J. F. (2004). Associations of location and perceived environmental attributes with walking in neighborhoods. *American Journal of Health Promotion, 18*(3), 239–242.

Ilic, D., & Maloney, S. (2014). Methods of teaching medical trainees evidence-based medicine: A systematic review. *Medical Education, 48*, 124–135.

Jamal, F., Bonell, C., Harden, A., & Lorenc, T. (2015). The social ecology of girls' bullying practices: Exploratory research in two London schools. *Sociology of Health & Illness, 37*, 731–744.

Kellar, S. P., & Kelvin, E. (2013). *Munro's statistical methods for health care research*. Philadelphia, PA: Wolters Kluwer/Lippincott Williams & Wilkins.

Kennedy, H. P., Rousseau, A. L., & Kane Low, L. (2003). An exploratory metasynthesis of midwifery care. *Midwifery, 19*(3), 203–214.

Kohn, L. T., Corrigan, J. M., & Donaldson, M. S. (Eds.). (1999). *To err is human: Building a safer health system*. Washington, DC: Committee on Quality of Health Care in America, Institute of Medicine.

Korhonen, A., Hakulinen-Vitanen, T., Jylhä, V., & Holopainen, A. (2013). Meta-synthesis and evidence-based health care: A method for systematic review. *Scandinavian Journal of Caring Sciences, 27*, 1027–1034.

Kuhn, T. S. (1970). *The structure of scientific revolutions*. Chicago, IL: University of Chicago Press.

Lanuzza, D. M. (1999). Research and practice. In M. A. Mateo & K. T. Kirchoff (Eds.), *Using and conducting nursing research in the clinical setting* (2nd ed., pp. 2–12). Philadelphia, PA: Saunders.

Levin, R., & Chang, A. (2014). Tactics for teaching evidenced-based practice: Determining the level of evidence of a study. *Worldviews on Evidence-Based Nursing, 11*(1), 75–78.

Maggio, L. A., & Kung, J. Y. (2014). How are medical students trained to locate biomedical information to practice evidence-based medicine? A review of the 2007–2012 literature. *Journal of the Medical Library Association, 102*(3), 184–191. doi:10.3163/1536-5050.102.3.008

Marckmann, G., Schmidt, H., Sofaer, N., & Strech, D. (2015). Putting public health ethics into practice: A systematic framework. *Frontiers in Public Health, 3*, 1–7.

McDonald, L. (Ed.). (2004). Florence Nightingale and the foundations of public health care, as seen through her collected works. Retrieved from http://www.uoguelph.ca/~cwfn/nursing/dalpaper.htm

Melnyk, B. M., Gallagher-Ford, L., Long, L. E., & Fineout-Overholt, E. (2014). The establishment of evidence-based practice competencies for practicing registered nurses and advanced practice nurses in real-world clinical settings: Proficiencies to improve healthcare quality, reliability, patient outcomes and costs. *Worldviews on Evidence-Based Nursing, 11*(1), 5–15.

Miller, S., & Skinner, J. (2012). Are first-time mothers who plan home birth more likely to receive evidence-based care? A Comparative study of home and hospital care provided by the same midwives. *Birth, 39*(2), 135–144.

Mishler, E. G. (1984). *The discourse of medicine: Dialectics of medical interviews.* Norwood, NJ: Ablex.

Mitchell, C., Lawton, E., Morton, C., McCain, C., & Main, E. (2014). California pregnancy-associated mortality review: Mixed methods approach for improved case identification, cause of death analyses and translation of findings. *Maternal and Child Health Journal, 18,* 518–526.

National Institutes of Health. (2001). *Highlight significance and innovation.* Bethesda, MD: Office of Behavioral and Social Sciences Research, National Institutes of Health. Retrieved from http://www.niaid.nih.gov/researchfunding/grant/strategy/pages/3significance.aspx

Nightingale, F. (1859/1957). *Notes on nursing: What it is and what it is not.* Philadelphia, PA: Lippincott.

Owens, D. K., Lohr, K. N., Atkins, D., Treadwell, J. R., Reston, J. T., Bass, E. B., . . . Helfand, M. (2010). AHRQ Series Paper 5: Grading the strength of a body of evidence when comparing medical interventions—Agency for Healthcare Research and Quality and the Effective Health-Care Program. *Journal of Clinical Epidemiology, 63*(5), 513–523.

Palazzo, M. O. (2015). Transformation by design. Nursing workforce innovation and reduction strategies in turbulent times of change. *Nursing Administration Quarterly, 39*(2), 164–171.

Polit, D. F., & Beck, C. T. (2012). *Nursing research: Generating and assessing evidence for nursing practice* (9th ed.). New York, NY: Lippincott Williams & Wilkins.

Quine, W. V. (1952). *From a logical point of view* (2nd ed.). Cambridge, MA: Harvard University Press.

Sackett, D. L., Haynes, R. B., Guyatt, G. H., & Tugwell, P. (2000). *Clinical epidemiology and science for clinical medicine* (2nd ed.). Boston, MA: Little, Brown.

Sackett, D. L., Strauss, S. E., Richardson, W. S., Rosenberg, W., & Haynes, R. B. (2000). *Evidence-based medicine: How to practice and teach EBM.* New York, NY: Churchill Livingstone.

Sandelowski, M., Docherty, S., & Emden, C. (1997). Qualitative metasynthesis: Issues and techniques. *Research in Nursing & Health, 20,* 365–371.

Schaffer, M. A., Sandau, K. E., & Diedrick, L. (2013). Evidence-based practice models for organizational change: Overview and practical applications. *Journal of Advanced Nursing 69*(5), 1197–1209. doi:10.1111/j.1365-2648.2012.06122.x

Sehon, S. R., & Stanley, D. E. (2003). A philosophical analysis of the evidence-based medicine debate. *BMC Health Services Research, 3*(14). Retrieved from http://www.biomedcentral.com/1472-6963/3/14

Smith, R., & Rennie, D. (2014). Evidence-based medicine: An oral history. *Journal of the American Medical Association, 311*(4), 365–367.

Speziale, H. J. S., & Carpenter, D. R. (2003). *Qualitative research in nursing: Advancing the humanistic imperative* (3rd ed.). New York, NY: Lippincott Williams & Wilkins.

Stetler, C. B. (2001). Updating the Stetler model of research utilization to facilitate evidence-based practice. *Nursing Outlook, 49,* 272–279.

Straus, S. E., Richardson, W. S., Glasziou, P., & Haynes, R. B. (2010). *Evidence-based medicine: How to practice and teach it* (4th ed.). New York, NY: Churchill Livingstone.

Strauss, A., & Corbin, J. (1998). *Basics of qualitative research: Techniques and procedures for developing grounded theory* (2nd ed.). Thousand Oaks, CA: Sage.

Tashakkori, A., & Teddlie, C. (1998). *Mixed methodology: Combining qualitative and quantitative approaches.* Thousand Oaks, CA: Sage.

U.S. Preventive Services Task Force (USPSTF). (2015). United States Preventive Services Task Force methods and processes. Retrieved from http://www.uspreventiveservicestaskforce.org/Page/Name/grade-definitions

van Manen, M. (1990). *Researching lived experience: Human science for an action sensitive pedagogy.* Albany, NY: State University of New York Press.

APPENDIX 3-A

Sources of Research Evidence

Online Access to the Evidence Base: Databases

Evidence Collection	Contents	Locations
PubMed	Free access to more than 24 million citations across biomedical literature, most with abstract access.	http://www.ncbi.nlm.nih.gov/pubmed
Cumulative Index to Nursing and Allied Health Literature (CINAHL)	Nursing and allied health journal citations, available via EBSCO host with proxy access.	http://www.ebscohost.com/biomedical-libraries/the-cinahl-database
EMBASE	International biomedical database covering journals and conference publications, available with proxy access.	http://www.elsevier.com/online-tools/embase
Google Scholar	Free search of literature across multiple disciplines and sources. Can coordinate with library proxies to provide full-text links.	http://scholar.google.com
Database of Abstracts of Reviews of Effects (DARE)	Details of systematic reviews covering healthcare interventions and health services organization. Includes critical commentary on reliability of evidence.	http://www.crd.york.ac.uk/crdweb
Cochrane Library	Free, full-text systematic reviews focusing on health care and health policy.	http://www.cochranelibrary.com

(continues)

Online Access to the Evidence Base: Preappraised Evidence Sources

Evidence Collection	Contents	Locations
American College of Physicians (ACP) Journal Club	Subscription. International content selected against criteria for scientific merit and relevance to medical practice. Offers commentary on clinical application of findings.	http://www.acpjc.org
Clinical Evidence	Subscription. International content. Systematic overviews of harms and benefits of treatments.	http://www.clinicalevi dence.bmj.com
DynaMed	Subscription. Point-of-care reference for clinical decision making. Provides summaries, resources, and overall conclusions updated daily.	http://www.ebscohost .com/dynamed/aboutUs .php
UpToDate	Subscription. Clinical decision support reference with summaries, resources, and evidence-based recommendations for range of clinical topics.	http://www.uptodate.com
National Guideline Clearinghouse	Free. Current guidelines for evidence-based treatment. Initiative of the Agency for Healthcare Research and Quality (AHRQ).	http://www.guideline.gov
TRIP	Free. This meta-search engine includes results from journals, Cochrane reviews, clinical guidelines, and other websites on various clinical topics.	http://www.tripdatabase .com

Reproduced from Carlson, N. S. (2014). Current resources for evidence-based practice. *Journal of Midwifery & Women's Health, 59*(6), 660–665.

Health Assessment and Promotion

CHAPTER 4

Health Promotion

Kathryn Osborne

The leading causes of death for women in the United States are related to modifiable, behavioral risk factors (Centers for Disease Control and Prevention [CDC], 2015a). Smoking-related illnesses kill an average of 173,940 women each year (CDC, 2008). An increasing number of women are also experiencing morbidity and mortality as a result of being overweight or obese. More than 64% of all American women were overweight between the years 2009 and 2012, and more than half of these women were obese (National Center for Health Statistics [NCHS], 2014). In addition to causing premature death and disability, illnesses related to just these modifiable behavioral risk factors lead to annual medical expenditures of more than $300 billion in the United States (Hammond & Levine, 2010; Healthy People 2020, 2015a). Health promotion and disease prevention must be priorities to improve the overall health of the nation and to reduce the spending of our limited healthcare dollars on illnesses related to modifiable risk factors.

HEALTH PROMOTION: A NATIONAL INITIATIVE

The 1979 Surgeon General's report *Healthy People* set the stage for the development of a national initiative that is founded on scientific evidence and focuses on disease prevention. One year after the *Healthy People* report, *Healthy People 2000: National Health Promotion and Disease Prevention Objectives* established health objectives for use by state and local agencies and private organizations in the development of plans to move the U.S. population toward improved levels of wellness. *Healthy People*

is designed to measure changes in health status over time and identifies 10-year national objectives for improving the health of all Americans (Healthy People 2020, 2010).

Healthy People 2010 expanded the content found in the aforementioned documents and established a set of health-related objectives for the nation to achieve in the new millennium. The primary goals of *Healthy People 2010* were to increase quality and years of healthy life and to eliminate health disparities (Healthy People 2020, 2015b). By the year 2010, the nation had either met or moved forward toward the targets for 71% of the *Healthy People 2010* goals (Healthy People 2020, 2010).

In December 2010, the U.S. Department of Health and Human Services announced the *Healthy People 2020* goals and objectives for the nation. The overarching goals of *Healthy People 2020* are as follows:

- Attain high-quality, longer lives free of preventable disease, disability, injury, and premature death
- Achieve health equity, eliminate disparities, and improve the health of all groups
- Create social and physical environments that promote good health for all
- Promote quality of life, healthy development, and healthy behaviors across all lifestyles (Healthy People 2020, 2010)

Healthy People 2020 was devised using a framework based on the determinants of health, with particular focus on social determinants (Healthy People 2020, 2010). Determinants of health comprise a range of personal, social, economic, and environmental factors that influence health status and that fall under several broad categories, including policy making, social factors, health services, individual behavior, biology, and genetics. Four foundational health measures are being used to monitor the progress of *Healthy People 2020* initiatives: (1) general health status, (2) health-related quality of life and well-being, (3) determinants of health, and (4) disparities. Currently *Health People 2020* identifies 39 topic areas to be addressed, and others are evolving (**Box 4-1**).

The membership of the *Healthy People* initiative consists of both private- and public-sector groups, including the U.S. Department of Health and Human Services, state and local health departments, and hundreds of private-sector groups and organizations. Members of the initiative periodically assess the health status of the nation and evaluate the effectiveness of specific interventions (Healthy People 2020, 2010).

Healthy People 2010 identified multiple objectives that were associated with each of the indicators that reflect the major health concerns in the United States. *Healthy People 2020* maintained some of these as focus areas and added other new focus areas for the 2020 program (see **Box 4-1**). Clinicians are encouraged to utilize the objectives in establishing local programs focused on

---

BOX **4-1** *Healthy People 2020* **Focus Areas**

- Access to quality health services
- Adolescent health[a]
- Arthritis, osteoporosis, and chronic back conditions
- Blood disorders and blood safety[a]
- Cancer
- Chronic kidney disease
- Dementias, including Alzheimer's disease[a]
- Diabetes
- Disability and health
- Early and middle childhood[a]
- Educational and community-based programs
- Environmental health
- Family planning
- Food safety
- Genomics[a]
- Global health[a]
- Health communication and health information technology
- Health-related quality of life and well-being[a]
- Healthcare-associated infections[a]
- Hearing and other sensory or communication disorders

- Heart disease and stroke
- HIV
- Immunization and infectious disease
- Injury and violence prevention
- Lesbian, gay, bisexual, and transgender health[a]
- Maternal, infant, and child health
- Medical product safety
- Mental health and mental disorders
- Nutrition and weight status
- Occupational safety and health
- Older adults[a]
- Oral health
- Physical activity
- Preparedness[a]
- Public health infrastructure
- Respiratory diseases
- Sexually transmitted infections
- Sleep health[a]
- Social determinants of health[a]
- Substance abuse
- Tobacco use
- Vision

[a] A new focus area addressed in *Healthy People 2020*.
Healthy People 2020. (2010). About Healthy People. ODPHP Publication No. B0132. Retrieved from http://www.healthypeople.gov/2020/About-Healthy-People

the improvement of the health of communities. More information about these objectives—and specifically ways in which they may be applied to the delivery of women's health care—can be found at http://www.healthypeople.gov.

As the United States continues to deal with the financial realities of health care, it is becoming increasingly clear to policy makers, clinicians, and insurance underwriters alike that allocating healthcare dollars for health promotion and disease prevention has significant benefits. The United States spent $2.7 trillion on health care in 2011, or 17.9% of the nation's gross domestic product (NCHS, 2014). In 2010, almost half of the total U.S. healthcare budget was spent on just 5% of the population: individuals whose healthcare expenses were primarily related to expensive chronic conditions, many of which are preventable (Kaiser Family Foundation, 2015). Healthcare costs have continued to rise such that in 2012 the dollar amount spent on health care per U.S. resident was about $8,895, more than twice the amount spent per capita in 1995 (World Bank, 2015).

The Affordable Care Act

The 2010 passage of the Patient Protection and Affordable Care Act (ACA) signaled additional congressional support for health promotion. Key provisions of the ACA established a mandate for every American to carry health insurance and increased access to health insurance through Medicaid expansion and the creation of health insurance exchanges/marketplaces, where both individuals and employers can purchase lower-cost health insurance policies. Moreover, the ACA includes multiple reforms relative to individual and group health insurance policies that are sold on and off the exchanges. Among those reforms is a mandate that all insurance policies sold on and off an exchange must include, at a minimum, an essential health benefits package with no cost sharing (through deductibles or copayments) to the individual. Included in the essential health benefits package are the preventive health services that are recommended by the U.S. Preventive Services Task Force. (For a more detailed discussion of this organization, see Chapter 7.)

Preventive Health Services for Women Under the ACA

In addition to coverage of the screening and counseling services recommended by the USPSTF, the ACA includes provisions that require all individual and group health insurance policies (sold on and off the exchanges) to provide coverage for several preventive services with no cost sharing to the individual (Kaiser Family Foundation, 2014). In regard to preventive health services for women, the following essential health benefits must be covered:

- Well-woman physical examinations (with recommended counseling, screening, and immunizations)
- Contraceptives and related services
- Breastfeeding support (including breast pumps and other supplies)
- Maternity and newborn care

Clinicians should remain aware that a small percentage of women are covered under "grandfathered policies," which are exempt from requirements for no cost-sharing coverage of these preventive health services. Furthermore, Medicaid is not subject to the same requirements, although the ACA includes incentives for individual states to include the same preventive health services covered under Medicaid at no cost sharing to the individual (Kaiser Family Foundation, 2013).

Moving away from the traditional medical focus on the treatment of illness to health care that includes health promotion and disease prevention is an important step in the quest for cost containment (Meunier, 2009). The looming question is, "How can a healthcare delivery system that is illness centered undergo a paradigm shift to focus on wellness?" At the federal level, implementation of *Healthy People 2020* and the Affordable Care Act has brought about initial changes in the priority placed on health promotion and disease prevention, but much work is yet to be done to achieve this shift in paradigm. Clinicians are taking initial steps in this direction by clarifying the definitions of *health* and *prevention*. The multidisciplinary nature of healthcare delivery creates an opportunity for variations in these definitions.

DEFINING HEALTH

Many organizations and specialty groups have their own standard definition of health. Perhaps the broadest of these definitions is that established by the World Health Organization (WHO) in 1948: "Health is a state of complete physical, mental and social well-being and not merely the absence of disease or infirmity." To some, this definition may appear to make health unattainable. Yet, when health is viewed through a holistic lens, this definition begins to make sense. A holistic view of health includes its assessment in the context of physical, mental, and social well-being. Health, as defined in various contexts, can be achieved even in the presence of illness. For example, a young woman who has been HIV positive for 5 years may feel a sense of physical, mental, and social well-being if she is being cared for in a healthcare delivery system that addresses her healthcare needs in a holistic fashion. The presence of a disease state does not exclude her from being considered healthy according to the WHO definition of health.

Nursing is a discipline that focuses on health and wellness. Consequently, numerous nursing theorists have proposed definitions of health. Perhaps one of the most well known is that developed by Martha Rogers (1970), who theorized that the study of human beings would yield meaningful theories and concepts only when their wholeness is perceived. Rogers's perception has served as a springboard for the development of a myriad of nursing definitions of health, each of which uses a holistic lens, viewing human beings as whole persons, encompassing mind, body, and spirit.

Madeleine Leininger, expanding on the work of earlier nurse theorists, has provided a conceptual framework for nursing care. She proposes that caring is the essence of nursing and theorizes that, while it may be expressed in different ways, caring is universal across cultures (Leininger, 1985). Supporting this theory are reports that the cultural beliefs of patients influence their perceptions of health, and outcomes of care are improved when the patient's definition of health is considered and care is provided within the patient's cultural context (Fisher & Owen, 2008).

Applying Leininger's theory of transcultural caring to earlier definitions of health, one could conclude that proper health care requires a consideration of the whole person and must include knowledge and appreciation for the cultural context of the individual. This view provides a definition of health that is patient specific and includes the individual patient's cultural perceptions of health. Health promotion, then, encompasses a wide range of services that are delivered within the cultural context of the patient and that promote the general health and well-being of individuals and the communities in which they live.

DEFINING PREVENTION

The delivery of healthcare services aimed at the prevention of physical and mental illness and disease is defined on three levels:

- Primary prevention: These services focus on preventing disease in susceptible populations (Meunier, 2009). Examples of primary preventive efforts include health education and counseling, and targeted immunization.
- Secondary prevention: These services focus on the early detection of disease states and subsequent prompt treatment that will reduce the severity and limit the short- and long-term sequelae of the disease (Shi & Singh, 2004). Routine laboratory screening is an example of secondary prevention.
- Tertiary prevention: These services limit disability and promote rehabilitation from clinical disease states (Shi & Singh, 2004).

The rest of this chapter focuses on primary preventive efforts in healthcare delivery.

COUNSELING AND EDUCATION AS PREVENTIVE STRATEGIES

Clinicians are in a prime position to offer information that provides their patients with the tools needed to maintain a healthy lifestyle and assist in altering behaviors that may cause harm or illness. Women often seek information during their yearly physical examination that can guide them in making lifestyle changes and confirm that their current practices are an effective means of maintaining health. However, episodic visits may offer more frequent opportunities for providing health promotion and disease prevention information. Many women seek health care only from providers who specialize in women's health, such as midwives and obstetrician-gynecologists. Given this reality, it is essential that women's healthcare providers use each patient encounter as an opportunity for the provision of preventive health services.

In 1984, the U.S. Public Health Service convened the U.S. Preventive Services Task Force (USPSTF). One of the goals of the USPSTF was to examine the evidence regarding the effective use of preventive services to reduce morbidity and mortality rates. After examining the use and effectiveness of hundreds of preventive services, the USPSTF identified four categories—counseling interventions, screening tests, immunizations, and chemoprophylaxis—for which evidence supported the realization of significant health benefits. In 2003, the Institute of Medicine (IOM) issued a report mandating that "all health professionals should be educated to deliver patient-centered care as members of an interdisciplinary team, emphasizing evidence-based practice, quality improvement approaches and informatics" (p. 3). Further, Sackett, Strauss, Richardson, Rosenberg, and Haynes (2000) defined the elements of evidence-based practice as "the integration of the best research evidence with clinical expertise and patient values" (p. 1).

Consistent with this definition of evidence-based practice, and in keeping with the basic tenets of evidence-based practice, the USPSTF continues to seek out and appraise the evidence regarding effective counseling interventions using well-established rating schemas. It provides recommendations that are intended to be integrated with the clinician's own expertise and experience, as well as with the patient's preference and values, to guide professional decision making and practice (USPSTF, 2014a). The USPSTF's commitment to including the patient's preferences and values in shared decision making is reflected in the 2012 revision of its recommendations for using preventive services in clinical practice. Under the revised recommendation schema, the USPSTF (2014a) recommends that decisions to use services for which the balance of benefits is similar to the balance of harm (little or no net benefit) should be made based upon professional judgment and patient preference. It also recommends that clinicians use every patient interaction as an opportunity to participate in counseling and education. See Chapter 7 for a detailed discussion of the USPSTF.

EFFECTIVE COUNSELING INTERVENTIONS FOR HEALTHY, ASYMPTOMATIC WOMEN

Patient education and counseling are important components of primary health care and have been identified as a primary responsibility for nurses (American Nurses Association, n.d.). Much of that education and counseling is individualized, conducted as part of a plan aimed at managing specific problems or conditions. Described in this section are the USPSTF's counseling recommendations for use in women's health and primary care settings. **Table 4-1** summarizes the recommendations to which the USPSTF has assigned a grade of A or B, and which must therefore be covered by insurance policies sold on and off the health insurance exchanges with no cost sharing.

Breastfeeding

Healthy People 2020 (2015c) has established goals for the proportion of infants ever breastfed (81.9%), breastfed for 6 months (60.6%), and breastfed for 1 year (34.1%). While breastfeeding rates in the United States have improved since the inception of *Health People 2000*, work remains to be done to meet the 2020 goals. In 2006, 74% of infants were ever breastfed, 43.5% of infants were breastfed at 6 months, and 22.7% were breastfed at 1 year (Healthy People 2020, 2015c).

In its review of the evidence, the USPSTF identified significant benefits of breastfeeding for infants and children as well as for women who breastfeed. As a result, it recommends interventions (including counseling) to promote and support breastfeeding during pregnancy and the postpartum period (USPSTF, 2014b). See Chapter 32 for a discussion of interventions that promote and support breastfeeding.

TABLE 4-1	Grade A and B Counseling Recommendations of the U.S. Preventive Services Task Force

Topic	Target Population	Recommendation Summary
Alcohol misuse	Women engaged in risky or hazardous drinking	Brief behavioral counseling intervention to reduce alcohol misuse
Breastfeeding	All pregnant women	Counseling interventions during pregnancy and the postpartum period to promote and support breastfeeding
Diet and exercise	Women with cardiovascular risk factors	Offer or refer women with cardiovascular risk factors for intensive behavioral counseling to promote a healthy diet and increased physical activity
Falls prevention	Women age 65 and older at increased risk for falls	Falls prevention counseling including recommendations for exercise or physical therapy and vitamin D supplementation
Sexually transmitted infections	All sexually active adolescents and all women at increased risk for infection	Intensive behavioral counseling to prevent sexually transmitted infections
Skin cancer	Adolescents and young women age 10–24 who have fair skin	Counseling with recommendations to minimize exposure to ultraviolet radiation
Tobacco use	All pregnant and nonpregnant women	Ask all women about tobacco use and provided cessation counseling and interventions for those who use tobacco

Data from U.S. Preventive Services Task Force (USPSTF). (2014b). The guide to clinical preventive services—2014. Retrieved from http://www.uspreventiveservicestaskforce.org/Page/Name/tools-and-resources-for-better-preventive-care.

Diet and Exercise

The recommendations for diet and exercise counseling have changed over time with the emergence of new evidence. In the second edition of *Guide to Clinical Preventive Services*, the USPSTF (1996) recommended that all women be counseled to limit the amount of fat and cholesterol in their diet and to devise plans for diet and regular exercise that balanced caloric intake with energy expenditures. In 2003, it amended those recommendations after reviewing more recent research and concluded that there was insufficient evidence to advise either for or against routine dietary counseling or behavioral counseling to promote a healthy diet

and physical activity for patients in primary care settings (USPSTF, 2003, 2004).

More recently, the USPSTF has identified evidence to support the provision of dietary counseling for certain populations. Recommendations for diet and exercise counseling in patients who are at increased risk for cardiovascular disease are described later in this chapter. For patients without those risk factors, the USPSTF recognizes that there is a strong correlation between diet/exercise and cardiovascular disease. However, based on the available evidence at the time of the last review (2012), it found that the benefits associated with routinely counseling all patients in primary care settings about diet and exercise were very small; consequently, the USPSTF recommended that rather than incorporating diet and exercise counseling into the care of all patients, clinicians may choose to selectively provide this counseling when appropriate. The potential harms associated with the provision of this counseling are related to the missed opportunity to spend time during the patient encounter providing counseling with greater benefits (USPSTF, 2012). This recommendation is currently being updated. Readers are advised to check the website of the USPSTF for more recent recommendations.

Falls in Older Adults

Falls among older adults are a serious public health problem. One of every three adults age 65 and older experiences a fall each year. Approximately 2.4 million adults were treated in emergency rooms for nonfatal injuries sustained in a fall during 2012, leading to total direct medical costs of approximately $30 billion (CDC, 2014a). Among older adults who are injured in a fall, 20% to 30% suffer long-term consequences that include difficulty living independently and early death (CDC, 2014a). As the population of older adults continues to grow, the costs and suffering associated with falls in older adults will only become worse. Therefore, the USPSTF (2014b) recommends providing falls prevention counseling to all community-dwelling adults age 65 and older who are at increased risk for falls.

Risk factors associated with falls include older age (65 years and older), history of previous falls, and history of difficulty with mobility (USPSTF, 2014b). A quick way to assess fall risk (the *Get-Up-and-Go Test*) is to ask a woman to rise from a sitting position in an armchair, walk 10 feet, turn around, and return to a seated position in the chair. Women who take longer than 10 seconds to accomplish this task may be considered at increased risk for falls (USPSTF, 2014b). Counseling for falls prevention should include recommendations for moderate- to vigorous-intensity aerobic exercise (75–150 minutes per week), muscle-strengthening activities twice a week, and balance training at least 3 days each week. The USPSTF also recommends vitamin D supplementation; the American Geriatrics Society (AGS, 2015) recommends 800 IU

per day. The USPSTF found insufficient evidence and therefore makes no recommendation about counseling older adults at risk for falls about discontinuing certain medications, vision correction, or home hazard reduction, although these are all measures recommended by AGS (2015).

Motor Vehicle Safety

Motor vehicle accidents (MVAs) are the leading cause of death for people ages 5 to 34 and one of the leading causes of death for adults of all ages. More than 2 million adults are treated in emergency departments each year as a result of motor vehicle accidents, at an estimated cost of $70 billion in medical expenses and time away from work (CDC, 2011).

Counseling recommendations regarding seat belt use have also evolved since the early work of the USPSTF. The earliest recommendations were to advise all women about the proper use and placement of lap and shoulder restraints and to avoid riding with an alcohol-impaired driver or driving while alcohol impaired. Legislative efforts and community-based interventions over the past decade have resulted in high rates of seat belt use among people of all ages; an estimated 85% of all adults in the United States currently use seat belts (CDC, 2011). The USPSTF found no well-conducted research that evaluated the effect of counseling in the primary care setting on seat belt use. It also did not find any research addressing the impact of counseling in the primary care setting on driving while under the influence of alcohol or riding with an impaired driver. Nevertheless, strong evidence suggests that seat belt laws and enforcement strategies have resulted in increased use of these restraints. Consequently, the USPSTF (2014b) recognizes the important role of primary care providers in promoting community-based interventions but makes no recommendation for or against counseling patients in the primary care setting about seat belt use.

Skin Cancer

The most common type of cancer in the United States is skin cancer, and the most deadly form—melanoma—is usually caused by excessive exposure to ultraviolet (UV) light (CDC, 2015b). The USPSTF (2014b) recommends that all fair-skinned adolescent girls and women ages 10 to 24 be counseled to minimize exposure to UV light. In the absence of sufficient evidence to weigh the balance of benefits against harms, it makes no recommendation relative to counseling women older than age 24 on this topic.

Women at increased risk of developing skin cancer include those with light-colored hair and eyes, freckling, and a history of frequent burning when exposed to the sun. Measures to minimize UV exposure include wearing hats and protective clothing, using sunblock with a SPF of at least 15, limiting time in the sun (particularly between the hours of 10 a.m. and 3 p.m.), and avoiding the use of tanning beds (CDC, 2015b; USPSTF, 2014b). In addition to counseling adolescents and young women about how to minimize UV exposure, counseling strategies that include a description of the effects of UV light on skin appearance, such as early aging, have been particularly effective (USPSTF, 2014b).

COUNSELING INTERVENTIONS FOR WOMEN WITH ADDITIONAL RISK FACTORS

The counseling interventions described thus far have been those that are recommended for all women regardless of existing symptoms or risk factors. In addition to establishing these guidelines, the USPSTF has made recommendations regarding counseling interventions for women with certain risk factors for disease. See Chapter 7 for an in-depth discussion of recommendations related to screening for risk factors.

Alcohol Misuse: Interventions for Women Who Engage in Risky or Hazardous Drinking

Screening women for risky or hazardous drinking behavior is described in Chapter 7. For women age 18 and older who screen positive for alcohol misuse, the USPSTF recommends the use of brief (6–15 minutes) multicontact behavioral counseling interventions aimed at changing unhealthy drinking behaviors. In the absence of sufficient evidence to weigh the balance of benefits against harms, it makes no recommendation

regarding screening and counseling for adolescents (USPSTF, 2014b).

The brief intervention for at-risk drinkers recommended by the National Institute on Alcohol Abuse and Alcoholism (NIAAA) is based on the five A's framework: Ask, Advise, Assess, Assist, and Arrange follow-up. After the screening identification of women who engage in risky or hazardous drinking, clinicians should begin the intervention by describing their conclusions and making recommendations for change. Steps should be taken to assess the women's readiness to change and establish plans for follow-up. **Figure 4-1** provides a detailed description of a brief intervention for women at risk for drinking disorder (NIAAA, 2005).

Diet and Exercise: Interventions for Women at Increased Risk for Cardiovascular Disease

Heart disease is the leading cause of death for women in the United States (CDC, 2015a). Once thought of as a man's disease, heart disease is now gender neutral, killing as many women each year as men (CDC, 2015c). Several of the key risk factors for heart disease can be modified with dietary changes. These modifiable risk factors include high levels of low-density lipoprotein (LDL) cholesterol, diabetes, and overweight and obesity; poor diet and physical inactivity are stand-alone risk factors for heart disease (CDC, 2015c).

The USPSTF (2015a) recommends that all women who are overweight or obese and have additional risk factors for cardiovascular disease be offered or referred for high-intensity behavioral counseling to promote a healthful diet and physical activity. The counseling strategies that appear to be most effective are very intensive, occur in group or individual settings, and require frequent contact (by phone or face to face) over 6 months to 1 year. Counseling and education also appear to be most effective when conducted by healthcare providers who specialize in dietary and exercise counseling, such as dieticians and exercise physiologists. It is possible that these services can be provided in primary care settings, but when time and additional personnel are not available women should be referred for specialty care.

FIGURE 4-1   How to conduct a brief intervention for at-risk drinking.

HOW TO CONDUCT A BRIEF INTERVENTION
FOR AT-RISK DRINKING (no abuse or dependence)

Step 3 Advise and Assist

- **State your conclusion and recommendation clearly** and relate them to medical concerns or findings.

- **Gauge readiness to change drinking habits.**

Is patient ready to commit to change?

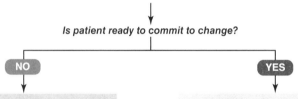

NO

- **Restate your concern.**
- **Encourage reflection.**
- **Address barriers to change.**
- **Reaffirm your willingness to help.**

YES

- **Help set a goal.**
- **Agree on a plan.**
- **Provide educational materials.**
  (See http://www.niaaa.nih.gov/guide.)

Step 4 At Follow-up: Continue Support

REMINDER: Document alcohol use and review goals each visit.

Was patient able to meet and sustain drinking goal?

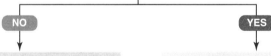

NO

- **Acknowledge that change is difficult.**
- **Support positive change** and address barriers.
- **Renegotiate goal and plan;** consider a trial of abstinence.
- **Consider engaging significant others.**
- **Reassess diagnosis if patient is unable to either cut down or abstain.**

YES

- **Reinforce and support continued adherence** to recommendations.
- **Renegotiate drinking goals** as indicated (e.g., if the medical condition changes or if an abstaining patient wishes to resume drinking).
- **Encourage to return** if unable to maintain adherence.
- **Rescreen** at least annually.

Note: This is a portion of a multistep program in *A Pocket Guide for Alcohol Screening and Brief Intervention*. Step 1 is intended to screen for heavy drinking and Step 2 is intended to assess for alcohol use disorders.
Reproduced from National Institute on Alcohol Abuse and Alcoholism (NIAAA). (2005). How to conduct a brief intervention. Retrieved from http://pubs.niaaa.nih.gov/publications/Practitioner/pocketguide/pocket_guide7.htm.

Risky Sexual Behavior

The USPSTF (2014b) recommends high-intensity behavioral counseling to prevent sexually transmitted infections (STIs) in all sexually active adolescents and all sexually active adult women at increased risk for STIs. Adult women at increased risk for STIs include those with current STIs or infections within the past year and women with multiple current sexual partners. Counseling should be based on individual risk factors, which can be assessed during a careful drug and sexual history (see Chapters 6 and 20), as well as on local information about the epidemiologic risks for STIs. Clinicians who work in practices located in high-prevalence areas should consider all sexually active women in nonmonogamous relationships to be at increased risk of STIs.

Patients identified as being at increased risk for the acquisition of an STI need to receive information about risk factors and ways to reduce their likelihood of infection. Such measures include abstinence, maintaining a mutually monogamous sexual relationship with a partner who is not infected, regular use of latex condoms, and avoiding sexual interaction with individuals who are at increased risk for STIs (USPSTF, 2014b). The USPSTF found little evidence to support the effectiveness of brief, individual counseling sessions in the primary care setting and no evidence supporting abstinence-only education. In contrast, strong evidence suggests that moderate- to high-intensity counseling, delivered in multiple individual or group sessions (with a total duration of 2 or more hours), results in a statistically significant reduction in STIs (USPSTF, 2014c).

Women who are at increased risk for STIs should be advised to use a condom with every sexual encounter and to avoid anal intercourse. Women who use condoms should be advised to use them in accordance with the manufacturer's recommendations. Measures to reduce the chance of infection when a partner will not use a condom should also be discussed—for example, use of the female condom. All women who are at increased risk for STIs should be offered screening and counseled to receive the hepatitis B vaccine; in addition, all adolescent and young women should be counseled about the appropriateness of the human papillomavirus vaccine (USPSTF, 2014c).

In light of the fact that almost half of all pregnancies in the United States each year are unintended (CDC, 2013), any discussion regarding counseling women about sexual behavior would be incomplete without addressing contraceptive counseling. The USPSTF does not address contraceptive counseling in its recommendations for clinical preventive services. However, the CDC (2013) recommends counseling all women who are sexually active with male partners about effective contraceptive methods (see Chapter 11). Counseling should be based on information obtained from a detailed sexual history, as discussed in Chapters 6 and 20.

Some researchers have suggested that preconception counseling should be integrated into women's routine health visits (Elsinga et al., 2008). Certainly, strong evidence supports the idea that general wellness counseling serves to improve pregnancy outcomes (CDC, 2013; Elsinga et al., 2008). However, clinicians should demonstrate sensitivity and an understanding and respect for an individual's preferences when initiating preconception counseling. It is important to keep in mind that some women will choose not to conceive, and not all women who conceive will choose to continue the pregnancy.

Tobacco Use

Tobacco use is the leading preventable cause of death in the United States. Recent morbidity and mortality figures reveal that an average of 183,300 women die from smoking-related illnesses each year (CDC, 2014b), and lung cancer is the leading cause of cancer death among women (CDC, 2014c). The USPSTF strongly recommends that clinicians offer counseling on interventions that aid in smoking cessation to patients who use tobacco. Evidence demonstrates that interventions such as screening, brief behavioral counseling, and the use of pharmacotherapeutics can increase the number of patients who attempt to quit and remain abstinent for 1 year, and that for nonpregnant women combined pharmacotherapy and counseling is more effective than either component used alone (USPSTF, 2014d).

While a single brief encounter may potentially offer some benefit, repeated sessions of longer duration are more effective. Similar to counseling women about alcohol misuse, a framework provided by the "five A's" is an effective way in which to engage women who smoke in discussion about cessation:

- Ask about tobacco use
- Advise to quit through clear personalized messages
- Assess willingness to quit
- Assist to quit
- Arrange follow-up and support (USPSTF, 2014b)

To prevent initiation of tobacco use, the USPSTF (2014b) also recommends behavioral counseling interventions for all adolescents and school-aged children. Effective strategies include face-to-face individual counseling, group counseling, printed materials, telephone and mobile device messaging, and messages sent through the U.S. mail. Regardless of the methods used or the frequency of counseling, the strategies that appear to be most effective include the provision of age-appropriate information about the consequences of tobacco use, the impact of social pressure, warnings about tobacco marketing, and effective ways to say "no" to tobacco use. Counseling aimed at providing parents with tools to help their children remain tobacco free has also been effective (USPSTF, 2014e).

IMMUNIZATION GUIDELINES AND RECOMMENDATIONS

In addition to counseling interventions to assist patients in making healthy lifestyle choices and changes, primary prevention includes the delivery of targeted immunizations. Immunizations play an important role in the prevention of infectious diseases, many of which are debilitating and, in some cases, may prove fatal. As has been true since the inception of *Healthy People 1990*, *Healthy People 2020* recognizes the effectiveness of immunizations as a strategy to significantly reduce the incidence of vaccine-preventable disease and identifies immunization status as one of the leading health indicators by which to measure the health of the nation (Healthy People 2020, 2015d). The USPSTF also acknowledges the importance of immunizations as a primary preventive measure. Since 1996, it has deferred to the CDC's Advisory Committee on Immunization Practices (ACIP) regarding

evidence-based recommendations and guidelines for clinicians (USPSTF, 2015b).

Primary care clinicians are in a key position to implement policies to improve the immunization status of women in the United States. However, evidence suggests many of these clinicians fail to provide appropriate preventive care services, including the administration of immunizations, to women in the outpatient setting. In a study examining the preventive health services delivered to 4,683 women age 65 and older, researchers found that almost half of the participants had not receive the recommended immunizations for their age group. Conversely, many of the women in the sample population had received cervical cancer screening well past the age at which such screening is considered to be beneficial (Schonberg, Leveille, & Marcantonio, 2008). The authors concluded that few older women receive the appropriate preventive health measures: Cancer screening, from which older women likely do not benefit, is often provided, whereas immunizations, from which they may benefit, are not.

Roughly 42,000 adults and 300 children die in the United States each year as a result of vaccine-preventable disease (Healthy People 2020, 2015d). Although the number of children and adults who receive the recommended vaccines each year has improved over the past 3 decades, vaccine rates in the United States, particularly for adults, remain suboptimal (CDC, 2012). Women present for health care for multiple reasons including contraceptive counseling, yearly physical examinations, prenatal care, preconception care, urgent care, and care for chronic conditions. Each of these encounters should be considered an opportunity to provide preventive health services for women, including the administration of recommended vaccines.

The current immunization guidelines for women who are considered to have complete vaccine coverage are summarized in **Table 4-2**; catch-up vaccine schedules for women who are not fully immunized can be found on the CDC website (http://www.cdc.gov). As the human papillomavirus vaccine is relatively new, issues surrounding its use remain somewhat controversial and are discussed further in Chapter 20. When considering appropriate vaccination schedules for women, it is important to note that the measles, mumps, and rubella (MMR);

TABLE 4-2 | Recommended Vaccination Schedule for Women

Age-Related Recommendations

Vaccine	11–12 Years	13–18 Years	19–26 Years	27–49 Years	50–59 Years	60–64 Years	≥ 65 Years
Hepatitis A	2 doses for children at increased risk for infection if not previously immunized	2 doses for women with chronic liver disease or who receive clotting factor concentrates, women who use illegal drugs, and women who have occupational or travel exposure to hepatitis A					
Hepatitis B	3 doses beginning at birth; ages 11–18 if not previously immunized	3 doses for women who have not been previously immunized and those with risk factors for infection: end-stage renal disease, HIV infection, chronic renal disease, occupational and/or household exposure, travel exposure, IV drug use, increased STI risk					
Human papillomavirus (HPV)	3 doses	3 doses for all women age 13–26 not previously immunized	Not recommended				
Influenza	Adolescent girls and women of all ages should receive 1 dose of flu vaccine annually during flu season. Live vaccine should not be administered during pregnancy or to women with certain risk factors. See the CDC recommendations for vaccine types to use for women across the life span.						
Meningococcal	1 dose at age 11–12 if not previously immunized with booster at age 16	1 dose for women older than age 18 at increased risk for infection: first-year college students living in dormitories, military recruits, microbiologists exposed to Neisseria meningitidis, and women traveling to epidemic areas. See the CDC recommendations for certain adults who may need a second dose.					
Measles, mumps, and rubella (MMR)[a]	2 doses for those not previously immunized	1 or 2 doses for certain populations at increased risk[a] Contraindicated in pregnancy					
Pneumococcal (polysaccharide)	1 dose for women with risk factors for infection: chronic lung and cardiovascular diseases, diabetes mellitus, chronic renal and liver disease, asplenia, chronic alcoholism, cochlear implant, and immunocompromise. A booster dose may be necessary based on risk factors and type of vaccine administered (PCV13 or PPSV23).					1 dose for all women 65 years or older

Age-Related Recommendations

Vaccine	11–12 Years	13–18 Years	19–26 Years	27–49 Years	50–59 Years	60–64 Years	≥ 65 Years
Tetanus, diphtheria (Td)/tetanus, diphtheria, pertussis (Tdap)	1 time dose of Tdap for those who have received the primary immunization series followed by Td booster every 10 years. Pregnant women should receive one dose of Tdap with each pregnancy, preferably at 27–36 weeks' gestation.						
Varicella	2 doses for all women and girls without evidence of immunity (previous infection or vaccination) Contraindicated in pregnancy						
Zoster (herpes)	Not recommended				1 dose for all women 60 years or older		

[a] In the absence of a contraindication, women born during or after 1957 should receive one dose of MMR unless there is documented evidence of receipt of one or more previous doses; a history or measles, mumps, and/or rubella based on healthcare provider diagnosis; or laboratory evidence of immunity. A second dose of MMR is recommended for women who (1) have been exposed to measles or mumps, or who live in an outbreak area; (2) are students in postsecondary education institutions; (3) work in a healthcare facility; (4) plan international travel; or (5) were vaccinated previously with killed or unknown measles vaccine. Unvaccinated women born before 1957 without evidence of mumps immunity and who work in healthcare settings should receive one dose of MMR; administering a second dose during an outbreak should be strongly considered. Rubella immunity should be determined for all women of childbearing age; those without evidence of immunity should receive the MMR vaccine upon completion or termination of pregnancy and before discharge from the healthcare facility. MMR vaccine is contraindicated in pregnancy.
Modified from Centers for Disease Control and Prevention (CDC). (2015d). Immunization schedules. Retrieved from http://www.cdc.gov/vaccines/schedules.

herpes zoster; and varicella vaccines are contraindicated for women who are pregnant or who are immunocompromised, including some women with HIV infection (CDC, 2015d). It is also important to note that **Table 4-2** is a brief listing of vaccines and does not include the multiple footnotes that are included in the CDC recommendations and that must be taken into consideration when deciding upon appropriate vaccine administration for certain at-risk women across the life span.

CONCLUSION

This chapter has examined definitions of health and prevention, and the utilization of those definitions in the provision of primary preventive services, both as a national initiative and for individual clinicians. Readers are encouraged to use this information, in conjunction with frequently updated guidelines available from the USPSTF, CDC, and other organizations (which can often be found online), in the development of management plans addressing the total healthcare needs of women across the life span. The current edition of the *Guide to Clinical Preventive Services* (USPSTF, 2014b) is available online and can be downloaded from the following website: http://www.uspreventiveservicestaskforce.org/Page/Name/tools-and-resources-for-better-preventive-care. The USPSTF provides additional tools for clinicians including the USPSTF Electronic Preventive Services Selector (the ePSS app), which can be downloaded to most electronic mobile devices from the same website. Given that the recommendations for preventive services are frequently updated in response to the ongoing work of the USPSTF, readers are advised to use ePSS or consult the website of the USPSTF regularly for changes.

References

American Geriatrics Society (AGS). (2015). AGS clinical practice guideline: Prevention of falls in older persons. Retrieved from http://www.americangeriatrics.org/health_care_professionals/clinical_practice/clinical_guidelines_recommendations/prevention_of_falls_summary_of_recommendations

American Nurses Association. (n.d.). What nurses do. Retrieved from http://www.nursingworld.org/EspeciallyForYou/What-is-Nursing/Tools-You-Need/RNsAPNs.html

Centers for Disease Control and Prevention (CDC). (2008). Smoking-attributable mortality, years of potential life lost, and productivity losses—United States, 2000–2004. *Morbidity and Mortality Weekly Report, 57*(45), 1226–1228. Retrieved from http://www.cdc.gov/mmwr/preview/mmwrhtml/mm5745a3.htm

Centers for Disease Control and Prevention (CDC). (2011). Adult seat belt use. Retrieved from http://www.cdc.gov/vitalsigns/seatbeltuse/index.html

Centers for Disease Control and Prevention (CDC). (2012). *Epidemiology and prevention of vaccine-preventable diseases* (12th ed.). Washington, DC: Public Health Foundation. Retrieved from http://www.cdc.gov/vaccines/pubs/pinkbook/index.html

Centers for Disease Control and Prevention (CDC). (2013). Unintended pregnancy prevention. Retrieved from http://www.cdc.gov/reproductivehealth/UnintendedPregnancy

Centers for Disease Control and Prevention (CDC). (2014a). Costs of falls among older adults. Retrieved from http://www.cdc.gov/HomeandRecreationalSafety/Falls/fallcost.html

Centers for Disease Control and Prevention (CDC). (2014b). Tobacco-related mortality. Retrieved from http://www.cdc.gov/tobacco/data_statistics/fact_sheets/health_effects/tobacco_related_mortality/index.htm#women

Centers for Disease Control and Prevention (CDC). (2014c). Lung cancer incidence trends among men and women—United States, 2005–2009. *Morbidity and Mortality Weekly Report, 63*(1), 1–5. Retrieved from http://www.cdc.gov/mmwr/preview/mmwrhtml/mm6301a1.htm

Centers for Disease Control and Prevention (CDC). (2015a). Leading causes of death in females United States, 2011. Retrieved from http://www.cdc.gov/women/lcod/index.htm

Centers for Disease Control and Prevention (CDC). (2015b). Skin cancer. Retrieved from http://www.cdc.gov/cancer/skin

Centers for Disease Control and Prevention (CDC). (2015c). Women and heart disease. Retrieved from http://www.cdc.gov/dhdsp/data_statistics/fact_sheets/fs_women_heart.htm

Centers for Disease Control and Prevention (CDC). (2015d). Immunization schedules. Retrieved from http://www.cdc.gov/vaccines/schedules

Elsinga, J., de Jong-Potjer, L., van der Pal-de Bruin, K., le Cessie, S., Assendelft, W., & Buitendijk, S. (2008). The effect of preconception counseling on lifestyle and other behaviour before and during pregnancy. *Women's Health Issues, 18*, S117–S125. http://dx.doi.org/10.1016/j.whi.2008.09.003

Fisher, P., & Owen, J. (2008). Empowering interventions in health and social care: Recognition through "ecologies of practice." *Social Science & Medicine, 67*, 2063–2071.

Hammond, R. A., & Levine, R. (2010). The economic impact of obesity in the United States. *Diabetes, Metabolic Syndrome and Obesity : Targets and Therapy, 3*, 285–295. http://doi.org/10.2147/DMSOTT.S7384

Healthy People 2020. (2010). About Healthy People. ODPHP Publication No. B0132. Retrieved from http://www.healthypeople.gov/2020/About-Healthy-People

Healthy People 2020. (2015a). Tobacco: Overview and impact. Retrieved from https://www.healthypeople.gov/2020/leading-health-indicators/2020-lhi-topics/Tobacco

Healthy People 2020. (2015b). History and development of *Healthy People*. Retrieved from http://www.healthypeople.gov/2020/about/History-and-Development-of-Healthy-People

Healthy People 2020. (2015c). Maternal, infant and child health. Retrieved from http://www.healthypeople.gov/2020/topics-objectives/topic/maternal-infant-and-child-health/objectives

Healthy People 2020. (2015d). Immunizations and infectious disease. Retrieved from https://www.healthypeople.gov/2020/topics-objectives/topic/immunization-and-infectious-diseases

Institute of Medicine (IOM). (2003). *Health professions education: A bridge to quality.* Washington, DC: National Academies Press.

Kaiser Family Foundation. (2013). Summary of the Affordable Care Act. Retrieved from http://kff.org/health-reform/fact-sheet/summary-of-the-affordable-care-act

Kaiser Family Foundation. (2014). Preventive services covered by private health plans under the Affordable Care Act. Retrieved from http://kff.org/health-reform/fact-sheet/preventive-services-covered-by-private-health-plans

Kaiser Family Foundation. (2015). Concentration of health care spending in the U.S. population, 2010. Retrieved from http://kff.org/health-costs/slide/concentration-of-health-care-spending-in-the-u-s-population-2010

Leininger, M. M. (1985). Transcultural care diversity and universality: A theory of nursing. *Nursing and Health Care, 6*, 209–212.

Meunier, Y. A. (2009). Healthcare: The case for the urgent need and widespread use of preventive medicine in the U.S. [Report]. *Internet Journal of Healthcare Administration, 6*.2. Retrieved from http://ispub.com/IJHCA/6/2/13517

National Center for Health Statistics (NCHS). (2014). *Health, United States, 2013: With special feature on prescription drugs.* Hyattsville, MD: Author. Retrieved from http://www.cdc.gov/nchs/data/hus/hus13_InBrief.pdf

National Institute on Alcohol Abuse and Alcoholism (NIAAA). (2005). How to conduct a brief intervention. Retrieved from http://pubs.niaaa.nih.gov/publications/Practitioner/pocketguide/pocket_guide7.htm

Rogers, M. E. (1970). *An introduction to the theoretical basis of nursing.* Philadelphia, PA: Davis.

Sackett, D. L., Strauss, S. E., Richardson, W. S., Rosenberg, W., & Haynes, R. B. (2000). *Evidence-based medicine: How to practice and teach EBM.* New York, NY: Churchill Livingston.

Schonberg, M., Leveille, S., & Marcantonio, E. (2008). Preventive health care among older women: Missed opportunities and poor targeting. *American Journal of Medicine, 121*(11), 974–981.

Shi, L., & Singh, D. (2004). *Delivering health care in America: A systems approach* (3rd ed.). Sudbury, MA: Jones and Bartlett.

U.S. Preventive Services Task Force (USPSTF). (1996). *Guide to clinical preventive services* (2nd ed.). Baltimore, MD: Williams & Wilkins. Retrieved from http://www.ncbi.nlm.nih.gov/books/NBK15435

U.S. Preventive Services Task Force (USPSTF). (2003, 2004). *Guide to clinical preventive services, third edition: Periodic updates.* Washington, DC: Author.

U.S. Preventive Services Task Force (USPSTF). (2012). Healthful diet and physical activity for cardiovascular disease prevention in adults: Behavioral counseling. Retrieved from http://www.uspreventiveservicestaskforce.org/Page/Topic/recommendation-summary/healthful-diet-and-physical-activity-for-cardiovascular-disease-prevention-in-adults-behavioral-counseling

U.S. Preventive Services Task Force (USPSTF). (2014a). Grade definitions. Retrieved from http://www.uspreventiveservices taskforce.org/Page/Name/grade-definitions

U.S. Preventive Services Task Force (USPSTF). (2014b). The guide to clinical preventive services—2014. Retrieved from http://www.uspreventiveservicestaskforce.org/Page/Name/tools-and-resources-for-better-preventive-care

U.S. Preventive Services Task Force (USPSTF). (2014c). Final recommendation statement: Sexually transmitted infections: Behavioral counseling. Retrieved from http://www.uspreventiveservicestaskforce.org/Page/Document/RecommendationStatementFinal/sexually-transmitted-infections-behavioral-counseling1

U.S. Preventive Services Task Force (USPSTF). (2014d). Final recommendation statement: Tobacco use in adults and pregnant women: Counseling and interventions. Retrieved from http://www.uspreventiveservicestaskforce.org/Page/Document/RecommendationStatementFinal/tobacco-use-in-adults-and-pregnant-women-counseling-and-interventions

U.S. Preventive Services Task Force (USPSTF). (2014e). Final recommendation statement: Tobacco use in children and adolescents: Primary care interventions. Retrieved from http://www.uspreventiveservicestaskforce.org/Page/Document/RecommendationStatementFinal/tobacco-use-in-children-and-adolescents-primary-care-interventions

U.S. Preventive Services Task Force (USPSTF). (2015a). Final recommendation statement: Healthful diet and physical activity for cardiovascular disease prevention in adults with cardiovascular risk factors: Behavioral counseling. Retrieved from http://www.uspreventiveservicestaskforce.org/Page/Document/RecommendationStatementFinal/healthy-diet-and-physical-activity-counseling-adults-with-high-risk-of-cvd

U.S. Preventive Services Task Force (USPSTF). (2015b). Immunizations for adults. Retrieved from http://www.uspreventive servicestaskforce.org/BrowseRec/ReferredTopic/232

World Bank. (2015). Health expenditure per capita. Retrieved from http://data.worldbank.org/indicator/SH.XPD.PCAP?page=3

World Health Organization (WHO). (1948). WHO definition of health. Retrieved from http://www.who.int/about/definition/en/print.html

CHAPTER 5

Gynecologic Anatomy and Physiology

Deana Hays

Nicole R. Clark

The editors acknowledge Nancy J. Hughes, Nancy M. Steele, and Suzanne M. Leclaire, who were the authors of the previous edition of this chapter.

The women's health movement encourages women to be knowledgeable about their bodies, to appreciate the unique form and function of the female body, and to take responsibility for caring and making decisions about their bodies that will positively affect their health. This chapter reviews female anatomy and physiology in terms of how they directly affect gynecologic health and well-being.

Female anatomy and physiology are often referred to as reproductive anatomy and physiology. Gynecology is defined as the branch of medicine dealing with the study of diseases and treatment of the female reproductive system. Regardless of whether a woman is pregnant or ever intends to reproduce, her gynecologic care has historically focused on reproduction. This example of naming provides insight into why women often continue to be essentialized to reproductive functions by clinicians.

The authors of this chapter assume the reader has had basic human anatomy and physiology content. Readers requiring a more in-depth discussion are referred to general anatomy and physiology references.

PELVIC ANATOMY

Pelvic Bones and Pelvic Joints

The pelvis is composed of (1) two hip bones called the innominate bones (also known as *ox coxae*),

(2) the sacrum, and (3) the coccyx. The innominate bones consist of the pubis, the ischium, and the ilium, all of which are fused together at the acetabulum (Corton, 2012). The ilium comprises the posterior and upper portion of the innominate bone, forming what is known as the iliac crest. It articulates with the sacroiliac joint posteriorly, and together with its ligaments is the major contributor to pelvic stability. The pubic bones articulate anteriorly with the symphysis pubis and, with their inferior angles from the descending rami, form the important bony landmark of the pubic arch (**Figure 5-1**). The ischial spines are bony prominences that are clinically important because they are used as landmarks when performing pudendal blocks and in other medical procedures such as sacrospinous ligament suspension (Anderson & Gendry, 2007). The ischial spines are also used to assess progression of fetal descent during childbirth.

The sacrum and the coccyx shape the posterior portion of the pelvis. The sacrum is formed by the fusion of the five sacral vertebrae, which includes the important bony landmark of the sacral promontory, and joins the coccyx at the sacrococcygeal symphysis. The coccyx is formed by the fusion of four rudimentary vertebrae, is usually movable, and is itself a key bony landmark. The true pelvis constitutes the bony passageway through which the fetus must maneuver to be born vaginally.

The best-known classification of the female pelvis is the Caldwell–Moloy (1933) classification,

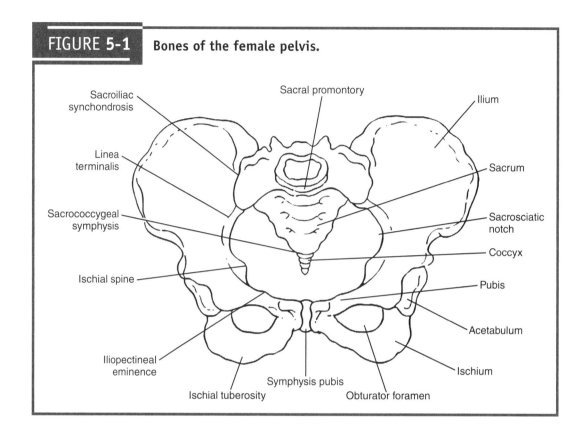

FIGURE 5-1 Bones of the female pelvis.

which includes four basic pelvic types: gynecoid, android, anthropoid, and platypelloid (**Figure 5-2**). Each pelvic type is classified in accordance with the characteristics of the posterior segment of the inlet. The development of this classification resulted in the realization that most pelves are not pure types but rather a mixture of types (Kolesova & Vetra, 2012).

Pelvic Support

Pelvic support structures include not only the muscles and connective tissue of the pelvic floor, but also the fibromuscular tissue of the vaginal wall and endopelvic connective tissue (Richter & Varner, 2007). The piriformis and obturator internus muscles and their fasciae form part of the walls of the pelvic cavity. The piriformis muscle originates at the front of the sacrum, near the third and fourth sacral foramina. This muscle leaves the pelvis by passing laterally through the greater sciatic foramen and inserts in the upper border of the greater trochanter of the femur. The origin of the obturator internus muscle includes the pelvic surfaces of the ilium and ischium and the obturator membrane. It exits the pelvis through the lesser sciatic foramen, where it attaches to the greater trochanter of the hip, enabling it to function in external hip rotation (Anderson & Gendry, 2007; Corton, 2012).

The deep perineal space is a pouch that lies superiorly to the perineal membrane (**Figure 5-3**). This deep space is continuous with the pelvic cavity and contains the compressor urethrae and urethrovaginal sphincter muscles, the external urethral sphincter, parts of the urethra and vagina, branches of the pudendal artery, and the dorsal nerve and vein of the clitoris (Corton, 2012). The perineal membrane (also known as the urogenital diaphragm, although this label is a misnomer) is a sheet made up of dense

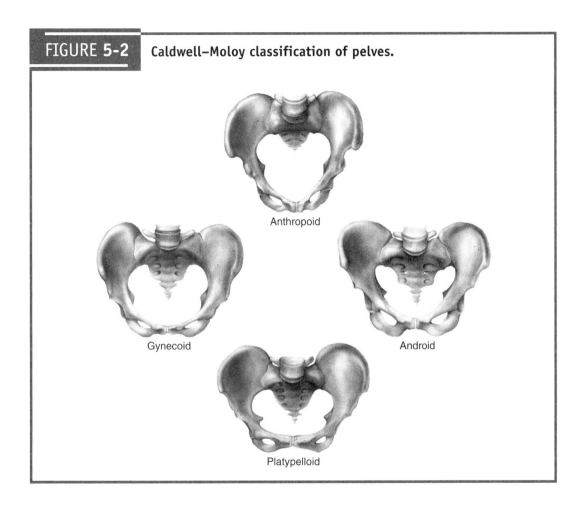

FIGURE 5-2 Caldwell–Moloy classification of pelves.

Anthropoid

Gynecoid

Android

Platypelloid

fibrous tissue that spans the opening of the anterior pelvic outlet. The perineal membrane attaches to the side walls of the vagina and provides support to the distal vagina and urethra by attaching these structures to the bony pelvis (Corton, 2012).

The levator ani muscle is a critical component of pelvic support; indeed, it is often considered the most important muscle of the pelvic floor (Corton, 2012). Normally this muscle is in a constant state of contraction, providing support for all of the abdominopelvic contents against intra-abdominal pressures. The levator ani muscle is actually a complex unit of several muscles with different origins, insertions, and functions. The pubococcygeus, puborectalis, and iliococcygeus are the primary components making up this muscle. The pubococcygeus is further divided into the pubovaginalis, puboperinealis, and puboanalis.

The levator ani and coccygeus muscles form the pelvic floor, and the related fascia form a supportive sling for the pelvic contents. The muscle fibers insert at various points in the bony pelvis and form functional sphincters for the vagina, rectum, and urethra. The origin of the levator ani muscle is the pubic bone and the adjacent fascia of the obturator internus muscle. Various portions of this muscular sheet insert on the coccyx (the anococcygeal rapine) and the perineal body, which is a fibrous band lying between the vagina and the rectum. The different sections of the levator ani muscular sheet are subdivided based on the exact origin and insertion of the fibers:

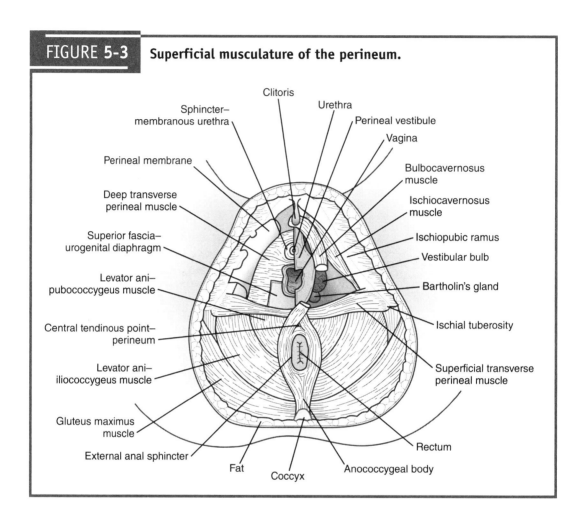

FIGURE 5-3 Superficial musculature of the perineum.

- The levator prostatae or sphincter vaginae fibers form the sling around the vagina and originate from the posterior surface of the pubis; they insert in the perineal body.
- The puborectalis fibers are important in maintaining fecal continence; they originate from the posterior surface of the pubis and form a sling around the rectum.
- The pubococcygeus fibers originate from the posterior surface of the pubis and insert into the anococcygeal rapine.
- The iliococcygeus fibers originate from the obturator internus fascia and the ischium and insert into the anococcygeal rapine.

The fan-shaped coccygeus muscle lies anterior to the sacrospinous ligament, originates from the ischial spine, inserts into the lower part of the sacrum and coccyx, and works synergistically to aid the levator ani muscle. The transverse perinei are small straplike muscles that help support the pelvic viscera. They originate from the ischial tuberosity, pass by the genitalia, and insert in the central tendon at the midline. The bulbocavernosus muscles aid in strengthening the pelvic diaphragm and in constricting the urinary and vaginal openings. Their muscle fibers originate in the perineal body and surround the vaginal openings as the muscle fibers pass forward to insert into the pubis. The ischiocavernous muscle contracts to cause erection of the clitoris during sexual arousal. Its muscle fibers originate in the tuberosities of the ischium and continue at an angle to insert next to the bulbocavernosus muscle (Anderson & Gendry, 2007; Corton, 2012).

FEMALE GENITALIA

Dr. Nelson Soucasaux, a Brazilian gynecologist, has devoted much of her writing to the traditionally typical and symbolic aspects of women's sexual organs, and the importance these views have in influencing our understanding of women's nature. According to Soucasaux (1993a, 1993b), historically it was believed that the key to understanding the female psyche was having a deeper understanding of woman's genital functions. By tradition, a woman's uterus was considered "the fundamental organ" and was synonymous with her genital organs.

This conception depicted a woman's wholeness to be totally related to her genitals, of which the most important was her uterus. Consequently, there was little appreciation for female genitalia.

This section describes the multiple organs and anatomic structures that constitute a woman's gynecologic anatomy, which are shown in a midsagittal view in **Figure 5-4** and **Color Plate 1**. Equally important to the discussion of women's gynecologic anatomy are the multiple nongenital peripheral anatomic structures involved in female sexual responses, such as salivary and sweat glands, cutaneous blood vessels, and breasts.

External Genital Anatomy

Vulva

The vulva is the externally visible outer genitalia (**Figure 5-5** and **Color Plate 2**). It includes the mons pubis, labia minora, labia majora, clitoris, urinary meatus, vaginal opening, and corpus

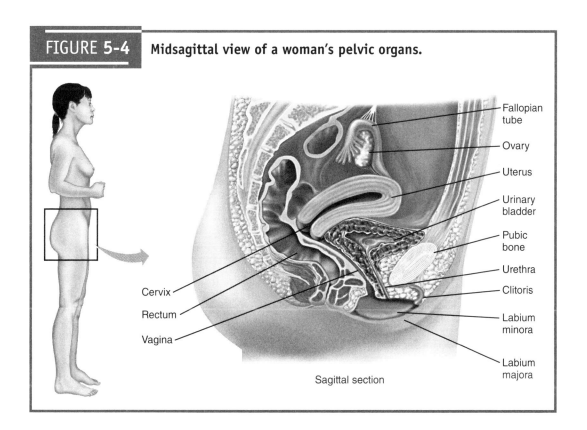

FIGURE 5-4 **Midsagittal view of a woman's pelvic organs.**

Fallopian tube
Ovary
Uterus
Urinary bladder
Pubic bone
Urethra
Clitoris
Labium minora
Labium majora

Cervix
Rectum
Vagina

Sagittal section

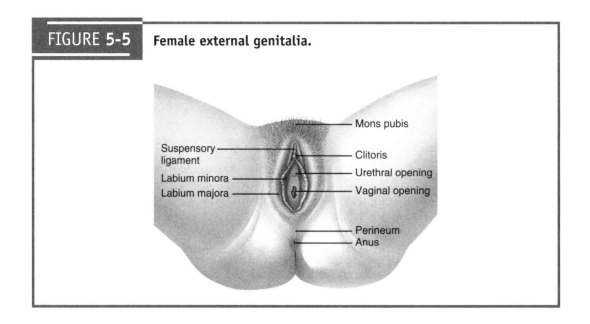

FIGURE 5-5 Female external genitalia.

Mons pubis

Suspensory ligament

Clitoris

Urethral opening

Labium minora

Labium majora

Vaginal opening

Perineum

Anus

spongiosum erectile tissue (vestibular bulbs) of the labia minora and perineum. The vestibule is inside the labia minora and outside the hymen. On each side of the vestibule is a Bartholin's gland, which secretes lubricating mucus into the introitus during sexual excitement. The mons pubis is the mound-like fatty tissue that covers and protects the symphysis pubis. During puberty, genital hair growth covers this pad of tissue.

The labia majora are fused anteriorly with the mons veneris, or anterior prominence of the symphysis pubis, and posteriorly with the perineal body or posterior commissure. They assist in keeping the vaginal introitus closed, which in turn helps prevent infection. The labia minora are surrounded by the labia majora and are smaller, nonfatty folds covered by non-hair-bearing skin laterally and by vaginal mucosa on the medial aspect. The anterior aspect of the labia minora forms the prepuce of the clitoris and also assists in enclosing the opening of the urethra and the vagina.

Women's vulva vary in size, related to the amount of adipose tissue, length, and pigment color of the labia minora or majora, which may be light pink, dark pink, shades of gray, peach, brown, or black. There is also considerable variation in the size of the labia minora in women of reproductive age. The labia minora are usually more prominent in children and women who are postmenopausal (Katz, 2012).

Clitoris

The clitoris is a sensitive organ that is typically described as the female homologue of the penis in the male, particularly in terms of its erogenous function (Puppo, 2013). During the early 1800s, a respected English gynecologist, Isaac Baker Brown, theorized that habitual clitoral stimulation was the cause of the majority of women's diseases because it caused an overexcitement of a woman's nervous system. As a result, clitorectomy came into favor as a means to rid women of ailments believed to be caused by clitoral stimulation (Duffy, 1963; Hall, 1998). Fortunately, this theory has long been refuted, and the practice of clitorectomy in the Western world is rare.

Anatomically, the clitoris is formed from the genital tubercle (Bradshaw, 2012; Martini, Timmons, & Tallitsch, 2011). It is 1.5 to 2 cm in length, consists of two crura and two corpora cavernosa, and is covered by a sensitive rounded tubercle known as the glans (Anderson & Gendry, 2007; Katz, 2012).

The clitoris is a small, sensitive organ that consists of two paired erectile chambers and is located at the superior portion of the vestibule (Katz, 2012). These chambers are composed of endothelial-lined lacunar spaces, trabecular smooth muscle, and trabecular connective tissue; they are surrounded by a fibrous sheath, the tunica albuginea. The paired corpus spongiosum (bilateral vestibular bulbs) unite ventrally to the urethral orifice to form a thin strand of spongiosus erectile tissue connection (pars intermedia) that ends in the clitoris as the glans (Martini et al., 2011). The clitoris is capped externally by the glans, which is covered by a clitoral hood formed in part by the fusion of the upper part of the two labia minora.

The clitoris has numerous nerve endings and contains tissue that fills with blood when the woman is sexually aroused. The blood supply to this organ includes the dorsal and clitoral cavernosal arteries, which arise from the iliohypogastric pudendal bed. The autonomic efferent motor innervation occurs via the cavernosal nerve of the clitoris arising from the pelvic and hypogastric plexus (Bradshaw, 2012; Katz, 2012).

The labia minora, together with the clitoris, play a critical role in sexual activity. Because of their rich nerve and vascular supply, they are easily sensitized and become engorged with blood during sexual arousal. This vascular erectile tissue is capable of becoming significantly enlarged and tense during sexual excitement. In addition to the great quantity of erectile tissue in the clitoris, erectile tissue is found inside the labia majora and minora, around the vulvovaginal opening, and along the lower third of the vagina. A very small quantity of this tissue can also be found in the vaginal walls and along the urethra. Age-associated female sexual dysfunction from decreased clitoral sensitivity may be associated with histologic changes in clitoral cavernosal erectile tissue (Katz, 2012).

Periurethral Glands

Two Skene's (paraurethral) glands open directly into the vulva and are adjacent to the distal urethra (Katz, 2012). The Skene's glands, which release mucus, form a triangular area of mucous membrane surrounding the urethral meatus from the clitoral glans to the vaginal upper rim or caruncle (Martini et al., 2011).

Bartholin's or Greater Vestibular Glands

The pea-sized Bartholin's glands are located at about the 4 and 8 o'clock positions in the vulvovaginal area, just beneath the fascia. Each gland has an approximately 2-cm duct that opens into a groove between the labia minora and hymen. The glands, which are made of columnar cells that secrete clear or whitish mucus, are stimulated during sexual arousal (Corton, 2012). If the Bartholin's ducts are blocked, infection can occur, resulting in cyst formation that can lead to the development of an abscess requiring surgical incision and drainage.

Internal Genital Anatomy

Urethra

The urethra is a short conduit, approximately 3 to 5 cm long, extending from the base of the bladder and exiting externally to the vestibule (Katz, 2012). The urethral mucosa is composed of stratified transitional epithelium near the urinary bladder; the rest of this structure is lined by a stratified squamous epithelium (Katz, 2012; Martini et al., 2011). In women, the urethra passes through the urogenital diaphragm, which is a circular band of skeletal muscle that forms the sphincter urethrae, better known as the external urethral sphincter (Martini et al., 2011). For a woman to urinate, this sphincter must be voluntarily relaxed—its typical state is contraction.

Ovaries

The paired ovaries resemble a large almond in terms of their size and configuration; they are located near the lateral walls of the pelvic cavity (Katz, 2012; Martini et al., 2011) Each ovary measures approximately 1.5 cm × 2.5 cm × 4 cm and weighs 3 to 6 gm (Katz).

The ovaries produce gametes (also known as ova) and the sex hormones known as estrogen and progesterone. The color and texture of these organs change with a woman's age and reproductive stage. The ovaries in a nulliparous woman are situated on a shallow depression called the ovarian fossa, located on either side of the uterus in the upper pelvic cavity. Several ligaments support the ovaries. The broad ligament is the principal supporting membrane of a woman's internal genital organs, including the fallopian tubes and uterus.

The remaining ligaments include the mesovarium, a posterior extension of the broad ligament; the ovarian ligament, which is anchored to the uterus; and a suspensory ligament, which is attached to the pelvic wall. The outermost layer of the ovary is composed of a thin layer of cuboidal epithelial cells called the germinal epithelium. Immediately below this epithelial layer is the tunica albuginea, which is made up of collagenous tissue (Katz, 2012).

The ovaries comprise three parts:

- An outer cortical region (cortex), which contains germinal epithelium with oogonia and ovarian follicles that number approximately 400,000 at the initiation of puberty (Halvorson, 2012a)
- The medullary region (medulla), which consists of connective tissue, myoid-like contractile cells, and interstitial cells
- A hilum, which is the point of entrance for all of the ovarian vessels and nerves (Halvorson, 2012b; Katz, 2012)

Two ovarian arteries that arise from the aorta descend in the retroperitoneal space and cross in front of the psoas muscles and internal iliac vessels (Katz, 2012). They enter the infundibulopelvic ligaments, finally reaching the mesovarium found in the broad ligament. The ovarian blood supply enters through the hilum, and venous return occurs through a venous plexus, which collects blood from the adnexal region and drains into the vena cava on the right and the renal vein on the left.

Innervation of the ovaries is accomplished by sympathetic and parasympathetic fibers of the ovarian plexus that descend along the ovarian vessels. These nerves supply the ovaries, broad ligaments, and uterine tube. The parasympathetic fibers in the ovarian plexus arise from the vagus nerves. The nerve fibers to the ovaries innervate only the vascular networks, and not the stroma (Katz, 2012). Because the ovaries and surrounding peritoneum are sensitive to pain and pressure, it is important to take great care when examining the ovaries during the bimanual examination.

Fallopian Tubes

The fallopian tubes (also known as the oviducts) are paired narrow muscular tubes that extend approximately 10 cm from each cornu of the body of the uterus, outward to their openings near the ovaries. Each fallopian tube includes four segments:

- The pars interstitialis (intramural portion) penetrates the uterine wall. It contains the fewest mucosal folds, with the myometrium contributing to its muscularis.
- The isthmus, the narrow segment adjacent to the uterine wall, contains few mucosal folds.
- The middle segment, known as the ampulla, is the widest and longest segment. It contains extensive branched mucosal folds and is the most common site of fertilization.
- The infundibulum, the funnel-shaped distal segment, opens near the ovary but is not attached to it (Katz, 2012). Very fine fingerlike fronds of its mucosal folds, known as fimbriae, project from the opening toward the ovary to help direct the oocyte into the lumen of the fallopian tube.

The inner surface of each fallopian tube is covered by fine hairlike structures called cilia that help to move ova, when they are released from the ovaries, along the tube and into the cavity of the uterus. The fallopian tube extends medially and inferiorly from the infundibulum into the superior-lateral cavity of the uterine opening (Katz, 2012).

The wall of the fallopian tube is composed of three layers: mucosa, muscularis, and serosa. The internal mucosa includes the lamina propria and ciliated columnar epithelium, which consists primarily of two main cell types. On the surface, the abundant ciliated columnar cells beat in waves toward the uterus, aiding in egg transport. Shorter, mucus-secreting peg cells are interspersed among the ciliated cells. These cilia propel the film they produce toward the uterus, help transport the ovum, and hinder bacterial access to the peritoneal cavity. The muscularis—the middle layer of the fallopian tube wall—contains both inner circular and outer longitudinal smooth muscle layers. Its wavelike contractions move the ovum toward the uterus. The outer covering of the fallopian tubes is the serosa; this lubricative layer is part of the visceral peritoneum (Corton, 2012; Katz, 2012).

The ovarian and uterine arteries supply blood to the fallopian tubes. The uterine veins, which parallel the path of the arteries, provide the venous drainage from this area. Sympathetic and parasympathetic innervation to the fallopian tubes from the hypogastric plexus and pelvic splanchnic nerves regulates the activity of the smooth muscles and blood vessels (Corton, 2012).

Uterus

The uterus is a muscular, inverted, pear-shaped, hollow, thick-walled organ that opens to the vagina at the cervix and then widens toward the top where the uterine tubes enter. Its anatomic regions include the fundus, body, and cervix (**Figure 5-6** and **Color Plate 3**). The fundus is the uppermost dome-shaped extension of the uterine body, located above the point of entry of the fallopian tubes. The body is the enlarged main portion. The cervix is the downward constricted extension of the uterus that opens into the vagina.

The uterus is located anteriorly between the urinary bladder and posteriorly between the sigmoid colon and the rectum. When the bladder is empty, the uterus angles forward over the bladder. As the bladder fills, the uterus is lifted dorsally and may become retroflexed, pressing against the rectum.

The nulliparous uterus is approximately 8 cm long, 5 cm wide, and 2.5 cm thick, and weighs approximately 40 to 50 gm (Katz, 2012).

The uterine wall of the fundus and body consists of three layers: the endometrium, the myometrium, and the serosa (also known as the adventitia). The uterine mucosa layer consists of simple columnar epithelium supported by a lamina propria. Simple tubular glands extend from the luminal surface into the lamina propria. The stratum functionale is the temporary layer at the luminal surface that responds to ovarian hormones by undergoing cyclic thickening and shedding. The stratum basale is the deeper, thinner, permanent layer that contains the basal portions of the endometrial glands; this layer is retained during menstruation. The epithelial cells lining these glands divide and cover the raw surface of exposed endometrium that occurs during menstruation.

The endometrium receives a double blood supply. In the middle of the myometrium, a pair of uterine arteries branch to form the arcuate arteries. These arteries then bifurcate into two sets

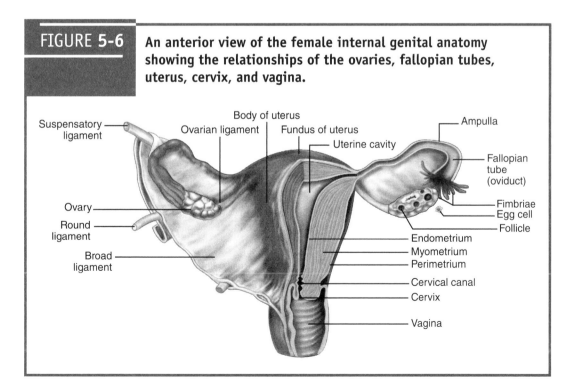

FIGURE 5-6 **An anterior view of the female internal genital anatomy showing the relationships of the ovaries, fallopian tubes, uterus, cervix, and vagina.**

Suspensatory ligament

Body of uterus

Ovarian ligament

Fundus of uterus

Uterine cavity

Ampulla

Fallopian tube (oviduct)

Fimbriae

Egg cell

Follicle

Ovary

Round ligament

Broad ligament

Endometrium

Myometrium

Perimetrium

Cervical canal

Cervix

Vagina

of arteries: straight arteries to the stratum basale and coiled arteries to the functionalis. The double blood supply to the endometrium is important in the cyclic shedding of the functionalis; the straight arteries are retained during this process, while the coiled arteries are lost (Anderson & Gendry, 2007).

The myometrium is composed of four poorly defined layers of smooth muscle that are thickest at the top of the uterus. The middle layers contain the abundant arcuate arteries. The outer layer of the uterus consists of two types of outer coverings: A cap of serosa covers the fundus, and the body is surrounded by an adventitia of loose connective tissue (Anderson & Gendry, 2007).

Structurally, the cervix is made mostly of dense connective tissue, is usually 2.5 to 3 cm in length, and is covered interiorly by a mucus-secreting ciliated epithelium at the upper regions and by stratified squamous epithelium at the vaginal end. The opening of the cervix into the vagina occurs at almost a right angle to the long axis of the vagina. Uterine blood supply is provided via the uterine and ovarian arteries, with venous return traveling via the uterine veins. The hypogastric and ovarian nerve plexuses supply sympathetic and parasympathetic fibers as well as carry uterine afferent sensory fibers on their way to the spinal cord at T11 and T12 (Anderson & Gendry, 2007; Katz, 2012).

Vagina

The vagina is a thin-walled tube extending from the external vulva to the cervix. Its walls are normally in apposition and flattened, but can extend (stretch) greatly, as observed during childbirth. The length of the vaginal walls varies greatly but on average the anterior vaginal length is 6 to 9 cm and the posterior vaginal length is 8 to 12 cm (Corton, 2012; Katz, 2012). The upper portion of the vagina encircles the vaginal portion of the cervix. The vagina touches the empty bladder on the ventral and superior surface. Inferiorly, it adheres to the posterior wall of the urethra and opens adjacent to the labia minora.

The internal mucosal layer of the vagina contains traverse folds, known as rugae. This muscular canal extends from the midpoint of the cervix to its opening located between the urethra and the rectum. The mucous membrane lining the vagina and musculature is continuous with the uterus.

The vaginal walls can be easily separated because their surfaces are normally moist, lubricated by a basal vaginal fluid.

The vaginal wall is composed of three layers: mucosa, muscle, and adventitia. Vaginal epithelium is stratified squamous epithelium supported by a thick lamina propria. The lamina propria has many thin-walled blood vessels that contribute to diffusion of vaginal fluid across the epithelium. The lamina propria of the mucosa contains many elastic fibers as well as a dense network of blood vessels, lymph nodes, and nerve supply. To a much lesser degree than seen in the skin, this epithelium undergoes hormone-related cyclic changes, including slight keratinization of the superficial cells during the menstrual cycle (Corton, 2012). The epithelium has no glands, so it does not secrete mucus. Release of estrogen causes the epithelium to thicken, differentiate, and accumulate glycogen. Vaginal bacteria metabolize the glycogen to lactic acid, causing the typically low pH of the vaginal environment.

Loose connective tissue containing many elastic fibers is found underneath the vaginal epithelium, which has a subdermal layer rich in capillaries. This rich vascular supply is the source for vaginal moisture during sexual stimulation (Soper, 2007).

Within the epithelium lie the smooth muscles of the muscularis, which are oriented longitudinally on the outer layer and as circular bundles on the inner layer. The outer layer—the adventitia—consists of dense connective tissue with many elastic fibers, which provides structural support for the vagina. It also contains an extensive nerve supply and venous capillaries. The adventitia is elastic and rich in collagen, provides structural support to the vagina, and allows for expansion of the vagina during intercourse and childbirth.

The upper two-thirds of the vagina receives efferent innervation through the uterovaginal plexus, which contains both sympathetic and parasympathetic fibers. The pelvic splanchnic nerves provide the parasympathetic efferent input to the uterovaginal plexus. The proximal two-thirds of the vagina is innervated via the uterovaginal plexus. The lower vagina receives autonomic efferent innervation from the pudendal nerve. The distal one-third of the vagina has primarily somatic sensation; this innervation arises from the pudendal nerve and is carried to the sacral spinal cord (Katz, 2012).

BREAST ANATOMY AND PHYSIOLOGY

In Western society, it often seems that a woman's breasts have two functions or roles: one that is sexual, and one that is maternal. The breasts are visible social sex symbols, and they are often a key source of a woman's anxiety about her body. Breasts often define women in both the public and private eye.

The breasts—that is, the mammary glands—are large, modified sebaceous glands contained within the superficial fascia of the chest wall located over the pectoral muscles (Katz & Dotters, 2012). Each consists of a nipple, lobes, ducts, and fibrous and fatty tissue (**Color Plate 4**). Each breast is composed of 12 to 20 lobes of glandular tissue. The number of lobes is not related to the size of the breast. The lobes branch to form 10 to 100 lobules per lobe, which are in turn subdivided into many secretory alveoli. These glands are connected together by a series of ducts. The alveoli produce milk and other substances during lactation. Each lobe empties into a single lactiferous duct that travels out through the nipple. As a result, there are 15 to 20 passages through the nipple, resulting in just as many openings in the nipple.

Fatty and connective tissues surround the lobes of glandular tissue. The amount of fatty tissue depends on many factors, including age, the percentage of body fat relative to total body weight, and heredity. Cooper's ligaments connect the chest wall to the skin of the breast, giving the breast its shape and elasticity (Katz & Dotters, 2012). The size of the nonpregnant breasts reflects the amount of adipose tissue in the breast rather than the amount of glandular tissue. The secretory nature of the breasts develops during pregnancy.

The nipple and areola are located near the center of each breast; the areola is the pigmented area surrounding the nipple. These areas usually have a color and texture that differ from those of the adjacent skin. Notably, the color of the nipple–areolar complex varies and darkens during pregnancy and lactation. The consistency of the nipple and areola may range from very smooth to wrinkled and bumpy. The size of the nipples and areolae also varies a great deal from woman to woman, and some size variation between a woman's breasts is normal. The nipple and areola are made of smooth muscle fibers and feature a thick network of nerve endings.

The areola is populated by numerous oil-producing Montgomery's glands. These glands may form raised bumps and be responsive to a woman's menstrual cycle. They protect and lubricate the nipple during lactation.

The nipple usually protrudes out from the surface of the breast. Some nipples project inward or are flat with the surface of the breast. Neither flat nor inverted nipples appear to negatively affect a woman's ability to breastfeed.

Reproductive hormones are vital to the development of the breast during puberty and lactation. Prolactin (PRL) and growth hormone (GH) from the anterior lobe of the pituitary stimulate mammary gland development. These hormones are aided by human placental lactogen from the placenta, which stimulates the mammary gland ducts to become active during pregnancy. Estrogen promotes the growth of the gland and ducts, while progesterone stimulates the development of milk-producing cells. Prolactin, which is released from the anterior pituitary, stimulates milk production. Oxytocin, which is released from the posterior pituitary in response to suckling, causes milk ejection from the lactating breast.

The lymphatic system in the breast is abundant and empties the breast tissue of excess fluid. Lymph nodes along the pathway of drainage monitor for foreign bodies such as bacteria or viruses. Although the main flow moves toward the axilla and anterior axillary nodes, lymph drainage has been shown to pass in all directions from the breast (Martini et al., 2011).

MENSTRUAL CYCLE PHYSIOLOGY

The initiation of menstruation, called menarche, usually happens between the ages of 12 and 15. Menstrual cycles typically continue to age 45 to 55, when menopause occurs. Many women find themselves reluctant to discuss the existence and normality of menstruation. The word *menstruation* has been replaced by a variety of euphemisms, such as *the curse*, *my period*, *my monthly*, *my friend*, *the red flag*, or *on the rag*.

Most women experience deviations from the average menstrual cycle during their reproductive years. As a result, it is not uncommon for women to display certain preoccupations regarding their menstrual bleeding, not only in relation to the regularity of its occurrence, but also in regard to the characteristics of the flow, such as volume, duration, and associated signs and symptoms. Unfortunately, society has encouraged the notion that a woman's normalcy is based on her ability to bear children. This misperception has understandably forced women to worry over the most miniscule changes in their menstrual cycles. Indeed, changes in menstruation are one of the most frequent reasons why women visit their clinician.

Numerous patterns in the secretion of estrogens and progesterone are possible; in fact, it is difficult to find two cycles that are exactly the same. Studies that include women of different ethnicities, occupations, genetics, nutritional status, and age have demonstrated that the length and duration of the menstrual cycle vary widely (Assadi, 2013; Johnson et al., 2013; Karapanou & Papadimitriou, 2010).

Menarche is the most readily evident external event that indicates the end of one developmental stage and the beginning of a new one. It is now believed that body composition is critically important in determining the onset of puberty and menstruation in young women (Ferin & Lobo, 2012). The ratio of total body weight to lean body weight is probably the most relevant factor, and individuals who are moderately obese (i.e., 20–30% above their ideal body weight) tend to have an earlier onset of menarche (Johnson et al., 2013). Widely accepted standards for distinguishing what are regular versus irregular menses, or normal versus abnormal menses, are generally based on what is considered average and not necessarily typical for every woman. According to these standards, the normal menstrual cycle is 21 to 35 days with a menstrual flow lasting 4 to 6 days, although a flow for as few as 2 days or as many as 8 days is still considered normal (Ferin & Lobo, 2012).

The amount of menstrual flow varies, with the average being 50 mL; nevertheless, this volume may be as little as 20 mL or as much as 80 mL. Generally, women are not aware that anovulatory cycles and abnormal uterine bleeding (changes in bleeding outside of normal; see Chapter 24) are common after menarche and just prior to menopause (Ferin & Lobo, 2012; Fritz & Speroff, 2011). Menstrual cycles that occur during the first 1 to 1.5 years after menarche are frequently irregular due to the immaturity of the hypothalamic–pituitary–ovarian axis (Fritz & Speroff, 2011).

The Hypothalamic–Pituitary–Ovarian Axis

Hypothalamus

The hypothalamus controls anterior pituitary functions via the secretion of releasing and inhibiting factors. Together with the pituitary, it manages the production of hormones that serve as chemical messengers for the regulation of the gynecologic system. The hypothalamus initially releases gonadotropin-releasing hormone (GnRH) in a pulsatile manner. On average, the frequency of GnRH secretion is once per 60 to 100 minutes during the early follicular phase, increases to once per 60 to 70 minutes during the middle of the menstrual cycle, and then decreases during the luteal phase (McCartney & Marshall, 2014). The release of GnRH stimulates the pituitary gland to produce follicle-stimulating hormone (FSH) and luteinizing hormone (LH). Two other hormones necessary for gynecologic health, estrogen and progesterone, are secreted by the ovaries at the command of FSH and LH.

Pituitary Gland

The oval-shaped, pea-sized pituitary gland is located in a small depression in the sphenoid bone of the skull. It is controlled by the hypothalamus, which secretes releasing factors into a special blood vessel network (hypothalamic–hypophyseal portal system) that feeds the pituicytes (McCartney & Marshall, 2014). These releasing factors either stimulate or inhibit the release of pituitary hormones that travel via the circulatory system to target organs.

The anterior pituitary synthesizes seven hormones:

- Growth hormone (GH)
- Thyroid-stimulating hormone (TSH)
- Adrenocorticotropin (ACTH)
- Melanocyte-stimulating hormone (MSH)
- Prolactin (PRL)
- Follicle-stimulating hormone (FSH)
- Luteinizing hormone (LH)

FSH and LH (both gonadotropins) are responsible for regulating gynecologic organ activities. FSH targets the ovaries, where it stimulates the growth and development of the primary follicles and results in the production of estrogen and progesterone. The release of FSH from the pituitary is governed by a negative feedback mechanism involving these steroids. In contrast, LH targets the developing follicle within the ovary; it is responsible for ovulation, corpus luteum formation, and hormone production in the ovaries. Prolactin is responsible for preparing the mammary gland for lactation and brings about the synthesis of milk (McCartney & Marshall, 2014; Molitch, 2014).

Ovaries and Uterus
Complex changes occur in the ovaries and the endometrium as a result of the cyclic fluctuations of gonadotropic hormones. The endometrium emulates the activities of the ovaries; thus whatever happens in the uterus during the menstrual cycle is precisely correlated with whatever is occurring in the ovaries. The objective of the ovarian cycle is to produce an ovum, while the objective of the endometrial cycle is to prepare a site to nourish and maintain the ovum if it becomes fertilized. The ovarian cycle includes three distinct phases: the follicular phase, ovulation, and the luteal phase. The endometrial cycle can be divided into the proliferative phase, the secretory phase, and menstruation (Fritz & Speroff, 2011).

Hormonal Feedback System

The menstrual cycle is influenced by a complex interaction of hormones. In particular, the monthly rhythmic functioning of the menstrual cycle depends on the changing concentrations of gonadotropic hormones. The release of LH and FSH from the pituitary depends on the secretion of GnRH from the hypothalamus, which is modulated by the feedback effects of estrogen and progesterone. The hormones LH and FSH, in turn, play important roles in stimulating secretion of estrogen and progesterone.

Almost all hormones are released in short pulses at intervals of 60 to 90 minutes throughout most of the menstrual cycle, with these pulses decreasing in frequency closer to menstruation. Steroid hormones modulate the frequency and amplitude

of the pulse, which varies throughout the cycle (Fritz & Speroff, 2011); see **Color Plate 5**.

As noted earlier, under normal physiologic conditions, GnRH pulses stimulate the release of FSH and LH. As a result of this gonadotropic hormone stimulation, the ovarian follicles develop and produce estrogen. As the amount of estrogen in the circulation increases and reaches the pituitary gland, it affects the amount of FSH and LH secreted, albeit without significantly affecting the pulse frequency (negative feedback).

When the estrogen level becomes high enough, the negative feedback effect on the pituitary is reversed. Now estrogen causes a midcycle positive feedback effect on the pituitary, which results in a surge of LH and FSH and causes ovulation. Under LH influence, the ruptured follicle becomes the corpus luteum and secretes progesterone. Although the presence of progesterone reduces the frequency of the hypothalamic GnRH pulses, the amount of LH released from the pituitary is proportionally increased to sustain the corpus luteum and the production of progesterone. In the absence of pregnancy, the corpus luteum degenerates, progesterone levels decline, and menstruation occurs. The GnRH pulses return to the frequency associated with the beginning of the follicular phase and a new cycle begins (Ferin & Lobo, 2012).

The Ovarian Cycle

The ovarian cycle comprises three phases: follicular, ovulatory, and luteal.

Follicular Phase
The follicular phase is characterized by the development of ovarian follicles and usually lasts from day 1 (first day of menses) to day 14 of the ovarian cycle. Folliculogenesis begins during the last few days of the previous menstrual cycle and continues until the release of the mature follicle at ovulation. The decrease in estrogen production by the corpus luteum and the dramatic fall of inhibin levels allow the FSH level to rise during the last few days of the menstrual cycle. During days 1 through 4 of the menstrual cycle, a cohort of primary follicles is recruited from a pool of nonproliferating follicles in response to the increased concentration of FSH (Fritz & Speroff, 2011). Follicles that have enough granulosa cells will develop receptors for estrogen

and FSH on the cells of the granulosa layers, and LH receptors on the theca cells. The primary role of FSH is to induce the development of increased receptors on the granulosa cells and thereby stimulate estrogen production. The preliminary role of LH is to stimulate the cells' production of androgen that will be converted to estrogen by the granulosa layers.

Between cycle days 5 and 7, only one dominant follicle from the cohort of recruited follicles is destined to ovulate during the next menstrual cycle. As menses progresses, FSH levels decline due to the negative feedback of estrogen and the negative effects of the peptide hormone inhibin, which is secreted by the granulosa and theca cells of the developing follicle (Fritz & Speroff, 2011; Halvorson, 2012b). The decrease in FSH level promotes a more androgenic microenvironment within the adjacent follicles. By the eighth day of the cycle, the dominant follicle (Graafian follicle) is producing more estrogen than the total amount produced by the other developing follicles. In response to the dominant follicle's combined production of estrogen and FSH, LH receptors develop on its outermost granulosa layers. The dominant follicle continues to flourish and gradually moves toward the surface of the ovary (see **Color Plate 6**). The Graafian follicle contains the ovum and is surrounded by a layer of granulosa cells, which are themselves surrounded by the specialized theca interna and theca externa cells.

An oocyte maturation inhibitor (OMI) in the follicular fluid suppresses the final maturation of the dominant follicle until the time of ovulation. The OMI's suppressive effects end hours before the LH surge that causes ovulation (Halvorson, 2012b).

Ovulatory Phase
Ovulation is the process whereby the mature ovum is released from the follicle (Halvorson, 2012b). It occurs approximately 10 to 12 hours after the LH peak—that is, when the highest level of LH is attained. Ovulation and the subsequent conversion of the follicle to the corpus luteum are dependent on an increased level of estrogen and the LH surge, which marks the beginning of the rapid rise of LH. During the mid-follicular phase, the dominant follicle's FSH levels diminish, but estrogen levels

continue to increase. At the end of the follicular phase, estrogen reaches a blood level of approximately 200 picograms per milliliter (pg/mL); this concentration may be maintained for as long as 50 hours (Fritz & Speroff, 2011; Halvorson, 2012b). At this critical time, the high estrogen level initiates a positive feedback of LH, generating the preovulatory LH surge. The LH surge, which begins 34 to 36 hours prior to ovulation and provides a relatively accurate predictor for timing ovulation, is responsible for many changes in the follicle selected for rupture.

Initially the nuclear membrane around the oocyte breaks down, the chromosomes progress through the rest of the first meiotic division, and the egg moves on to the secondary stage. Meiosis ceases at this time and will be initiated again only if the ovum is fertilized. The LH surge stimulates luteinization of the granulosa cells as well as synthesis of progesterone. Progesterone, in turn, enhances the positive feedback effect of estrogen on the LH surge and is responsible for promoting enzyme activity in the follicular fluid capable of digesting the follicle wall. High levels of LH and progesterone cause the synthesis of prostaglandins and proteolytic enzymes such as collagenase and plasmin. Although the exact mechanism underlying this process is unknown, the activated proteolytic enzymes and prostaglandins digest collagen in the follicular wall, leading to an explosive release of the ovum (oocyte), along with the zona pellucida and corona radiate surrounding it. At ovulation, the ovum is expelled and drawn up by the ciliated fimbriae of the fallopian tube to initiate its migration through the oviduct (Ferin & Lobo, 2012; Fritz & Speroff, 2011).

New information about the timing of the LH surge and ovulation is available now because of the amount of data collected by many clinicians during in vitro fertilization. The LH surge has a tendency to occur around 3 a.m. in more than two-thirds of women, and ovulation has been found to occur primarily in the morning during the spring months and primarily during the evening during autumn and winter (Fritz & Speroff, 2011). In the Northern Hemisphere, from July to February, approximately 90% of women will ovulate between 4 and 7 p.m. During the spring, 50% of women will ovulate between midnight and 11 a.m. (Fritz & Speroff, 2011, p. 228).

Luteal Phase

Under the influence of LH, the follicle's granulosa cells that are left in the ruptured follicle become enlarged, undergo luteinization, and form the corpus luteum. The corpus luteum continues to function for approximately 8 days after ovulation. It secretes increased progesterone and some estrogen that start the negative feedback loop to the hypothalamus and pituitary gland, preventing further ovulation within the current cycle. In the absence of a fertilized ovum, luteal cells degenerate, causing a decline in estrogen and progesterone levels, and the corpus luteum regresses to become the corpus albicans. As a result of the regression of the corpus luteum, estrogen and progesterone levels decrease rapidly, removing the negative feedback effect. FSH and LH then begin to increase once again to initiate the next menstrual cycle (Ferin & Lobo, 2012; Fritz & Speroff, 2011).

The Endometrial Cycle

The endometrial cycle has three phases: proliferative, secretory, and menstrual.

Proliferative Phase

The proliferative phase is influenced by estrogen and entails the regrowth of endometrium after the menstrual bleed. It starts on about the fourth or fifth day of the cycle and usually lasts approximately 10 days, ending with the release of the ovum. The proliferative phase involves changes in the endometrium, myometrium, and ovaries. These cyclic changes, which result from fluctuations in gonadotropin and estrogen levels, are characterized by progressive mitotic growth of the deciduas functionalis in response to increasing levels of estrogen secreted by the ovary. They occur in preparation for implantation of the fertilized ovum.

At the beginning of the proliferative phase, the endometrium is relatively thin and the endometrial glands are straight, narrow, and short. As the phase progresses, the glands become long and tortuous. The endometrium becomes thicker as a result of the glandular hyperplasia and growth of the stroma. The endometrium proliferates from 4 to 12 mm in height and increases eightfold in thickness in preparation for implantation of the fertilized ovum (Ferin & Lobo, 2012).

Secretory Phase

The secretory phase begins at ovulation. When part of a 28-day cycle, it usually lasts from day 15 (the day after ovulation—the exact cycle day will vary with cycle length) to day 28. This phase does not take place if ovulation has not occurred. It tends to be the most constant phase, in terms of time.

During the secretory phase, the glands of the endometrium become more tortuous and dilated and fill with secretions, primarily as a result of increased progesterone production. The endometrium becomes thick, cushiony, and nutritive in preparation for implantation of the fertilized ovum. In the absence of implantation, the corpus luteum shrinks, and progesterone and estrogen levels subsequently decrease. The endometrium begins to regress toward the end of the secretory phase. By days 25 to 26, progesterone and estrogen withdrawal results in increased tortuous coiling and constriction of the spiral arterioles in the thinning layer.

Until the last decade, it was believed that decreased blood flow to the superficial endometrial layers resulted in tissue ischemia and resulting menses. The end of menses was believed to be caused "by longer and more intense waves of vasoconstriction, combined with coagulation mechanisms activated by vascular stasis and endometrial collapse, aided by rapid re-epithelization mediated by estrogen from the emerging new follicular cohort" (Fritz & Speroff, 2011, p. 595). Newer studies do not support the theory that menstruation results from vascular events. Rather, the current theory suggests that menstruation is initiated by enzymatic autodigestion of the functional layer of the endometrium, which is triggered by estrogen–progesterone withdrawal (Fritz & Speroff, 2011). As estrogen and progesterone levels fall during the days prior to menses, lysosomal membranes become destabilized, such that the enzymes within them are released into the cytoplasm of the epithelial, stromal, and endothelial cells and into the intercellular space. These enzymes are proteolytic: They digest the cells surrounding them as well as surface membranes. Their actions result in platelet deposition, release of prostaglandins, vascular thrombosis, extravasation of red blood cells, and tissue necrosis in the vascular endothelium (Ferin & Lobo, 2012). Enzymatic action progressively degrades the endometrium and eventually disrupts the capillaries and venous system just under the endometrial surface, causing interstitial hemorrhage and dissolution of the surface membrane and allowing blood to escape into the endometrial cavity (Fritz & Speroff, 2011). This degeneration continues and extends to the functional layer of the endometrium, where rupture of the basal arterioles contributes to the bleeding. The concepts about how the menstrual flow ceases remain unchanged.

Menstrual Phase

The menstrual phase begins with the initiation of menses and lasts 4 to 6 days. Prostaglandins initiate contractions of the uterine smooth muscle and sloughing of the degraded endometrial tissue, leading to menstruation. The composition of menstrual fluid comprises desquamated endometrial tissue, red blood cells, inflammatory exudates, and proteolytic enzymes. Because some of the clotting factors ordinarily found in blood are lysed by lysosomal enzymes in the uterus, menstrual blood does not clot (Ferin & Lobo, 2012; Fritz & Speroff, 2011). For 3 to 5 days, 20 to 80 mL (on average) of blood loss occurs. Approximately 2 days after the start of menstruation, estrogen stimulates the regeneration of the surface endometrial epithelium, while concurrent simultaneous endometrial shedding is occurring.

Changes in Organs Due to Cyclic Changes

Cervix

After menstruation, the cervical mucus is scant and viscous. During the late follicular phase, it becomes clear, copious, and elastic. The quantity of cervical mucus increases 30-fold compared to the early follicular phase and can stretch to at least 6 cm (Ferin & Lobo, 2012; Fritz & Speroff, 2011). The cervical mucus during this time is clear and stretchable (spinnbarkeit). It displays a characteristic ferning appearance during the ovulatory period if observed under a microscope.

After ovulation, when progesterone levels are high, the cervical mucus once again becomes thick, viscous, opaque, and decreased in amount. This thick mucus is hostile and impenetrable to the sperm. The increased viscosity also reduces the risk of ascending infection at the time of possible implantation.

Increased estrogen levels promote stromal vascularization and edema and relax the myometrial fibers that supply the cervix. Activated collagenase causes the tightly bound collagen bundles to form a loose matrix, triggering the cervix to become softer a few days prior to and at ovulation. The external cervical os everts prior to ovulation. Progesterone causes the cervical muscle to retract, the collagen matrix to tighten, and the cervix to become firmer (Fritz & Speroff, 2011; Halvorson, 2012b).

Fallopian Tube Mobility

Estrogen stimulates epithelial cell activity, resulting in increased cilia movement and secretions in the uterine tubes. These special effects assist ovum mobility along the fallopian tube following ovulation. Progesterone reverses these effects, thereby inhibiting the peristaltic activity of the fallopian tube smooth muscle.

Vagina

The changes in hormonal levels of estrogen and progesterone have characteristic effects on the vaginal epithelium. This information becomes important when cervical cells are examined under the microscope, as their morphologic differences can be related to specific stages of the menstrual cycle. During the early follicular phase, exfoliated vaginal epithelial cells have vesicular nuclei and are basophilic. They appear flatter than the corresponding cells in the later phases owing to the influence of progesterone, which causes them to become folded and clumped. The pH of the vagina responds to cyclical changes as estrogen stimulates the growth of lactobacilli. Lactobacilli metabolize glycogen from cervical secretions, producing lactic acid that decreases the vaginal pH to a level that assists in protecting the gynecologic tract against opportunistic pathogens (Fritz & Speroff, 2011; Halvorson, 2012b).

References

Anderson, J., & Gendry, R. (2007). Anatomy and embryology. In J. Berek (Ed.), *Berek and Novak's gynecology* (14th ed., pp. 75–127). Philadelphia, PA: Lippincott Williams & Wilkins.

Assadi, S. N. (2013). Is being a health-care worker a risk factor for women's reproductive system. *International Journal of Preventive Medicine, 4*(7), 852–857.

Bradshaw, K. (2012). Anatomic disorders. In B. L. Hoffman, J. O. Schorge, J. I. Schaffer, L. M. Halvorson, K. D. Bradshaw, F. G. Cunningham, & L. E. Calver (Eds.), *Williams gynecology* (2nd ed., pp. 481–505). New York, NY: McGraw-Hill.

Caldwell, W. E., & Moloy, H. C. (1933). Anatomical variations in female pelvic bones and their effect on labor with a suggested classification. *American Journal of Obstetrics & Gynecology, 26*, 479–482.

Corton, M. (2012). Anatomy. In B. L. Hoffman, J. O. Schorge, J. I. Schaffer, L. M. Halvorson, K. D. Bradshaw, F. G. Cunningham, & L. E. Calver (Eds.), *Williams gynecology* (2nd ed., pp. 918–947). New York, NY: McGraw-Hill.

Duffy, J. (1963). Masturbation and clitoridectomy. *Journal of the American Medical Association, 186*(3), 246–248. doi:10.1001/jama.1963.63710030028012

Ferin, M., & Lobo, R. (2012). Reproductive endocrinology. In G. Lentz, R. Lobo, D. Gershenson, & V. Katz (Eds.), *Comprehensive gynecology* (6th ed., pp. 67–95). Philadelphia, PA: Mosby Elsevier.

Fritz, M., & Speroff, L. (2011). *Clinical gynecologic endocrinology and infertility*. Philadelphia, PA: Lippincott Williams & Wilkins.

Hall, L. A. (1998). The other in the mirror: Sex, Victorians, and historians. Retrieved from http://www.lesleyahall.net/sexvict.htm

Halvorson, L. M. (2012a). Amenorrhea. In B. L. Hoffman, J. O. Schorge, J. I. Schaffer, L. M. Halvorson, K. D. Bradshaw, F. G. Cunningham, & L. E. Calver (Eds.), *Williams gynecology* (2nd ed., pp. 440–459). New York, NY: McGraw-Hill.

Halvorson, L. M. (2012b). Reproductive endocrinology. In B. L. Hoffman, J. O. Schorge, J. I. Schaffer, L. M. Halvorson, K. D. Bradshaw, F. G. Cunningham, & L. E. Calver (Eds.), *Williams gynecology* (2nd ed., pp. 400–439). New York, NY: McGraw-Hill.

Johnson, W., Choh, A., Curran, J., Czerwinski, S. A., Bellis, C., Dyer, T. D., & Demerath, E. (2013). Genetic risk for earlier menarche also influences peripubertal body mass index. *American Journal of Physical Anthropology, 150*, 10–20.

Karapanou, O., & Papadimitriou, A. (2010). Determinants of menarche. *Reproductive Biology and Endocrinology, 5*(1), 115–123.

Katz, V. (2012). Reproductive anatomy. In V. Katz, G. Lentz, R. Lobob, & D. Gershenson (Eds.), *Comprehensive gynecology* (6th ed., pp. 39–65). Philadelphia, PA: Mosby Elsevier.

Katz, V., & Dotters, D. (2012). Breast diseases. In V. Katz, G. Lentz, R. Lobo, & D. Gershenson (Eds.), *Comprehensive gynecology* (6th ed., pp. 301–334). Philadelphia. [A: Mosby Elsevier.

Kolesova, O., & Vetra, J. (2012). Female pelvic types and age differences in their distribution. *Papers on Anthropology, 21*, 147–154.

Martini, F., Timmons, M. J., & Tallitsch, R. (2011). *Human anatomy* (7th ed.). San Francisco, CA: Benjamin Cummings.

McCartney, C. R., & Marshall, J. C. (2014). Neuroendocrinology of reproduction. In J. F. Strauss & R. L. Barbien (Eds.), *Reproductive endocrinology: physiology, pathophysiology, and clinical management* (7th ed., pp. 3–26.) Philadelphia, PA: Saunders.

Molitch, M. (2014). Prolactin in human reproduction. In J. F. Strauss & R. L. Barbien (Eds.), *Reproductive endocrinology: physiology, pathophysiology, and clinical management* (7th ed., pp. 45–65). Philadelphia, PA: Saunders.

Puppo, V. (2013). Anatomy and physiology of the clitoris, vestibular bulbs, and labia minora with a review of the female orgasm and the prevention of female dysfunction. *Clinical Anatomy, 26*(1), 134–152.

Richter, H., & Varner, R. (2007). Pelvic organ prolapse. In J. Berek (Ed.), *Berek and Novak's gynecology* (14th ed., pp. 897–934). Philadelphia, PA: Lippincott Williams & Wilkins.

Soper, D. (2007). Genitourinary infections and sexually transmitted diseases. In J. Berek (Ed.), *Berek and Novak's gynecology* (14th ed., pp. 541–559). Philadelphia, PA: Lippincott Williams & Wilkins.

Soucasaux, N. (1993a). Archetypal aspects of the female genitals. *Museum of Menstruation & Women's Health*. Retrieved from http://www.mum.org/sougenit.htm

Soucasaux, N. (1993b). Psychosomatic and symbolic aspects of menstruation. *Museum of Menstruation & Women's Health*. Retrieved from http://www.mum.org/psychos.htm

CHAPTER 6

Gynecologic History and Physical Examination

Stephanie Tillman
Frances E. Likis

The editors acknowledge Deborah Narrigan, who was the author of the previous edition of this chapter.

Gynecologic care occurs for two main reasons: to enhance or maintain health and to identify and treat a problem of the gynecologic system. This chapter presents the core knowledge and skill base for the gynecologic health history and physical examination. Often this examination is embedded within a clinical visit that has a wider focus on primary care screening and counseling (see Chapters 4 and 7). In other circumstances, it is the base examination for a visit centered on an identified concern, such as a sexual assault (see Chapter 14), which may require further evaluation than is detailed in this text. The gynecologic examination is modifiable and individualizable to every patient, every time.

Considerations of and approach to this examination must acknowledge the cultural, social, historical, and personal sensitivity of discussion and examination of the body parts involved. A woman's breasts or chest, vagina, rectum, and corresponding body parts are experienced outside of a healthcare environment in myriad contexts, including overt sexualization, consensual intercourse, and sexual assault, and they are lived personally as intimate and private spaces. Particularly for women, the objectification and experience of the private body can be a very public and involuntary one, so the onus of acknowledging and diminishing these factors is on the clinician, given the power differentials between care provider and care seeker, and providers' role in holistically caring for those women whom they serve. Importantly, the clinician should state explicitly that the care seeker at any point can stop an examination, ask for a change in method, decline a recommendation, or request a chaperone. This acknowledges the care seeker's control and creates space in which the individual knows that her words and bodily responses will be heard and respected.

For the purpose of this chapter, as is the titled purpose of this text, the referenced individual will be identified as a woman. Healthcare providers whose scope of practice focuses on vaginas, cervices, uteri, ovaries, and chests or breasts and their corresponding physiologic body systems may see people who do not identify with the terms *woman* or *female*, or whose gender expressions, sexual orientations, and sexual identities do not match with this terminology or a provider's presumed understanding of those terms. See Chapter 9 for further information about lesbian, bisexual, and queer (LBQ) women, as well as transgender and gender-nonconforming (TGNC) people, and considerations for their care.

HEALTH HISTORY

The purpose of the health history is to establish a relationship with a woman while learning about her health. To a great extent, taking a health history means listening to a woman's story. Both the content and manner of what she conveys provide important information for a clinician's understanding of what an individual woman wants and needs. To optimize health history taking, several environmental and logistical arrangements should be consistently in place. These include providing a comfortable and private setting, scheduling an appropriate amount of time, and choosing the optimal format and staff member for obtaining the health history.

Privacy is an essential component for obtaining the health history. Ideally, the room or office where the history is taken will have a door that can be closed so no noise or traffic interrupts the interview. A closed door ensures confidentiality and conveys the clinician's intent to offer the woman undivided attention. The woman should remain fully clothed. The clinician and the woman should be seated a comfortable distance from each other, preferably face to face, without furniture or electronics between them. This seating arrangement promotes a conversational, rather than a confrontational or hierarchical, approach. Especially in the age of the electronic health record, each clinician should find a way to minimize use of the computer during the history taking. If an interpreter is present, he or she should be seated so that all three persons can see and hear one another.

Generally, the optimal way to gather the health history is to interview the woman alone, because distractions are minimized and privacy is ensured. If the woman prefers to have a spouse, friend, or other person with her, however, she should have this choice. If young children are present, a second adult should be available to attend to them.

If the woman has another person present during the health history, it is essential that at some point the woman be given the opportunity to speak privately with the clinician. This practice is advisable for handling topics that either clinician or woman find sensitive, such as the sexual health history, safety at home, and mental health concerns. It also allows the clinician to ensure that the choice to have the other adult present was made freely by the woman. For adolescents accompanied by parents or guardians, this policy is particularly important. Regarding the latter, always commend parental involvement and care, but authoritatively establish and separate the provider relationship, while following state and national guidelines. For example, the provider could say to the parent, "Thank you for coming today. As a provider, it is so important to see parents involved. I would like to obtain the family history while you are here, and then complete the remainder of the visit alone, so that we can begin to develop our care relationship together." For resources related to minors' consent and access to services, see the Guttmacher Institute's (2015) website.

Schedule an appropriate amount of time to allow a woman being seen for an initial visit to tell her story in an unhurried manner. This approach generally yields a rich and pertinent database. Structure the interview around standard questions (**Boxes 6-1**, **6-2**, and **6-3**) but encourage responses to be open ended, and allow the flow to be flexible based on individual responses and needs. As much as possible, pose questions that allow open-ended responses, such as "Tell me about your sexual partners," "Describe your periods," and "How do you feel your overall health is right now?"

Listen intently. This involves maintaining eye contact, nodding along with understanding of facts and concerns, asking follow-up questions that pertain specifically to the visit at hand, and responding with words of empathy or excitement as appropriate. During a busy clinic day, the provider's focus may be on many tasks and concerns. Every woman deserves the full attention of the provider during her visit, and providers must find ways to refocus and ensure complete attention during each visit. If support staff calls the provider away from the conversation or there is an emergency that interrupts the examination, the provider must again refocus completely on the task at hand when reentering the room. Language such as "I apologize for the interruption. I always fully dedicate my attention to everyone I serve, and in an emergency my attention is refocused to that concern. Know that I would do the same for you in an emergency, so thank you for your patience," assures the woman that she has your attention and your focus is intentional.

If the topic veers off from the presumed focus, carefully steer the conversation back to the original concern. A suggested phrase to do so might be "I am so glad you brought that up today. If we are not able to address that during this visit, I will make a note for us to focus on it next time." Interject only for specific clarification or to bring the woman back to the topic if she seems to be digressing too far.

BOX 6-1 General Health History

Reason the woman is seeking care
(chief concern)

History of present illness/concern
(see **Box 6-2**)

General medical history
- Current health conditions
- Previous serious illnesses
- Past hospitalizations
- Prior surgical procedures
- Immunization status

Mental health history
- Diagnoses and treatment
- History of self-harm practices and/or suicidal or homicidal thoughts
- Current concerns (depression screening)

Medications and allergies
- Current medications
- Over-the-counter (OTC) medications, including vitamins and complementary therapies
- Medication and other allergies

Substance use
- Alcohol
- Tobacco
- Cannabis
- Illegal drugs
- Misuse of OTC or prescribed medications

Family health history
- Illnesses and causes of death of first-degree relatives
- Congenital malformations and unexplained intellectual and developmental disabilities

Social history
- Education
- Hobbies
- Long-term life plans
- Partner(s)
- Living companions (children, family, roommates)
- Support system

Occupation and finances
- Current employment
- Occupational safety
- Military service
- Financial security

Safety
- Personal
- Home
- Community
- Sexual (current and historical)

Personal habits
- Health maintenance: exercise, sleep, nutrition, hydration
- Ongoing health maintenance

Abbreviation: OTC, over-the-counter.

If the provider recognizes a need to refocus the visit during the history taking, allow questions to follow that path as indicated. The reality of time pressure in ambulatory care settings may make an allocation of 20 to 30 minutes for obtaining a health history seem like a luxury, but it should be considered a key to excellent care. Many clinicians posit that 90% of the information needed for accurate diagnosis comes directly from the health history.

A variety of formats may be used for obtaining the health history, ranging from a self-administered questionnaire to a conversation between the clinician and the woman, with information recorded in a prepared format. The trade-offs required for each of these alternatives are obvious. Disadvantages to self-administered health questionnaires include the possibilities that answers to items may be omitted, questions may be misunderstood, or terms may be unfamiliar to the respondent. In addition, the entire questionnaire will require visual and verbal review by a nurse or the clinician to fill in missing information and clarify answers. Advantages include that some persons may disclose information more freely on sensitive topics in writing than if asked verbally, and the total time for this procedure may be less than if all information is obtained

---

BOX 6-2 History of Present Illness/Concern: OLDCARTS

Onset: When did the concern or symptoms begin? What were the circumstances at that time? Have you had this before?

Location: Where are the symptoms located physically?

Duration: How long have you had the symptoms?

Characteristics: Describe the concern or symptoms. In the case of pain, is it sharp, stabbing, dull, radiating, burning?

Associated symptoms: What other symptoms happen at the same time as the primary concern?

Relieving factors: What makes your symptoms better or worse? What have you tried already to change or solve the symptoms? How effective have those strategies been?

Timing: When do the symptoms happen? Are they constant or do they occur only during certain times or activities (e.g., during particular points in the menstrual cycle or during sex)?

Severity: How much is the concern affecting your daily quality of life? In the case of pain, try to rate it on a scale of no pain (0) to the worst pain imaginable (10).

---

in an interview. Regardless of which staff person is responsible for obtaining the health history, whoever conducts the interview should be skilled at putting the woman at ease, and in conveying respectful attention through his or her verbal style and behavior.

All providers should attempt to use common language rather than medical terminology when phrasing questions or describing the examination. Many practices record data on average number of years of schooling completed, and for clinics in underserved areas, this average may be in the elementary school years with an equivalent reading ability. All attempts must be made to provide language, consent, and resources at a woman's level of understanding.

General Health History

Initially the interviewer briefly introduces herself or himself, states the purposes of the interview, and invites questions from the woman at any point during the visit. The interviewer proceeds next to checking basic demographic information, which is less personal and helps to put the woman at ease.

Reason the Woman Is Seeking Care/Chief Concern

Asking, "How may I help you today?" or "What brought you here today?" are good ways to begin addressing the chief concern. Encourage the woman to describe the problem or reason for the visit in her own words—for example, "I think I want to change from pills to an IUD."

History of Present Illness/Concern

When the woman has finished describing why she is seeking care, the interviewer will need to obtain additional details about the reason for the visit. To maximize understanding of the woman's concern, the clinician should be sure he or she has answers to all relevant questions related to her concern. The acronym OLDCARTS (**Box 6-2**), often used related to pain, covers a full conversation around any reported concern. Historically, the term *history of present illness* (HPI) references the purpose of the visit, though when the woman describes her reason for seeking care it may be related to health maintenance or a concern that might not be defined as illness.

General Medical History

The woman will need to list any significant health conditions she has had in her lifetime, including all hospitalizations and surgical procedures. Many people omit common surgeries, such as cesarean births, tubal ligations, and breast reduction or enhancement. In addition, the interviewer should ask about specific illnesses that occur frequently, such as diabetes, hypertension, respiratory illnesses, and infectious diseases. A review of adult immunizations is also necessary. Depending on the

---

BOX 6-3 Gynecologic Health History

Menstrual history

- Age at menarche
- Date of last normal menstrual period (LMP)
- Cycle length, duration, and flow
- Any menstrual irregularities or symptoms associated with menses

Pregnancy history

- Gravida and para (see **Box 6-4**)
- Course of pregnancies: date, duration, type of birth, complications (pregnancy, birth, and postpartum), newborn's sex and weight, and whether the child is currently alive and well
- For abortions (induced or spontaneous), ectopic pregnancies, blighted ovum, and molar pregnancies: gestational age, management, and complications

History of vaginal and sexually transmitted infections

- Previous vaginal infections and sexually transmitted infections
- Treatments received, frequency of infections, and complications

Genital hygiene

- Vaginal or rectal douching frequency, medication or solutions used, reasons for douching
- Hair maintenance
- Piercings
- Other products: creams, lubricants, specialty soaps, scented pads or tampons

Gynecologic procedures and surgeries

- Type of procedure or surgery, date, indication, complications, and outcome

Urologic and rectal health

- Occurrence and frequency of infections
- Urinary or bowel incontinence
- Other abnormal symptoms

Cervical cancer screening

- Date of last testing
- History of an abnormal result, and if so, follow-up and results since then

Sexual health

- Sexual orientation and gender identity
- Current sexual relationship(s): number of partners (current, in the past 6 months, and lifetime), sexual practices, safer sex practices
- Sexual satisfaction and orgasm
- Types of intercourse: oral, anal, vaginal, other
- Pain with sex
- Sexual concerns

Contraceptive use

- Present contraceptive method: type, duration used, satisfaction, side effects, and consistency of use
- Previous contraceptive use: method(s), duration of use, satisfaction, side effects, and reasons for discontinuing

Abnormal symptoms

- Pelvic pain, bleeding unrelated to menstruation, and other symptoms

---

population, specifically asking certain questions may be important to ensure an accurate history.

Mental Health History

Inquire about any current concerns related to mental health. Discuss any current or past diagnoses, and treatment related to them, including medications, inpatient care, or outpatient therapy. Ask specifically about self-harm practices, such as cutting, and past or current suicidal or homicidal thoughts. For the last two, if the woman responds "yes" to current suicidal or homicidal ideation, further questioning must follow to elucidate intent, plan, and access to means. Immediate action must be taken for anyone responding positively to suicidal or homicidal ideation, usually by calling emergency services. Often, a prescreening questionnaire can be helpful in asking specific questions related to daily struggles or general symptoms, such as appetite, hunger, and how others perceive the woman's mental health.

Medications and Allergies

Review all medications the woman is currently taking, including over-the-counter (OTC) preparations, vitamins, supplements, and complementary therapies (e.g., herbs, homeopathics, probiotics), as well as reasons for their use. If the woman cannot recall the name of a medication she is using, encourage her to bring the package to the next visit. Intrauterine devices (IUDs) and implants are often not included in reported medication lists, so if the woman is at risk for pregnancy based on her sexual activity and partners, inquire about current contraceptive use. Obtain information on any allergic responses to medications, foods, the environment, or other substances.

Substance Use

Perhaps the easiest way to proceed with this topic is to inquire about each substance separately, beginning with legal substances, such as alcohol, tobacco, and, depending on the state, cannabis, and then moving to illegal drugs and misuse of OTC and prescribed medications. Ask about the amount and type of each substance used per day or week. See Chapter 8 for further discussion of screening for alcohol misuse. Ask if the woman has smoked or is currently smoking, the daily number of cigarettes or joints, the length of time smoked, the number of attempts at quitting, and interest in quitting now. For cannabis, ask if the woman is using it specifically for anxiety, depression, hunger, nausea, or other underlying symptoms, which may be addressed separately or adequately managed with legal cannabis use. For illegal drugs, inquire about types, amount, route, and frequency of use. Depending on the community, using common street drug names may provide the patient with additional entrée into the provider's knowledge and comfort base. Finally, asking if there are any medications used outside of their prescription or designation

provides information about misuse of accessible medications.

For interviewers new to the process, positive answers to these questions may elicit surprise or concern, but this is not the time to intervene with counseling. The interviewer needs to stay focused on gathering information. As with all information sought during the history taking, specific facts become part of a broader picture of a clinician's approach to care provision; therefore, an environment of nonjudgment is imperative to encourage comfort with sharing the truth, including with legal drug misuse or illegal drug use.

Family Health History

Gather information about first-degree relatives: parents, grandparents, siblings, and children. A family tree or narrative can be recorded, and information on serious illnesses and causes of death for each of these individuals should be obtained. In addition, occurrences of congenital malformations, unexplained intellectual and developmental disabilities, or other disabilities should be covered to offer clues to possible inherited diseases. Note that for many cancers, such as breast, uterine, and ovarian, the affected family member's age of diagnosis may impact the patient's own screening recommendations.

Social History

Ask the woman about her highest educational level attained, hobbies, and long-term life plans. Review relationships, including spouses, partners, sexual relationships, and current family or family planning, as well as her current support system.

Occupation and Finances

Ask about current employment, concerns about safety or hazardous conditions at work, employment stability, physical safety, and body mechanics. Ask if the woman has ever served in the military as this puts her at risk for health concerns, including post-traumatic stress disorder, traumatic brain injury, and military sexual trauma (American Academy of Nursing, 2015). Reviewing financial security, including ability to cover housing and food costs, is imperative to understand the need to connect individuals with further care resources. Logistics related to healthcare provision are also important, including insurance concerns and barriers to seeking care, the latter of which may range from transportation issues to childcare needs.

Safety

Safety issues—primarily the use of seat belts in motor vehicles, and helmets with bicycle or motorcycle use—should be assessed, as well as presence of firearms in the woman's household and sense of security in the home or lived community. Current or past intimate partner violence, sexual assault, incest, emotional abuse, and/or reproductive coercion are essential components to review to fully assess needs around healthy sexual and intimate relationships. All individuals deserve to be asked at every visit about personal and bodily safety. As the provider relationship develops, more information may be disclosed with time that was not revealed at the first history taking session. See Chapters 4, 7, and 13 for more information about intimate partner violence.

Personal Habits

Ask the woman about her exercise, sleep, self-care, and nutrition patterns. A 24-hour dietary recall and asking "What do you drink when you're thirsty?" can provide a snapshot into the woman's common meals, drinks, and snacks. Ongoing health maintenance, such as dental care, eye examinations, massage, Reiki, acupuncture, and mental health support, can be screened with general questions, such as "What other health or personal care-related appointments have you had in the past year?"

Gynecologic Health History

The gynecologic health history elicits significant details that provide the essential background for a concern-focused visit, as well as for a health maintenance visit for a well woman. The standard topics for this health history are listed in **Box 6-3**. Specific points that should be included about each topic follow.

Menstrual History

The menstrual history is usually the first topic in the gynecologic history and should cover the following information: age at menarche; date when the last normal menstrual period (LMP) began; length of the cycle, counting from the first day of one menses until the first day of the next menses; average

number of days of menses; characteristics of the menstrual flow; regularity of cycles; and description of any irregularities or accompanying symptoms. In general, cycles range from 21 to 35 days, and menses last from 4 to 7 days. If the woman is perimenopausal, document the most recent menstrual cycle and note whether the cycles are regularly irregular (e.g., every 3 months) or irregularly irregular (unpredictable). If she is postmenopausal, document the month and year of last menses, and note the pertinent negative of "no vaginal bleeding since menopause."

Pregnancy History

Begin by asking the woman the total number of times she has been pregnant. Then ask her to describe each pregnancy in chronologic order. As the woman explains her pregnancy history, the interviewer will make written notes and complete the GTPAL five-digit numeric summary description of pregnancies (**Box 6-4**).

Specific information to obtain for each pregnancy includes the year it occurred; its duration; the type of birth (spontaneous vaginal birth, assisted vaginal birth, or cesarean); complications (during pregnancy, during birth, or postpartum); sex and weight of the newborn; and whether the

---

BOX 6-4 Recording Pregnancy History: GTPAL System

Gravida or pregnancy: the total number of pregnancies the woman has had (this number should total the TPAL numbers)

Term births: those occurring from 37 to 42 weeks' gestation

Preterm births: those occurring after the point of viability, which is usually interpreted as gestational age greater than 20 weeks and less than 37 weeks and/or fetal weight greater than 500 gm

Abortions: spontaneous and induced prior to 20 weeks' gestation

Living children

child is currently alive and well. The category of abortion includes information about induced abortions, spontaneous abortions, ectopic pregnancies, blighted ovum, and molar pregnancies. For these pregnancies, record details of gestational age, management (e.g., spontaneous, medication, aspiration, dilation and curettage, dilation and evacuation, laparoscopic removal), and any complications.

History of Vaginal and Sexually Transmitted Infections

Ask which types of infections, if any, the woman has had; which treatments she has received; how frequently each infection has occurred; and what, if any, complications have occurred. Naming each infection specifically may promote recall or disclosure. Discuss any known pelvic inflammatory disease (PID) diagnosis. Ask the woman the number of sexual partners she has at present, has had over the past 6 months, and has had during her lifetime. Inquire if she is sexually active with persons who present high risk for sexually transmitted infections (STIs) and whether she uses condoms. Further individualization of screening recommendations may result from the disclosed information. Detailed assessment of sexual risk is described in Chapter 20.

Genital Hygiene

Ask about frequency, medication or solutions used, and reasons for douching. Discuss hair maintenance and piercings, including any related problems. Review any creams, lubricants, specialty soaps, scented pads or tampons, wipes, or sprays.

Gynecologic Procedures and Surgeries

Include information on minor procedures, such as endometrial biopsy, laparoscopic examination, and cyst or abscess drainage, as well as surgeries, including tubal ligation or hysterectomy. The information needed includes the year in which the procedure or surgery was performed, indication, significant complications, and outcome. Obtaining pertinent medical records may also be useful if detailed information is needed.

If serving populations for whom female genital cutting is a known practice, include questions related to this procedure, which is also referred to as female circumcision or female genital mutilation

---

BOX 6-5 Female Genital Cutting

Female genital cutting, also called female circumcision and female genital mutilation, comprises "all procedures that involve partial or total removal of the external female genitalia, or other injury to the female genital organs for nonmedical reasons" (World Health Organization [WHO], 2014). There are four major types of female genital cutting:

- Clitoridectomy: Partial or total removal of the clitoris and/or the prepuce
- Excision: Partial or total removal of the clitoris and the labia minora, with or without excision of the labia majora
- Infibulation: Narrowing of the vaginal orifice with creation of a covering seal by cutting and repositioning the labia minora and/or the labia majora, with or without excision of the clitoris
- Other: All other harmful procedures to the female genitalia for nonmedical purposes, such as pricking, piercing, incising, scraping, and cauterization (WHO, 2014)

Long-term sequelae of female genital cutting include recurrent urinary tract infections, dermoid cysts, infertility, and obstetric complications (United Nations Children's Fund, 2013; WHO, 2014).

Modified from United Nations Children's Fund. (2013). *Female genital mutilation/cutting: A statistical overview and exploration of the dynamics of change.* New York, NY: Author; World Health Organization (WHO). (2014). *Female genital mutilation.* Fact sheet No. 241. Geneva, Switzerland: Author. Retrieved from http://www.who.int/mediacentre/factsheets /fs241/en.

(**Box 6-5** and **Figure 6-1**). For many women, this procedure may be normalized and thus not listed unless specifically asked. Additionally, "mutilation" may not be how the woman identifies with the process or the outcome, and is a pejorative term about someone's private anatomy. Thus asking

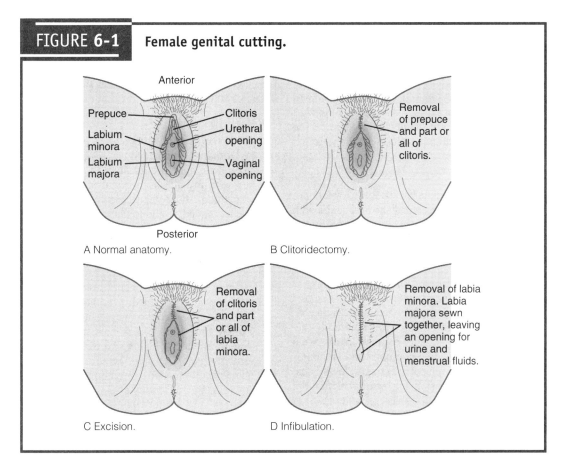

FIGURE **6-1** **Female genital cutting.**

Anterior

Prepuce
Clitoris
Labium minora
Urethral opening
Labium majora
Vaginal opening

Posterior

A Normal anatomy.

Removal of prepuce and part or all of clitoris.

B Clitoridectomy.

Removal of clitoris and part or all of labia minora.

C Excision.

Removal of labia minora. Labia majora sewn together, leaving an opening for urine and menstrual fluids.

D Infibulation.

about being "cut" or "circumcised" is typically more linguistically and culturally appropriate. If vaginal alterations are noted in the examination that were not mentioned in the history, the provider should stop the examination and revisit this section of the history with care.

Women may not disclose during the health history that they have been cut for a variety of reasons, including fear that the clinician will disapprove or respond negatively to this information. If a woman does disclose that her genitals were cut, that information may be shared while describing associated complications noted previously. A woman may also provide this information in response to an open-ended question such as "Is there anything else you would like me to know about your health background before we begin your examination?" It is important for the clinician to ask when the

cutting occurred, whether the woman has previously had a pelvic examination, and if she is experiencing symptoms of long-term sequelae.

The extent of cutting will be determined during the inspection of the external genitalia. A pediatric speculum and single-digit bimanual examination may be necessary for pelvic examination. A special form for recording health history and physical findings relevant to female genital cutting can be helpful (see Campbell, 2004, for a sample form).

Urologic and Rectal Health
Urologic topics include the occurrence and frequency of urinary tract infections, incontinence, and other abnormal symptoms (e.g., urinary frequency, dysuria). Rectal topics include incontinence, constipation, hemorrhoids, bloody stools, and pain with defecation.

Cervical Cancer Screening

Ask if the woman has had previous cervical cancer screening. If so, find out the approximate date of the last test and if the results were abnormal. For a woman who has had an abnormal cervical cancer screening result, ask what follow-up occurred and if subsequent screening results have been normal. Check the most recent guidelines to know if the screening is up-to-date per recommendations and based on her history.

Sexual Health

Ask if the woman is sexually active. If so, ask her to describe her sexual partners, if she is satisfied with her sexual function, and if she or her partner(s) have any sexual concerns. Do not presume gender identity, expression, or sexual orientation solely from a description of sexual partners: Follow up these answers with further questions that would directly pertain to her healthcare provision and provider understanding as needed (see Chapter 9). It is unacceptable to provide care differently due to someone's gender identity, expression, or sexual orientation. Use objective language and standardize history taking for all patients, regardless of sex, gender identity, expression, and sexual orientation. Additional information about assessment of sexual health can be found in Chapter 10.

Contraceptive Use

The contraceptive history is obtained from women who engage in sex that can lead to pregnancy. If relevant, ask if the woman or her partner is currently using a contraceptive method, if she is satisfied with the method or desires a change, or if she has questions about her current method. Discussing past methods used may be relevant depending on the woman's reason for the visit. Additionally, many women use contraceptive methods for menstrual regulation or other indications. Consider using "contraception" rather than "birth control" or "family planning" to be more all-encompassing of reasons people use these medications. Finally, use of emergency contraception, including frequency of use, may provide further information about contraceptive need, pregnancy risk, and cycle irregularities.

Abnormal Symptoms

Problems such as pelvic pain should be fully described, noting their relationship in time with the menstrual cycle, and any association with sexual activity, tampon use, or other factors. Additionally, any vaginal bleeding not related to menstruation should be fully described. See Chapters 24 and 28 for detailed information about the assessment of bleeding and pelvic pain.

Final Steps

Closure of the health history should include offering the woman the chance to add comments or ask questions. One approach is simply to say, "I have finished with my questions about your health. Is there anything I have omitted or not covered, or that you would like to add to help me better understand your health or concerns today?"

Once the clinician has completed taking the health history, the next step is to begin to examine, sort, and prioritize the information gathered and to decide which further assessment measures, such as laboratory tests, are needed. It is often helpful at this time to summarize the findings and offer tentative answers to questions or concerns posed by the woman about her health. An example would be to say, "Based on what you have described, let's talk about recommended screening tests, physical examination, and laboratory evaluations, and then you can ask any further questions based on the conclusions we come to together before we continue the rest of the visit." This type of statement emphasizes the woman and clinician's partnership in her care.

In charting, note pertinent positives and negatives in the review of systems and health history. Documentation should include language such as "Reports itching," "Describes pain in certain sexual positions," or "No odor or burning," rather than "Denies pain with urination," which suggests provider suspicion of truth in the history telling. If during the history taking the woman indicates she does not desire a portion or portions of the physical examination, document this as "Declines breast examination" or "Prefers pelvic examination to be included at a different visit," rather than "Refused bimanual examination," which indicates a negative connotation to patient consent to procedures. Clinicians should be cognizant of verbal or documented language that diminishes concerns, devalues presented facts, patronizes emotional or mental health reports, or otherwise calls into question the validity of a report. If there is concern for withheld historical information or a woman's preferred process that differs from a clinician's recommendations, document this in the note's "Plan" section, detailing education provided, consent process reviewed and the outcomes, and future considerations.

PHYSICAL EXAMINATION FOR A GYNECOLOGIC VISIT

Evaluating a new patient usually includes performing a physical examination. The details and description of the techniques, such as auscultation, are beyond the scope of this chapter. Readers are referred to textbooks on physical examination for a review of maneuvers, equipment, and organization of the examination (Ball, Dains, Flynn, Solomon, & Stewart, 2015; Bickley, 2013; Jarvis, 2016). This text assumes that the age range for patients will extend from adolescence through the older adult. Gynecologic care for children requires specialized pediatric skills that go beyond the scope of this chapter.

What constitutes a complete physical examination in the ambulatory gynecology or primary care setting is not standardized. It is customary to evaluate major organ systems briefly and carefully, but not exhaustively. For example, the cardiovascular examination would include complete auscultation of the heart and evaluation of circulation by noting skin color, but would usually omit other maneuvers, such as checking carotid bruits or palpation of the precordium. When deciding what to include in the physical examination, novice clinicians may want to use the following principle as a guideline: Be able to state the rationale for including or excluding any assessment maneuver or particular feature of any organ system. If a rationale for performing a maneuver and obtaining the specific information that maneuver provides can be stated, then including it would be justified.

If family members or partners were present during the history taking portion of the visit, ask the woman if she would like to proceed with the physical examination portion with or without those individuals present. Keep in mind that evidence of physical violence, identifying past or current experiences of sexual abuse, and an opportunity to speak with the woman alone are all possible

components of the physical examination. Even if the woman requested for people to stay for the history taking, offer again for them to leave for the physical examination to give another opportunity for privacy. For women who may currently be experiencing physical or sexual abuse by those in the room, be attentive for deference to questions, positive or negative communications, guarding during physical interactions, or any other sign that might trigger an intuitive response to request others to leave the room during the examination. A suggestion for language in this circumstance would be, "If it's okay with you, I would prefer to begin your examination with an assistant in the room to help with tools." If the woman does not interject and say something like, "That's okay" or "I'd rather they stayed," turn to look at other individuals in the room and say, "Would you mind waiting in the waiting room, and once the physical examination is over, I'll have you come back in as we finish the visit?'

Before beginning any component of the physical examination, providers must consider offering an internal reflection of power as well as a verbal acknowledgment and discussion. Phrases such as "You are in complete control of this examination. If at any point you feel uncomfortable, want me to stop, or have questions, please let me know. I will stop at any point if you ask me to or if I feel that your body is telling me to," remind the provider and inform the woman of her ability to stop or change the examination at any time. A woman's mere presence for an examination or evaluation does not indicate consent for every component a provider might consider routine. Particularly for individuals with a history of sexual assault, many of whom may not report it during the history taking, this verbal transfer of power and reminder that the word "stop" is respected in the healthcare space is essential. For women with a known sexual assault history, providers must take extra caution regarding language, transfer of power, ensuring comfort, validating consent, and considering the presence of a chaperone for both the woman's comfort and the provider's documentation. Given that many women will experience a sexual assault attempt or completed rape in their lifetime, but often do not report that event legally or during the history taking portion of the examination, intentional language and physical examination approaches should be standardized and sensitive to this issue for every individual. This must be considered routine and is part of feministic, humanistic, individualized care that intentionally includes informed consent throughout the entire process, as all care should.

General Physical Examination

The order of the examination presented here assumes the woman is sitting up to begin the examination. This description proceeds from head to toe, rather than by system.

1. *Physical measurements.* Obtain and review height, weight, blood pressure, pulse, and temperature (if indicated) before performing the physical examination. Height and weight are most useful when converted to the body mass index (BMI) using **Table 6-1**. Both BMI and blood pressure should be considered screening tools (see Chapter 7 for further discussion).
2. *General appearance.* Observe the woman for posture; striking or obvious characteristics or limitations; general emotional state; and appropriateness of dress, speech pattern, and social interaction during the visit.
3. *Eyes, ears, nose, and throat.* Inspect the physical health of the eyes, nose, and ears. Examination of the ears with the otoscope and examination of the eyes with the ophthalmoscope may be performed as indicated. The oropharynx examination includes inspection of the lips, teeth, and gums for dental health, and visualization of the oral cavity for mucosal color, lesions, and tonsillar edema or exudates.
4. *Neck.* Note range of motion and palpate lymph nodes in the neck and clavicular area.
5. *Thyroid.* Palpate the gland and isthmus.
6. *Chest and lungs.* Auscultate the posterior, lateral, and anterior lobes.
7. *Spine.* Palpate the vertebral column, and inspect the skin.
8. *Kidneys.* Check costovertebral tenderness.
9. *Reflexes.* Elicit patellar and additional reflexes as indicated.
10. *Peripheral circulation and varicosities.* Inspect legs and feet.

The woman then reclines and the examination continues:

11. *Heart.* Auscultate.
12. *Breasts and axillary lymph nodes.* See the next section.
13. *Abdomen.* Inspect the skin, palpate superficially and deeply in all quadrants, and palpate inguinal lymph nodes.

Breast Examination

Despite ongoing controversy regarding the efficacy of breast self-examination, clinical breast examination performed by health professionals remains a part of the general physical examination (see Chapter 7 for further discussion of breast cancer screening). It is relatively simple and quick, with only two types of maneuvers being performed: inspection and palpation. Conditions that promote ease and accuracy in findings are also simple. Adequate lighting helps to reveal subtle variations in skin texture and color. Adequate exposure, or having the woman disrobe to the waist, allows simultaneous observation and comparison of both breasts. For those initially hesitant about this method, explaining why this exposure is needed and employing an approach that is gentle but focused on the examination will convey the clinician's concern and respect.

Breast Inspection

This maneuver begins with the woman sitting, usually on the examining table, with arms relaxed at her sides, and the examiner standing facing her. Look at each breast and compare them for size, symmetry, contour, skin color, texture, venous patterns, and lesions. Lift the breast with fingertips to inspect the lower and lateral aspects. Breasts vary in shape, and frequently one will be slightly larger than the other. Skin texture should be smooth, contours uninterrupted bilaterally, and venous patterning similar in both breasts. Benign lesions, such as nevi, if longstanding, unchanged, and nontender, are considered normal findings. Ask the woman about the history of these skin changes during the examination to clarify as needed.

Next, inspect the nipples and areolae. The areolae should be round or oval and nearly equal in configuration bilaterally with a smooth surface. Color ranges from pink to black. Montgomery's

TABLE 6-1 Body Mass Index

Height (inches)	Normal						Overweight					Obese										Extreme Obesity														
BMI	19	20	21	22	23	24	25	26	27	28	29	30	31	32	33	34	35	36	37	38	39	40	41	42	43	44	45	46	47	48	49	50	51	52	53	54
												Body Weight (pounds)																								
58	91	96	100	105	110	115	119	124	129	134	138	143	148	153	158	162	167	172	177	181	186	191	196	201	205	210	215	220	224	229	234	239	244	248	253	258
59	94	99	104	109	114	119	124	128	133	138	143	148	153	158	163	168	173	178	183	188	193	198	203	208	212	217	222	227	232	237	242	247	252	257	262	267
60	97	102	107	112	118	123	128	133	138	143	148	153	158	163	168	174	179	184	189	194	199	204	209	215	220	225	230	235	240	245	250	255	261	266	271	276
61	100	106	111	116	122	127	132	137	143	148	153	158	164	169	174	180	185	190	195	201	206	211	217	222	227	232	238	243	248	254	259	264	269	275	280	285
62	104	109	115	120	126	131	136	142	147	153	158	164	169	175	180	186	191	196	202	207	213	218	224	229	235	240	246	251	256	262	267	273	278	284	289	295
63	107	113	118	124	130	135	141	146	152	158	163	169	175	180	186	191	197	203	208	214	220	225	231	237	242	248	254	259	265	270	278	282	287	293	299	304
64	110	116	122	128	134	140	145	151	157	163	169	174	180	186	192	197	204	209	215	221	227	232	238	244	250	256	262	267	273	279	285	291	296	302	308	314
65	114	120	126	132	138	144	150	156	162	168	174	180	186	192	198	204	210	216	222	228	234	240	246	252	258	264	270	276	282	288	294	300	306	312	318	324
66	118	124	130	136	142	148	155	161	167	173	179	186	192	198	204	210	216	223	229	235	241	247	253	260	266	272	278	284	291	297	303	309	315	322	328	334
67	121	127	134	140	146	153	159	166	172	178	185	191	198	204	211	217	223	230	236	242	249	255	261	268	274	280	287	293	299	306	312	319	325	331	338	344
68	125	131	138	144	151	158	164	171	177	184	190	197	203	210	216	223	230	236	243	249	256	262	269	276	282	289	295	302	308	315	322	328	335	341	348	354
69	128	135	142	149	155	162	169	176	182	189	196	203	209	216	223	230	236	243	250	257	263	270	277	284	291	297	304	311	318	324	331	338	345	351	358	365
70	132	139	146	153	160	167	174	181	188	195	202	209	216	222	229	236	243	250	257	264	271	278	285	292	299	306	313	320	327	334	341	348	355	362	369	376
71	136	143	150	157	165	172	179	186	193	200	208	215	222	229	236	243	250	257	265	272	279	286	293	301	308	315	322	329	338	343	351	358	365	372	379	386
72	140	147	154	162	169	177	184	191	199	206	213	221	228	235	242	250	258	265	272	279	287	294	302	309	316	324	331	338	346	353	361	368	375	383	390	397
73	144	151	159	166	174	182	189	197	204	212	219	227	235	242	250	257	265	272	280	288	295	302	310	318	325	333	340	348	355	363	371	378	386	393	401	408
74	148	155	163	171	179	186	194	202	210	218	225	233	241	249	256	264	272	280	287	295	303	311	319	326	334	342	350	358	365	373	381	389	396	404	412	420
75	152	160	168	176	184	192	200	208	216	224	232	240	248	256	264	272	279	287	295	303	311	319	327	335	343	351	359	367	375	383	391	399	407	415	423	431
76	156	164	172	180	189	197	205	213	221	230	238	246	254	263	271	279	287	295	304	312	320	328	336	344	353	361	369	377	385	394	402	410	418	426	435	443

Reproduced from National Heart, Lung, and Blood Institute. (n.d.). Body mass index table. Retrieved from http://www.nhlbi.nih.gov/health/educational/lose_wt/BMI/bmi_tbl.pdf.

tubercles—very small sebaceous glands—may be seen as slightly raised fleshy protuberances and are a common finding. The nipples also should be equal or nearly equal in size. Most nipples are everted. If one or both are inverted, ask if inversion has been a lifelong characteristic. A newly inverted nipple suggests pathology. A second abnormal finding to note is nipple retraction or a flattening of the nipple. Look also at the orientation of the nipples. If one points in a different direction from the other, this may be caused by the presence of malignant tissue in the breast. The color of the nipples should be the same as the areolae, while the surface may be smooth or wrinkled and should be without discharge. Supernumerary or extra nipples may also be seen. They are benign, usually small, and commonly mistaken as moles. They may occur anywhere along a vertical line from the axilla to the inner thigh and are usually unilateral.

The last step in inspection in the sitting position is to have the woman change positions slightly so that the contour and symmetry of the breasts can be assessed completely. The three positions for examination while seated are arms over the head, hands pressed against the hips, and leaning forward at the waist.

Seated Breast Palpation
The woman remains sitting with arms resting freely at her sides. The examiner remains standing facing her. Cover the other breast for warmth and comfort. Palpate all four quadrants for nodules and lumps. Use the finger pads because they are more sensitive to touch than the fingertips. Do a complete light palpation, followed by a deep palpation. Be aware that a firm transverse ridge of compressed tissue is often found along the lower edge of the breast. It comprises the inframammary ridge and is a normal finding. For large breasts, it may be helpful to place one hand beneath the breast to stabilize it while palpating with the other hand (**Figure 6-2**). Press firmly enough to get a good sense of underlying tissue but not so firmly that the tissue is compressed against the rib cage. Rotate the fingers in a clockwise or counterclockwise direction. Palpating systematically is key to performing a complete examination. Two patterns commonly used for breast palpation are concentric circles starting from the outer edge and spiraling

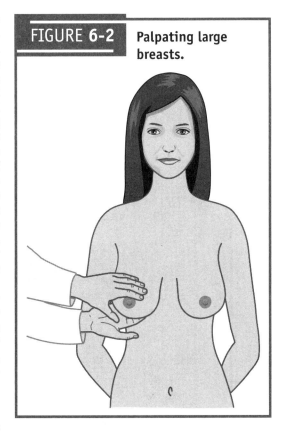

FIGURE 6-2 Palpating large breasts.

inward to the nipple, and top to bottom in vertical strips. For this latter pattern begin at the top, palpate downward and then upward, working gradually over the entire breast. Either pattern is acceptable as long as the entire breast is palpated. Note any discomfort or pain that the woman mentions or responds to physically with a change in facial expression or body movement.

Breast tissue in adult women feels dense, firm, and elastic. Prior to and during menstruation, some women experience cyclical tenderness, swelling, and nodularity. If a mass is felt, note the location, size, shape, consistency, tenderness, mobility, and demarcation of borders.

The tail of Spence—breast tissue that extends from the upper outer quadrant toward the axilla—must also be palpated because most malignancies develop in the upper outer quadrant (VanMeter & Hubert, 2014). This is best done by having the woman raise her arms over her head while the examiner

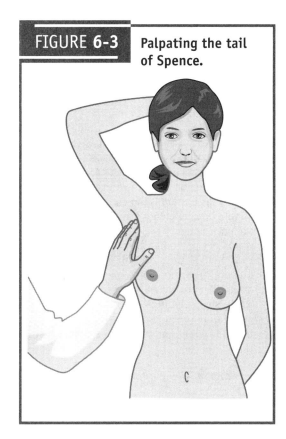

FIGURE 6-3   **Palpating the tail of Spence.**

gently compresses the tissue where it enters the axilla between thumb and fingers (**Figure 6-3**).

Examination of Lymph Nodes
While the woman is still sitting, include evaluation of the lymph nodes along with the breast examination. Have the woman sit with arms flexed at the elbow. The examiner stands facing the woman, but slightly off center. If beginning with the right axilla, use the left hand. Reach deeply into the axillary hollow and press firmly upward with the palmar surfaces of the fingers. Then bring the fingers downward to gently roll the soft tissue against the chest wall. Be sure to examine not only the apex, but also the central and medial aspects along the rib cage, the lateral aspect along the medial surface of the arm, the anterior wall along the pectoral muscles, and the posterior wall along the border of the scapula. Repeat this procedure with the other axilla. Axillary lymph nodes are usually

not palpable in adults. The supraclavicular area should also be palpated. Hook the fingers over the clavicle and rotate them over the entire supraclavicular area.

Supine Breast Palpation
Breast palpation now continues with the woman supine. Place a small pillow or folded towel under the shoulder before beginning the examination of the breast on that side. Use the same palpation technique and pattern for the supine position as for the sitting position. Repeat the examination with the woman's arm at her side. This repetition aids in a complete palpation because breast tissue shifts with different positions. After the entire breast is palpated, the nipple should also be gently palpated. Compress the nipple between thumb and index finger to inspect for discharge. This usually causes the nipple to become erect, and may be momentarily painful.

For the beginning practitioner, explaining the component of each examination while performing it not only ensures a complete review, but also engages the woman in her care and informs her of parts of her anatomy or concerning abnormalities. Once this examination becomes second nature, many clinicians simultaneously perform the breast examination and discuss components of the evaluation the woman may do during her self-examination.

Abbreviated forms of the breast examination may include a seated breast inspection and palpation only in the supine position. Each practitioner modifies the examination according to the individual woman, time per visit, concerning symptoms or history, and if an abnormality is identified.

Pelvic Examination

The pelvic examination customarily concludes the physical examination. The description offered here assumes the reader is familiar with the anatomy of the pelvic structures, and particularly the anatomy of the gynecologic organs, both internal and external (see Chapter 5). A few features of these structures, such as their size and relative locations, as well as their common findings, are particularly pertinent to performing this examination easily and successfully.

Few experiences that women encounter in the evaluation of their health are as intimate—and, therefore, as potentially anxiety producing—as the pelvic examination. All clinicians who perform this type of examination have the professional responsibility to carry it out proficiently, promptly, and respectfully. Each woman brings her own past experiences and her own needs to the present examination. Specific conditions that generally enhance the experience include the following:

- Before starting the examination, and at several points during, explain in general what you are going to do prior to beginning.
- Use language that can be understood by the woman. Use common words, not medical terms. Some women prefer to have the entire process explained to them throughout the procedure, whereas others prefer to be in conversation about something other than the examination itself. Clinicians must respect the woman's preferences and adjust approaches to the examination for each individual.
- Ask the woman if she has any concerns or questions.
- Never talk lightly or make jokes about genitalia or the examination. This is entirely inappropriate.
- Maintain ability for eye contact during the examination as much as possible, recognizing that women from many cultural groups may not return eye contact. Raising the head of the examination table slightly allows continued face-to-face visualization, and typically does not interfere with the cervical evaluation.
- If the examiner encounters an unexpected finding, conscious attempts should be made to avoid expressing surprise in facial expression or voice. If feasible, wait until the end of the examination to discuss the finding. If assistance is needed from another health professional to evaluate an abnormal or unexpected finding, briefly explain the finding and the reason for a second examiner's assessment.
- Assure the woman that the examination will proceed as gently as possible and ask her to indicate if and when she feels discomfort.
- Be sure the examination room is a comfortable temperature.

- Ensure privacy for this examination, including closing the door as well as a curtain if available. Minimize interruptions by fellow staff, such as knocking or calling through the closed door.
- Invite the woman to have someone accompany her for support during the examination if she desires.
- The clinician may or may not have an assistant. Regardless of the clinician's sex or gender, consider having an assistant present as a legal protection for both woman and clinician. This is customary if the clinician is male, but should be considered for all clinicians and all patients.
- If this is the woman's first genital and pelvic examination, it is both informative and empowering at this point in the physical examination to review the process from start to finish, including demonstrating the tools commonly used, discussing external and internal components, and answering any questions.

Preparing and Beginning the Pelvic Examination

1. Ask if the woman would like to go to the bathroom before starting the examination. Bimanual examination can be very uncomfortable with a full bladder or rectum. A full bladder also makes palpation of pelvic organs difficult. Finally, depending on how long the woman has waited for the provider in the waiting room or in the examination room, she may not have had access to a bathroom for quite a while and offering her time to do so acknowledges this fact.
2. Offer the woman the option of a drape. It provides some privacy and warmth and may facilitate her relaxing, but some women may find it intrusive or unnecessary. Its use is optional.
3. Raise the top portion of the examination table to at least 30° and have a pillow at the head of the table. These measures add to the woman's comfort and make it easier for the clinician to maintain eye contact with her once the examination is in progress.
4. Assist the woman into the lithotomy position, first helping stabilize her feet in the footrests

or on the supportive pull-out table. Place the back of one hand at the bottom edge of the table and instruct her to move down, being sure her buttocks are slightly beyond the edge of the examination table. This detail is important to allow correct positioning of the speculum.

5. After making sure that all examination materials are prepared and within easy reach, wash your hands. Seat yourself on a stool so you are at eye level with the perineum. Don latex or nonlatex gloves (depending on clinician or patient allergy) and start the examination.

6. Ask the woman to separate her legs. Never try to force her legs open, even by pressing gently. It is sometimes helpful to touch the outside of the woman's knees or thighs and ask her to open her legs toward the examiner's hands. Using language such as "Relax your knees out to the side like an open book" might give the woman a visual cue if she is having a difficult time understanding the provider's direction. Additionally, many women are uncomfortable at the very beginning of the examination. After utilizing all description options, often the clinician needs to simply wait for the woman to be ready. Suggesting, "I will know that you are ready once you are in position. Take your time, and let me know if you have any questions," again gives the woman the power to start the examination when ready.

7. Adjust the light so it illuminates the perineal and vaginal area.

8. The pelvic examination is intrusive. Wait a moment until both the examiner and the woman are ready, and then tell the woman that the examination will begin. Start with a firm touch with the back of one gloved hand on one of the woman's lower thighs, and then move the examining hand along the thigh toward the external genitalia. If the woman prefers the examination described throughout, helpful language might include "You will feel my hand on your thigh, then on the outside of your vagina. I will be examining just on the outside first. Let me know if anything is uncomfortable or painful."

9. If the woman becomes tense or upset during the examination, stop and ask if there is anything she needs or anything you can do

differently. Tell her the examination will not continue until she is at ease. Then make any adjustments that will ensure her comfort with the examination before continuing. If during external examination the woman has significant discomfort or pain, or if the clinician visualizes the vaginal muscles clamping closed, she may have vulvodynia, pelvic pain, or a history of forced vaginal entry. Consider delaying further examination until another visit. If the examination is for general health maintenance rather than for a specific concern, or if further evaluation and testing can be done without vaginal entry, consider adjusting the examination appropriately.

Inspection and Palpation of External Genitalia, Vaginal Orifice, and Accessory Glands

1. Proceed with inspection in order so as not to repeat touching unnecessarily. Many clinicians use a clockwise approach to ensure a complete examination and minimize repetition. Utilize a consistent pressure throughout the examination to avoid light touch or a poking sensation.

2. Inspect, and then palpate the mons pubis, labia majora, and perineum, noting the pattern of hair distribution, size and shape of the labia, and presence of lesions, scars, rashes, erythema, discharge, discoloration, or piercings.

3. Separate the labia majora, inspect and palpate the labia minora, and inspect the urethral orifice and clitoris. Note the anatomic placement of the urethral opening and inspect for clitoral enlargement. There is no need to palpate the clitoris or the underlying clitoral body as part of this examination.

4. Inspect the vaginal introitus (opening) for presence or absence of the hymen and hymenal tags and shape of the opening; note swelling, discharge, irregular growths, nevi, or lesions. Be careful to not mistake a hymen for a vaginal septum. If a septum is noted, a bimanual examination must be considered prior to speculum examination to determine the extent of the septum, if there are possibly two complete vaginas or cervices or uteri that may need evaluation, and whether consultation is necessary.

5. Insert the index and third fingers to the second joint into the vagina, and press down gently

against the posterior vaginal wall, encouraging the woman to relax the perineal muscle to assist with comfort during the examination and visualization of the vaginal orifice. To assess for pelvic organ prolapse (POP), ask the woman to cough or bear down. If she has a cystocele (**Figure 6-4**), the anterior vaginal wall will bulge with this maneuver. Observe also for rectocele (**Figure 6-5**), or bulging of the posterior vaginal wall; this is a far less common finding. Cystoceles, rectoceles, and uterine prolapse are typically graded on their position in the vagina as related to the hymenal ring or the vaginal introitus (**Box 6-6**). Early stages of POP, including of the uterus, may not be symptomatic and thus are undetected by history taking. Detailing changes in vaginal tone and appropriate pelvic organ suspension in the documentation of the visit is important for considerations of stable or worsening condition during future evaluations.

6. To assess the tone of the perineal muscles, ask the woman to tighten her muscles around your vaginal examining fingers. This maneuver also ensures appropriate Kegel exercises, and the woman should be instructed toward grasping the examining fingers if she pushes outward during this portion of the examination.

7. Palpate the Bartholin's glands by inserting the index finger of the examining hand about 2 cm into the vagina near the perineum, turning the hand laterally, and gently palpating the tissue behind the vaginal wall between the thumb and index finger on one side; then, after rotating the examining hand, palpate in the same manner on the other side of the vagina. Healthy Bartholin's glands are not palpable, but if they are inflamed this maneuver will elicit notable pain. If a cyst is present, a fluctuant, nontender mass will be palpable. If an abscess is present, the site of the mass will be tender and warm. Many clinicians omit this portion of the examination unless a specific concern is identified.

8. Palpation of the Skene's glands, which lie immediately lateral to the urethral meatus, is performed by turning the examining hand upward, inserting the index finger into the vagina to the second knuckle, pressing gently upward, and then pulling this finger outward

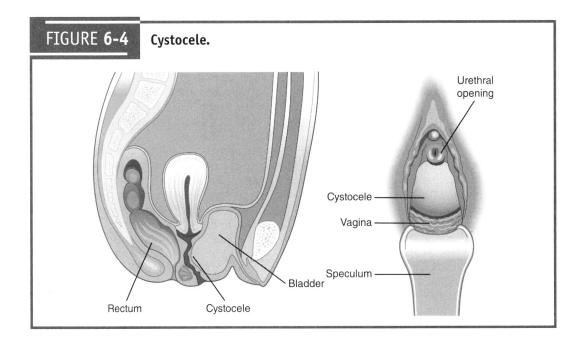

FIGURE 6-4   **Cystocele.**

Urethral opening

Cystocele

Vagina

Speculum

Bladder

Rectum   Cystocele

FIGURE 6-5 Rectocele.

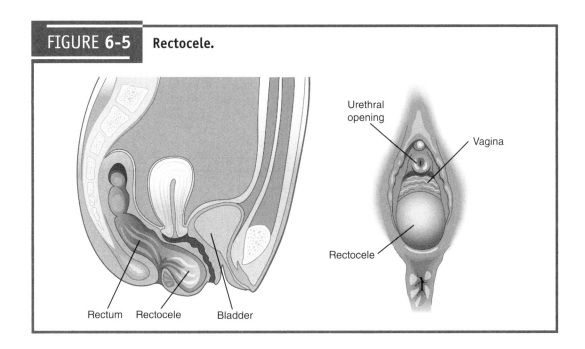

Urethral opening

Vagina

Rectocele

Rectum Rectocele Bladder

BOX 6-6 Pelvic Organ Prolapse Quantification (POP-Q)[a]

Stage 0: No prolapse

Stage I: Most distal portion of the prolapse is > 1 cm above the level of the hymen

Stage II: Most distal portion of the prolapse is ≤ 1 cm proximal to or distal to the plane of the hymen

Stage III: Most distal portion of the prolapse is > 1 cm below the plane of the hymen

Stage IV: Complete eversion of the total length of the vagina

[a] Assessment is performed while the woman strains as if she is having a bowel movement.

Data form Bump, R. C., Mattiasson, A., Bo, K., Brubaker, L. P., DeLancey, J. O. L., Klarskov, P., . . . Smith, A. R. B. (1996). The standardization of terminology of female pelvic organ prolapse and pelvic floor dysfunction. *American Journal of Obstetrics & Gynecology, 175,* 10–17.

while pressing against the vaginal tissue. Discharge at the urethral meatus with palpation of the Skene's glands usually indicates infection. This examination lasts only about 10 seconds, but usually causes pain. Many clinicians omit this portion of the examination unless a specific concern is identified, such as for a thorough examination for gonorrhea.

Note that steps 4 through 8 may be performed with the bimanual examination, according to the clinician's preference and the woman's comfort.

Speculum Examination

It is essential that clinicians become familiar with how the speculum operates before performing this examination. This preparation ensures women do not experience inadvertent pain caused by its incorrect use. Each clinician must also decide which hand to use for holding the speculum—a decision that is based entirely on personal preference. One hand should be kept "clean" to reach for tools and specimens and avoid contamination, while the other hand is utilized solely for examination. These can be distinguished as the "room" and "woman" hands, respectively. If the hands become cross-contaminated, the clinician should replace one or both gloves before the examination proceeds.

Importantly, speculum examination should be utilized as needed, such as for evaluation of vaginal or pelvic pain or cervical cytology screening. This examination is not required annually, nor is it a necessary component of every examination for symptomatic evaluation if there is no concern or symptom for which a speculum examination would provide further information. As noted in the appendices, vaginal swabs for microscopy or STI testing can be completed with a clinician swab collected without speculum insertion or with a self-swab collected by the woman. Speculum examination, as with all components of any examination, should be used intentionally and to garner specific information and assist in overall health determination.

1. Select the appropriate type (Graves or Pederson) and size (pediatric, small, medium or standard, or large) of speculum (**Figure 6-6**). For most parous women, the standard Graves speculum is used. For women with significant pelvic or genital adipose tissue, lax vaginal walls, or grand multiparity, the large Graves speculum will not only allow the best visualization but will also be more comfortable. The wider blade size of the large Graves speculum more effectively holds the vaginal walls open, permitting visualization of the cervix. For individuals who are pre-coitarche but still require an internal examination, nulliparas, postmenopausal women, transgender men on testosterone, or transgender women with neovaginas, the Pederson speculum is the usual choice. Its blades are the same length as those of the Graves speculum, but are narrower and flat rather than curved. A pediatric speculum may also be considered for these individuals. This shape and size minimizes pressure on the anterior and posterior vaginal walls, promoting a more comfortable examination. Plastic and metal speculum are equally clean and effective, and their availability is often according to provider or clinic preference (**Figure 6-6**).

2. Warm the speculum by running it under warm tap water, or equip the examination table drawer with a heating pad where specula can be stored. Lubricate the end of the speculum blades with water or a small amount (one teaspoon) of water-soluble gel. Wetting the speculum with water instead of lubricating it with water-soluble gel has been thought to be necessary to ensure optimal collection of specimens for cervical cytology. Multiple studies examining this practice have found that using a small amount of gel on the speculum does not interfere with cervical cytology specimens or results and decreases discomfort of the speculum insertion (Amies, Miller, Lee, & Koutsky, 2002; Harer, Valenzuela, & Lebo, 2002; Pergialiotis et al., 2015; Simavli, Kaygusuz, Kinay, & Cukur, 2014).

3. With the thumb and fourth finger of one hand, separate the labia majora to visualize the introitus, then place the index and third fingers slightly inside the vagina. Tell the woman she will feel some pressure, then press these two fingers downward. Ask the woman to try and relax these muscles downward, to facilitate comfort during the examination. For some women, this placement may be on the hymenal ring and actually increase discomfort. If so, advance the pressure internally by 1 cm, press downward, and try to encourage relaxation a second time. The very close proximity of the urethra and the pubic bone to the anterior vaginal wall can lead to distinct discomfort when the speculum or examining fingers enter and exit the vagina. This maneuver allows for good visualization of the opening of the vagina. With the other hand, grasp the speculum with index finger over the top of the proximal end of the anterior blade and the other fingers around the handle. This position allows control of the blades as the speculum is inserted.

4. Insert the speculum into the vagina at an oblique angle, and place it on top of the fingers at the perineum. Remove the fingers at the perineum. Keeping the blades closed, let them advance internally following the direction of the vagina until the blades are all the way in the vagina, pressing posteriorly throughout

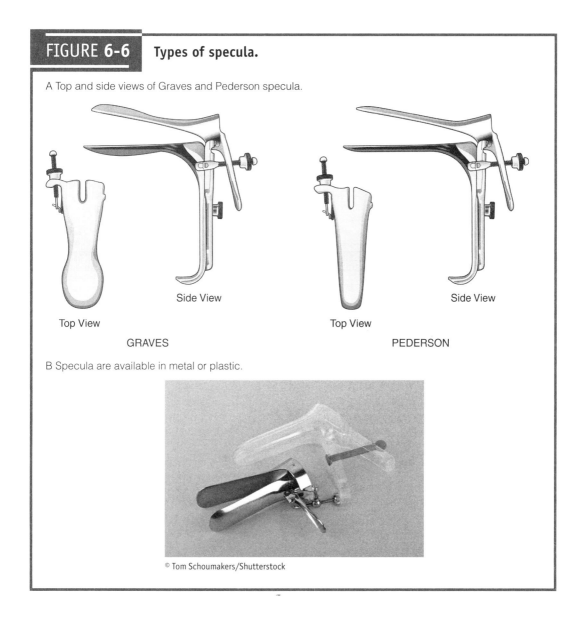

FIGURE 6-6 Types of specula.

A Top and side views of Graves and Pederson specula.

Side View

Top View

GRAVES

Side View

Top View

PEDERSON

B Specula are available in metal or plastic.

© Tom Schoumakers/Shutterstock

the insertion (**Figure 6-7**). The length of the blades is 6 to 7 inches, which matches the average length of the vagina. Remember that when lying supine, a woman's vagina inclines posteriorly about 45° downward from the vaginal opening toward the sacrum. Keeping the blades at this angle also avoids pressure on

the urethra and pubic bone, thereby minimizing discomfort.

5. Rotate the speculum horizontally and, once inserted completely into the posterior fornix, open the blades by pressing firmly and steadily on the thumbpiece. The cervix should come into view between the blades at the end of the

FIGURE 6-7 Speculum insertion and placement.

A Insertion.

B Placement.

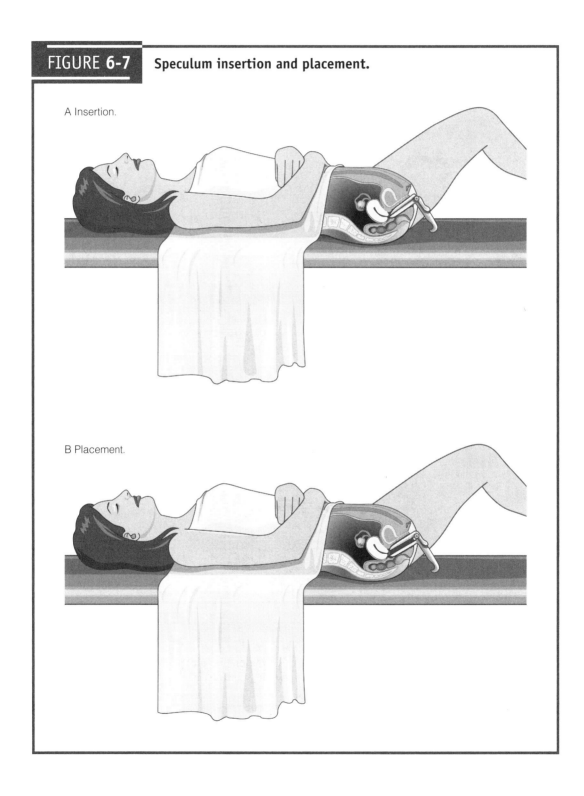

vagina. If it is not immediately visible with the blades wide open, relax the pressure on the thumbpiece, allowing the blades to close. Then reposition the speculum. Slide the speculum partially away from the posterior fornix, redirect the blades at a slightly different angle, and reinsert it obliquely. Open the blades; the cervix should now come into view. Adequate cervical visualization is essential for obtaining any specimens from the cervix. Depending on the position of the uterus, the position of the cervix may be very posterior or anterior. With a clear plastic speculum, if the os is visualized during speculum insertion, continue to insert the speculum to the posterior fornix to visualize the vaginal walls as part of the examination, but retract the speculum and direct the opening of the blades toward the os to avoid discomfort and unnecessary repositioning with the blades already opened.

6. Once the cervix is visualized, manipulate the speculum a little farther into the vagina so that the cervix is well exposed. If using a metal speculum, tighten the screw on the thumbpiece. If using a plastic speculum, click the upper blade onto the notch of the handle. Describing the noise the speculum might make before starting the insertion may facilitate the woman's comfort at this point in the examination; otherwise, the noise of the screw or the plastic clicking might be disconcerting. The speculum should remain in place so that both hands can be removed, making it possible for the examiner to handle other equipment.

Depending on the individual's anatomy and vaginal tone, this may or may not be possible, and a clinical chaperone or assistant may facilitate maintaining the speculum's position as needed.

Inspect the cervix for color, position, size, surface characteristics, shape of the os, and discharge. The cervix is remarkable for the vast variety of shapes, sizes, and appearances that are within the range of health. The color should be pink. Symmetric, circumscribed erythema around the os is a normal finding caused by exposing, or everting, the columnar epithelium lining of the endocervical canal. This eversion results from pressure of the speculum blades against the anterior and posterior fornices. Knowledge of cervical anatomy is important to document normal findings versus abnormalities, including presence of the squamocolumnar junction, ectropion, and transformation zone based on age, phase of the menstrual cycle, pregnancy, menarche, menopause, and malignancy.

The position of the cervix correlates to the position of the uterus. The most common position of the cervix is posterior, indicating an anteverted uterus. The cervix should be located in the midline; significant deviation may indicate a pelvic mass or adhesions. The diameter of the cervix is approximately 2 to 3 cm, and its length is approximately 3 cm. The os of a nulliparous woman is small and round, while a multiparous os is usually a horizontal slit or may be irregular or stellate (**Figure 6-8**).

FIGURE 6-8   **Variations of the cervical os.**

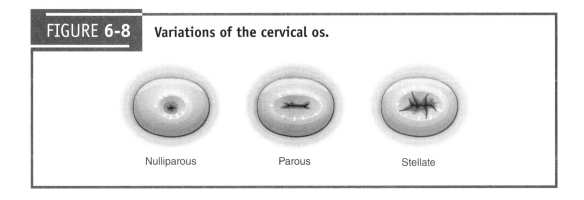

Nulliparous   Parous   Stellate

The surface should be smooth. Nabothian cysts may be seen as small white or yellow, raised areas; these retention cysts of endocervical glands are a normal variation (see Chapter 26). Note any friable tissue, a strawberry appearance, abnormal coloration such as a blue or purple tinge, granular areas, or red or white patchy areas. Note any discharge, and determine if its source is vaginal, which is far more common than a cervical origin. Note the color and consistency of the discharge. Normal vaginal discharge is odorless, creamy or clear, and thick or thin, depending on time in the menstrual cycle.

Three types of specimens are frequently collected at this point in the speculum examination: cervical cells for cytology screening; a vaginal or endocervical sample for gonorrhea, chlamydia, and trichomoniasis testing; and vaginal secretions for microscopy (see the chapter appendices for information on these procedures). In some laboratories, the same cervical sample is used for cytology screening and gonorrhea, chlamydia, and trichomoniasis testing. If separate cervical samples are collected for these tests, the optimal order for collecting these specimens is unknown because no evidence exists to guide this choice. Vaginal swabs are the preferred specimen type for such testing, even when a full pelvic examination is performed (Papp, Schachter, Gaydos, & Van Der Pol, 2014).

7. To begin removing a metal speculum, loosen the screw on the thumbpiece, but press on it to keep the blades open as the speculum is withdrawn from around the cervix. If using a plastic speculum, press on the thumbpiece to release it from the notch that has kept the anterior blade open. Once the cervix is no longer within the speculum blades, release most of the pressure on the thumbpiece, and rotate the speculum back to the oblique angle. Depending on the vaginal anatomy, the cervix may not release easily from within the blades. If this occurs, use the speculum handle as a lever and gently lift and lower the speculum body while slowly retracting the blades, until the cervix releases. The pulling and compression of the cervix into the vaginal canal as the speculum is removed often causes significant discomfort at this point of the examination if not given careful attention and patience.

As the speculum is withdrawn, inspect the vaginal walls. Note the color, surface characteristics, and secretions. Vaginal mucosa should be almost the same color as the cervix, and the surface should be moist and smooth or rugated. Normal discharge will appear thin, clear or cloudy, and odorless.

After inspection, continue to remove the speculum. Release all pressure on the thumbpiece; the blades will close themselves. Taking care not to pinch the vaginal mucosa, quickly and completely withdraw the speculum in an upward direction, but with downward pressure, similar to that used during insertion. This maneuver provides the most comfort for the woman, and avoids unintentional and unnecessary pressure against the urethra and suprapubic bone.

8. Deposit the speculum in an appropriate container.

Bimanual Examination

Inform the woman that the next step is examining her gynecologic organs internally (**Figure 6-9**). This examination is most easily done with the examiner standing.

As with the speculum examination, the bimanual component of the examination is included for specific clinical reasons. This examination is not required annually for pelvic health screening for asymptomatic women, nor is it a necessary component of every examination for symptomatic evaluation if there is no concern or symptom for which an internal examination would provide further information. The bimanual examination, as with all components of any examination, should be used intentionally and to garner specific information and assist in overall health determination.

1. Remove the glove from one hand, and lubricate the index and middle fingers of the gloved hand. Generally the dominant hand is gloved and used for the internal examination, but this is a clinician preference. If the remaining gloved hand was used for instruments and tools during specimen collection, put on a new glove to avoid introducing foreign

FIGURE 6-9 Bimanual examination.

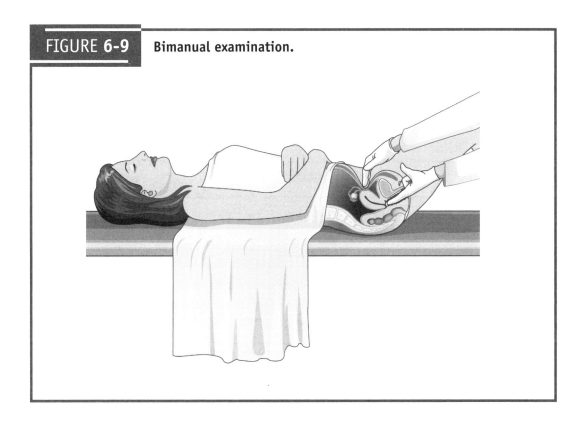

bacteria into the vaginal canal. Using the thumb and fourth finger, separate the labia to visualize the vaginal introitus. Place the index and third fingers just inside the vaginal orifice, press downward and encourage the woman to relax her perineum as much as possible, and gently insert the fingers, maintaining posterior pressure, to the posterior fornix.

2. Rotate the hand superiorly, or palm-up. As the examination continues, be careful of where the thumb of the examining hand is resting. Avoid touching the clitoris or the underlying clitoral body, which is usually very sensitive. Once the hand is rotated superiorly, consciously extend the thumb as far laterally as possible to avoid unconsciously folding it medially and inadvertently resting it on the clitoris during the examination.

3. Locate and palpate the end of the cervix with the palmar surface of the examining fingers, then run the examining fingers around the circumference of the cervix to feel the size, length, shape, and consistency. A nonpregnant cervix will be firm, like the tip of the nose, while during pregnancy it is softer. A multiparous cervix may allow easy palpation inside the external os. Note nodules, surface texture, and position.

4. Assess for cervical motion tenderness by grasping the cervix gently between the examining fingers, moving it from side to side once, and observing the woman for any expression of pain or discomfort. The cervix should move 1 to 2 cm laterally without discomfort. Painful cervical movement suggests a pelvic inflammatory process.

5. Begin palpation of the uterus by placing the ungloved hand on the abdomen, halfway between the umbilicus and the pubis at the midline. Place the intravaginal fingers in front of the cervix in the anterior fornix. Palms should be facing each other, with one internally on the

anterior vaginal wall and the other externally on the abdomen. Slowly slide the abdominal hand down toward the pubis, pressing downward and forward with the flat surface of all four fingers. At the same time, press upward with the vaginal fingers. This combination of abdominal and vaginal pressure will feel as if the two hands are pressing against each other. The uterus is relatively mobile, usually inclines forward at about 45°, and is essentially flat. It measures approximately 5 to 8 cm long, 3.5 to 5 cm wide, and 2 to 3 cm thick. If the uterus is anteflexed or anteverted (**Figure 6-10**), the fundus will be palpable between the fingers of the two hands at the level of the pubis. Movement of the uterus during palpation may cause discomfort. At this point, stating, "It is normal to feel pressure or a sensation of movement during this evaluation," normalizes this sensation and aids the woman

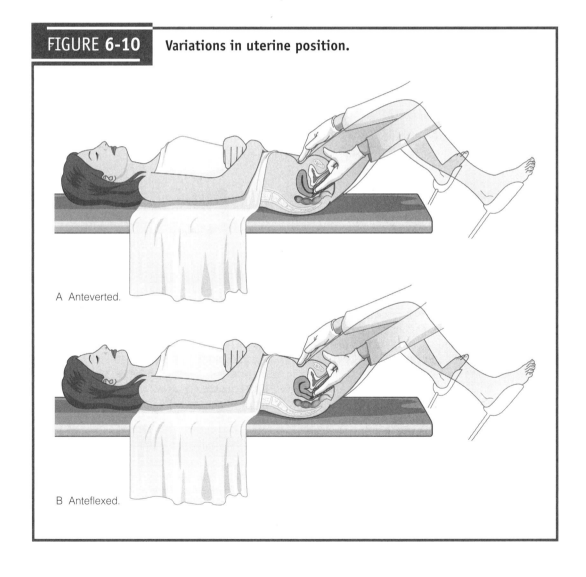

FIGURE 6-10 **Variations in uterine position.**

A Anteverted.

B Anteflexed.

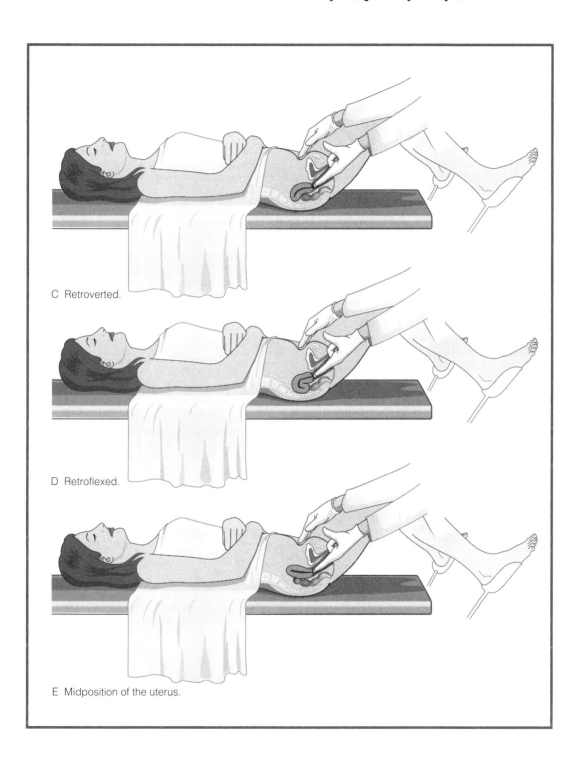

C Retroverted.

D Retroflexed.

E Midposition of the uterus.

in differentiating it from pain, which must be noted if present.

6. If the uterus cannot be palpated with the maneuver described in step 5, keeping the hand palm-up, place the vaginal fingers together in the posterior fornix with the abdominal hand at the pubis. Press firmly downward with the abdominal fingers. With the vaginal fingers turned upward, press up against the cervix moving it inward. If the uterus is retroverted (**Figure 6-10**), the fundus should be palpable with this maneuver.

7. If the uterus still is not palpated, move the vaginal fingers to the sides of the cervix, one on each side, pressing the cervix inward as far as possible. Then move one finger on top and the other beneath the cervix, continuing to press inward, while pressing down with the abdominal fingers. If the uterus is in the midposition (**Figure 6-10**), it is not possible to palpate the fundus with the abdominal hand. Confirm the location of the uterus as midline, regardless of its anterior, midposition, or posterior position. Also palpate the uterus for size, contour, and consistency. It should feel smooth, firm, round, and flat. It should be mobile in the anterior–posterior plane. This examination should not cause pain, although a sensation of pressure is common.

8. Continue the bimanual examination by palpating the ovaries and surrounding area, called the adnexae. This term refers to the areas lateral to the uterus, which are taken up by the broad ligaments, as well as to the structures located there. Move the abdominal hand to the right lower quadrant. The vaginal fingers remain facing upward. Now place both fingers in the right lateral fornix. Press deeply inward and upward toward the abdominal hand. At the same time, with the abdominal hand, sweep the flat surface of the fingers deeply inward and obliquely down toward the pubis. Palpate the entire area in this manner, repeating this sweeping movement, while at the same time the vaginal fingers press upward, inward, and slide downward (**Figure 6-11**). This maneuver is then repeated on the left side.

Often normal ovaries are difficult to palpate because they are small, sometimes positioned deep in the pelvis, or obscured by the presence of abdominal adipose tissue or tense abdominal muscles. If palpable, they are about $3 \times 2 \times 1$ cm, smooth and firm. If the ovaries are palpable, this examination usually causes momentary moderate pain when the ovaries are located. Usually no other adnexal structures are palpable. However, palpable ovaries in postmenopausal women are reason for concern and require follow-up. If the ovaries are not felt after thorough palpation with one or two sweeps, the examination is normal in the absence of any clinical signs or symptoms, and does not require repeating or further pressure or palpation.

9. Once the adnexal examination is completed, remove the intravaginal fingers, and take off and discard the examination glove. If this is the conclusion of the pelvic examination (i.e., rectovaginal examination is not being performed), help the woman to sit up. Give her a moment to adjust her position and become comfortable, and then offer her tissues to wipe excess secretions and lubricant. Leave the examining room to allow her privacy and time to dress. Tell her you will discuss your findings with her after she is clothed.

Rectovaginal Examination

This part of the pelvic examination allows palpation to a depth of an additional 2.5 cm, facilitating a more complete evaluation of some pelvic structures (**Figure 6-12**). Such an examination is perhaps most useful if the uterus is retroflexed or retroverted. It is usually an uncomfortable examination, but once mastered, can be very rapidly completed. Many clinicians omit this examination because the vaginal examination allows for sufficient palpation of gynecologic organs and because digital rectal examination to collect a stool sample for fecal occult blood testing is an unacceptable screening strategy for colorectal cancer screening (Levin et al., 2008). Especially in asymptomatic women, this examination may be eliminated as part of routine screening and health maintenance.

Rectal examinations were previously used for cervical dilation checks in labor, and many

FIGURE **6-11**   **Adnexal examination.**

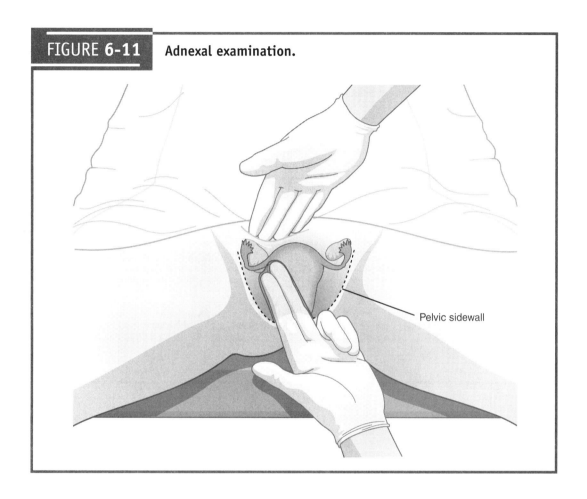

Pelvic sidewall

practitioners continue to utilize this examination for women who may experience difficult vaginal examinations, for pediatric pelvic examination, or for those women for whom an evaluation for a rectovaginal fistula is necessary. Learning to perform a gentle rectal examination is an important skill for any clinician, though it should be utilized sparingly and with full consent from the individual.

1. Before beginning, tell the woman that the rectum and vagina will be briefly examined. Inform her that this may be uncomfortable and may also cause a sensation similar to that of having a bowel movement. Assure her that she will not have one.

2. Put an examination glove on one hand, and lubricate the index and third fingertips with water-soluble gel. Place the third finger against the anus, ask the woman to bear down, and insert this finger into the rectum just past the sphincter. Palpate the anorectal junction and rotate the examining finger to sweep over the anterior and then posterior rectum that can be reached above the sphincter. Note sphincter tone, which should be moderate. The mucosal surfaces should feel smooth and uninterrupted.

3. Now also insert the index finger of the examining hand into the vagina as far as it will go. Palpate the septum between the rectum and posterior vaginal wall for thickness. Ask the woman to bear down, which will bring the

FIGURE 6-12   Rectovaginal examination.

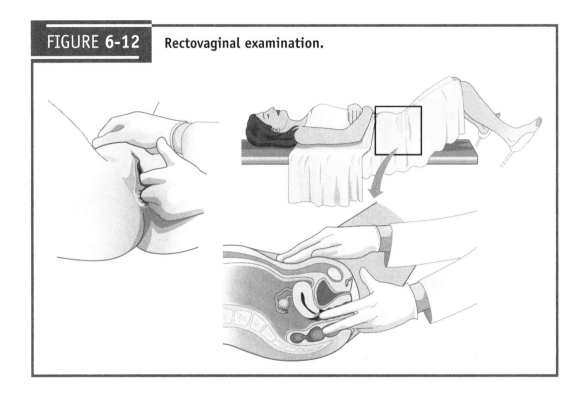

uterus about 1 cm closer to your examining finger. Place the vaginal finger in the posterior fornix. With the other hand, press firmly on the abdomen just above the pubis. The posterior surface of the uterus should be palpable, especially if it is retroverted. If the findings of the adnexal examination were questionable, repeat that examination as described previously.

4. Gently remove the examining fingers, inspect for secretions, and prepare a specimen for fecal occult blood testing if indicated. Remove and discard gloves, and help the woman to sit up. Give her a moment to adjust her position and become comfortable, and then offer her tissues to wipe excess secretions and lubricant. Leave the examining room to allow her privacy and time to dress. Tell her you will discuss your findings with her after she is clothed.

CONCLUSION: SUMMING UP AND DOCUMENTING FINDINGS

It is incredibly important to take the time to review normal and abnormal findings from the examination. Describe expected findings as "normal" or "healthy." If any abnormal findings occurred, they should be explained appropriately. The clinician should gauge how much detailed explanation, description, and thoughts on treatment, management, or follow-up should be presented based on the individual woman's desire for information and the degree of severity of the finding. If the clinician is not sure of the implications of the finding, it is reasonable to say so, but also assure the woman that consultation with another health professional will be sought promptly, and that a more complete explanation and plan will be forthcoming.

Encourage women to voice their concerns, questions, and reactions to the examination. Ask, "How are you feeling?" to welcome both physical and emotional responses to the examination. Attention to these issues demonstrates the clinician's commitment to understanding and responding to the individual woman. Discuss ways the woman may contact the provider after the examination with any recollected health history, new questions, or follow-up needs.

The final clinical responsibility for this step in management is concise and accurate documentation of findings in the woman's record. Clinicians should balance medically accurate documentation of the physical examination and recommendations with more personal information. Find space in the note or the medical record to include social aspects, including the woman's individual goals, upcoming life plans such as school or celebrations, names of family members or relationships, and other aspects to the examination that will remind you of her unique character and will continue to build on the provider relationship with each subsequent visit.

References

American Academy of Nursing. (2015). Have you ever served in the military? Retrieved from http://www.haveyoueverserved.com

Amies, A. E., Miller, L., Lee, S., & Koutsky, L. (2002). The effect of vaginal speculum lubrication on the rate of unsatisfactory cervical cytology diagnosis. *Obstetrics & Gynecology, 100,* 899–892.

Ball, J. W., Dains, J. E., Flynn, J. A., Solomon, B. S., & Stewart, R. W. (2015). *Seidel's guide to physical examination* (8th ed.). St Louis, MO: Elsevier.

Bickley, L. S. (2013). *Bates' guide to physical examination and history taking* (11th ed.). Philadelphia, PA: Lippincott Williams & Wilkins.

Bump, R. C., Mattiasson, A., Bo, K., Brubaker, L. P., DeLancey, J. O. L., Klarskov, P., ... Smith, A. R. B. (1996). The standardization of terminology of female pelvic organ prolapse and pelvic floor dysfunction. *American Journal of Obstetrics & Gynecology, 175,* 10–17.

Campbell, C. C. (2004). Care of women with female circumcision. *Journal of Midwifery & Women's Health, 49,* 364–365.

Guttmacher Institute. (2015). State level adolescents resources. Retrieved from https://www.guttmacher.org/statecenter/adolescents.html

Harer, W. B., Valenzuela, G., & Lebo, D. (2002). Lubrication of the vaginal introitus and speculum does not affect Papanicolaou smears. *Obstetrics & Gynecology, 100*(5), 887–888.

Jarvis, C. (2016). *Physical examination and health assessment* (7th ed.). St. Louis, MO: Elsevier.

Levin, B., Lieberman, D. A., McFarland, B., Smith, R. A., Brooks, D., Andrews, K. S., ... Winawer, S. J. (2008). Screening and surveillance for the early detection of colorectal cancer and adenomatous polyps, 2008: A joint guideline from the American Cancer Society, the US Multi-Society Task Force on Colorectal Cancer, and the American College of Radiology. *Gastroenterology, 134*(5), 1570–1595.

National Heart, Lung, and Blood Institute. (n.d.). Body mass index table. Retrieved from http://www.nhlbi.nih.gov/health/educational/lose_wt/BMI/bmi_tbl.pdf

Papp, J. R., Schachter, J., Gaydos, C. A., & Van Der Pol, B. (2014). Recommendations for the laboratory-based detection of *Chlamydia trachomatis* and *Neisseria gonorrhoeae*—2014. *Morbidity and Mortality Weekly Report, 63*(2), 1–19.

Pergialiotis, V., Vlachos, D. G., Rodolakis, A., Thomakos, N., Christakis, D., & Vlachos, G. D. (2015). The effect of vaginal lubrication on unsatisfactory results of cervical smears. *Journal of Lower Genital Tract Disease, 19*(1), 55–61.

Simavli, S., Kaygusuz, I., Kinay, T., & Cukur, S. (2014). The role of gel application in decreasing pain during speculum examination and its effects on Papanicolaou smear results. *Archives of Gynecology and Obstetrics, 289*(4), 809–815.

United Nations Children's Fund. (2013). *Female genital mutilation/cutting: A statistical overview and exploration of the dynamics of change.* New York, NY: Author.

VanMeter, K. C., & Hubert, R. J. (2014). *Gould's pathophysiology for the health professions.* (5th ed.). St. Louis, MO: Saunders.

World Health Organization (WHO). (2014). *Female genital mutilation.* Fact sheet No. 241. Geneva, Switzerland: Author. Retrieved from http://www.who.int/mediacentre/factsheets/fs241/en

APPENDIX 6-A

Cervical Cytology Screening

The goal of this test is to obtain adequate cells from the cervical squamocolumnar junction (SCJ) for cytology screening. The SCJ, or transformation zone, where columnar endocervical epithelium and squamous ectocervical epithelium meet, is where most cervical cancers arise.

For many years, specimens were collected using a special wooden spatula (Ayer spatula), sometimes in conjunction with a cotton-tipped swab. The conventional method of preparing the sample for cytology is the Papanicolaou (Pap) smear, which entails applying the specimen to a glass slide. Limitations of this method of specimen collection and preparation are well documented. They include not obtaining sufficient endocervical cells for adequate laboratory cytologic evaluation; unavoidably leaving much of the cellular sample on the collection device when transferring the materials to the glass slide; and obscured detection of abnormal cells due to the presence of blood, mucus, air-drying, or other artifacts on the slide. Newer specimen collection devices and liquid-based preparation methods have been developed to try to overcome these limitations and improve cervical cytology screening.

More recent specimen collection devices include endocervical brushes, a broom device that can simultaneously sample the ectocervix and endocervix, and extended-tip spatulas (**Figure 6A-1**). The use of cotton-tipped swabs is no longer recommended. Endocervical brushes plus spatulas, brooms, and extended-tip spatulas are all effective. Use the ectocervical device first when two devices are used (Massad et al., 2013).

Liquid-based methods for cervical cytology screening (ThinPrep, SurePath) allow for more complete removal of cellular material by rinsing the sampling devices in a liquid medium. Cells for cytologic examination are removed from the medium via a filtering process that minimizes the presence of obscuring artifacts. However, liquid-based methods are neither more sensitive nor more specific

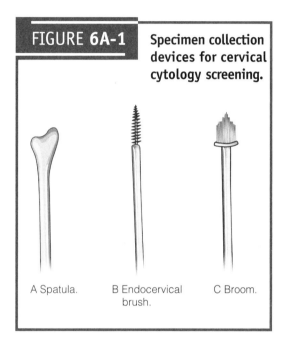

FIGURE 6A-1 Specimen collection devices for cervical cytology screening.

A Spatula.   B Endocervical brush.   C Broom.

than the conventional Pap test for detecting cervical intraepithelial neoplasia (Arbyn et al., 2008; Siebers et al., 2009). An advantage of liquid-based cytology methods is that the sample can also be used to test for human papillomavirus (HPV) deoxyribonucleic acid (DNA), chlamydia, gonorrhea, and trichomoniasis. This eliminates the need for a second visit for a woman who has a cytologic abnormality that warrants HPV DNA testing. A disadvantage of liquid-based methods is their higher cost compared to the conventional (Pap) cytology method. Additionally, liquid-based cytology is not considered diagnostic for trichomoniasis. If this test is positive for trichomoniasis, a nucleic acid amplification test (NAAT) should follow to confirm the presence of this infection (see **Appendix 6-B**). These considerations, and the failure of scientific evidence to establish clear superiority of one method over the other, have led multiple organizations to recommend that use of conventional cytology or liquid-based cervical cytology is acceptable (American College of Obstetricians and Gynecologists, 2012, reaffirmed 2015; Saslow et al., 2012; U.S. Preventive Services Task Force, 2012). Procedures for both conventional and liquid-based methods for cervical cytology screening using the different specimen collection devices are described in the next section. See Chapter 7 for cervical cancer screening recommendations.

CONVENTIONAL METHOD FOR CERVICAL CYTOLOGY SCREENING

1. Assemble the necessary materials: a labeled container for one or two standard microscope slides, slides, spatula, endocervical brush, and canister of fixative.
2. Tell the woman the Pap smear will be performed and she may feel slight pressure or discomfort, which is caused primarily from the contact of the sampling devices with the endocervix.
3. Visualize the cervix, using the speculum examination procedure described in this chapter.
4. Pick up the spatula, and insert the longer end into the cervical os. Press and rotate the spatula 360°, making sure it stays in direct contact with the inner surface of the cervical os (**Figure 6A-2**).

5. Pick up the glass slide, press the spatula flat against the surface, and smear the spatula across the slide (**Figure 6A-3**). Turn the spatula over, and spread the secretions from the second side of the spatula onto the slide. Discard the spatula. Some clinicians prefer to proceed to step 6 and place samples from the spatula and endocervical brush onto the slide after both specimens have been collected.
6. Insert the endocervical brush so that the bristles are fully in the cervical os, and rotate the brush 180° to 360°, which is one-half to one turn (**Figure 6A-4**).
7. Pick up the glass slide (or the second glass slide if using two) and, with firm pressure, roll the bristles of the endocervical brush across the slide surface (**Figure 6A-3**). If using one slide, recommendations vary as to whether to keep the spatula and endocervical brush samples separate (placing one on each half of the slide), or whether to place the endocervical

FIGURE 6A-3 Preparation of the glass slide for cervical cytology screening.

FIGURE 6A-2 Obtaining cervical cells with a spatula.

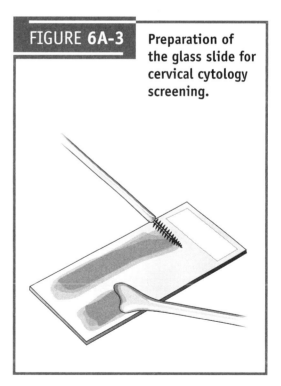

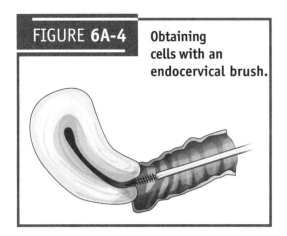

FIGURE **6A-4** Obtaining cells with an endocervical brush.

5. Place the spatula into the vial and swirl vigorously 10 times to mix the specimen and the medium (**Figure 6A-5**). Remove and discard the spatula.
6. Collect the specimen with the endocervical brush as described in step 6 for the conventional method.
7. Place the endocervical brush into the vial and swirl vigorously 10 times to mix the specimen and the medium (**Figure 6A-5**). Discard the endocervical brush.
8. Screw the lid tightly and securely onto the vial.
9. Proceed as described in step 9 for the conventional method.

Specimen Collection with the Broom Device

1. Assemble the necessary materials: labeled vial of liquid medium and broom device. Take the lid off the vial.
2. Prepare the woman as described in step 2 for the conventional method.
3. Visualize the cervix as described in step 3 for the conventional method.

brush sample over the spatula sample. Clinicians should consult their laboratory for the preferred preparation method. Discard the endocervical brush.
8. Spray fixative promptly onto the slide, holding the container about 12 inches away from the slide. Allow the sample to air-dry for a few minutes before placing the slide in the transport container.
9. Continue the speculum examination or prepare to collect additional specimens.

Note that an assistant, if present, can hold the slides for the clinician and apply the fixative.

LIQUID-BASED METHODS FOR CERVICAL CYTOLOGY SCREENING

Specimen Collection with the Spatula and Endocervical Brush

1. Assemble the necessary materials: labeled vial of liquid medium, spatula, and endocervical brush. Take the lid off the vial.
2. Prepare the woman as described in step 2 for the conventional method.
3. Visualize the cervix as described in step 3 for the conventional method.
4. Collect a specimen with the spatula as described in step 4 for the conventional method.

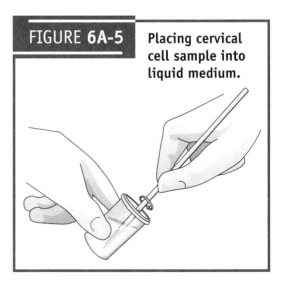

FIGURE **6A-5** Placing cervical cell sample into liquid medium.

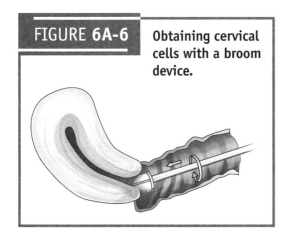

FIGURE 6A-6 **Obtaining cervical cells with a broom device.**

4. Insert the central bristles of the broom into the endocervical canal deep enough to allow the shorter bristles to fully contact the ectocervix (**Figure 6A-6**). Push gently, and rotate the broom in a clockwise direction five times.
5. Place the broom into the vial and press firmly to the bottom of the vial so that the bristles of the broom are forced apart. Swirl vigorously 10 times to mix the specimen and the medium (**Figure 6A-5**). Remove and discard the broom.
6. Screw the lid tightly and securely onto the vial.
7. Proceed as described in step 9 for the conventional method.

References

American College of Obstetricians and Gynecologists. (2012, reaffirmed 2015). Screening for cervical cancer. Practice Bulletin No. 131. *Obstetrics & Gynecology, 120*(5), 1222–1238.

Arbyn, M., Bergeron, C., Klinkhamer, P., Martin-Hirsch, P., Siebers, A. G., & Bulten, J. (2008). Liquid compared with conventional cervical cytology: A systematic review and meta-analysis. *Obstetrics & Gynecology, 111*(1), 167–177.

Massad, L. S., Einstein, M. H., Huh, W. K., Katki, H. A., Kinney, W. K., Schirrman, M., . . . Lawson, H. W. (2013). 2012 updated consensus guidelines for the management of abnormal cervical cancer screening tests and cancer precursors. *Journal of Lower Genital Tract Disease, 17*(5), S1–S27.

Saslow, D., Solomon, D., Lawson, H. W., Killackey, M., Kulasingam, S., Cain, J., . . . Myers, E.R. (2012). American Cancer Society,

American Society for Colposcopy and Cervical Pathology, and American Society for Clinical Pathology screening guidelines for the prevention and early detection of cervical cancer. *Journal of Lower Genital Tract Disease, 16*(3), 175–204.

Siebers, A. G., Klinkhamer, P. J. J. M., Grefte, J. M. M., Massuger, L. F. A. G., Vedder, J. E. M., Beijers-Broos, A., . . . Arbyn, M. (2009). Comparison of liquid-based cytology with conventional cytology for detection of cervical cancer precursors: A randomized controlled trial. *Journal of the American Medical Association, 302*(16), 1757–1764.

U.S. Preventive Services Task Force. (2012). Screening for cervical cancer: U.S. Preventive Services Task Force recommendation statement. *Annals of Internal Medicine, 156*(12), 880–891.

Screening for *Chlamydia trachomatis*, *Neisseria gonorrhoeae*, and *Trichomonas vaginalis* Infections

The nucleic acid amplification test (NAAT) is the recommended method for detecting gynecologic tract infections with *Chlamydia trachomatis*, *Neisseria gonorrhoeae*, and *Trichomonas vaginalis* (Centers for Disease Control and Prevention [CDC], 2014, 2015). *C. trachomatis*, *N. gonorrhoeae*, and

T. vaginalis cultures should be reserved for specific indications, such as supporting research activities and monitoring resistance to treatment regimens. In women, NAATs can be performed on vaginal swabs, endocervical swabs, or urine specimens. Vaginal swabs are the preferred sample type for

---

FIGURE 6B-1 | **Vaginal swab collection.**

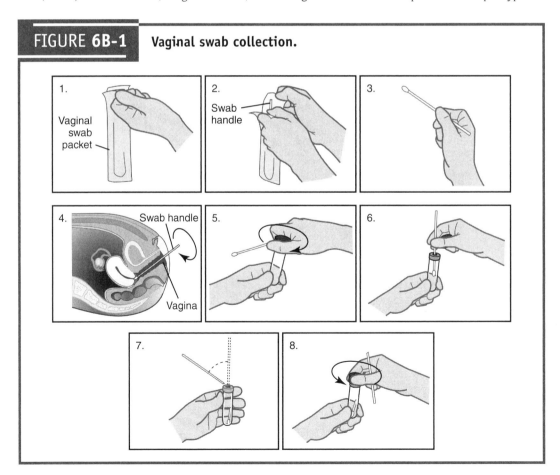

C. trachomatis and *N. gonorrhoeae* NAATs. Endocervical swabs are acceptable if a pelvic examination is indicated. A urine specimen is also acceptable but may detect fewer infections when compared with vaginal and endocervical swabs (CDC, 2014). Vaginal swabs, endocervical swabs, and urine specimens are acceptable for *T. vaginalis* testing, and detection is similar among all three sample types (CDC, 2015). Several commercial NAAT products are available, including many that test for *C. trachomatis, N. gonorrhoeae,* and *T. vaginalis* from the same sample. Clinicians should follow the manufacturer's instructions when using these products.

To collect a vaginal swab specimen, the swab is inserted into the vagina about 2 inches past the introitus and gently rotated for 10 to 30 seconds (**Figure 6B-1**). The swab should touch the walls of the vagina to absorb moisture. The swab is then withdrawn and placed into the transport medium. The sample may be self-collected by the woman or obtained by the clinician, and self-obtained vaginal swabs are as accurate as or more accurate than clinician-obtained specimens (Hobbs et al., 2008). A speculum examination is thus not required for this form of testing, and should be considered only if other vaginal or cervical evaluation is needed beyond NAAT testing for these infections.

To collect an endocervical swab specimen, visualize the cervix using the speculum examination procedure earlier described in this chapter. Remove all secretions and discharge from the cervix with a large swab. Insert the swab supplied by the manufacturer 1 to 2 cm into the cervical os, rotate it firmly at least twice against the walls of the canal, and allow it to remain in the os for the time recommended by the manufacturer. Withdraw the swab and place it into the transport medium.

References

Centers for Disease Control and Prevention (CDC). (2014). Recommendations for the laboratory-based detection of *Chlamydia trachomatis* and *Neisseria gonorrhoeae*—2014. *Morbidity and Mortality Weekly Report, 51*(RR-15), 1–27. Retrieved from http://www.cdc.gov/mmwr/Preview/mmwrhtml/rr5115a1.htm

Centers for Disease Control and Prevention (CDC). (2015). Sexually transmitted diseases treatment guidelines, 2015. *Morbidity and Mortality Weekly Report, 64*(3), 1–137.

Hobbs, M. M., van der Pol, B., Totten, P., Gaydos, C. A., Wald, A., Warren, T.,...Martin, D. H. (2008). From the NIH: Proceedings of a workshop on the importance of self-obtained vaginal specimens for detection of sexually transmitted infections. *Sexually Transmitted Diseases, 35*(1), 8–13.

Preparing a Sample of Vaginal Secretions for Microscopic Examination

Vaginal secretions and exudates can be directly examined with a microscope to aid in the diagnosis of vaginal and sexually transmitted infections (see Chapters 19 and 20). Immediately after obtaining the vaginal secretions (whether by clinician collection or a woman's self-swab as described in **Appendix 6-B**), mix one sample with normal saline solution, and a second sample with a 10% solution of potassium hydroxide (KOH). *Candida albicans*, *Trichomonas vaginalis*, clue cells (epithelial cells with indistinct borders due to adherent bacteria) associated with bacterial vaginosis, and white blood cells can be seen in normal saline solution. Microscopy has poor sensitivity for *T. vaginalis* detection; NAAT testing is recommended if trichomoniasis is suspected (see **Appendix 6-B** and Chapter 19) (CDC, 2015). Potassium hydroxide lyses trichomonads, white blood cells, and most bacteria, making visualization of *Candida* species easier. The presence of an amine or fishy odor with the addition of KOH to the vaginal secretions should be noted (whiff test), and is associated with, but not diagnostic for, bacterial vaginosis and trichomoniasis.

The CDC (2001) offers the following directions for collecting and preparing these specimens for microscopic examination:

1. Assemble the necessary materials: one or two standard glass microscope slides and cover slips, nonsterile cotton-tipped swabs, saline solution, and potassium hydroxide (KOH) solution. Some clinicians also use a small test tube.

2. Using a dropper or single-use blister pack of the solutions, place two to three large drops of saline on one slide and KOH on the second slide. Alternatives include the use of one slide (put drops of both solutions separately on it), or the test tube method (place drops of saline in a test tube and drops of KOH on a slide).

3. Obtain a specimen of vaginal discharge by either swabbing the vaginal walls and posterior fornix with a cotton-tipped swab or by sampling from the concave surfaces of the speculum blade after the speculum has been removed.

4. Mix the sample of the discharge with the drops of saline and KOH on the slides. Be sure to put the sample in the saline before the KOH, and keep the saline and KOH solutions separate. If using the test tube method, immerse the swab in the test tube, and then use the swab to apply the premixed specimen onto a dry slide.

5. Cover each specimen with a glass cover slip. Avoid trapping air bubbles under the cover slip, which makes the microscopic examination more difficult. Put one edge of the cover slip into the mixed specimen, and then lower the cover slip onto the specimen. Proceed as soon as possible to microscopic examination of the slide.

References

Centers for Disease Control and Prevention (CDC). (2001). Appendix ML-B: Commonly used stat tests—saline and 10% KOH wet mounts, vaginal pH. Program operations guidelines for STD prevention: Medical and laboratory services. Retrieved from http://www.cdc.gov/std/program/medlab.pdf

Centers for Disease Control and Prevention (CDC). (2015). Sexually transmitted diseases treatment guidelines, 2015. *Morbidity and Mortality Weekly Report, 64*(3), 1–137.

Anorectal Cytology Screening

For individuals who test positive for human papillomavirus (HPV) infection on cervical cytology and engage in receptive anal intercourse, recommendations for anogenital care include anal cytology screening (Slama, Sehnal, Dusek, Zima, & Cibula, 2015). HPV is a systemic infection that can cause cervical and anal cancerous changes (Palefsky, 2013; Santoso, Long, Crigger, Wan, & Haefner, 2010; Stier et al., 2015). Similar to cervical cytology screening, anal cytology screening is utilized to determine the existence and degree of cellular changes. Depending on geographic location and insurance coverage, the clinician should ensure full availability of services before implementing anal cytology screening into clinical practice and subsequently possibly needing anoscopy diagnostic follow-up. Additionally, as research on anal cytology screening and anoscopy is relatively new at the timing of this writing, check the most recent guidelines for recommendations.

The procedure to obtain anorectal cytology samples to screen for anal cancer proceeds as follows (Newman, 2005; University of California San Francisco Anal Dysplasia Clinic, 2014):

1. Request that the woman not insert anything in the rectum 24 hours prior to the examination. This includes douches, enemas, lubricants, toys, or engaging in receptive sex.

2. The sample is obtained without direct internal visualization, meaning no speculum is used.

3. Clinicians may utilize lateral or lithotomy position, either of which may be offered to increase comfort during collection.

4. Alert the woman that the specimen will be collected without lubricant, as it can obscure results. Moisten the tip of Dacron cotton swab with water to facilitate insertion and promote comfort. The Dacron swab is preferred over a cotton swab attached to a wooden base, as the latter may break and splinter.

5. Separate the buttocks with the nondominant hand.

6. With the dominant hand, insert the Dacron swab 5 to 6 cm into the rectal canal. Rotate the swab 360° while applying firm and consistent pressure laterally. Continue to rotate while slowly retracting and removing the swab. Continuing to rotate the swab during retraction ensures collection of cells from the transition zone.

7. Prepare the sample to send to the laboratory as described in **Appendix 6-A**: steps 7 and 8 of liquid cervical cytology collection (preferred) or steps 7 through 9 for conventional collection (acceptable).

References

Newman, E. (2005). Procedural advice for performing anal Pap smears [Letter to the editor]. *American Family Physician, 71,* 1879.

Palefsky, J. (2013). *Epidemiology of HPV and anal cancer* [PowerPoint slides]. Presented at the American Society for Colposcopy and Cervical Pathology High Resolution Anoscopy Course. Retrieved from http://www.asccp.org/Portals/9/docs/1%20Epidemiology%20of%20HPV%20and%20Anal%20Cancer.pdf

Santoso, J. T., Long, M., Crigger, M., Wan, J. Y., & Haefner, H. K. (2010). Anal intraepithelial neoplasia in women with genital intraepithelial neoplasia. *Obstetrics & Gynecology, 116,* 578–582.

Slama, J., Sehnal, B., Dusek, L., Zima, T., & Cibula, D. (2015). Impact of risk factors on prevalence of anal HPV infection in women with simultaneous cervical lesions. *Neoplasma, 62,* 308–315.

Stier, E. A., Sebring, M. C., Mendez, A. E., Fatimata, S., Trimble, D. D., & Chiao, E. Y. (2015). Prevalence of anal human papillomavirus infection and anal HPV-related disorders in women: A systematic review. *American Journal of Obstetrics & Gynecology, 213*(3), 278-309.

University of California San Francisco Anal Dysplasia Clinic. (2014). Obtaining a specimen for anal cytology. Retrieved from http://www.analcancerinfo.ucsf.edu/obtaining-specimen-anal-cytology

CHAPTER 7

Periodic Screening and Health Maintenance

Kathryn Osborne

Secondary preventive services are those services that enable early identification of risk factors or diagnosis of disease conditions in asymptomatic patients. The initial step in secondary prevention is assessment, which includes obtaining the patient's medical history, performing a physical examination, and evaluating data from laboratory tests. A comprehensive patient history is one of the most valuable screening tools available to the clinician. It affords the clinician an opportunity to receive detailed information about the patient and an opportunity to establish a therapeutic relationship with the patient. The patient's health history forms the basis for determining disease entities for which the patient is at risk and, therefore, requires further screening. A management plan is developed once risk factors are identified and should include measures that focus on reducing the short- and long-term consequences of any identified risks.

Cost containment continues to be critically important in today's healthcare environment, so it is imperative that clinicians make decisions about testing and treatment that are based on current evidence. It is the professional responsibility of every clinician to make healthcare delivery decisions that contain costs. As part of this responsibility, only tests and treatments with proven benefits should be used. Rather than conducting a battery of yearly, routine laboratory tests on every patient, the most effective approach to periodic screening is to individualize decisions about preventive health services by combining the best evidence with each patient's unique needs and circumstances (U.S. Preventive Services Task Force [USPSTF], 2014a).

In 1984, the U.S. Public Health Service gathered together a panel of experts to examine the efficacy of preventive health services including screening tests, counseling, immunizations, and chemoprevention. That panel—the USPSTF—remains active today and currently includes 16 experts from various private-sector specialty groups. It has the following mission:

- "Evaluate the benefits and harms of preventive services in healthy populations based on age, gender, and risk factors for disease
- Make recommendations about which preventive services should be incorporated routinely into primary care practice
- In making its recommendations, assess
  - The quality of evidence supporting a specific preventive service
  - The magnitude of net benefit in providing the service" (Agency for Healthcare Research and Quality, 2014)

The initial findings of the USPSTF were published in 1989 as the *Guide to Clinical Preventive Services*. These findings were updated in 1996 and included the evaluation of more than 200 clinical services. The current edition (2014a) is available online as a guide for clinicians and can be downloaded from the following website: http://www.ahrq.gov/professionals/clinicians-providers/guidelines-recommendations/guide/index.html. The USPSTF also provides the USPSTF Electronic

Preventive Services Selector (the ePSS app), which can be downloaded to most electronic mobile devices at http://epss.ahrq.gov/PDA/index.jsp. Given that the work of the USPSTF is ongoing, and recommendations are frequently updated, readers are advised to use ePSS or look for updates on the USPSTF website on a regular basis.

HEALTH MAINTENANCE: A NATIONAL PRIORITY

Passage of the Patient Protection and Affordable Care Act (ACA) marked a change in U.S. national health policy relative to maintaining health through the delivery of preventive health services. Coupled with a requirement for every U.S. citizen to carry health insurance, key objectives of the ACA are to expand Medicaid coverage to all individuals with incomes that amount to 138% of the federal poverty level (FPL) and to make lower-cost health insurance available for purchase (for those who do not qualify for Medicaid) on health insurance market places (exchanges). Also included in the ACA are provisions that affect insurance coverage of and reimbursement for health services. One such provision is that all individual and group insurance policies, whether sold on government-sponsored exchanges or privately (outside the exchanges), must include a predefined Essential Health Benefits Package. The Essential Health Benefits Package includes coverage of all preventive health services that receive an A or B rating from the USPSTF at no cost sharing (i.e., deductibles or copayments) to the individual (Kaiser Family Foundation, 2013). It is, therefore, incumbent upon all clinicians to remain aware of preventive services covered under qualified health plans, meaning those that have received a grade of A or B from the USPSTF.

The intent of the USPSTF is to provide clinicians with a framework for decision making about the provision of preventive health services that is based on an extensive review of existing evidence for each preventive service. The current recommendation scheme assigns a letter grade to each recommendation that serves as a guide for informed and shared decision making. The grade that each service is assigned reflects the net benefit (benefits minus harms) as well as the quality of evidence upon which each recommendation is made (USPSTF, 2014b). The services designated as "essential" are those that the USPSTF recommends because there is a high (grade A) or moderate (grade B) degree of certainty that the net benefit from the service is substantial (grade A) or moderate to substantial (grade B). Services designated as grade C are those that the USPSTF has found to have such a small net benefit that they are not recommended for routine use in target populations, although grade C services may be justified for some individual patients (USPSTF, 2014b).

The USPSTF recommends against the use of grade D services—those for which there is a moderate or high degree of certainty that the service has no net benefit or that harms associated with the service outweigh the benefits. Services for which the USPSTF found insufficient evidence to either recommend for or against receive an "I Statement" and no recommendation for use or nonuse. This designation indicates that the USPSTF could not assess the magnitude of benefits or harms with any degree of certainty.

The USPSTF updated its grade definitions in 2012 to reflect the periodic need to make screening decisions that are individualized based on patients' unique circumstances (**Table 7-1**). **Table 7-2** explains the level of certainty relative to the net benefits of testing.

The screening recommendations of the USPSTF described here are intended for the general population of women who do not have signs or symptoms of disease or risk factors for specific disease entities. Lopez, Mathers, Ezzati, Jamison, and Murray (2006) define a risk factor as "an attribute or exposure which is causally associated with an increased probability of a disease or injury" (p. 467). When no risk factors are found for a particular disease, a woman is considered not at risk for that disease. However, women may experience changes in various aspects of their lives over time, and occasionally such changes are accompanied by developing risk factors. When that happens, there is a concomitant change in their risk status. For example, a 30-year-old woman who is not at increased risk for breast cancer experiences a change in risk status when she turns 40. The clinician must be aware of the various risk factors that may alter the risk status of individual women so that additional screening is obtained when needed.

TABLE 7-1	U.S. Preventive Services Task Force Grade Definitions and Suggestions for Practice

Grade	Definition	Suggestions for Practice
A	The USPSTF recommends the service. There is high certainty that the net benefit is substantial.	Offer or provide this service.
B	The USPSTF recommends the service. There is high certainty that the net benefit is moderate or there is moderate certainty that the net benefit is moderate to substantial.	Offer or provide this service.
C	The USPSTF recommends selectively offering or providing this service to individual patients based on professional judgment and patient preferences. There is at least moderate certainty that the net benefit is small.	Offer or provide this service for selected patients depending on individual circumstances.
D	The USPSTF recommends against the service. There is moderate or high certainty that the service has no net benefit or that the harms outweigh the benefits.	Discourage the use of this service.
I Statement	The USPSTF concludes that the current evidence is insufficient to assess the balance of benefits and harms of the service. Evidence is lacking, of poor quality, or conflicting, and the balance of benefits and harms cannot be determined.	Read the clinical considerations section of the USPSTF Recommendation Statement. If the service is offered, patients should understand the uncertainty about the balance of benefits and harms.

Reproduced from U.S. Preventive Services Task Force (USPSTF). (2014c). U.S. Preventive Services Task Force grade definitions. Retrieved from http://www.uspreventiveservicestaskforce.org/Page/Name/grade-definitions.

This chapter focuses on the recommendations of the USPSTF that have received a grade of A or B and provides a brief summary of these evidence-based recommendations. The USPSTF recommendations and guidelines developed by other professional groups are provided so that clinicians may compare and contrast the recommendations from each group (**Table 7-3**). The USPSTF's *Guide to Clinical Preventive Services,* which is available online, provides a more detailed description of the research underlying these recommendations and highlights the implications that the recommendations have for clinical practice. The *Guide to Clinical Preventive Services* also provides detailed information for screening recommendations that have received a grade of C, D, or I—that is, screening tests that are not recommended for routine use or for which there is insufficient evidence to make a recommendation for or against their use.

TABLE 7-2	Levels of Certainty Regarding Net Benefit

Level of Certainty[a]	Description
High	The available evidence usually includes consistent results from well-designed, well-conducted studies in representative primary care populations. These studies assess the effects of the preventive service on health outcomes. This conclusion is therefore unlikely to be strongly affected by the results of future studies.
Moderate	The available evidence is sufficient to determine the effects of the preventive service on health outcomes, but confidence in the estimate is constrained by such factors as: • The number, size, or quality of individual studies. • Inconsistency of findings across individual studies. • Limited generalizability of findings to routine primary care practice. • Lack of coherence in the chain of evidence. As more information becomes available, the magnitude or direction of the observed effect could change, and this change may be large enough to alter the conclusion.
Low	The available evidence is insufficient to assess effects on health outcomes. Evidence is insufficient because of: • The limited number or size of studies. • Important flaws in study design or methods. • Inconsistency of findings across individual studies. • Gaps in the chain of evidence. • Findings not generalizable to routine primary care practice. • Lack of information on important health outcomes. More information may allow estimation of effects on health outcomes.

[a] The USPSTF defines certainty as "likelihood that the USPSTF assessment of the net benefit of a preventive service is correct." The net benefit is defined as benefit minus harm of the preventive service as implemented in a general, primary care population. The USPSTF assigns a certainty level based on the nature of the overall evidence available to assess the net benefit of a preventive service.
Reproduced from U.S. Preventive Services Task Force (USPSTF). (2014c). U.S. Preventive Services Task Force grade definitions. Retrieved from http://www.uspreventiveservicestaskforce.org/Page/Name/grade-definitions.

GRADE A AND B SCREENING RECOMMENDATIONS FOR ALL WOMEN

Alcohol Misuse

The USPSTF (2014a) assigns a "B" recommendation to screening all adults age 18 and older (including pregnant women) for alcohol misuse; screening adolescents younger than age 18 has been assigned an "I Statement." Historically, research regarding the effects of alcohol on humans and animals has been conducted on males. Only recently has the research focus changed in an attempt to discover the effects of alcohol use on females. An initial finding of these studies is that smaller quantities of alcohol can result in more severe damage to women (National Institute on Alcohol Abuse and Alcoholism [NIAAA], 2013a). Alcohol consumption is considered hazardous for a woman who has either more than seven drinks per week or more than three drinks per day. This is considerably lower than the threshold for males. The *Diagnostic and Statistical Manual, Fifth Edition* (DSM-5; the most recent edition) combines the two alcohol-related disorders that have historically been separately

TABLE 7-3	A Comparison of Screening Recommendations		
	U.S. Preventive Services Task Force	American College of Obstetricians and Gynecologists	American Cancer Society	Other Groups
Cervical cancer	Pap test every 3 years for all women aged 21–65 (grade: A). Co-testing with Pap test and HPV testing for women aged 30–65 who wish to extend the screening interval (grade: A). Recommends against screening women younger than age 21. Recommends against screening women older than age 65 if they have had adequate prior screening and are otherwise not at risk for cervical cancer. Recommends against screening women who have had a total hysterectomy for benign disease.	Cervical cytology alone, every 3 years beginning at age 21 until age 29. Co-testing with Pap test and HPV testing every 5 years for women aged 30–65 with no history of cervical cancer who are not immunocompromised, not infected with HIV, and have no history of in utero exposure to diethylstilbestrol. Screening with Pap test alone, every 3 years, for women without risk factors is also acceptable. Women with any of the aforementioned risk factors have unique screening needs. Women who are HIV positive should have cervical cytology testing every 6 months after diagnosis and then annually after two consecutive normal results.	Pap test every 3 years for all women aged 21–29. Co-testing with Pap test and HPV testing every 5 years for women aged 30–65. While this is the preferred method of screening for this age group, Pap test every 3 years is acceptable. Recommends against screening women younger than age 21. Recommends against HPV testing for women aged 21–29 unless necessary after an abnormal Pap test. Recommends against screening women older than age 65 who have had adequate prior testing and normal results.	

(continues)

TABLE 7-3	A Comparison of Screening Recommendations (*continued*)		
	U.S. Preventive Services Task Force	**American College of Obstetricians and Gynecologists**	**American Cancer Society**	**Other Groups**
Cervical cancer (*continued*)	Recommends against screening women younger than age 30 with HPV testing alone or with Pap test.	Screening should be discontinued in women with a history of hysterectomy for reasons other than carcinoma. Women with a history of CIN 2 or 3 should have routine age-based screening for 20 years following post-treatment surveillance. In the absence of a history of cervical cancer, all screening should be discontinued after age 65 in women with adequate negative prior screening results.	Recommends against screening women who have had a hysterectomy for benign disease. Women who have been diagnosed with serious cervical precancerous lesions should be tested for at least 20 years following their diagnosis regardless of age.	
Breast cancer	Mammogram every 2 years for women aged 50–74 (grade: B). Decisions regarding biennial screening for women aged 40–49 should be made on an individual basis (grade: C).	CBE every 1–3 years for women aged 20–39 and yearly for women age 40 and older. Annual mammogram for all women age 40 and older.	Mammogram and CBE every year beginning at age 40 and continuing for as long as the woman is in good health. CBE every 3 years for women aged 20–39.	

Insufficient evidence to recommend for or against screening after age 74 (I Statement). Recommends against teaching self-breast examination (grade: D).	BSE should be considered for women of all ages at high risk for breast cancer. Breast self-awareness is recommended for women of all ages regardless of risk factors.	Recommend that women know how their breasts normally feel and identify breast self-examination as an option for women starting at age 20.	
Elevated cholesterol Total cholesterol, HDL, and LDL for women age 45 and older who are at increased risk for coronary heart disease (grade: A) and for women aged 20–45 who are at increased risk for coronary artery disease (grade: B).	Lipid profile assessment every 5 years beginning at age 45. Screening is recommended for women aged 19–44 based on risk factors.		The National Cholesterol Education Program (sponsored by NIH) recommends screening all adults older than age 20 with total cholesterol, LDL, HDL, and triglycerides every 5 years.
Osteoporosis Recommends routine screening for osteoporosis with bone density measurements for all women age 65 and older and screening younger women who are at increased risk (grade: B).	Concurs with the National Osteoporosis Foundation.		The National Osteoporosis Foundation recommends screening all women age 65 and older, and younger postmenopausal women who have had a fracture or who have one or more risk factors for osteoporosis.

(continues)

TABLE 7-3 A Comparison of Screening Recommendations (*continued*)

	U.S. Preventive Services Task Force	American College of Obstetricians and Gynecologists	American Cancer Society	Other Groups
Colorectal cancer	Screen all women aged 50–75 for colorectal cancer using FOBT, sigmoidoscopy, or colonoscopy (grade: A). Screening decisions for women aged 76–85 should be made individually based on risk factors (grade: C). Recommends against screening adults older than 85 years of age (grade: D).	Recommends colorectal cancer screening beginning at age 50 years for average-risk women and at age 45 for African American women. Decisions to screen younger women are made based on risk factors. The recommended method of screening is colonoscopy every 10 years. Discuss various screening methods with patients and choose the method most likely to be completed; abnormal findings of any treatment method must be followed with diagnostic colonoscopy. Routine screening may be discontinued at age 75.	Starting at age 50: colonoscopy every 10 years *or* flexible sigmoidoscopy every 5 years *or* double-contrast barium enema every 5 years or CT colonography every 5 years. Colonoscopy should be done following positive flexible sigmoidoscopy, barium enema, and/or CT colonography.	The American Academy of Family Physicians has recommendations similar to ACS.

Ovarian cancer	Recommends against routine screening with tumor markers, ultrasound, or pelvic examination (grade: D).	No techniques have proven to be effective in the routine screening of asymptomatic low-risk women for ovarian cancer. Clinicians should remain vigilant for signs and symptoms of disease. May recommend transvaginal ultrasound or CA 125 for certain women at high risk for epithelial ovarian cancer.	No recommended screening for ovarian cancer. Women and clinicians should remain alert for signs and symptoms of ovarian cancer, which may include: • Bloating • Pelvic or abdominal pain • Trouble eating or feeling full quickly • Urinary symptoms such as urgency • Fatigue • Upset stomach • Back pain • Painful intercourse • Constipation
IPV	Screen all women of childbearing age for IPV.	Periodically screen all adolescents and women for IPV and reproductive and sexual coercion. Screen all pregnant women at the first prenatal visit and periodically during pregnancy and postpartum.	The American Academy of Family Physicians advises healthcare providers to remain alert for signs of family violence at every patient encounter.

Abbreviations: ACS, American Cancer Society; BSE, breast self-examination; CA, cancer antigen; CBE, clinical breast examination; CIN, cervical intraepithelial neoplasia; CT, computerized tomography; FOBT, fecal occult blood test; HDL, high-density cholesterol; HIV, human immunodeficiency virus; HPV, human papillomavirus; IPV, intimate partner violence; LDL, low-density cholesterol; NIH, National Institutes of Health.

Data from American Cancer Society (ACS). (2014). American Cancer Society guidelines for the early detection of cancer. Retrieved from http://www.cancer.org/healthy/findcancerearly /cancerscreeningguidelines/american-cancer-society-guidelines-for-the-early-detection-of-cancer; American Cancer Society (ACS). (2015). Ovarian cancer. Retrieved from http://www .cancer.org/cancer/ovariancancer/detailedguide/index; American College of Obstetricians and Gynecologists. (2013). *Well-woman care: Assessments and recommendations*. Washington, DC: Author; U.S. Preventive Services Task Force (USPSTF). (2014a). The guide to clinical preventive services 2014. Retrieved from http://www.uspreventiveservicestaskforce.org/Page /Name/tools-and-resources-for-better-preventive-care.

defined—alcohol abuse and alcohol dependence—into a single disorder—alcohol use disorder (AUD). AUD has three subclassifications: mild, moderate, and severe. Women who consume more than seven drinks per week or three drinks per day are considered at risk for developing AUD (NIAAA, 2013b).

A variety of effective alcohol misuse screening tools are available, and many of these can be found at the NIAAA website (http://www.niaaa.nih.gov). To screen for alcohol misuse, the USPSTF (2014a) recommends using either the AUDIT or Abbreviated AUDIT-C instrument, or asking a single question about alcohol use such as "How many times in the past year have you had four or more drinks in a day?" Each of these approaches has been found to have adequate sensitivity and specificity for detecting alcohol misuse and can be easily applied in primary care settings (USPSTF, 2014a).

Cervical Cancer

The USPSTF assigns an "A" recommendation to screening all women aged 21 to 65. for cervical cancer. The recommended screening test is the Papanicolaou test, commonly called a Pap test. The recommended screening interval for Pap test alone is every 3 years. For women aged 30 to 65 who would like to lengthen the screening interval, the USPSTF (2014a) assigns an "A" recommendation to co-testing with a combination of Pap test and human papillomavirus (HPV) testing every 5 years. It found that the harms or potential harms outweigh the benefits and therefore recommends *against* ("D" recommendation) the following practices:

- Screening women younger than age 21
- Screening women older than 65 years who have been screened adequately and who are not at increased risk for cervical cancer
- Screening women who have had a hysterectomy with removal of the cervix and have no history of high-grade precancerous lesions or cervical cancer
- Screening women younger than age 30 with HPV testing either with Pap test or alone (USPSTF, 2014a)

Chlamydia and Gonorrhea Infection

The USPSTF (2015c) assigns a "B" recommendation to screening all sexually active women age 24 years and younger, and women older than 24 who are at an increased risk for a sexually transmitted infection (STI), for chlamydia and gonorrhea. The most significant risk factor for infection is age. Adolescents and women through 24 years of age are at highest risk for developing these STIs. Additionally, women at increased risk of infection include African American and Hispanic women, women with a history of STIs, those with new or multiple sexual partners, women who exchange sex for money or drugs, and those in nonmonogamous relationships who do not use condoms consistently. In addition to individual risk factors, chlamydia and gonococcal infections are seen more frequently in particular communities. Clinicians should be aware of prevalence rates of infection in the communities in which they practice (USPSTF, 2015c). The USPSTF recommends using nucleic acid amplification tests (NAATs) to diagnose chlamydia and gonorrhea infections, both of which can be tested using the same specimen.

Depression

Screening recommendations for depression have been recently updated and now reflect a recognition of the benefits associated with screening pregnant and postpartum women. The Task Force assigns a "B" recommendation to screening all adults for depression, including women who are pregnant or postpartum (USPSTF, 2016). Screening for depression is an important aspect of women's health care because women are at an increased risk for developing clinical depression. Notably, women are 70% more likely than men to develop clinical depression (National Institute of Mental Health, 2011).

A variety of depression screening tools are available. The most commonly used screening tools are self-administered questionnaires that have been previously validated, such as versions of the Patient Health Questionnaire (PHQ), the Geriatric Depression Scale for older adults, and the Edinburgh Postnatal Depression Scale (EPDS) for postpartum and pregnant women (USPSTF, 2016). Perhaps the easiest tool to use in primary care settings is the PHQ-2 wherein a woman is asked about her ability to find pleasure in activities she usually enjoys and whether or not she has felt down, depressed, or hopeless. Women who elicit a positive screen should be further evaluated by clinicians who are skilled in the diagnosis and treatment of depressive disorders (USPSTF, 2016). The Task Force was unable to determine the optimal screening frequency but suggests that clinicians screen all adults who have not been previously screened and rescreen based on clinical judgment and the existence of risk factors for depression (USPSTF, 2016).

Height and Weight

The USPSTF assigns a "B" recommendation to screening all adults and adolescents for obesity. The body mass index (BMI) is the recommended method of identifying women at increased risk for morbidity and mortality from excessive weight. It is calculated by dividing a woman's weight in kilograms by her height in meters squared. Overweight is defined as having a BMI in the range of 25 to 29.9. Anyone with a BMI of 30 or greater is classified as obese. Patients should be counseled on the importance of maintaining a healthy diet and regular exercise (USPSTF, 2014a).

Hypertension

The Task Force assigns an "A" recommendation to screening adults 18 years and older for hypertension; the routine screening of children and adolescents has been assigned an "I statement." The recommended screening test for hypertension is a blood pressure measurement obtained in the healthcare provider's office using a sphygmomanometer (USPSTF, 2015b). Initial screening should be conducted using the mean of two blood pressure measurements, obtained with the patient in a seated position, with at least 5 minutes between measurements. The Task Force also recommends confirming a diagnosis of hypertension with ambulatory blood pressure monitoring or blood pressure measurements taken in the patient's home. Recommendations for the treatment of hypertension are consistent with the Joint National Committee on Prevention (JNC8) hypertension guidelines, which were published in 2013 and include changes in the threshold for both systolic and diastolic readings that are based on age and

the existence of comorbidities. Under the 2013 guidelines, the goal blood pressure for patients age 60 or older, who do not have chronic kidney disease or diabetes, is less than 150/90; the goal for all other adults regardless of age or comorbidities is less than 140/90 (Page, 2014).

HIV Infection

The USPSTF (2014a) assigns an "A" recommendation to screening all adolescents and adults aged 15 to 65 years for HIV; younger adolescents and older adults at increased risk for infection and all pregnant women should also be screened. It found insufficient evidence to recommend a screening interval, though the recommendation is to obtain a one-time screen for all patients aged 15 to 65 to identify existing disease, with follow-up testing based on risk factors (USPSTF, 2015c). The recommended screening test for HIV is the serum repeatedly reactive immunoassay with confirmation using Western blot or immunofluorescent assay. When rapid HIV testing is used, conventional methods must be used to confirm initial positive findings (USPSTF, 2015c).

Intimate Partner Violence

The USPSTF assigns a "B" recommendation to screening all women of childbearing age (14–46) for intimate partner violence (IPV). Several screening tools have been found to have high levels of sensitivity and specificity for identifying IVP, including the *Hurt, Insult, Threaten, Scream* (HITS); *Humiliation, Afraid, Rape, Kick* (HARK); and *Slapped, Threatened, and Throw* (STaT) instruments. Each of these tools includes three to four questions and can be self-administered.

According to the Centers for Disease Control and Prevention (2014a), in the United States more than one in four women have experienced IPV. Women presenting with symptoms or injuries should receive detailed documentation of their injuries, medical treatment, counseling referrals, and a list of community resources that provide shelter and protection. See Chapter 20 for more information on IPV and Chapter 14 for more information on sexual assault.

Rubella Immunity

Previous recommendations of the USPSTF relative to screening for rubella immunity were based on the findings and recommendations of the CDC with regard to immunizations. Those recommendations have not been updated since 1996 and are currently considered "inactive"; the USPSTF has decided not to review the evidence and update the recommendations. However, the USPSTF's 1996 recommendations are consistent with the current recommendations of the CDC, which call for obtaining serologic confirmation of rubella immunity for all women of childbearing age and vaccinating nonpregnant women who are not immune. Pregnant women who are not immune to rubella should be vaccinated immediately postpartum (CDC, 2015b).

Tobacco Use

The USPSTF assigns an "A" recommendation to screening all adults for tobacco use. The recommended approach is to implement the "five A's" behavioral counseling framework (described in the Chapter 4), which begins with questions about tobacco use (USPSTF, 2015c). In 2012, an estimated 15.8% of U.S. women smoked cigarettes (CDC, 2014b). The USPSTF recommends implementing interventions to promote smoking cessation in all patients who use tobacco. Scientific evidence demonstrates that patients who quit using tobacco are likely to realize substantial overall health benefits, regardless of the number of years of tobacco use, and that even brief interventions are effective at increasing quit rates (USPSTF, 2015c).

GRADE A AND B SCREENING RECOMMENDATIONS FOR OLDER WOMEN

The screening recommendations described thus far have applied primarily to all women, regardless of age. For several disease entities, however, age is a significant risk factor. Therefore, as women age, some additional screening recommendations apply.

Breast Cancer

Screening mammography every 2 years for women age 50 to 74 years receives a "B" recommendation from the USPSTF (2014a). There is insufficient evidence to weigh the benefits or harms of screening mammograms after the age of 74 (I Statement). Recommendations for a biennial screening mammogram prior to age 50 should be made on an individual basis, and the clinician should take into account the patient's beliefs and values about benefits and harms (grade C). Clinicians should also be aware that the U.S. Department of Health and Human Services used the 2002 recommendations to identify breast cancer screening covered (with no cost sharing) under the ACA. The 2002 recommendations (grade B) called for screening mammography, with or without clinical breast examination, every 1 to 2 years beginning at age 40 (USPSTF, 2014a).

The USPSTF recommends against teaching breast self-examination (BSE) because there is no evidence to support it (grade D). Additionally, it concluded that there is a lack of evidence that clinical breast examination (CBE) has any effect on breast cancer mortality and that not enough evidence is available to assess its benefits and harms beyond a screening mammography in women age 40 years and older (I statement). Furthermore, the USPSTF states that there is not enough evidence to determine the benefits and risks of either digital mammography or magnetic resonance imaging (MRI) versus the standard film mammography as to which provides the best screen for disease (I Statement). Some evidence suggests that CBE and BSE may actually increase the likelihood of further testing and biopsy while doing little to improve outcomes (USPSTF, 2014a). Refer to Chapter 15 for a more in-depth discussion of breast cancer.

Colorectal Cancer

The USPSTF (2014a) recommends screening all adults aged 50 to 75 for colorectal cancer (grade A). It suggests that earlier initiation of screening for women with any of the following characteristics may also be reasonable:

- History of colorectal cancer in a first-degree relative at a younger age or multiple affected first-degree relatives
- Rare genetic disorders such as familial adenomatous polyposis or hereditary nonpolyposis colorectal cancer
- Inflammatory bowel disease

Recommended screening tests include yearly high-sensitivity fecal occult blood testing (FOBT), flexible sigmoidoscopy every 5 years in combination with FOBT every 3 years, or colonoscopy every 10 years. Each of these options has advantages and disadvantages for the patient and the practice setting. Clinicians should discuss the risks and benefits of each screening test, and include patient preference in choosing a screening method. Clinicians who provide health care for women who require screening should familiarize themselves with the risks, costs, and benefits of the various screening options. The USPSTF assigns a C grade to screening women older than 76 to 85 and recommends against screening individuals older than 85. Further, it found insufficient evidence to assess the benefits and harms of screening with fecal DNA testing and computerized tomography colonography (CTC) and has assigned these methods an "I Statement" (USPSTF, 2014a).

Hepatitis C Virus Infection

The USPSTF (2014a) recommends hepatitis C infection screening (grade B) for all adults born between 1945 and 1965, and for all individuals at increased risk for infection. The risks of infection for those born between 1945 and 1965 are related to blood transfusions received prior to universal screening of donated blood (which began in 1992) or other risk factors for infection. Additional risk factors for hepatitis C infection include past or current IV or intranasal drug use, long-term hemodialysis, incarceration, being born to an infected mother, getting a tattoo at an unregulated establishment, and other exposure through percutaneous means. The recommended screening test is anti-HCV antibody testing and confirmation with polymerase chain reaction (PCR) testing. Women screened because their only risk factor was date of birth need just a one-time screen; women with additional risk factors should be screened periodically (USPSTF, 2014a).

Lipid Disorders

The USPSTF assigns an "A" recommendation to routinely screening women 45 years of age and older for lipid disorders only if they are at increased risk for coronary heart disease (CHD). Screening cholesterol levels in women aged 20 to 44 with preexisting risk factors for coronary artery disease receives a "B" recommendation. The USPSTF (2014a) makes no recommendation—either for or against—routinely screening women age 20 and older who are not at increased risk for coronary heart disease. Increased risk is defined by the USPSTF as the presence of any one of the following risk factors:

- Diabetes
- Previous personal history of CHD or noncoronary atherosclerosis
- Family history of cardiovascular disease before age 50 in male relatives or age 60 in female relatives
- Tobacco use
- Hypertension
- Obesity (BMI $\geq$ 30)

The recommended screening tool is a serum measurement of total cholesterol, low-density lipoprotein (LDL) cholesterol, and high-density lipoprotein (HDL) cholesterol with the patient either fasting or nonfasting. The optimal frequency of screening is unknown; however, the USPSTF recommends screening every 5 years for the general population, more frequently for individuals with high normal lipid levels, and less frequently for those with repeatedly low levels. All women should receive counseling about the benefits of a healthy diet (low in saturated fats and high in fruits and vegetables), regular exercise, and maintaining a healthy weight (USPSTF, 2014a).

Osteoporosis

Screening women age 65 and older for osteoporosis receives a "B" recommendation from the USPSTF (2014a). Screening younger women who have a 10-year fracture risk of 9.3% or greater also receives a "B" recommendation. Risk for fracture is best assessed using a validated screening tool such as the Fracture Risk Assessment instrument (FRAX). Factors associated with increased risk for the development of osteoporosis include low body weight (BMI < 21), cigarette smoking, family history of osteoporosis, increased alcohol intake, and white race. The best predictor of hip fracture is bone density testing using dual-energy x-ray absorptiometry (DXA) of the hip and lumbar spine (USPSTF, 2014a). Optimal frequency of screening has not been studied, but evidence suggests it may take up to 2 years to identify changes in bone density and longer to improve fracture risk prediction. Women in whom osteoporosis is identified should be counseled on the risks and benefits of various treatment options (USPSTF, 2015c). See Chapter 12 for further information about osteoporosis.

SPECIAL POPULATIONS

In addition to the previously discussed screening recommendations for healthy women across the life span, the USPSTF has made recommendations for the screening of pregnant women that are addressed elsewhere in this text. It has also made the following recommendations for women with special circumstances that are often seen in primary care settings.

BRCA-Related Cancer

The USPSTF has assigned a "B" recommendation to screening women for *BRCA*-related cancer, but *only* for women with a family history associated with an increased risk for *BRCA* gene mutations. It recommends against screening women without familial risk factors for *BRCA*-related cancer (grade D). Risk factors include a family history of any of the following:

- Breast cancer diagnosed before age 50
- Bilateral breast cancer
- Breast and ovarian cancer
- Breast cancer in one or more male family members
- Multiple cases of breast cancer in the family
- One or more family members with two types of *BRCA*-related cancer
- Ashkenazi Jewish ethnicity

Following the identification of one or more of these risk factors by a primary care provider, women should be referred to a qualified healthcare provider for genetic counseling, additional screening, and, for some women, testing for *BRCA* mutations (USPSTF, 2014a). See Chapter 27 for a more in-depth discussion of gynecologic cancers.

Hepatitis B

The USPSTF (2015c) recommends screening all adolescents and adults at increased infection risk for hepatitis B virus (HBV) infection (grade B). Screening all pregnant women at the first prenatal visit receives an "A" recommendation. Women at increased risk for infection include those born in a country with high HBV prevalence rates, those who have never received HBV vaccine, HIV-positive women, household contacts or sexual partners of persons infected with HBV, and women who use intravenous (IV) drugs. The CDC also recommends screening women on hemodialysis and women on cytotoxic or immunosuppressive therapy. The recommended screening test is the hepatitis B surface antigen (HBsAg) with confirmation of initially reactive tests. There was insufficient evidence to determine appropriate screening intervals for nonpregnant women at increased risk for infection. Decisions regarding repeat testing should be made based on clinical judgment (USPSTF, 2015c).

Lung Cancer

The USPSTF (2014a) recommends lung cancer screening for all asymptomatic women aged 55 to 80 with a 30 pack per year smoking history who have either quit smoking within the past 15 years or who currently smoke (grade B). The recommended approach is yearly screening with low-dose computed tomography (CT). Screening should be discontinued 15 years after smoking cessation.

Syphilis

The USPSTF (2015c) has assigned an "A" recommendation to screening all persons at increased risk and all pregnant women for syphilis infection. Women at increased risk for infection include commercial sex workers and those who exchange sex for drugs, women who live in correctional facilities, and women who engage in high-risk sexual behavior. Recommended screening tests include the Venereal Disease Research Laboratory (VDRL) and rapid plasmin regain (RPR) test. The USPSTF recommends against screening nonpregnant women who are not at increased risk for infection (grade D).

Type 2 Diabetes Mellitus

In 2014, more than 1.4 million adults in the United States were newly diagnosed with diabetes (CDC, 2015a). When adjusted for age and gender, the incidence of new diabetes diagnoses in 2014 was 10 per 1,000 for women between the ages of 45 and 64 and 11.1 per 1,000 for women between the ages of 65 and 79 (CDC, 2015a). The USPSTF has recently revised its recommendations for screening women for type 2 diabetes mellitus (DM) and now assigns a "B" recommendation to screening all adults between the ages of 40 and 70 who are overweight or obese (BMI > 25); earlier screening may be considered for adults with additional risk factors for type 2 DM. It also recommends that all patients with abnormal blood glucose levels be offered or referred for intensive behavioral counseling to promote physical activity and a healthy diet. (USPSTF, 2015a). Screening tests for DM include fasting plasma glucose, 2-hour postload plasma glucose, and hemoglobin A_{1C}. The optimal screening interval is unclear, although the strongest evidence suggests that rescreening adults with normal blood glucose levels every 3 years is a reasonable approach (USPSTF, 2015a).

ADDITIONAL OBSERVATIONS

The screening recommendations discussed in this chapter are intended for healthy, asymptomatic women unless otherwise specified. Healthcare providers are advised to remain alert for signs and symptoms or changes in health history that suggest the need for testing beyond the recommended screening described here. As noted earlier, the gynecologic history and physical examination provide excellent opportunities to gather important screening information about the patient. Answers to a few direct questions and close attention during the physical examination can give the clinician important information and should always be part of a routine patient encounter.

References

Agency for Healthcare Research and Quality (AHRQ). (2014). USPSTF mission. Retrieved from http://www.ahrq.gov/professionals/quality-patient-safety/quality-resources/tools/ppip/ppipslides/ppiplongsl18.html

American Cancer Society (ACS). (2014). American Cancer Society guidelines for the early detection of cancer. Retrieved from http://www.cancer.org/healthy/findcancerearly/cancerscreeningguidelines/american-cancer-society-guidelines-for-the-early-detection-of-cancer

American Cancer Society (ACS). (2015). Ovarian cancer. Retrieved from http://www.cancer.org/cancer/ovariancancer/detailedguide/index

American College of Obstetricians and Gynecologists. (2013). *Well-woman care: Assessments and recommendations.* Washington, DC: Author.

Centers for Disease Control and Prevention (CDC). (2014a). National data on intimate partner violence, sexual violence, and stalking. Retrieved from http://www.cdc.gov/violenceprevention/pdf/nisvs-fact-sheet-2014.pdf

Centers for Disease Control and Prevention (CDC). (2014b). Current cigarette smoking among adults—United States, 2005–2012. Retrieved from http://www.cdc.gov/mmwr/preview/mmwrhtml/mm6302a2.htm?s_cid=mm6302a2_w

Centers for Disease Control and Prevention (CDC). (2015a). Diabetes public health resource: Incidence and age at diagnosis. Retrieved from http://www.cdc.gov/diabetes/statistics/incidence_national.htm

Centers for Disease Control and Prevention (CDC). (2015b). Recommended adult immunization schedule – United States – 2015.

Retrieved from http://www.cdc.gov/vaccines/schedules/downloads/adult/adult-combined-schedule.pdf

Kaiser Family Foundation. (2013). Summary of the Affordable Care Act. Retrieved from http://kff.org/health-reform/fact-sheet/summary-of-the-affordable-care-act

Lopez, A., Mathers, C., Ezzati, M., Jamison, D., & Murray, C. (2006). *Global burden of disease and risk factors.* Washington, DC: Oxford University Press & World Bank.

National Institute on Alcohol Abuse and Alcoholism (NIAAA). (2013a). Women and alcohol. Retrieved from http://pubs.niaaa.nih.gov/publications/womensfact/womensFact.pdf

National Institute on Alcohol Abuse and Alcoholism (NIAAA). (2013b). Alcohol use disorder: A comparison between *DSM-IV* and *DSM-5*. Retrieved from http://pubs.niaaa.nih.gov/publications/dsmfactsheet/dsmfact.htm

National Institute of Mental Health. (2011). Depression. Retrieved from http://www.nimh.nih.gov/health/topics/depression/index.shtml

Page, M.R. (2014). The JNC8 hypertension guidelines: An in-depth guide. Retrieved from http://www.ajmc.com/publications/evidence-based-diabetes-management/2014/january-2014/The-JNC-8-Hypertension-Guidelines-An-In-Depth-Guide

U.S. Preventive Services Task Force (USPSTF). (1996). *Guide to clinical preventive services* (2nd ed.). Baltimore, MD: Williams & Wilkins.

U.S. Preventive Services Task Force (USPSTF). (2014a). The guide to clinical preventive services 2014. Retrieved from http://www.uspreventiveservicestaskforce.org/Page/Name/tools-and-resources-for-better-preventive-care

U.S. Preventive Services Task Force (USPSTF). (2014b). Update on methods: How to read the new recommendation statement. Retrieved from http://www.uspreventiveservicestaskforce.org/Page/Name/update-on-methods-how-to-read-the-new-recommendation-statement

U.S. Preventive Services Task Force (USPSTF). (2014c). U.S. Preventive Services Task Force grade definitions. Retrieved from http://www.uspreventiveservicestaskforce.org/Page/Name/grade-definitions

U.S. Preventive Services Task Force (USPSTF). (2015a). Final update summary: Abnormal blood glucose and type 2 diabetes mellitus: Screening. Retrieved from http://www.uspreventiveservicestaskforce.org/Page/Document/UpdateSummaryFinal/screening-for-abnormal-blood-glucose-and-type-2-diabetes

U.S. Preventive Services Task Force. (2015b). Final update summary: High blood pressure in adults: Screening. Retrieved from http://www.uspreventiveservicestaskforce.org/Page/Document/UpdateSummaryFinal/high-blood-pressure-in-adults-screening

U.S. Preventive Services Task Force (USPSTF). (2015c). Published recommendations. Retrieved from http://www.uspreventiveservicestaskforce.org/BrowseRec/Index

U.S. Preventive Services Task Force (USPSTF). (2016). Final recommendation statement: Depression in adults: Screening. Retrieved from http://www.uspreventiveservicestaskforce.org/Page/Document/RecommendationStatementFinal/depression-in-adults-screening

CHAPTER 8

Women's Health After Bariatric Surgery

Amy Pondo

The editors acknowledge Janet Graham, who was the author of the previous edition of this chapter.

INTRODUCTION

Obesity in the United States is a major health concern because more than one-third of adults are considered obese (Mechanick et al., 2013). The Centers for Disease Control and Prevention (CDC, 2015b) reports that 34.9% of adults and 17% of children between the ages of 2 and 19 years are obese. By 2030, approximately 65 million more adults are expected to be classified as obese (Willis & Sheiner, 2013). Women who are obese outnumber men by almost a 3:1 ratio; obesity in women requires special considerations related to their reproductive health, given that the majority of individuals undergoing bariatric surgery are women of reproductive age (Magdaleno, Pereira, Chaim, & Turato, 2012; Maggard-Gibbons, 2014; Scholtz, Le Roux, & Balen, 2010).

DESCRIPTION

Diet and exercise—the traditional approaches to treating obesity—have met with only limited success in treating morbid obesity (Amsalem, Aricha-Tamir, Levi, Shai, & Sheiner, 2014). Consequently, bariatric surgery is often considered the best choice for sustained weight loss (Lier, Biringer, Hove, Stubhaug, & Tangen, 2011; Musella et al., 2012; Scholtz et al., 2010). Between 1994 and 2004, the number of weight-loss surgeries performed in the United States increased more than 10-fold. Buchwald and Oien (2013)

have reported that the largest number of bariatric surgeries on a worldwide basis take place in the United States and Canada, although it appears that the number of U.S. individuals having weight loss surgery has now plateaued at approximately 113,000 cases annually (Livingston, 2010). Because the number of women having bariatric surgery is significant, it is highly likely that clinicians providing health care for women will have patients who have had or are contemplating having a bariatric surgical procedure.

Obesity is defined in terms of body mass index (BMI); BMI is calculated as weight in kilograms divided by height in meters squared. Weight is considered normal or healthy if the BMI falls between 18.5 and 24.9 (CDC, 2015a). Individuals with a BMI of 40 or greater are considered extremely obese and meet the criteria for weight-loss surgery if they have no coexisting medical problems and the surgical risk is not deemed to be excessive (Mechanick et al., 2013). A person would also meet the criteria for surgery if her BMI was 35 or greater and was accompanied by a high-risk comorbid disease such as hypertension or diabetes for which bariatric surgery is considered a valid treatment.

Bariatric surgical procedures are classified into three categories: malabsorptive, restrictive, and combined restrictive and malabsorptive. Each procedure can be performed by laparoscopy or laparotomy. Advancements in surgical technique allow for more than 90% of bariatric surgeries to be done laparoscopically (Schroeder, Garrison, & Johnson, 2011).

Malabsorptive surgeries bypass parts of the digestive system with some reduction of the stomach pouch to limit the amount of food eaten at one time, with the main goal of decreasing the calories and fat the body is able to absorb. Restrictive bariatric surgeries produce a small stomach pouch, so that the individual feels full after ingesting very little food. The reduced size of the stomach pouch also slows digestion, producing a longer feeling of satiation. Combined procedures provide a small stomach pouch for reduced intake and also bypass parts of the digestive system, thereby decreasing absorption of calories and fat.

The bariatric surgical procedures most commonly performed in the United States include the roux-en-Y, sleeve gastrectomy, and adjustable gastric banding. The biliopancreatic bypass, with or without a duodenal switch, has decreased in popularity, but is still performed in the United States for some extremely obese patients (Bennett, Mehta, & Rhodes, 2007; Schroeder et al., 2011).

The roux-en-Y gastric bypass (RYGB)—a combined restrictive and malabsorptive procedure—is the most frequently performed type of bariatric surgery (see **Color Plate 7**). A small gastric pouch, approximately 15 to 20 mL in volume, is created by dividing the stomach. The jejunum is then resected and a gastrojejunostomy is created with the small gastric pouch, bypassing the larger portion of the stomach and upper portion of the small intestine. Potential complications associated with the RYGB procedure include anastomotic leak, pulmonary embolism, gastro-gastric fistula, internal hernia, incisional hernia, wound infection, marginal ulcer, malnutrition, dumping syndrome, and vitamin/mineral deficiencies (Bennett et al., 2007; Schroeder et al., 2011).

The sleeve gastrectomy (sleeve) is a restrictive procedure that was traditionally performed as part of a stepwise approach to malabsorptive procedures, such as the biliopancreatic bypass with or without duodenal switch (see **Color Plate 8**). In 2009, the sleeve was accepted as a stand-alone procedure by the American Society for Metabolic and Bariatric Surgery and it has been gaining popularity ever since. This surgery entails resection of the body and fundus of the stomach, leaving the pylorus intact. The remaining stomach is long and narrow, resembling a tube, allowing only small amounts of intake and providing quick satiety (Schroeder et al., 2011). Potential complications and risks associated with sleeve gastrectomy include staple line leak, pulmonary embolism, incisional hernia, wound infection, malnutrition, and vitamin/mineral deficiencies.

The adjustable gastric banding is also considered a restrictive procedure (see **Color Plate 9**). In this procedure, a flexible, adjustable band is placed around the upper portion of the stomach. The band is attached to a port that is placed subcutaneously, allowing access to add or remove saline as needed. Adjustments to the band cause a restriction of the upper stomach, resulting in a reduction in the amount of intake required for satiety. The rapid feeling of satiety reduces calorie intake (Bennett et al., 2007; Schroeder et al., 2011). Potential complications and risks associated with adjustable gastric banding include band slippage, band erosion, esophageal dilatation, bleeding, pulmonary embolism, incisional hernia, wound infection, and vitamin/mineral deficiencies.

The biliopancreatic bypass, with or without duodenal switch (BP/DS), is a combination procedure that is being done less frequently than the aforementioned procedures (see **Color Plate 10**). The BP/DS includes a sleeve gastrectomy with preservation of the pyloric sphincter. A long RYGB is then constructed. The ileum is also divided and an enteroenterostomy is formed to create an alimentary limb and common channel. The new routing does not allow for adequate digestion, thus decreasing the nutrients, calories, and fat absorbed, and subsequently inducing weight loss (Bennett et al., 2007). Potential complications and risks associated with BP/DS include anastomotic leak, respiratory complications, stomal ulceration, wound-related complications, incisional hernia, malnutrition, and vitamin/mineral deficiencies.

Bariatric surgery necessitates a change in eating habits, the consistency and amounts of food that can be ingested, and the need for supplementation of vitamins and minerals. Clinicians who provide care to women who have undergone bariatric surgery should be knowledgeable about the types of surgery available, the possible complications from each type of surgery, and the subsequent care that each woman may require.

ASSESSMENT

History

When a woman who has had bariatric surgery presents for gynecologic or maternity care, a careful and thorough history should be obtained. Obesity has been shown to evoke negative responses from clinicians. Some clinicians may attribute negative personal characteristics to women who are or have been obese, simply because they are obese (Anderson et al., 2001; Foster & Hirst, 2014). This attitude could manifest itself in a subtle, unintentional bias against women who struggle with obesity. Clinicians need to strive to be nonjudgmental and accepting of their patients, regardless of the patient's current or past body habitus.

In addition to the routine health history information, the health history of a woman who has had bariatric surgery should include the following elements:

- Date of bariatric surgery
- Type of bariatric surgery
- Last follow-up visit with bariatric surgeon
- Maximum amount of weight lost and current weight
- Dietary habits and restrictions
- Medications, including vitamin and mineral supplementation
- Menstrual history, including any problems or irregularities before or after the bariatric surgery
- Contraception use
- Psychological history

Physical Examination

The initial physical examination should include a complete assessment. If it has been several years since the bariatric surgery or logistical problems (e.g., long distances, lack of health insurance) have prevented follow-up, presentation to the clinician may be the woman's only interaction with the healthcare system. Vital clues to the woman's overall health may be observed during the assessment of body systems that are not usually included during a gynecologic visit. For example, a neurologic assessment may reveal abnormalities commonly associated with a vitamin B_{12} deficiency; assessment of the integumentary system may reveal symptoms of anemia or deficiencies in fat-soluble vitamins; and the abdominal examination may alert the clinician to hernia formation near the surgical site or cholelithiasis, which are both frequently noted complications following bariatric surgery (Goritz & Duff, 2014). A physical examination of a woman who has had bariatric surgery may also take longer, so it is important to allow enough time for the clinician to complete the initial assessment.

If the woman is of childbearing age, it is important to assess her contraception needs. Interestingly, research has shown that 65% of bariatric surgeons refer their patients for initiation of contraception, while 35% do not know how their patients obtain contraception (Chor, Chico, Ayloo, Roston, & Kominiarek, 2015). These numbers illustrate the importance of advising women who have undergone bariatric surgery and who are of childbearing age about contraception options.

General Diagnostic Testing

Monitoring nutritional status through laboratory studies should be strongly considered, especially if the woman plans to become or is pregnant upon presentation. If the woman has not followed up with her bariatric surgeon in an extended amount of time, it is extremely prudent for the clinician to obtain a full laboratory evaluation. Important laboratory tests to consider as part of the annual gynecologic visit of a postbariatric surgery patient include a complete blood count, albumin, serum vitamin B_{12}, iron, ferritin level, phosphorus, calcium, folate, homocysteine level, thiamine, zinc, and 25-hydroxyvitamin D level (Boan, 2005; McSherry, 2012; Smith, 2005). The following labs should also be considered, especially in patients who have undergone RYGB and BP/DS procedures: copper; selenium; vitamins A, B_2, B_6, C, E, and K; and niacin (Gadgil et al., 2014; McSherry, 2012; O'Donnell, 2011). If an abnormality is noted in any of these laboratory tests, treatment needs to be initiated, along with follow-up at more frequent intervals. Laboratory testing should routinely be done yearly, at a minimum, for all postbariatric surgery patients.

PREVENTION

Vitamin deficiency is one of the most common complications after bariatric surgery and can easily be prevented. Current clinical guidelines state that postoperative patients who have undergone RYGB or sleeve gastrectomy should take the following supplements on a daily basis: 2 adult multivitamins plus minerals, 1,200 to 1,500 mg of elemental calcium citrate in divided doses (including dietary intake), and at least 3,000 international units of vitamin D. Supplemental vitamin B_{12} should be added as needed to maintain normal levels. Women who have undergone adjustable gastric banding should take the following supplementation daily: 1 adult multivitamin plus minerals, 1,200 to 1,500 mg of elemental calcium citrate in divided dose (including dietary intake), and at least 3,000 international units of vitamin D (Mechanick et al., 2013).

MANAGEMENT

Iron and calcium absorption occurs primarily in the duodenum. Therefore, women who have had most of the stomach, duodenum, and upper intestine bypassed are not able to absorb much of the iron and calcium they ingest. For this reason, iron deficiency is of particular concern among menstruating women who have undergone bariatric surgery. These deficiencies can usually be controlled with proper diet and vitamin and mineral supplementation. Adequate fluid intake—especially water intake—should be emphasized because of the constipating properties of iron and calcium supplements.

Bone density studies should be done for all women who are post bariatric surgery, and especially for women who are in menopause and those who have limited capacity for weight-bearing activity, to assess for bone loss. Malabsorptive surgeries alter bone metabolism and can lead to osteomalacia and osteoporosis (Kerner, 2014). Long-term use of proton-pump inhibitors (PPIs) postoperatively also may contribute to changes in bone health. Daily supplementation with calcium and vitamin D is crucial for these women. In addition, weight-bearing exercise for both the upper and lower extremities can help reduce the severity of bone loss. Bisphosphonates, which are frequently prescribed for osteoporosis, may not be well tolerated after bariatric surgery because of the woman's smaller (surgically altered) stomach pouch. The clinician needs to assess the risks and benefits to decide whether a woman who is post bariatric surgery, and has osteoporosis, will benefit more from the available intravenous or subcutaneous medications to treat her osteoporosis.

Women who have had bariatric surgery, and have not followed up with their surgeon in a year or more, should be strongly encouraged to do so. This referral is most important if the woman presents with severe malnutrition, vitamin deficiencies, nausea, vomiting, or abdominal pain, as such complications may require surgical intervention. Referral to a nutritionist may be an appropriate option if the woman is not reporting complications, but reports poor food choices or recurrent weight gain.

PATIENT EDUCATION

Overall, it is important to educate women on the importance of follow-up with their bariatric surgeon on a regular basis. Vitamin and mineral supplementation is also of utmost importance, as well as maintaining a well-balanced diet. Compliance with recommendations for supplementation helps to avoid deficiencies in the short- and long-term postoperative time periods. Refraining from pregnancy is also important throughout the recommended time period (refer to the fertility and pregnancy section of this chapter)—a consideration that should be reviewed with all women of childbearing age. Activity and exercise education should be discussed at every encounter the women has with a clinician as well. Lifestyle modifications are imperative for long-term weight management, even after bariatric surgery.

SPECIAL CONSIDERATIONS

Fertility and Pregnancy

Infertility related to ovarian dysfunction and anovulation is a common problem among women who are obese (Deitel, 1998; McCook, Reame, & Thatcher, 2005; Raymond, 2005; Whited, Bersoux, Jadoon-Khamash, & Mayer, 2015). A diagnosis often related to both menstrual abnormalities and increased risk of infertility is polycystic ovary syndrome (PCOS); as many as 6% to 10% of women of reproductive age may have PCOS (Jamal et al., 2012). In addition, one-third to one-half of women who are obese have irregular menstrual cycles, and this condition worsens in direct proportion to increased weight (Nelson & Fleming, 2007). Weight loss is considered first-line therapy for treatment of infertility in women who are obese. In many cases, infertility and a desire for pregnancy may be the impetus for bariatric surgery.

A waiting period of 12 to 24 months between bariatric surgery and pregnancy is recommended (Dao, Kuhn, Ehmer, Fisher, & McCarty, 2006; Goritz & Duff, 2014; Mechanick et al., 2013; Shuster & Vasquez, 2005). Following weight-loss surgery, a woman may experience a rapid weight loss that puts her in a relative catabolic state during the first 12 to 18 months after surgery—a condition that increases the potential for nutritional deficits in both mother and fetus if she becomes pregnant. Indeed, the early postbariatric surgery adjustment phase is often characterized by rapid weight loss, frequent vomiting, and inability to ingest appropriate calories or nutrients, all of which may threaten the sustainability of a pregnancy.

A woman who experienced infertility prior to surgery may resume ovulation with a relatively small weight loss, which can lead to an unplanned pregnancy soon after bariatric surgery. As little as a 5% to 10% weight reduction can lead to improvements in PCOS, thereby improving fertility (Chor et al., 2015; Jamal et al., 2012). Weight loss prior to pregnancy also reduces the risk of complications of pregnancy (Scholtz et al., 2010). Pregnancy rates for adolescents who have had bariatric surgery are double the rate in the general adolescent population, suggesting that this population is particularly in need of contraceptive counseling (Roehrig, Xanthakos, Sweeney, Zeller, & Inge, 2007).

Attention should be paid to iron, folic acid, fat-soluble vitamins, and vitamin B_{12} levels in postbariatric surgery women, but it is strongly recommended to evaluate for a wide array of nutrient deficiencies. At a minimum, daily supplementation with iron, folate, calcium, and multivitamins is strongly encouraged during pregnancy (Magdaleno et al., 2012). Ideally, all women who have undergone bariatric surgery and are potentially fertile should be placed on folic acid supplements, regardless of whether they choose to use contraception.

The clinician should offer appropriate contraceptive options, especially if gynecologic care is provided within the first 18 months after bariatric surgery and there is a potential for pregnancy. Some controversy persists regarding the efficacy of combined oral contraceptives (COCs) in women who have undergone a RYGB. If the bariatric surgery has a malabsorptive component, nonoral administration of contraceptive hormones should be considered (Merhi, 2007), as the limited size of the stomach and lack of enzymes or stomach digestive acids may limit the absorption of COCs. Backup of COCs with barrier methods should be discussed with women who are fertile or who may become fertile soon after weight loss begins. If a woman who is post bariatric surgery has a comorbid condition such as hypertension, COC use may also exacerbate blood pressure elevations. Estrogen-containing contraceptive pills are known to increase the incidence of gallstones—also a frequent complication after bariatric surgery (Goritz & Duff, 2014).

Intrauterine contraception (IUC) can provide long-term contraceptive benefits without triggering digestive problems. Other contraceptive options that bypass the digestive system include progestin-based methods such as the depot medroxyprogesterone injection (DMPA, Depo-Provera) and the subdermal progestin implant (Implanon). However, DMPA may promote weight gain, making it an unpopular choice among women who are trying to lose weight. Implanon has not been studied in women who are significantly overweight, so its efficacy is unknown in the obese population. The combined estrogen and progestin vaginal ring may also provide contraception while bypassing the digestive system. Although the cervical cap and the diaphragm do not affect the digestive system, rapid weight loss could alter the efficacy of these methods if the woman's cervix or vaginal walls change size. This alteration in physiology would necessitate frequent fittings to adapt to the weight changes.

Consideration of the woman's cultural and religious background, as well as current or potential health problems, is necessary when discussing contraception. Chapter 11 provides additional information about contraceptive options.

Pregnancy presents some distinct challenges for women who have undergone bariatric surgery. For example, malabsorption related to the bypassing of segments of the bowel where nutrients are absorbed may put both mother and fetus at risk for nutrient deficiencies (Gadgil et al., 2014; Goritz & Duff, 2014; Maggard-Gibbons, 2014). In addition, the increased nausea and vomiting experienced by many pregnant women may disrupt an adjustable gastric band's placement or put the pregnant woman at an even higher risk for protein malnutrition (Patel, Colella, Esaka, Patel, & Thomas, 2007). Best practice clinical guidelines for directing the care of women who become pregnant after bariatric surgery remain unclear. Therefore, clinicians need to gather the best evidence and use it as a guide when providing prenatal care for women who have undergone bariatric surgery.

Although bariatric surgery can increase some risks during pregnancy, the benefits of the sustained weight loss are significant and may even make it feasible for the woman to become pregnant. Surgical weight loss has been shown to improve fertility (Maggard-Gibbons, 2014) as well as decrease the incidence of hypertensive disorders, gestational diabetes, and large for gestational age infants. Although some research has identified a link between bariatric surgery and an increased risk of small for gestational age infants and decreased gestation length, no corresponding increase in preterm births has been identified (Johansson et al., 2015).

Tables 8-1, **8-2**, and **8-3** provide guidelines that are evidence-based interpretations of currently available literature for nutritional counseling, laboratory testing, and weight management for women who become pregnant after having bariatric surgery (Graham, 2007). Using Stetler et al.'s (1998) criteria and taking into consideration the level of evidence found in the studies reviewed, only reasonable recommendations (in light of low risk) or pragmatic recommendations (in light of high need and/or based on national experts' opinions) can be made. The recommendations used to support the use of a practice deemed reasonable are based on

TABLE 8-1	Daily Recommendations for Nutritional Management

Nutrition Need	R/P	Recommendation
Protein	R	65–70 gm or 1.5 gm per kg weight
Vitamin B_{12}	R	500–1,000 mcg crystalline per day
Folic acid	R	400 mcg per day
Vitamin A	R	No more than 10,000 international units per day
Vitamin D	R	1,000 international units per day
Prenatal vitamins	R	One daily; check vitamins A and D content
Calcium citrate	R	1,200–2,000 mg calcium citrate per day
Carbohydrates	P	No more than 130 gm per day Avoid high sugar and simple carbohydrates
Iron	R	40–65 mg ferrous fumerate daily
Vitamin C	P	Usual RDA; take with iron to increase iron's absorption
Fluids	R	Minimum of 64 oz per day; no fluids 15 min before or 90 min after meals
Thiamine	R	50 mg per day
Fats	P	Polyunsaturated, omega-3

Abbreviations: P, pragmatic; R, reasonable; RDA, recommended daily allowance.

TABLE 8-2 Recommended Laboratory Studies to Evaluate Nutritional Status

Timing	R/P	Laboratory Testing
Initial prenatal visit	P	Complete blood count, albumin, serum B_{12}, serum iron, ferritin level, phosphorus, calcium, folic acid, homocysteine level, 25-hydroxy-vitamin D level, vitamin A, zinc, parathyroid hormone
Monthly	P	Iron level and check all other laboratory indices that were previously found to be deficient until they are at an adequate level

Abbreviations: P, pragmatic; R, reasonable.

TABLE 8-3 Recommendations for Weight Management and Monitoring

Weight Management	R/P	Monitoring
Timing of pregnancy after surgery	P	No less than 12 months or until stable
BMI	P	Measure at beginning of pregnancy
Weight gain	R	Individualize based on BMI: BMI 25–29.9: 15–25 pounds BMI > 30: 11–20 pounds
Weight monitoring	R	Every prenatal visit
Weight loss	P	Not recommended

Abbreviations: BMI, body mass index; P, pragmatic; R, reasonable.

limited but suggestive research-based evidence combined with low risk for the persons using that recommendation. All of the recommendations are based on national expert opinion, local expert opinion, and/or high need for recommendations in a given area (Goritz & Duff, 2014; Stetler et al., 1998; UCSF Medical Center, 2015).

Close nutritional monitoring of the woman who has had bariatric surgery should continue into the postpartum period.

Mental Health

A relationship between obesity and psychological disorders is thought to exist, but it is uncertain whether psychopathology is a cause or a consequence of extreme obesity (Sarwer, Wadden, & Fabricatore, 2005). Depression and anxiety, in particular, are disorders identified in patients suffering from morbid obesity (Andersen et al.,

2010). Some research suggests that patients who have undergone bariatric surgery have high rates of psychiatric disorders in comparison to obese patients not seeking bariatric surgery or patients undergoing other types of surgeries (Greenberg, Sogg, & Perna, 2009). Mental health disorders are not considered a contraindication for bariatric surgery, but should be carefully reviewed when considering risks versus benefits of the surgery and overall outcomes (Greenberg et al., 2009).

Researchers have also documented that a large number of patients who present for bariatric surgery have a preexisting eating disorder such as binge eating (Boan, 2005). Some epidemiologic studies have shown that mood disorders antedate weight problems. Often mood disorders tend to be recurrent, such that the individual who overeats or binge eats may be overeating in response to depression, which in turn results in weight gain (Kalarchian et al., 2007).

A controversial theory—and one that remains unproven—suggests that bariatric surgery may enable a patient to lose weight, only to then have the patient transfer food addiction to some other harmful addiction. Kalarchian et al. (2007) have also speculated that substance abuse and weight problems may have a shared diathesis. These researchers propose that eating behaviors increase when substance abuse is minimal and, conversely, that the risk of substance abuse behaviors may increase when eating behaviors are decreased. The symptom substitution theory may also explain the transferred additions. This theory states that without treating the underlying cause of the addiction, the termination of a particular symptom will be replaced by a substitute symptom (Conason et al., 2013). The incidence of alcohol use disorders has been shown to increase in postbariatric surgery patients, likely for this reason. Notably, those individuals with a preexisting alcohol use disorder are likely to present with symptoms postoperatively. The highest incidence of alcohol use disorders is reported in postoperative year 2, with the largest number of cases following RYGB procedures. It is unclear if bariatric surgery itself is a risk factor for alcohol use disorders (King et al., 2012).

An increased risk of suicide among patients following bariatric surgery has been identified as well (Anderson, 2007). Increased risk for suicide has been associated with coexisting alcohol use disorders and diabetes (Mitchell et al., 2013). Retrospective studies have shown as much as a 58% increase in the rate of suicide among patients who have undergone bariatric surgery compared to individuals who are obese and did not have weight-loss surgery (Adams et al., 2007). Postoperative years 2 and 3 have been identified as the times of highest risk for suicide—accounting for 30% and 70% of these events, respectively (Mitchell et al., 2013). Given this risk, it is vitally important that the psychological assessment include questions related to suicidal ideation in any patient evidencing symptoms of depression or alcohol use disorders.

The clinician has a role in assessing the mental health status and needs of all women who present for gynecologic care. The familiarity between women and their clinicians can provide a trusting atmosphere in which to undertake mental health assessments. In fact, the clinician may be the first health professional a woman reaches out to when she has mental health problems.

Mental health assessments may take various forms: having the woman answer a questionnaire focused on mental health status, asking direct questions during the history and physical examination, and observing the woman's affect, mood, and appearance during the visit. If a woman who is post bariatric surgery has a past history of depression or other mental health diagnosis, careful attention should be paid to her mental health needs, especially after the first postsurgical year has passed. Studies suggest that women who are post bariatric surgery may experience recurrent weight gain as a result of the psychosocial improvements that occurred in the first 6 to 18 postoperative months (Sarwer et al., 2005). In contrast, weight gain or lack of adherence to prescribed postbariatric health regimens may indicate depression or other mood disorders (Aguilera, 2014). If the gynecologic patient is suspected to have psychosocial disorders, the clinician should refer her to a mental health specialist.

Improvement in body image is a positive mental health benefit after bariatric surgery. Less pain and fatigue associated with weight loss may also improve quality of life. In addition, many women report increased marital satisfaction and improved sexual functioning after successful weight-loss surgery (Sarwer et al., 2005).

CONCLUSION

Bariatric surgery is an increasingly popular, viable, and sustainable weight-loss method for women with severe obesity. Clinicians who serve women in a general or gynecology practice need to be aware of the types of weight-loss surgeries available, the nutrient deficiencies that commonly occur after such surgery, and the side effects that women may experience post bariatric surgery. Clinicians must also pay careful attention to the psychosocial needs of women who have undergone weight-loss surgery.

References

Adams, T. D., Gress, R. E., Smith, S. C., Halverson, R. C., Simper, S. C., Rosamond, W. D., . . . Hunt, S. C. (2007). Long-term mortality after gastric bypass surgery. *New England Journal of Medicine, 357*, 753–761.

Aguilera, M. (2014). Post-surgery support and the long-term success of bariatric surgery. *Practice Nursing, 20*(4), 455–459.

Amsalem, D., Aricha-Tamir, B., Levi, I., Shai, D., & Sheiner, E. (2014). Obstetric outcomes after restrictive bariatric surgery: What happens after 2 consecutive pregnancies? *Surgery for Obesity and Related Diseases, 10*, 445–449.

Andersen, J. R., Aasprang, A., Bergsholm, P., Sletteskog, N., Våge, V., & Natvig, G. K. (2010). Anxiety and depression in association with morbid obesity: Changes with improved physical health after duodenal switch. *Health and Quality of Life Outcomes, 8*, 52–58.

Anderson, C., Peterson, C. B., Fletcher, L., Mitchell, J. E., Thuras, P., & Crow, S. J. (2001). Weight loss and gender: An examination of physician attitudes. *Obesity Research, 9*(4), 257–263.

Anderson, P. (2007). Higher-than-expected suicide rate following bariatric surgery. Retrieved from http://www.medscape.org/viewarticle/564994

Bennett, J. M. H., Mehta, S., & Rhodes, M. (2007). Surgery for morbid obesity. *Postgraduate Medical Journal, 83*, 8–15.

Boan, J. (2005, April). Post-op management for bariatric surgery. *Clinical Advisor*, 30–35.

Buchwald, H., & Oien, D. M. (2013). Metabolic/bariatric surgery worldwide 2011. *Obesity Surgery, 23*, 427–436.

Centers for Disease Control and Prevention (CDC). (2015a). Defining adult overweight and obesity. Retrieved from http://www.cdc.gov/obesity/adult/defining.html

Centers for Disease Control and Prevention (CDC). (2015b). Overweight and obesity: Data and statistics. Retrieved from http://www.cdc.gov/obesity/data/index.html

Chor, J., Chico, P., Ayloo, S., Roston, A., & Kominiarek, M. A. (2015). Reproductive health counseling and practices: A cross-sectional survey of bariatric surgeons. *Surgery for Obesity and Related Diseases, 11*, 187–192.

Conason, A., Teixeira, J., Hsu, C. H., Puma, L., Knafo, D., & Geliebter, A. (2013). Substance use following bariatric weight loss surgery. *Journal of the American Medical Association, 148*(2), 145–150.

Dao, T., Kuhn, J., Ehmer, D., Fisher, T., & McCarty, T. (2006). Pregnancy outcomes after bariatric surgery. *American Journal of Surgery, 192*(6), 762–766.

Deitel, M. (1998). Pregnancy after bariatric surgery. *Obesity Surgery, 8*, 1–4.

Foster, C. E., & Hirst, J. (2014). Midwives' attitudes towards giving weight-related advice to obese pregnant women. *British Journal of Midwifery, 22*(4), 254–262.

Gadgil, M. D., Chang, H. Y., Richards, T. M., Gudzune, K. A., Huizinga, M. M., Clark, J. M., & Bennett, W. L. (2014). Laboratory testing for and diagnosis of nutritional deficiencies in pregnancy before and after bariatric surgery. *Journal of Women's Health, 23*(2), 129–137.

Goritz, T., & Duff, E. (2014). Bariatric surgery: Comprehensive strategies for management in primary care. *Journal for Nurse Practitioners, 10*(9), 687–693.

Graham, J. E. (2007). *Guidelines for prenatal care for post-bariatric women: An integrative review* [Unpublished doctoral dissertation]. Oakland University, Rochester, MI.

Greenberg, I., Sogg, S., & Perna, F. M. (2009). Behavioral and psychological care in weight loss surgery: Best practice update. *Obesity, 17*(5), 880–884.

Jamal, M., Gunay, Y., Capper, A., Eid, A., Heitshusen, D., & Samuel, I. (2012). Roux-en-Y gastric bypass ameliorates polycystic ovary syndrome and dramatically improves conception rates: A 9-year analysis. *Surgery for Obesity and Related Diseases, 8*, 440–444.

Johansson, K., Cnattingius, S., Näslund, I., Roos, N., Lagerros, Y. T., Granath, F., . . . Neovius, M. (2015). Outcomes of pregnancy after bariatric surgery. *New England Journal of Medicine, 372*(9), 814–825.

Kalarchian, M. A., Marcus, M. D., Levine, M. D., Courcoulas, A. P., Pilkonis, P. A., Ringham, R. M., & Rofey, D. L. (2007). Psychiatric disorders among bariatric surgery candidates: Relationship to obesity and functional health status. *American Journal of Psychiatry, 164*, 328–334.

Kerner, J. (2014). Nutrition support after bariatric surgery. *Support Line, 35*(3), 9–21.

King, W. C., Chen, J. Y., Mitchell, J. E., Kalarchian, M. A., Steffen, K. J., Engel, S. G., . . . Yanovski, S. Z. (2012). Prevalence of alcohol use disorders before and after bariatric surgery. *Journal of the American Medical Association, 307*(23), 2516–2525.

Lier, H. Ø., Biringer, E., Hove, O., Stubhaug, B., & Tangen, T. (2011). Quality of life among patients undergoing bariatric surgery: Associations with mental health: A 1 year follow-up study of bariatric surgery patients. *Health and Quality of Life Outcomes, 9*, 79–88.

Livingston, E. H. (2010). The incidence of bariatric surgery has plateaued in the U.S. *American Journal of Surgery, 200*, 378–385.

Magdaleno, R., Jr., Pereira, B. G., Chaim, E. A., & Turato, E. R. (2012). Pregnancy after bariatric surgery: A current view of maternal obstetrical and perinatal challenges. *Archives of Gynecology and Obstetrics, 285*, 559–566.

Maggard-Gibbons, M. (2014). Optimizing micronutrients in pregnancies following bariatric surgery. *Journal of Women's Health, 23*(2), 107.

McCook, J. G., Reame, N. E., & Thatcher, S. S. (2005). Health related quality of life issues in women with polycystic ovarian syndrome. *Journal of Obstetric, Gynecologic, and Neonatal Nursing, 34*(1), 12–20.

McSherry, R. L. (2012). Bariatric surgery: Nutritional considerations for patients. *Nursing Standard, 26*(49), 41–48.

Mechanick, J. I., Youdim, A., Jones, D. B., Garvey, W. T., Hurley, D. L., McMahon, M. M., . . . Brethauer, S. (2013). Clinical practice guidelines for preoperative nutritional, metabolic, and nonsurgical support of the bariatric surgery patient—2013 update: Cosponsored by American Association of Clinic Endocrinologists, the Obesity Society, and American Society for Metabolic & Bariatric Surgery. *Obesity, 21*, S1–S27.

Merhi, Z. O. (2007). Challenging oral contraception after weight loss by bariatric surgery. *Gynecology Obstetric Investigation, 64*, 100–102.

Mitchell, J. E., Crosby, R., de Zwaan, M., Engel, S., Roerig, J., Steffen, K., . . . Wonderlich, S. (2013). Possible risk factors for increased suicide following bariatric surgery. *Obesity, 21*(4), 665–672.

Musella, M., Milone, M., Bellini, M., Sosa Fernandez, L. M., Leongito, M., & Milone, F. (2012). Effect of bariatric surgery on obesity-related infertility. *Surgery for Obesity and Related Diseases, 8*, 445–449.

Nelson, S. M., & Fleming, R. F. (2007). The preconceptual contraception paradigm: Obesity and infertility. *Human Reproduction, 22*(4), 912–915.

O'Donnell, K. (2011). Severe micronutrient deficiencies in RYGB patients: Rare but potentially devastating. *Practical Gastoenterology, XXXV*(11), 13–27.

Patel, J. A., Colella, J. J., Esaka, E., Patel, N. A., & Thomas, R. L. (2007). Improvement in infertility and pregnancy outcomes after weight loss surgery. *Medical Clinics of North America, 91*(3), 515–528.

Raymond, R. H. (2005). Hormonal status, fertility, and pregnancy before and after bariatric surgery. *Critical Care Nursing Quarterly, 28*(3), 263–268.

Roehrig, H. R., Xanthakos, S. S., Sweeney, J., Zeller, M. H., & Inge, T. H. (2007). Pregnancy after gastric bypass surgery in adolescents. *Obesity Surgery, 17*, 873–877.

Sarwer, D. B., Wadden, T. A., & Fabricatore, A. N. (2005). Psychosocial and behavioral aspects of bariatric surgery. *Obesity Research, 13*(2014), 639–648.

Scholtz, S., Le Roux, C., & Balen, A. H. (2010). The role of bariatric surgery in the management of female fertility. *Human Fertility, 13*(2), 67–71.

Schroeder, R., Garrison, J. M., & Johnson, M. S. (2011). Treatment of adult obesity with bariatric surgery. *American Family Physician, 84*(7), 805–814.

Shuster, M., & Vasquez, N. A. (2005). Nutritional concerns related to roux-en-Y gastric bypass. *Critical Care Nursing Quarterly, 28*(3), 227–260.

Smith, B. L. (2005). Bariatric surgery: It's no easy fix. *RN, 6*(6), 58–63.

Stetler, C. B., Morsi, D., Rucki, S., Broughton, S., Corrigan, B., Fitzgerald, J.,...Sheridan, E. A. (1998). Utilization-focused integrative reviews in a nursing service. *Applied Nursing Research, 11*(4), 195–206.

UCSF Medical Center. (2015). Dietary guidelines after bariatric surgery. Retrieved from http://www.ucsfhealth.org/education/dietary_guidelines_after_gastric_bypass

Whited, M. H., Bersoux, S., Jadoon-Khamash, E., & Mayer, A. P. (2015). Great expectations: Pregnancy after bariatric surgery. *Journal of Women's Health, 24*(3), 250–251.

Willis, K., & Sheiner, E. (2013). Bariatric surgery and pregnancy: The magical solution? *Journal of Perinatal Medicine, 41*, 133–140.

CHAPTER 9

Lesbian, Bisexual, Queer, and Transgender Health

Simon Adriane Ellis

The editors acknowledge Linda A. Bernhard, who was the author of the previous edition of this chapter.

INTRODUCTION

Health, and specifically gynecologic health, is experienced in the context of each person's life. It is experienced biologically, psychosocially, sexually, and spiritually by all people, including people of all sexual orientations and gender identities. However, not all people enjoy the same access to compassionate, informed gynecologic health care. This chapter considers the special gynecologic health care needs of lesbian, bisexual, and queer (LBQ) women, as well as transgender and gender-nonconforming (TGNC) people. Using a feminist approach to unpack health disparities, this chapter will "examine the connections between disadvantage and health, and the distribution of power in the process of . . . health" (Rogers, 2006, p. 351) to gain an understanding of the realities and needs of LBQ and TGNC people.

The U.S. population includes approximately 5.1 million LBQ women, of whom an estimated 350,000 are transgender women (Center for American Progress & Movement Advancement Project, 2015). These communities are diverse, with people of color being more likely to identify as LBQ or TGNC than their white peers (Center for American Progress & Movement Advancement Project, 2015; Ranji, Beamesderfer, Kates, & Salganicoff, 2014). Additionally, more than 900,000 LBQ and TGNC women in the United States are immigrants, approximately 30% of whom are undocumented and living without basic social and legal protections (Center for American Progress & Movement

Advancement Project, 2015). Thus the LBQ and TGNC communities represent a large and dynamic segment of the U.S. population with a wide range of gynecologic and other health needs.

Despite great improvements since the late 1980s, the research base on LBQ and TGNC health remains limited, and a number of barriers hinder the collection of accurate and nuanced data on this population (Institute of Medicine, 2011). Nevertheless, understanding of the healthcare needs and life experiences of LBQ and TGNC people has been greatly improved since 2010, with the publication of several landmark surveys and reports by Lambda Legal (2010), the Institute of Medicine (2011), and the Washington National Center for Transgender Equality and National Gay and Lesbian Task Force (Grant et al., 2011). In addition, professional organizations in gynecologic health have affirmed the importance of access to quality health care for women of all sexual orientations (American College of Nurse-Midwives, 2014; American College of Obstetricians and Gynecologists, 2012) and transgender people (American College of Nurse-Midwives, 2012; American College of Obstetricians and Gynecologists, 2011).

GENDER AND SEXUALITY CONCEPTS

There are no official definitions for *lesbian, bisexual, queer, transgender*, or *gender nonconforming*. Indeed, definitions and labels are constantly evolving and highly complex. Some argue that definitions are inherently problematic when it comes to sexual

161

orientation and gender identity. FORGE, an organization that serves TGNC people and their loved ones, articulates this as the *terms paradox*: Terms are meaningless in that there is no consensus on their definitions, yet they are crucial in that clinicians must ascertain the terms each person uses to define themselves and reflect them back when providing care (FORGE, 2012). The simplest way to think of this is that people are who they say they are, and clinicians should be respectful of this self-identification in the language they use when communicating with and about the people they serve.

For purposes of clarity, this section outlines some very basic terms and concepts used in this chapter. **Box 9-1** summarizes these terms and concepts.

Definitions

First, it is important to emphasize that sexual orientation and gender identity are two separate concepts. Similarly, sex and gender are two separate concepts. *Sex* is a designation based on one's chromosomes and genitalia. While sex is often thought as a binary consisting only of male or female, in reality there are a great number of *intersex* people whose chromosomes and genitals fall somewhere in between these two designations. In this chapter, people assigned female sex at birth are described as *natal females*, and people assigned male sex at birth are described as *natal males*. *Gender* is a social construct that assigns roles and attributes to people based on their natal sex.

Both sexual orientation and gender identity are understood as having a number of components. Sexual orientation is composed of attraction, identity, and behavior (Fenway Institute, 2009). Sexual *attraction* refers to whom, if anyone, a person desires sexually or fantasizes about, and may be described as sexual preference or desire. Sexual *identity* refers to individuals' inner understanding of themselves in regard to sexual orientation and the words they use to describe themselves as sexual beings. Sexual *behavior* refers to individuals' sexual partners, as well as the sexual activities in which they engage. All people have all three components. In some people the three components will be more or less the same, while in other people they will differ.

Lesbian has historically been used to refer to the sexual orientation of natal females who are attracted to natal female sexual partners; a better definition might be people with a female gender identity who are attracted to other people with a female gender identity. *Bisexual* people are attracted to those with both male and female gender identities. *Queer* is a reclaimed word that is used as an umbrella term to describe all people with non-heterosexual gender identities. The use of queer or related terms, such as *pansexual*, allows people to describe their sexual orientation outside of a binary gender construct. Additionally, some people identify as *asexual*, and experience little to no sexual attraction or desire for sexual activity.

Like sexual orientation, gender identity is composed of three components: natal sex, identity, and expression. *Natal sex*, as described earlier, refers to the label that was placed on a person by the clinician at birth. Gender *identity* refers to one's inner understanding of themselves in regard to gender. *Expression* refers to one's dress, mannerisms, and other factors that communicate gender cues to the outside world. In any given person, these components may be the same, or they may differ significantly. It is important to remember that a person's sexual orientation does not define that individual's gender identity, and vice versa.

Transgender is an umbrella term used to describe those persons whose gender identity is in some way different from their natal sex assigned at birth. A large number of related terms describe this same concept; this chapter uses the term *transgender* for clarity. A *transgender woman* is a natal male who has a female gender identity. A *transgender man* is a natal female who has a male gender identity. These are examples of binary gender identities, in which one identifies as male or female, but not both or neither. In reality, a great number of people do not comfortably identify within this binary gender framework. These people may identify as somewhere between male and female, as both male and female, or as having no gender at all. A great number of terms are used to describe this relationship to the social construct of gender; for purposes of clarity, this chapter uses the term *gender nonconforming*. *Gender affirmation* refers to any process that strives to better align one's gender expression, social perception, or physical appearance with one's gender identity. Examples include medical interventions to change secondary

BOX 9-1 Gender and Sexual Orientation Terminology

Asexual: A person who experiences little to no sexual attraction or desire for sexual activity

Binary gender: A concept of gender that recognizes only two dichotomous gender identities, male and female

Bisexual: A person who is attracted to people with both male and female gender identities

Cisgender: A person whose gender identity is the same as their natal sex

Gay: A person with a male gender identity who is primarily attracted to other people with a male gender identity; historically used as an umbrella term for all non-heterosexual people

Gender: A social construction assigning roles and attributes to a person based on their natal sex

Gender affirmation: Any process that strives to better align gender expression, social perception, or physical appearance with gender identity

Gender expression: Outward expression of gender or gender identity

Gender identity: Internal understanding of oneself in regard to gender

Gender nonconforming: A person who identifies as somewhere between male and female, both male and female, or having no gender

Intersex: People whose chromosomes are neither XX nor XY, or whose genitals are ambiguous or incongruent with chromosomal makeup

Lesbian: A person with a female gender identity who is primarily attracted to other people with a female gender identity

Man: A person who identifies as male, regardless of natal sex

Natal female: Assigned female at birth based on appearance of genitalia

Natal male: Assigned male at birth based on appearance of genitalia

Natal sex: Sex designation assigned at birth based on appearance of genitalia

Nonbinary gender: A concept of gender that recognizes gender as existing on a spectrum rather than as a dichotomy

Pansexual: A person who is attracted to people of all gender identities, not limited to those with binary gender identities

Queer: Umbrella term to describe all people with non-heterosexual gender identities; historically used as a derogatory slur by those outside of the lesbian, gay, bisexual, transgender, and gender-nonconforming communities, and still experienced as derogatory by many community members

Sex: A designation based on chromosomes and genitalia

Sexual orientation: A concept describing one's sexual attraction, identity, and behavior

Transgender: Umbrella term used to describe all people whose gender identity is in some way different from their natal sex

Transgender woman: A natal male who has a female gender identity

Transgender man: A natal female who has a male gender identity

Woman: A person who identifies as female, regardless of natal sex

sex characteristics, and requesting the use of one's preferred name and pronoun in social interactions. The term *cisgender* refers to a non-transgender person—someone whose gender identity matches their natal sex.

Complexities of Identity and Behavior

The fact that identity does not always mirror behavior—and both identity and behavior are fluid over time—makes understanding the healthcare needs of LBQ and TGNC people complex. Clinically, one cannot make assumptions about a patient's sexual behaviors based on identity alone. For example, research has shown that few people who describe themselves as lesbians have had zero lifetime male sexual partners, and in many studies more than 30% of self-identified lesbians reported having a recent male partner (Abdessamad, Yudin, Tarasoff, Radford, & Ross, 2013; Estrich, Gratzer, & Hotton, 2014; Gorgos & Marrazzo, 2011; Muzny, Sunesara, Martin, & Mena, 2011). Similarly, in one study of 669 women attending a sexually transmitted infection (STI) clinic in Chicago, 2.5% of straight-identified women reported having a female sexual partner within the past 90 days (Estrich et al., 2014). These data, however, are complicated by the fact that few studies provide information on whether transgender men and women were reported as "male" or "female" partners.

Like behavior, identity is fluid over time. In general, LBQ women demonstrate greater fluidity in sexual identity than their male and heterosexual peers; this is particularly true for bisexual people (Mock & Eibach, 2012; Ott, Corliss, Wypij, Rosario, & Austin, 2011). Early research has also found significant fluidity in the sexual orientation of TGNC people, regardless of whether they seek out medical or surgical gender affirmation (Auer, Fuss, Höhne, Stalla, & Sievers, 2014).

Assumptions about the desire for gender affirmation in TGNC people are equally as problematic as assumptions about sexual behavior based on identity. Historically, it has been assumed that all TGNC people have a binary gender identity and desire full social, legal, medical, and surgical gender affirmation. Recent studies have challenged this assumption. In a study of 292 TGNC adults, the majority identified as "genderqueer,"

and greater than 70% identified with more than one gender identity (Kuper, Nussbaum, & Mustanski, 2012). Similarly, the most commonly indicated sexual orientations were "pansexual" and "queer." The same study found a great deal of variation in desires for medical and surgical gender affirmation. For example, almost one-third of participants did not plan to ever take gender-affirming hormones, and more than half did not plan to ever have genital surgery. These data indicate that it is critical for clinicians to base their assessments and care plans on behavior, current anatomy, and patient goals rather than on assumptions based on identity.

SOCIAL AND LEGAL CONTEXT

Minority Stress

It is widely accepted that LBQ women and TGNC people experience interpersonal and institutional discrimination. Minority stress theory—which has primarily been utilized to understand the experiences of people of color, LBQ women, and gay men—provides a critical tool for examining the impact of everyday discrimination experiences on the physical and emotional health of marginalized communities. The building blocks of minority stress are microaggressions: "brief, daily assaults on minority individuals, which can be social, environmental, verbal or nonverbal, as well as intentional or unintentional" (Balsam, Molina, Beadnell, Simoni, & Walters, 2011, p. 163) and "communicate hostile, derogatory, or negative slights" (McCabe, Dragowski, & Rubinson, 2013, p. 10). As will be explored in this chapter, healthcare experiences are rife with microaggressions for LBQ women and TGNC people. Microaggressions play an important role in maintaining institutionalized systems of oppression. In the case of LBQ and TGNC communities, microaggressions uphold heteronormativity and cisgender normativity.

Heteronormativity is the societal institutionalization of a dichotomy where one group of people—in this case, heterosexuals—is valued, and another group of people—in this case, LBQ women and gay men—is devalued and oppressed. *Cisgender normativity* similarly places value on cisgender people, and devalues and oppresses TGNC people. Related concepts are *homophobia*, the irrational fear or hatred of anything that challenges heteronormativity, including non-heterosexual people themselves, and *transphobia*, the irrational fear or hatred of anything that challenges cisgender normativity, including TGNC people themselves. *Heterosexism* describes the belief that heterosexuality is the best sexual orientation, and that all people should be heterosexual.

Microaggressions affect all aspects of physical and emotional well-being (Balsam et al., 2011; Frost, Lehavot, & Meyer, 2015; Grant et al., 2011; Lick, Durso, & Johnson, 2013). In a New York–based study of 396 lesbian and bisexual women and gay men, participants who had experienced a discrimination event were three times more likely to have a physical health problem between the baseline point and 1-year follow-up (Frost et al., 2015). In the National Transgender Discrimination Survey, a 2011 landmark national study of 6,000 TGNC people that culminated in a report aptly titled *Injustice at Every Turn*, 63% of participants reported experiencing discriminatory events significant enough to impact quality of life and emotional and financial stability; 23% had experienced a "catastrophic" level of discrimination (Grant et al., 2011). Note, however, that minority stress differs from routine daily stress that is unrelated to discrimination, in that the former sustains higher-than-average levels of stress, is chronic regardless of life improvements and social advancements, and is nonmodifiable by the individual person (Blosnich, Lee, & Horn, 2011).

People who inhabit multiple marginalized identities, such as LBQ women and TGNC people who are also people of color or have a disability, experience exponentially increased levels of minority stress. This can be understood using the framework of intersectionality, which "asserts that social categories are only meaningful in combination . . . [challenging] the notion that we can understand individual experiences by examining a single aspect of one's identity" (McGarrity, 2014, p. 383). Using this more nuanced, whole-person view, it is clear that people who experience multiple layers of oppression and microaggressions are more likely to suffer negative physical and emotional impacts from these stressors; these individuals may also be torn between aspects of

their identity that are often in conflict with each other (Balsam et al., 2011).

Social and Familial Supports

For many LBQ women and TGNC people, living openly as one's authentic self comes at a high social cost or, in some cases, is not possible. Studies have shown significant levels of family rejection after disclosure of an individual's sexual orientation and/or gender identity. In a large national survey of LBQ women, TGNC people, and gay men conducted by Pew Research Center (2013), 39% of the respondents had experienced family rejection. In the National Transgender Discrimination Survey, 57% of participants reported family rejection (Grant et al., 2011). This finding is particularly significant given that "family acceptance had a protective effect against many threats to well-being including health risks such as HIV infection and suicide" (Grant et al., 2011, p. 7), and family rejection is a frequently cited cause of youth homelessness (Durso & Gates, 2012).

Rejection of LBQ and TGNC people is common not only at a family level, but also at a community and spiritual level. For example, 29% of survey participants in the Pew Research Center (2013) study had felt unwelcome in a place of worship.

Not surprisingly, then, many LBQ and TGNC people choose not to disclose their sexual orientation or gender identity in a number of social and familial settings. In the Pew Research Center (2013) survey, 34% of participants had not disclosed their sexual orientation or gender identity to their mother, and 39% had not disclosed it to their father. Of those who had, most found this discussion very difficult. Interestingly, the same study found that bisexual women were significantly less likely to disclose their sexual orientation: 71% of lesbian participants stated that "all or most of the important people" in their life were aware of their sexual orientation, while only 29% of bisexual women made the same assertion. Lesbians were also more likely than their bisexual peers to perceive their sexual orientation as a positive force in their lives.

For LBQ and TGNC people of color, as well as for those from religious backgrounds that prohibit homosexuality, issues of family and community acceptance may be more complicated. In a study of 701 Chinese, Korean, and Vietnamese daughters of immigrant parents, 18% of the sample identified as lesbian or bisexual, and these participants often noted rejection by family members as well as their larger cultural community (Lee & Hahm, 2012). African American TGNC women who participated in community-engaged research noted dual experiences of discrimination in different communities they inhabited: Many experienced homophobia within their families and communities of origin, as well as racism within the larger gay, LBQ, and TGNC community (Kubicek et al., 2013).

In response to these struggles, resilient LBQ and TGNC people are well versed in creating supportive familial and social structures of their own. The language of the community reflects this—the term *family* is a common insider term that is used to denote community membership. Historically, the gay bar has been the foremost social structure and safe place where LBQ and TGNC people have gathered as "chosen family" and community. While LBQ and TGNC people certainly have many social options today, this has not always been the case. In the past, "the gay bar . . . acted as the conduit between identity and having a community for that identity. [It was] 'the only place': the only place to meet, socialize, and most importantly, be one's self" (Addison, 2014). This feeling of the bar or club as community space continues to permeate LBQ and TGNC culture today, and looks different within different communities (Blosnich et al., 2011; Kubicek et al., 2013).

Legal Protections and Vulnerabilities

LBQ and TGNC communities have a complicated relationship to the law, in that their rights change frequently and vary drastically by geographic location within the United States, and community divisions have historically presented significant barriers to the pursuit of equity. In the past, the same couple might be legally married in their home state but considered legal strangers in another state. Even within the same state, rights granted may come and go with referendums and Supreme Court decisions. Approximately one-fourth of all LBQ and TGNC people in the United States live in what can be considered "low-equality states" based on the presence or absence of protective employment, relationship, adoption, and school bullying legislation; another 25% live in "medium-equality states" (Center for American Progress & Movement Advancement

Project, 2015). Equally troubling is the issue of in-community divisions between gay, LBQ, and TGNC people, which have hampered social change efforts. A classic example of this was an unsuccessful push in 2006—backed by the prominent organization Human Rights Campaign (HRC)—to pass the Employment Non-Discrimination Act (ENDA) by removing all protections for TGNC people.

A great deal of in-community debate has surrounded the issue of same-sex marriage as well. While many LBQ and TGNC people do not seek marriage or are critical of marriage as a legal and social institution, the presence or absence of marriage equality still has significant implications for LBQ and TGNC people and their children. In a landmark decision on June 26, 2015, the U.S. Supreme Court ruled that bans on same-sex marriage were unconstitutional; this decision in effect legalized same-same marriage nationwide (Supreme Court of the United States, 2015). Until the date of this ruling, same-sex marriage had been prohibited in 13 states (Human Rights Campaign, 2015), and most states in which same-sex marriage was legal had endured a barrage of legal struggles to get, maintain, or regain this right for all committed couples. This legal back-and-forth caused a great deal of distress and anxiety for couples living in affected states (Hatzenbuehler, McLaughlin, Keyes, & Hasin, 2010), and marriage discrimination was recognized as having a deleterious health impact on LGB and TGNC people (American College of Obstetricians and Gynecologists, 2013).

Parenting status for nonbiological parents, such as lesbian mothers or TGNC parents whose partners gave birth to their children, is significantly impacted by marriage status. The ability to foster or adopt children is also affected by marriage status, gender identity, and sexual orientation. Prior to legalization of same-sex marriage, nonbiological parents were considered legal strangers to their children in a number of states, and lacked the ability to make legal and health decisions for their own children (Center for American Progress & Movement Advancement Project, 2015). While the passage of federal marriage-equality legislation has provided a great deal of reassurance to nonbiological parents, its true impact on parenting status and the ability to foster or adopt children remains to be seen. Same-sex couples who are not married continue to lack the presumed parenting rights enjoyed by their unmarried heterosexual peers. Moreover, while marriage theoretically offers de facto protection regardless of sexual orientation or gender identity, some states have sought workarounds to allow for continued parental status discrimination. As of October 2015, two states allowed child welfare agencies to refuse joint adoption based on religious objections (Family Equality Council, 2015). One state prohibited LGB and TGNC people from adopting children out of its foster care system, and another state placed specific restrictions on fostering by LGB and TGNC parents (Family Equality Council, 2015).

LBQ and TGNC people are also at risk of being denied the right to be with their partners in times of health crisis, or the right to make medical decisions on behalf of their incapacitated partners. A notable example of this limitation occurred in 2006, when a Seattle woman was denied access to her dying wife's bedside by social workers and healthcare personnel; she was allowed into her wife's hospital room only when a biological family member arrived and granted her access (Chansanchair, 2015). In response to this and other incidents, President Barack Obama issued a memorandum in 2010 stating that all patients should be able to choose who visits them in the hospital and who is authorized to make healthcare decisions on their behalf (Obama, 2010). Nonetheless, only 25% of healthcare entities responding to the Human Rights Campaign's 2014 Health Equity Index survey stated that they trained employees on medical decision making for gay, LBQ, and TGNC couples (Hanneman, 2014). Issues of citizenship are also more complicated for gay, LBQ, and TGNC couples, and many couples who are unable to marry live under threat of deportation.

In the first large-scale study using matched controls, the U.S. Department of Housing and Urban Development concluded in 2013 that housing discrimination against gay and LBQ couples occurs throughout the country (Friedman, Reynolds, & Scovill, 2013). In the National Transgender Discrimination Survey, 19% of TGNC people reported being refused a home or apartment based on their gender identity, and 11% stated that they had been evicted at some point for the same reason (Grant et al., 2011). As of October 2015, 28 states lacked housing laws that prohibit discrimination based

on sexual orientation or gender identity, and three other states offered only partial legal protection from housing discrimination (Human Rights Campaign, 2015).

Employment discrimination takes a particularly heavy toll on LBQ and TGNC communities. In the Pew Research Center's 2013 survey, 21% of participants reported having been treated unfairly by their employer specifically because of their sexual orientation or gender identity. In another study, 16% of LBQ women stated that they had been fired at some point because of their sexual orientation, and 62% reported enduring disparaging jokes in the workplace (Center for American Progress & Movement Advancement Project, 2015). Among TGNC people, reported rates of employment termination due to their gender identity ranged from 26% to 36%; more than half reported workplace harassment or being turned down for a job for the same reason (Center for American Progress & Movement Advancement Project, 2015; Grant et al., 2011). As of October 2015, only 20 states had comprehensive employment laws that prohibited discrimination based on sexual orientation or gender identity; another 4 states offered partial legal protection, and 27 states offered no legal protections (Human Rights Campaign, 2015).

Finally, a large body of evidence reveals that violence is a pressing concern in LBQ and TGNC communities. Protections from violence and harassment can be assessed in several ways; legislation regarding hate crimes and bullying is a particularly useful marker. As of October 2015, 20 states lacked legislation that defines violence based on sexual orientation or gender identity as a hate crime, and 30 states lacked laws against bullying of students based on sexual orientation and gender identity (Human Rights Campaign, 2015).

Economic Inequality

Interpersonal and institutionalized homophobia, transphobia, and heterosexism directly impact the economic stability of gay, LBQ, and TGNC people and families (Blosnich, Farmer, Lee, Silenzio, & Bowen, 2014; Grant et al., 2011; Ranji et al., 2014). This effect is compounded for LBQ and TGNC women, and for people of color, because they face additional forms of oppression and threats to their economic stability. In fact, the presence or absence of legal protections in a geographic region of the United States has been shown to correspond with the percentage of LBQ and TGNC women who are living in poverty (Center for American Progress & Movement Advancement Project, 2015).

Overall, LBQ and TGNC people are more likely to be poor than their heterosexual counterparts (Ranji et al., 2014). Bisexual women are significantly more likely to be poor than both heterosexual and lesbian women (Przedworski, McAlpine, Karaca-Mandic, & VanKim, 2014); transgender women are 3.8 times more likely to be poor than non-transgender, heterosexual women (Center for American Progress & Movement Advancement Project, 2015). Among LBQ and transgender women in same-sex relationships, African American couples are three times more likely and Latina couples two times more likely to be poor than their white peers (Center for American Progress & Movement Advancement Project, 2015).

TGNC communities demonstrate particularly alarming trends in regard to poverty when education is considered. In 2011, TGNC people were four times more likely to have an annual income of less than $10,000 per year, regardless of educational attainment (Grant et al., 2011). Additionally, as a result of high rates of family rejection, school bullying, and employment discrimination, many TGNC people are driven to work in the underground economy, performing dangerous work such as selling drugs or transactional sex to obtain housing, food, and other basic necessities (Grant et al., 2011).

Violence and Harassment

Hate-based harassment and violence are significant threats to the safety and well-being of LBQ and TGNC people; additionally, issues such as intimate partner violence (IPV) are often inadequately addressed among this population. Gay, LBQ, and TGNC people report high levels of harassment and assault in places of public accommodation, such as retail stores and buses, and in interactions with law enforcement (Grant et al., 2011; Pew Research Center, 2013). In data on hate violence collected from 13 U.S. states as well as Puerto Rico, gay, LBQ, and TGNC people represented 86% of hate violence victims in 2013; people of color, regardless of sexual orientation, accounted for 59% of all hate violence victims (Ahmed & Jindasurat, 2014).

The picture is particularly bleak for transgender women. In 2015, 21 transgender women were murdered in the United States (Kellaway & Brydum, 2016). This alarming statistic is consistent with data that demonstrate high levels of violence and murder against transgender women, and particularly transgender women of color—67% of all hate-crime homicide victims in 2013 were transgender women of color (Ahmed & Jindasurat, 2014).

Gay and LBQ violence survivors generally, and TGNC violence survivors specifically, cannot count on law enforcement officials to protect their safety or dignity when reporting hate crimes. In 2013, more than half of gay, LBQ, and TGNC survivors chose not to report acts of hate violence to the police. Of those who did, many met with some form of hostility or misconduct, including arrest and physical violence. Transgender women were 6 times more likely and transgender men 5.2 times more likely than other survivors to experience physical police violence after a hate crime (Ahmed & Jindasurat, 2014).

IPV is likely underreported in LBQ and TGNC communities, largely due to isolation, fear of having to disclose one's sexual orientation or gender identity, and fear of discrimination at the hands of service providers and law enforcement. Nonetheless, data show that rates of IPV are likely the same among gay, LBQ, and TGNC couples as among heterosexual couples (National Center for Victims of Crime & National Coalition of Anti-Violence Programs, 2010). Bisexual women are particularly affected by IPV: They are more likely than both heterosexual and lesbian women to experience physical, sexual, and emotional violence by an intimate partner, and sexual violence by any perpetrator (Walters, Chen, & Breiding, 2013). Most IPV service agencies are underprepared to meet the needs of LBQ and TGNC survivors. This lack of cultural competency is apparent in the paucity of outreach, staff training, and LBQ- and TGNC-specific policies. For example, 93% of legal and social services agencies responding to a 2010 survey stated that they had not received adequate training to support transgender victims of violence (National Center for Victims of Crime & National Coalition of Anti-Violence Programs, 2010).

BARRIERS TO HEALTH CARE

LBQ women and TGNC people experience significant barriers to health care, including financial barriers, lack of insurance, historical trauma, lack of clinician knowledge, and restrictive healthcare systems, infrastructure, and policies. By all measures, these barriers are increased for those who experience multiple forms of oppression, such as people of color, people with low incomes, and people with disabilities. This section briefly explores some of the factors that contribute to disparities in access to needed healthcare services.

Financial Barriers

LBQ women and TGNC people are less likely to have insurance and to be able to afford healthcare services than their heterosexual and cisgender peers. While 9.8% of the general population of cisgender women is uninsured, 21% of lesbians, 27% of bisexual women, and 35% of transgender women are uninsured (Center for American Progress & Movement Advancement Project, 2015). LBQ and TGNC women who have low to moderate incomes are also more likely than their peers to have medical debt (Center for American Progress & Movement Advancement Project, 2015). This is explained in part by the fact that many employers deny insurance benefits for same-sex partners who are not legally married, and Medicaid eligibility rules may exclude women in same-sex partnerships (Center for American Progress & Movement Advancement Project, 2015; Przedworski et al., 2014). Inability to afford healthcare services leads to significantly increased rates of delaying necessary care (Blosnich et al., 2014; Grant et al., 2011; Ward, Dahlhamer, Galinsky, & Joestl, 2014).

Historical Trauma

Historical trauma describes the "cumulative emotional and psychological wounding over the life span and across generations emanating from massive group experiences" (Walls & Whitbeck, 2012, p. 416). Historical trauma theory is grounded in the experiences of people of color and, in particular, the Native American experience of genocide. This theory provides a useful lens for examining the impact today of homophobia and transphobia experienced within the

healthcare system by previous generations. When LBQ or TGNC persons present for health care, those individuals carry the weight of not only their personal experiences of mistreatment within the healthcare system, but also the cumulative pain and mistreatment experienced by their predecessors. As a result, LBQ women and TGNC people tend to expect discrimination in healthcare settings, regardless of whether they have directly experienced such bias themselves.

This legacy of trauma influences healthcare utilization behaviors and patient–clinician rapport and is supported by current research. In a large national survey of gay, LBQ, and TGNC healthcare experiences conducted by Lambda Legal (2010), participants frequently cited fear of being discriminated against if they chose to seek health care. More than half of TGNC participants and almost 10% of gay and LBQ participants believed they would be refused care because of their sexual orientation and gender identity. Similarly, 73% of TGNC respondents and 28.5% of gay and LBQ participants anticipated being treated differently by healthcare professionals. Actual experiences corroborated these expectations, with more than half of gay and LBQ respondents and 70% of TGNC participants reporting some form of discrimination in healthcare settings, including being refused care, blamed for their health concerns, and treated with physical roughness. In addition, 2% of TGNC people report being physically assaulted in a healthcare setting (Grant et al., 2011). The healthcare climate can be filled with multiple safety threats, including harassment and assault by fellow patients.

Clinician Knowledge

Lack of understanding of the specific needs of LBQ and TGNC people is another significant barrier to health care, particularly for TGNC people (Institute of Medicine, 2011). This is unsurprising, as clinicians typically must work hard to find opportunities to learn about LBQ and TGNC health. A survey of 132 allopathic and osteopathic medical schools in the United States and Canada revealed that the median teaching time dedicated to gay, LBQ, and TGNC content during the entire course of medical education was 5.0 hours; 33.3% of schools did not allocate any teaching time to this content, and 6.8% had no content at all (Obedin-Maliver et al., 2011).

Fewer than one-fourth of medical schools offered clinical rotations that focused on care for gay, LBQ, and TGNC patients (Obedin-Maliver et al., 2011). An earlier survey of medical students found that increased exposure to gay, LBQ, and TGNC patients resulted in greater knowledge and improvement in clinician attitudes (Sanchez, Rabatin, Sanchez, Hubbard, & Kalet, 2006).

Patient experiences confirm this glaring lack of clinician knowledge. Half of TGNC people report having to teach their clinician how to care for them, and this number is even higher for participants who have undergone gender-affirming hormone therapy (Grant et al., 2011). In a small focus group investigating gay, LBQ, and TGNC patients' perspectives on clinician behaviors, participants articulated a desire for clinicians to be aware of the dynamics of power and privilege in the healthcare system, use clear communication and language regarding sexual health, put in the effort to make a clinic space truly welcoming and safe, and demonstrate an understanding of insurance coverage issues for gender-affirming care (Rounds, McGrath, & Walsh, 2013).

Healthcare Systems and Infrastructure

Inequities in healthcare systems and infrastructure set the tone for all LBQ and TGNC patient experiences. Often, these inequities are experienced as microaggressions long before a patient ever meets the clinician. Such disparities might include being misgendered on the phone during the scheduling process, being asked to fill out forms that cannot accommodate one's sexual orientation or gender identity, finding a lack of relevant artwork and literature in the healthcare setting lobby, or having a partner being ignored or referred to as a "friend." In addition to creating negative experiences and impacting health-seeking behavior in the future, heterosexist healthcare systems limit the quality and scope of care provided by even well-intentioned clinicians.

The electronic medical record (EMR) is at the heart of many accessibility problems within healthcare systems. Most EMR systems are not equipped to track sexual orientation, gender identity, and related concerns accurately or in adequate detail. These deficits, in effect, render LBQ and TGNC patients invisible to their clinicians, and

this invisibility denies access to the specific care needed to reduce healthcare disparities (Callahan, Hazarian, Yarborough, & Sánchez, 2014). One very obvious example is the inability to differentiate sex from gender in the EMR, and the inability of most systems to easily track preferred name and pronoun. Being called by an incorrect pronoun in a healthcare setting negatively affects patient satisfaction and future health-seeking behaviors. Patient safety is also threatened because public incidents of misgendering increase the risk of harassment or assault by fellow patients (Deutsch et al., 2013). In addition, these EMR-related limitations hinder clinicians' ability to plan appropriate health screening (Callahan et al., 2014; Deutsch et al., 2013).

Healthcare facility policies are also critical to equity in healthcare environments. In its most recent annual survey of healthcare facility policies and procedures relating to LGBQ and TGNC patients, the Human Rights Campaign found that many such facilities do not have a comprehensive gay, LBQ, and TGNC patient nondiscrimination policy, and 16% lack equal visitation policies (Hanneman, 2014).

Restrictive Policies for Gender-Affirming Health Care

As has already been explored in this section, healthcare systems and infrastructure are particularly punishing of TGNC people. Since the advent of gender identity clinics in the mid-1960s, restrictive policies have been the standard in TGNC health. The first gender identity clinic to open in the United States was so restrictive in its care policies that only 24 of the first 2,000 patients who applied for care met the eligibility criteria (Beemyn, 2014). Through such policies, healthcare and mental health clinicians have been placed in a gatekeeping role that erodes rapport and creates significant obstacles to care.

For example, until 2011 either a 3-month "real life experience" or an extensive course of psychotherapy was required to be eligible for gender-affirming hormone therapy. The required duration of therapy presented an insurmountable financial barrier for many patients, and the "real life experience" was an often-dangerous path to care in which TGNC people were required to "present full time" as their affirmed gender without any benefit of physical changes from hormones, regardless of whether this practice was safe in their home community. This is inconsistent with standards of informed consent for all other medically necessary health services.

While eligibility for treatment has become more accessible over time, insurance policies continue to be quite restrictive, despite the fact that gender-affirming health care is recognized as medically necessary. As of October 2015, 42 states allowed insurance exclusions for TGNC healthcare services or refused to provide these services as a health benefit to state employees; an additional 3 states offered only partial access to health care (Human Rights Campaign, 2015). Even in states that have a ban on such exclusions, accessing the full range of gender-affirming services remains difficult.

In the face of this lack of access, many TGNC people are unable to tolerate their gender dysphoria and take health care into their own hands by self-administering hormones (Makadon, Mayer, Potter, & Goldhammer, 2010) or using non-medical-grade silicone injections to create changes to body shape without surgery (Wilson, Rapues, Jin, & Raymend, 2014). Both of these self-managed interventions have significant health consequences that could be avoided with adequate access to care.

HEALTH DISPARITIES

While this book is dedicated to gynecologic health, a feminist understanding of health recognizes that all health is interconnected, and it is important to look at the whole person when providing any type of specialized care. For example, mental health status and substance abuse directly affect STI risk behaviors. Overall, heterosexual women are more likely than their LBQ and TGNC peers to report good health (Przedworski et al., 2014; Ward et al., 2014). When asked about their general health, lesbian and bisexual women report higher rates of asthma, hepatitis, and urinary tract infections (Lick et al., 2013). Specific health concerns vary by race both within and between sexual orientations. As with social markers of well-being, health outcomes across the board are worse for people of color. This section explores key aspects of health that may be addressed in a gynecologic visit or annual examination.

Mental Health

Minority stress theory posits that LBQ women and TGNC people experience higher rates of mental distress than their heterosexual peers. This supposition is supported by data demonstrating higher rates of suicide and mental health concerns—particularly suicidal ideation, depression, and anxiety—in LBQ women than in heterosexual women (Cochran & Mays, 2015; Miranda et al., 2010; Ward et al., 2014). One large study of pooled data from the Behavior Risk Factor Surveillance System from 2001 to 2008 was less clear on this correlation, showing increased rates of mental distress in the short term, but no difference in the long term; however, this study did identify a significant difference in limitation of activities based on mental distress (Blosnich et al., 2014). Data from studies of LBQ women from different ethnic groups have supported higher levels of emotional distress in communities of color. In a 2012 study, suicidal ideation was two to three times higher among lesbian and bisexual Asian American women than among heterosexual Asian American women (Lee & Hahm, 2012). Data from the 2003 to 2009 Washington State Behavioral Risk Factor Surveillance System also demonstrated higher risk of mental distress in bisexual Latina women (Kim & Fredriksen-Goldsen, 2012).

Similar trends hold within TGNC communities. In the National Transgender Discrimination Survey, 41% of participants reported that they had attempted suicide compared to 1.6% of the general population at the time, and this rate was even higher with specific experiences of discrimination (Grant et al., 2011). A 3-year prospective study of 230 transgender women in New York found rates of depression that were five times the rates for the general population (Nuttbrock et al., 2013).

Reassuringly, results of several small studies have been supportive of the hypothesis that gender-affirming hormone therapy improves mental health outcomes (Gómez-Gil et al., 2012; Keo-Meier et al., 2015; Murad et al., 2010). In the first case-controlled prospective study of the impact of gender-affirming hormone therapy on psychosocial functioning, transgender men demonstrated poor psychosocial functioning compared to male and female cisgender controls at baseline, but were functioning as well as controls after 3 months of hormone therapy (Keo-Meier et al., 2015).

Body Image and Body Composition

In recent years, much political, social, and scientific exploration has focused on issues of body image, body weight, and health. Feminist and social justice voices have encouraged a movement toward body acceptance and body positivity that celebrates, rather than punishes, diversity in body size and encourages health, rather than weight loss. At the same time, the medical community is slowly coming to recognize the inefficacy of body weight, body mass index (BMI), and adiposity as accurate measures of current and future health (Bacon & Aphramor, 2011; Dias et al., 2013; Roberson et al., 2014). Weight-based discrimination has been identified as a barrier to health care for many women regardless of sexual orientation, and it is common for women to delay gynecologic care specifically for this reason (Fikkan & Rothblum, 2012).

Research findings vary as to whether LBQ women are protected from the social pressure to be thin that is well recognized as a driving force of body dissatisfaction and disordered eating in heterosexual women. A qualitative study of 21 lesbians found that younger lesbian women did not perceive any difference in body satisfaction between themselves and their heterosexual peers. Older lesbians, in contrast, perceived themselves as more critical of heteronormative standards regarding thinness and were more accepting of a range of body sizes and shapes (Roberts, Stuart-Shor, & Oppenheimer, 2010). Another qualitative study in the United Kingdom found that all lesbian participants felt negatively impacted by pressure to be thin from media and other social outlets; no participants felt relief of this body dissatisfaction after coming out as lesbian (Huxley, Clarke, & Halliwell, 2014). A 2013 qualitative study of lesbian college students did find lower internalization of social pressures to become thinner as well as greater interest in muscularity compared to heterosexual peers; however, this did not correspond with a decrease in body dissatisfaction or disordered eating (Yean et al., 2013). Some evidence suggests that LBQ women in general are more accepting of a variety of body shapes and sizes in others (Markey & Markey, 2013).

Actual body size and weight status in LBQ women vary significantly by race and a number of other factors. Overall, data suggest that LBQ women are more likely to be overweight, to be obese, or to experience "steep weight-gain trajectories" in adulthood (Blosnich et al., 2014; Jun et al., 2012; Ward et al., 2014). Overweight is more common in white and African American lesbians than in Latina and Asian American lesbian women (Deputy & Boehmer, 2014).

Research on body image and body composition in TGNC people is less robust. Data suggest that rates of disordered eating and body weight and shape dissatisfaction are higher in TGNC people compared to cisgender people (Diemer, Grant, Munn-Chernoff, Patterson, & Duncan, 2015; Vocks, Stahn, Loenser, & Legenbauer, 2009), and that this phenomenon is often related to the desire to suppress or accentuate specific gender characteristics (Ålgars, Alanko, Santtila, & Sandnabba, 2012). At least one study has demonstrated improvement of body image with gender-affirming surgery in transgender women (Gómez-Gil et al., 2012). A single health center study of 100 TGNC people with an average of 10 years on gender-affirming hormone therapy found that 24% of transgender men and 22% of transgender women participants were overweight, and 14% of all TGNC participants were obese (Wierckx et al., 2012).

Substance Use

Cultural context is important to understanding substance use within LBQ and TGNC communities. Environments such as bars and club scenes have long offered safe spaces for gay, LBQ, and TGNC people to find community, mentorship, and family. While they provide needed social supports and relief from homophobic microaggressions, these environments also pose risks related to alcohol and drug use, tobacco use, violence, and unsafe sexual behaviors (Blosnich et al., 2011; Kubicek et al., 2013).

Multiple studies demonstrate that LBQ women and TGNC people smoke at higher rates than their heterosexual and cisgender peers (Blosnich et al., 2014; Farmer, Jabson, Bucholz, & Bowen, 2013; Przedworski et al., 2014; Ward et al., 2014). Some research has also shown an increase in tobacco-associated illness in LBQ women (Blosnich et al., 2011). Similarly, alcohol and substance abuse rates are higher in LBQ women and TGNC people than in their heterosexual and cisgender peers; this relationship has held true in studies specific to Asian American and Latina LBQ women as well (Kim & Fredriksen-Goldsen, 2012; Lee & Hahm, 2012).

Data from the 2009–2011 American College Health Association National College Health Assessment II found higher lifetime use of alcohol and most drugs in lesbian women versus heterosexual women, including recreational use of prescription drugs. Unlike in other studies, patterns of alcohol use were the same between lesbian and heterosexual women, but lesbians were more likely to report serious negative consequences associated with alcohol use (Kerr, Ding, & Chaya, 2014). The same study found that bisexual women had higher lifetime use of all drugs versus heterosexual women, and higher lifetime use of most drugs versus lesbian women.

Binge drinking, in particular, is notably high in LBQ women when compared to their heterosexual peers (Blosnich et al., 2014; Miranda et al., 2010; Przedworski et al., 2014; Ward et al., 2014). TGNC people frequently cite alcohol use as a current or past coping strategy for dealing with microaggressions, violence, and other experiences of discrimination (Grant et al., 2011).

Cardiovascular Health

Most research agrees that LBQ women and TGNC people have higher risk factors for cardiovascular disease; however, data are sparse on whether these risks translate into actual increases in morbidity and mortality. Data from the 2008–2009 wave of the National Longitudinal Study of Adolescent Health found a difference in risk factors, but no difference in biomarkers of cardiovascular risk, between heterosexual women and their lesbian and bisexual peers (Hatzenbuehler, McLaughlin, & Slopen, 2013). Similarly, a 2013 study of hypertension in young people found no differences in prevalence among lesbian, bisexual, and heterosexual women (Everett & Mollborn, 2013).

Data from the 2001–2008 National Health and Nutrition Examination Surveys were analyzed using the Framingham General Cardiovascular Risk Score, and a "vascular age" was established for participants. This study revealed an increased rate of "vascular aging" among LBQ women; disparities in aging were even more pronounced when women who identified as heterosexual (but had

at least one female partner in their lifetime) were removed, implying that minority stress may be of clinical significance in cardiovascular health (Farmer et al., 2013).

Data are scarcer when it comes to TGNC people who have undergone gender-affirming therapy. The few long-term studies conducted to date have been preliminarily reassuring. A 1997 landmark study of 1,109 TGNC people with a cumulative total of 10,152 patient-years of gender-affirming hormone therapy revealed no serious morbidity or mortality in transgender men; thromboembolic events did occur in transgender women but were reduced when estradiol was administered by transdermal patch in those older than 40 (Van Kesteren, Asscheman, Megens, & Gooren, 1997). Subsequent studies confirmed these findings and demonstrated that most morbidity and mortality seen in transgender women were unrelated to hormone therapy, although thromboembolic events and transient ischemic attacks (TIAs) did occur at higher rates than in natal males or females not using hormonal medications (Asscheman et al., 2011; Wierckx et al., 2012). Current, but not past, use of ethinyl estradiol (which is no longer the standard of care for gender affirmation) was associated with an increased rate of cardiovascular death.

It is worth noting that in all cases, transgender men have been underrepresented in research on TGNC health.

Endocrine Function

While the exact prevalence of polycystic ovary syndrome (PCOS) in the United States is unclear due to wide variations in diagnostic criteria, the general prevalence in young women is likely in the range of 10% to 20% (El Hakim & Wardle, 2010; March et al., 2010). In the past, it was believed that LBQ women have higher rates of endocrine disorders, such as PCOS, than the general population of women. This is concerning because of the potential complications associated with PCOS, including infertility, insulin resistance, dyslipidemia, and metabolic syndrome (see Chapter 25). In a 2004 study of 254 lesbian women and 364 heterosexual women, a significant difference in PCOS rates was seen: 38% in lesbian participants and 14% in heterosexual participants (Agrawal et al., 2004). However, two larger, more recent studies did not find a statistically significant increase in PCOS rates in lesbian women (De Sutter et al., 2008; Smith et al., 2011).

Very limited data exist on rates of PCOS in transgender men, and the studies that collected these data have significant limitations in their design. In a 1993 study of 16 transgender men who had not been exposed to exogenous androgen therapy, 50% of participants demonstrated signs and symptoms of PCOS, and all but one were formally diagnosed with this condition by ultrasound (Balen, Schachter, Montgomery, Reid, & Jacobs, 1993). In a similar study of 69 Japanese transgender men who had never undergone gender-affirming hormone therapy, 58% of participants were diagnosed with PCOS, and 39% demonstrated hyperandrogenism (Baba et al., 2007).

Ikeda et al. (2013) completed a small retrospective case-control study that compared histologic changes associated with PCOS between 11 transgender men taking testosterone and a control group. Several histologic changes that are common in PCOS were noted in transgender male participants, but none met the diagnostic criteria for PCOS. There was no way to assess whether these changes had occurred prior to or after initiation of gender-affirming hormone therapy.

Additional research is needed to understand the true rates of PCOS in LBQ women and transgender men, and to determine whether these rates are of clinical significance.

Vaginal and Sexually Transmitted Infections

When assessing for STI risk, sexual behavior—rather than sexual orientation or gender identity—is the most important concern. Sexual partners and sexual behaviors are what determine a person's risk for contracting and transmitting STIs.

Although both LBQ women and clinicians have long thought that transmission of STIs and vaginal infections between natal female partners is unlikely, that myth has been debunked in recent decades. Research has demonstrated that human papillomavirus (HPV) (Marrazzo, Koutsky, Kiviat, Kuypers, & Stine, 2001), bacterial vaginosis (BV) (Gorgos & Marrazzo, 2011; Marrazzo, Thomas, Agnew, & Ringwood, 2010; Marrazzo, Thomas, & Ringwood, 2011), gonorrhea and chlamydia (Singh,

Fine, & Marrazzo, 2011), and herpes simplex virus (HSV) (Marrazzo, Stine, & Wald, 2003) can all be sexually transmitted between natal females. In addition, case reports suggest that trichomoniasis (Kellock & O'Mahony, 1996), syphilis (Campos-Outcalt & Hurwitz, 2002), and human immunodeficiency virus (HIV) (Chan et al., 2014) can be transmitted as well.

Natal female-to-female transmission is not the only concern for this population; as discussed earlier, many lesbian-identified women have recent and past histories of sex with natal males. For transgender men who undergo gender-affirming hormone therapy, atrophic changes to the vaginal mucosa mimic those seen in postmenopausal women. This transformation is clinically significant in that atrophic vaginal tissue is more friable and subject to lacerations, creating routes for STI transmission (Minkin, 2010). Transgender women face a number of challenges that contribute to high rates of STI acquisition, including higher rates of HIV and syphilis (Centers for Disease Control and Prevention [CDC], 2013; Solomon et al., 2014).

It is likely that STI rates are underreported in LBQ women and TGNC people, as clinicians often neglect to ask about sex of intimate partners, and reporting structures make it difficult to directly track LBQ women and TGNC people in case reports (Teti & Bowleg, 2011). Similarly, cases of STIs in this population may not be identified due to clinician bias in screening recommendations (Estrich et al., 2014). Overall, LBQ women and transgender men report low rates of barrier (e.g., condoms, gloves, dental dams) use (Estrich et al., 2014; Feldman, Romine, & Bockting, 2014; Reisner, Perkovich, & Mimiaga, 2010; Rowen et al., 2013; Timm, Reed, Miller, & Valenti, 2011), and bisexual women and TGNC people tend to have a higher number of sexual partners than their lesbian and heterosexual peers (Estrich et al., 2014; Feldman et al., 2014). In addition, Asian American and African American LBQ women and TGNC people have increased risk factors for STI acquisition (Lee & Hahm, 2012; Muzny et al., 2011; Thoma, Huebner, & Rullo, 2013; Timm et al., 2011).

Bacterial vaginosis is more common in LBQ women than in heterosexual women (Gorgos & Marrazzo, 2011; Marrazzo et al., 2010), and in African American LBQ women than in their white counterparts (Muzny, Sunesara, Austin, Mena, & Schwebke, 2013). To date, researchers have been unable to determine causal and preventative factors for BV transmission in LBQ women (Gorgos & Marrazzo, 2011). Associated risk factors have also been difficult to pinpoint. In one study, recent new partner and sharing of penetrative vaginal sex toys were associated with BV (Marrazzo et al., 2010), while in another study toy sharing was not associated with BV but douching, age at sexual debut, and a number of partner factors were (Muzny et al., 2013). A randomized trial focused on reducing exchange of vaginal fluid between natal female partners was successful in greatly increasing glove use during digital intercourse, but this was not associated with any change in BV persistence (Marrazzo et al., 2011).

Understanding of neovaginal flora in transgender women is limited. Prior to a study in 2014, it was believed that the neovagina, which is typically created using a penile inversion technique during gender-affirming surgery, did not produce or maintain lactobacilli, contributing to an elevation in neovagina pH and development of BV (Petricevic et al., 2014; Weyers et al., 2009). However, a study using molecular detection techniques identified lactobacilli similar to those found in natal females in the majority of the 63 study participants (Petricevic et al., 2014). The clinical significance of neovaginal pH and lactobacilli has not yet been determined, and clinicians' approach should include an understanding that the neovagina is a blind-ended skin-lined pouch, rather than a mucosa-lined structure connected to secretory glands and reproductive organs. This means, for example, that the neovagina is not capable of self-cleansing; thus douching is typically required to prevent discharge resulting from accumulated exudate, lubricant, semen, and other material.

Transmission of HIV is of great concern to LBQ women and TGNC people. HIV transmission between natal females is possible but rare (Chan et al., 2014). However, sex with natal males remains a common source of transmission to LBQ women and TGNC people, with transgender women being the most commonly affected population. TGNC people accounted for the highest percentage of new HIV infections in 2010, and 99% of TGNC people with new infections were transgender women

(CDC, 2013). For TGNC people, having cisgender male sex partners, whether they are romantic partners or clients in the case of transactional sex work, is the strongest predictor of unprotected sex and subsequent risk of HIV exposure (Feldman et al., 2014). In a study of 1,229 TGNC adults, 33.3% of transgender women and 17.1% of transgender men reported sex with a cisgender male within the past 3 months (Feldman et al., 2014). Additionally, 32.2% of transgender women and 15.8% of transgender men in the same study reported recent anal or vaginal intercourse without a condom. In a small study of sexual health in transgender men, 43.8% reported unprotected sex with a cisgender male within the past year (Reisner et al., 2010).

Experiencing discrimination that affects economic stability is also a risk factor for HIV infection. In the National Transgender Discrimination Survey, HIV rates were more than twice as high in TGNC participants who had lost a job due to discrimination (Grant et al., 2011). Discrimination that forces TGNC people to work in the underground economy has a double impact on HIV exposure. Transactional sex work not only involves frequent intercourse with natal males, but also is often accompanied by financial incentives to forego condom use as well as coping strategies, such as drug use, that further increase HIV risk. Outside of a small handful of studies, very little is known about HIV, STIs, and sexual health in transgender men (CDC, 2013; Reisner, Lloyd, & Baral, 2013). In the few studies that have been conducted to address these questions, HIV prevalence in transgender men ranged from 0% to 10%; nevertheless, only two studies confirmed HIV status with serum testing (Reisner et al., 2013).

Clinicians should counsel their patients about ways to prevent the spread of STIs and encourage all patients to be tested regularly. LBQ women and TGNC people should know their own and their partners' HIV status, and use barriers consistently and correctly. Condoms can be used for intercourse and with penetrative sex toys. Sex toys should be cleaned regularly according to the manufacturer's instructions. Gloves can be used during digital sex; removing gloves before touching one's one genitals helps prevent transmission of vaginal fluid from one partner to another. Dental dams can be used as a barrier for vaginal oral sex, although many people find them too small or difficult to use. Clinicians can suggest using clear plastic wrap instead. Special care should be taken to provide clear, nonjudgmental, and relevant information on sexual health to patients who are engaged in transactional sex.

Gynecologic Cancers

Like any other individuals, LBQ women and TGNC people should be screened for cancers based on the organs that are present. As is discussed further in this section, rates of such screening are lower in this population, often because common entry points to health care are less frequently utilized. This section discusses cancer and screening rates for breast, cervical, and ovarian cancer.

Breast Cancer

In the early 1990s, the issue of breast cancer in lesbians was thrown into the spotlight when Suzanne Haynes at the National Cancer Institute stated that lesbians had a one in three risk of developing breast cancer, compared to the one in eight or nine risk for the general population of women at that time. Haynes's analysis was not based in empiric research, but rather on assumptions regarding higher rates of nulliparity, delayed childbirth, alcohol use, and overweight in lesbian women. In contemporary discussion of breast cancer risk factors in LBQ women and transgender men, these risk factors—as well as lower rates of breastfeeding, higher rates of smoking, and minority stress—continue to be cited as potentially concerning in relation to breast cancer risk within this population (Cochran & Mays, 2012; Meads & Moore, 2013; Zaritsky & Dibble, 2010).

To date, however, no studies have definitively determined whether LBQ women are at higher risk for breast cancer. The data remain quite mixed on this issue. A systematic review of research from the United States, the United Kingdom, and Denmark revealed a number of problems related to the accuracy of existing data: All studies found were small and/or had significant limitations in study design or data reporting, and no studies reported incidence (Meads & Moore, 2013). In the nine studies that reported prevalence, the findings were mixed: Two reported higher prevalence in lesbian and bisexual women as compared to heterosexual women, four found no difference in prevalence, and three did not provide sufficient data to justify their findings (Meads & Moore, 2013). Interestingly, one small study of quality of life in breast cancer survivors found no difference between lesbian women and heterosexual women when data were adjusted for income and education (Jabson, Donatelle, & Bowen, 2011). Based on these findings, the authors suggested further inquiry into the relationship between minority stress and resilience, hypothesizing that the experience of coping with daily microaggressions may have facilitated improved coping skills during breast cancer diagnosis and treatment. Data from the Nurses' Health Study II demonstrated only small disparities in mammogram screening based on sexual orientation overall, although lower mammography rates were seen in Latina and Asian American women regardless of sexual orientation (Austin et al., 2013).

There are no data on mammography rates, efficacy, or screening parameters in TGNC people, and data on breast cancer rates in this population are sparse. Mammography and clinical breast examinations may be more difficult to access for TGNC people secondary to lack of clinician knowledge and refusal of claims by insurance companies that perceive regular screening as incongruent with natal sex or current gender marker. Two studies of long-term impacts of gender-affirming hormone therapy revealed no cases of breast cancer in a cumulative total of 1,866 transgender women and 343 transgender men (Van Kesteren et al., 1997; Wierckx et al., 2012). Another study revealed one confirmed case and one likely case of breast cancer in a sample of 2,307 transgender women, and one confirmed case in a sample of 795 transgender men (Gooren, van Trotsenburg, Giltay, & van Diest, 2013). A more recent retrospective chart review examined breast cancer rates in 5,135 veterans receiving gender-affirming care through the Veterans Health Administration. A total of seven cases of breast cancer were noted in transgender men, two in transgender women, and one in a gender-nonconforming natal male who had not undergone hormone therapy (Brown & Jones, 2014). Although the authors of all these studies cautiously concluded that gender-affirming hormone therapy does not increase breast cancer risk in either transgender men or transgender women, the data are likely flawed by underdetection, often do not account for surgery status, and are not statistically significant in many cases. Additional rigorous research is needed to understand breast cancer risk and appropriate screening schedules in both LBQ women and TGNC people.

Cervical Cancer

Both risk factors and protective factors for cervical cancer are common in LBQ women and transgender men. Many of the risk factors for breast cancer described previously are also risk factors for cervical cancer. However, nulliparity and lack of combined oral contraceptive pill (OCP) use are protective factors, and these are common in this population (Zaritsky & Dibble, 2010).

While evidence is lacking as to whether LBQ women and transgender men have increased or decreased prevalence of cervical cancer, data support decreased cervical cytology screening rates in LBQ women versus heterosexual women (Charlton et al., 2014; Waterman & Voss, 2013) and transgender men versus LBQ and heterosexual women (Peitzmeier, Khullar, Reisner, & Potter, 2014). In large part, this pattern may reflect the fact that this population does not frequently access the most common entry points to gynecologic care: contraceptive management and STI screening (Agénor, Krieger, Austin, Haneuse, & Gottlieb, 2014; Charlton et al., 2014). Additionally, cervical cytology screening rates are influenced by both clinician and patient beliefs that LBQ women and transgender men are at low risk for HPV infection and cervical cancer (Charlton et al., 2014). Factors that increase the likelihood of routine screening include affordable care, a welcoming clinical environment, and accurate information and referrals from clinicians (Tracy, Schluterman, & Greenberg, 2013).

Pelvic examinations may be emotionally and physically difficult to tolerate for LBQ women and transgender men who do not receive penetrative vaginal sex. For transgender men, additional barriers to comfort with pelvic examinations include body dysphoria and atrophic changes that occur with testosterone therapy (Peitzmeier, Reisner, Harigopal, & Potter, 2014). Abnormal cervical cytology results are common in transgender men, possibly due to both physiologic changes to the endocervix with testosterone therapy, and discomfort

with the examination on the part of both clinicians and patients (Peitzmeier, Reisner et al., 2014). The American Society for Colposcopy and Cervical Pathology does not yet offer tailored clinical guidance on this issue. Further, insurance companies may reject claims for seemingly gender-incongruent examinations and laboratory tests. As with breast cancer, existing long-term research has suggested no increased risk of ovarian and cervical cancer in transgender men who undergo gender-affirming hormone therapy, but these data have significant limitations in study design and reporting (Wierckx et al., 2012).

Ovarian Cancer

Very limited data are available regarding ovarian cancer rates in LBQ women and transgender men. This population does have potential risk factors for ovarian cancer, including fewer pregnancies, less frequent use of combined oral contraceptives, and higher rates of smoking. Results of a retrospective study of risk factors for ovarian cancer revealed some differences in these risks between lesbian and heterosexual women (Dibble, Roberts, Robertson, & Paul, 2002). A later study confirmed higher rates of nulliparity and discussed disproportionate obesity in LBQ women as a risk factor for ovarian cancer (Zaritsky & Dibble, 2010). In considering these data, it is important to remember that an assumption of increased prevalence cannot be made based on the presence of risk factors alone.

Preconception and Pregnancy Experiences

Historically, LBQ women and TGNC people have been expected to forego parenthood. In relationships in which no partner produces sperm, there are certainly obstacles to overcome in regard to becoming parents. Nevertheless, recent surveys have suggested that parenting is a common experience in this population, with half of LBQ women of childbearing age (Center for American Progress & Movement Advancement Project, 2015) and more than half of TGNC people (Grant et al., 2011) stating that they are raising children. Many routes to parenthood are possible, including pregnancy (which may include collaborative reproduction, see Chapter 18), adoption, fostering, and surrogacy, and LBQ women and TGNC people use all of these routes. Although no studies to date have specifically addressed abortion experiences within this population, it is clear that LBQ women and transgender men do experience unintended pregnancy and subsequent abortion as a result of both consensual sex and sexual assault.

Several qualitative studies provide rich insight into the experiences of LBQ women seeking preconception care. Yager et al. (2010) examined the preconception experiences of LBQ women who were trying to conceive. Many participants described this process as difficult, emotionally stressful, and exhausting. While most participants in this study had positive experiences with clinicians, they expected to have negative experiences and, therefore, had some level of distress before engaging in care.

A study of 60 LBQ women in the United States, the United Kingdom, Canada, and Australia found that most participants' conception experiences involved assistance from clinicians as well as significant financial costs and investments in "lifestyle and behavior change" in preparation for trying to conceive (Peel, 2010). More than one-fourth of the participants reported experiencing "heterosexism, homophobia, or prejudice" in the course of receiving preconception and miscarriage management care.

The financial burden of trying to conceive is often exacerbated by limited insurance coverage for procreative management services, such as insemination and assisted reproductive technology. Some insurance companies provide coverage of these services for heterosexual couples but not for LBQ or TGNC couples (Center for American Progress & Movement Advancement Project, 2015).

To date, two studies have been published on TGNC people's experiences of conception and pregnancy following social and/or medical gender affirmation. Both of these studies found isolation to be a key theme in participants' experiences (Ellis, Wojnar, & Pettinato, 2014; Light, Obedin-Maliver, Sevelius, & Kerns, 2014). In addition, some participants experienced intense body dysphoria and detachment during pregnancy, while others felt more connected, "whole," and embodied during their pregnancy. Ellis et al. (2014) identified the preconception period as the time of participants' greatest time of distress and least involvement with health care. Participants in both studies expected negative

experiences with clinicians, including rudeness, denial of care, and being treated as "other." In one instance, a clinician called Child Protective Services on a patient, believing he would be an unfit parent based on his gender identity (Light et al., 2014).

Interestingly, in the Light et al. study (2014), unintended pregnancy was experienced by 50% of participants who had not undergone gender-affirming hormone therapy and 25% of those who had. These data point to an unmet need for preconception care and contraceptive management for TGNC people, as well as culturally responsive and accessible pregnancy and abortion care.

CULTURALLY RESPONSIVE CARE

LBQ women and TGNC people will feel most comfortable and safe in healthcare environments when they think that their sexuality or gender identity is *not* an issue and will not be the primary focus on their treatment. To create such a culture in their care settings, clinicians must educate themselves about the health needs and concerns of this population, and create environments that are welcoming, nonthreatening, and normalized to people of all gender identities and sexual orientations. **Box 9-2** identifies resources that clinicians can use to provide culturally responsive care for LBQ women and TGNC people.

First, clinicians should consider the physical environment. Having images of all types of people and families as well as reading materials designed for people of all sexual orientations and gender identities in the waiting area sends an immediate message to LBQ women and TGNC people that they are welcome and recognized. Transgender men, in particular, have reported feeling uncomfortable and out of place in obstetric or gynecologic waiting rooms (Ellis et al., 2014). An inclusive non-discrimination policy should be easily found on the healthcare setting's website and should be physically posted at the facility itself (Hanneman, 2014; New York City Bar, Lambda Legal, & Human Rights Campaign Foundation, 2013). Whenever possible, healthcare settings should have at least one single-stall, gender-neutral restroom available for patient use, and all settings should have a restroom policy that clearly states all patients are welcome to use the restroom consistent with their gender identity,

BOX 9-2 Resources for Clinicians

Policy Guidance and Staff Training

Creating Equal Access to Quality Health Care for Transgender Patients: Transgender-Affirming Hospital Policies
New York City Bar, Lambda Legal, and Human Rights Campaign
http://www.lambdalegal.org/publications/fs_transgender-affirming-hospital-policies

Providing Welcoming Services and Care for LGBT People: A Learning Guide for Health Care Staff
National LGBT Health Education Center
http://www.lgbthealtheducation.org/wp-content/uploads/Learning-Guide.pdf

Webinars and Continuing Education

Clinically Competent and Culturally Proficient Care for Transgender and Gender Nonconforming Patients
Cardea Services
http://www.cardeaservices.org/training/providing-culturally-proficient-services-to-transgender-and
  -gender-nonconforming-people.html

Cultural Competence Webinar Series
Gay and Lesbian Medical Association
http://www.glma.org/index.cfm?fuseaction=Page.viewPage&pageId=1025&grandparentID=534
  &parentID=940

If You Have It, Check It: Overcoming Barriers to Cervical Cancer Screening with Patients on the Female-to-Male Transgender Spectrum
National LGBT Health Education Center
http://www.lgbthealtheducation.org/wp-content/uploads/Overcoming-Barriers-to-Cervical-Cancer
  -Screening.pdf

Learning Modules
National LGBT Health Education Center
http://www.lgbthealtheducation.org/training/learning-modules

Transgender Healthcare Protocols

Clinical Practice Guidelines for the Endocrine Treatment of Transsexual Persons
Endocrine Society
http://press.endocrine.org/doi/pdf/10.1210/jc.2009-0345

Primary Care Protocol for Transgender Patient Care
University of California San Francisco Center of Excellence for Transgender Health
http://transhealth.ucsf.edu/trans?page=protocol-00-00

Standards of Care for the Health of Transsexual, Transgender, and Gender Nonconforming People
World Professional Association for Transgender Health
http://www.wpath.org/uploaded_files/140/files/Standards%20of%20Care,%20V7%20Full%20Book.pdf

regardless of transition status (New York City Bar et al., 2013).

LBQ women and TGNC people will also feel more comfortable when intake forms are inclusive of them, and EMR systems track key data in a manner that allows for a smooth flow at point of care. For example, the options of married, single, widowed, and divorced have historically been inadequate for LBQ and TGNC people in committed long-term relationships who were not legally allowed to marry. While same-sex marriage is now legal across the United States, many LBQ and TGNC people remain in long-term partnerships without pursuing marriage. Similarly, simply asking if sex partners are "men, women, or both" prevents patients from giving accurate information on sexual practices if they are sexually active with TGNC people. The resource *Creating Equal Access to Quality Health Care for Transgender Patients: Transgender-Affirming Hospital Policies* provides excellent guidelines on intake form questions regarding gender identity, as well as TGNC patient rooming guidelines for facilities that offer inpatient care (New York City Bar et al., 2013).

All clinicians and staff must be required to check the patient's preferred name and pronoun before each patient interaction—whether this encounter involves placing a phone call, retrieving a patient from the waiting room, or having a clinical visit. Patients should be allowed to indicate gender-neutral pronouns such as "they/them" or "ze/zir" if this is their preference.

Prior to each clinical visit, the clinician must review the patient's sexual history and surgical history thoroughly. Having EMR functionality to keep a simple inventory of anatomy present is very helpful and allows for appropriate STI screening and preventive care (Deutsch et al., 2013).

All clinicians and staff must be fully trained to be sensitive to the needs of LBQ and TGNC patients, and to maintain their confidentiality and protect their privacy. An excellent resource for staff training is *Providing Welcoming Services and Care for LGBT People: A Learning Guide for Health Care Staff* (National LGBT Health Education Center, 2015). For clinicians, being educated includes having knowledge about both the provision and content of care. To educate themselves about the content of health care for LBQ women and TGNC

people, clinicians should read current research and other literature about LBQ and TGNC health, or attend conferences. The annual conference of the Gay and Lesbian Medical Association provides a wide spectrum of educational content. The National Transgender Health Summit is a semi-annual conference that provides both beginner- and advanced-level training in TGNC clinical care, and the Philly Trans* Health Conference and Gender Odyssey are annual events that host clinician education tracks.

Clinicians must also be willing to search for relevant clinical information, rather than simply dismiss questions that LBQ and TGNC patients might ask or assume no data are available. Clinicians should be familiar with resources such as the Gay and Lesbian Medical Association's *Cultural Competence Webinar Series*, Cardea's *Clinically Competent and Culturally Proficient Care for Transgender and Gender Nonconforming Patients* independent learning series, and the National LGBT Health Education Center's *Learning Modules*. All of these resources are available as online, on-demand webinars. Critical resources specific to TGNC health include the *Center of Excellence for Transgender Health Primary Care Protocols* (Center of Excellence for Transgender Health, 2011), *WPATH Standards of Care for the Health of Transsexual, Transgender, and Gender Nonconforming People* (World Professional Association for Transgender Health, 2012), and the Endocrine Society's *Clinical Practice Guidelines for the Endocrine Treatment of Transsexual Persons* (Hembree et al., 2009).

Regarding the provision of care, clinicians must use good communication skills. Specifically, they must use open, gender-neutral language. This consideration is particularly critical for clinicians in gynecologic and settings, who typically operate under the assumption that their patients will be both heterosexual and female identified. Clinicians should ask about important relationships, including whom the patient defines as family and partner(s). When a family member or partner is present with the patient, they should be included in the discussion and care as appropriate. Screening for IPV should be consistent with that used in all patients.

Clinicians should use a nonthreatening, nonjudgmental approach, and work specifically to build trust and make LBQ and TGNC patients feel at ease, comfortable, and safe. The clinician is responsible for setting the tone for the encounter. If the clinician is relaxed, that attitude will help the patient to relax. Clinicians should encourage disclosure of sexual orientation or gender identity when it is relevant to the presenting need. They may also disclose their own identity status, especially if they are LBQ or TGNC themselves and believe that disclosure of this fact will facilitate rapport.

To avoid patients believing that the clinician is unable to see them as a whole person—rather than as just a sexual orientation or gender identity—clinicians should always consider the full range of physical and psychosocial health problems for which the individual may be seeking care, and explain why they are asking the questions they ask. It is critical that clinicians resist the urge to ask questions out of curiosity alone. While clinicians may feel that they are connecting with LBQ or TGNC patients by asking numerous questions about the patient's coming out or transition experience, these questions are likely to feel intrusive and inappropriate to the patient who is seeking care for an unrelated issue. When left unchecked, curiosity can constitute a significant barrier to care regardless of clinician intent.

As for all patients, comfort in the examination room is important for LBQ and TGNC people. For those who have not been in a healthcare environment for a long time (or ever) since coming out about their sexual orientation or gender identity, the examination room can be particularly threatening. Examinations should be based on anatomy and organs present, not on the perceived gender of a patient. As mentioned earlier, pelvic examinations in particular can be both physically and emotionally painful for LBQ women and TGNC people. As yet, evidence-based guidance is not available on reducing pain and increasing the likelihood of obtaining adequate cervical samples for cytology screening when this is the case, particularly in transgender men taking testosterone. However, strategies that may be effective include a short course of vaginal estradiol prior to the examination, application of a topical anesthetic such as lidocaine at the time of examination, use of as small a speculum as possible, and use of an adequate amount of water-based lubricant (Bernstein, Peitzmeier, Potter, & Reisner, 2015). Collecting multiple endocervical

samples using several different types of collection instruments (i.e., broom, brush, and spatula) may also increase the likelihood of obtaining an adequate sample for cytology.

Encouraging the patient to have a support person present may also be helpful in making the patient comfortable. It may be necessary to meet with the patient several times with all clothes on before enough rapport has been built to allow for breast/chest or pelvic examinations. In some cases, patients may require anxiety medication or other support to tolerate these examinations.

Finally, clinicians should be aware of community resources and referrals, such as peer support groups and recovery programs, as well as mainstream culturally sensitive referrals. Clinicians who have created an inclusive and welcoming culture in their clinics should advertise their services in both LBQ- and TGNC-specific media and mainstream media, as well as with local community organizations. Within such a small community, LBQ and TGNC people are likely to talk freely about both good and bad experiences with clinicians and institutions. When the community finds a "good" clinician with a positive attitude toward LBQ women and TGNC people, others will go to that clinician. Open communication will allow for initial good experiences, and will also create space for patients to discuss any concerns that come up in the course of their care, allowing for positive experiences moving forward.

NEEDS OF SPECIFIC POPULATIONS
Youth

For all people, youth is a time of heightened safety and health risks, due to developmentally appropriate experimentation, boundary testing, and searching for successful coping strategies. Gay, LBQ, and TGNC youth face specific additional challenges that are similar to those of their adult peers. In a 2005–2007 survey of youth from 15 different regions in the United States, gay, LBQ, and TGNC participants reported higher rates of substance use, tobacco use, early intercourse, multiple recent sex partners, substance abuse at time of sexual intercourse, and sedentary lifestyle (Rosario et al., 2014). These findings are consistent with data from other studies, in which gay, LBQ, and TGNC youth showed higher rates of substance use and dependence than their heterosexual peers (Goldberg, Strutz, Herring, & Halpern, 2013; Keuroghlian, Shtasel, & Bassuk, 2014). Risky sexual behavior and negative reproductive outcomes are also more common among lesbian and bisexual girls than among heterosexual girls (Riskind, Tornello, Younger, & Patterson, 2014). Additionally, rates of major depression, suicidality, and suicide attempts are higher in gay, LBQ, and TGNC youth (Keuroghlian et al., 2014).

Gay, LBQ, and TGNC youth account for 30% to 45% of services accessed by homeless and street-involved youth, and they cite family rejection as the primary reason for their homelessness (Durso & Gates, 2012; Keuroghlian et al., 2014). In one study, 68% reported rejection and 54% reported abuse within their family of origin (Durso & Gates, 2012). In another study, the mean age of becoming homeless was 14 years old (Keuroghlian et al., 2014). Youth are particularly vulnerable to the negative sequelae of family rejection because, being minors with limited legal and financial autonomy, they cannot easily escape violence and harassment that are occurring within their own homes. Living in the streets may be the only immediate solution to their dilemma.

Regardless of their housing status, LBQ and TGNC youth are at increased risk of violence compared to their peers. Youth who are even *perceived* as being LBQ or TGNC are often victims of violence, regardless of actual sexual orientation or gender identity. Schools are rife with homophobic and transphobic bullying. Half of LBQ girls and three-fourths of TGNC youth have reported feeling unsafe in school due to sexual orientation or gender identity; a great number of these individuals reported harassment, physical assault, and sexual assault while at school (Center for American Progress & Movement Advancement Project, 2015; Grant et al., 2011). In a survey of school counselors, 16% stated that they observed homophobic or transphobic harassment on at least a monthly basis (McCabe et al., 2013). Casual use of homophobic phrases (e.g., "That's so gay") in the school environment is common and not limited to students; counselors reported frequently hearing staff members making such comments in front of students (McCabe et al., 2013).

Self-reports from TGNC people are consistent with these observations by school counselors. In the National Transgender Discrimination Survey, 31% of respondents reported bullying by teachers or staff between kindergarten and twelfth grade; 5% reported physical assault and 3% reported sexual assault by teachers or staff during this same time period. Rates of harassment by teachers and staff were greatest among Latino/a and mixed-race respondents (Grant et al., 2011). As with abuse in families of origin, the available remedies to this harassment are limited by imbalances of power between youth and the adults and systems that are charged with their care. Many students drop out to avoid harassment, or are expelled for factors related to their sexual orientation or gender identity.

LBQ and TGNC youth who access homeless shelters and drop-in centers are challenged by many of the same risks faced in the school environment, as well as the risk of exploitation by adults accessing services in the same spaces. The chance of emotional harassment and physical or sexual assault increases when youth are required to share sleeping areas, showers, or restrooms with people of a different gender identity—for example, a transgender girl being forced to use the boys' bathroom and shower area (Keuroghlian et al., 2014). Due to the dangers of shelter environments, homeless gay, LBQ, and TGNC youth are three times more likely than their peers to seek shelter with a stranger, which exposes them to additional risks for sexual exploitation (Keuroghlian et al., 2014). Overall, homeless gay, LBQ, and TGNC youth are 70% more likely than their peers to engage in transactional sex (Keuroghlian et al., 2014). This is particularly true for African American, mixed-race, and TGNC youth (Walls & Bell, 2011).

Older Adults

In 2014, there were an estimated 3 million gay and LBQ older adults (older than age 65) living in the United States (Hillman & Hinrichsen, 2014). Older people, and especially older women, often experience age discrimination. Older LBQ women and TGNC people also experience sexism, heterosexism, transphobia, and other forms of oppression such as racism.

Overall, gay, LBQ, and TGNC older adults have more concerns about aging than do their heterosexual peers (Gabrielson, 2011). Typical social and familiar supports, such as having a partner in older age or having adult children, are less likely to be in place for these older adults than their heterosexual and cisgender peers, and family rejection may separate LBQ and TGNC older adults from extended family support systems and a "crisis support network" (Gabrielson, 2011; Hillman & Hinrichsen, 2014).

Data from the 2003–2010 Washington State Behavioral Risk Surveillance System indicate higher rates of disability, mental health concerns, tobacco use, and binge drinking in this group of older adults versus their heterosexual peers (Fredriksen-Goldsen, Kim, Barkan, Muraco, & Hoy-Ellis, 2013). These disparities could be related to surviving an era in which the risk of homophobic violence and harassment was very high, as well as a long duration of exposure to minority stress (Fredriksen-Goldsen et al., 2013; Hillman & Hinrichsen, 2014).

Gay, LBQ, and TGNC older adults are two times more likely to live in poverty than their heterosexual counterparts. This is due to both higher lifetime poverty rates for these populations and Medicaid and Social Security regulations that penalize same-sex couples (Center for American Progress & Movement Advancement Project, 2015). Medicaid rules that protect spouses from impoverishment secondary to their partner's medical expenses do not extend to unmarried same-sex couples and, in some states, to those who are married. Similarly, Social Security spousal benefits are not available to most unmarried same-sex couples (Center for American Progress & Movement Advancement Project, 2015). It remains to be seen if equity in partner benefits will be achieved in the future as a result of legalization of same-sex marriage nationwide.

Many LBQ and TGNC older adults turn to the "chosen family" they have created over the course of their lifetime for emotional, logistical, and financial support as they age. For some, however, this is not possible. As survivors of the AIDS epidemic, many older adults may have lost a large proportion of their community and chosen family (Hillman & Hinrichsen, 2014). Even when good social supports are in place, LBQ and TGNC older adults are particularly vulnerable to abuse, neglect, and poverty. In institutional settings, rates of older adult abuse are higher among gay, LBQ, and TGNC residents (Hillman & Hinrichsen, 2014). As a result, many older adults stay independently housed as long as possible; losing the ability to stay at home is equated to losing the ability to exercise control over one's safety, and often the ability to live authentically as well. When transfer to a care setting is imminent, many older adults feel forced to "go back into the closet." Some have described using a number of strategies to conceal their sexual orientation, including hiding treasured mementos of a partner who has passed away, actively pretending to be heterosexual, and even legally changing the person's last name to that of the partner to present the couple as siblings and request a shared housing placement (Hillman & Hinrichsen, 2014). In response to this, a number of gay, LBQ, and TGNC retirement communities and housing programs have begun to appear across the United States.

People with Disabilities

All people with disabilities face barriers to health care, but this difficulty in accessing needed care is compounded for LBQ women and TGNC people. The term *disability* refers to a wide range of physical, emotional, and intellectual differences, including both visible disabilities, such as deafness and mobility challenges, and more invisible disabilities, such as intellectual disabilities, mental health problems, and chronic illness. Disabilities may be lifelong or acquired, and vary in their impact on activities of daily living.

The prevalence of disabilities may be higher among LBQ women and TGNC people than in the general population (Fredriksen-Goldsen, Kim, & Barkan, 2012; Siordia, 2014). LBQ women and TGNC people with disabilities share common challenges and vulnerabilities faced by heterosexual people with disabilities, as well as common challenges and vulnerabilities faced by other LBQ women and TGNC people. Many people with disabilities experience violence; in 2013, for example, 31.62% of all hate violence in the United States was perpetuated against people with disabilities. Of these victims, 36.78% had a physical disability and 50% had a mental health disability (Ahmed & Jindasurat, 2014). In a study of college students with and without auditory deficits, students who were deaf or hard of hearing *and* gay, LBQ, or TGNC identified were more likely than other students to experience interpersonal violence; this was especially true for physical violence and emotional abuse (Porter & McQuiller Williams, 2013).

Of particular concern regarding gynecologic health is the fact that many clinicians are hesitant to discuss sexuality with people who have physical or intellectual disabilities or a chronic illness, or perceive these people as being nonsexual (Dune, 2012; Noonan & Gomez, 2011). When people with disabilities are seen as potentially sexual, they are usually assumed to be heterosexual (Noonan & Gomez, 2011). As is true for all people, incorrect clinician assumptions regarding sexual behaviors may lead to inappropriate screening and assessment for sexual health, and can increase the risk of undiagnosed STIs. Additionally, LBQ and TGNC people with disabilities who rely on caregivers for activities of daily living or social support often face denial of access to sexual information and sexual expression (Noonan & Gomez, 2011). Consequently, it is incumbent upon clinicians to not only provide the same quality of care for LBQ women and TGNC people with disabilities as they offer to all patients, but also actively initiate discussion of sexual health and provide accurate, accessible information that supports a full range of sexual expression.

CONCLUSION

This chapter has described some of the unique health needs of LBQ women and TGNC people. Much more needs to be understood about the healthcare needs of this population, and the research base in this area is growing. Clinicians must strive to provide culturally responsive care to their LBQ and TGNC patients. Given that health professionals' education continues to lag behind in clinical content relevant to care of LBQ women and TGNC people, ensuring that they meet this standard will require concerted effort and advocacy on the part of clinicians.

References

Abdessamad, H. M., Yudin, M. H., Tarasoff, L. A., Radford, K. D., & Ross, L. E. (2013). Attitudes and knowledge among obstetrician-gynecologists regarding lesbian patients and their health. *Journal of Women's Health, 22*(1), 85–93. doi:10.1089/jwh.2012.3718

Addison, B. (2014). LGBT history: The gay bar as church. *Long Beach Post*. Retrieved from http://lbpost.com/lgbt/2000003213-the-gay-bar-as-church-local-academic-explores-gay-bars-as-religious-experience-in-book

Agénor, M., Krieger, N., Austin, S. B., Haneuse, S., & Gottlieb, B. R. (2014). Sexual orientation disparities in Papanicolaou test use among US women: The role of sexual and reproductive health services. *American Journal of Public Health, 104*(2), e68–e73. doi:10.2105/AJPH.2013.301548

Agrawal, R., Sharma, S., Bekir, J., Conway, G., Bailey, J., Balen, A. H., & Prelevic, G. (2004). Prevalence of polycystic ovaries and polycystic ovary syndrome in lesbian women compared with heterosexual women. *Fertility and Sterility, 82*(5), 1352–1357. doi:10.1016/j.fertnstert.2004.04.041

Ahmed, O., & Jindasurat, C. (2014). *Lesbian, gay, bisexual, transgender, queer and HIV-affected hate violence 2013*. New York, NY: National Coalition of Anti-Violence Programs.

Ålgars, M., Alanko, K., Santtila, P., & Sandnabba, N. K. (2012). Disordered eating and gender identity disorder: A qualitative study. *Eating Disorders, 20*, 300–311. doi:10.1080/10640266.2012.668482

American College of Nurse-Midwives. (2012). *Position statement: Transgender/transsexual/gender variant health care*. Silver Spring, MD: Author.

American College of Nurse-Midwives. (2014). *Position statement: Health care for all families*. Silver Spring, MD: Author.

American College of Obstetricians and Gynecologists. (2011). Committe opinion: Health care for transgender individuals. *Obstetrics & Gynecology, 118*(6), 1454–1458. doi:10.1097/AOG.0b013e31823ed1c1

American College of Obstetricians and Gynecologists. (2012). Committee opinion: Health care for lesbian and bisexual women. *Obstetrics & Gynecology, 119*(5), 1077–1080. doi:10.1300/J291v01n03_07

American College of Obstetricians and Gynecologists. (2013). Committee opinion: Marriage equality for same-sex couples. *Obstetrics & Gynecology, 122*(3), 729–732. doi:10.1097/01.AOG.0000433995.46087.cc

Asscheman, H., Giltay, E. J., Megens, J. A. J., De Ronde, W., Van Trotsenburg, M. A. A., & Gooren, L. J. G. (2011). A long-term follow-up study of mortality in transsexuals receiving treatment with cross-sex hormones. *European Journal of Endocrinology, 164*, 635–642. doi:10.1530/EJE-10-1038

Auer, M. K., Fuss, J., Höhne, N., Stalla, G. K., & Sievers, C. (2014). Transgender transitioning and change of self-reported sexual orientation. *PLoS ONE, 9*(10). doi:10.1371/journal.pone.0110016

Austin, S. B., Pazaris, M. J., Nichols, L. P., Bowen, D., Wei, E. K., & Spiegelman, D. (2013). An examination of sexual orientation group patterns in mammographic and colorectal screening in a cohort of U.S. women. *Cancer Causes and Control, 24*, 539–547. doi:10.1007/s10552-012-9991-0

Baba, T., Endo, T., Honnma, H., Kitajima, Y., Hayashi, T., Ikeda, H., . . . Saito, T. (2007). Association between polycystic ovary syndrome and female-to-male transsexuality. *Human Reproduction, 22*(4), 1011–1016. doi:10.1093/humrep/del474

Bacon, L., & Aphramor, L. (2011). Weight science: Evaluating the evidence for a paradigm shift. *Nutrition Journal*, *10*(9), 1–13. doi:10.1186/1475-2891-10-9

Balen, A. H., Schachter, M. E., Montgomery, D., Reid, R. W., & Jacobs, H. S. (1993). Polycystic ovaries are a common finding in untreated female to male transsexuals. *Clinical Endocrinology*, *38*(3), 325–329. doi:10.1111/j.1365

Balsam, K. F., Molina, Y., Beadnell, B., Simoni, J., & Walters, K. (2011). Measuring multiple minority stress: The LGBT People of Color Microaggressions Scale. *Cultural Diversity & Ethnic Minority Psychology*, *17*(2), 163–174. doi:10.1037/a0023244

Beemyn, G. (2014). *Transgender history in the United States: A special unabridged version of a book chapter from Trans Bodies, Trans Selves* (L. Erickson-Schroth, Ed.). New York, NY: Oxford University Press. Retrieved from http://www.umass.edu/stonewall/uploads/listWidget/32733/trans%20hist%20ebook.pdf

Bernstein, I., Peitzmeier, S., Potter, J., & Reisner, S. (2015). *If you have it, check it: Overcoming barriers to cervical cancer screening with patients on the female-to-male transgender spectrum*. Boston, MA: National LGBT Health Education Center.

Blosnich, J. R., Farmer, G. W., Lee, J. G. L., Silenzio, V. M. B., & Bowen, D. J. (2014). Health inequalities among sexual minority adults: Evidence from ten U.S. states, 2010. *American Journal of Preventive Medicine*, *46*(4), 337–349. doi:10.1016/j.amepre.2013.11.010

Blosnich, J., Lee, J. G. L., & Horn, K. (2011). A systematic review of the aetiology of tobacco disparities for sexual minorities. *Tobacco Control*, *22*, 66–73. doi:10.1136/tobaccocontrol-2011-050181

Brown, G. R., & Jones, K. T. (2014). Incidence of breast cancer in a cohort of 5,135 transgender veterans. *Breast Cancer Research and Treatment*, *149*, 191–198. doi:10.1007/s10549-014-3213-2

Callahan, E. J., Hazarian, S., Yarborough, M., & Sánchez, J. P. (2014). Eliminating LGBTIQQ health disparities: The associated roles of electronic health records and institutional culture. *LGBT Bioethics: Visability, Disparities, and Dialogue, Special Report, Hastings Center Report 44*, *5*, 48–52. doi:10.1002/hast.371

Campos-Outcalt, D., & Hurwitz, S. (2002). Female-to-female transmission of syphilis: A case report. *Sexually Transmitted Diseases*, *29*, 119.

Center for American Progress & Movement Advancement Project. (2015). *Paying an unfair price: The financial penalty for LGBT women in America*. Washington, DC: Author.

Center of Excellence for Transgender Health. (2011). *Primary care protocols for transgender patient care*. San Francisco, CA: University of California, San Francisco, Department of Family and Community Medicine.

Centers for Disease Control and Prevention (CDC). (2013). HIV among transgender people. Retrieved from http://www.cdc.gov/hiv/risk/transgender

Chan, S. K., Thornton, L. R., Chronister, K. J., Meyer, J., Wolverton, M., Johnson, C. K., . . . Sullivan, V. (2014). Likely female-to-female sexual transmission of HIV—Texas, 2012. *Morbidity and Mortality Weekly Report*, *63*(10), 209–212.

Chansanchair, A. (2015). The end of an ordinary life. *Seattle Post-Intelligencer*. Retrieved from http://www.seattlepi.com/local/article/The-end-of-an-ordinary-life-1301899.php

Charlton, B. M., Corliss, H. L., Missmer, S. A., Frazier, A. L., Rosario, M., Kahn, J. A., & Austin, S. B. (2014). Influence of hormonal contraceptive use and health beliefs on sexual orientation disparities in Papanicolaou test use. *American Journal of Public Health*, *104*(2), 319–325. doi:10.2105/AJPH.2012.301114

Cochran, S. D., & Mays, V. M. (2012). Risk of breast cancer mortality among women cohabiting with same sex partners: Findings from the National Health Interview Survey, 1997–2003. *Journal of Women's Health*, *21*(5), 528–533. doi:10.1089/jwh.2011.3134

Cochran, S. D., & Mays, V. M. (2015). Mortality risks among persons reporting same-sex sexual partners: Evidence from the 2008 General Social Survey—National Death Index data set. *American Journal of Public Health*, *105*(2), 358–364. doi:10.1055/s-0029-1237430

Deputy, N. P., & Boehmer, U. (2014). Weight status and sexual orientation: Differences by age and within racial and ethnic subgroups. *American Journal of Public Health*, *104*(1), 103–109. doi:10.2105/AJPH.2013.301391

De Sutter, P., Dutré, T., Vanden Meerschaut, F., Stuyver, I., Van Maele, G., & Dhont, M. (2008). PCOS in lesbian and heterosexual women treated with artificial donor insemination. *Reproductive Biomedicine Online*, *17*(3), 398–402. doi:10.1016/S1472-6483(10)60224-6

Deutsch, M. B., Green, J., Keatley, J., Mayer, G., Hastings, J., & Hall, A. M. (2013). Electronic medical records and the transgender patient: Recommendations from the World Professional Association for Transgender Health EMR Working Group. *Journal of the American Medical Informatics Association*, *20*, 700–703. doi:10.1136/amiajnl-2012-001472

Dias, I. B. F., Panazzolo, D. G., Marques, M. F., Paredes, B. D., Souza, M. G. C., Manhanini, D. P., . . . Kraemer-Aguiar, L. G. (2013). Relationships between emerging cardiovascular risk factors, z-BMI, waist circumference and body adiposity index (BAI) on adolescents. *Clinical Endocrinology*, *79*(5), 667–674. doi:10.1111/cen.12195

Dibble, S. L., Roberts, S. A., Robertson, P. A., & Paul, S. M. (2002). Risk factors for ovarian cancer: Lesbian and heterosexual women. *Oncology Nursing Forum*, *29*(1), E1–E7.

Diemer, E. W., Grant, J. D., Munn-Chernoff, M. A., Patterson, D. A., & Duncan, A. E. (2015). Gender identity, sexual orientation, and eating-related pathology in a national sample of college students. *Journal of Adolescent Health*, *57*(2), 1–6. doi:10.1016/j.jadohealth.2015.03.003

Dune, T. M. (2012). Sexuality and physical disability: Exploring barriers and solutions in healthcare. *Sexuality and Disability*, *30*(2), 247–255. doi:10.1007/s11195-012-9262-8

Durso, L. E., & Gates, G. J. (2012). *Serving our youth: Findings from a national survey of services providers working with lesbian, gay, bisexual and transgender youth who are homeless or at risk of becoming homeless*. Los Angeles, CA: Williams Institute, True Colors Fund, & Palette Fund.

El Hakim, E. A., & Wardle, P. (2010). Polycystic ovary syndrome. *Practice Nurse*, *40*(1), 21–24.

Ellis, S. A., Wojnar, D. M., & Pettinato, M. (2014). Conception, pregnancy, and birth experiences of male and gender variant gestational parents: It's how we could have a family. *Journal of Midwifery & Women's Health*, *60*(1), 62–69. doi:10.1111/jmwh.12213

Estrich, C. G., Gratzer, B., & Hotton, A. L. (2014). Differences in sexual health, risk behaviors, and substance use among women by sexual identity: Chicago, 2009–2011. *Sexually Transmitted Diseases*, *41*(3), 194–199. doi:10.1097/OLQ.0000000000000091

Everett, B., & Mollborn, S. (2013). Differences in hypertension by sexual orientation among U.S. Young adults. *Journal of Community Health*, *38*, 588–596. doi:10.1007/s10900-013-9655-3

Family Equality Council. (2015). Equality maps: Joint adoption laws. Retrieved from http://www.familyequality.org/get_informed/equality_maps/joint_adoption_laws

Farmer, G. W., Jabson, J. M., Bucholz, K. K., & Bowen, D. J. (2013). A population-based study of cardiovascular disease risk in sexual-minority women. *American Journal of Public Health*, *103*(10), 1845–1850. doi:10.2105/AJPH.2013.301258

Feldman, J., Romine, R. S., & Bockting, W. O. (2014). HIV risk behaviors in the U.S. transgender population: Prevalence and predictors in a large Internet sample. *Journal of Homosexuality*, *61*, 1558–1588. doi:10.1080/00918369.2014.944048

Fenway Institute. (2009). *Ending invisibility: Better care for LGBT populations*. Boston, MA: Author.

Fikkan, J. L., & Rothblum, E. D. (2012). Is fat a feminist issue? Exploring the gendered nature of weight bias. *Sex Roles*, *66*(9–10), 575–592. doi:10.1007/s11199-011-0022-5

FORGE. (2012). Terms paradox. Retrieved from http://forge-forward .org/2012/06/terms-paradox

Fredriksen-Goldsen, K. I., Kim, H. J., & Barkan, S. E. (2012). Disability among lesbian, gay, and bisexual adults: Disparities in prevalence and risk. *American Journal of Public Health*, *102*(1), 16–22. doi:10.2105/AJPH.2011.300379

Fredriksen-Goldsen, K. I., Kim, H.-J., Barkan, S. E., Muraco, A., & Hoy-Ellis, C. P. (2013). Health disparities among lesbian, gay, and bisexual older adults: Results from a population-based study. *American Journal of Public Health*, *103*(10), 1802–1809. doi:10.2105/AJPH.2012.301110

Friedman, S., Reynolds, A., & Scovill, S. (2013). *An estimate of housing discrimination against same-sex couples*. Washington, DC: U.S. Department of Housing and Urban Development.

Frost, D. M., Lehavot, K., & Meyer, I. H. (2013). Minority stress and physical health among sexual minority individuals. *Journal of Behavioral Medicine*, *38*, 1–8. doi:10.1007/s10865-013-9523-8

Gabrielson, M. L. (2011). "We have to create family": Aging support issues and needs among older lesbians. *Journal of Gay & Lesbian Social Services*, *23*, 322–334. doi:10.1080/10538720.2011. 562803

Goldberg, S., Strutz, K. L., Herring, A. A., & Halpern, C. T. (2013). Risk of substance abuse and dependence among young adult sexual minority groups using a multidimensional measure of sexual orientation. *Public Health Reports*, *128*, 144–152.

Gómez-Gil, E., Zubiaurre-Elorza, L., Esteva, I., Guillamon, A., Godás, T., Cruz Almaraz, M., . . . Salamero, M. (2012). Hormone-treated transsexuals report less social distress, anxiety and depression. *Psychoneuroendocrinology*, *37*(5), 662–670. doi:10.1016/ j.psyneuen.2011.08.010

Gooren, L. J., van Trotsenburg, M. A. A., Giltay, E. J., & van Diest, P. J. (2013). Breast cancer development in transsexual subjects receiving cross-sex hormone treatment. *Journal of Sexual Medicine*, *10*, 3129–3134. doi:10.1111/jsm.12319

Gorgos, L. M., & Marrazzo, J. M. (2011). Sexually transmitted infections among women who have sex with women. *Clinical Infectious Diseases*, *53*(suppl 3). doi:10.1093/cid/cir697

Grant, J. M., Mottet, L. A., Tanis, J., Harrison, J., Herman, J. L., & Keisling, M. (2011). *Injustice at every turn: A report of the National Transgender Discrimination Survey*. Washington, DC: National Center for Transgender Equality & National Gay and Lesbian Task Force.

Hanneman, T. (2014). *Healthcare equality index 2014*. Washington, DC: Human Rights Campaign.

Hatzenbuehler, M. L., McLaughlin, K. A., Keyes, K. M., & Hasin, D. S. (2010). The impact of institutional discrimination on psychiatric disorders in lesbian, gay, and bisexual populations: A prospective study. *American Journal of Public Health*, *100*(3), 452–459. doi:10.2105/AJPH.2009.168815

Hatzenbuehler, M. L., McLaughlin, K. A., & Slopen, N. (2013). Sexual orientation disparities in cardiovascular biomarkers among

young adults. *American Journal of Preventive Medicine*, *44*(6), 612–621. doi:10.1016/j.amepre.2013.01.027

Hembree, W. C., Cohen-Kettenis, P., Delemarre-van de Waal, H. A., Gooren, L. J., Meyer, W. J., III, Spack, N. P., . . . Montori, V. M. (2009). Endocrine treatment of transsexual persons: An endocrine society clinical practice guideline. *Journal of Clinical Endocrinology and Metabolism*, *94*, 3132–3154. doi:10.1210/jc.2009-0345

Hillman, J., & Hinrichsen, G. A. (2014). Promoting an affirming, competent practice with older lesbian and gay adults. *Professional Psychology: Research and Practice*, *45*(4), 269–277. doi:10.1037/ a0037172

Human Rights Campaign. (2015). Maps of state laws & policies. Retrieved from http://www.hrc.org/state_maps

Huxley, C. J., Clarke, V., & Halliwell, E. (2014). A qualitative exploration of whether lesbian and bisexual women are "protected" from sociocultural pressure to be thin. *Journal of Health Psychology*, *19*, 273–284. doi:10.1177/1359105312468496

Ikeda, K., Baba, T., Noguchi, H., Nagasawa, K., Endo, T., Kiya, T., & Saito, T. (2013). Excessive androgen exposure in female-to-male transsexual persons of reproductive age induces hyperplasia of the ovarian cortex and stroma but not polycystic ovary morphology. *Human Reproduction*, *28*(2), 453–461. doi:10.1093/ humrep/des385

Institute of Medicine. (2011). *The health of lesbian, gay, bisexual, and transgender people: Building a foundation for better understanding*. Washington, DC: National Academies Press.

Jabson, J. M., Donatelle, R. J., & Bowen, D. J. (2011). Relationship between sexual orientation and quality of life in female breast cancer survivors. *Journal of Women's Health*, *20*(12), 1819–1824. doi:10.1089/jwh.2011.2921

Jun, H.-J., Corliss, H. L., Nichols, L. P., Pazaris, M. J., Spiegelman, D., & Austin, S. B. (2012). Adult body mass index trajectories and sexual orientation. *American Journal of Preventive Medicine*, *42*(4), 348–354. doi:10.1016/j.amepre.2011.11.011

Kellaway, M., & Brydum, S. (2016, January). The 21 trans women killed in 2015. *The Advocate*. Retrieved from http://www .advocate.com/transgender/2015/07/27/these-are-trans -women-killed-so-far-us-2015

Kellock, D., & O'Mahony, C. P. (1996). Sexually acquired metronidazole-resistant trichomoniasis in a lesbian couple. *Genitourinary Medicine*, *72*(1), 60–61. doi:10.1136/sti.72.1.60

Keo-Meier, C. L., Herman, L. I., Reisner, S. L., Pardo, S. T., Sharp, C., & Babcock, J. C. (2015). Testosterone treatment and MMPI-2 improvement in transgender men: A prospective controlled study. *Journal of Consulting and Clinical Psychology*, *83*(1), 143–156.

Kerr, D. L., Ding, K., & Chaya, J. (2014). Substance use of lesbian, gay, bisexual and heterosexual college students. *American Journal of Health Behavior*, *38*(6), 951–962.

Keuroghlian, A. S., Shtasel, D., & Bassuk, E. L. (2014). Out on the street: A public health and policy agenda for lesbian, gay, bisexual, and transgender youth who are homeless. *American Journal of Orthopsychiatry*, *84*(1), 66–72. doi:10.1037/h0098852

Kim, H. J., & Fredriksen-Goldsen, K. I. (2012). Hispanic lesbians and bisexual women at heightened risk or health disparities. *American Journal of Public Health*, *102*(1), 9–16. doi:10.2105/ AJPH.2011.300378

Kubicek, K., Beyer, W. H., McNeeley, M., Weiss, G., Omni, L. F. T. U., & Kipke, M. D. (2013). Community-engaged research to identify house parent perspectives on support and risk within the House and Ball scene. *Journal of Sex Research*, *50*(2), 1–12. doi:10.1080 /00224499.2011.637248

Kuper, L. E., Nussbaum, R., & Mustanski, B. (2012). Exploring the diversity of gender and sexual orientation identities in an online sample of transgender individuals. *Journal of Sex Research, 49,* 244–254. doi:10.1080/00224499.2011.596954

Lambda Legal. (2010). *When health care isn't caring: Lambda Legal's survey on discrimination against LGBT people and people living with HIV.* New York, NY: Author.

Lee, J., & Hahm, H. C. (2012). HIV risk, substance use, and suicidal behaviors among Asian American lesbian and bisexual women. *AIDS Education and Prevention, 24*(6), 549–563. doi:10.1521/aeap.2012.24.6.549

Lick, D. J., Durso, L. E., & Johnson, K. L. (2013). Minority stress and physical health among sexual minorities. *Perspectives on Psychological Science, 8,* 521–548. doi:10.1177/1745691613497965

Light, A. D., Obedin-Maliver, J., Sevelius, J. M., & Kerns, J. L. (2014). Transgender men who experienced pregnancy after female-to-male gender transitioning. *Obstetrics & Gynecology, 124*(6), 1120–1127. doi:10.1097/AOG.0000000000000540

Makadon, H. J., Mayer, K. H., Potter, J., & Goldhammer, H. (2010). *The Fenway guide to lesbian, gay, bisexual, and transgender health.* Philadelphia, PA: American College of Physicians.

March, W. A., Moore, V. M., Willson, K. J., Phillips, D. I. W., Norman, R. J., & Davies, M. J. (2010). The prevalence of polycystic ovary syndrome in a community sample assessed under contrasting diagnostic criteria. *Human Reproduction, 25*(2), 544–551. doi:10.1093/humrep/dep399

Markey, C. N., & Markey, P. M. (2013). Gender, sexual orientation, and romantic partner influence on body image: An examination of heterosexual and lesbian women and their partners. *Journal of Social and Personal Relationships, 31*(2), 162–177. doi:10.1177/0265407513489472

Marrazzo, J. M., Koutsky, L. A., Kiviat, N. B., Kuypers, J. M., & Stine, K. (2001). Papanicolaou test screening and prevalence of genital human papillomavirus among women who have sex with women. *American Journal of Public Health, 91*(6), 947–952. doi:10.1097/00128360-200201000-00017

Marrazzo, J. M., Stine, K., & Wald, A. (2003). Prevalence and risk factors for infection with herpes simplex virus type-1 and -2 among lesbians. *Sexually Transmitted Diseases, 30,* 890–895.

Marrazzo, J. M., Thomas, K. K., Agnew, K., & Ringwood, K. (2010). Prevalence and risks for bacterial vaginosis in women who have sex with women. *Sexually Transmitted Diseases, 37*(5), 335–339. doi:10.1097/OLQ.0b013e3181ca3cac

Marrazzo, J. M., Thomas, K. K., & Ringwood, K. (2011). A behavioural intervention to reduce persistence of bacterial vaginosis among women who report sex with women: Results of a randomised trial. *Sexually Transmitted Infections, 87,* 399–405. doi:10.1136/sti.2011.049213

McCabe, P. C., Dragowski, E. A., & Rubinson, F. (2013). What is homophobic bias anyway? Defining and recognizing microaggressions and harassment of LGBTQ youth. *Journal of School Violence, 12,* 7–26. doi:10.1080/15388220.2012.731664

McGarrity, L. A. (2014). Socioeconomic status as context for minority stress and health disparities among lesbian, gay, and bisexual individuals. *Psychology of Sexual Orientation and Gender Diversity, 1*(4), 383–397.

Meads, C., & Moore, D. (2013). Breast cancer in lesbians and bisexual women: Systematic review of incidence, prevalence and risk studies. *BMC Public Health, 13,* 1127. doi:10.1186/1471-2458-13-1127

Minkin, M. J. (2010). Sexually transmitted infections and the aging female: Placing risks in perspective. *Maturitas, 67*(2), 114–116. doi:10.1016/j.maturitas.2010.05.003

Miranda, K., Pace, D. A., Cintron, R., Rodrigues, J. C. F., Fang, J., Smith, A., . . . Moreno, S. N. J. (2010). Sexually transmitted

disease (STD) diagnoses and mental health disparities among women who have sex with women screened at an urban community center, Boston, Massachusetts, 2007. *Sexually Transmitted Disease, 37*(1), 1358–1375. doi:10.1111/j.1365-2958.2010.07165.x. Characterization

Mock, S. E., & Eibach, R. P. (2012). Stability and change in sexual orientation identity over a 10-year period in adulthood. *Archives of Sexual Behavior, 41*(3), 641–648. doi:10.1007/s10508-011-9761-1

Murad, M. H., Elamin, M. B., Garcia, M. Z., Mullan, R. J., Murad, A., Erwin, P. J., & Montori, V. M. (2010). Hormonal therapy and sex reassignment: A systematic review and meta-analysis of quality of life and psychosocial outcomes. *Clinical Endocrinology, 72,* 214–231. doi:10.1111/j.1365-2265.2009.03625.x

Muzny, C. A., Sunesara, I. R., Austin, E. L., Mena, L. A., & Schwebke, J. R. (2013). Bacterial vaginosis among African American women who have sex with women. *Sexually Transmitted Diseases, 40*(9), 751–755. doi:10.1097/OLQ.0000000000000004

Muzny, C. A., Sunesara, I. R., Martin, D. H., & Mena, L. A. (2011). Sexually transmitted infections and risk behaviors among African American women who have sex with women: Does sex with men make a difference? *Sexually Transmitted Diseases, 38*(12), 1118–1125. doi:10.1097/OLQ.0b013e31822e6179

National Center for Victims of Crime & National Coalition of Anti-Violence Programs. (2010). *Why it matters: Rethinking victim assistance for lesbian, gay, bisexual, transgender, and queer victims of hate violence and intimate partner violence.* Washington, DC: Authors.

National LGBT Health Education Center. (2015). *Providing welcoming services and care for LGBT people: A learning guide for health care staff.* Boston, MA: Author.

New York City Bar, Lambda Legal, & Human Rights Campaign Foundation. (2013). *Creating equal access to quality health care for transgender patients: Transgender-affirming hospital policies.* New York, NY/Washington, DC: Authors.

Noonan, A., & Gomez, M. T. (2011). Who's missing? Awareness of lesbian, gay, bisexual and transgender people with intellectual disability. *Sexuality and Disability, 29*(2), 175–180. doi:10.1007/s11195-010-9175-3

Nuttbrock, L., Bockting, W., Rosenblum, A., Hwahng, S., Mason, M., Macri, M., & Becker, J. (2013). Gender abuse and major depression among transgender women: A prospective study of vulnerability and resilience. *American Journal of Public Health, 104*(11), 1–8. doi:10.2105/AJPH.2013.301545

Obama, B. (2010). Presidential memorandum: Hospital visitation. Retrieved from http://www.whitehouse.gov/the-press-office/presidential-memorandum-hospital-visitation

Obedin-Maliver, J., Goldsmith, E. S., Stewart, L., White, W., Brenman, S., Wells, M., . . . Lunn, M. R. (2011). Lesbian, gay, bisexual, and transgender-related content in undergraduate medical education. *Journal of the American Medical Association, 306*(9), 971–977. doi:10.1001/jama.2011.1255.ABSTRACT

Ott, M. Q., Corliss, H. L., Wypij, D., Rosario, M., & Austin, S. B. (2011). Stability and change in self-reported sexual orientation identity in young people: Application of mobility metrics. *Archives of Sexual Behavior, 40*(3), 519–532. doi:10.1007/s10508-010-9691-3

Peel, E. (2010). Pregnancy loss in lesbian and bisexual women: An online survey of experiences. *Human Reproduction, 25*(3), 721–727. doi:10.1093/humrep/dep441

Peitzmeier, S. M., Khullar, K., Reisner, S. L., & Potter, J. (2014). Pap test use is lower among female-to-male patients than non-transgender women. *American Journal of Preventive Medicine, 47*(6), 808–812.

Peitzmeier, S. M., Reisner, S. L., Harigopal, P., & Potter, J. (2014). Female-to-male patients have high prevalence of unsatisfactory Paps compared to non-transgender females: Implications for cervical cancer screening. *Journal of General Internal Medicine*, *29*(5), 778–784. doi:10.1007/s11606-013-2753-1

Petricevic, L., Kaufmann, U., Domig, K. J., Kraler, M., Marschalek, J., Kneifel, W., & Kiss, H. (2014). Molecular detection of *Lactobacillus* species in the neovagina of male-to-female transsexual women. *Scientific Reports*, *4*(3746), 1–4. doi:10.1038/srep03746

Pew Research Center. (2013). *A survey of LGBT Americans: Attitudes, experiences and values in changing times*. Washington, DC: Author.

Porter, J. L., & McQuiller Williams, L. (2013). Dual marginality: The impact of auditory status and sexual orientation on abuse in a college sample of women and men. *Journal of Aggression, Maltreatment & Trauma*, *22*(1999), 577–589. doi:10.1080/10926771.2013.805175

Przedworski, J. M., McAlpine, D. D., Karaca-Mandic, P., & VanKim, N. A. (2014). Health and health risks among sexual minority women: An examination of 3 subgroups. *American Journal of Public Health*, *104*(6), 1045–1047. doi:10.2105/AJPH.2013.301733

Ranji, U., Beamesderfer, A., Kates, J., & Salganicoff, A. (2014). *Health and access to care and coverage for lesbian, gay, bisexual , and transgender individuals in the U.S.* Menlo Park, CA: Henry J. Kaiser Family Foundation.

Reisner, S. L., Lloyd, J., & Baral, S. (2013). *Technical report: The global health needs of transgender populations*. Arlington, VA: USAID's AIDS Support and Technical Assistance Resources, AIDSTAR-Two, Task Order 2.

Reisner, S. L., Perkovich, B., & Mimiaga, M. J. (2010). A mixed methods study of the sexual health needs of New England transmen who have sex with nontransgender men. *AIDS Patient Care and STDs*, *24*(8), 501–513. doi:10.1089/apc.2010.0059

Riskind, R. G., Tornello, S. L., Younger, B. C., & Patterson, C. J. (2014). Sexual identity, partner gender, and sexual health among adolescent girls in the United States. *American Journal of Public Health*, *104*(10), 1957–1963. doi:10.2105/AJPH.2014.302037

Roberson, L. L., Aneni, E. C., Maziak, W., Agatston, A., Feldman, T., Rouseff, M., . . . Nasir, K. (2014). Beyond BMI: The "metabolically healthy obese" phenotype and its association with clinical/subclinical cardiovascular disease and all-cause mortality: A systematic review. *BMC Public Health*, *14*(1), 14. doi:10.1186/1471-2458-14-14

Roberts, S. J., Stuart-Shor, E. M., & Oppenheimer, R. A. (2010). Lesbians' attitudes and beliefs regarding overweight and weight reduction. *Journal of Clinical Nursing*, *19*, 1986–1994. doi:10.1111/j.1365-2702.2009.03182.x

Rogers, W. A. (2006). Feminism and public health ethics. *Journal of Medical Ethics*, *32*(6), 351–354. doi:10.1136/jme.2005.013466

Rosario, M., Corliss, H. L., Everett, B. G., Reisner, S. L., Austin, S. B., Buchting, F. O., & Birkett, M. (2014). Sexual orientation disparities in cancer-related risk behaviors of tobacco, alcohol, sexual behaviors, and diet and physical activity: Pooled youth risk behavior surveys. *American Journal of Public Health*, *104*(2), 245–254. doi:10.2105/AJPH.2013.301506

Rounds, K. E., McGrath, B. B., & Walsh, E. (2013). Perspectives on provider behaviors: A qualitative study of sexual and gender minorities regarding quality of care. *Contemporary Nurse*, *44*(1), 99–110. doi:10.5172/conu.2013.44.1.99

Rowen, T. S., Breyer, B. N., Lin, T. C., Li, C. S., Robertson, P. A., & Shindel, A. W. (2013). Use of barrier protection for sexual activity among women who have sex with women. *International Journal of Gynecology and Obstetrics*, *120*(1), 42–45. doi:10.1016/j.ijgo.2012.08.011

Sanchez, N. F., Rabatin, J., Sanchez, J. P., Hubbard, S., & Kalet, A. (2006). Medical students' ability to care for lesbian, gay, bisexual, and transgendered patients. *Family Medicine*, *38*(1), 21–27.

Singh, D., Fine, D. N., & Marrazzo, J. M. (2011). *Chlamydia trachomatis* infection among women reporting sexual activity with women screened in family planning clinics in the Pacific Northwest, 1997 to 2005. *American Journal of Public Health*, *101*(7), 1284–1290. doi:10.2105/AJPH.2009.169631

Siordia, C. (2014). Disability estimates between same- and different-sex couples: Microdata from the American Community Survey (2009–2011). *Sexuality and Disability*, *33*(1), 107–121. doi:10.1007/s11195-014-9364-6

Smith, H. A., Markovic, N., Matthews, A. K., Danielson, M. E., Kalro, B. N., Youk, A. O., & Talbott, E. O. (2011). A comparison of polycystic ovary syndrome and related factors between lesbian and heterosexual women. *Women's Health Issues*, *21*(3), 191–198. doi:10.1016/j.whi.2010.11.001

Solomon, M. M., Mayer, K. H., Glidden, D. V, Liu, A. Y., McMahan, V. M., Guanira, J. V, . . . Grant, R. M. (2014). Syphilis predicts HIV incidence among men and transgender women who have sex with men in a preexposure prophylaxis trial. *Clinical Infectious Diseases*, *59*, 1020–1026. doi:10.1093/cid/ciu450

Supreme Court of the United States. *Case of Obergefell et al. v. Hodges, Director, Ohio Department of Health, et al.* (2015).

Teti, M., & Bowleg, L. (2011). Shattering the myth of invulnerability: Exploring the prevention needs of sexual minority women living with HIV/AIDS. *Journal of Gay & Lesbian Social Services*, *23*, 69–88. doi:10.1080/10538720.2010.538009

Thoma, B., Huebner, D., & Rullo, J. (2013). Unseen risks: HIV-related risk behaviors among ethnically diverse sexual minority adolescent females. *AIDS Education and Prevention*, *25*(6), 535–541. doi:10.1521/aeap.2013.25.6.535

Timm, T. M., Reed, S. J., Miller, R. L., & Valenti, M. T. (2011). Sexual debut of young black women who have sex with women: Implications for STI/HIV risk. *Youth & Society*, *45*(2), 167–183. doi:10.1177/0044118X11409445

Tracy, J. K., Schluterman, N. H., & Greenberg, D. R. (2013). Understanding cervical cancer screening among lesbians: A national survey. *BMC Public Health*, *13*, 442. doi:10.1186/1471-2458-13-442

Van Kesteren, P., Asscheman, H., Megens, J., & Gooren, L. (1997). Mortality and morbidity in transsexual subjects treated with cross-sex hormones . *Clinical Endocrinology*, *47*(3), 337–342.

Vocks, S., Stahn, C., Loenser, K., & Legenbauer, T. (2009). Eating and body image disturbances in male-to-female and female-to-male transsexuals. *Archives of Sexual Behavior*, *38*(3), 3640377.

Walls, M. L., & Whitbeck, L. B. (2012). Advantages of stress process approaches for measuring historical trauma. *American Journal of Drug and Alcohol Abuse*, *38*(5), 416–420. doi:10.3109/00952990.2012.694524

Walls, N. E., & Bell, S. (2011). Correlates of engaging in survival sex among homeless youth and young adults. *Journal of Sex Research*, *48*(5), 423–436. doi:10.1080/00224499.2010.501916

Walters, M. L., Chen, J., & Breiding, M. J. (Eds.). (2013). *The National Intimate Partner and Sexual Violence Survey (NISVS): 2010 findings on victimization by sexual orientation*. Atlanta, GA: National Center for Injury Prevention and Control, Centers for Disease Control and Prevention. doi:10.1037/e541522013-001

Ward, B. W., Dahlhamer, J. M., Galinsky, A. M., & Joestl, S. S. (2014). Sexual orientation and health among U.S. adults: National Health Interview Survey, 2013. *National Health Statistics Reports*, (77), 1–12.

Waterman, L., & Voss, J. (2013). HPV, cervical cancer risks, and barriers to care for lesbian women. *Nurse Practitioner*, *40*(1), 46–53.

Weyers, S., Verstraelen, H., Gerris, J., Monstrey, S., Santiago, G. D. S. L., Saerens, B., . . . Verhelst, R. (2009). Microflora of the penile skin-lined neovagina of transsexual women. *BMC Microbiology*, *9*, 102. doi:10.1186/1471-2180-9-102

Wierckx, K., Mueller, S., Weyers, S., Van Caenegem, E., Roef, G., Heylens, G., & T'Sjoen, G. (2012). Long-term evaluation of cross-sex hormone treatment in transsexual persons. *Journal of Sexual Medicine*, *9*, 2641–2651. doi:10.1111/j.1743-6109.2012.02876.x

Wilson, E., Rapues, J., Jin, H., & Raymend, H. F. (2014). The use and correlates of illicit silicone or "fillers" in a population-based sample of transwomen, San Francisco, 2013. *Journal of Sexual Medicine*, *11*(7), 1717–1724. doi:10.1111/jsm.12558

World Professional Association for Transgender Health. (2012). *Standards of care for the health of transsexual, transgender, and gender nonconforming people* (7th ed.). Minneapolis, MN: Author.

Yager, C., Brennan, D., Steele, L. S., Epstein, R., & Ross, L. E. (2010). Challenges and mental health experiences of lesbian and bisexual women who are trying to conceive. *Health & Social Work*, *35*, 191–200.

Yean, C., Benau, E. M., Dakanalis, A., Hormes, J. M., Perone, J., & Timko, C. A. (2013). The relationship of sex and sexual orientation to self-esteem, body shape satisfaction, and eating disorder symptomatology. *Frontiers in Psychology*, *4*(887), 1–11. doi:10.3389/fpsyg.2013.00887

Zaritsky, E., & Dibble, S. (2010). Risk factors for reproductive and breast cancers among older lesbians. *Journal of Women's Health*, *19*(1), 125–131.

CHAPTER 10

Sexuality and Sexual Health

Phyllis Patricia Cason

The editors acknowledge Catherine Ingram Fogel, who was the author of the previous edition of this chapter.

Humans are inherently sexual beings, and sexual health is an essential component of health care. When sex is voluntary, wanted, pleasurable, and noncoercive—which the World Health Organization (WHO) and the Centers for Disease Control and Prevention (CDC) define as a basic right of all women—it is healthy. When freely engaged in, sex can have numerous health benefits, including improving cardiovascular health, affording protection from fatal coronary events with no increase in risk of strokes, and extending the life span (Bassett, Bourbonnais, & McDowell, 2007; Buettner, 2008; Davey Smith, 2010; Drory, 2002; Ebrahim et al., 2002; Jannini, Fisher, Bitzer, & McMahon, 2009; Lindau & Gavrilova, 2010; Palmore, 1982; Seldin, Friedman, & Martin, 2002). In women, increased frequency of orgasm has been shown to increase their pain threshold and to protect against mortality (Levin, 2007; Seldin et al., 2002). Healthy sex is positively associated with higher levels of happiness and life satisfaction and also supports immune function (Davison, Bell, LaChina, Holden, & Davis, 2009). For couples, maintaining a positive sex life is associated with a healthier relationship that is more likely to remain intact (Kaschak & Tiefer, 2001; Sprecher & Cate, 2004). In laboratory studies, intimate physical contact with another person has been shown to stimulate oxytocin release, which is associated with wide-ranging health advantages (Imanieh, Bagheri, Alizadeh, & Ashkani-Esfahani, 2014; Murrell, 1995).

While healthy sex can deliver these benefits, sexual health is not viewed as an essential component of health care by many women and even by some clinicians. Women often have questions or concerns about their sexual health and function, and they may express these concerns to their clinicians. Women have the right to receive nonjudgmental, open, and direct communication, counseling, and therapy from clinicians regarding sexual health and concerns (sexual concerns are addressed in more detail in Chapter 16). Clinicians see women from a variety of socioeconomic and religious backgrounds and may care for women from countries around the world. In all aspects of care for women, considerations of the "whole patient" are paramount; this is nowhere more critical than when approaching a woman regarding her sexuality and sexual health.

This chapter seeks to develop a solid knowledge base about women's sexuality and sexual health for use in clinical practice. Beginning with and interweaving definitions and discussion of commonly used terminology, it goes on to cover sexual health and practices, sexual desire, sexual anatomy and physiology, and sexual response. The chapter aims to provide clinicians with tools to support women in achieving the goals they establish for their own sexuality by delineating three cornerstones to sexual health, which are critical for the experience of healthy, pleasurable sex: sexual self-knowledge, sexual agency, and strength in pelvic muscles. Information on sexual assessment is presented, and the chapter concludes with information about sexual health for specific populations as well as influences of culture on sexuality.

DEFINITIONS OF KEY TERMS

Increasingly, a plethora of terms are being used to describe various aspects of human sexuality, sexual health, the sexual rights of individuals, gender identity, and sexual orientation. WHO (2006) has created working definitions for sexuality, sexual health, and sexual rights, which it has offered as a contribution to ongoing discussions about sexual health (**Box 10-1**). The CDC and the Health Resources and Services

---

BOX 10-1 Definitions of Sexuality, Sexual Health, and Sexual Rights

Sexuality

Sexuality is a central aspect of being human throughout life and encompasses sex, gender identities and roles, sexual orientation, eroticism, pleasure, intimacy, and reproduction. Sexuality is experienced and expressed in thoughts, fantasies, desires, beliefs, attitudes, values, behaviors, practices, roles, and relationships. While sexuality can include all of these dimensions, not all of them are always experienced or expressed. Sexuality is influenced by the interaction of biological, psychological, social, economic, political, cultural, ethical, legal, historical, religious, and spiritual factors. (WHO, 2006, p. 5)

Sexual Health

Sexual health is a state of physical, emotional, mental, and social well-being in relation to sexuality; it is not merely the absence of disease, dysfunction, or infirmity. Sexual health requires a positive and respectful approach to sexuality and sexual relationships, as well as the possibility of having pleasurable and safe sexual experiences, free of coercion, discrimination, and violence. For sexual health to be attained and maintained, the sexual rights of all persons must be respected, protected and fulfilled. (WHO, 2006, p. 5)

- Sexual health is a state of well-being in relation to sexuality across the life span that involves physical, emotional, mental, social, and spiritual dimensions.
- Sexual health is an inextricable element of human health and is based on a positive, equitable, and respectful approach to sexuality, relationships, and reproduction that is free of coercion, fear, discrimination, stigma, shame, and violence.
- Sexual health includes the ability to understand the benefits, risks, and responsibilities of sexual behavior; the prevention of disease and other adverse outcomes; and the possibility of fulfilling sexual relationships.
- Sexual health is impacted by socioeconomic and cultural contexts (including policies, practices, and services) that support healthy outcomes for individuals and their communities. (U.S. Department of Health and Human Services, 2012, p. 41)

Sexual Rights

Sexual rights embrace human rights that are already recognized in national laws, international human rights documents, and other consensus statements. They include the right of all persons, free of coercion, discrimination, and violence, to the highest attainable standard of sexual health, including access to sexual and reproductive healthcare services; seek, receive, and impart information related to sexuality; sexuality education; respect for bodily integrity; choose their partner; decide to be sexually active or not; consensual sexual relations; consensual marriage; decide whether or not, and when, to have children; and pursue a satisfying, safe and pleasurable sexual life. The responsible exercise of human rights requires that all persons respect the rights of others. (WHO, 2006, p. 5)

Definitions reproduced from U.S. Department of Health and Human Services. (2012). CDC/HRSA Advisory Committee on HIV, Viral Hepatitis, and STD Prevention and Treatment; May 8–9, 2012; Atlanta, Georgia. Record of the proceedings. Retrieved from http://www.cdc.gov/maso/facm/pdfs/CHACHSPT/20120508_CHAC.pdf; World Health Organization (WHO). (2006). *Defining sexual health: Report of a technical consultation on sexual health, 28–31 January 2002, Geneva.* Geneva, Switzerland: Author. Retrieved from http://www.who.int/reproductivehealth/publications/sexual_health/defining_sexual_health.pdf?ua=1.

Administration (U.S. Department of Health and Human Services, 2012) have also developed a definition of sexual health (**Box 10-1**). In further recognition of the notion that sexual rights are essential to achieve sexual health, the World Association for Sexual Health (2014) issued *The Declaration of Sexual Rights* in 1999, which was subsequently revised in 2014.

Clinicians must understand and be sensitive to language related to gender identity and sexual orientation. It is important to remember that while the terms *gender* and *sex* are used often interchangeably, they are not synonymous. Definitions for these terms and concepts can be found in Chapter 9.

Female sexuality is defined as the integrated, unique expression of self that includes the physiologic and psychological processes inherent in sexual development. The complex process known as sexuality is coordinated by the neurologic, vascular, muscular, and endocrine systems (Basson & Baram, 2011). It encompasses an individual's values, attitudes, behaviors, physical appearance, beliefs, emotions, personality, and social and cultural orientations. Sexuality is a fundamental component of a woman's life and is interwoven with her reproductive functioning.

The unique human quality that is sexuality has several dimensions, including sexual desire, presentation of self as a sexual being, sexual orientation, and sexual lifestyles and relationships. Sexuality involves a wide range of behaviors including fantasy, self-stimulation, noncoital pleasuring, erotic stimuli other than touch, communication about needs and desires, and the ability to define what is wanted and pleasurable in a relationship (Fogel & Woods, 2008). Sexual expression is influenced by ethical, cultural, moral, and spiritual factors and is demonstrated differently at different times—alone, with one partner, or with many partners. A woman's sexuality is not limited by age, attractiveness, partner availability or participation, or sexual orientation (Bergner, 2013).

Sexual lifestyles and relationships provide the pattern and context for an individual's sexuality. To be valuable as a resource to their patients regarding their sexuality, clinicians need to avoid making assumptions about any aspect of a woman's sexual lifestyles and relationships. The most frequently acknowledged pattern for women is heterosexual, marital monogamy, which is assumed to be the most desirable status by many societies. Many individuals, however, may identify as lesbian, bisexual, queer, pansexual, or asexual (see Chapter 9 for definitions of these terms and concepts). Rather than classical monogamy, in which partners marry as virgins and are sexually exclusive throughout their lives (Scheff, 2014), individuals may choose celibacy, serial monogamy, or nonmonogamy.

Celibacy involves the conscious choice to abstain from sexual activity, and it can be chosen within the context of a relationship or by a woman not currently in a relationship. Individuals may view this choice positively, as a means of giving their time and energy and total attention to other activities. Alternatively, celibacy may be involuntary, as when a woman is between relationships or when her partner is ill. Celibacy often refers to lack of sexual activity with another person, but it is helpful to understand how a woman defines it for herself because masturbation is also sexual activity.

Serial monogamy is a pattern of conducting one monogamous relationship, which is then followed by another monogamous relationship. The rules that determine which behaviors are and are not allowed within a couple's monogamous relationship are unique to that dyad, and it is best if the two people agree on their understanding of those rules. Much recent work within the field of couples therapy centers on "redefinitions" of monogamy and emphasizes the benefits of clear communication regarding expectations of monogamy.

Individuals who are nonmonogamous (polyamorous) elect to participate in sexual activity with one or more concurrent partners. Nonmonogamy may be chosen by committed couples, including individuals who are married, who have sex with other individuals or couples.

SEXUAL HEALTH AND PRACTICES

For many people, sexual health is not something that is considered until its absence is noticed. In clinical situations, sexual health is frequently an undefined default state, devoid of any positive connotations, that describes the absence of infection, cancer, sexual violence, coercion, unintended pregnancy, or abnormal pregnancy. In contrast, when considered from a sex-positive position, the definition of sexual health encompasses far more than the lack of negatives. A working definition that moves forward toward the more sex-positive end of the spectrum would include the acknowledgment that satisfying sexual activity stemming from sexual agency and sexual self-knowledge is both healthy and desirable.

Definitions of sexual health and sexual practices may contain value-laden terms that are subject to different interpretations. In many cases, cultural norms dictate what is acceptable or normal behavior (Joyal, Cossette, & Lapierre, 2015). Because it is not always easy to distinguish between aberrant and merely unconventional practices, clinicians must be aware of how they define normal and abnormal sexual practices. Is the sexual practice consensual? Does a particular behavior put the person or her partner(s) at risk? If so, in what way, and is that risk one they understand and are willing to take? Is anyone else harmed by the behavior?

In general, unless the answer to one of these questions indicates the potential for coercion or unacceptable risk, a clinician must examine his or her own biases before interacting judgmentally with a patient. Sexual behaviors and practices that have been labeled as paraphilias (also known as sexual perversion or sexual deviation) in some generations and cultures are considered normative in others. For example, until recently homosexuality was considered a paraphilia and given a medical diagnosis, and it is still considered a perversion in many societies. Another example is BDSM—a shortened acronym used to refer to some combination of bondage, discipline, dominance, submission, sadism, and masochism. These terms are listed in *The Diagnostic and Statistical Manual of Mental Disorders, Fifth Edition* (DSM-5; American Psychiatric Association, 2013) as paraphilias, yet studies suggest that BDSM practitioners have favorable psychological characteristics and no increase in sexual or psychological difficulties compared to non-BDSM practitioners (Pascoal, Cardoso, & Henriques, 2015; Richters, de Visser, Rissel, Grulich, & Smith, 2008; Wismeijer & van Assen, 2013).

SEXUAL DESIRE

Possibly even more nuanced than gender and sexual behavior is the understanding of desire. Sexual desire has been defined as the motivation to engage in sexual acts. However, this motivation is molded by a continuum of biology, psychology, and society (Mark, Herbenick, Fortenberry, Sanders, & Reece, 2014; Pfaus, 2009; Pfaus et al., 2012). Clearly, biology drives humans to have sex to reproduce; however, a multitude of other factors come into play with sexual desire (Georgiadis, Kringelbach, & Pfaus, 2012).

The concept of sexual desire in general, and female desire in particular, is neither well defined nor well researched. Each individual (clinicians, individuals, and researchers) defines desire in their own unique way. For some, the focus is on physical drive; for others, the key element is a sense of emotional craving or heightened subtle sense of excitement. Perhaps because of the elusive nature of desire or the fact that desire was thought to lie outside the realm of what can be measured with science, sex researchers until recently studied behavior rather than the feelings, such as desire, that motivate behavior. William Masters and Virginia Johnson's research, which included filming research participants having sex, focused on sexual function (Masters & Johnson, 1966). Sexologists in the 1970s began examining what women want, rather than their sexual behaviors; however, with the advent of the HIV/AIDS epidemic, prevention of infection became the paramount concern. It was not until the late 1990s that full-scale research into desire resumed when pharmaceutical companies began attempting to develop a female equivalent of sildenafil (Viagra), a medication to treat men's erectile dysfunction (Bergner, 2013).

Sexual desire is shaped by a variety of factors, including familial and cultural rules. These forces mold how desire is perceived and experienced and what is considered acceptable versus taboo. Historically, these social norms have differed for men and women, sometimes shifting or blending over time. Women, in particular, have been perceived in some cultural or societal contexts as asexual and therefore "pure at heart." In contrast, in other contexts, they have been viewed as evil temptresses.

These perceptions, in turn, can affect an individual woman's experience of herself as a sexual person and her ability to experience desire and sexual arousal. In some societies, women act intensely aroused and active during sex; in others, they have no concept of orgasm. In fact, women in some settings, when told about orgasm, do not even believe it exists, as anthropologists discovered in some parts of Nepal (Schwartz & Rutter, 1998).

What individuals desire may be highly correlated with early conditioning. A woman's view of herself as a female and her presentation as a sexual being form in early childhood and evolve throughout her life as life circumstances shape her identity (Alexander, LaRosa, Bader, & Garfield, 2007). New research is sharpening the understanding of the effects that early sexual experience can have on sexual desire later in life. Groundbreaking laboratory experiments with rats and voles have shown that positive, pleasurable early sexual experiences condition, through this positive feedback, preferences for partner characteristics, place, smell, and even clothing choices. In addition, endogenous opioid activation forms the chemical/emotional basis of positive sexual conditioning and sexual reward (Pfaus, 2009; Pfaus et al., 2012).

In the United States, the current emphasis on female desire is relatively new. Since the introduction of the oral contraceptive pill in 1960 and the sexual liberation "revolution" that followed in the 1960s and 1970s, the cultural expectation for women in the United States has become, to a greater or lesser degree, that they are sexual beings. Many books and articles have been written discussing the intricacies of this societal understanding and its impact upon female sexuality. For today's practicing clinician, an understanding of the changing perception of woman's sexual desire, and the context within which that perception has developed, is important. This is particularly helpful for comprehending and evaluating the debate that is currently raging among feminist researchers and authors, sexual medicine specialists, and pharmaceutical companies over female desire and how it is represented in the media. In their own practices, clinicians may interact with women who have questions or concerns about their own levels of desire and may need help exploring how cultural or societal expectations may be influencing

these concerns or limiting their own expression of desire before rushing to a discussion of potential disorders. See Chapter 16 for information on assessment and management of alterations in sexual desire.

SEXUAL SELF-KNOWLEDGE

Early experiences, combined with myriad socioeconomic and cultural factors, strongly impact the first cornerstone to sexual health: self-knowledge. *Self-knowledge* is a woman's ability both to understand her own arousal and its physical manifestation and to recognize her own desire and preferences. It is the ability for a woman to be fluent in the language of her own body. With self-knowledge, if she is feeling lubrication or engorgement, a woman can correctly interpret those sensations as arousal. By the same token, if she is feeling an increase in lubrication due to sexual arousal, she will not mistake the sensation as vaginal discharge or interpret engorgement as irritation or discomfort. If she detects a need for more lubrication, she knows to have some nearby (Herbenick et al., 2011; Jozkowski et al., 2013).

Genital sexual arousal has measurable objective components, which were observed by Masters and Johnson and include swelling of the clitoral erectile tissue, production of lubricating secretions from the Bartholin's glands, and other vaginal lubrication. Arousal also has subjective components, not least of which is the subjective experience of each of these objective changes as well as the less easily measured range of emotions related to arousal. The matching of the objective signs—for example, measured engorgement—with the subjective experience of arousal is called *concordance* or *coherence*. Laboratory studies of engorgement using a vaginal plethysmograph, which is a probe placed in the vagina to measure blood flow, have shown that these measurements can correlate very poorly with a woman's subjective experience of arousal (Chivers & Timmers, 2012). In contrast, males generally have fairly good concordance (Chivers, Seto, Lalumiere, Laan, & Grimbos, 2010), probably because they have visual feedback—in the form of an erection—that they are experiencing arousal.

For women, concordance may be associated with higher levels of satisfaction with sex, although the data on this relationship are mixed. One study did find significantly positive concordance estimates for frequently orgasmic women (Adams, Haynes, & Brayer, 1985). Research has demonstrated that instructing a woman to focus on physical cues, specifically genital blood flow, during sexual fantasy increases both her self-reported and measured genital sexual responses (Prause, Barela, Roberts, & Graham, 2013).

The subjective experience of sexual arousal is not uniquely related to experience of physiological response and is mediated by additional cognitive and emotional mechanisms. Women may demonstrate low sexual interoceptive awareness as a result of interpretations of the physiologic responses based on preferences. In other words, a woman may screen out perception of physical sensations not consistent with what she thinks is appropriate or based on her sexual desires. Information used to appraise one's emotional state of sexual arousal is influenced by one's attitudes, beliefs, and values regarding sexuality, as well as immediate contextual factors. For example, physiologic arousal in reaction to a stimulus that is not deemed appropriate may be filtered either consciously or unconsciously.

A similar phenomenon was identified in a study in which women and men were attached to fake lie detector tests and asked questions about their sexual behavior (Fisher, 2013). The men in this study answered questions about casual sex and number of partners the same way regardless of whether they were attached to the fake electrodes. Interestingly, the women who were not attached to the electrodes reported significantly fewer partners than the women who believed they had a compelling reason (the lie detector machine) to tell the truth. In fact, the women hooked up to the fake polygraph reported the same sexual behavior as the men in this study. These findings indicate self-reports of sexual behavior may not be entirely accurate.

Concordance is essentially a laboratory assessment; it is an interesting finding that helps individuals appreciate the importance of focusing on physical cues as sensations of arousal. Nevertheless, it is merely one small data point in the complex and critically important realm of sexual self-knowledge. Sexual self-knowledge encompasses layers upon layers of information that by most accounts build over the course of a woman's lifetime. As a woman matures, by attending to her own sexual interests and responses, she catalogs all that she learns about what and who she finds erotic, how she likes to be touched, what is arousing, and what creates orgasm. Thus, while the popular media often stresses that individuals' sexual prime is associated with youth, maturity can bring both sexual self-knowledge and the capability of greater intimacy, leading to sex that is better than that experienced in younger years (Schnarch, 2009).

Sexual Anatomy and Physiology

A woman's understanding of her own sexual anatomy is an important precursor to sexual self-knowledge, the ability to gain sexual arousal and satisfaction, and communication of her needs to her partner(s). All too often, information about even the most accessible portion of a woman's sexual anatomy—the clitoral complex—may be incomplete or lacking altogether. Traditionally, many women's definition and understanding of the clitoris have been limited to what is actually merely the head of the clitoris. In fact, the clitoral complex is vast and incorporates the shaft, the crura, vestibular bulbs, and the neural plexus across much of the introitus and lower vagina (Federation of Feminist Women's Health Centers, 1991; van Anders, Hipp, & Kane Low, 2013). And, while erect penises are familiar concepts to many, clitoral erections tend to be unrecognized. Yet, the size of clitoral erections can range from 10 to 20 cm (4–7.9 inches), with the clitoral body itself extending from 2 to 4 cm (0.8–1.6 inches) and attaining a width of from 1 to 2 cm (0.39–0.79 inches). When stimulated, the crura can swell to 5 to 9 cm (2–3.5 inches), and the bulbs' length can vary from 3 to 7 cm (1.2–2.8 inches).

The G-Spot

A recent review looked at histologic data from the literature that demonstrated the existence of discrete anatomic structures within the anterior vaginal wall composed of erectile tissue (Jannini et al., 2010). This region, while containing erectile tissue, has not been found to be a constant and can be highly variable from woman to woman. It has been shown to demonstrate dynamic changes during digital and penile stimulation. Other experts argue critically, and sometimes vehemently, against this so-called G-spot. Although a huge amount of data (not always of good quality) has been accumulated in the last 60 years, there is not consensus on the existence of a discrete G-Spot (Jannini et al., 2010).

Female Ejaculation

Clinicians may be asked by a woman if it is normal to experience involuntary emission of fluid during sexual arousal or orgasm (also known as female ejaculation or squirting). It is important to get a sense from the woman if this is a welcome or concerning experience. While it is likely that large amounts of fluid are the result of coital urinary incontinence, the amount that a woman may report can vary from less than 0.3 mL to more than 150 mL. Smaller amounts of fluid may reflect vaginal hyperlubrication or fluid produced by the Bartholin's glands or by the Skene's glands; these structures are also referred to as the female prostate and are able to produce some amount of prostate-specific antigen (PSA). The fluid is sometimes described as looking like watered-down or fat-free milk.

Until recently, there were many reports of female ejaculation and squirting, but fewer than 20 women had participated in controlled laboratory studies during which they emitted fluid in a laboratory setting that was then analyzed. Those studies showed that the emitted fluid had a varied biochemical makeup but was mostly similar to dilute urine, albeit sometimes containing significant amounts of PSA (Pastor, 2013). A subsequent study of women reporting larger volumes of squirting utilized pre- and post-emission ultrasonographic bladder monitoring and biochemical analyses. This investigation indicated that squirting is essentially the involuntary emission of urine during sexual activity, and that the emitted fluid contains only a marginal amount of prostatic secretions (Tennfjord et al., 2015).

Sexual Response in Women

Sexual response involves both capacity (i.e., what someone is capable of experiencing) and activity (i.e., what she actually experiences). Emotion and physiology are interwoven within the sexual response cycle (Salonia et al., 2010). Traditionally the Masters and Johnson (1966) model of sexual response, as adapted by Kaplan (1979), has been used to explain sexual response in both women and men. Masters and Johnson began the modern movement toward an understanding of the sexual response cycle, and their description focuses on physiologic responses to stimuli. They identified two principal physiologic responses to sexual stimulation: vasocongestion and muscle tension. These responses are represented differently throughout the phases of the sexual response cycle. Later authorities incorporated both biologic and psychological components of sexual response (American Psychiatric Association, 2013; Kaplan, 1979).

The traditional female sexual response cycle as described by Masters and Johnson and Kaplan, when modified to include the element of consent (Chalker, 1994), consists of four sequential phases: desire, excitement, orgasm, and resolution. The desire phase consists of sexual fantasy, thoughts, and awareness that sexual stimulation is wanted, albeit without physiologic changes. Vasocongestion, muscle tension, and other physiologic changes build, peak and release, and then resolve during the excitement, orgasm, and resolution phases, respectively. During this cycle, progression occurs from a subjective sense of anticipation and pleasure to release and finally to relaxation.

Basson (2000) describes an alternative model of female sexual response that is less linear than the traditional model. Basson's model is based on the theory that women are not motivated toward sexual activity by predominantly physical urges (**Figure 10-1**). In this model, women move from a sexually neutral state to seeking sexual stimuli when they sense either an opportunity to be sexual or a partner's need, or when they have an awareness of one or more of the potential benefits of sexual activity. Sexual desire may be experienced as a craving for sexual sensations for their own sake, a desire to experience physical and subjective arousal, or possibly a release of sexual tension. According to this model, sexual desire is a response rather than a spontaneous event. Although a woman may experience spontaneous desire in the form of sexual dreams, thoughts, or fantasies, she is more likely to be at a baseline neutral state at the onset of a partner experience (Basson, 2000). Many sexually satisfied individuals do not experience spontaneous

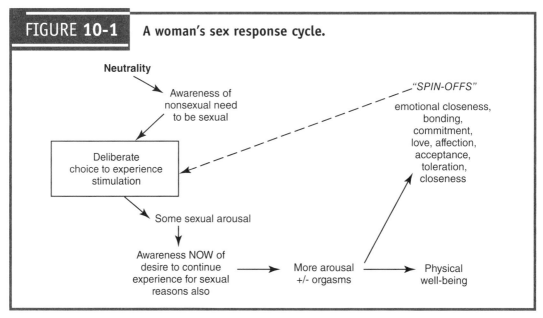

FIGURE **10-1**   **A woman's sex response cycle.**

Reproduced from Basson, R. (2000). The female sexual response: A different model. *Journal of Sex & Marital Therapy, 26*, 51–65. Reproduced by permission of Taylor & Francis, Ltd., http://www.informaworld.com. © 2000.

sexual desire (Basson et al., 2004). Rather, sexual arousal and responsive sexual desire may occur simultaneously after the decision to experience sexual stimulation. While Basson's model has gained significant traction since its introduction, it is based on her years of experience as a therapist rather than on data collected in clinical studies. One valuable facet of Basson's theories is the concept that one need not be aroused or actively desiring sex to engage in fully satisfying sexual activity.

SEXUAL AGENCY

Another cornerstone of sexual health is sexual agency. Sexual agency is the concept that an individual has control over her or his own sexuality. Given the realities of sexual coercion and abuse, clinicians often emphasize the skills a woman needs to allow her to say no to unwanted sexual activity. This means supporting a woman in her ability to set limits on whether she engages in sexual activity, the type of sexual activity she engages in, and

the timing of that activity. Safer sex practices (e.g., condom use) may require negotiation. Clinicians can assist women by providing interactive counseling conversations, active listening, and other tools to support sexual agency in women's interactions with their partners.

In the more positive realm, sexual agency encompasses a woman's ability to say yes to wanted sexual activity. Agreeing to wanted sex can be challenging in an environment where sexual activity may be stigmatized, regulated, or have unintended consequences; even highly desired, pleasurable sex between consenting adults can result in transmission of sexually transmitted infections (STIs) or unintended pregnancy. Developing sexual agency includes making increasingly conscious choices regarding one's own sexuality, sexual behavior, and sexual activity, including increasing the ability to say yes to wanted sex.

Historically, women have faced negative societal messages about female sexuality. These messages range from relatively benign stereotyped images that teach that women have sex solely to please their partner, to extremes such as punishment by death for a woman who openly expresses her sexuality or is caught being sexual. Sex-negative family attitudes and conditioning can have a negative impact on a woman's ability to enjoy sex (Peixoto & Nobre, 2014).

In the face of these constraints, a clinician can be a valuable resource for a woman by utilizing active listening skills and asking open-ended questions designed to clarify negative conditioning about sex. In this way a woman can be assisted to sort out her own values around her sexuality and make conscious choices that are consistent with these values. Examples of these skills include rephrasing (also called paraphrasing): "So, I hear you saying that you feel like you have gotten some pretty strong negative impressions about masturbation from your mom. Do I have that right?" or "It sounds like, on the one hand, you really enjoy it when your partner performs oral sex on you, and, on the other hand, you feel a bit embarrassed about it. Am I hearing that correctly?"

Finally, sexual agency includes the ability to initiate sexual interaction or activity, either partnered or solo. This encompasses a woman's ability to initiate the type, timing, and range of sexual activity that she wants. Traditionally, women have been at best considered passive partners in sexual encounters or at worst relegated to an assortment of sex-negative roles regarding sex. Given these constraining messages, it can be challenging for a woman to overcome familial, cultural, religious, or societal expectations to gain enough sexual agency to initiate sexual activity. In addition to these barriers, women who initiate sexual interaction run the risk of feeling disappointment, rejection, or worse, as there is always the possibility that a partner might not be available or might not agree to engage in sex or the type of sex that the woman initiating the encounter was seeking. Women also experience, and therefore may be legitimately wary of, societal stigma, such as being termed promiscuous or a slut, in response to taking an active role in sex.

Clinicians can assist women to gain sexual agency by supporting their efforts to initiate satisfying sexual encounters. This support can be accomplished by using active listening and rephrasing or paraphrasing, as described previously, with the goal

being to ask open-ended questions designed to help a woman clarify what has worked well for her in terms of initiating sexual encounters in the past.

When proffering information or education about sexual health topics, an additional tool that a clinician can use is to sandwich the information between two questions, so that the discussion remains centered on the particular woman rather than the clinician merely reciting advice. This process, which is called making an information sandwich, is helpful when a clinician has a piece of valuable information to share. For example, a clinician might say, "It sounds like you're saying that you feel like you are being pushy when you initiate sex with your partner. Are there any things you have tried in the past that work?" Then, after the woman has replied and the clinician has rephrased what she has said, the clinician can offer a piece of information: "Sometimes people in relationships who are less interested in sexual interactions at a given time in the relationship begin feeling interested when their partner frames sexual feedback in positive ways rather than in negative terms." Then, a clinician would follow this statement with another question.

When discussing sexuality with women who are in partnered sexual relationships, one of the important pieces of information for a clinician to share is the benefit of framing information regarding preferences and giving positive feedback to a partner while minimizing critical feedback when appropriate. For example, a woman might say, "I love it when you do . . ." rather than "Don't do that." However, sometimes saying "Don't do that" is appropriate from a standpoint of safety and agency.

STRENGTH IN PELVIC MUSCLES

Another cornerstone to sexual health is awareness of, control over, and strength in the pelvic muscles—the ones that are under conscious control and are collectively referred to as the *pelvic floor* (more fully described in Chapter 5). There are many benefits to strengthening and having control over the pelvic musculature. Pelvic floor control can decrease urinary incontinence and prevent pelvic organ prolapse. Control over the muscles distributed throughout a woman's vagina and her introitus can also aid sexual health and pleasure multiple ways. In the case of a woman who chooses to have penetration as part of her sexual activity, she can relax the muscles to facilitate various types of penetration. She can also relax the musculature to accommodate various positions. A woman can tighten these muscles to help protect her from deep dyspareunia if she experiences sensitivity deep in the pelvis or has a retroverted or retroflexed uterus. Because the muscles surrounding the introitus and anus create a figure-eight shape that fully enshrouds and supports the clitoral complex, a woman can contract these muscles to increase the physical stimulation to her clitoral complex (Braekken, Majida, Ellstrom Engh, & Bo, 2015; Citak et al., 2010; Lowenstein, Gruenwald, Gartman, & Vardi, 2010; Martinez, Ferreira, Castro, & Gomide, 2014; Sacomori & Cardoso, 2015).

A clinician can assess a woman's pelvic musculature during any visit that includes a pelvic examination (Herderschee, Hay-Smith, Herbison, Roovers, & Heineman, 2011; Peschers, Gingelmaier, Jundt, Leib, & Dimpfl, 2001). Most of the earliest data on the benefits of Kegel exercises utilized biofeedback machines for training women to identify and gain control of their pelvic muscles (Taylor & Henderson, 1986). During a biofeedback session, a woman relaxes and contracts the muscles in her pelvic floor, with the feedback helping her to differentiate these muscles from her abdominal, thigh, and buttocks muscles. With time and feedback, she can also isolate the muscles that control the perianal region from her vaginal musculature. Biofeedback remains the gold standard for assessment and training of pelvic musculature to this day.

Clinician feedback can substitute for a biofeedback machine, when that is not an option, in an office visit. To assess a woman's current ability to identify and control her pelvic floor muscles, while also assessing their strength, a clinician inserts one or two fingers into a woman's vagina, just as one would for a bimanual pelvic examination, and asks the woman to grip the clinician's fingers with her vaginal muscles. The clinician can simultaneously grasp the woman's fingers in her own to reflect and transmit the information that the clinician gains during the examination to the woman. The clinician can note the baseline tone, control, and strength in the chart to compare these values with those obtained at future follow-up visits. Instruction in how to perform Kegel exercises should be given during the first visit. See Chapter 22 for more information on Kegel exercises.

Kegel exercises can also be helpful for women who are pre-orgasmic and are interested in exploring ways to experience orgasm. To heighten her awareness of her sensual responses, a woman must give herself the time to explore these feelings and, to the greatest extent possible, banish the "self-critic" that might be hovering around her. Distraction can easily interrupt her focus and prevent orgasm. Often, distraction is worse with a partner, but even when a woman is alone, her distraction can prevent orgasm.

VIBRATORS

Vibrators and other sex toys and aids can be a valuable adjunct to the cornerstones of sexual health. Exploration with a vibrator or sex toy can provide a pathway to experiencing or improving arousal and/or orgasm, whether a woman uses it for masturbation or with a partner. Clinicians should normalize vibrator use by telling women how common it is; 53% of women in a nationally representative study report having used vibrators (Herbenick et al., 2009). Referring to vibrators as sex accessories or sexual enhancements may also make women feel more comfortable with their use. Clinicians can also help women by having knowledge of factors that women should consider in vibrator selection, such as types (e.g., external/clitoral, internal, and combined external and internal stimulation); materials (e.g., silicone, sealed ceramics, stainless steel, medical-grade plastics); shapes; sizes; strength of vibration, including range of settings and speeds; power source (e.g., disposable battery, rechargeable); and volume.

Women may express concern that they will become dependent on a vibrator. A clinician can use active listening skills to understand the full context of the concern that the woman has expressed. For example, she may feel shame about her inability to orgasm with her partner, or perhaps her partner has expressed feelings of inadequacy. One piece of information that may be helpful for a woman to hear is that once her body has gained the ability to go from arousal to orgasm, it becomes easier to reach orgasm consistently.

Women may also have concerns about the chemical makeup of vibrators or other sex toys.

The least allergenic and safest sex toys are made from 100% silicone, sealed ceramics, stainless steel, or medical-grade plastics. One way to determine if a sex toy is potentially unsafe is the "smell test." Toys that give off any detectable chemical or plastic type of smell (which often include less expensive sex toys) may contain phthalates. Phthalates are a group of chemicals used to make plastics more flexible and harder to break, but some of them have been shown to affect the reproductive systems of laboratory animals (CDC, 2015).

ASSESSMENT OF SEXUAL HEALTH

To provide excellent-quality sexual health care, clinicians should spend some time becoming aware of their own biases. When providing sexual health care, it is essential not to make assumptions about a woman's sexual attitudes or behavior. Additionally, clinicians need to know how medical diagnoses and their treatment affect sexual health.

History

The sexual history is the first step in providing excellent sexual health care. Clinicians comfortable introducing topics of sexual health will establish a positive tone before beginning. Rapport and sufficient time for sensitive discussions are helpful before soliciting information that women may consider highly personal or intimate. Choose a private place where the woman can be comfortable and interruptions can be minimized. Have the woman remain dressed and sit at eye level with her. Such measures foster a sense of acceptance and respect for the woman and reduce her possible feelings of intimidation.

It is essential for clinicians to take care to monitor their own verbal and nonverbal responses to guard against negative reactions, which are easily conveyed. Usually more information is obtained by beginning with open-ended questions and allowing a woman to tell her story in the way she is most comfortable. If a woman begins to drift off-topic or the interview is becoming too lengthy, a clinician can redirect the discussion by utilizing rephrasing or paraphrasing rather than interrupting.

It is best to begin with less threatening material, such as a woman's pregnancy history or childhood sexual education, and move to more sensitive topics such as her current sexual practices. Questions about an individual's sexual education history (e.g., How did you learn about sex?) can proceed to personal attitudes and beliefs about sexuality and then on to sexual behaviors.

Avoid using excessive medical terminology during an interview; both the clinician and the woman need to know the meanings of any terms used. Avoid euphemisms such as *slept with* or the term *sexually active* in favor of specific terms (e.g., oral sex, vaginal sex, anal sex). Ask one question at a time, and allow the woman enough time to answer. Statistical questions such as "How many times a week do you have sex?" are not helpful. Instead, ask a woman if she is satisfied with how frequently she has sex. Rather than asking whether a particular sexual experience has occurred (e.g., "Have you ever had sex without a condom?"), which tends to cause people to respond, "No," it is better to ask how many times the experience has occurred. This technique suggests that the experience is normal. Techniques such as universalizing or prefacing questions by comments such as "Many people . . ." or "Other women I have talked with have said . . ." may make a woman feel more comfortable when answering sensitive questions. In assisting a woman to clarify the degree of satisfaction with her sex life, a clinician can ask her about her present relationship with respect to sexual communication, affection, and sexual needs met.

When taking a sexual history, it is most useful to focus on behaviors, practices, and a woman's perception of her sexual experiences rather than on labels about sexual orientation. In terms of building rapport between patient and clinician, it is helpful to hear how a woman defines her own sexual orientation. Direct inquiry concerning sexual orientation establishes that a clinician is open to a range of sexual orientations; however, it is more helpful when taking a sexual history to ask detailed questions about what someone did sexually, when, and with whom, and how those experiences fit into the woman's goals for her sexual life. For example, a woman who self-identifies as a lesbian may have penile–vaginal intercourse. When discussing strategies to promote sexual health, it is more relevant to be clear on the details of sexual practices than to assign labels.

Often, a sexual history includes questions designed to elicit risk for STIs, pregnancy, and intimate partner violence. For example, the CDC (n.d.) has established an excellent set of sexual history questions (the "Five P's") designed to address this aspect of sexual health. The Five P's are a list of possible relevant sexual history questions pertaining to partners, practices, protection from STIs, past history of STIs, and prevention of pregnancy. See Chapter 20 for a complete list of the questions in the Five P's.

If a woman has already brought up sexual topics or issues regarding her sexual life, the following introduction may not be necessary. If a clinician plans to bring up sensitive topics proactively, however, it may be helpful to prepare for the discussion. For example, a clinician can say, "I am going to ask you a few questions about your sexual health and sexual practices. I understand that these questions are very personal, but they are important for your overall health." The clinician could add, "Just so you know, I ask these questions of all my adult patients, regardless of age, gender, or marital status. Like the rest of our visits, this information is kept in strict confidence" (CDC, n.d.). Alternatively, a clinician might take a neutral, straightforward approach: "At this point in the exam, I generally ask some questions regarding your sexual life. Will that be okay?" A woman will be assured that a clinician is listening, and able to be of assistance by asking

> direct questions in a professional, straightforward, reassuring, and empathic manner. Use a direct approach with inquiry initiated in a neutral tone, using nonjudgmental, open-ended questions. The quest for details must be balanced by sensitivity to the patient's concerns and feelings as the information is collected and the interview proceeds. Let the story unfold, in the available time, carefully guiding her rather than unnecessarily interrupting while mechanistically pursuing a predetermined list of questions. (Althof, Rosen, Perelman, & Rubio-Aurioles, 2013, pp. 29–30)

Use the term *partner* when asking about the patient's sexual relationships (Althof et al., 2013). Once a woman has designated a word for her partner, such as *girlfriend*, *husband*, or *sweetie*, the clinician can then follow her lead and use the same term.

Box 10-2 contains examples of open-ended questions clinicians can use when taking a history

---

BOX 10-2 Examples of Sexual Health Assessment Questions

- Do you masturbate?
- Are you having sex of any kind with anyone?
- If no, have you ever had sex of any kind with another person?
- If yes, how many sex partners do you have currently?
- What kind of sex are you having (vaginal, oral, anal)?
- Tell me how things are going for you with your sexual relationship.
- Are you satisfied with the quality of your sexual life? If not, what might make it better? *or* In what ways are you not satisfied?
- Is sex pleasurable for you?
- Do you use any form of lubrication during sex? *or* What kind of lubrication do you use during sex?
- Have you ever had an orgasm/climax? Have you had an orgasm with a partner? By yourself?
- What ways have you worked out to ask or show your partner what you like sexually?
- Do you feel comfortable initiating sex with your partner?
- How is it for you when your sexual partner initiates sex?
- Are there any sexual problems or concerns that you would like to discuss with me today?
- Sometimes people who _____ (e.g., have just given birth, are diagnosed with cancer, are on chemotherapy, are dealing with fertility issues, have diabetes, have hypertension, have depression, are on this medication you are taking) have sexual issues. Have you experienced this?
- Many women around the time of menopause (or after menopause) tell me that they have vaginal dryness or sometimes discomfort or even pain in their vaginal area. Have you experienced this?

focused on an individual's sexual life. In addition, much of the information gained from a complete medical and gynecologic history pertains to sexual health. See Chapter 6 for further information on history taking. Detailed assessment of risk for STIs can be found in Chapter 20. Assessment and management of sexual concerns is addressed in Chapter 16.

Physical Examination and Diagnostic Studies

A physical examination or laboratory test may at times be indicated by history, the reason for seeking care (such as dyspareunia or symptoms of an STI), treatment goals, or need for referral. Physical examination and diagnostic studies to be considered in the evaluation of sexual concerns can be found in Chapter 16.

SPECIAL CONSIDERATIONS

Sexual concerns and dysfunction are addressed elsewhere in this text (see Chapter 16). However, it bears mentioning here that there are specific circumstances, such as certain medical conditions and medications, and particular times in a woman's life when she could benefit from proactive questioning and support regarding her sexual life. Some of the most vulnerable times include adolescence, pregnancy, postpartum, midlife, and older adulthood. Brief discussions of these considerations are included here to guide clinicians' treatment approaches. In addition, clinicians should be sensitive to the impacts that major life changes, such as changes in relationship or financial status or death of a loved one, can have on sexual health.

Medical Factors

Medical diagnoses, especially common ones such as diabetes and depression, can negatively impact a person's sexual life in a variety of ways (Basson & Schultz, 2007). In addition, some of the medications used to treat common medical conditions can have negative sexual effects (see Chapter 16). Because a given individual's response to a particular medication can vary, the clinician needs to ask a woman about any effects she may be having. When doing so, it is better to avoid saying, "Are you doing well on this medication?" Instead,

it is preferable to say something like "Some people taking this medication report a change in their sexual response or sexual feelings. Now that I mention this, do you think you have noticed any differences?"

A clinician can be a valuable resource to a woman who is taking a medication or who has a medical condition that may affect her sexuality. Similarly, clinicians can be immensely helpful in caring for women with cancer or surviving cancer, particularly those with breast or gynecologic cancers; women who are recovering from surgery; and women struggling with fertility issues by addressing possible sexual challenges, in addition to the health challenges.

Adolescents

Adolescence, which is generally defined as the ages from 12 to 19 years, is a period of rapid physical change and potentially stressful psychosocial demands, including awareness of and changes in sexual feelings. It is also a time when preferences are being formed and early sexual experiences contribute significantly to preference conditioning. The development of adolescent sexuality focuses on five aspects:

- Physical changes of puberty and their relationship to self-esteem and body image
- Learning about normal bodily functions and sensual and sexual responses and needs
- Developing one's sense of gender identity and comfort with one's sexual orientation
- Learning about sexual and romantic relationships
- Developing a personal sexual value system (Masters, Johnson, & Kolodney, 1995)

The proportion of adolescents who have had sex increases with age, from fewer than 2% at age 12 to 16% of 15-year-olds, 33% of 16-year-olds, 48% of 17-year-olds, 61% of 18-year-olds, and 71% of 19-year-olds. The timing of first sex varies little by gender. The average age at which young people have sex for the first time is 17 (Guttmacher Institute, 2014).

The most common reason adolescents do not have sex is that it is against their religion or morals (cited by 38% of females and 31% of males). The other most common reasons why adolescent females say they do not have sex are that they do not want to get pregnant or have not found the right person yet.

Most adolescents (70% of females and 56% of males) have their first sexual experience with a steady partner; 16% of females and 28% of males first have sex with someone whom they have just met or who is just a friend. Among young women aged 18 to 24 years who had sex before age 20, 11% describe their first sex as unwanted (Guttmacher Institute, 2014).

Adolescent sexual activity rates are similar in the United States and Europe; however, European adolescents have substantially lower pregnancy rates due to their higher use of contraception overall and their tendency to use the most effective contraceptive methods. Between 2006 and 2008, 8% of females aged 18 to 19 years reported they were lesbian or bisexual, and 12% reported any same-sex sexual experience (Guttmacher Institute, 2014).

Adolescents are planting the seeds for a lifetime of ever-expanding sexual self-knowledge and increasing sexual agency. Clinicians can support adolescents by proactively addressing issues of pleasure and agency in addition to engaging them in discussions about protection from STIs and unintended pregnancy. Adolescents will benefit from detailed information about female sexual anatomy and diagrams of the clitoral complex. Clinicians should ensure that adolescents understand the concept that the most likely route to learning how to orgasm is with masturbation or a partner's hands or mouth rather than with penile–vaginal intercourse.

Pregnant and Postpartum Women

Changes associated with pregnancy, postpartum, and lactation offer an opportunity to discuss sexuality and provide education for a childbearing couple's changing needs (Leeman & Rogers, 2012; Ribeiro et al., 2014).

Women may experience changes in sexual function with each trimester of pregnancy. During the first trimester, common symptoms, such as nausea and vomiting, breast tenderness, and fatigue, may impact a woman's desire for sex. It may be a time when a couple is feeling particularly close, being intimate, and enjoying nesting. Some women and some couples have anxiety about the pregnancy, which can impact their sexual activity. In the

second trimester, women often express heightened desire as they feel better. Even so, it is helpful if the clinician asks the woman about her feelings regarding the changes in her body, including increasing weight and body image. The third trimester can be associated with physical discomfort related to increasing size, especially when a woman is near term. Fears about the effects of intercourse on pregnancy maintenance and harming the fetus may decrease sexual interest or pleasure at any time during pregnancy.

During the postpartum period, sleep loss, exhaustion, and physical discomforts, including dyspareunia, are common (Declercq, Sakala, Corry, Applebaum, & Herrlich, 2014). Women may notice marked vaginal dryness associated with decreased levels of estrogen; this dryness may persist until ovulatory cycles resume. Although vaginal dryness is more common among women who are breastfeeding, it can occur in any postpartum woman, and affected women will benefit from the use of a lubricant to prevent dyspareunia (Herbenick et al., 2011; Jozkowski et al., 2013). Vaginal estrogen therapy may also be appropriate for women who are breastfeeding (Palmer & Likis, 2003).

Relationship dynamics between a couple change with the addition of a newborn to the family. These changes can herald some of the most precious moments in a couple's life together, yet also have the potential for setting the couple up for alienation. For example, a partner may feel shut out of the mother–infant dyad. Clinicians can act proactively during this time of vulnerability by asking detailed and open-ended questions about how things are unfolding and offering targeted suggestions or information to address the particular issues that a woman describes. For example, explaining that breastfeeding women may experience arousal when they breastfeed and have let-down with orgasm can help a lactating woman normalize her experience (Polomeno, 1999).

Midlife Women

In midlife (40–60 years of age), women's sexuality is as varied as are women themselves. For women who have been having positive sexual experiences throughout their lives with the cornerstones to sexual health in place, this time of life can be one of great sexual satisfaction, as increased self-knowledge, sexual agency, and capacity for intimacy intertwine with the mastery they and their partner(s) may have developed. For some women, a decreased concern of becoming pregnant may increase sexual desire and lessen inhibitions. This may also be a time of relationship transition and changing family dynamics as children grow up and leave the household.

During this time, fluctuations and the eventual decrease in estrogen levels can affect the vulvar and vaginal mucosa. *Genitourinary syndrome of menopause* (GSM) is a new term that replaces the older terms *vulvovaginal atrophy* (VVA) and *atrophic vaginitis*. The GSM term was created by a consensus panel because the prior nomenclature inadequately described the range of symptoms associated with physical changes of the vulva and vagina (Portman & Gass, 2014). One of the most effective ways to maintain healthy vaginal tissue in the perimenopause and after menopause is consistent sexual activity (Leiblum, Bachmann, Kemmann, Colburn, & Swartzman, 1983; North American Menopause Society, 2013). Other therapies for GSM are discussed in Chapter 12.

Older Women

During older adulthood (after age 65), women continue to be sexual beings and enjoy sexual activity. The prevailing cultural view of older women as asexual beings has the potential to negatively affect sexual expression and activity, and can become a self-fulfilling prophecy (Nappi & Lachowsky, 2009; Ringa, Diter, Laborde, & Bajos, 2013). Further, the current cultural emphasis on youth, beauty, and thinness contributes to societal expectations about asexuality in older women. Happily, when cornerstones to sexual health have been in place, this time of life can continue the sexual satisfaction that occurred in midlife; the health benefits of sexual activity become increasingly evident. In addition to cardiovascular benefits (Buettner, 2008; Davey Smith, 2010; Drory, 2002, Levin, 2007; Seldin et al., 2002), sexual activity helps maintain the integrity of vulvar and vaginal tissues by preventing thinning (North American Menopause Society, 2013). Strength and control over pelvic muscles prevents and improves urinary incontinence and pelvic organ prolapse (Herderschee et al., 2011).

Influences of Culture

Restrictive family upbringing or a belief that expressions of intimacy or sexuality are shameful or taboo may contribute to a woman's inability to express herself sexually. Religion also influences sexual attitudes, beliefs, and values, and can exert a strong influence throughout a person's life. Some religious proscriptions may contribute to sexual concerns or problems. For example, a view that sexual intercourse is acceptable only for procreation may raise concerns when pleasurable sensations are felt. Accepting or rejecting premarital sex, allowing or limiting contraception to prevent pregnancy, beliefs about monogamy for men and women, and condoning or rejecting homosexuality are examples of religious influences in a woman's life.

Society and culture are inextricably interwoven with sexuality and influence it as much as physiology and psychology do. Society defines what sexual behavior is, identifies the norms for that behavior, and guides the behavior of the individuals in a given culture. In part, women form their ideas of what is sexually appropriate and desirable from years of cultural scripting. These scripts are frequently different for men and women, and can be the basis for many of the issues women experience in sexual relationships. The notions that men who are sexually aggressive are "macho" or "studs" and that sexually aggressive women are "whores" and "easy" are examples of such cultural beliefs. In addition, sex role stereotypes often prescribe that men initiate sexual activity and women exercise control.

Sexual myths are common in every culture and society, and they are a source of sexual misinformation. Often they interfere with women reaching full sexual agency. Examples include the ideas that women's needs are secondary to men's, that large amounts of sexual stimulation are needed to arouse a woman, and that when a woman says "no" she does not really mean it (Peixoto & Nobre, 2014). Other sexual myths are specific to older women, such as statements that older women are not interested in or capable of sexual expression, physically unattractive, and sexually undesirable.

A specific behavior may be defined as desirable by one cultural group and evil by another. Different views often exist regarding premarital, extramarital, and marital sex; appropriate sexual positions; accepted foreplay activities; and duration of coitus.

CONCLUSION

Sexual health can contribute substantially to a woman's overall health throughout her life. A trusted clinician who has a good rapport with a woman is in a unique position to support her in achieving the cornerstones to sexual health: sexual self-knowledge, sexual agency, and control over the pelvic musculature. It is essential for clinicians who are caring for women to provide a nonjudgmental, supportive approach so that women are comfortable in discussing whatever issues they may have regarding their sexuality and can get accurate information and counseling. By fostering communication and, when needed, making appropriate referrals to other health professionals, clinicians can help each woman to achieve and enjoy her own version of sexuality.

References

Adams, A. E., III, Haynes, S. N., & Brayer, M. A. (1985). Cognitive distraction in female sexual arousal. *Psychophysiology, 22*(6), 689–696.

Alexander, L. L., LaRosa, J. H., Bader, H., & Garfield, S. (2007). *New dimensions in women's health* (4th ed.). Sudbury, MA: Jones and Bartlett.

Althof, S. E., Rosen, R. C., Perelman, M. A., & Rubio-Aurioles, E. (2013). Standard operating procedures for taking a sexual history. *Journal of Sexual Medicine, 10*(1), 26–35.

American Psychiatric Association. (2013). *Diagnostic and statistical manual of mental disorders* (5th ed.). Washington, DC: Author.

Bassett, R., Bourbonnais, V., & McDowell, I. (2007). Living long and keeping well: Elderly Canadians account for success in aging. *Canadian Journal of Aging, 26*(2), 113–126. doi:10.3138/cja .26.2.113

Basson, R. (2000). The female sexual response: A different model. *Journal of Sex & Marital Therapy, 26*, 51–65.

Basson, R., & Baram, D. A. (2011). Sexuality, sexual dysfunction, and sexual assault. In J. S. Berek (Ed.), *Berek and Novak's gynecology* (15th ed., pp. 313–349). Philadelphia, PA: Lippincott Williams & Wilkins.

Basson, R., Leiblum, S., Brotto, L., Derogatis, L., Fourcroy, J., Fugl-Meyer, K.,...Schultz, W. W. (2004). Revised definitions of women's sexual dysfunction. *Journal of Sexual Medicine, 1*, 40–48.

Basson, R., & Schultz, W. W. (2007). Sexual sequelae of general medical disorders. *Lancet, 369*, 409–424.

Bergner, D. (2013). *What do women want? Adventures in the science of female desire.* New York, NY: HarperCollins.

Braekken, I. H., Majida, M., Ellstrom Engh, M., & Bo, K. (2015). Can pelvic floor muscle training improve sexual function in women with pelvic organ prolapse? A randomized controlled trial. *Journal of Sexual Medicine, 12*(2), 470–480. doi:10.1111/jsm.12746

Buettner, D. (2008). *The blue zones: 9 lessons in living longer from the people who have lived the longest.* Washington, DC: National Geographic Society.

Centers for Disease Control and Prevention (CDC). (n.d.). A guide to taking a sexual history. Retrieved from http://www.cdc.gov /std/treatment/sexualhistory.pdf

Centers for Disease Control and Prevention (CDC). (2015). Phthalates fact sheet. Retrieved from http://www.cdc.gov/biomonitoring /Phthalates_FactSheet.html

Chalker, R. (1994). Updating the model of female sexuality. *Sexuality Information and Education Council of the United States, 22*, 1–6.

Chivers, M. L., Seto, M. C., Lalumiere, M. L., Laan, E., & Grimbos, T. (2010). Agreement of self-reported and genital measures of sexual arousal in men and women: A meta-analysis. *Archives of Sexual Behavior, 39*(1), 5–56.

Chivers, M. L., & Timmers, A. D. (2012). Effects of gender and relationship context in audio narratives on genital and subjective sexual response in heterosexual women and men. *Archives of Sexual Behavior, 41*(1), 185–197. doi:10.1007/s10508-012-9937-3

Citak, N., Cam, C., Arslan, H., Karateke, A., Tug, N., Ayaz, R., & Celik, C. (2010). Postpartum sexual function of women and the effects of early pelvic floor muscle exercises. *Acta Obstetrica et Gynecologica Scandinavica, 89*(6), 817–822. doi:10.3109/ 00016341003801623

Davey Smith, G. (2010). Pearls of wisdom: Eat, drink, have sex (using condoms), abstain from smoking and be merry. *International Journal of Epidemiology, 39*(4), 941–947.

Davison, S. L., Bell, R. J., LaChina, M., Holden, S. L., & Davis, S. R. (2009). The relationship between self-reported sexual satisfaction and general well-being in women. *Journal of Sexual Medicine, 6*(10), 2690–2697. doi:10.1111/j.1743 -6109.2009.01406.x

Declercq, E. R., Sakala, C., Corry, M. P., Applebaum, S., & Herrlich, A. (2014). Major survey findings of Listening to Mothers III: New mothers speak out: Report of national surveys of women's childbearing experiences conducted October–December 2012 and January–April 2013. *Journal of Perinatal Education, 23*(1), 17–24. doi:10.1891/1058-1243.23.1.17

Drory, Y. (2002). Sexual activity and cardiovascular risk. *European Heart Journal Supplements, 4*, H13–H18.

Ebrahim, S. M., M., Shlomo, Y.B., McCarron, P., Frankel S., Yarnell J., & Davey Smith, G. (2002). Sexual intercourse and risk of ischaemic stroke and coronary heart disease: The Caerphilly study. *Journal of Epidemiology and Community Health, 56*, 99–102.

Federation of Feminist Women's Health Centers. (1991). *A new view of a woman's body.* Los Angeles, CA: Feminist Health Press.

Fisher, T. D. (2013). Gender roles and pressure to be truthful: The bogus pipeline modifies gender differences in sexual but not non-sexual behavior. *Sex Roles, 68*(7/8), 401.

Fogel, C. I., & Woods, N. F. (2008). Women's sexuality. In C. I. Fogel & N. F. Woods (Eds.), *Women's health care in advanced practice nursing* (pp. 295–312). New York, NY: Springer.

Georgiadis, J. R., Kringelbach, M. L., & Pfaus, J. G. (2012). Sex for fun: A synthesis of human and animal neurobiology. *Nature Reviews Urology, 9*(9), 486–498. doi:10.1038/nrurol.2012.151

Guttmacher Institute. (2014). American teens' sexual and reproductive health fact sheet. Retrieved from https://www.guttmacher.org/pubs/FB-ATSRH.pdf

Herbenick, D., Reece, M., Hensel, D., Sanders, S., Jozkowski, K., & Fortenberry, J. D. (2011). Association of lubricant use with women's sexual pleasure, sexual satisfaction, and genital symptoms: A prospective daily diary study. *Journal of Sexual Medicine, 8,* 202–212.

Herbenick, D., Reece, M., Sanders, S., Dodge, B., Ghassemi, A., & Fortenberry, J. D. (2009). Prevalence and characteristics of vibrator use by women in the United States: Results from a nationally representative study. *Journal of Sexual Medicine, 6*(7), 1857–1866.

Herderschee, R., Hay-Smith, E. J., Herbison, G. P., Roovers, J. P., & Heineman, M.J. (2011). Feedback or biofeedback to augment pelvic floor muscle training for urinary incontinence in women. *Cochrane Database of Systematic Reviews, 7,* CD009252. doi:10.1002/14651858.CD009252

Imanieh, M. H., Bagheri, F., Alizadeh, A. M., & Ashkani-Esfahani, S. (2014). Oxytocin has therapeutic effects on cancer: A hypothesis. *European Journal of Pharmacology, 741,* 112–123. doi:10.1016/j.ejphar.2014.07.053

Jannini, E. A., Fisher, W. A., Bitzer, J., & McMahon, C. G. (2009). Is sex just fun? How sexual activity improves health. *Journal of Sexual Medicine, 6*(10), 2640–2648. doi:10.1111/j.1743-6109.2009.01477.x

Jannini, E. A., Whipple, B., Kingsberg, S. A., Buisson, O., Foldes, P., & Vardi, Y. (2010). Who's afraid of the G-spot? *Journal of Sexual Medicine, 7*(1 pt 1), 25–34. doi:10.1111/j.1743-6109.2009.01613.x

Joyal, C. C., Cossette, A., & Lapierre, V. (2015). What exactly is an unusual sexual fantasy? *Journal of Sexual Medicine, 12*(2), 328–340. doi:10.1111/jsm.12734

Jozkowski, K. N., Herbenick, D., Schick, V., Reece, M., Sanders, S. A., & Fortenberry, J. D. (2013). Women's perceptions about lubricant use and vaginal wetness during sexual activities. *Journal of Sexual Medicine, 10*(2), 484–492.

Kaplan, H. (1979). *Disorders of sexual desire and other new concepts and techniques in sex therapy.* New York, NY: Brunner/Mazel.

Kaschak, E., & Tiefer, L. (2001). *A new view of women's sexual problems.* Binghampton, NY: Haworth Press.

Leeman, L. M., & Rogers, R. G. (2012). Sex after childbirth: Postpartum sexual function. *Obstetrics & Gynecology, 119*(3), 647–655. doi:10.1097/AOG.0b013e3182479611

Leiblum, S., Bachmann, G., Kemmann, E., Colburn, D., & Swartzman, L. (1983). Vaginal atrophy in the postmenopausal woman: the importance of sexual activity and hormones. *Journal of the American Medical Association, 249,* 2195–2198.

Levin, R. J. (2007). Sexual activity, health and well-being: The beneficial roles of coitus and masturbation. *Sexual and Relationship Therapy, 22*(1), 135–148. doi:10.1080/14681990601149197

Lindau, S. T., & Gavrilova, N. (2010). Sex, health, and years of sexually active life gained due to good health: Evidence from two US population based cross sectional surveys of ageing. *BMJ, 340,* c810. doi:10.1136/bmj.c810

Lowenstein, L., Gruenwald, I., Gartman, I., & Vardi, Y. (2010). Can stronger pelvic muscle floor improve sexual function? *International Urogynecology Journal, 21*(5), 553–556. doi:10.1007/s00192-009-1077-5

Mark, K., Herbenick, D., Fortenberry, D., Sanders, S., & Reece, M. (2014). The object of sexual desire: Examining the "What" in "What do you desire?" *Journal of Sexual Medicine, 11*(11), 2709–2719. doi:10.1111/jsm.12683

Martinez, C. S., Ferreira, F. V., Castro, A. A. M., & Gomide, L. B. (2014). Women with greater pelvic floor muscle strength have better sexual function. *Acta Obstetrica et Gynecologica Scandinavica, 93*(5), 497–502. doi:10.1111/aogs.12379

Masters, W., & Johnson, V. (1966). *The human sexual response cycle.* Boston, MA: Little, Brown.

Masters, W. H., Johnson, V. E., & Kolodney, R. C. (1995). *Human sexuality* (5th ed.). New York, NY: HarperCollins.

Murrell, T. G. C. (1995). The potential for oxytocin (OT) to prevent breast cancer: A hypothesis. *Breast Cancer Research and Treatment, 35,* 225–229.

Nappi, R. E., & Lachowsky, M. (2009). Menopause and sexuality: Prevalence of symptoms and impact on quality of life. *Maturitas, 63*(2), 138–141. doi:10.1016/j.maturitas.2009.03.021

North American Menopause Society. (2013). Management of symptomatic vulvovaginal atrophy: 2013 position statement of the North American Menopause Society. *Menopause, 20*(9), 888–902.

Palmer, A. R., & Likis, F. E. (2003). Lactational atrophic vaginitis. *Journal of Midwifery & Women's Health, 48,* 282–284.

Palmore, E. B. (1982). Predictors of the longevity difference: a 25-year follow-up. *Gerontologist, 22,* 513–518.

Pascoal, P. M., Cardoso, D., & Henriques, R. (2015). Sexual satisfaction and distress in sexual functioning in a sample of the BDSM community: A comparison study between BDSM and non-BDSM contexts. *Journal of Sexual Medicine, 12*(4), 1052–1061. doi:10.1111/jsm.12835

Pastor, Z. (2013). Female ejaculation orgasm vs. coital incontinence: A systematic review. *Journal of Sexual Medicine, 10*(7), 1682–1691. doi:10.1111/jsm.12166

Peixoto, M. M., & Nobre, P. (2014). Dysfunctional sexual beliefs: A comparative study of heterosexual men and women, gay men, and lesbian women with and without sexual problems. *Journal of Sexual Medicine, 11*(11), 2690–2700. doi:10.1111/jsm.12666

Peschers, U. M., Gingelmaier, A., Jundt, K., Leib, B., & Dimpfl, T. (2001). Evaluation of pelvic floor muscle strength using four different techniques. *International Urogynecology Journal and Pelvic Floor Dysfunction, 12*(1), 27–30.

Pfaus, J. G. (2009). Pathways of sexual desire. *Journal of Sexual Medicine, 6*(6), 1506–1533. doi:10.1111/j.1743-6109.2009.01309.x

Pfaus, J. G., Kippin, T. E., Coria-Avila, G. A., Gelez, H., Afonso, V. M., Ismail, N., & Parada, M. (2012). Who, what, where, when (and maybe even why?) How the experience of sexual reward connects sexual desire, preference, and performance. *Archives of Sexual Behavior, 41*(1), 31–62. doi:10.1007/s10508-012-9935-5

Polomeno, V. (1999). Sex and breastfeeding: An educational perspective. *Journal of Perinatal Education, 8*(1), 30–40.

Portman, D. J., & Gass, M. L. (2014). Genitourinary syndrome of menopause: New terminology for vulvovaginal atrophy from the International Society for the Study of Women's Sexual Health and the North American Menopause Society. *Menopause, 21*(10), 1063–1068.

Prause, N., Barela, J., Roberts, V., & Graham, C. (2013). Instructions to rate genital vasocongestion increases genital and self-reported sexual arousal but not coherence between genital and self-reported sexual arousal. *Journal of Sexual Medicine, 10*(9), 2219–2231.

Ribeiro, M. C., Nakamura, M. U., Torloni, M. R., Scanavino, M. T., do Amaral, M. L. S., Puga, M. E. S., & Mattar, R. (2014). Treatments of female sexual dysfunction symptoms during pregnancy: A systematic review of the literature. *Sexual Medicine Review, 2,* 1–9.

Richters, J., de Visser, R. O., Rissel, C. E., Grulich, A. E., & Smith, A. M. (2008). Demographic and psychosocial features of participants in bondage and discipline, "sadomasochism" or dominance and submission (BDSM): Data from a national survey. *Journal of Sexual Medicine, 5*(7), 1660–1668. doi:10.1111/j.1743-6109.2008.00795.x

Ringa, V., Diter, K., Laborde, C., & Bajos, N. (2013). Women's sexuality: From aging to social representations. *Journal of Sexual Medicine, 10*(10), 2399–2408. doi:10.1111/jsm.12267

Sacomori, C., & Cardoso, F. L. (2015). Predictors of improvement in sexual function of women with urinary incontinence after treatment with pelvic floor exercises: A secondary analysis. *Journal of Sexual Medicine, 12*(3), 746–755. doi:10.1111/jsm.12814

Salonia, A., Giraldi, A., Chivers, M. L., Georgiadis, J. R., Levin, R., Maravilla, K. R., & McCarthy, M. M. (2010). Physiology of women's sexual function: Basic knowledge and new findings. *Journal of Sexual Medicine, 7*(8), 2637–2660. doi:10.1111/j.1743-6109.2010.01810.x

Scheff, E. A. (2014). Seven forms of non-monogamy. *Psychology Today.* Retrieved from https://www.psychologytoday.com/blog/the-polyamorists-next-door/201407/seven-forms-non-monogamy

Schnarch, D. (2009). *Passionate marriage: Love, sex, and intimacy in emotionally committed relationships.* New York, NY: W. W. Norton.

Schwartz, P., & Rutter, V. (1998). *The gender of sexuality.* Thousand Oaks, CA: Pine Forge Press.

Seldin, D. R., Friedman, H. S., & Martin, L. R. (2002). Sexual activity as a predictor of life-span mortality risk. *Personality and Individual Differences, 33*(3), 409–425.

Sprecher, S., & Cate, R. H. (2004). Sexual satisfaction and sexual expression as predictors of relationship satisfaction and stability. In J. H. Harvey, A. Wenzel, & S. Sprecher (Eds.), *The handbook of sexuality in close relationships* (pp. 235–256). Mahwah, NJ: Erlbaum.

Taylor, K., & Henderson, J. (1986). Effects of biofeedback and urinary stress incontinence in older women. *Journal of Gerontological Nursing, 12*(9), 25–30.

Tennfjord, M. K., Hilde, G., Staer-Jensen, J., Siafarikas, F., Engh, M. E., & Bo, K. (2015). Coital incontinence and vaginal symptoms and the relationship to pelvic floor muscle function in primiparous women at 12 months postpartum: A cross-sectional study. *Journal of Sexual Medicine.* [Epub ahead of print]. doi:10.1111/jsm.12836

U.S. Department of Health and Human Services. (2012). CDC/HRSA Advisory Committee on HIV, Viral Hepatitis, and STD Prevention and Treatment; May 8–9, 2012; Atlanta, Georgia. Record of the proceedings. Retrieved from http://www.cdc.gov/maso/facm/pdfs/CHACHSPT/20120508_CHAC.pdf

van Anders, S. M., Hipp, L. E., & Kane Low, L. (2013). Exploring co-parent experiences of sexuality in the first 3 months after birth. *Journal of Sexual Medicine, 10*(8), 1988–1999. doi:10.1111/jsm.12194

Wismeijer, A. A., & van Assen, M. A. (2013). Psychological characteristics of BDSM practitioners. *Journal of Sexual Medicine, 10*(8), 1943–1952. doi:10.1111/jsm.12192

World Association for Sexual Health. (2014). The declaration of sexual rights. Retrieved from http://www.worldsexology.org/wp-content/uploads/2013/08/declaration_of_sexual_rights_sep03_2014.pdf

World Health Organization (WHO). (2006). *Defining sexual health: Report of a technical consultation on sexual health, 28–31 January 2002, Geneva.* Geneva, Switzerland: Author. Retrieved from http://www.who.int/reproductivehealth/publications/sexual_health/defining_sexual_health.pdf?ua=1

CHAPTER 11

Contraception

Patricia Aikins Murphy

Caroline M. Hewitt

Cynthia Belew

The editors acknowledge Katherine Morgan and Frances E. Likis, who were coauthors of the previous edition of this chapter.

Contraceptive management is often a challenging undertaking, but providing family planning services offers clinicians the opportunity to empower people by helping them to make choices that can truly alter their life courses. There are more than 62 million women of reproductive age in the United States, and approximately 7 in 10 of these women—nearly 43 million women—are sexually active and do not want to become pregnant (Guttmacher Institute, 2014). The average woman in the United States desires two children and, therefore, must use contraception for approximately 3 decades of her life.

Sixty-four percent of U.S. women of reproductive age who use contraception choose reversible methods (Guttmacher Institute, 2014). Contraception is highly effective at preventing unwanted pregnancy. Women who use contraceptives consistently and correctly account for only 5% of all unintended pregnancies. In contrast, approximately 18% of women at risk of unintended pregnancy who use contraceptives but do so inconsistently account for 41% of unintended pregnancies; the 14% of women at risk of unintended pregnancy who do not use contraceptives at all or have a gap in use of 1 month or longer account for the remaining (54%) unintended pregnancies (Guttmacher Institute, 2014).

Avoidance of unintended pregnancy is critical to the health of women, families, and society. Its personal impact on the health of the woman and her offspring is evident in the increased rates of preterm birth, low-birth-weight infants, and infant mortality associated with unintended pregnancy. Higher rates of maternal anxiety and depression are also seen with unintended pregnancies (Gipson, Koenig, & Hindin, 2008).

When it comes to contraception, the challenge lies in helping each woman choose the method that best meets her needs and providing education so that she can use the chosen method correctly and consistently. The importance of the healthcare provider's role in guiding women to select the best option for their needs and in educating women on correct use cannot be overstated. Most women report that they do not feel very knowledgeable about the contraceptive options that are available to them and that they do not receive in-depth counseling on how to use their selected option. In addition, some women feel pressured by their provider to select a certain method. Indeed, there is a sorry history of reproductive coercion aimed at women who were deemed to be at high risk of unintended pregnancy and were pressured (and in some cases mandated by courts) to adopt long-acting methods of contraception (Gomez, Fuentes, & Allina, 2014). Policies and counseling designed to steer women toward a particular method ignore the unique needs of the individual woman and undermine her autonomy. Family planning policies and encounters reflect the racial inequality of the larger society. In particular, African American and Latina women report experiencing race-based discrimination when they seek family planning services (Kossler et al., 2011; Thorburn & Bogart, 2005). Providers must make efforts to be aware of their own implicit biases and to stay informed about the social and political contexts of family planning to ensure that all women can choose freely from all contraceptive options, which is one aspect of reproductive justice. The growing movement for reproductive justice goes beyond the focus on access and individual choice to analysis of the social, economic, and structural constraints on women's reproductive decisions (Asian Communities for Reproductive Justice, n.d.).

A woman who is pressured into choosing a certain method is more likely to feel ambivalent about its use, leading to higher rates of inconsistent use and discontinuation. Likewise, clients' dissatisfaction with their interactions with care providers and lack of continuity of providers are other factors connected with inconsistent method use (Frost & Darroch, 2008). Ambivalence about pregnancy is yet another factor underlying inconsistent method use (Frost & Darroch, 2008).

Support for developing a reproductive life plan is a key element of high-quality family planning care and may assist women to clarify their goals and use contraception more consistently (Files et al., 2011). Many women report misconceptions about the risk of conception from unprotected sex as well as the effectiveness and safety of contraceptive options (American College of Nurse-Midwives, 2013; Biggs & Foster, 2013). Improved knowledge may encourage more consistent and effective contraceptive use. Specifically, overestimation of contraceptive risk and underestimation of health benefits are common and must be addressed. The small risks associated with contraception for most women are dwarfed by the health risks of unintended pregnancy. In addition, use of hormonal contraceptive methods may actually protect future fertility by decreasing the risk of endometriosis, ectopic pregnancy, pelvic inflammatory disease (PID), and abortion-related complications. Hormonal methods also decrease the risk of ovarian, endometrial, and colon cancer (Maguire & Westhoff, 2011).

Unfortunately, there is no perfect contraceptive method—one that requires no effort, never fails, has no side effects, is easily affordable, and can be reversed immediately. The good news, however, is that more contraceptive options are available now than ever before. Contraceptive users today want more than efficacy from a method. They desire a method that is safe, convenient, and cost effective, and that has few side effects. How a method affects a woman's life—from side effects such as daily spotting to the need to remember to do something every day—may be a major determinant in consistency of use. In addition, knowledge about the noncontraceptive health benefits of some methods is increasing; this background enables women to make contraceptive choices that can have positive implications for their health. Most therapeutic uses of contraception are not approved by the U.S. Food and Drug Administration (FDA), although many are supported by evidence gathered through research studies. Clinicians frequently prescribe medications for conditions other than those for which they have FDA approval, and this off-label use is within the scope of prescriptive authority when a sound rationale and evidence are used (FDA, 2014b).

Contraceptive counseling should never be guided by a clinician's biases about what is best for a particular woman. Rather, the best method for any woman is the one that she wants and is motivated to use. Clinicians should present all of the choices that are reasonable (i.e., those that are acceptable in light of the individual history) and assist each woman to find her own best option. In doing so, clinicians should rely only on evidence-based contraindications to avoid unnecessarily restricting contraceptive options when determining whether the woman's history makes a particular method acceptable. The *U.S. Medical Eligibility Criteria for Contraceptive Use* (Centers for Disease Control and Prevention [CDC], 2010) is helpful in determining whether a woman is a candidate for a particular method (see **Appendix 11-A** for these guidelines). In addition, evidence-based guidance on how to use contraceptive methods appropriately is available in the *U.S. Selected Practice Recommendations for Contraceptive Use* (CDC, 2013b).

A thorough knowledge of the contraceptive methods available, including their mechanisms of action (see **Appendix 11-B**), is imperative for providing contraceptive counseling that leads to a fully informed choice. Women usually use contraception in the context of a relationship, so their partners may need education as well. A woman may at times need supportive counseling to negotiate contraceptive issues within her relationship.

In 2014, the CDC and the U.S. Department of Health and Human Services issued national quality standards for provision of family planning services (Gavin et al., 2014). These recommendations define which services should be offered in a family planning visit and give primary care providers the information they need to improve the quality of family planning services.

This chapter provides an overview of the various methods of contraception. Data on efficacy and effectiveness, safety and side effects, noncontraceptive benefits, and the advantages and disadvantages of each method are presented. A full discussion of contraceptive counseling and management is beyond the scope of this chapter, but interested readers are referred to the bibliography at the end of the chapter, which suggests resources for further research.

CONTRACEPTIVE EFFICACY AND EFFECTIVENESS

The effectiveness of contraceptive methods is described in several ways. *Efficacy*, sometimes referred to as "method failure" or "perfect use" failure rates, is how well a method works inherently. Efficacy describes the likelihood that an unintended pregnancy will occur even when the method is used consistently and exactly as prescribed. In most research studies, pregnancies that result from inconsistent use or incorrect use are not included in "method failure" rates. *Effectiveness*, also termed "user failure" or "typical use" failure rates, is how well a method works in actual practice. Effectiveness describes all unintended pregnancies that occur if a method is not used properly, such as in the case of inconsistent or incorrect use. The terms *efficacy* and *effectiveness* are often used interchangeably when discussing contraception.

Not all contraceptive failures qualify as "user failures." Indeed, all contraceptive methods have inherent failure rates. Unintended pregnancies may occur even with highly effective methods such as sterilization (**Table 11-1**). Methods that are highly dependent on user consistency may have higher failure rates, but not all unintended pregnancies

occur as a result of user errors. Clinicians should avoid implying that unintended pregnancies are the user's fault.

In addition to inherent method efficacy and consistent and correct use of a method, several other factors affect contraceptive failure rates. Most failures are concentrated in early usage. More fertile women will have earlier failures, and women who use contraception incorrectly or inconsistently will get pregnant sooner. In addition, older women are less fecund (able to get pregnant) than younger women; thus any method used by younger women will have a higher failure rate than when the same method is used by older women. Other factors contributing to contraceptive success include the fertility of the male partner, the motivation to avoid pregnancy (as opposed to simply wanting to space pregnancies), relationship status, and frequency of sexual intercourse.

NONHORMONAL METHODS

The nonhormonal contraceptive methods can be grouped into three general categories:

- Physiologic methods: abstinence, coitus interruptus, lactational amenorrhea method (breastfeeding), and fertility awareness-based (FAB) methods
- Barrier methods: male condoms, vaginal barrier methods, and spermicides
- Permanent contraception (sterilization): male and female

One additional contraceptive method that does not contain hormones—the copper intrauterine device (IUD)—is covered in the section on intrauterine contraception. The physiologic and barrier reversible nonhormonal contraceptive options generally require motivated users, and most of these methods necessitate taking action with every act of sexual intercourse. In general, their efficacy is less than that of hormonal methods, but these options do not have systemic side effects. In addition, many barrier methods do not require involvement of a clinician. Nonhormonal methods may also be chosen because they fit within the woman's cultural beliefs. The permanent contraceptive options—that is, male and female sterilization—are the only permanent forms of contraception and require certainty that future childbearing is not desired.

Physiologic Methods

Abstinence

Abstaining from penile–vaginal intercourse is the only certain way to avoid pregnancy. Abstinence is most often practiced in conjunction with FAB methods or prior to becoming sexually active. Although abstinence is generally promoted as the method of choice for adolescents, counseling should include all contraceptive options.

Efficacy and Effectiveness Abstinence is 100% effective at preventing pregnancy.

Safety and Side Effects There are no contraindications to or side effects from using abstinence.

Noncontraceptive Benefits There are no noncontraceptive benefits of abstinence.

TABLE 11-1	Percentage of Women Experiencing an Unintended Pregnancy During the First Year of Typical Use and the First Year of Perfect Use of Contraception, and the Percentage Continuing Use at the End of the First Year, United States

Method	% of Women Experiencing an Unintended Pregnancy Within the First Year of Use		% of Women Continuing Use at 1 Year[c]
	Typical Use[a]	Perfect Use[b]	
No method[d]	85	85	
Spermicides[e]	28	18	42
Fertility awareness-based methods	24		47
Standard Days method[f]		5	
TwoDay method[f]		4	
Ovulation method[f]		3	
Symptothermal method[f]		0.4	
Withdrawal	22	4	46
Sponge			36
Parous women	24	20	
Nulliparous women	12	9	
Condom[g]			
Female	21	5	41
Male	18	2	43
Diaphragm[h]	12	6	57
Combined pill and progestin-only pill	9	0.3	67
Evra patch	9	0.3	67
NuvaRing	9	0.3	67
Depo-Provera	6	0.2	56

(continues)

Method	% of Women Experiencing an Unintended Pregnancy Within the First Year of Use		% of Women Continuing Use at 1 Year[c]
	Typical Use[a]	Perfect Use[b]	
Intrauterine contraceptives			
Paragard (copper T)	0.8	0.6	78
Mirena (levonorgestrel)	0.2	0.2	80
Implanon	0.05	0.05	84
Female sterilization	0.5	0.5	100
Male sterilization	0.15	0.10	100

Emergency contraception: Emergency contraceptive pills or insertion of a copper intrauterine contraceptive after unprotected intercourse substantially reduces the risk of pregnancy.[i]

Lactational amenorrhea method (LAM): LAM is a highly effective, *temporary* method of contraception.[j]

[a] Among *typical* couples who initiate use of a method (not necessarily for the first time), the percentage who experience an accidental pregnancy during the first year if they do not stop use for any other reason. Estimates of the probability of pregnancy during the first year of typical use for spermicides, withdrawal, fertility awareness-based methods, the diaphragm, the male condom, the oral contraceptive pill, and Depo-Provera are taken from the 1995 National Survey of Family Growth corrected for underreporting of abortion; see the text for the derivation of estimates for the other methods.

[b] Among couples who initiate use of a method (not necessarily for the first time) and who use it *perfectly* (both consistently and correctly), the percentage who experience an accidental pregnancy during the first year if they do not stop use for any other reason. See the text for the derivation of the estimate for each method.

[c] Among couples attempting to avoid pregnancy, the percentage who continue to use a method for 1 year.

[d] The percentages becoming pregnant in columns (2) and (3) are based on data from populations where contraception is not used and from women who cease using contraception in order to become pregnant. Among such populations, about 89% become pregnant within 1 year. This estimate was lowered slightly (to 85%) to represent the percentage who would become pregnant within 1 year among women now relying on reversible methods of contraception if they abandoned contraception altogether.

[e] Foams, creams, gels, vaginal suppositories, and vaginal film.

[f] The ovulation and TwoDay methods are based on evaluation of cervical mucus. The Standard Days Method avoids intercourse on cycle days 8 through 19. The symptothermal method is a double-check method based on evaluation of cervical mucus to determine the first fertile day and evaluation of cervical mucus and temperature to determine the last fertile day.

[g] Without spermicides.

[h] With spermicidal cream or jelly.

[i] ella, Plan B One-Step, and Next Choice are the only dedicated products specifically marketed for emergency contraception. The label for Plan B One-Step (1 dose is 1 white pill) says to take the pill within 72 hours after unprotected intercourse. Research has shown that all of the brands listed here are effective when used within 120 hours of unprotected sex. The label for Next Choice (1 dose is 1 peach pill) says to take one pill within 72 hours after unprotected intercourse and another pill 12 hours later. Research has shown that both pills can be taken at the same time with no decrease in efficacy or increase in side effects and that they are effective when used within 120 hours after unprotected sex. The Food and Drug Administration has in addition declared the following 19 brands of oral contraceptives to be safe and effective for emergency contraception: Ogestrel (1 dose is 2 white pills); Nordette (1 dose is 4 light-orange pills); Cryselle, Levora, Low-Ogestrel, Lo/Ovral, or Quasense (1 dose is 4 white pills); Jolessa, Portia, Seasonale, or Trivora (1 dose is 4 pink pills); Seasonique (1 dose is 4 light-blue-green pills); Enpresse (1 dose is 4 orange pills); Lessina (1 dose is 5 pink pills); Aviane or LoSeasonique (1 dose is 5 orange pills); Lutera or Sronyx (1 dose is 5 white pills); and Lybrel (1 dose is 6 yellow pills).

[j] However, to maintain effective protection against pregnancy, another method of contraception must be used as soon as menstruation resumes, the frequency or duration of breastfeeds is reduced, bottle feeds are introduced, or the baby reaches 6 months of age.

Reproduced from Trussell, J., & Guthrie, K. A. (2011). Choosing a contraceptive: Efficacy, safety, and personal considerations. In R. A. Hatcher, J. Trussell, A. L. Nelson, W. Cates, D. Kowal, & M. S. Policar (Eds.), *Contraceptive technology* (20th ed., pp. 45–74.). New York, NY: Ardent Media.

Advantages and Disadvantages Abstinence is readily available and completely effective. Abstinence prevents sexually transmitted infections (STIs), including infection with the human immunodeficiency virus (HIV) via penile–vaginal transmission, but users must be cautioned to avoid other sexual practices (e.g., oral sex and anal sex) that put them at risk for STIs (see Chapter 20). The major disadvantage of abstinence is that it is unrealistic for most couples in long-term relationships to use abstinence exclusively for an extended period of time.

Coitus Interruptus

Coitus interruptus, also known as withdrawal, is the removal of the penis from the vagina prior to ejaculation. Coitus interruptus prevents pregnancy by keeping sperm from entering the vagina. While only 3% of women in the United States using contraception employ coitus interruptus as their primary method, 60% of women in the 2010 National Survey of Family Growth report having used withdrawal at some time in their lives (Daniels & Mosher, 2013).

Efficacy and Effectiveness The theoretical efficacy of coitus interruptus is high, but the estimated typical use failure rate is around 22% (**Table 11-1**; Trussell, 2011). The long-held belief that preejaculatory fluid contains sperm, which could theoretically cause pregnancy even if withdrawal were used correctly, has been subjected to small clinical studies, with conflicting results (Killick, Leary, Trussell, & Guthrie, 2011; Zukerman, Weiss, & Orvieto, 2003).

Safety and Side Effects There are no contraindications to or side effects from using coitus interruptus.

Noncontraceptive Benefits There are no noncontraceptive benefits of coitus interruptus.

Advantages and Disadvantages Coitus interruptus is readily available, requires no supplies or cost, and is user controlled. Couples can use coitus interruptus intermittently when other methods are unavailable. Disadvantages include the need to use this method with every act of intercourse, and the need to exert the self-discipline and control necessary to stop intercourse. Coitus interruptus does not prevent STI transmission because penile–vaginal contact occurs, and HIV and other STIs can be present in pre-ejaculatory fluid. Women who use coitus interruptus should be educated about emergency contraception as a backup method.

Lactational Amenorrhea Method

Infant suckling during breastfeeding increases maternal prolactin levels, which in turn inhibit ovulation; this is the physiologic basis of the lactational amenorrhea method (LAM) of contraception. Three conditions must be met for LAM to be effective: (1) exclusive or near-exclusive breastfeeding, (2) amenorrhea, and (3) infant younger than 6 months (Kennedy & Trussell, 2011). Breastfeeding education and support are beneficial for women using LAM.

Efficacy and Effectiveness Breastfeeding is an extremely effective method of contraception if the conditions for its use are met (**Table 11-1**). Failures typically occur when breastfeeding is nonexclusive or after the infant reaches 6 months of age. In these instances, the likelihood of ovulation increases and the woman may be unaware of her return to fertility.

Safety and Side Effects There are no contraindications to LAM, but breastfeeding is not recommended for women who are HIV positive in countries such as the United States where infant formula is accessible, or for women who are taking medications that could be harmful to the infant. The only side effects of LAM are those associated with breastfeeding, such as sore nipples and mastitis.

Noncontraceptive Benefits Women who breastfeed their infants have decreased risk of ovarian, endometrial, and breast cancers (Anderson, Schwab, & Martinez, 2014; Cramer, 2012). Breastfeeding also has numerous benefits for infant health.

Advantages and Disadvantages LAM is readily available, free, and can be used immediately postpartum. The disadvantages of LAM are that it is available only to women who are breastfeeding, its duration of use is limited, and women may have difficulty sustaining the patterns of breastfeeding required to maintain contraceptive effectiveness. In addition, LAM does not provide protection from STIs.

Fertility Awareness-Based Methods

FAB methods involve determining when a woman is most fertile during each month and using either abstinence or barrier contraception during that time to prevent pregnancy. The "fertile window" or time when intercourse is most likely to result in pregnancy comprises the 5 days before plus the day of ovulation (Smoley & Robinson, 2012). FAB methods are also referred to as natural family planning and the rhythm method. Among women in the United States who use contraception, 1% use FAB methods (Daniels & Mosher, 2013).

The fertile window can be identified with calendar methods or by using signs and symptoms of ovulation. Calendar methods require counting the days in the menstrual cycle. In the calendar FAB method, the woman records the length of 6 to 12 menstrual cycles and determines the longest and shortest cycles. She then uses that information to identify the first (days in shortest cycle minus 18) and last (days in longest cycle minus 11) fertile days each month. Calculations must be updated with each cycle (Smoley & Robinson, 2012). Because this method requires careful calculations that can be confusing, the Standard Days Method (SDM) was developed as a simpler calendar method. Women using the SDM are advised to use abstinence or a barrier contraceptive on days 8 to 19 of the menstrual cycle. A color-coded set of beads called CycleBeads can be used in conjunction with the SDM to help women keep track of their fertile window (http://www.cyclebeads.com). The SDM is recommended for women whose cycles are 26 to 32 days in length (Smoley & Robinson, 2012). There are also now apps for smartphones and tablets that can be used to track cycles for the FAB method (for example, http://www.dottheapp.com).

The postovulation method is another variation on the calendar method. With this method, the woman subtracts 14 days from her average cycle length to predict the day of ovulation. Abstinence or a barrier method is used during the first half of the cycle until the fourth morning after the predicted day of ovulation. This method requires the longest period of abstinence or use of additional contraception.

Signs and symptoms of ovulation include a rise in the basal body temperature (BBT) and changes in cervical mucus. The BBT increases at the time of ovulation and remains elevated for the rest of the cycle. Using BBT charting in conjunction with the postovulation observations is beneficial, but predicting the fertile period with BBT is difficult because ovulation has already occurred once the rise in temperature is observed.

The Billings ovulation method uses assessment of cervical mucus to determine the fertile window. Women check daily for the increased, clear, stretchy, slippery cervical secretions associated with ovulation. The fertile time lasts from the day when ovulatory cervical secretions are first observed until 4 days after they are last observed (Smoley & Robinson, 2012).

The TwoDay Method is a simplified version of the ovulation method. The woman checks daily for cervical secretions and is considered fertile any day that she has cervical secretions present or had them present the day before (Smoley & Robinson, 2012).

The symptothermal method involves observing multiple indicators of the fertile window; the most common combination is assessment of cervical mucus and daily BBT charting. The cervical secretions can be used to identify the beginning of the fertile window, and the BBT can be used to detect the end. Some women using the symptothermal method also assess cervical position and signs of ovulation (e.g., mittelschmerz).

Home ovulation tests originally used for women with infertility (e.g., Clearblue Easy Fertility Monitor) can be used in conjunction with the calendar, ovulation, or symptothermal methods to improve their effectiveness (Leiva et al., 2014).

The detailed information required for patient education about FAB methods is beyond the scope of this chapter. Readers are referred to the websites listed in **Box 11-1** for further information, including training courses for clinicians.

Efficacy and Effectiveness The theoretical efficacy of FAB methods varies according to the specific technique used (**Table 11-1**). The typical use failure rate reflects the difficulty of using these methods correctly and consistently. A Cochrane

BOX 11-1 **Websites for Fertility Awareness-Based Methods Information**

Institute for Natural Family Planning:
http://www.marquette.edu/nursing
/natural-family-planning
Billings Ovulation Method:
http://www.boma-usa.org
Creighton Model:
http://www.creightonmodel.com
Couple to Couple League:
http://ccli.org
Institute for Reproductive Health:
http://irh.org/focus-areas/family_planning
Taking Charge of Your Fertility:
http://www.ovusoft.com

review, which was updated in 2012, concluded that the comparative efficacy of FAB methods of contraception remains unknown (Grimes, Gallo, Grigorieva, Nanda, & Schulz, 2004). Researchers at the Institute for Reproductive Health have demonstrated typical use effectiveness rates of 88% and 86% for the SDM and the TwoDay Method, respectively, and they have developed extensive resources for teaching these methods to providers, community health workers, and women (Institute for Reproductive Health, 2015).

Safety and Side Effects There are no health concerns with the use of FAB methods, but certain circumstances or conditions complicate their use. These factors include the postpartum period, breastfeeding, having an abortion immediately before their use, recent menarche or perimenopause when cycles may be irregular, medications that alter the regularity of cycles or fertility signs, vaginal discharge, irregular vaginal bleeding, and conditions associated with elevated body temperature (CDC, 2010). There are no side effects of FAB methods.

Noncontraceptive Benefits The principles of FAB methods can also be used to conceive when couples decide they want children.

Advantages and Disadvantages Women may have to pay for FAB methods training or supplies (e.g., basal body thermometer, CycleBeads), but there is no ongoing cost unless a barrier contraceptive is used during the fertile window. These methods are user controlled and may be the only acceptable form of contraception for members of some religions and cultures. Disadvantages include the need for detailed education, ongoing attention to identifying the fertile window, and abstaining from intercourse or using an additional contraceptive method several days each month. FAB methods do not protect either partner from STIs, and users should be educated about emergency contraception.

Barrier Methods

All barrier methods are coitus dependent. They must be applied at the time of intercourse, before any penile penetration, and ideally before any genital contact to avoid disruption in sex play. This requirement may be a problem for some couples due to the need to plan ahead, or for others who find application disruptive. Couples can be taught to make application or insertion of the barrier method part of their sex play. The coitus-dependent nature of barrier methods may be an advantage for couples who have infrequent intercourse.

Although these methods are less effective in preventing pregnancy than contemporary hormonal or intrauterine methods, interest in barrier contraception is on the rise again. This trend partly reflects the hormone-free aspects of barrier methods, but largely indicates recognition of their potential role as dual protection against pregnancy and STIs, including HIV. The cervix is the point of entry for many sexually transmitted pathogens. Protecting the cervix via chemical or physical barriers is an expanding area of research in the prevention of STIs. Finally, barrier contraceptives can be used by most people because contraindications to the use of these methods are rare (CDC, 2010).

Male Condoms

The male condom is a thin sheath that is placed over the erect penis. It serves as a barrier to pregnancy by trapping seminal fluid and sperm and offers protection against STIs. In fact, early descriptions of condom use in the 1500s emphasized the condom's role in protection from syphilis and other diseases (Tone, 2001).

Latex condoms are manufactured and packaged with a rolled rim, designed to be applied to the tip of the penis and then rolled down over the erect penis. It is important to note that there is a right side and a wrong side when the condom is rolled up; applying the condom with the wrong side out will prevent it from being placed properly, and potentially contaminate the outside of the condom with seminal fluid. Minor design changes over the years to this rolled-rim construction have included enlarged tips to contain ejaculated fluid (**Figure 11-1**), as well as variety in colors, sizes, flavors, and textured surfaces that are purported to enhance sexual pleasure. Some condoms add lubricants as well, including spermicidal lubricants.

Nonlatex condoms were developed in response to several concerns about latex. These condoms are made of polyurethane or a latex-like material called styrene ethylene butylene styrene (SEBS). Nonlatex condoms are odorless, colorless, and nonallergenic. They transmit body heat better and have a looser fit, theoretically allowing more sensitivity. They can be used with any lubricant and do not usually deteriorate with the use of oil-based lubricants or under adverse storage conditions. Nonlatex condoms appear to have twice the odds of breakage or slippage during intercourse or withdrawal compared to latex condoms (Festin, 2013). Many users prefer the nonlatex condoms over latex, and these preferences may translate into more consistent use of condoms. Consistent use and consumer familiarity with and education about the product may reduce the higher rates of breakage and slippage with this method that have been reported in studies.

Efficacy and Effectiveness When used correctly and consistently, latex condoms are an effective form of contraception (**Table 11-1**). Condom failures are commonly related to breakage of the condom, or slippage during intercourse or while removing the condom. In general, pregnancy rates for nonlatex condoms are slightly higher than the corresponding rates for latex condoms, but within the range considered acceptable for barrier methods. As noted, nonlatex condoms have higher reported rates of breakage and slippage than latex condoms. It is unclear whether this difference is related to the product or to a lack of familiarity with the product.

Safety and Side Effects Latex condoms should not be used by persons with known latex allergies. Some women report genital irritation and discomfort

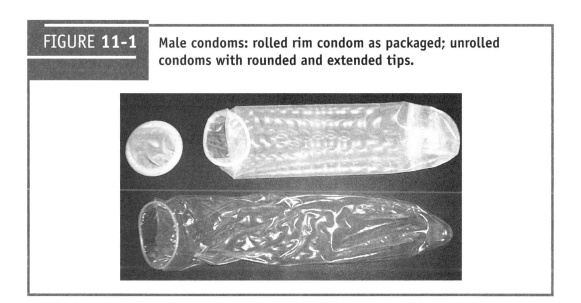

| FIGURE 11-1 | Male condoms: rolled rim condom as packaged; unrolled condoms with rounded and extended tips. |

TABLE 11-2	Advantages and Disadvantages of Barrier Methods[a]

Advantages	Disadvantages
Nonhormonal	Require planning
Do not require daily action	Require application at the time of intercourse and may be interruptive
Some are available without prescription	
Some offer protection against STIs	Breakage or slippage of barrier methods at time of intercourse may increase risk of unintended pregnancy

[a]All women relying on barrier or coitus-dependent methods should be aware of emergency contraception and be offered an advance prescription.

from the use of condoms, an issue that may be related either to the condom or to concomitant lubricant use. Some condoms are lubricated with a spermicide (nonoxynol-9 [N-9]) that may produce genital irritation in some women (see the section on spermicides). One study of a polyurethane condom evaluated genital irritation in both men and women. Although no differences were observed among the men in each group, the female partners in the polyurethane group had significantly less genital pain, pruritus, and vaginal pain than their counterparts in the latex condom group (Steiner, Dominik, Rountree, Nanda, & Dorflinger, 2003).

Noncontraceptive Benefits Condoms are routinely recommended for their noncontraceptive benefit of protection from STIs. Consistent use of latex condoms in sexually active HIV-serodiscordant couples can result in an 80% reduction in the incidence of HIV infection (Weller & Davis, 2002). Condoms also offer statistically significant protection against gonorrhea, chlamydia, herpes simplex virus (HSV) type 2, and syphilis, and they may protect women from trichomoniasis (CDC, 2013a). While condoms do not appear to offer protection against human papillomavirus (HPV) infection, their use is associated with higher rates of cervical intraepithelial neoplasia regression and cervical HPV infection clearance (CDC, 2013a).

Advantages and Disadvantages Condoms have the advantage of being widely available on an over-the-counter basis, without the need for clinician visit or prescription. The nonlatex condoms tend to be more expensive than their latex counterparts. The effectiveness of condoms is coitus dependent (**Table 11-2**). Correct use is critical to prevent breakage, slippage, and resultant unintended pregnancy. A potential disadvantage of using condoms as a contraceptive method is that they are male controlled. Women who are in relationships where they cannot negotiate condom use with their partners need a method they can control.

Spermicides
Spermicides are chemical barriers that are used either alone or in conjunction with a physical barrier (such as a condom, diaphragm, or sponge) to prevent pregnancy. The most common spermicides currently marketed in the United States contain N-9. This product may be formulated as a gel, cream, foam, suppository, foaming tablet, or film, and is generally provided in 50- to 150-milligram (mg) dosages. Other spermicidal compounds are available in other countries, such as octoxynol-9, benzalkonium chloride, and menfegol. Fewer than 0.5% of women report use spermicides as their primary method of contraception (Daniels & Mosher, 2013).

Efficacy and Effectiveness Studies comparing N-9 in various formulations (vaginal contraceptive film, foaming tablets, suppositories, and gels), each used without condoms or other physical barriers, showed typical use pregnancy rates over 6 months that ranged from 10% to 15% to a high of 28% (Raymond, Chen, Luoto, & Group, 2004)

(**Table 11-1**). These rates are higher than those for other barrier contraceptives. Formulations containing at least 100 mg of N-9 are associated with lower unintended pregnancy rates. Although the effectiveness of spermicides used as a sole agent is less than that of other contraceptive methods, spermicide use is more effective than using no method at all.

Safety and Side Effects N-9 is a surfactant, and surfactants can disrupt cell membranes. By extension, it was envisioned that the surfactant in this product would also act against pathogenic organisms and protect the user against gonorrhea, chlamydia, herpes, and syphilis. Studies from the late 1980s suggested that N-9 could inactivate HIV and other STIs. However, more recent studies have shown that N-9 is an irritant to both animal and human tissue. Frequent use is associated with increased reports of vaginal irritation. As an irritant, N-9 has the potential to disrupt or damage epithelial tissue in both the vagina and the rectum. The risk of this disruption increases with frequency of use and dose. Because intact tissue is the first defense against infection, use of N-9 could, therefore, potentially increase the risk of transmission of infection by causing microabrasions in the epithelium. In addition, strong evidence indicates that N-9 does not reduce STIs among sex workers or women attending STI clinics. In fact, some research suggests that N-9 use can even increase the risk of HIV acquisition in high-risk women (Van Damme et al., 2002; Wilkinson, Ramjee, Tholandi, & Rutherford, 2002).

Recommendations for the use of N-9 were developed in 2001 by a World Health Organization (WHO) task force (WHO/CONRAD, 2001):

- N-9 should not be used for purposes of STI protection.
- N-9 should not be used by women who engage in multiple daily acts of intercourse.
- N-9 should not be used by women at high risk for HIV acquisition.
- N-9 should not be used rectally.

The *U.S. Medical Eligibility Criteria for Contraceptive Use* classifies spermicides as category 4 methods for women at high risk for HIV infection and as category 3 methods for women with HIV/AIDS.

For women at low risk of HIV acquisition, however, N-9 products can be a valid contraceptive option (CDC, 2010).

The likelihood of women who use N-9 for contraception developing specific genitourinary symptoms after 6 to 7 months of use is 13% to 17% for a yeast infection, 8% to 12% for bacterial vaginosis, 19% to 27% for vulvovaginal irritation, and 11% to 15% for urinary tract symptoms (but only 3% to 6% for culture-proven urinary tract infection). The likelihood of irritation and other genitourinary symptoms in the male partner ranges from 6% to 14% after 6 to 7 months of use. In the studies that produced these findings, there was no comparison group to indicate whether these rates are higher than, lower than, or the same as the rates in the general population of sexually active women using contraception (Raymond et al., 2004). However, the reported rates are high enough to warrant counseling women to report symptoms so that they can be evaluated, diagnosed, and properly treated.

Noncontraceptive Benefits Despite concerns about the potential for cervicovaginal epithelial disruption with N-9-based spermicides, vaginally applied chemical barriers remain appealing. This attraction stems largely from their potential to provide dual protection—they can be both spermicidal and microbicidal. Woman-controlled, vaginally applied, lubricating microbicides offer great potential for protection against STIs, including HIV. Microbicide development and clinical trials are ongoing.

Advantages and Disadvantages Spermicides containing N-9 are widely available as over-the-counter products and do not require a prescription or clinician visit. Thus they are readily accessible to women who need personally controlled, discreet, low-cost contraception. The effectiveness of spermicides is coitus dependent (**Table 11-2**). Disadvantages include the low contraceptive effectiveness and the potential for symptoms of cervicovaginal irritation. As noted earlier, women who engage in multiple daily acts of intercourse or who are at high risk for STIs should avoid use of spermicides containing N-9.

Diaphragms

The traditional contraceptive diaphragm is a shallow dome-shaped cup that is inserted in the vagina to cover the cervix. Currently, fewer than 1% of women in the United States using contraception use the diaphragm (Guttmacher Institute, 2014).

Efficacy and Effectiveness The contraceptive efficacy of the diaphragm is similar to that of the male condom (**Table 11-1**). Traditional diaphragms are designed to be used in conjunction with a spermicide. The only study comparing differences in the contraceptive effectiveness of a diaphragm depending on whether spermicide is used was underpowered and, therefore, could not reach firm conclusions (Bounds, Guillebaud, Dominik, & Dalberth, 1995).

During sexual excitement, the upper part of the vagina expands; thus, diaphragms and other devices that might be in contact with the vaginal walls during fitting may no longer provide a complete physical barrier to sperm migration during intercourse. Theoretically, an additional and important function of the diaphragm would be to maintain spermicide in contact with the cervical os, thereby ensuring that sperm are trapped by the chemical barrier.

Safety and Side Effects The spermicide side effects discussed earlier in this chapter may also be experienced by diaphragm users. The *U.S. Medical Eligibility Criteria for Contraceptive Use* classifies the diaphragm as a category 3 or 4 method for women with HIV/AIDS or at high risk of HIV infection; this is solely due to concerns about the spermicide (CDC, 2010).

The diaphragms available in the United States as of this writing are made of silicone and can be used by women with latex allergies. Water-based products (rather than those containing silicone) are recommended for women who wish to use a lubricant with silicone diaphragms. Irritation or even abrasions of the vaginal mucosa have been noted in women with improperly sized diaphragms or prolonged retention of the diaphragm in the vagina. Although no clear association with toxic shock syndrome has been demonstrated, diaphragms and other contraceptive barrier devices should not be left in the vagina for more than 24 hours, and their use during menses is discouraged.

Urinary tract infections are more common in diaphragm users than among women using hormonal contraceptives. Two factors may explain this phenomenon. The first is mechanical: The rim of the diaphragm may exert pressure against the urethra, which might be perceived as frequency, dysuria, or incomplete bladder emptying, and may lead to infection. The second factor is that the spermicides used with the diaphragm can alter normal vaginal flora and may increase the likelihood of *Escherichia coli* bacteriuria (Hooton et al., 2000; Schreiber, Meyn, Creinin, Barnhart, & Hillier, 2006).

Noncontraceptive Benefits The diaphragm has possible or theoretical value in protecting the cervix from infection, but data demonstrating such a protective effect are not currently available. The only barrier methods known to reduce STIs are male and female condoms.

Advantages and Disadvantages Diaphragms are user-controlled, nonhormonal contraceptive methods that are needed only at the time of intercourse (**Table 11-2**). One of the diaphragms currently available in the United States comes in multiple sizes, varying in diameter (**Figure 11-2**). This device must be fit by a clinician and requires a prescription to purchase. A new one-size-fits-all diaphragm is also available in the United States by prescription (Kessel, n.d.).

As a result of the need for a clinician visit, diaphragms have a higher initiation cost than condoms, but can be used for years with proper care. The only additional cost is the spermicide that must be used with the diaphragm. Diaphragms are washable and reusable. Proper use is important. Users should be counseled on the timing of insertion and removal, use of spermicide, appropriate care of the device, and need for periodic reevaluation of the size.

Cervical Caps

Cervical caps are cuplike devices that cover the cervix. Smaller than diaphragms, they maintain their position over the cervix by suction, adhering to the cervix, or via a design that uses vaginal walls for support. Caps were long popular in Europe, where several types of caps were available. However, most of these are no longer being manufactured

FIGURE **11-2**   Diaphragms.

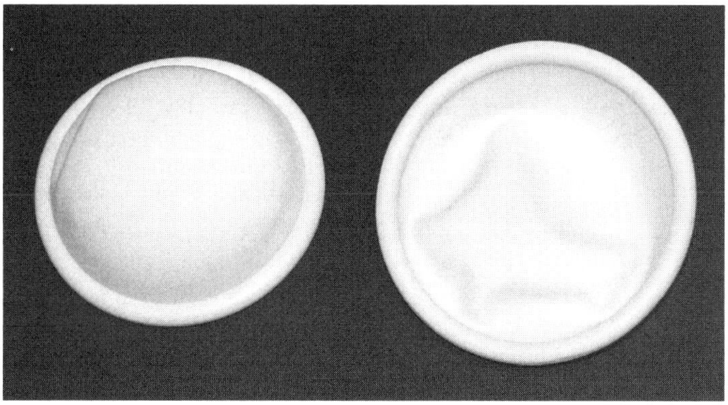

FIGURE **11-3**   The FemCap.

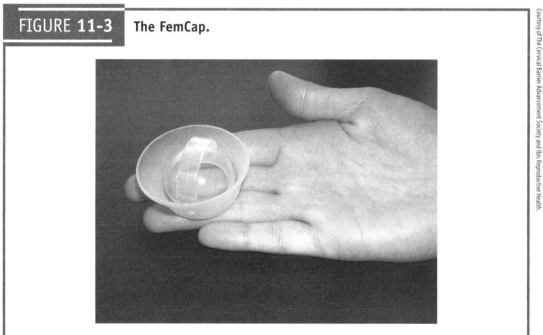

Courtesy of The Cervical Barrier Advancement Society and Ibis Reproductive Health.

(Cervical Barrier Advancement Society, n.d.). The FemCap is the only cervical cap device available in the United States.

The FemCap is made of silicone and has a design like an inverted sailor's cap (**Figure 11-3**). The dome covers the cervix, and the longer side of the brim fits into the back of the vagina. Three sizes are available, and selection is determined by pregnancy and birth history (the 22-cm FemCap is for women who have never been pregnant; the 26-cm FemCap is for women who have had a miscarriage, abortion, or cesarean birth; the 30-cm

FemCap is for women who have had a vaginal birth). The FemCap can be worn for as long as 48 hours, but, as with all vaginal devices, should not be used during menses. The device is designed to be used with a thin layer of spermicide around the outer brim.

Efficacy and Effectiveness The FemCap was not as effective in preventing pregnancy as the traditional diaphragm in clinical studies; the extrapolated annual failure rates slightly exceed 20% (Gallo, Grimes, & Schulz, 2002). Cervical caps may be less effective in women who have had children than in those who have not.

Safety and Side Effects In a randomized trial comparing FemCap to the traditional diaphragm, FemCap users had significantly fewer urinary tract infections (7.5%) than those in the diaphragm group (12.4%). In this same study, there were no differences in vaginitis, irritation, dysmenorrhea, or Pap test changes between the groups (Mauck, Callahan, Weiner, & Dominik, 1999).

Noncontraceptive Benefits The cervical cap has possible or theoretical value in protecting the cervix from infection, but there are no data to support this benefit. The only barrier methods known to reduce STIs are male and female condoms.

Advantages and Disadvantages Cervical caps are coitus dependent (**Table 11-2**) and may be appropriate for women who do not want or cannot use hormonal contraception. The latex-free FemCap is appropriate for women who have, or whose partners have, latex allergies. Insertion and removal of cervical caps may be complex for some women; these women will need additional teaching and counseling to use this contraceptive method consistently and correctly. In a comparative study, more insertion and removal problems were noted with FemCap than with the traditional diaphragm. Approximately 10% to 15% of research participants could not be fit with the FemCap or were unable to insert or remove it (Mauck et al., 2006).

Caps require an initial cost for fitting and purchase, but should last for approximately 2 years with proper care. Ongoing costs include the purchase of spermicides. The FemCap website

(http://www.femcap.com) provides detailed information about obtaining this device.

Vaginal Sponges

The Today sponge is a single-use, soft, absorbent, polyurethane device that contains approximately 1,000 mg of N-9 spermicide; when moistened, the sponge gradually releases 125 to 150 mg of spermicide over 24 hours of use (**Figure 11-4**). Its primary contraceptive effectiveness derives from the gradual release of spermicide, but it also provides a physical barrier to the cervix and absorbs semen. The vaginal sponge can be used for multiple episodes of coitus over 24 hours without inserting more spermicide.

Efficacy and Effectiveness Typical use pregnancy rates are somewhat higher among parous women who use contraceptive sponges than among women who use diaphragms, although rates for nulliparous women are similar (**Table 11-1**).

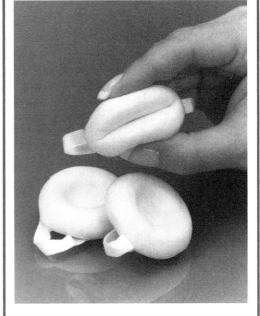

FIGURE 11-4   The Today Sponge.

Courtesy of Mayer Laboratories, Inc.

Safety and Side Effects Women who use the vaginal sponge tend to discontinue use of their method at higher rates than women who use the diaphragm; more than 40% of the women who used both methods stopped using the vaginal sponge in research studies. Allergic-type reactions, such as dermatitis, erythema, irritation, and vaginal itching, were more common with the sponge, although they occurred in only 4% of users (Kuyoh, Toroitich-Ruto, Grimes, Schulz, & Gallo, 2003).

Four cases of toxic shock syndrome among users of the sponge were reported in 1983. These were associated with recent childbirth, use of the method for more than 24 hours, and/or difficult removal with fragmentation of the sponge. Given the number of sponges sold during that time, experts estimated that the risk of toxic shock syndrome was extremely low—approximately 10 cases per year per 100,000 women using sponges ("Leads from the *MMWR*: Toxic-Shock Syndrome and the Vaginal Contraceptive Sponge," 1984).

Noncontraceptive Benefits There are no data to suggest that the contraceptive sponge has value in protecting the cervix from infection; the only barrier methods known to reduce STIs are male and female condoms.

Advantages and Disadvantages The sponge shares the advantages and disadvantages of other nonhormonal barrier, coitus-dependent methods (**Table 11-2**). It does not require a clinician visit or fitting and is available on an over-the-counter basis. Its single-use application may prove more expensive over time than methods that can be reused.

Female Condoms
The female condom is a barrier device designed to protect the cervix, vagina, and part of the vulva and perineum. It was developed as an alternative to male condoms to give women a nonprescription barrier contraceptive method that they could control and that would reduce their exposure to STIs.

The female condom available in the United States is a sheath made from a nitrile polymer, which is soft and smooth, and quickly warms to body temperature (**Figure 11-5**). A small ring at the closed end of the sheath is inserted high in

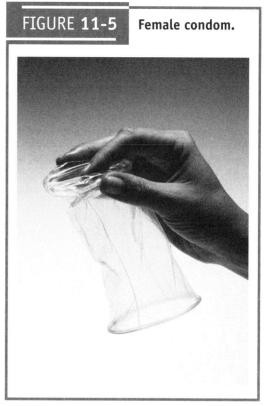

| FIGURE **11-5** | **Female condom.** |

the vagina. A larger ring rests outside the vagina against the vulva and acts as a guide during penetration. This ring also maintains the sheath covering the full length of the vagina and prevents it from "bunching up" inside the vagina. The sheath is coated with a silicone-based, nonspermicidal lubricant, and women can use additional lubricant as well.

The female condom should not be used simultaneously with a male condom, as this practice increases the risk of breakage. It should not be used with the diaphragm, cervical cap, or contraceptive vaginal ring, as the inner ring of the female condom fits into the same place by the cervix as those methods.

Efficacy and Effectiveness The effectiveness of the female condom in preventing pregnancy is in the same range as that of other barrier methods (**Table 11-1**).

Safety and Side Effects Female condoms are made of a synthetic rubber called nitrile and so do not present problems for people with latex allergies.

Noncontraceptive Benefits The female condom can protect against some STIs.

Advantages and Disadvantages The female condom is a nonhormonal, female-controlled method that is available as an over-the-counter product. The results of a randomized crossover trial suggested that most users prefer the male condom to the female condom (Kulczycki, Kim, Duerr, Jamieson, & Macaluso, 2004). The population in this study, however, may not be representative of women who desire female-controlled barrier methods and protection from STIs.

Some women find the female condom difficult to insert, although this problem decreases with proper education (Beksinska, Smit, Greener, Piaggio, & Joanis, 2015). Although it is a female-controlled method, male partner cooperation may still be necessary for consistent use; the partner's lack of acceptance is often cited as a reason for discontinuation. Female condoms can be used only once, and are more expensive than male condoms, so this method can be costly over time.

Permanent Contraception

Permanent contraception, or sterilization, is one of the most prevalent contraceptive methods in the United States. People choose sterilization when they are sure they do not want any children or any more children. Among married U.S. individuals aged 15 to 44, 21.1% of women report having undergone female sterilization and 13.1% of men report having undergone male sterilization. The percentage of women reporting female sterilization increases with age, from 2.6% of women aged 15 to 24 to 34.1% of those aged 40 to 44. The same is true for vasectomy, which is reported by 1.0% of men aged 25 to 29 and 26.5% of those aged 40 to 44. Approximately 600,000 tubal occlusions and 200,000 vasectomies are performed annually in the United States (American College of Obstetricians and Gynecologists, 2013; Anderson et al., 2012).

Female Sterilization

Female sterilization involves permanently blocking the fallopian tubes, which prevents sperm from ascending the reproductive tract and thereby meeting and fertilizing an egg released from the ovary. Female sterilization can be performed postpartum, post abortion, or as an "interval" procedure unrelated to pregnancy. Few sterilization procedures in the United States are performed in conjunction with abortion; approximately half are done postpartum, and half are interval procedures. The surgical approaches employed include laparoscopy, mini-laparotomy, transcervical or hysteroscopic methods, and procedures concurrent with a cesarean birth (Gizzo et al., 2014).

A variety of methods exist for occluding the fallopian tubes, including unipolar or bipolar electrocoagulation; mechanical occlusion using clips, rings, or bands; and ligation or salpingectomy, using one of several techniques. Procedures other than transcervical methods are generally effective immediately.

The only FDA-approved transcervical sterilization method (Essure) is performed via hysteroscopy and can be done in an office setting. Essure involves placement of micro-inserts of metal and fibers into the fallopian tubes. After placement, tissue grows into the insert or matrix, effectively blocking the tubes. A hysterosalpingogram (HSG) must be performed 3 months after the procedure to confirm tubal occlusion, and women must continue to use reliable contraception until sterilization effectiveness is confirmed with HSG (Zite & Borrero, 2011).

Efficacy and Effectiveness Tubal sterilization is a highly effective contraceptive method (**Table 11-1**). Although its overall failure rate is low, failures do occur and are more frequent in women who are younger at the time of sterilization. Failure rates are similar to those of other highly effective, long-term contraceptive methods such as the progestin implant and intrauterine contraception. In a study that estimated the probability of pregnancy over 10 years after three different female sterilization procedures (hysteroscopic, laparoscopic silicone rubber band application, and laparoscopic bipolar coagulation), the authors concluded that pregnancy probability at 1 year and cumulatively over 10 years is expected to be higher in women having hysteroscopic sterilization as compared to laparoscopic sterilization (Gariepy, 2014). Many experts recommend timing an interval procedure during the follicular phase of the menstrual cycle and using a highly sensitive pregnancy test prior to surgery to reduce the risk of pregnancies that are conceived but not recognized before sterilization is performed.

Safety and Side Effects Sterilization is a very effective method of contraception, but when pregnancy does occur after tubal sterilization, the risk of ectopic pregnancy is high. In the largest study of sterilization, one-third of all post-sterilization pregnancies were ectopic (Peterson et al., 1997). A recent Australian study estimated the rates of ectopic pregnancy after tubal sterilization to be between 2.4 and 2.9 per 1,000 procedures. The rate was 3.5 times higher in women sterilized before the age of 28 years than in women sterilized after age 33 (Malacova, Kemp, Hart, Jama-Alol, & Preen, 2014). Other risks are related to the surgical procedures used and include infection, hemorrhage, anesthesia complications, and surgical trauma or injury. The likelihood of these complications is very low, with such events occurring in fewer than 1% of all procedures. The transcervical sterilization methods avoid the risks of abdominal incisions and anesthesia.

A "post-tubal syndrome" has been described, which typically includes increased dysmenorrhea and abnormalities in the menstrual cycle. Most authorities believe such symptoms are more likely related to discontinuing hormonal contraceptives, or simply getting older and entering perimenopause. There is no consistent evidence of a true post-tubal syndrome within the first 2 years after the procedure (Peterson, 2008).

Noncontraceptive Benefits There is a decreased risk of ovarian cancer following tubal sterilization. In addition, studies have shown a lower risk of PID among women who have been sterilized compared to women who have not undergone sterilization (Bartz & Greenberg, 2008). The reasons for this effect are not entirely clear but could be related to mechanical blockage of the ascending spread of pathologic organisms.

Advantages and Disadvantages Tubal sterilization is a highly effective permanent method of contraception, and one that is well suited to women who do not desire future fertility. The surgical procedures are expensive, however, and insurance coverage for them varies. Additional barriers to access include requirements for a waiting period after signing consent and minimum age requirements. Studies in the United States suggest that women who have been sterilized are less likely to return for annual checkups or to use other preventive health services such as Pap tests. They are also less likely to use condoms for prevention of STIs (Pruitt, von Sternberg, Velasquez, & Mullen, 2010; Whitehouse, Montealegre, Follen, Scheurer, & Aagaard, 2014). Counseling for women contemplating or undergoing sterilization should include the continued need for preventive health services.

The younger the woman is at the time of her sterilization, the more likely she is during subsequent years to express regret about having the procedure. Younger women are also more likely to inquire about or seek a reversal of the procedure than older women (Curtis, Mohllajee, & Peterson, 2006).

Male Sterilization
Male sterilization, or vasectomy, cuts or blocks both the right and left vas deferens—that is, the small tubes that carry sperm from the testes to become part of the seminal fluid. Three techniques are used for occlusion of the vas deferens: vasectomy, vassal occlusion, and vassal injection. Vasectomy is the most common.

Sperm account for only 5% of the semen that is produced by the prostate and other glands; thus, there is only a minimal decrease in the amount of seminal fluid following male sterilization. Vasectomies have no effect on sex drive, male hormone production, or sexual function.

Vasectomy—one of the three techniques used for occlusion of the vas deferens—includes two approaches, and both can be performed in an outpatient setting. The conventional vasectomy requires one midline or two lateral incisions in the scrotum. The vas is lifted out through the incision and occluded using one of a variety of methods, such as ligation, cautery, excision of a segment of the vas, or application of clips. The opening is then sutured. With the "no-scalpel" method, the skin of the scrotum is pierced and the vas exposed and blocked through an opening so small it does not require stitches. A systematic review showed that the no-scalpel approach resulted in less bleeding, hematoma, infection, and pain as well as a shorter operation time than the traditional incision technique, with no difference in effectiveness (Cook, Pun, Gallo, Lopez, & Van Vliet, 2014).

Vasectomy is not immediately effective. Sperm are continually produced and transported through the male reproductive tract, so some sperm will continue to be present distal to the site of the vasectomy. Generally, it takes between 15 and 20 ejaculations to clear all sperm from the reproductive tract and be assured of contraception. The current recommendation is for men to wait 3 months, rather than a specific number of ejaculations, before relying on vasectomy (CDC, 2013b). Men are usually advised to have a follow-up visit and examination of ejaculate to ensure the absence of sperm before they stop using other contraceptive methods.

Efficacy and Effectiveness A systematic review estimated the failure rate of vasectomy to be less than 1%, which is similar to the rate associated with female sterilization (Sharlip et al., 2012) (**Table 11-1**).

Safety and Side Effects Most men will experience some degree of postoperative discomfort; infection and scrotal hematoma occur on rare occasions. Some men experience chronic testicular pain after vasectomy, but only a small percentage (3% or fewer) report pain that negatively affects their life or causes them to regret having had the procedure. Antisperm antibodies are more common among men who have had vasectomies than the general population, although this condition does not appear to be associated with any adverse health consequences. Vasectomy does not increase the risk of prostate cancer (Sharlip et al., 2012).

Noncontraceptive Benefits No benefits other than contraception have been demonstrated to date for vasectomy.

Advantages and Disadvantages Vasectomy is a simple procedure that is less complicated and less costly than female sterilization for couples wishing permanent contraception. As is true with tubal sterilization, regret may occur with certain unanticipated life changes. Reversal has a better chance of success when performed within 10 years of vasectomy; pregnancy rates decrease as the interval between vasectomy and reversal increases (Michielsen & Beerthuizen, 2010; Roncari & Hou, 2011). Men need to be counseled that vasectomy does not prevent STIs.

HORMONAL METHODS

The FDA's approval of combined oral contraceptives (COCs) in 1960 marked a revolutionary change in reproductive rights and responsibilities for women around the world. For the first time, women had access to a nearly 100% effective form of contraception that did not require the participation of the male partner and was independent of the act of coitus. COCs (or "the Pill") are some of the best-studied and most widely used medications available today; they remain the most popular form of reversible contraception in the United States (Guttmacher Institute, 2014).

Two types of hormonal contraceptives are available: those that contain progestin (progestin-only) and those that contain progestin and estrogen (combined). Progestin, the synthetic version of the endogenous hormone progesterone, is highly effective alone as a contraceptive, but may cause irregular bleeding. The addition of estrogen to progestin in combined methods results in more predictable bleeding patterns due to stabilization of the endometrium. Estrogen as a single agent for contraception requires doses that may cause unacceptable risks of serious side effects, such as thromboembolic events and endometrial hyperplasia. The synergistic activity of estrogen and progestin makes it possible to combine these hormones in lower doses to produce successful contraception than would be possible using either hormone alone (Wallach & Grimes, 2000).

Combined contraceptive methods currently available in the United States include COCs, the patch, and the vaginal ring. Progestin methods include progestin-only pills, the depot medroxyprogesterone acetate injection, the sub-dermal implant, and three levonorgestrel-containing IUDs. The implant and IUDs are discussed in the section on long-acting reversible contraception.

Both progestin and estrogen inhibit the hypo-thalamic–pituitary–ovarian axis and subsequent steroidogenesis. Progestins have several contraceptive effects, including preventing the luteinizing hormone (LH) surge and thereby inhibiting ovulation; thickening the cervical mucus, which inhibits sperm penetration and transport; changing the motility of the fallopian tubes so that transport of sperm or ova is impaired; and causing the endometrium to become atrophic, although it is unknown whether these changes are sufficient to prevent implantation in the rare event that fertilization occurs. Estrogen suppresses the production of follicle-stimulating hormone (FSH), thereby preventing the selection and emergence of a dominant follicle.

The primary mechanism of action of all hormonal contraceptive methods, with the exception of progestin-only pills (POPs) and the levonorgestrel intrauterine systems (LNG-IUSs), is preventing ovulation (see **Appendix 11-B**). Other contraceptive effects of progestin represent secondary mechanisms to prevent pregnancy should ovulation occur. POPs and the LNG-IUSs do not consistently inhibit ovulation, and their primary mechanism of action is thickening the cervical mucus.

In the past, a barrier to contraception use has been the requirement for a pelvic examination prior to initiation of hormonal methods. Researchers have demonstrated that provision of oral contraceptives without a mandatory pelvic examination does not place women at higher risk of cervical cancer (CDC, 2013b).

None of the hormonal methods provide STI protection. For this reason, it is important to stress the concomitant use of barrier methods in women who are at risk of exposure to STIs.

Many popular myths exist regarding the health risks of hormonal methods, and the healthcare provider must be proactive in educating clients about the noncontraceptive benefits of these methods. Future fertility may be preserved through the decreased risk of pelvic inflammatory disease and ectopic pregnancy associated with the use of hormonal methods (Li et al., 2014; Schindler, 2010).

Other benefits of hormonal methods include a decreased risk of several cancers (colon, ovarian, and endometrial) as well as a decreased risk of the serious diseases of endometriosis, adenomyosis, rheumatoid arthritis, and asthma. Protection against ovarian and uterine cancer may persist as long as 28 years after discontinuation of use of these methods (Schindler, 2010; Vessey & Yeates, 2013). The preservation of bone density that occurs in ever-users of COCs may persist up to age 80 (Wei et al., 2011). The LNG-IUSs are connected with a 50% decreased risk of cervical cancer (Castellsagué et al., 2011).

The use of COCs is not associated with an increase the risk of breast cancer (Vessey & Yeates, 2013), and this lack of association is also seen in carriers of the *BRCA1* and *BRCA2* mutations (Cibula et al., 2010). An increased risk of cervical cancer is seen in long-term COC users, though this risk returns to normal after cessation of use (Hannaford et al., 2007). Although an increased risk of a rare type of liver tumor is connected with COC use, the decreased risk of other, more common cancers may lead to an overall decrease in cancer-related mortality (Hannaford et al., 2007).

During the first few postpartum weeks, the risk of venous thromboembolism (VTE; deep vein thromboses and pulmonary emboli) is greatly elevated in all women; consequently, estrogen-containing contraceptives are contraindicated during this time. Progestin-only methods may be initiated immediately postpartum.

Combined Hormonal Methods

Early formulations of COCs contained unnecessarily high doses of hormones: 80 to 100 micrograms (mcg) of either ethinyl estradiol or mestranol and 1 to 5 mg of progestins. Since the 1970s, the trend has been toward lower-dose formulations that are equally effective, are safer, and have a better side-effect profile. In addition to improving COC formulations, alternative delivery systems for combined contraception have been developed that allow women to avoid a daily dosing schedule. These alternative delivery systems include the combined contraceptive patch and vaginal ring. This section begins by providing information about COCs, which is then followed by a discussion of the patch and the vaginal ring.

Combined Oral Contraceptives

Since the milestone introduction of COCs in the United States in 1960, many formulations of COCs have been developed. Each is unique while its patent protection remains in force; once the patent expires, however, generic formulations tend to outnumber the brand-name products, so the same formulation may have several names. COCs are classified as monophasic or multiphasic (biphasic, triphasic, or quadphasic), depending on whether the dosage of hormones is constant or varies. There is no evidence that either monophasic or multiphasic formulations are a superior choice.

Most of the COCs available today contain 10 to 35 mcg of ethinyl estradiol, although a few COCs contain 50 mcg of ethinyl estradiol or mestranol, the methyl ether of ethinyl estradiol. Approximately 30% of mestranol is lost when it is converted to ethinyl estradiol; thus a 50-mcg mestranol pill is bioequivalent to a 35-mcg ethinyl estradiol pill. Estradiol valerate is found in the new quadphasic COC.

COCs also contain one of several different progestins. The progestins are often referred to as belonging to the first, second, or third generation. With the exception of drospirenone, all progestins in COCs available in the United States are derived from C-19 androgens. These derivatives are classified into two categories: (1) the estranes, or chemical derivatives of norethindrone (norethindrone, norethindrone acetate, and ethynodiol diacetate), and (2) the gonanes, or chemical derivatives of norgestrel (norgestrel, its active isomer levonorgestrel, desogestrel, and norgestimate). Members of these categories differ in terms of both their bioavailability and their half-life. Caution should be exercised when comparing the potency or purported androgenicity of the various types of progestins by category. Rather, formulations should be judged on the clinical response of the woman.

Drospirenone, the only non-testosterone-derived progestin, is an analogue of the diuretic spironolactone. Drospirenone has a mild potassium-sparing diuretic effect, necessitating that potassium levels be checked during the first cycle in women using angiotensin-converting enzyme (ACE) inhibitors, chronic daily nonsteroidal anti-inflammatory drugs (NSAIDs), angiotensin-II receptor antagonists, potassium-sparing diuretics, heparin, or aldosterone antagonists. Women with conditions that predispose them to hyperkalemia should not use COCs containing drospirenone.

The initial choice of a particular COC should be made with the goal of providing the woman with safe, effective contraception. All low-dose (less than 50 mcg) COCs meet this requirement, so it is reasonable to provide a woman with whatever formulation is most cost effective, or whatever pill she requests by name.

Instructions contained in the pill package insert include options for a Sunday start, a first-day start, and a day 5 start. All of these options are based on the principle that as long as COCs are begun within the first 5 days of the menses, there is contraceptive protection in the first cycle. The Sunday start has been the traditional approach in the United States, because the appearance of COC packages often reflects that regimen, and the withdrawal bleed does not usually occur on the weekend, which couples may find preferable. The advantage of the first-day start is that no backup contraceptive method is required in the first cycle. Women are advised to use additional contraception, such as condoms, with the regimens having other starting points for the first 7 days.

An increasingly popular alternative approach is to utilize a "quick start" by beginning the pill regardless of where the woman is in her menstrual cycle, if pregnancy is excluded and with additional contraception for the first 7 days. Instructions are given to take a pregnancy test in 2 to 3 weeks if unprotected sex occurred during the cycle. This practice has been shown to increase continuation rates for COCs and is not associated with an increased incidence of adverse bleeding patterns (CDC, 2013b).

With the traditional cyclic schedule, women take 21 to 24 days of active COCs, followed by 4 to 7 days of inactive pills or no pills. During the hormone-free interval, bleeding from the withdrawal of estrogen and progestin occurs. This is technically a withdrawal bleed, rather than menses, and is based primarily on convention rather than on science. Extended (omitting the hormone-free interval for two or more cycles) and continuous (omitting the hormone-free interval indefinitely) COC regimens are becoming increasingly popular, both for medical indications and convenience. Monophasic pills are generally preferred for this use.

Efficacy and Effectiveness COCs require the woman's daily adherence to the dosing schedule, which can be compromised by many factors, resulting in a gap between efficacy and effectiveness (**Table 11-1**). Based on U.S. data related to pill use, it appears that approximately 9% of women will become pregnant unintentionally due to incorrect pill use (Trussell, 2011). Common reasons for COC failure include not starting a new pack on time, missing pills, "taking a break" from the pill, and discontinuing the pill in response to normal side effects. The counseling and education provided by the clinician are critical to the ultimate success of the woman in avoiding unwanted pregnancy.

The most important pills to take in each cycle are the first and last active COCs, which ensure that the hormone-free interval does not exceed 7 days. During the hormone-free interval, pituitary stimulation of the ovaries by FSH is likely to resume and follicular development may begin in many women. Immature follicles stimulated during the hormone-free phase generally regress once the hormonal pills are resumed, and 7 consecutive days of pill use have been shown to be sufficient in suppressing any follicular function. Hormone-free intervals of less than 7 days have become increasingly standard (CDC, 2013b). Patient instructions must stress the importance of starting a new pack on time and not taking more than 7 days off of the active pills. If a woman does extend the hormone-free interval beyond 7 days, she should be instructed to abstain from intercourse or use additional contraception until 7 consecutive pills have been taken.

Missing pills is almost universal among women who choose COCs for contraception. Missing a random pill now and then is unlikely to lead to a method failure. Unfortunately, this fact may lead to complacency regarding the importance of daily adherence to the schedule, as women come to believe that inconsistent pill use is adequate. The probability of pill failure increases with repeated missed pills, however. This issue is complicated by the fact that instructions for women who miss a pill can be confusing. Current recommendations are as follows: If one pill is missed and is less than 48 hours late, take the late or missed pills as soon as possible and continue taking the remaining pills at the usual time. No backup method or emergency contraception is needed. If two or more consecutive hormonal pills have been missed and it is more 48 hours or more since a pill should have been taken, take the most recent pill as soon as possible (any other missed pills should be discarded). Continue taking the remaining pills at the usual time and use a backup method or avoid sexual intercourse until hormonal pills have been taken for 7 consecutive days. If pills were missed during the last week of hormonal pills, finish the remaining hormonal pills and start new pill pack the following day. Emergency contraception should be considered if pills were missed during the first week and sexual intercourse occurred during last 5 days (CDC, 2013b).

Many women incorrectly believe that temporarily discontinuing or "taking a break from" COCs is beneficial. It is important to convey to women that the hormones found in the pill do not accumulate in the body, and the occurrence of a withdrawal bleed indicates that the endometrium is responding to the absence of hormones. There are no differences in the long-term fertility of women who use the pill intermittently and those who use the pill for many years.

Nearly half of all women who begin taking oral contraceptives discontinue their use before the end of 1 year; the most commonly reported reasons for discontinuation in a recent study were side effects and difficulty obtaining contraception (Stuart, Secura, Zhao, Pittman, & Peipert, 2013). A misunderstanding about the management of side effects may compound this dissatisfaction. Clear information about the side effects commonly encountered during the first three cycles of pill use should be given. Whenever a woman begins a new COC, she should be advised to contact the clinician prior to discontinuing the pills if she experiences unwanted side effects. In such a case, a different pill may be substituted without interrupting effective contraception. Many references are available to assist the clinician in fine-tuning COC formulations to each woman's needs (see the bibliography at the end of this chapter).

A number of medications can modify the effectiveness of COCs. Pharmacologic mechanisms that alter medication metabolism include induction of liver enzymes, alterations in sex hormone-binding globulin (SHBG), and medications that alter the first-pass effect in the gut. Medications that can reduce the effectiveness of COCs include antiretroviral therapy, rifampin, griseofulvin, and some anticonvulsants (e.g., carbamazepine, phenytoin, barbiturates, primidone, topiramate, oxcarbazepine, lamotrigine), as well as some over-the-counter herbal supplements such as St. John's wort (CDC, 2010). Broad-spectrum antibiotics have been blamed for COC failures, although pharmacologic evidence to support this assertion is lacking. Given the prevalence of antibiotic use, any pill failures are more likely to be coincidence or to be associated with missed pills. Women who are concerned about reduced COC efficacy while on antibiotics can shorten or eliminate the use of the placebo pills in the pill pack or use an additional contraceptive, but it is not necessary to routinely recommend these precautions.

Safety and Side Effects COCs are among the most extensively studied medications available and are known to be extremely safe for healthy women. Many of the side effects associated with COCs are bothersome but not dangerous; however, serious complications are possible and are the basis of contraindications to COC use. These contraindications may be related to the direct effects of the hormonal ingredient, as in breast cancer, or they may result from hormonal effects on other systems, as in thromboembolism. The *U.S. Medical Eligibility Criteria for Contraceptive Use* (see **Appendix 11-A**) provides an evidence-based guide to the contraindications to COC use. One must always weigh the risks of pregnancy in relation to the risks associated with contraceptive use.

All COCs increase the risk of VTE. The level of this risk appears to be related to the dose of estrogen and is greatest for women with known clotting disorders, such as factor V Leiden, or a family history of thrombosis. The various progestin components may contribute to the risk of VTE to a differing degree; however, the difference between pills is small, and the studies showing their relative risks have been subject to methodological errors (Fritz & Speroff, 2011). A recent large multinational study reported incidence of VTE to be similar among users of drospirenone-containing,

levonorgestrel-containing, and other progestin-containing COCs (Dinger, Bardenheuer, & Heinemann, 2014). COCs containing less than 50 mcg of estrogen do not appear to increase the risk of arterial thrombosis (myocardial infarction or stroke) in healthy, nonsmoking women, including women older than 40 years. COCs may increase blood pressure in some women through an increase in plasma angiotensin. Because hypertension is a cofactor in the development of cardiovascular disease, blood pressure should be monitored in COC users.

Metabolic effects of COCs may include development of benign hepatocellular adenomas, although this side effect is very rare with the low-dose pills. There does not appear to be an association between these benign tumors and the development of liver cancer. Low-dose COCs appear to create negligible changes in insulin levels or glucose levels and have no effect on the development of diabetes. There is no difference in weight gain in pill users versus nonusers in large studies; however, a few women may experience an anabolic response to COCs, though they are able to lose weight once the oral contraceptive is discontinued (Fritz & Speroff, 2011).

History of COC use, regardless of duration, does not affect breast cancer risk. Women who are currently taking COCs have a slightly increased risk of developing breast cancer; however, this risk is small and may represent a detection bias, as pill users are more likely to receive regular screening (Fritz & Speroff, 2011). Some studies have noted an increase in the incidence of cervical cancer in COC users. It is difficult to determine whether this finding reflects a true increase or results from the fact that women who use COCs have more sexual partners, HPV infections, and Pap tests, the latter of which causes detection bias (Fritz & Speroff, 2011).

Mood changes and changes in libido have been noted among COC users and may respond to a change in the pill formulation. Depression, although rare, may justify the use of alternative methods of contraception. Other side effects specific to estrogen include nausea, cervical ectopy and leukorrhea, telangiectasis, chloasma (darkening of sun-exposed skin), growth of breast tissue (ductal tissue or fat deposition), increased cholesterol content within the bile (which can lead to gallstones), benign hepatocellular adenomas, and changes in the clotting cascade. Effects specific to the androgenic impact of progestins include increased appetite and subsequent weight gain, mood changes and depression, fatigue, complexion changes, changes in carbohydrate metabolism, increased low-density lipoprotein (LDL) and decreased high-density lipoprotein (HDL) cholesterol, decreased libido, and pruritus. Effects that can be either estrogen or progestin related include headaches, hypertension, and breast tenderness. Many of the side effects that women associate with COCs occur either during the 7 hormone-free days or appear to be associated with the demise of follicles recruited during the hormone-free interval (Sulak, Scow, Preece, Riggs, & Kuehl, 2000). In some cases, a trial of extended use may be recommended to improve the symptoms that women experience at predictable times in their pill cycles.

Grimes and Schulz (2011) have suggested that counseling women that they might have side effects such as headaches, nausea, breast pain, and mood changes may be unethical. The prevalence of these nonspecific symptoms is high in the general population of reproductive-age women, and several trials show no difference in these side effects when an oral hormonal contraceptive is compared with placebo. If women are told to expect troublesome side effects, these symptoms may occur simply because of the power of suggestion. Given that high-quality evidence indicates that the frequency of nonspecific side effects is no greater with COCs than with inert pills, optimistic counseling should be the norm.

Noncontraceptive Benefits The noncontraceptive benefits of COCs are numerous and often underappreciated (American College of Obstetricians and Gynecologists, 2010; Maguire & Westhoff, 2011). Some evidence indicates that the relative risk of ovarian cancer is decreased by 20% for each 5 years of COC use (Havrilesky et al., 2013). This reduction in risk persists more than 30 years after pills are discontinued, although the extent of risk reduction diminishes somewhat with time (Beral, Doll, Hermon, Peto, & Reeves, 2008). Likewise, COC use reduces the risk of endometrial cancer by approximately 50%. This risk lessens with increasing duration of use and persists for as long as 20 years after the COCs are stopped (Vessey & Yeates, 2013). Women on COCs also experience lower rates of PID requiring

hospitalization, fewer ectopic pregnancies, and a lower incidence of endometriosis. These conditions are the most common causes of infertility; thus the pill helps preserve fertility—not by conservation of ovulation, but rather through prevention of causes of subfertility. Other well-documented noncontraceptive benefits of the pill include menstrual-related effects (discussed in the next paragraph), improvement in acne and hirsutism, and reduced incidence of benign breast conditions. Older studies demonstrated a reduced risk of developing functional ovarian cysts while women were on COCs, but this effect is less profound with the lower doses of hormones in currently used COCs (Maguire & Westhoff, 2011).

In addition to being effective contraceptive methods, COCs have many other therapeutic uses. For example, they regulate menstrual cycles and are useful in the management of abnormal bleeding patterns. While taking COCs, women experience lighter "periods" (withdrawal bleeds) that may treat or improve anemia. COCs can also be an effective treatment for mittelschmerz, dysmenorrhea, endometriosis, premenstrual symptoms, and the vasomotor symptoms of perimenopause (American College of Obstetricians and Gynecologists, 2010). Women who experience catamenial conditions—those that rise and fall in synchronicity with the menstrual cycle, such as menstrual migraines—may also find that COCs improve those conditions. Decreasing the number of withdrawal bleeding episodes per year may further diminish these problems.

Advantages and Disadvantages COC use is unrelated to coitus. Most women in the United States are familiar with the instructions for COC use, and this method is widely available in pharmacies and clinics. Confidence in the product is high due to the fact it has been on the market for more than 50 years and has been continually researched. Additionally, more than 30 different formulations of COCs are available, allowing for individualization based on response to the products.

The obvious disadvantage of COCs is the need for daily pill taking. The ongoing cost of the method can be problematic as well. Particularly for young women, lack of privacy may also be an issue. Finally, some women experience side effects with COCs that they are unable to tolerate.

Combined Contraceptive Patch and Vaginal Ring
The contraceptive patch (the original Ortho Evra has been discontinued by the manufacturer for business reasons [FDA, 2014a]; a generic version, Xulane, is still available) and vaginal ring (Nuva-Ring) share many similarities with COCs, yet have some distinct differences. The patch and ring utilize delivery systems that allow for simpler dosing than daily pill taking. Both methods avoid the first-pass metabolism of COCs, allowing for lower-dose administration and potentially avoiding interactions with other medications.

The patch releases 20 mcg per day of ethinyl estradiol and 150 mcg per day of the progestin norelgestromin, the active metabolite of norgestimate. These active ingredients are rapidly absorbed and reach therapeutic serum concentrations within 24 to 48 hours. The thin, beige patch, which is approximately the size of a matchbook, is applied by the woman and worn for 1 week at a time. The patch is changed weekly on the same day of the week for 3 weeks, and then no patch is worn for 1 week to allow for a withdrawal bleed. As with COCs, no more than 7 days should pass between removal of the last patch and the beginning of the next patch cycle. The patch can be worn on the buttocks, upper arm, abdomen, and anywhere on the upper torso except the breasts (**Figure 11-6**).

The vaginal ring is colorless and flexible, with an outer diameter of about 2 inches (**Figure 11-7**). It releases 15 mcg per day of ethinyl estradiol and 120 mcg per day of the progestin etonogestrel, the active metabolite of desogestrel. The active ingredients of the ring rapidly diffuse across the mucous membrane of the vagina and reach a steady state in the serum. The ring is left in place in the vagina for 21 days and then removed for 1 week, allowing for a withdrawal bleed. The ring provides a steady delivery of hormones, which leads to a very low serum concentration—approximately half of the serum concentration found with a 35-mcg COC.

Efficacy and Effectiveness The patch and the vaginal ring have the same theoretical efficacy and typical use failure rates as COCs (**Table 11-1**). There is less opportunity for user error with the patch and ring, however, as these methods need not be remembered daily. Each patch continues to emit hormones at therapeutic levels for at least 9 days (Nanda, 2011).

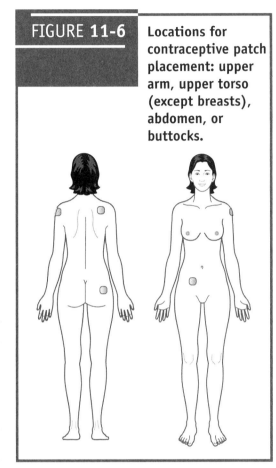

FIGURE 11-6 Locations for contraceptive patch placement: upper arm, upper torso (except breasts), abdomen, or buttocks.

The hormones emitted by the ring also remain at therapeutic levels after 3 weeks; therefore, there is also some margin of error if women forget to change the products on time. Extended (omitting the patch/ring-free week for two or more cycles) and continuous (omitting the patch/ring-free week indefinitely) use of the patch and ring, as with COCs, is becoming increasingly common (CDC, 2013b).

The patch is effective only if it is completely attached to the skin; even partial detachment necessitates replacement. The exact placement of the ring in the vagina is not critical to its efficacy. Although previous studies suggested increased failure rates of the patch in women who weigh more than 198 pounds, more recent research does not support this finding (Westhoff, Reinecke, Bangerter, & Merz, 2014).

FIGURE 11-7	Combined contraceptive ring (NuvaRing).

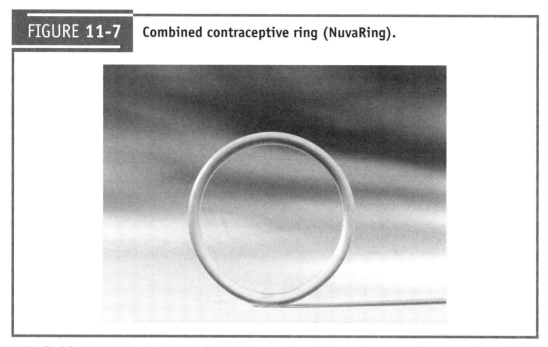

Safety and Side Effects   The *U.S. Medical Eligibility Criteria for Contraceptive Use* (CDC, 2010) currently specifies the same criteria for COCs, the patch, and the ring except in women who have undergone malabsorptive bariatric surgery procedures (see **Appendix 11-A** and Chapter 8). It is theoretically possible that the nonoral delivery systems may result in different safety and side-effect profiles, but to date no evidence has been published to support this hypothesis. Clinicians are cautioned to not presume the patch and ring are "safer" than COCs. A woman who is not a candidate for COCs should not be given the patch or ring either.

The patch has been associated with heightened concern about an increased risk of VTE. In 2005, a warning was added to the label of the patch that includes the following statement:

The pharmacokinetic (PK) profile for the ORTHO EVRA® patch is different from the PK profile for oral contraceptives in that it has higher steady state concentrations and lower peak concentrations. Area under the time–concentration curve (AUC) and average concentration at steady state for ethinyl estradiol (EE) are approximately 60% higher in women using ORTHO EVRA® compared with women using an oral contraceptive containing 35 mcg of EE. In contrast, peak concentrations for EE are approximately 25% lower in women using ORTHO EVRA®. It is not known whether there are changes in the risk of serious adverse events based on the differences in PK profiles of EE in women using ORTHO EVRA® compared with women using oral contraceptives containing 30–35 mcg of EE. Increased estrogen exposure may increase the risk of adverse events, including venous thromboembolism. ("Ortho Evra Prescribing Information," 2014)

Studies have produced conflicting results on this topic. While hormone levels with the patch are typically higher than those with COCs, the clinical implications of these pharmacokinetic findings are unclear and do not necessarily indicate any increased risk of serious side effects. A recent FDA advisory committee concluded that the benefits of the patch (e.g., pregnancy prevention) outweigh the risk of VTE (FDA, 2011).

In general, the side effects of the patch and the vaginal ring are very similar to those of COCs, such as breakthrough bleeding and nausea. In addition, the patch and ring have some unique side effects related to their delivery systems. In studies of the patch, approximately 20% of participating women experienced some skin irritation at the site of application, but fewer than 3% discontinued use for this reason (Lopez, Grimes, Gallo, Stockton, & Schulz, 2013). The ring may be felt during intercourse, although this is not commonly cited as a reason for discontinuation. Although there is no increase in cervical cytologic changes with the vaginal ring, increased incidence of vaginitis and leukorrhea has been noted (Ahrendt et al., 2006).

Noncontraceptive Benefits It is theoretically plausible that the noncontraceptive benefits of COCs may be realized with the patch and ring as well, because these methods affect the hypothalamic–pituitary–ovarian axis in the same way as COCs; however, epidemiologic studies to support this theory are lacking. Caution must be exercised in attributing the same long-term benefits of COCs to the patch and ring in the absence of published evidence of this effect.

Advantages and Disadvantages The intrinsic advantage of the patch and ring is the avoidance of daily dosing, which may lead to greater effectiveness. A specific advantage of the vaginal ring is the lack of visible evidence of its use, which may appeal to some women, particularly adolescents, who want to keep their contraceptive use private. The patch may appeal to women who are not comfortable with vaginal placement, but desire a non-daily method of contraception.

One current disadvantage of the patch and ring is that only one formulation of each method is available. The development of a variety of products may allow for individual variations in response to hormones, and patch color choices may appeal to some women as well. These methods are also associated with ongoing costs. A final disadvantage of the patch and the ring is that both methods still contain large amounts of active ingredients upon their disposal. The presence of these chemicals has prompted environmental concerns about the effect of high doses of estrogen and progestin seeping into the water supply. In the future, a recommendation may be issued to place the used devices into a biohazard waste container instead of landfills.

Progestin-Only Methods

Progestin-only contraceptives are used continuously; there is no hormone-free interval, as occurs with combined methods. These contraceptive methods have minimal effects on coagulation factors, blood pressure, or lipid levels and are generally considered safer for women who have contraindications to estrogen, such as cardiovascular risk factors, migraine with aura, or a history of VTE. In spite of this belief, the product labeling for some progestin-only products mimics the labeling for products containing estrogen. The *U.S. Medical Eligibility Criteria for Contraceptive Use* (CDC, 2010; see **Appendix 11-A**) can be used to identify appropriate candidates for progestin-only contraception.

Progestin-only contraceptives do not provide the same cycle control as methods containing estrogen, and unscheduled bleeding is common with all progestin-only methods. Typically, unscheduled bleeding occurs most frequently during the first 6 months of method use, with a substantial number of users becoming amenorrheic by 12 months of use (Hubacher, Lopez, Steiner, & Dorflinger, 2009). Overall blood loss decreases over time, making progestin-only methods protective against iron-deficiency anemia. With appropriate counseling, many women see amenorrhea as a benefit of these methods.

All progestin-only methods are likely to improve menstrual symptoms, including dysmenorrhea, menorrhagia, premenstrual syndrome, and anemia (Burke, 2011). The thickening of cervical mucus seen with progestin methods is protective against PID.

Progestin-only contraceptives include the progestin-only pill (POP), an injection, an implant, and three progestin-containing intrauterine devices. The implant and devices are covered in the section on long-acting reversible contraception.

Progestin-Only Pills

The POPs or "mini-pills" available in the United States contain 0.35 mg of norethindrone. Each pill contains active ingredients; there is no hormone-free interval, as occurs with COCs. POPs must be taken not only daily, but also at the same time each day.

Efficacy and Effectiveness Sparse data exist on the efficacy of POPs, but this property is thought to be lower than that of COCs (Grimes, Lopez, O'Brien, & Raymond, 2013). POPs do not suppress ovulation as reliably as COCs, but rather rely primarily on the contraceptive effect of thickened cervical mucus. The onset of cervical mucus thickening occurs 2 to 4 hours after a POP is taken and persists for 22 hours after each dose. For this reason, if intercourse generally occurs in the morning or evening, the POP should be taken at midday (Zieman, Hatcher, & Allen, 2015). In a woman who ovulates while taking the POP, taking the pill as few as 3 hours late may allow the cervical mucus to return to its fertile state and render the contraceptive effect temporarily void. When POPs are used in combination with lactation, the effectiveness of the two methods is nearly 100%.

Safety and Side Effects POPs have the fewest contraindications of all hormonal methods. In one survey, only 1.6% of women had contraindications to the pills (White et al., 2012). Contraindications to POP use can be found in **Appendix 11-A**. Unscheduled bleeding and spotting are the side effects most commonly associated with POPs. Decreased effectiveness of POPs is possible when these agents are used in combination with rifampin or rifabutin (CDC, 2010).

Noncontraceptive Benefits Noncontraceptive benefits are described in the introduction to the "Progestin-Only Methods" section. The reductions in ovarian and endometrial cancer rates seen with COCs have not been reported with POPs.

Advantages and Disadvantages Each package of POPs contains one type of pill (versus two or more types in a package of COCs), so there may be less confusion about which pill is to be taken. POPs are a safe method for many women who cannot take estrogen for medical reasons. Similarly, women who are sensitive to even low-estrogen pills, as manifested by nausea, breast tenderness, or hypertension, but who still want an oral contraceptive, may do well on POPs. POPs are preferable to COCs for lactating women because they do not cause adverse effects on the volume or quality of breastmilk (Raymond, 2011b). Some recent research has suggested that COCs given as early as 2 weeks postpartum do not adversely affect breastfeeding performance (Espey et al., 2012); however, the 2011 update to the *U.S. Medical Eligibility Criteria for Contraceptive Use* classified COC use in breastfeeding women who have no other risk factors for venous thromboembolism in category 4 up to 21 days postpartum, in category 3 from 21 to 29 days postpartum, and in category 2 from 30 days postpartum on (CDC, 2011). The contraceptive effect ends immediately upon discontinuation of POPs.

Disadvantages of POPs, other than the side effects previously mentioned, include the need for careful adherence to the dosing schedule. Utilizing an alarm or watch that beeps daily at the same time may enhance compliance.

Progestin Injection

The depot medroxyprogesterone acetate (DMPA) injection (Depo-Provera) has been approved as a method of contraception only since 1995, although clinical trials with this agent were conducted in the 1960s and 1970s, and the medication was used for the treatment of endometriosis and as an off-label contraceptive prior to FDA approval. DMPA is a synthetic progestogen and a member of the pregnane family, but it differs from the estrane and gonane progestins found in oral contraceptives. DMPA is a powerful inhibitor of the hypothalamic–pituitary axis at the level of the hypothalamus (Bartz & Goldberg, 2011).

DMPA is given as either a 150-mg intramuscular injection or a 104-mg subcutaneous injection that can be self-administered. Either injection is given every 13 weeks. Intramuscular DMPA must be provided by a trained healthcare professional, which requires that the woman make regular visits for injections. Self-administration of the subcutaneous formulation is feasible and increases this method's convenience for women who find it difficult to get to a clinician's office. The subcutaneous formulation provides a dose that is 30% lower and a reduction in peak blood levels by 50%; however, it is more expensive because is it provided in a proprietary delivery system. Researchers are investigating the efficacy of lower doses and subcutaneous administration of the current intramuscular DMPA formulation (Shelton & Halpern, 2014). Lower doses may reduce the metabolic side effects of weight gain and glucose intolerance. Ovulatory suppression with this method often lasts longer than 13 weeks; however, because the contraceptive effect expires at this point in a minority of women, all women are instructed to return for repeat doses at 13-week intervals (CDC, 2013b).

Although prescribing information advises that the first DMPA injection should be given during the first 5 days of the menses or postpartum (if not breastfeeding), the *U.S. Selected Practice Recommendations for Contraceptive Use* advises that DMPA can be initiated at any time it is reasonably certain that the woman is not pregnant. This includes immediately postpartum or post abortion (CDC, 2013b). In other situations, it is reasonable to provide the injection once pregnancy has been ruled out and, if circumstances warrant, advise the woman to take a highly sensitive pregnancy test 2 to 3 weeks after the first injection, as amenorrhea may be interpreted as a normal effect of the method. If DMPA is given in early pregnancy, it does not appear to stimulate fetal anomalies or miscarriage (it was previously used to prevent miscarriage); nevertheless, it is important to detect pregnancy as soon as possible to facilitate entry to prenatal care or abortion care. Women given DMPA "off cycle" (outside the previously mentioned ideal parameters for initiation of the method) should be instructed to use a barrier method for the first 7 days while the serum levels are reaching adequate concentrations. The same instructions apply to women who are late for their injections. If she has engaged in unprotected intercourse in the previous 5 days, a woman should be offered emergency contraception as well.

Efficacy and Effectiveness The failure rates for DMPA are listed in **Table 11-1**. The differences between theoretical efficacy and typical use probably reflect the pattern of women not returning on time for subsequent injections.

Safety and Side Effects Like other progestin-only methods, DMPA is safer than combination products overall and can be used by women who

are not candidates for estrogen contraceptives. **Appendix 11-A** provides a complete list of contraindications and precautions regarding DMPA use.

In 2004, the following warning was added to the DMPA label:

> *Women who use Depo-Provera Contraceptive Injection may lose significant bone mineral density. Bone loss is greater with increasing duration of use and may not be completely reversible. It is unknown if use of Depo-Provera Contraceptive Injection during adolescence or early adulthood, a critical period of bone accretion, will reduce peak bone mass and increase the risk for osteoporotic fracture in later life. Depo-Provera Contraceptive Injection should not be used as a long-term birth control method (i.e., longer than 2 years) unless other birth control methods are considered inadequate.* ("Depo-Provera [Medroxyprogesterone Acetate Injectable Suspension]," n.d.)

Experts have called for removal of the FDA warning, citing abundant evidence that the effects of DMPA on bone density are considerably less than originally believed (American College of Obstetricians and Gynecologists, 2014a). While bone mineral density (BMD) does decrease during DMPA use, a systematic review of the literature determined that this decline in BMD reverses after DMPA discontinuation (American College of Obstetricians and Gynecologists, 2014a). This pattern is similar to the BMD changes seen in women who breastfeed. Changes in BMD are an intermediate outcome, but the truly important clinical outcome is fracture risk. Studies examining fracture risk in low-risk women who previously used DMPA are not yet available (American College of Obstetricians and Gynecologists, 2014a).

The American College of Obstetricians and Gynecologists does not recommend restricting DMPA initiation or duration of use based on concerns about BMD. Likewise, use of DMPA is not considered an indication for BMD screening or initiation of medications to prevent osteoporosis, such as estrogen, bisphosphonates, or selective estrogen receptor modulators (American College of Obstetricians and Gynecologists, 2014a; Kaunitz, Arias, & McClung, 2008). All women, regardless of contraceptive method, should be counseled about osteoporosis prevention, including adequate intake of calcium and vitamin D via diet and/or supplements.

Uncertainty exists regarding the impact of DMPA use on the risk of HIV acquisition and transmission (Crook et al., 2014; Polis et al., 2014). Recently, the CDC issued an update to the *U.S. Medical Eligibility Criteria for Contraceptive Use*, noting the inconclusive evidence and calling for more research. The guidelines do not restrict the use of DMPA for women at risk of HIV exposure, but advise that women using progestin-only injectable contraception be strongly advised to use HIV-preventive measures (CDC, 2012).

Some researchers have reported that the 150-mg intramuscular dose of DMPA impairs glucose tolerance and that women with borderline glucose tolerance may have an increased risk of developing diabetes when using DMPA (Xiang, Kawakubo, Kjos, & Buchanan, 2006).

As with all progestin-only methods, side effects associated with DMPA include changes in bleeding patterns, with breakthrough bleeding and spotting occurring in the majority of women in the first 6 months of use. After 12 months of use, approximately 40% to 50% of women will have become amenorrheic, with this rate increasing to 80% after 5 years of use (Bartz & Goldberg, 2011). With appropriate counseling, many women see amenorrhea as a benefit of DMPA.

Use of DMPA is associated with an increase of approximately 2 kg of body weight at 12 months of use (Lopez, Edelman, et al., 2013). Given that obesity and its attendant health risks are already at epidemic proportions, counseling about healthy weight management is essential for all women, with close attention being paid to this issue in women using DMPA. Other side effects reported in a small minority of women on DMPA include depression, headache, decreased libido, and dizziness (Bartz & Goldberg, 2011).

Noncontraceptive Benefits Noncontraceptive benefits of DMPA include a reduction in the number of seizures in women with epilepsy and seizure disorders (Bartz & Goldberg, 2011). DMPA is not affected by the anticonvulsant medications, making it ideal for the woman with seizure disorders who does not want to become pregnant (CDC, 2010).

DMPA is also associated with a reduction in sickle cell crises in women with sickle cell disease (Bartz & Goldberg, 2011). DMPA is not affected by any medications except aminoglutethimide, which is used to treat Cushing's disease.

As is the case with all hormonal contraceptive options, women have less menorrhagia and less dysmenorrhea with DMPA. Ectopic pregnancy, PID, and endometriosis are decreased in DMPA users—outcomes that are protective of future fertility.

Advantages and Disadvantages Advantages of DMPA include its high degree of efficacy and long-term nature and its noninterference with coitus. For women who want to keep their contraceptive choice private, there is no visible evidence of DMPA use. DMPA has long been used to achieve amenorrhea in women with mental disabilities who cannot manage their menses.

The long-term nature of DMPA may also be considered a disadvantage, as the contraceptive effect may not cease immediately upon discontinuation. The time to return of ovulation varies widely, ranging from 15 to 49 weeks after the last injection (Paulen & Curtis, 2009). DMPA requires intramuscular injections be provided by a trained healthcare professional, which requires that the woman make regular visits for injections. The subcutaneous formulation might improve continuation of contraception among women who find it difficult to get to a clinician's office. However, there remains the possibility of allergic reaction to either the progestin or the vehicle used for injection, or vagal reactions to the injection itself. Like all hormonal methods, DMPA does not provide any protection from STIs.

LONG-ACTING REVERSIBLE CONTRACEPTION

Long-acting reversible contraception (LARC), which includes IUDs and subdermal implants, refers to methods that prevent pregnancy for extended periods of time with no effort from the user. As LARC removes the factors of user consistency and error from the contraceptive equation, its effectiveness is the highest of all contraceptive methods. If 10% of U.S. women aged 20 to 29 years switched from oral contraception to LARC, it is estimated that total healthcare costs of unintended pregnancy would be reduced in this country by $288 million per year (Trussell et al., 2013). LARC methods also have high satisfaction and continuation rates compared with other methods (Dickerson et al., 2013).

Barriers to use of LARC include provider lack of training in insertion and persistent misperceptions about safety. In addition, although LARC is more cost effective than most other methods over time, the high initial cost is a barrier to access.

The ease of use, high efficacy, and privacy provided by LARC methods are particularly relevant considerations for adolescent women. Adolescent women using pills, the patch, or the ring may have as much as a 20-fold increase in contraceptive failure compared to their peers using LARC methods (Winner et al., 2012). The American College of Obstetricians and Gynecologists, WHO, and the CDC all support the use of LARC methods in women younger than age 20.

Progestin Implant

The subdermal progestin implant is among the most effective methods of contraception, and American College of Obstetricians and Gynecologists (2011) recommends that this LARC be offered as a first-line method and its use encouraged among most women as a contraceptive option. The single-rod etonogestrel implant (Nexplanon) available in the United States is 40 mm long and 2 mm in diameter and contains 68 mg of etonogestrel that is released slowly over 3 years (**Figure 11-8**). Etonogestrel is the active metabolite of desogestrel. Training of clinicians is needed to ensure appropriate placement and skilled removal of the implant. Removing the etonogestrel implant is reported to be easier than was the case with the previously used multiple-rod systems for several reasons: It is a single rod, slightly larger in size than the multiple-rod systems, and made of ethylene vinyl acetate, which is less flexible than the Silastic used to make older rods.

The implant should be inserted during the first 7 days of the menses, postpartum, or post abortion, to avoid pregnancy in the first cycle. After removal of the implant, etonogestrel levels are undetectable in most women within 1 week, and ovulation generally returns within 6 weeks (Raymond, 2011a).

Efficacy and Effectiveness
The failure rates for the progestin implant are listed in **Table 11-1**. Its high rate of effectiveness is related to the intrinsic efficacy of the product and the fact that once inserted, there is no room for user error.

FIGURE 11-8 Single-rod etonogestrel implant (Implanon).

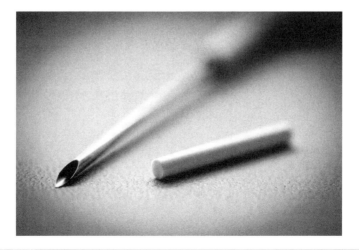

Safety and Side Effects

Based on worldwide data, the progestin implant appears to be as safe as other progestin-only methods and is associated with similar side effects, such as irregular bleeding and amenorrhea (Grunloh, Casner, Secura, Peipert, & Madden, 2013). Unscheduled bleeding is more common and persistent in implant users than in LNG-IUS users and is the most common reason for discontinuation (Berenson, Tan, & Hirth, 2014). Because ovarian activity is not completely suppressed, persistent follicles and small ovarian cysts have been reported in a small percentage of implant users, although these generally resolve without treatment (Hidalgo et al., 2006; Raymond, 2011a). Side effects of the method include bruising and irritation at the insertion site, breast tenderness, and weight gain (Lopez, Edelman, et al., 2013).

Noncontraceptive Benefits

The implant can decrease dysmenorrhea and endometriosis symptoms (Raymond, 2011a).

Advantages and Disadvantages

Advantages of the subdermal progestin implant include the presence of highly effective contraception following a single insertion procedure. This contraceptive effect is immediately reversible upon removal of the device. The implant is discreet but palpable, providing reassurance to the woman that it is in place and has not migrated.

Intrauterine Contraception

The use of medical devices placed in the uterus to prevent pregnancy dates back to the early 1900s. Although the infection risk with early devices was high, design improvements led to a variety of IUDs becoming available in the 1960s and 1970s (Tone, 2001). Popular devices were generally made of inert plastic, with single filament threads that protruded through the cervix into the vagina.

The one memorable exception to this design was the Dalkon Shield, which was introduced in 1970. This device quickly became associated with a high risk of pelvic infection and infertility. It had a multifilament tail enclosed in a sheath; when the strings were cut, the protective sheath was compromised and bacteria could ascend into the uterus inside the sheath (Nelson, 2000). Although other IUDs did not have the same design flaw, the adverse publicity and lawsuits associated with the Dalkon Shield tainted all IUDs, and these devices fell out of favor in the United States during the late 1970s.

Recent developments in design and scientific review of the risks and benefits associated with intrauterine contraception have led to a revival of interest in this contraceptive method. IUDs are still underused due the high initial cost, lack of provider training in insertion, and misperceptions on the part of both healthcare providers and the public about safety (Yoost, 2014). Recognizing that IUDs represent a highly efficacious and effective form of LARC, American College of Obstetricians and Gynecologists (2011) recommends intrauterine contraception be offered as a first-line method and its use encouraged among most women as an option.

Four intrauterine contraceptives are available in the United States, though others are used in other countries.

The copper IUD (T380A, Paragard) is a T-shaped device of polyethylene with copper wire wound around the stem and arms (**Figure 11-9**). A monofilament polyethylene thread is attached to a ball on the end of the stem. The copper adds spermicidal and other effects that allow the device to be smaller than a plain plastic device. The primary contraceptive effect is provided by the reaction to having a foreign body in the reproductive tract—specifically, a sterile inflammatory response that has spermicidal effects (Alvarez et al., 1988).

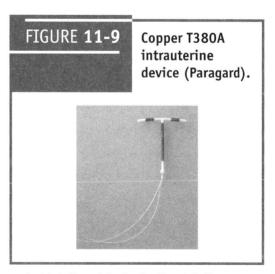

| FIGURE **11-9** | Copper **T380A** intrauterine device (Paragard). |

Reprinted with permission from Teva Women's Health.

Three IUDs containing levonorgestrel are also available: Mirena, Skyla, and Liletta (Eisenberg et al., 2015). These T-shaped IUDs feature a reservoir that releases levonorgestrel at varying doses; they contain no copper (**Figure 11-10**). After insertion, Mirena releases levonorgestrel at a rate of 20 mcg per day, Skyla at 14 mcg per day, and Liletta at 18 to 19 mcg per day. Daily release rates decline over the time as the device remains in place. The local delivery of progestin produces thickening of the cervical mucus and an endometrial reaction, in addition to the foreign body reaction. The LNG-IUS also has a monofilament thread. Ovulation is suppressed in some women with this device, particularly in the first year after its placement, but most cycles are ovulatory (American College of Obstetricians and Gynecologists, 2011). Skyla is the smallest device and may be easier to insert for women with cervical stenosis or small uterine cavities; Liletta is available at a lower cost to public health clinics.

The copper IUD is effective for at least 10 years, Mirena for at least 5 years, and Skyla and Liletta for at least 3 years. Preliminary research suggests that the devices may be effective past these time frames; however, these are the current FDA-approved limits (McNicholas, Maddipati, Zhao, Swor, & Peipert, 2015).

Insertion of an IUD may occur at any time during the menstrual cycle (American College of Obstetricians and Gynecologists, 2011). Many clinicians perform insertion of LNG-IUSs during menses to be certain the woman is not pregnant. Insertion of the copper IUD will serve as emergency contraception. Postabortion, postplacental (within 10 minutes after expulsion of the placenta), and postpartum (at least 4 weeks postpartum) insertion may also be performed. The procedures for copper IUD and LNG-IUS insertion differ and are beyond the scope of this chapter. The manufacturers provide insertion training for clinicians and can be contacted via their websites (http://www.paragard.com, http://www.mirena -us.com, http://www.skyla-us.com, and http:// www.liletta.com).

Effectiveness and Efficacy

Intrauterine contraception is extremely effective (**Table 11-1**). In a cohort of more than 58,000 IUD users, the pregnancy rate per 100 woman-years was 0.06 for copper IUDs and 0.52 for LNG-IUSs (Heinemann, Reed, Moehner, & Do Minh, 2015a). Pregnancy may occur if partial or complete expulsion of the IUD occurs. The expulsion rate ranges from 2% to 10%, with most expulsions occurring in

---

FIGURE 11-10   **Levonorgestrel intrauterine system (Mirena).**

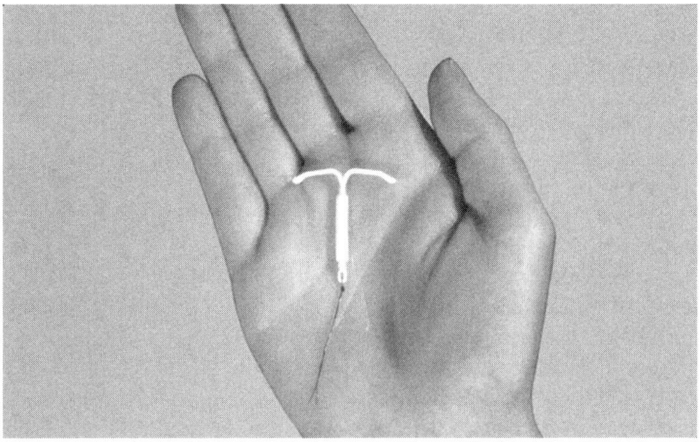

the first 3 months after insertion of the device. While expulsion may be associated with cramping or bleeding, it may also go unnoticed. Women should be encouraged to check periodically for the strings to ensure the device is still in place.

Safety and Side Effects

Despite the negative experience associated with the Dalkon Shield, contemporary intrauterine contraceptives with monofilament threads are very safe for most women (see **Appendix 11-A**). Questions about their safety center on infection, future fertility, ectopic pregnancy, and risk of uterine perforation. A transient increase in infection rates occurs in the first 20 days after insertion, likely due to the insertion process or preexisting infection (American College of Obstetricians and Gynecologists, 2011), with this risk reported to range from 1 to 10 cases per 1,000 women. The risk of infection returns to baseline thereafter. Antibiotic prophylaxis for insertion is not necessary (American College of Obstetricians and Gynecologists, 2011). The FDA has removed recommendations against use of intrauterine contraceptives in women with more than one sexual partner. STI screening may occur on the day of insertion, and insertion may take place without waiting for results (American College of Obstetricians and Gynecologists, 2011). If pelvic infection occurs, it can be treated without removing the IUD (CDC, 2013b). The cervical mucus barrier and atrophic endometrium created by the LNG-IUS may actually protect the user from PID.

Use of an IUD does not increase the rate of infertility (Hubacher, Lara-Ricalde, Taylor, Guerra-Infante, & Guzman-Rodriguez, 2001). Actual rates of ectopic pregnancy are among IUD users are up to 10-fold lower than in nonusers, but if the method fails the resulting pregnancies are more likely to be ectopic (Sivin & Batar, 2010).

Perforation of the uterus during insertion of an IUD occurs at a rate of 1 in 1,000 and is usually a benign event (Heinemann, Reed, Moehner, & Do Minh, 2015b). The risk of perforation is higher in postpartum and breastfeeding women.

Previous concerns about the use of IUDs in nulliparous women have largely been put to rest. Today, in fact, intrauterine contraception for adolescents is promoted by several professional organizations as the best means to reduce unintended pregnancy in young women (American College of Obstetricians and Gynecologists, 2011, 2012; CDC, 2010).

The most common side effects associated with the copper IUD are bleeding and dysmenorrhea, although some reports describe no increased severity of dysmenorrhea with use of the copper IUD (Lindh & Milsom, 2013). Menstrual blood loss increases by as much as 50% with copper IUDs, as can the duration of the menses. NSAIDs can be used to treat excessive bleeding (CDC, 2013b).

Unscheduled bleeding is common with the three LNG-IUSs. As the duration of use increases, menstrual flow declines and amenorrhea often develops. Counseling prior to insertion of the device may help reduce anxiety about the irregular bleeding. Women should be told that the bleeding does not represent hormonal fluctuations, but rather the shedding of the endometrial lining as an atrophic state is achieved.

Other side effects linked to LNG-IUSs include lower abdominal pain, complexion changes, back pain, breast tenderness, headaches, mood changes, and nausea, although all of these effects decline with time, and they are noted in only a minority of women. In general, few hormonal side effects are observed with the low dose of progestin found in intrauterine contraceptives. As with other progestin-only methods, benign functional ovarian cysts are common, occurring in 8% to 12% of LNG-IUS users. Most cysts are asymptomatic and resolve spontaneously (Nahum, Kaunitz, Rosen, Schmelter, & Lynen, 2015).

Noncontraceptive Benefits

LNG-IUSs have many noncontraceptive benefits. Menstrual flow is reduced by as much as 90% (Dean & Schwarz, 2011), and the device is FDA approved to treat heavy menstrual bleeding. The LNG-IUS can be used to treat idiopathic menorrhagia as well as heavy menstrual bleeding associated with perimenopause, uterine fibroids, and adenomyosis; it may also be useful in the treatment of endometrial hyperplasia, endometriosis, and dysmenorrhea (American College of Obstetricians and Gynecologists, 2011). Reduced risks of endometrial cancer and cervical cancer are seen in IUD users (Castellsagué et al., 2011). The progestin in the device is sufficient to protect the endometrium as a component of hormone therapy. IUDs can be inserted in women's late reproductive years and then left in place through the transition to menopause.

Advantages and Disadvantages

Intrauterine contraception has the advantage of providing long-term contraception that is not coitus dependent and does not require adjustments to daily activities (such as remembering to take a pill every day). Contemporary intrauterine contraception options have effectiveness rates that are comparable to those of sterilization. Unlike permanent sterilization, however, intrauterine contraception offers the added advantage of being rapidly reversible, making this method ideal for young women who desire long-term contraception. IUDs are also discreet and private methods. Copper and levonorgestrel-containing IUDs are effective contraceptive methods for women who have contraindications to estrogen-containing contraceptives. The reduced bleeding with the LNG-IUS can lead to substantial savings in the cost of sanitary products.

There can be a high upfront cost for intrauterine contraception. The copper IUD and LNG-IUS cost several hundred dollars, and a visit to a skilled clinician is needed for their insertion. Many clinicians also require a pre-insertion visit to test for infections, and a post-insertion visit after the first menses to ensure the device has not been expelled. However, these are long-term contraceptives with no additional costs; thus they are among the least expensive methods over time.

EMERGENCY CONTRACEPTION

Sperm can live for up to 5 days in the female reproductive tract, and pregnancy can occur with intercourse 5 days prior to ovulation. The highest risk of pregnancy is in the 48 hours immediately preceding ovulation (Wilcox, Dunson, & Baird, 2000). However, due to the uncertainty of ovulation timing, emergency contraception is offered if unprotected intercourse (UPI) occurs at any time in the menstrual cycle.

The Yuzpe, levonorgestrel, and ulipristal acetate emergency contraceptive pill (ECP) regimens as well as the copper IUD may all be used within 120 hours of UPI. The Yuzpe and levonorgestrel methods have a dramatic decline in their effectiveness with time and should be used as soon as possible after an event of UPI.

The Yuzpe regimen consists of combined ECPs that must contain at least 100 mcg of ethinyl estradiol and 0.50 mg of levonorgestrel, repeated in 12 hours. A dedicated combined ECP product is not available in the United States, but numerous COCs can be used as combined ECPs (see **Table 11-1**, footnote i). COCs containing norgestrel are preferable to those with norethindrone, as failure rates are slightly higher with norethindrone (Zieman et al., 2015). Because the high dose of ethinyl estradiol causes unpleasant side effects, this regimen has largely fallen out of favor.

Until recently, the most widely used emergency contraception method was levonorgestrel ECPs, which contain either a 1.5-mg single dose (Plan B One-Step) or two doses of 0.75 mg taken 12 hours apart (Next Choice and Plan B). Women can take both doses in the two-dose products (Next Choice and Plan B) as a single dose. Levonorgestrel ECPs are available over the counter to women and men age 17 and older; women 16 and younger need a prescription to obtain them. Levonorgestrel ECPs are more effective than the Yuzpe regimen and have fewer side effects.

Ulipristal acetate (ella), a selective progesterone receptor modulator provided as a single 30-mg dose, is the most effective oral emergency contraception method. The effectiveness of this medication does not decline within the 120-hour window after UPI, as is the case for levonorgestrel and combined ECPs (Fine et al., 2010). Ulipristal acetate is available only by prescription.

The copper IUD can be inserted as long as 5 days after unprotected intercourse. Some contraceptive guidelines recommend its use up to 7 days after UPI (Dunn et al., 2013). This method is rarely utilized as emergency contraception in the United States; however, recent evidence suggests some women might choose the copper IUD if it is offered as an option (Turok et al., 2011). It has the advantage of being highly effective in obese women and providing ongoing contraception.

Efficacy and Effectiveness

Factors influencing the risk of pregnancy when ulipristal acetate or levonorgestrel is used for emergency contraception include body mass index (BMI), the day of the cycle, and further intercourse during the same menstrual cycle after use of emergency contraception (Glasier et al., 2011).

Women with a BMI greater than 30 have a 2- to 40-fold higher risk of pregnancy after ECP use. Levonorgestrel may be completely ineffective at reducing pregnancy risk in obese women. The efficacy of levonorgestrel and ulipristal acetate further vary according to the stage of the cycle.

Levonorgestrel and ulipristal acetate inhibit ovulation in 96% and 100% of cycles, respectively, when used prior to the onset of the LH surge (Brache, Cochon, Deniaud, & Croxatto, 2013). However, if given after the onset of the LH surge, these medications inhibit ovulation in 14% and 79% of cycles, respectively (Glasier, 2013). Levonorgestrel is no more effective than placebo when used in the critical 5 days preceding ovulation. The risk of pregnancy with ulipristal acetate use is half that seen with use of levonorgestrel (Glasier, 2014).

Both levonorgestrel and ulipristal acetate delay ovulation. If women have repeated acts of UPI after using ECPs, they are at a 4-fold increased risk of pregnancy compared with women who do not have further intercourse within the same cycle.

The copper IUD is by far the most effective of emergency contraception methods, with a pregnancy rate of approximately 1 in 1,000 cases in which it is used for this purpose (Cheng, Che, & Gulmezoglu, 2012).

Safety and Side Effects

Levonorgestrel ECPs, combined ECPs, and ulipristal acetate should not be given to women with a known or suspected pregnancy; there are no other contraindications to their use. The long history of use of levonorgestrel indicates little risk exists if it is inadvertently taken in early pregnancy. There is less experience with ulipristal acetate, although no reasons for concern were raised in the clinical trials. The usual contraindications and precautions for ongoing COC and POP use do not apply to ECPs (CDC, 2010), but the usual contraindications and precautions to copper IUD use do apply when using this method for emergency contraception (see **Appendix 11-A**). Neither the copper IUD nor oral emergency contraception methods are considered abortifacients (American College of Obstetricians and Gynecologists, 2014b).

Combined ECPs frequently cause nausea and vomiting, which can be reduced by giving an antiemetic, such as promethazine, prior to treatment. Spotting, changes in next menses, headache, breast tenderness, and mood changes can also occur. These same side effects are sometimes noted with levonorgestrel ECPs but are much less frequent and less severe with this option (Zieman et al., 2015). Headache, dysmenorrhea, nausea, and abdominal pain are the most frequently observed side effects with ulipristal acetate (Fine et al., 2010; Glasier et al., 2010). The copper IUD can cause the side effects discussed in the section on intrauterine contraception.

Advantages and Disadvantages

Emergency contraception is the only contraceptive method that can be used after intercourse. It cannot be used as an ongoing method of contraception, however, and it provides no STI protection. Access to emergency contraception remains limited because only one method—levonorgestrel ECPs—is available without prescription—and even then it is available only to women 17 and older. Clinicians can increase access to emergency contraception by providing advance prescriptions to all women of reproductive age for ulipristal acetate. Studies have shown that having ECPs at home increases the likelihood that they will be used when needed and does not promote sexual risk taking (Glasier & Baird, 1998; Raine, Harper, Leon, & Darney, 2000). Providing emergency contraception prescriptions over the phone as needed is another way to increase access.

Bibliography

Centers for Disease Control and Prevention (CDC). (2010). U S. medical eligibility criteria for contraceptive use, 2010: Adapted from the World Health Organization medical eligibility criteria for contraceptive use, 4th edition. *Morbidity and Mortality Weekly Report Recommendations and Reports, 59*(RR-4), 1–86.

Centers for Disease Control and Prevention (CDC). (2011). Update to CDC's U.S. medical eligibility criteria for contraceptive use, 2010: Revised recommendations for the use of contraceptive methods during the postpartum period. *Morbidity and Mortality Weekly Report, 60*(26), 878–883.

Centers for Disease Control and Prevention (CDC). (2012). Update to CDC's U.S. medical eligibility criteria for contraceptive use, 2010: Revised recommendations for the use of hormonal contraception among women at high risk for HIV infection or infected with HIV. *Morbidity and Mortality Weekly Report, 61*(24), 449–452.

Centers for Disease Control and Prevention (CDC). (2013). U.S. selected practice recommendations for contraceptive use, 2013: Adapted from the World Health Organization selected practice recommendations for contraceptive use, 2nd edition. *Morbidity and Mortality Weekly Report Recommendations and Reports, 62*(RR-05), 1–60.

Dickey, R. P. (2014). *Managing contraceptive pill patients* (15th ed.). Dallas, TX: EMIS Medical.

Fritz, M. A., & Speroff, L. (2011). *Clinical gynecologic endocrinology and infertility* (8th ed.). Baltimore, MD: Lippincott Williams & Wilkins.

Hatcher, R. A., Trussell, J., Nelson, A. L., Cates, W., Kowal, D. & Policar, M. (Eds.). (2011). *Contraceptive technology* (20th ed.). New York, NY: Ardent Media.

Office of Population Research and the Association of Reproductive Health Professionals. (2015). The emergency contraception web site. Retrieved from http://www.not-2-late.com

Speroff, L., & Darney, P. D. (2010). *A clinical guide for contraception* (5th ed.). Baltimore, MD: Lippincott Williams & Wilkins.

Zieman, M., Hatcher, R., & Allen, A. (2015). *Managing contraception: 2015–2016*. Atlanta, GA: Bridging the Gap Communications.

References

Ahrendt, H. J., Nisand, I., Bastianelli, C., Gomez, M. A., Gemzell-Danielsson, K., Urdl, W., . . . Milsom, I. (2006). Efficacy, acceptability and tolerability of the combined contraceptive ring, NuvaRing, compared with an oral contraceptive containing 30 microg of ethinyl estradiol and 3 mg of drospirenone. *Contraception, 74*(6), 451–457. doi:10.1016/j.contraception.2006.07.004

Alvarez, F., Brache, V., Fernandez, E., Guerrero, B., Guiloff, E., Hess, R., . . . Zacharias, S. (1988). New insights on the mode of action of intrauterine contraceptive devices in women. *Fertility and Sterility, 49*(5), 768–773.

American College of Nurse-Midwives. (2013). Our Moment of Truth 2013 survey of women's health care experiences and perceptions: Spotlight on family planning and contraception. Retrieved from http://ourmomentoftruth.midwife.org/acnm/files/ccLibraryFiles/Filename/000000003461/2013%20ACNM%20Contraception%20Survey%20-%20Executive%20Summary.pdf

American College of Obstetricians and Gynecologists. (2010). ACOG Practice Bulletin No. 110: Noncontraceptive uses of hormonal contraceptives. *Obstetrics & Gynecology, 115*(1), 206–218. doi:10.1097/AOG.0b013e3181cb50b5

American College of Obstetricians and Gynecologists. (2011). ACOG Practice Bulletin No. 121: Long-acting reversible contraception: Implants and intrauterine devices. *Obstetrics & Gynecology, 118*(1), 184–196. doi:10.1097/AOG.0b013e318227f05e

American College of Obstetricians and Gynecologists. (2012). Committee Opinion No. 539: Adolescents and long-acting reversible contraception: Implants and intrauterine devices. *Obstetrics & Gynecology, 120*(4), 983–988. doi:10.1097/AOG.0b013e3182723b7d

American College of Obstetricians and Gynecologists. (2013). ACOG Practice Bulletin No. 133: Benefits and risks of sterilization. *Obstetrics & Gynecology, 121*(2 pt 1), 392–404. http://10.1097/01.AOG.0000426425.33845.b2

American College of Obstetricians and Gynecologists. (2014a). Committee Opinion No. 602: Depot medroxyprogesterone acetate and bone effects. *Obstetrics & Gynecology, 123*(6), 1398–1402. doi:10.1097/01.AOG.0000450758.95422.c8

American College of Obstetricians and Gynecologists. (2014b). *Facts are important: Emergency contraception (EC) and intrauterine devices (IUDs) are not abortifacients*. Washington, DC: Author.

Anderson, J. E., Jamieson, D. J., Warner, L., Kissin, D. M., Nangia, A. K., & Macaluso, M. (2012). Contraceptive sterilization among married adults: National data on who chooses vasectomy and tubal sterilization. *Contraception, 85*(6), 552–557. doi:10.1016/j.contraception.2011.10.009

Anderson, K. N., Schwab, R. B., & Martinez, M. E. (2014). Reproductive risk factors and breast cancer subtypes: A review of the literature. *Breast Cancer Research and Treatment, 144*(1), 1–10. doi:10.1007/s10549-014-2852-7

Asian Communities for Reproductive Justice. (n.d.). What is reproductive justice? http://strongfamiliesmovement.org/what-is-reproductive-justice

Bartz, D., & Goldberg, A. (2011). Injectable contraceptives. In R. A. Hatcher, J. Trussell, A. L. Nelson, W. Cates, D. Kowal, & M. S. Policar (Eds.), *Contraceptive technology* (20th ed., pp. 209–236). New York, NY: Ardent Media.

Bartz, D., & Greenberg, J. A. (2008). Sterilization in the United States. *Reviews in Obstetrics & Gynecology, 1*(1), 23–32.

Beksinska, M., Smit, J., Greener, R., Piaggio, G., & Joanis, C. (2015). The female condom learning curve: Patterns of female condom failure over 20 uses. *Contraception, 91*(1), 85–90. doi:10.1016/j.contraception.2014.09.011

Beral, V., Doll, R., Hermon, C., Peto, R., & Reeves, G. (2008). Ovarian cancer and oral contraceptives: Collaborative reanalysis of data from 45 epidemiological studies including 23,257 women with ovarian cancer and 87,303 controls. *Lancet, 371*(9609), 303–314. doi:10.1016/s0140-6736(08)60167-1

Berenson, A. B., Tan, A., & Hirth, J. M. (2014). Complications and continuation rates associated with 2 types of long-acting contraception. *American Journal of Obstetrics & Gynecology.* doi:10.1016/j.ajog.2014.12.028

Biggs, M. A., & Foster, D. G. (2013). Misunderstanding the risk of conception from unprotected and protected sex. *Women's Health Issues, 23*(1), e47–e53. doi:10.1016/j.whi.2012.10.001

Bounds, W., Guillebaud, J., Dominik, R., & Dalberth, B. T. (1995). The diaphragm with and without spermicide: A randomized, comparative efficacy trial. *Journal of Reproductive Medicine, 40*(11), 764–774.

Brache, V., Cochon, L., Deniaud, M., & Croxatto, H. B. (2013). Ulipristal acetate prevents ovulation more effectively than levonorgestrel: Analysis of pooled data from three randomized trials of emergency contraception regimens. *Contraception, 88*(5), 611–618. doi:10.1016/j.contraception.2013.05.010

Burke, A. E. (2011). The state of hormonal contraception today: Benefits and risks of hormonal contraceptives: Progestin-only contraceptives. *American Journal of Obstetrics & Gynecology., 205*(4, Suppl.), S14–S17. doi:10.1016/j.ajog.2011.04.033

Castellsagué, X., Díaz, M., Vaccarella, S., de Sanjosé, S., Muñoz, N., Herrero, R., . . . Bosch, F. X. (2011). Intrauterine device use, cervical infection with human papillomavirus, and risk of cervical cancer: A pooled analysis of 26 epidemiological studies. *Lancet Oncology, 12*(11), 1023–1031. doi:10.1016/s1470-2045(11)70223-6

Centers for Disease Control and Prevention (CDC). (2010). U.S. medical eligibility criteria for contraceptive use, 2010: Adapted from the World Health Organization medical eligibility criteria for contraceptive use, 4th edition. *Morbidity and Mortality Weekly Report Recommendations and Reports, 59*(RR-4), 1–86. Retrieved from http://www.cdc.gov/reproductivehealth/unintendedpregnancy/USMEC.htm

Centers for Disease Control and Prevention (CDC). (2011). Update to CDC's U.S. Medical eligibility criteria for contraceptive use, 2010: Revised recommendations for the use of contraceptive methods during the postpartum period. *Morbidity and Mortality Weekly Report, 60*(26), 878–883. Retrieved from http://www.cdc.gov/mmwr/preview/mmwrhtml/mm6026a3.htm

Centers for Disease Control and Prevention (CDC). (2012). Update to CDC's U.S. medical eligibility criteria for contraceptive use, 2010: Revised recommendations for the use of hormonal contraception among women at high risk for HIV infection or infected with HIV. *Morbidity and Mortality Weekly Report, 61*(24), 449–452. Retreived from http://www.cdc.gov/mmwr/preview/mmwrhtml/mm6124a4.htm

Centers for Disease Control and Prevention (CDC). (2013a, March 25). Condoms and STDs: Fact sheet for public health personnel. 2013. Retrieved from http://www.cdc.gov/condomeffectiveness/latex.html

Centers for Disease Control and Prevention (CDC). (2013b, October 6). U.S. selected practice recommendations for contraceptive use, 2013: Adapted from the World Health Organization selected practice recommendations for contraceptive use, 2nd edition. *Morbidity and Mortality Weekly Report Recommendations and Reports, 62*(RR-05), 1–60. Retrieved from http://www.cdc.gov/reproductivehealth/UnintendedPregnancy/USSPR.htm

Cervical Barrier Advancement Society. (n.d.). Cervical barriers. Retrieved from http://www.cervicalbarriers.org

Cheng, L., Che, Y., & Gulmezoglu, M. (2012). Interventions for emergency contraception. *Cochrane Database of Systematic Reviews, 8,* CD001324. doi:10.1002/14651858.CD001324.pub4

Cibula, D., Gompel, A., Mueck, A. O., La Vecchia, C., Hannaford, P. C., Skouby, S. O., . . . Dusek, L. (2010). Hormonal contraception and risk of cancer. *Human Reproduction Update, 16*(6), 631–650. doi:10.1093/humupd/dmq022

Cook, L. A., Pun, A., Gallo, M. F., Lopez, L. M., & Van Vliet, H. A. (2014). Scalpel versus no-scalpel incision for vasectomy. *Cochrane Database of Systematic Reviews, 3,* CD004112. doi:10.1002/14651858.CD004112.pub4

Cramer, D. W. (2012). The epidemiology of endometrial and ovarian cancer. *Hematology/Oncology Clinics of North America, 26*(1), 1–12. doi:10.1016/j.hoc.2011.10.009

Crook, A. M., Ford, D., Gafos, M., Hayes, R., Kamali, A., Kapiga, S., . . . McCormack, S. (2014). Injectable and oral contraceptives and risk of HIV acquisition in women: An analysis of data from the MDP301 trial. *Human Reproduction, 29*(8), 1810–1817. doi:10.1093/humrep/deu113

Curtis, K. M., Mohllajee, A. P., & Peterson, H. B. (2006). Regret following female sterilization at a young age: A systematic review. *Contraception, 73*(2), 205–210. doi:10.1016/j.contraception.2005.08.006

Daniels, K., & Mosher, W. D. (2013). Contraceptive methods women have ever used: United States, 1982–2010. *National Health Statistics Report, 62,* 1–15.

Dean, G., & Schwarz, E. B. (2011). Intrauterine contraceptives. In R. A. Hatcher, J. Trussell, A. L. Nelson, W. Cates, D. Kowal, & M. S. Policar (Eds.), *Contraceptive technology* (20th ed., pp. 147–191). New York, NY: Ardent Media.

Depo-Provera (medroxyprogesterone acetate injectable suspension). (n.d.). Retrieved from http://www.fda.gov/Safety/MedWatch/SafetyInformation/SafetyAlertsforHumanMedicalProducts/ucm154784.htm

Dickerson, L. M., Diaz, V. A., Jordon, J., Davis, E., Chirina, S., Goddard, J. A., . . . Carek, P. J. (2013). Satisfaction, early removal, and side effects associated with long-acting reversible contraception. *Family Medicine, 45*(10), 701–707.

Dinger, J., Bardenheuer, K., & Heinemann, K. (2014). Cardiovascular and general safety of a 24-day regimen of drospirenone-containing combined oral contraceptives: Final results from the International Active Surveillance Study of Women Taking Oral Contraceptives. *Contraception, 89*(4), 253–263. doi:10.1016/j.contraception.2014.01.023

Dunn, S., Guilbert, E., Burnett, M., Aggarwal, A., Bernardin, J., Clark, V., . . . Wagner, M. S. (2013). Emergency contraception: No. 280 (replaces No. 131, August 2003). *International Journal of Gynaecology and Obstetrics, 120*(1), 102–107.

Eisenberg, D. L., Schreiber, C. A., Turok, D. K., Teal, S. B., Westhoff, C. L., & Creinin, M. D. (2015). Three-year efficacy and safety of a new 52-mg levonorgestrel-releasing intrauterine system. *Contraception, 92*(1), 10–16.

Espey, E., Ogburn, T., Leeman, L., Singh, R., Ostrom, K., & Schrader, R. (2012). Effect of progestin compared with combined oral contraceptive pills on lactation: A randomized controlled trial. *Obstetrics & Gynecology, 119*(1), 5–13. doi:10.1097/AOG.0b013e31823dc015

Festin, M. (2013). Non-latex versus latex male condoms for contraception (last revised: 1 April 2013). *The WHO Reproductive Health Library.* Retrieved from http://apps.who.int/rhl/fertility/contraception/cd003550_festinm_com/en

Files, J. A., Frey, K. A., David, P. S., Hunt, K. S., Noble, B. N., & Mayer, A. P. (2011). Developing a reproductive life plan. *Journal of Midwifery & Women's Health, 56*(5), 468–474. doi:10.1111/j.1542-2011.2011.00048.x

Fine, P., Mathe, H., Ginde, S., Cullins, V., Morfesis, J., & Gainer, E. (2010). Ulipristal acetate taken 48–120 hours after intercourse for emergency contraception. *Obstetrics & Gynecology, 115*(2 pt 1), 257–263. doi:10.1097/AOG.0b013e3181c8e2aa

Food and Drug Administration (FDA). (2011). Background document for joint meeting of the Advisory Committee for Reproductive Health Drugs and the Drug Safety and Risk Management Advisory Committee: NDA 21-180, Ortho Evra. Retrieved from http://www.fda.gov/downloads/AdvisoryCommittees

/CommitteesMeetingMaterials/Drugs/ReproductiveHealth DrugsAdvisoryCommittee/UCM282634.pdf

Food and Drug Administration (FDA). (2014a). Current and re-solved drug shortages and discontinuations reported to FDA. Retrieved from http://www.accessdata.fda.gov/scripts /drugshortages/

Food and Drug Administration (FDA). (2014b). "Off-label" and in-vestigational use of marketed drugs, biologics, and medical devices: Information sheet. Retrieved from http://www.fda.gov /RegulatoryInformation/Guidances/ucm126486.htm

Fritz, M. A., & Speroff, L. (2011). *Clinical gynecologic endocrinology and infertility* (8th ed.). Baltimore, MD: Lippincott Williams & Wilkins.

Frost, J. J., & Darroch, J. E. (2008). Factors associated with contracep-tive choice and inconsistent method use, United States, 2004. *Perspectives on Sexual and Reproductive Health, 40*(2), 94–104. doi:10.1363/4009408

Gallo, M. F., Grimes, D. A., & Schulz, K. F. (2002). Cervical cap versus diaphragm for contraception. *Cochrane Database of Systematic Reviews, 4*, CD003551. doi:10.1002/14651858.cd003551

Gariepy, A. M. (2014). Probability of pregnancy after sterilization: A comparison of hysteroscopic versus laparoscopic steriliza-tion: in reply. *Contraception, 90*(5), 557–558. doi:10.1016/j. contraception.2014.06.029

Gavin, L., Moskosky, S., Carter, M., Curtis, K., Glass, E., Godfrey, E., . . . Zapata, L. (2014). Providing quality family planning services: Recommendations of CDC and the U.S. Office of Population Affairs. *Morbidity and Mortality Weekly Report Rec-ommendations and Reports, 63*(RR-04), 1–54.

Gipson, J. D., Koenig, M. A., & Hindin, M. J. (2008). The effects of unintended pregnancy on infant, child, and parental health: A review of the literature. *Studies in Family Planning, 39*(1), 18–38.

Gizzo, S., Bertocco, A., Saccardi, C., Di Gangi, S., Litta, P. S., D'Antona, D., & Nardelli, G. B. (2014). Female sterilization: Up-date on clinical efficacy, side effects and contraindications. *Mini-mally Invasive Therapies & Allied Technologies, 23*(5), 261–270. doi:10.3109/13645706.2014.901975

Glasier, A. (2013). Emergency contraception: Clinical outcomes. *Contraception, 87*(3), 309–313. doi:10.1016/j.contraception. 2012.08.027

Glasier, A. (2014). The rationale for use of ulipristal acetate as first line in emergency contraception: Biological and clinical evi-dence. *Gynecological Endocrinology, 30*(10), 688–690. doi:10.310 9/09513590.2014.950645

Glasier, A., & Baird, D. (1998). The effects of self-administering emer-gency contraception. *New England Journal of Medicine, 339*(1), 1–4.

Glasier, A., Cameron, S. T., Blithe, D., Scherrer, B., Mathe, H., Levy, D., . . . Ulmann, A. (2011). Can we identify women at risk of pregnancy despite using emergency contraception? Data from randomized trials of ulipristal acetate and levonorgestrel. *Contra-ception, 84*(4), 363–367. doi:10.1016/j.contraception.2011.02.009

Glasier, A. F., Cameron, S. T., Fine, P. M., Logan, S. J., Casale, W., Van Horn, J., . . . Gainer, E. (2010). Ulipristal acetate ver-sus levonorgestrel for emergency contraception: A randomised non-inferiority trial and meta-analysis. *Lancet, 375*(9714), 555–562. doi:10.1016/s0140-6736(10)60101-8

Gomez, A. M., Fuentes, L., & Allina, A. (2014). Women or LARC first? Reproductive autonomy and the promotion of long-acting re-versible contraceptive methods. *Perspectives on Sexual and Re-productive Health, 46*(3), 171–175. doi:10.1363/46e1614

Grimes, D. A., Gallo, M. F., Grigorieva, V., Nanda, K., & Schulz, K. F. (2004). Fertility awareness-based methods for contracep-tion. *Cochrane Database of Systematic Reviews, 4*, CD004860. doi:10.1002/14651858.CD004860.pub2

Grimes, D. A., Lopez, L. M., O'Brien, P. A., & Raymond, E. G. (2013). Pro-gestin-only pills for contraception. *Cochrane Database of Systematic Reviews, 11*, CD007541. doi:10.1002/14651858.CD007541.pub3

Grimes, D. A., & Schulz, K. F. (2011). Nonspecific side effects of oral contraceptives: Nocebo or noise? *Contraception, 83*(1), 5–9. doi:10.1016/j.contraception.2010.06.010

Grunloh, D. S., Casner, T., Secura, G. M., Peipert, J. F., & Madden, T. (2013). Characteristics associated with discontinuation of long-acting reversible contraception within the first 6 months of use. *Obstetrics & Gynecology, 122*(6), 1214–1221. doi:10.1097/01. aog.0000435452.86108.59

Guttmacher Institute. (2014). Contraceptive use in the United States. Retrieved from http://www.guttmacher.org/pubs/fb_contr_use .html

Hannaford, P. C., Selvaraj, S., Elliott, A. M., Angus, V., Iversen, L., & Lee, A. J. (2007). Cancer risk among users of oral contraceptives: cohort data from the Royal College of General Practitioner's oral contraception study. *British Medical Journal, 335*(7621), 651. doi:10.1136/bmj.39289.649410.55

Havrilesky, L. J., Moorman, P. G., Lowery, W. J., Gierisch, J. M., Coeytaux, R. R., Urrutia, R. P., . . . Myers, E. R. (2013). Oral contraceptive pills as primary prevention for ovarian cancer: A systematic review and meta-analysis. *Obstetrics & Gynecology, 122*(1), 139–147. doi:10.1097/AOG.0b013e318291c235

Heinemann, K., Reed, S., Moehner, S., & Do Minh, T. (2015a). Com-parative contraceptive effectiveness of levonorgestrel-releasing and copper intrauterine devices: The European Active Surveil-lance Study for Intrauterine Devices. *Contraception, 91*(4), 280–283. doi:10.1016/j.contraception.2015.01.011

Heinemann, K., Reed, S., Moehner, S., & Do Minh, T. (2015b). Risk of uterine perforation with levonorgestrel-releasing and cop-per intrauterine devices in the European Active Surveillance Study on Intrauterine Devices. *Contraception, 91*(4), 274–279. doi:10.1016/j.contraception.2015.01.007

Hidalgo, M. M., Lisondo, C., Juliato, C. T., Espejo-Arce, X., Monteiro, I., & Bahamondes, L. (2006). Ovarian cysts in users of Implanon and Jadelle subdermal contraceptive implants. *Contraception, 73*(5), 532–536. doi:10.1016/j.contraception.2005.12.012

Hooton, T. M., Scholes, D., Stapleton, A. E., Roberts, P. L., Winter, C., Gupta, K., . . . Stamm, W. E. (2000). A prospective study of asymptomatic bacteriuria in sexually active young women. *New England Journal of Medicine, 343*(14), 992–997. doi:10.1056/ nejm200010053431402

Hubacher, D., Lara-Ricalde, R., Taylor, D. J., Guerra-Infante, F., & Guzman-Rodriguez, R. (2001). Use of copper intrauterine de-vices and the risk of tubal infertility among nulligravid women. *New England Journal of Medicine, 345*(8), 561–567.

Hubacher, D., Lopez, L., Steiner, M. J., & Dorflinger, L. (2009). Menstrual pattern changes from levonorgestrel subdermal implants and DMPA: Systematic review and evidence-based comparisons. *Con-traception, 80*(2), 113–118. doi:10.1016/j.contraception.2009.02.008

Institute for Reproductive Health. (2015). Family planning. Retrieved from http://irh.org/focus-areas/family_planning

Kaunitz, A. M., Arias, R., & McClung, M. (2008). Bone density re-covery after depot medroxyprogesterone acetate injectable contraception use. *Contraception, 77*(2), 67–76. doi:10.1016/j. contraception.2007.10.005

Kennedy, K., & Trussell, J. (2011). Postpartum contraception and lactation. In R. A. Hatcher, J. Trussell, A. L. Nelson, W. Cates, D. Kowal, & M. S. Policar (Eds.), *Contraceptive technology* (20th ed., pp. 483–511). New York, NY: Ardent Media.

Kessel. (n.d.). The new diaphragm fits me: Caya contoured dia-phragm. Retrieved from http://www.caya.eu/en

Killick, S. R., Leary, C., Trussell, J., & Guthrie, K. A. (2011). Sperm content of pre-ejaculatory fluid. *Human Fertility (Cambridge), 14*(1), 48–52. doi:10.3109/14647273.2010.520798

Kossler, K., Kuroki, L. M., Allsworth, J. E., Secura, G. M., Roehl, K. A., & Peipert, J. F. (2011). Perceived racial, socioeconomic, and gender discrimination and its impact on contraceptive choice. *Contraception, 84*(3), 273–279. doi:10.1016/j.contraception.2011.01.004

Kulczycki, A., Kim, D. J., Duerr, A., Jamieson, D. J., & Macaluso, M. (2004). The acceptability of the female and male condom: A randomized crossover trial. *Perspectives on Sexual and Reproductive Health, 36*(3), 114–119. doi:10.1363/psrh.36.114.04

Kuyoh, M. A., Toroitich-Ruto, C., Grimes, D. A., Schulz, K. F., & Gallo, M. F. (2003). Sponge versus diaphragm for contraception: A Cochrane review. *Contraception, 67*(1), 15–18.

Leads from the *MMWR:* Toxic-shock syndrome and the vaginal contraceptive sponge. (1984). *Journal of the American Medical Association, 251*(8), 1015–1016.

Leiva, R., Burhan, U., Kyrillos, E., Fehring, R., McLaren, R., Dalzell, C., & Tanguay, E. (2014). Use of ovulation predictor kits as adjuncts when using fertility awareness methods (FAMs): A pilot study. *Journal of the American Board of Family Medicine, 27*(3), 427–429. doi:10.3122/jabfm.2014.03.130255

Li, C., Zhao, W. H., Meng, C. X., Ping, H., Qin, G. J., Cao, S. J., . . . Zhang, J. (2014). Contraceptive use and the risk of ectopic pregnancy: A multi-center case-control study. *PLoS One, 9*(12), e115031. doi:10.1371/journal.pone.0115031

Lindh, I., & Milsom, I. (2013). The influence of intrauterine contraception on the prevalence and severity of dysmenorrhea: A longitudinal population study. *Human Reproduction, 28*(7), 1953–1960. doi:10.1093/humrep/det101

Lopez, L. M., Edelman, A., Chen, M., Otterness, C., Trussell, J., & Helmerhorst, F. M. (2013). Progestin-only contraceptives: Effects on weight. *Cochrane Database of Systematic Reviews, 7,* CD008815. doi:10.1002/14651858.CD008815.pub3

Lopez, L. M., Grimes, D. A., Gallo, M. F., Stockton, L. L., & Schulz, K. F. (2013). Skin patch and vaginal ring versus combined oral contraceptives for contraception. *Cochrane Database of Systematic Reviews, 4,* CD003552. doi:10.1002/14651858.CD003552.pub4

Maguire, K., & Westhoff, C. (2011). The state of hormonal contraception today: Established and emerging noncontraceptive health benefits. *American Journal of Obstetrics & Gynecology, 205*(4, Suppl.), S4–S8. doi:10.1016/j.ajog.2011.06.056

Malacova, E., Kemp, A., Hart, R., Jama-Alol, K., & Preen, D. B. (2014). Long-term risk of ectopic pregnancy varies by method of tubal sterilization: A whole-population study. *Fertility and Sterility, 101*(3), 728–734. doi:10.1016/j.fertnstert.2013.11.127

Mauck, C., Callahan, M., Weiner, D. H., & Dominik, R. (1999). A comparative study of the safety and efficacy of FemCap, a new vaginal barrier contraceptive, and the Ortho All-Flex diaphragm. The FemCap Investigators' Group. *Contraception, 60*(2), 71–80.

Mauck, C. K., Weiner, D. H., Creinin, M. D., Archer, D. F., Schwartz, J. L., Pymar, H. C., . . . Callahan, M. M. (2006). FemCap with removal strap: Ease of removal, safety and acceptability. *Contraception, 73*(1), 59–64. doi:10.1016/j.contraception.2005.06.074

McNicholas, C., Maddipati, R., Zhao, Q., Swor, E., & Peipert, J. F. (2015). Use of the etonogestrel implant and levonorgestrel intrauterine device beyond the U.S. Food and Drug Administration–approved duration. *Obstetrics & Gynecology, 125*(3), 599–604. doi:10.1097/aog.0000000000000690

Michielsen, D., & Beerthuizen, R. (2010). State-of-the art of nonhormonal methods of contraception: VI. Male sterilisation. *European Journal of Contraception & Reproductive Health Care, 15*(2), 136–149. doi:10.3109/13625181003682714

Nahum, G. G., Kaunitz, A. M., Rosen, K., Schmelter, T., & Lynen, R. (2015). Ovarian cysts: Presence and persistence with use of a 13.5mg levonorgestrel-releasing intrauterine system. *Contraception, 91*(5), 412–417. doi:10.1016/j.contraception.2015.01.021

Nanda, K. (2011). Contraceptive patch and vaginal contraceptive ring. In R. A. Hatcher, J. Trussell, A. L. Nelson, W. Cates, D. Kowal, & M. S. Policar (Eds.), *Contraceptive technology* (20th ed., pp. 343–369). New York, NY: Ardent Media.

Nelson, A. L. (2000). The intrauterine contraceptive device. *Obstetrics and Gynecology Clinics of North America, 27*(4), 723–740.

Ortho Evra Prescribing Information. (2014). Retrieved from http://www.janssen.com/us/sites/www_janssen_com_usa/files/products-documents/orthoevrapi_092014.pdf

Paulen, M. E., & Curtis, K. M. (2009). When can a woman have repeat progestogen-only injectables: Depot medroxyprogesterone acetate or norethisterone enantate? *Contraception, 80*(4), 391–408. doi:10.1016/j.contraception.2009.03.023

Peterson, H. B. (2008). Sterilization. *Obstetrics & Gynecology, 111*(1), 189–203. doi:10.1097/01.aog.0000298621.98372.62

Peterson, H. B., Xia, Z., Hughes, J. M., Wilcox, L. S., Tylor, L. R., & Trussell, J. (1997). The risk of ectopic pregnancy after tubal sterilization. U.S. Collaborative Review of Sterilization Working Group. *New England Journal of Medicine, 336*(11), 762–767.

Polis, C. B., Phillips, S. J., Curtis, K. M., Westreich, D. J., Steyn, P. S., Raymond, E., . . . Turner, A. N. (2014). Hormonal contraceptive methods and risk of HIV acquisition in women: A systematic review of epidemiological evidence. *Contraception, 90*(4), 360–390. doi:10.1016/j.contraception.2014.07.009

Pruitt, S. L., von Sternberg, K., Velasquez, M. M., & Mullen, P. D. (2010). Condom use among sterilized and nonsterilized women in county jail and residential treatment centers. *Women's Health Issues, 20*(6), 386–393. doi:10.1016/j.whi.2010.06.007

Raine, T., Harper, C., Leon, K., & Darney, P. (2000). Emergency contraception: Advance provision in a young, high-risk clinic population. *Obstetrics & Gynecology, 96*(1), 1–7.

Raymond, E. (2011a). Contraceptive implants. In R. A. Hatcher, J. Trussell, A. L. Nelson, W. Cates, D. Kowal, & M. S. Policar (Eds.), *Contraceptive technology* (20th ed., pp. 193–207). New York, NY: Ardent Media.

Raymond, E. (2011b). Progestin-only pills. In R. A. Hatcher, J. Trussell, A. L. Nelson, W. Cates, D. Kowal, & M. S. Policar (Eds.), *Contraceptive technology* (20th ed., pp. 237–247). New York, NY: Ardent Media.

Raymond, E. G., Chen, P. L., Luoto, J., & Group, S. T. (2004). Contraceptive effectiveness and safety of five nonoxynol-9 spermicides: a randomized trial. *Obstetrics & Gynecology, 103*(3), 430–439.

Roncari, D., & Hou, M. (2011). Female and male sterilization. In R. A. Hatcher, J. Trussell, A. L. Nelson, W. Cates, D. Kowal, & M. S. Policar (Eds.), *Contraceptive technology* (20th ed., pp. 435–482). New York, NY: Ardent Media.

Schindler, A. E. (2010). Non-contraceptive benefits of hormonal contraceptives. *Minerva Ginecologica, 62*(4), 319–329.

Schreiber, C. A., Meyn, L. A., Creinin, M. D., Barnhart, K. T., & Hillier, S. L. (2006). Effects of long-term use of nonoxynol-9 on vaginal flora. *Obstetrics & Gynecology, 107*(1), 136–143. doi:10.1097/01.AOG.0000189094.21099.4a

Sharlip, I. D., Belker, A. M., Honig, S., Labrecque, M., Marmar, J. L., Ross, L. S., . . . Sokal, D. C. (2012). Vasectomy: AUA guideline. *Journal of Urology, 188*(6, Suppl.), 2482–2491. doi:10.1016/j.juro.2012.09.080

Shelton, J. D., & Halpern, V. (2014). Subcutaneous DMPA: A better lower dose approach. *Contraception, 89*(5), 341–343. doi:10.1016/j.contraception.2013.10.010

Sivin, I., & Batar, I. (2010). State-of-the-art of non-hormonal methods of contraception: III. Intrauterine devices. *European Journal of Contraceptive & Reproductive Health Care, 15*(2), 96–112. doi:10.3109/13625180903519885

Smoley, B. A., & Robinson, C. M. (2012). Natural family planning. *American Family Physician, 86*(10), 924–928.

Steiner, M. J., Dominik, R., Rountree, R. W., Nanda, K., & Dorflinger, L. J. (2003). Contraceptive effectiveness of a polyurethane condom and a latex condom: A randomized controlled trial. *Obstetrics & Gynecology, 101*(3), 539–547.

Stuart, J. E., Secura, G. M., Zhao, Q., Pittman, M. E., & Peipert, J. F. (2013). Factors associated with 11-month discontinuation among contraceptive pill, patch, and ring users. *Obstetrics & Gynecology, 121*(2 pt 1), 330–336. http://10.1097/AOG.0b013e31827e5898

Sulak, P. J., Scow, R. D., Preece, C., Riggs, M. W., & Kuehl, T. J. (2000). Hormone withdrawal symptoms in oral contraceptive users. *Obstetrics & Gynecology, 95*(2), 261–266.

Thorburn, S., & Bogart, L. M. (2005). African American women and family planning services: Perceptions of discrimination. *Women & Health, 42*(1), 23–39.

Tone, A. (2001). *Devices and desires: A history of contraceptives in America.* New York, NY: Hill & Wong.

Trussell, J. (2011). Contraceptive failure in the United States. *Contraception, 83*(5), 397–404. doi:10.1016/j.contraception.2011.01.021

Trussell, J., & Guthrie, K. A. (2011). Choosing a contraceptive: Efficacy, safety, and personal considerations. In R. A. Hatcher, J. Trussell, A. L. Nelson, W. Cates, D. Kowal, & M. S. Policar (Eds.), *Contraceptive technology* (20th ed., pp. 45–74.). New York, NY: Ardent Media.

Trussell, J., Henry, N., Hassan, F., Prezioso, A., Law, A., & Filonenko, A. (2013). Burden of unintended pregnancy in the United States: Potential savings with increased use of long-acting reversible contraception. *Contraception, 87*(2), 154–161. doi:10.1016/j.contraception.2012.07.016

Turok, D. K., Gurtcheff, S. E., Handley, E., Simonsen, S. E., Sok, C., North, R., . . . Murphy, P. A. (2011). A survey of women obtaining emergency contraception: Are they interested in using the copper IUD? *Contraception, 83*(5), 441–446. doi:10.1016/j.contraception.2010.08.011

Van Damme, L., Ramjee, G., Alary, M., Vuylsteke, B., Chandeying, V., Rees, H., . . . Laga, M. (2002). Effectiveness of COL-1492, a nonoxynol-9 vaginal gel, on HIV-1 transmission in female sex workers: A randomised controlled trial. *Lancet, 360*(9338), 971–977.

Vessey, M., & Yeates, D. (2013). Oral contraceptive use and cancer: Final report from the Oxford-Family Planning Association contraceptive study. *Contraception, 88*(6), 678–683. doi:10.1016/j.contraception.2013.08.008

Wallach, M., & Grimes, D. A. (2000). *Modern oral contraception.* Totowa, NJ: Emron.

Wei, S., Venn, A., Ding, C., Foley, S., Laslett, L., & Jones, G. (2011). The association between oral contraceptive use, bone mineral density and fractures in women aged 50-80 years. *Contraception, 84*(4), 357–362. doi:10.1016/j.contraception.2011.02.001

Weller, S., & Davis, K. (2002). Condom effectiveness in reducing heterosexual HIV transmission. *Cochrane Database of Systematic Reviews, 1,* CD003255. doi:10.1002/14651858.cd003255

Westhoff, C. L., Reinecke, I., Bangerter, K., & Merz, M. (2014). Impact of body mass index on suppression of follicular development and ovulation using a transdermal patch containing 0.55-mg ethinyl estradiol/2.1-mg gestodene: A multicenter, open-label, uncontrolled study over three treatment cycles. *Contraception, 90*(3), 272–279. doi:10.1016/j.contraception.2014.04.018

White, K., Potter, J. E., Hopkins, K., Fernandez, L., Amastae, J., & Grossman, D. (2012). Contraindications to progestin-only oral contraceptive pills among reproductive-aged women. *Contraception, 86*(3), 199–203. doi:10.1016/j.contraception.2012.01.008

Whitehouse, K. C., Montealegre, J. R., Follen, M., Scheurer, M. E., & Aagaard, K. (2014). Sociodemographic factors associated with Pap test adherence and cervical dysplasia in surgically sterilized women. *Journal of Reproduction & Infertility, 15*(2), 94–104.

Wilcox, A. J., Dunson, D., & Baird, D. D. (2000). The timing of the "fertile window" in the menstrual cycle: day specific estimates from a prospective study. *British Medical Journal, 321*(7271), 1259–1262.

Wilkinson, D., Ramjee, G., Tholandi, M., & Rutherford, G. (2002). Nonoxynol-9 for preventing vaginal acquisition of HIV infection by women from men. *Cochrane Database of Systematic Reviews, 4,* CD003936. doi:10.1002/14651858.cd003936

Winner, B., Peipert, J. F., Zhao, Q., Buckel, C., Madden, T., Allsworth, J. E., & Secura, G. M. (2012). Effectiveness of long-acting reversible contraception. *New England Journal of Medicine, 366*(21), 1998–2007. doi:10.1056/NEJMoa1110855

World Health Organization (WHO)/CONRAD. (2001). *WHO/CONRAD technical ocnsultation on nonoxynol-9: Summary report.* Geneva, Switzerland: WHO.

Xiang, A. H., Kawakubo, M., Kjos, S. L., & Buchanan, T. A. (2006). Long-acting injectable progestin contraception and risk of type 2 diabetes in Latino women with prior gestational diabetes mellitus. *Diabetes Care, 29*(3), 613–617.

Yoost, J. (2014). Understanding benefits and addressing misperceptions and barriers to intrauterine device access among populations in the United States. *Patient Preference and Adherence, 8,* 947–957. doi:10.2147/ppa.s45710

Zieman, M., Hatcher, R., & Allen, A. (2015). *Managing contraception: 2015-2016.* Atlanta, GA: Bridging the Gap Communications.

Zite, N., & Borrero, S. (2011). Female sterilisation in the United States. *European Journal of Contraceptive & Reproductive Health Care, 16*(5), 336–340. doi:10.3109/13625187.2011.604451

Zukerman, Z., Weiss, D. B., & Orvieto, R. (2003). Does preejaculatory penile secretion originating from Cowper's gland contain sperm? *Journal of Assisted Reproduction and Genetics, 20*(4), 157–159.

Selected Medical Eligibility Criteria for Contraceptive Use

The *U.S. Medical Eligibility Criteria for Contraceptive Use* (CDC, 2010) is a comprehensive, evidence-based guide for determining whether women have relative or absolute contraindications to contraceptive methods. The *Medical Eligibility Criteria* uses the following four classification categories of whether a person can use or should not use a method:

- *Category 1*: a condition for which there is no restriction for the use of the contraceptive method
- *Category 2*: a condition where the advantages of using the method generally outweigh the theoretical or proven risks
- *Category 3*: a condition where the theoretical or proven risks usually outweigh the advantages of using the method
- *Category 4*: a condition that represents an unacceptable health risk if the contraceptive method is used

The following table is a summary of selected criteria for contraceptive use. The table is a quick reference and not inclusive of the full guidelines. Readers are referred to the complete *U.S. Medical Eligibility Criteria for Contraceptive Use* (available online; see the citation at the end of the appendix) for clarifications of category classification, complete references, and conditions and contraceptive methods that are not included in this table. Abbreviations for the methods in the table are as follows:

- *COC/P/R*: low-dose ($\leq$ 35 mcg ethinyl estradiol) combined oral contraceptives, patch, and vaginal ring
- *POP*: progestin-only pills
- *DMPA*: depot medroxyprogesterone acetate injection
- *Implant*: etonogestrel implant
- *Cu-IUD*: copper intrauterine device
- *LNG-IUD*: levonorgestrel intrauterine device

When there is a differentiation between the criteria for initiation and those for continuation of a method, these are noted with the abbreviations "I" and "C" next to the category number.

Personal Characteristics and Reproductive History

Condition	COC/P/R	POP	DMPA	Implant	Cu-IUD	LNG-IUD
Pregnancy						
Age	Menarche to < 40 = 1 ≥ 40 = 2	Menarche to > 45 = 1	Menarche to < 18 = 2 18–45 = 1 > 45 = 2	Menarche to > 45 = 1	Menarche to < 20 = 2 ≥20 = 1	Menarche to < 20 = 2 ≥ 20 = 1
Parity						
a. Nulliparous	1	1	1	1	2	2
b. Parous	1	1	1	1	1	1
Postpartum (breastfeeding women)						
a. < 21 days	4	2	2	2		
b. 21 to < 30 days						
i. With other risk factors for VTE (such as age ≥ 35 years, previous VTE, thrombophilia, immobility, transfusion at birth, BMI ≥ 30 kg/m², postpartum hemorrhage, postcesarean birth, preeclampsia, or smoking)	3–4	2	2	2		
ii. Without other risk factors for VTE	3	2	2	2		
c. 30–42 days						
i. With other risk factors for VTE (such as age ≥ 35 years, previous VTE, thrombophilia, immobility, transfusion at birth, BMI ≥ 30 kg/m², postpartum hemorrhage, postcesarean birth, preeclampsia, or smoking)	3–4	1	1	1		
ii. Without other risk factors for VTE	2	1	1	1		
d. > 42 days	2	1	1	1		

Condition	COC/P/R	POP	DMPA	Implant	Cu-IUD	LNG-IUD
Postpartum (nonbreastfeeding women)						
a. < 21 days	4	1	1	1		
b. 21–42 days						
i. With other risk factors for VTE (such as age ≥ 35 years, previous VTE, thrombophilia, immobility, transfusion at birth, BMI ≥ 30 kg/m^2, postpartum hemorrhage, postcesarean birth, preeclampsia, or smoking)	3–4	1	1	1		
ii. Without other risk factors for VTE	2	1	1	1		
c. > 42 days	1	1	1	1		
Postpartum (breastfeeding or nonbreastfeeding women, including postcesarean birth)						
a. < 10 minutes after delivery of the placenta					1	2
b. 10 minutes after delivery of the placenta to < 4 weeks					2	2
c. ≥ 4 weeks					1	1
d. Puerperal sepsis					4	4
Post abortion						
a. First trimester	1	1	1	1	1	1
b. Second trimester	1	1	1	1	2	2
c. Immediate postseptic abortion	1	1	1	1	4	4
Past ectopic pregnancy	1	2	1	1	1	1
History of pelvic surgery	1	1	1	1	1	1
Smoking						
a. Age < 35	2	1	1	1	1	1
b. Age ≥ 35						
i. < 15 cigarettes/day	3	1	1	1	1	1
ii. ≥ 15 cigarettes/day	4	1	1	1	1	1

(continues)

Condition	COC/P/R	POP	DMPA	Implant	Cu-IUD	LNG-IUD
Personal Characteristics and Reproductive History						
Obesity						
a. ≥ 30 kg/m² BMI	2	1	1	1	1	1
b. Menarche to < 18 years and ≥ 30 kg/m² BMI	2	1	2	1	1	1
History of bariatric surgery						
a. Restrictive procedures: decrease storage capacity of the stomach	1	1	1	1	1	1
b. Malabsorptive procedures: decrease absorption of nutrients and calories by shortening the functional length of the small intestine	COCs = 3 P/R = 1	3	1	1	1	1
Cardiovascular Disease						
Multiple risk factors for arterial cardiovascular disease (such as older age, smoking, diabetes, and hypertension)	3/4	2	3	2	1	2
Hypertension						
a. Adequately controlled hypertension	3	1	2	1	1	1
b. Elevated blood pressure levels (properly take measurements)						
i. Systolic 140–159 mm Hg or diastolic 90–99 mm Hg	3	1	2	1	1	1
ii. Systolic > 160 mm Hg or diastolic ≥ 100 mm Hg	4	2	3	2	1	2
c. Vascular disease	4	2	3	2	1	2
History of high blood pressure during pregnancy (where current blood pressure is measurable and normal)	2	1	1	1	1	1
DVT/PE						
a. History of DVT/PE, not on anticoagulant therapy						
i. Higher risk for recurrent DVT/PE (≥ 1 risk factor)	4	2	2	2	1	2
ii. Lower risk for recurrent DVT/PE (no risk factors)	3	2	2	2	1	2

Condition	COC/P/R	POP	DMPA	Implant	Cu-IUD	LNG-IUD
b. Acute DVT/PE	4	2	2	2	2	2
c. DVT/PE and established anticoagulant therapy for at least 3 months						
i. Higher risk for recurrent DVT/PE (≥1 risk factor)	4	2	2	2	2	2
ii. Lower risk for recurrent DVT/PE (no risk factors)	3	2	2	2	2	2
d. Family history (first-degree relatives)	2	1	1	1	1	1
e. Major surgery						
i. With prolonged immobilization	4	2	2	2	1	2
ii. Without prolonged immobilization	2	1	1	1	1	1
f. Minor surgery without immobilization	1	1	1	1	1	1
Known thrombogenic mutations (e.g., factor V Leiden; prothrombin mutation; protein S, protein C, and antithrombin deficiencies)	4	2	2	2	1	2
Superficial venous thrombosis						
a. Varicose veins	1	1	1	1	1	1
b. Superficial thrombophlebitis	2	1	1	1	1	1
Current and history of ischemic heart disease	4	I2/C3	3	I2/C3	1	I2/C3
Stroke (history of cerebrovascular accident)	4	I2/C3	3	I2/C3	1	2
Known hyperlipidemias (screening is *not* necessary for safe use of contraceptive methods)	2/3	2	2	2	1	2
Valvular heart disease						
a. Uncomplicated	2	1	1	1	1	1
b. Complicated (pulmonary hypertension, risk for atrial fibrillation, history of subacute bacterial endocarditis)	4	1	1	1	1	1
Peripartum cardiomyopathy						
a. Normal or mildly impaired cardiac function						
i. < 6 months	4	1	1	1	2	2
ii. ≥ 6 months	3	1	1	1	2	2
b. Moderately or severely impaired cardiac function	4	2	2	2	2	2

(continues)

Condition	COC/P/R	POP	DMPA	Implant	Cu-IUD	LNG-IUD
Rheumatic Diseases						
Systemic lupus erythematosus						
a. Positive (or unknown) antiphospholipid antibodies	4	3	3	3	1	3
b. Severe thrombocytopenia	2	2	I3/C2	2	I3/C2	2
c. Immunosuppressive treatment	2	2	2	2	I2/C1	2
d. None of the above	2	2	2	2	1	2
Rheumatoid arthritis						
a. On immunosuppressive therapy	2	1	2/3	1	I2/C1	I2/C1
b. Not on immunosuppressive therapy	2	1	2	1	1	1
Neurologic Conditions						
Headaches						
a. Nonmigrainous (mild or severe)	I1/C2	1	1	1	1	1
b. Migraine						
i. Without aura						
Age < 35	I2/C3	I1/C2	2	2	1	2
Age ≥ 35	I3/C4	I1/C2	2	2	1	2
ii. With aura (at any age)	4	I2/C3	I2/C3	I2/C3	1	I2/C3
Epilepsy	1	1	1	1	1	1
Depressive Disorders						
Depressive disorders	1	1	1	1	1	1
Reproductive Tract Infections and Disorders						
Vaginal bleeding patterns						
a. Irregular pattern without heavy bleeding	1	2	2	2	1	1
b. Heavy or prolonged bleeding (includes regular and irregular patterns)	1	2	2	2	2	I1/C2
Unexplained vaginal bleeding (suspicious for serious conditions)						
Before evaluation	2	2	3	3	I4/C2	I4/C2
Endometriosis	1	1	1	1	2	1
Benign ovarian tumors (including cysts)	1	1	1	1	1	1

Condition	COC/P/R	POP	DMPA	Implant	Cu-IUD	LNG-IUD
Severe dysmenorrhea	1	1	1	1	2	1
Gestational trophoblast disease						
a. Decreasing or undetectable β-hCG	1	1	1	1	3	3
b. Persistently elevated β-hCG levels or malignant disease	1	1	1	1	4	4
Cervical ectropion	1	1	1	1	1	1
Cervical intraepithelial neoplasia	2	1	2	2	1	2
Cervical cancer (awaiting treatment)	2	1	2	2	I4/C2	I4/C2
Breast disease						
a. Undiagnosed mass	2	2	2	2	1	2
b. Benign breast disease	1	1	1	1	1	1
c. Family history of cancer	1	1	1	1	1	1
d. Breast cancer						
i. Current	4	4	4	4	1	4
ii. Past and no evidence of current disease for 5 years	3	3	3	3	1	3
Endometrial hyperplasia	1	1	1	1	1	1
Endometrial cancer	1	1	1	1	I4/C2	I4/C2
Ovarian cancer	1	1	1	1	1	1
Uterine fibroids	1	1	1	1	2	2
Anatomic abnormalities						
a. That distort the uterine cavity					4	4
b. That do not distort the uterine cavity					2	2
PID						
a. Past PID (assuming no current risk factors of STIs)						
i. With subsequent pregnancy	1	1	1	1	1	1
ii. Without subsequent pregnancy	1	1	1	1	2	2
b. Current PID	1	1	1	1	I4/C2	I4/C2
STIs						
a. Current purulent cervicitis or chlamydial infection or gonorrhea	1	1	1	1	I4/C2	I4/C2
b. Other STIs (excluding HIV and hepatitis)	1	1	1	1	2	2
c. Vaginitis (including *Trichomonas vaginalis* and bacterial vaginosis)	1	1	1	1	2	2
d. Increased risk of STIs	1	1	1	1	I2-3/C2	I2-3/C2

(continues)

Condition	COC/P/R	POP	DMPA	Implant	Cu-IUD	LNG-IUD
HIV/AIDS						
High risk for HIV	1	1	1	1	2	2
HIV infection	1	1	1	1	2	2
AIDS	1	1	1	1	I3/C2	I3/C2
Clinically well on ARV therapy (see *ARV therapy* below)					2	2
Other Infections						
Schistosomiasis						
a. Uncomplicated	1	1	1	1	1	1
b. Fibrosis of the liver (if severe, see *cirrhosis*)	1	1	1	1	1	1
Tuberculosis						
a. Nonpelvic	1	1	1	1	1	1
b. Pelvic	1	1	1	1	I4/C3	I4/C3
Malaria	1	1	1	1	1	1
Endocrine Conditions						
Diabetes						
a. History of gestational disease	1	1	1	1	1	1
b. Nonvascular disease						
i. Non-insulin-dependent	2	2	2	2	1	2
ii. Insulin-dependent	2	2	2	2	1	2
c. Nephropathy/retinopathy/neuropathy	3/4	2	3	2	1	2
d. Other vascular disease or diabetes of more than 20 years' duration	3/4	2	3	2	1	2
Thyroid disorders						
a. Simple goiter	1	1	1	1	1	1
b. Hyperthyroid	1	1	1	1	1	1
c. Hypothyroid	1	1	1	1	1	1

Condition	COC/P/R	POP	DMPA	Implant	Cu-IUD	LNG-IUD
Gastrointestinal Conditions						
Inflammatory bowel disease (ulcerative colitis, Crohn's disease)	2/3	2	2	1	1	1
Gallbladder disease						
a. Symptomatic						
i. Treated by cholecystectomy	2	2	2	2	1	2
ii. Medically treated	3	2	2	2	1	2
iii. Current	3	2	2	2	1	2
b. Asymptomatic	2	2	2	2	1	2
History of cholestasis						
a. Pregnancy-related	2	1	1	1	1	1
b. Past COC-related	3	2	2	2	1	2
Viral hepatitis						
a. Acute or flare	I3-4/C2	1	1	1	1	1
b. Carrier	1	1	1	1	1	1
c. Chronic	1	1	1	1	1	1
Cirrhosis						
a. Mild (compensated)	1	1	1	1	1	1
b. Severe (decompensated)	4	3	3	3	1	3
Liver tumors						
a. Benign						
i. Focal nodular hyperplasia	2	2	2	2	1	2
ii. Hepatocellular adenoma	4	3	3	3	1	3
b. Malignant (hepatoma)	4	3	3	3	1	3
Anemias						
Thalassemia	1	1	1	1	2	1
Sickle cell disease	2	1	1	1	2	1
Iron-deficiency anemia	1	1	1	1	2	1

(continues)

Condition	COC/P/R	POP	DMPA	Implant	Cu-IUD	LNG-IUD
Solid Organ Transplantation						
Complicated: graft failure (acute or chronic), rejection, cardiac allograft vasculopathy	4	2	2	2	I3/C2	I3/C2
Uncomplicated	2	2	2	2	2	2
Drug Interactions						
ARV therapy						
a. Nucleoside reverse transcriptase inhibitors	1	1	1	1	I2-3/C2	I2-3/C2
b. Non-nucleoside reverse transcriptase inhibitors	2	2	1	2	I2-3/C2	I2-3/C2
c. Ritonavir-boosted protease inhibitors	3	3	1	2	I2-3/C2	I2-3/C2
Anticonvulsant therapy						
a. Certain anticonvulsants (phenytoin, carbamazepine, barbiturates, primidone, topiramate, oxcarbazepine)	3	3	1	2	1	1
b. Lamotrigine	3	1	1	1	1	1
Antimicrobial therapy						
a. Broad-spectrum antibiotics	1	1	1	1	1	1
b. Antifungals	1	1	1	1	1	1
c. Antiparasitics	1	1	1	1	1	1
d. Rifampicin or rifabutin therapy	3	3	1	2	1	1

Abbreviations: AIDS, acquired immune deficiency syndrome; ARV, antiretroviral; β-hCG, beta–human chorionic gonadotropin; BMI, body mass index; COC, combined oral contraceptive; DVT, deep venous thrombosis; HIV, human immunodeficiency virus; PE, pulmonary embolism; PID, pelvic inflammatory disease; STI, sexually transmitted infection; VTE, venous thromboembolism. Data from Centers for Disease Control and Prevention. (2010). U.S. medical eligibility criteria for contraceptive use, 2010: Adapted from the World Health Organization medical eligibility criteria for contraceptive use, 4th edition. *Morbidity and Mortality Weekly Report, 59*, 1–86. Retrieved from http://www.cdc.gov/reproductivehealth/unintendedpregnancy /USMEC.htm; Centers for Disease Control and Prevention. (2011). Update to CDC's U.S. *Medical Eligibility Criteria for Contraceptive Use, 2010:* Revised recommendations for the use of contraceptive methods during the postpartum period. *Morbidity and Mortality Weekly Report, 60*, 878–883; Centers for Disease Control and Prevention. (2012). Update to CDC's *U.S. Medical Eligibility Criteria for Contraceptive Use, 2010:* Revised recommendations for the use of hormonal contraception among women at high risk for HIV infection or infected with HIV. *Morbidity and Mortality Weekly Report, 61*, 449–452.

Primary Mechanisms of Action of Contraceptive Methods[a]

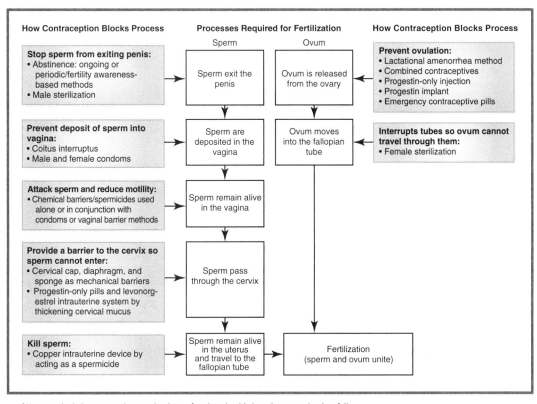

How Contraception Blocks Process

Stop sperm from exiting penis:
• Abstinence: ongoing or periodic/fertility awareness-based methods
• Male sterilization

Prevent deposit of sperm into vagina:
• Coitus interruptus
• Male and female condoms

Attack sperm and reduce motility:
• Chemical barriers/spermicides used alone or in conjunction with condoms or vaginal barrier methods

Provide a barrier to the cervix so sperm cannot enter:
• Cervical cap, diaphragm, and sponge as mechanical barriers
• Progestin-only pills and levonorgestrel intrauterine system by thickening cervical mucus

Kill sperm:
• Copper intrauterine device by acting as a spermicide

Processes Required for Fertilization

Sperm — Ovum

Sperm exit the penis

Ovum is released from the ovary

Sperm are deposited in the vagina

Ovum moves into the fallopian tube

Sperm remain alive in the vagina

Sperm pass through the cervix

Sperm remain alive in the uterus and travel to the fallopian tube

Fertilization (sperm and ovum unite)

How Contraception Blocks Process

Prevent ovulation:
• Lactational amenorrhea method
• Combined contraceptives
• Progestin-only injection
• Progestin implant
• Emergency contraceptive pills

Interrupts tubes so ovum cannot travel through them:
• Female sterilization

[a] Many methods have secondary mechanisms of action should the primary mechanism fail.
© Frances E. Likis.

CHAPTER 12

Menopause

Ivy M. Alexander
Kathryn P. Atkin
Linda C. Andrist

Menopause, which is often thought of as the closure of reproductive capability, has emerged as one of the predominant health issues for midlife women. A major reason that menopause is receiving so much attention is the increasing numbers of women reaching midlife. Approximately 2 million women reach menopause each year in the United States. It is estimated there were 50 million postmenopausal women in the United States in 2010, with approximately 45 million women being older than age 52, the average age of natural menopause in North America (North American Menopause Society [NAMS], 2014). The baby-boom generation—that is, people born between 1945 and 1960—is the largest middle-aged cohort ever recorded. With an estimated life expectancy of 81 years for women in the United States in 2010, many women will live one-third of their lives after menopause (Murphy, Xu, & Kochanek, 2013),

The emphasis on the end of reproduction ignores the myriad issues facing midlife women. Midlife brings with it many changes, such as children leaving home, illness or death of parents, and career changes. Transitions that accompany midlife include adjusting to the idea of mortality, adapting to changes in family relationships, becoming more authentic, and assessing and appreciating one's life experiences (Sampselle, Harris, Harlow, & Sowers, 2002).

During midlife, women continue to grow and develop psychologically. Increasingly, menopause is being appreciated as another life stage with potential for growth and development. The challenges experienced during this transition may serve as the basis for personal reflection and growth (Busch, Barth-Olofsson, Rosenhagen, & Collins, 2003).

MODELS OF WOMEN'S GROWTH AND DEVELOPMENT

Many researchers have elucidated women's unique growth and development over the life span. For example, Gilligan (1982) found that relationships were a priority for women. Jordan and colleagues (1991) found that women develop in relationship with others, such that development means increasing complexity, connection, and mutuality.

The major premise in many of the published works is the importance of recognizing variations in women's development based on culture, race, and socioeconomic variables. Collins (1990) highlighted the uniqueness of African American women's experiences. Likewise, Sampselle et al. (2002) conducted focus groups with 32 Caucasian and African American women who were in midlife, seeking to identify factors that enhanced their well-being and to determine whether these factors differed between the two groups. These researchers found that Caucasian participants were concerned about menopause as a sign of aging and the loss of youthful appearance, whereas the African American women were welcoming of menopause as a normal event. All of the women identified childbearing and child launching as major stages in women's lives. The potential for further personal development was enhanced by fewer childcare demands, and women felt few feelings of loss.

Quinn (1991) developed a theoretical model, known as "Integrating a New Me," through a qualitative study with 12 women. According to this model, women experience four processes:

- Tuning into me: The beginning of the awareness of entering perimenopause
- Facing a paradox of feelings: Both positive and negative feelings about situations such as getting older, reproduction, physical vulnerability, and uncertainty about the future
- Contrasting impressions: The processing of conflicting information, women developing their own symbolic meaning through integrating interactions with others, and their own self-appraisal
- Making adjustments: The changes and alterations that women make in response to their emotional, physical, and life changes in daily living

Arnold (2005) interviewed 23 women about the transition in moving from their 40s to their 50s. The women described these changes as "stepping out of the mold" of society's "rules" about how they should behave, and "letting go" of material things as well as previous expectations they had of themselves. One participant said, "I feel competent and no longer have to prove my abilities" (p. 641). "Walking in balance" was a theme that women described as "characterizing self as peaceful, accepting, and in line with their interests and needs" (p. 642). They described themselves as "moving in new directions," finding a new zest for life and interests for creative self-expression. At this stage of their lives, they were "redefining relationships" with family and particularly female friends. Finally, they expressed a freedom "to be" strong resourceful women.

Building on Sheehy's (1976, 1995) work, Wilmoth (1996) proposed a conceptual framework that includes disassembling, evaluating, and reassembling stages as means to find one's own truth. Disassembling entails taking apart our psychological lives and examining them from a new perspective. This phase includes a natural mourning process for lost youth, loss of procreative abilities, and lost opportunities, and is similar to Quinn's first process. The evaluation process that accompanies disassembling requires that women look into themselves to see who they are and whether they like themselves. Wilmoth argues that the context of each woman's experience depends on her lived experience and life situation—hence the variation in women's experiences. Reassembling incorporates a coming of age and a movement toward mastery.

Based on a longitudinal study, Ballard, Kuh, and Wadsworth (2001) described the menopause transition as a status passage, which includes five stages: (1) expectations of symptoms, (2) experience of symptoms and loss of control, (3) confirmation of the menopause, (4) regaining control, and (5) freedom from menstruation. All of the aforementioned models have three major phases in common: assessment, adjusting to change, and acceptance. It is noteworthy to mention that many researchers have found that menopause itself—that is, the cessation of menstruation—is just one event in the overall context of women's lives during midlife.

THE MEDICALIZATION OF MENOPAUSE: A HISTORICAL PERSPECTIVE

Menopause is a remarkable example of the medicalization of women's bodies. The biomedical model of the twentieth century perpetuated menopause as a deficiency disease (MacPherson, 1981) or endocrinopathy (Utian, 1987). Science attempted to establish hormone therapy (HT; **Table 12-1**) as the panacea for prevention of diseases in old age, and pharmaceutical corporations aggressively marketed their products as representing "the fountain of youth."

In 1938, researchers in England produced the first synthetic estrogen, diethylstilbestrol, which was heralded as the cure for menopause-related symptoms. Premarin, a medication introduced by Wyeth-Ayerst in 1942, was the first nonsynthetic estrogen produced from the urine of pregnant mares. Although this therapy was prescribed for many women, the use of HT did not increase significantly until the 1960s, particularly after the publication of *Feminine Forever* by gynecologist Robert Wilson (1966). The major message in this highly popular book—100,000 copies of which were sold in the first 7 months after its publication—was that

TABLE 12-1	Recommended Menopause Hormone Therapy Terminology[a]

Term	Abbreviation/Explanation
Estrogen therapy alone	ET
Estrogen–progestogen therapy	EPT
Menopause hormone therapy	MHT; encompassing term for ET/EPT
Progestogen	Encompassing term for progesterone and progestin

[a] The North American Menopause Society has urged clinicians, researchers, and the media to standardize terminology, which it considers essential for ensuring accurate communication. Note that the word *replacement* has been deleted from the terms *hormone replacement therapy* and *estrogen replacement therapy*.
Data from North American Menopause Society (NAMS). (2014). *Menopause practice: A clinician's guide* (5th ed.). Mayfield Heights, OH: Author.

after menopause women would become eunuchs with withered breasts and begin a "living decay" (p. 43). Estrogen use, which was then referred to as hormone replacement therapy (HRT), promised women the fountain of youth and was praised by Wilson as "one of the greatest biological revolutions in the history of civilization" (p. 16). Interestingly, Wilson's work was funded by the pharmaceutical manufacturers Ayerst, Searle, and Upjohn.

Between the years 1967 and 1975, sales of Premarin (conjugated equine estrogens [CEE]) tripled. By the time its association with endometrial cancer became known, Premarin was the fifth most popular drug in the United States. In 1975, researchers linked estrogen use with increased incidence of endometrial cancer, and the sales of Premarin dropped dramatically. In 1979, the National Institute on Aging convened a consensus conference and agreed that "women using estrogens should take them only for the shortest possible time, in the lowest possible dose," because HT increases the risk for endometrial cancer (U.S. Department of Health, Education, and Welfare, 1979, p. 1). Additionally, the committee concluded that HT was effective only for hot flashes and vaginal dryness (National Women's Health Network, 2000).

During the 1980s, epidemiologic data demonstrated that the addition of a progestogen to estrogen therapy (ET) lowered the risk of endometrial cancer. Once again, HT increased in popularity. When researchers demonstrated that HT could decrease the risk of osteoporosis in the early 1980s

(Weiss, Ure, Ballard, William, & Daling, 1980), the promotion of HT changed from an emphasis on symptom relief to a touting of its ability to prevent disease in old age. By the late 1980s, several observational studies had shown that HT was protective against heart disease. Indeed, until the release of the findings of the Women's Health Initiative (WHI) in 2002, clinicians continued recommending HT to nearly all postmenopausal women for long-term prevention of heart disease. The U.S. Preventive Services Task Force (USPSTF, 1996) made the recommendation in the 1990s that all women should be counseled about and consider preventive HT. It did not, however, offer a recommendation about whether women should actually take HT. Studies linking estrogen use and breast cancer were glossed over, and women were told that the risk of heart disease outweighed the risk of breast cancer. Studies were published linking the use of HT and reduced risk of Alzheimer's disease, memory loss, skin integrity, and colon cancer.

The WHI is the largest clinical trial ever to be conducted on health risks of postmenopausal women. As part of this study, nearly 17,000 women were randomized into HT or placebo groups between 1993 and 1998. The estrogen with progestogen therapy (EPT) arm of the study was halted in 2002, after a mean of 5.2 years of follow-up, because the health risks were found to outweigh the benefits. When interpreting these results, however, it is important to note the difference between relative risk and absolute risk. The WHI was designed to assess the disease prevention abilities of ET and EPT; as a result, the researchers tolerated a much lower level of risk when compared to treatment studies. Although the absolute risk of adverse outcomes with ET and EPT is low, the relative risk regarding disease prevention in the WHI caused greater concern, and those were the statistics revealed by the researchers (Santen et al., 2010). The deleterious outcomes of ET and EPT noted in the WHI included increased risks of breast cancer, coronary events, stroke, and pulmonary embolism (Rossouw et al., 2002). In March 2004, the estrogen arm of the study was also stopped because researchers found a relative increased risk of stroke. The study group reported that estrogen did not appear to increase or decrease heart disease or breast cancer (Anderson et al., 2004; National Institutes of Health [NIH], 2004).

Results from the WHI did confirm that ET prevents osteoporosis-related hip fractures and protects the spine and small bones against the development of osteoporosis. While CEE preparations are still indicated for the prevention of postmenopausal osteoporosis, they are not approved for the treatment of postmenopausal osteoporosis. Instead, most experts recommend the use of nonestrogen medications for these purposes (NAMS, 2014).

Many experts have pointed out the limitations of the WHI results, such as the age of participants. The mean age of women participating in the study was 63 years, which is significantly older than newly menopausal women. Several studies have suggested that older individuals respond differently to HT, likely due to the increasing atherosclerotic changes that occur with aging, which negatively impact risk for cardiovascular disease (CVD) (Goodman, 2012). Moreover, not only did the study fail to address quality of life issues for women with moderate to severe vasomotor symptoms related to menopause, but these women were actually excluded from the study. For these reasons, it remains difficult to evaluate differences in responses to HT between women who initiate HT before the cessation of menses and those who begin HT later in life (Wysocki, Alexander, Schnare, Moore, & Freeman, 2003). Finally, the study evaluated only CEE alone and CEE with medroxyprogesterone acetate (CEE/MPA), as they were the most commonly used HT formulations at that time (Manson, 2014).

Prior to the publication of the initial findings of the WHI, it was estimated that more than 40% of postmenopausal women in the United States were using HT (Manson et al., 2013). Women's use of postmenopausal HT declined shortly after the results of the WHI became public in 2002, and recent surveys indicate that between 50% and 80% of women now choose nonhormonal therapies for managing their menopause-related symptoms (NAMS, 2015a). This decline in use of HT can be attributed to the fact that many healthcare providers are now reluctant to prescribe HT, even to women with severe symptoms. Many of these providers did not understand that the WHI was a prevention study and that it is not appropriate to apply these results to the newly menopausal women with severe symptoms affecting quality of life (Duvall & Plourd, 2014).

In 2013, Manson et al. published extended post-intervention follow-up data from the WHI that stratified results by age, time since the onset of menopause, and other important variables to assess the benefit–risk balance of HT for chronic disease prevention in women. The results for women aged 50 to 59 years with recent onset of menopause (less than 10 years) as well as use of CEE in women with a prior hysterectomy revealed more favorable results. Indeed, Manson (2014) later reported "the quality-of-life benefits are likely to outweigh the risks for many women who seek treatment for symptoms in early menopause" (p. 921).

In contrast, Manson et al. (2013) concluded that the risks of CEE/MPA outweighed its benefits for chronic disease prevention. Although many of the risks and benefits dissipated after the intervention was stopped, an increased risk for breast cancer persisted post intervention in women who took CEE/MPA. There appeared to be more of a risk–benefit balance among women with a prior hysterectomy who took CEE—notably, a reduction in breast cancer was observed among this group (Anderson et al., 2012).

Age and timing since menopause were found to be important variables in subsequent analysis of the WHI data. Researchers found that HT had a harmful effect on risk for coronary heart disease (CHD) in women older than 60 years as well as in women who had a higher baseline risk for CVD. There appeared to be a neutral risk for CHD among younger women (50–59 years) who took CEE/MPA, and favorable results were observed among younger women taking CEE alone. Increased risks of stroke, venous thrombosis, gallstones, and urinary incontinence were observed among women taking both regimens, and results did not appear to differ based on the women's age. A growing body of evidence suggests that low-dose and transdermal estrogen formulations used in recently menopausal women carry fewer risks for venous thrombosis, stroke, and myocardial infarction (NAMS, 2012; Manson, 2014; Manson et al., 2013). In a review of the literature from 1990 to 2010, Goodman (2012) discussed the reduced risks of CVD and venous thromboembolic events (VTE) with transdermal estrogens compared to oral estrogens; the lower risks are attributable to avoidance of the first-pass metabolism of the liver as well as decreased hepatic protein synthesis with the transdermal formulations, which decrease levels of inflammatory and coagulation markers and reduce fibrinolysis. Nevertheless, more research is needed to elucidate these effects.

The Kronos Early Estrogen Prevention Study (KEEPS) is a double-blind, randomized controlled trial (RCT) that enrolled 729 recently menopausal women (within 3 years) to assess the impact of oral or transdermal estrogen on prevention of atherosclerosis and to determine if transdermal estrogen is equally effective and potentially safer than oral estrogen. The KEEPS data recently revealed beneficial results regarding cardiovascular safety in this population: Oral estrogen was associated with beneficial increases in high-density lipoprotein (HDL) and decreases in low-density lipoprotein (LDL) cholesterol, although both C-reactive protein levels and triglycerides increased in women receiving the oral therapy. Transdermal estrogen had no effect on cardiovascular markers. In addition, compared to placebo, oral and transdermal estrogen had no apparent effects on atherosclerosis progression. Transdermal estrogen was associated with an increase in libido, and oral estrogen was associated with an improvement in mood (Duvall & Plourd, 2014).

NAMS has released several position statements on the use of HT in menopausal women since 2004. In 2012, it published a position statement that further emphasized the benefit–risk ratio of HT based on the availability of more long-term data subsequent to the WHI. The 2012 statement includes specific recommendations for HT use (**Box 12-1**).

NAMS released an additional statement in 2015 noting that as many as 42% of women continue to experience severe vasomotor menopausal symptoms between 60 and 65 years of age, which can significantly impact their quality of life. With appropriate counseling regarding the risks of continuing HT beyond age 60, in some circumstances, with close clinical supervision, it may be appropriate to continue therapy with the lowest effective dose for women who continue to experience persistent symptoms (NAMS, 2015b).

The evolution of the use of HT for the prevention of disease has been challenged based on RCTs, epidemiologic, and observational data. The opening page of NAMS's 2014 publication *Menopause Practice: A Clinician's Guide*, *Fifth Edition,* begins with these words: "Menopause is a normal, physiological event …" (p. 1). This shift from the 1980s view of menopause as a pathologic condition, along with the increases in research focusing on women's experiences of menopause, indicates a paradigm shift is occurring, which is effectively dismantling the concept of "menopause as a disease." Nurse researchers, in particular, have demonstrated that menopause is a normal developmental stage in women's lives. Some women will need HT to increase their quality of life, but this practice is no longer standard treatment for all women during midlife.

NATURAL MENOPAUSE

Menopause is defined as the point in time in which there has been a cessation of menstruation for at least 12 consecutive months. Menopause occurs in response to normal physiologic changes in the hypothalamic–pituitary–ovarian axis (see Chapter 5 for a detailed description of the menstrual cycle). During the perimenopausal period, which spans approximately 2 to 8 years prior to the last menstrual period, and for the 12 months of amenorrhea preceding menopause, fewer ovarian follicles develop in each menstrual cycle. Anovulation is common during this period as the follicles that do develop are less responsive to follicle-stimulating hormone (FSH), and the ovaries produce less estradiol, progesterone, and androgens. Thus the usual negative

BOX 12-1 Recommendations for Hormone Therapy Use

- HT should be individualized, be based on the woman's health and personal risk factors, and take into account the woman's quality of life priorities.
- HT is not indicated for the sole purpose of preventing CVD. Beginning HT in women aged 50 to 59 years or within 10 years of menopause to treat menopause-related symptoms should not increase CHD risk. A growing body of evidence suggests that beginning ET during this time may decrease CHD risk.
- The recommended duration of therapy differs for ET versus EPT. Due to the established risk for breast cancer with EPT, therapy should be limited to 3 to 5 years. More flexibility with a longer duration of ET could be considered in the absence of adverse effects or known risk factors due to the more favorable safety profile of ET.
- ET is the most effective treatment for vulvar and vaginal atrophy, and low-dose, local ET is recommended when only vaginal symptoms are present.

- Women who are appropriate candidates for HT and have undergone premature or early menopause can use HT at least until the median age of menopause (age 52). Longer duration of therapy may be considered based on need for ongoing symptom management.
- Despite the fact that the WHI did not reveal an increased risk for breast cancer with ET, safety data are lacking to support the use of ET in breast cancer survivors.
- Transdermal and low-dose oral ET have been associated with a lower risk for VTE and stroke when compared to standard doses of oral estrogen, but RCTs are still needed to corroborate this relationship.
- HT is not recommended for prevention of cognitive aging or dementia.
- All women with an intact uterus receiving systemic estrogen should either receive systemic progestogen or have a LNG-IUS placed to decrease the risk of endometrial carcinoma.

Abbreviations: CHD, coronary heart disease; CVD, cardiovascular disease; ET, estrogen therapy; EPT, estrogen with progestogen therapy; HT, hormone therapy; LNG-IUS, levonorgestrel-releasing intrauterine system; RCT, randomized controlled trial; VTE, venous thromboembolism; WHI, Women's Health Initiative.
Data from North American Menopause Society (NAMS). (2012). The 2012 hormone therapy position statement of the North American Menopause Society. *Menopause, 19*(3), 257–271.

feedback effect from elevated estrogen and progesterone levels on hypothalamic production of gonadotropin-releasing hormone (GnRH) is lost, and the anterior pituitary production of FSH and luteinizing hormone (LH) continues. Irregular menstrual cycles—characterized by longer or shorter cycles, heavier or lighter flow, periods of amenorrhea, and worsening or newly developing premenstrual symptoms—are common during this time. Eventually, ovarian follicle production stops, estrogen and progesterone levels remain low, FSH and LH levels remain high, and menstruation ceases. The early postmenopausal period refers to the first 5 years following menopause when hormonal fluctuations often continue to occur. The late postmenopausal

period refers to 6 years after the final menstrual period through the remaining life span. This phase is marked by increasing genitourinary symptoms due to the reduced estrogen levels (Fritz & Speroff, 2011; Harlow et al., 2012; NAMS, 2014).

A woman is born with approximately 1.2 million ovarian follicles. Throughout her life, fewer than 500 of these follicles are used during ovulation; most are lost through atresia until menopause, when approximately 1,000 follicles remain. The decline in follicles occurs at a constantly increasing rate, with a more rapid decline noted with increasing age (NAMS, 2014).

Although it sounds like a smoothly functioning process, the perimenopausal transition is anything

---

BOX 12-2   Symptoms Associated with Perimenopause and Menopause

- Acne
- Arthralgia
- Asthenia
- Decreased libido
- Decreased vaginal lubrication
- Depression
- Dizziness
- Dry eyes
- Dry/thinning hair
- Dyspareunia
- Dysuria
- Fatigue
- Forgetfulness
- Formication
- Headache
- Hirsutism/virilization
- Hot flashes/flushes
- Irregular menses/bleeding
- Irritability/mood disturbances
- Mastalgia

- Myalgia
- Nervousness/anxiety
- Night sweats
- Nocturia
- Odor
- Palpitations
- Paresthesia
- Poor concentration
- Recurrent cystitis
- Recurrent vaginitis
- Skin dryness/atrophy
- Sleep disturbances/insomnia
- Stress urinary incontinence[a]
- Urinary frequency
- Urinary urgency
- Vaginal atrophy
- Vaginal/vulvar burning
- Vaginal/vulvar irritation
- Vaginal/vulvar pruritus

[a]Data are inconclusive.
Data from Alexander, I. M., Ruff, C., Rousseau, M. E., White, K., Motter, S., McKie, C., & Clark, P. (2003). Menopause symptoms and management strategies identified by black women [Abstract]. *Menopause, 10*(6), 601; Avis, N. E., Stellato, R., Crawford, S., Bromberger, J., Ganz, P., Cain, V., & Kagawa-Singer, M. (2001). Is there a menopausal syndrome? Menopausal status and symptoms across racial/ethnic groups. *Social Science and Medicine, 52*(3), 345–356; Greendale, G. A., Lee, N. P., & Arriola, E. R. (1999). The menopause. *Lancet, 353*(9152), 571–580; Jacobs Institute on Women's Health. (2003). Expert panel on menopause counseling. Retrieved from http://www.jiwh.org/menodownload.htm; McKinlay, S. M. (1996). The normal menopause transition: An overview. *Maturitas, 23*(2), 137–145.

---

but smooth for many women. Hormone levels can fluctuate wildly from day to day, causing many of the symptoms associated with the perimenopause and menopause transition (**Box 12-2**). Hormone fluctuation is related to many factors, including the reduced number of responsive ovarian follicles. Due to these fluctuations, measuring hormones during this time can be difficult to interpret and in most cases is not recommended (Shifren & Gass, 2014).

Contrary to popular belief, women continue to produce estrogen and androgens after menopause. Three types of estrogen exist:

- Estradiol (E_2), which is the most potent of the three, is the main estrogen produced during the reproductive years; it is present in low amounts in the postmenopausal years following peripheral conversion of androstenedione.
- Estriol (E_3) is secreted by the placenta and synthesized from androgens produced by the fetus during pregnancy. It is present in nonpregnant women in small amounts as a by-product of estradiol and estrone.
- Estrone (E_1), the weakest estrogen, is the primary estrogen present in postmenopausal women, children, and men. In the

postmenopausal period, estrone is produced by adipose conversion of androstenedione secreted by the adrenals (95%) and, to a lesser extent, the ovaries (5%), as well as by metabolism of estradiol.

The ovaries of postmenopausal women no longer produce estrogen or functional follicles after menopause; however, the corticostromal and hilar cells of the stromal tissue are steroidogenic and produce significant levels of both androstenedione and testosterone for many years. Circulating levels of androstenedione in postmenopausal women are approximately half those of premenopausal women. Conversely, circulating levels of testosterone remain relatively constant in women who are either premenopausal or postmenopausal, partly due to the presence of high FSH and LH levels, which stimulate the ovarian stromal tissues to increase their testosterone production (Fritz & Speroff, 2011; NAMS, 2014).

The age at natural menopause ranges from 40 to 58 years, with the average age of occurrence around 52 years. In several cross-sectional studies, the median age of menopause was estimated to be between 50 and 52 (Fritz & Speroff, 2011; NAMS, 2014). The age at menopause is difficult to predict for an individual woman, but does correlate with the age when her mother or older sisters experienced menopause (Cramer, Xu, & Harlow, 1995; de Bruin et al., 2001). A number of factors that may affect the age at menopause have been studied, such as parity, age at menarche, obesity, height, and oral contraceptive use (Bromberger et al., 1997; Cooper, Sandler, & Bohlig, 1999; Dvornyk et al., 2006; Gold et al., 2001; Santoro et al., 2007; Santoro et al., 2004; van Noord, Dubas, Dorland, Boersma, & te Velde, 1997).

Emerging data suggest that genetic factors may influence the age of menopause. Genome-wide association studies have had some success in revealing genetic determinants for menopause, and diagnosis of the fragile X mental retardation 1 (*FMR1*) premutation has been linked to an earlier age of menopause (He & Murabito, 2014; NAMS, 2014).

Current smoking has consistently been found to correlate with age at menopause. Specifically, women who smoke are likely to experience menopause 1 year earlier than women who do not (Sun et al., 2012).

Menstrual cycle changes—including length of cycle, amount of bleeding, and 2- and 3- month periods of amenorrhea—are associated with a shorter time to menopause (Garcia et al., 2005; Harlow et al., 2006). Cycle lengths less than 21 days have been associated with the early stages of the menopause transition (Van Voorhis, Santoro, Harlow, Crawford, & Randolph, 2008). A combination of symptoms—including irregular cycles, changed hormone levels, age, and smoking—was identified to be predictive in the Study of Women's Health Across the Nation (SWAN) (Santoro et al., 2007).

Body size has been identified as a contributing factor to the age at which women experience menopause due to the fact that body fat stores androstenedione and converts it to estrogen. Evidence has shown that undernourished women and vegetarians may experience an earlier menopause, whereas women with higher body weights often have more adipose tissue and may potentially experience a later menopause (Fritz & Speroff, 2011).

Cultural Considerations: Ethnicity and Age at Menopause

Ethnicity also may have an effect on age at menopause. A few studies have found that black women experience menopause slightly earlier than other women, with an average age at menopause of approximately 50 years (Bromberger et al., 1997; Palmer, Rosenberg, Wise, Horton, & Adams-Campbell, 2003). However, no significant difference in age at menopause was identified in black versus white women (average age = 51.4 years for both groups) in the SWAN study (Gold et al., 2001). Interestingly, the SWAN study did identify statistically significant differences in average age at menopause among Hispanic women (51.0 years) and Japanese American women (51.8 years), as compared with Caucasian women (51.4 years).

MENOPAUSE FROM OTHER CAUSES

Menopause can also occur due to several other causes (NAMS, 2014). Induced menopause occurs following either surgical excision of both ovaries (bilateral oophorectomy) or ovarian function ablation caused by medication, chemotherapy, or radiation. Although menstruation and fertility cease immediately following surgical menopause, both may persist for several months after ablative treatments are given.

Premature menopause is menopause that occurs before the age of 40; it is estimated to affect approximately 1% of women in the United States. It often follows the pattern of natural menopause and results in the permanent loss of menstruation and fertility.

Primary ovarian insufficiency (POI), previously referred to as premature ovarian failure (POF), also occurs in women younger than 40 years. Unlike premature menopause, POI is not always permanent. It is often associated with other health problems, such as autoimmune and genetic disorders.

Temporary menopause can occur at any age when normal ovarian function is lost and then resumes. This condition can be idiopathic, related to a disease entity, or induced by medications (NAMS, 2014).

Women who experience induced or premature menopause have early loss of fertility and often experience more severe symptoms. They are at greater risk for developing CVD, osteoporosis, and cognitive impairment with aging. They may also face significant health problems related to their underlying disease processes (NAMS, 2014).

DIAGNOSING MENOPAUSE

Menopause is actually a retrospective diagnosis because it is based on the clinical absence of menses for 12 consecutive months. Serial FSH testing that revealed sustained levels greater than 40 mIU/mL was used in the past to determine menopause status. However, serum FSH testing is no longer required or recommended for determining perimenopausal or menopausal status because FSH levels can return to normal and estrogen levels can unexpectedly rise high enough to trigger the LH surge needed for ovulation (NAMS, 2014).

The Stages of Reproductive Aging Workshop (STRAW) created a staging system in an attempt to standardize terminology when assessing reproductive aging in women. Researchers found that the proposed bleeding criteria established by the STRAW was a better indicator of the late menopausal transition than serum FSH levels. Based on

these criteria, women who are older than 45 years with periods of amenorrhea lasting for 60 days or more are considered to be in the late menopausal transition stage and are likely closer to menopause than women in the early menopause transition experiencing cycle irregularities of 7 days or greater (Harlow et al., 2012).

Anti-Müllerian hormone (AMH) has been identified as a marker of ovarian reserve, although serum blood tests for AMH have been used primarily among women seeking fertility assessment. Research has identified that AMH, which reflects the number of follicles, may be helpful in identifying when women can expect to be postmenopausal, with its level dropping to an undetectable point approximately 5 years before menopause. Limited data exist for the use of AMH testing among women outside of fertility assessment, and standardized assays using this test for prediction of menopause are lacking. For now, it is recommended that practitioners limit the use of this test to women seeking fertility assessment (NAMS, 2014; Shifren & Gass, 2014).

Perimenopause refers to the time when women begin to experience cycle irregularities as well as other menopause-related symptoms, such as hot flashes and vaginal dryness, and ends when the diagnosis of menopause is made after 12 months of amenorrhea. This period is often when women experience the most symptoms related to the menopause transition. Due to the potential for unexpected ovulation, women who are perimenopausal need to continue to use a reliable method of contraception. (See Chapter 11 for information about contraception.) Perimenopausal women experience a high rate of unintended pregnancies; an estimated 75% of pregnancies in women older than age 40 are unintended (Long, Faubion, MacLaughlin, Pruthi, & Casey, 2015).

Differential Diagnoses

Other health problems can mimic the symptoms of menopause and must also be considered when a woman presents with perimenopause- and menopause-related symptoms (NAMS, 2014). These diagnoses may include diabetes, hypertension, arrhythmias, thyroid disorders (hypothyroid or hyperthyroid), anemia, depression, tumors, or carcinoma.

| TABLE 12-2 | Examples of Differential Diagnoses That Have Symptoms Similar to Perimenopause and Menopause |

Diagnosis	Symptoms Similar to Perimenopause/ Menopause
Anemia	Fatigue Cognitive changes
Anovulation	Amenorrhea
Arrhythmias	Fatigue Palpitations
Arthritis	Joint aches/pain
Depression	Fatigue Moodiness Anxiety Sleep disturbances, insomnia
Diabetes	Fatigue Hot flashes/heat intolerance
Hyperprolactinemia	Menstrual cycle changes
Hypertension	Headaches
Hyperthyroidism	Sleep disturbance, insomnia Nervousness, irritability Heat intolerance
Hypothyroidism	Fatigue Dry skin Cognitive problems
Infections (viral illnesses, HIV, influenza, fever, tuberculosis, sexually transmitted infections)	Vasomotor symptoms Dyspareunia Cystitis symptoms Vaginitis
Pregnancy Spontaneous abortion Uterine fibroids Uterine polyps Endometriosis Adenomyosis Ovarian cysts Ovarian tumors	Menstrual changes Menorrhagia
Vulvar dystrophy	Vaginal atrophy Dyspareunia

A sample list of differential diagnoses is provided in **Table 12-2**. Medications, alcohol, or drug use can also cause many symptoms similar to those associated with perimenopause and menopause.

Each woman presenting with suspected menopause-related symptoms must be carefully evaluated with a thorough history, physical examination, and selective laboratory testing (such as a complete blood count, fasting glucose, serum thyroid-stimulating hormone [TSH] level, and prolactin level) to accurately identify the cause of her symptoms. Often a woman has several diagnoses to contend with at once, such as hypertension, diabetes, and menopause. Controlling her diabetes and hypertension may also reduce her menopause-related symptoms enough so that they no longer are bothersome for her.

PRESENTATION AND VARIATION OF THE MENOPAUSE EXPERIENCE

The experience of menopause is unique and personal. Some women have severe symptoms that disrupt all aspects of their lives, whereas others find menopause to be almost a "non-event" and report no bothersome symptoms. Most symptoms that do occur are related to reduced levels of estrogen and progesterone. Two types of estrogen receptors have been identified (alpha and beta), which are located in the cognitive and vasomotor centers of the brain, eyes, skin, heart, vascular system, gastrointestinal tract, breast tissue, urogenital tract, and bone. Progesterone receptors have been identified in the hypothalamus, pituitary, and vasomotor areas of the brain, as well as in the heart, vascular tissues, lung, breast, pancreas, gynecologic organs, and bones. As hormone levels rise and fall, related symptoms may develop. An individual woman's symptom experience may correlate with her body size, as adipose tissues store and convert androstenedione to estrogen (Fritz & Speroff, 2011). Additionally, women who are overweight or obese are more likely to experience hot flashes than women of normal weight (NAMS, 2014).

Both the type (**Box 12-2**) and severity of menopause-related symptoms can vary. Symptoms usually begin in the perimenopausal period and then gradually increase in severity during the early postmenopausal period, reaching a peak in the first 2 years after the final menstrual period. The symptoms women report most frequently are vasomotor in nature, including hot flashes, hot flushes, and sweats. Most symptomatic women will experience symptoms on average for as long as 5 years after menopause, and approximately one-third of women will experience these symptoms for 10 years or more (Freeman, Sammel, & Sanders, 2014).

Hot flashes are experienced as an intense heat sensation and may or may not be followed by sweating, which can be profuse. They are characterized by a measurable increase in skin temperature and conductance, which is followed by a decrease in core body temperature. Hot flushes are similar to hot flashes but include a flushing over the face and upper chest, most likely due to peripheral vascular dilation. Vasomotor symptoms that occur during the night are termed night sweats. Hot flashes occur concurrently with a surge in LH levels. Although the relationship between LH secretion and body temperature change is not well understood, the same mechanisms that trigger the hypothalamic event that causes the temperature increase also stimulate GnRH secretion and cause LH elevation (Fritz & Speroff, 2011). Many women feel cold following a hot flash owing to the reduction in core temperature; this effect is exacerbated if sweating is also present. Postmenopausal women are more sensitive to core temperature changes because their thermoneutral zone—the range of internally recognized normal core body temperature—narrows (Freedman & Blacker, 2002). Thus, when core temperature rises, they feel overly hot; conversely, when it falls, they feel overly chilled.

Sleep disruptions are also common among women both during the menopause transition and after it ends. Some of these sleep changes are related to normal aging, such as reduced time in sleep stages 3 (early deep sleep) and 4 (deep sleep and relaxation), more periods of brief arousal, and an overall decreased need for sleep, ranging from 6 to 9 hours among women (National Sleep Foundation, 2015). Hot flashes and sweats can further interrupt sleep (NAMS, 2014). Poor sleep is associated with somatic, mood, and cognitive symptoms as well as performance deficits. Women experiencing poor sleep may demonstrate an inability to concentrate, lethargy, fatigue, difficulty performing tasks, and a lack of motivation. Additionally, poor sleep has been linked to some chronic illnesses, such as cardiac disease and depression (NAMS, 2014).

Urogenital changes leading to atrophy affect all women, may cause vaginal dryness and dyspareunia, and can predispose women to urinary tract infections. The risk of urinary incontinence increases with age, but this condition is never considered normal. (See Chapter 22 for additional information on urinary incontinence.) Low estrogen has been suggested as a factor contributing to the increased prevalence of urinary incontinence among women of menopausal age; however, decreases in serum estradiol levels have not been shown to cause or worsen symptoms of urinary incontinence among women who are transitioning through menopause (Waetjen et al., 2011).

Many normal changes of aging can also affect sexual function in women, such as longer time to achieve vaginal lubrication and production of fewer vaginal secretions overall; reduced vaginal elasticity, pigment, rugation, and number of superficial epithelial cells, leading to increased petechiae and bleeding following minor trauma (including sexual activity); reduced lactobacilli populations, which increase pH and the risk of infection; and atrophy of adipose and collagen tissue in the vulva. Women may also experience lowered libido, lessened sexual activity, problems with their partner's sexual performance, or relationship problems that make them less interested in sex (Dennerstein, Dudley, & Burger, 2001; NAMS, 2014). Whatever the causes of dyspareunia or sexual dysfunction may be, this subject is often difficult for women to broach with their clinicians. Thus it is important for clinicians to ask women about sexual function and satisfaction, and remain open to the fact that sexual expression can take many forms. See Chapters 9, 10, and 16 for more information.

A woman's expectations for menopause may also affect her experience. These can range from no expectations, to positive or negative expectations, to uncertainty (Woods & Mitchell, 2008). Women with higher levels of perceived stress and negative attitudes toward menopause and aging are more likely to experience more severe symptoms (Nosek et al., 2010). Similarly, a woman's response to menopause can affect her experience. Many women view menopause as a natural life transition and may not be interested in any treatment options besides lifestyle changes. Others see it as a disruption of their lives and a sign of aging that they want to minimize as much as possible. Many women identify menopause as a time for reflection and reevaluation of their lives and health (Alexander et al., 2003; Woods & Mitchell, 2008).

Cultural Considerations: Ethnicity and Menopause-Related Symptoms

Cultural or racial background may have an effect on menopause-related symptoms. The SWAN study indicated that while Caucasian and Hispanic women reported the greatest number of psychosomatic symptoms, such as moodiness, headaches, and palpitations (Avis et al., 2001), the severity of vasomotor symptoms (hot flashes, sweats) was highest among African American women, followed by Hispanic, Caucasian, Chinese, and Japanese women (Gold et al., 2000). Vaginal dryness was more common among African American and Hispanic women, and Hispanic women were more likely to report urine leakage, forgetfulness, and heart pounding or racing than Caucasian women. However, Caucasian women were more likely to experience difficulty sleeping than women of other races (Gold et al., 2000). In the WHI, Hispanic women were more likely to have experienced urogenital symptoms such as dryness, irritation, discharge, and itching (Pastore, Carter, Hulka, & Wells, 2004).

Additionally, some symptoms may be more bothersome for certain women. For example, African American women have described a high degree of discomfort attributable to vaginal and body odor, sleep changes and night sweats, weight gain, moodiness, "rage," and irritability (Alexander et al., 2003). Asian women have reported more severe problems with joint pain and stiffness, especially in the neck, shoulders, and back (Gold et al., 2000).

MIDLIFE HEALTH ISSUES

Health risks change for women at midlife, partly due to the changed hormonal milieu and partly due to other normal aging processes. In particular, women at this point in life are at greater risk for developing heart disease, osteoporosis, and diabetes. Weight management is also a significant issue. See Chapter 7 for a full discussion of routine health screening for midlife women.

Overweight and Obesity

As women age, weight management often becomes a struggle. Although women tend to associate increased weight with menopause, it is not related specifically to hormonal changes but rather can be a natural part of aging. Women gain an average of 5 pounds at midlife (NAMS, 2014). This increase is partly due to the decrease in muscle mass that occurs with age and slows down the rate at which calories are burned, and partly due to a decrease in activity that often accompanies midlife. Maintaining one's weight through midlife usually requires both a reduction in caloric intake and an increase in activity.

Not only does weight often increase at midlife, but the distribution of body fat also changes. Adipose tissue tends to accumulate at the hips and thighs in younger women (the "pear"-shaped body). As women age, however, adipose tissue is redistributed and begins to accumulate at the waist (the "apple"-shaped body). Abdominal adiposity and weight gain at midlife are significant issues. This concern relates not only to the potentially negative body-image concerns for women, but also to the link between maintaining an ideal body weight and a decreased risk for CVD and diabetes. The American Heart Association (AHA, 2011) recommends dietary and lifestyle modifications to maintain or achieve an optimal body mass index (BMI) of 18.5 to 24.9 kg/m^2 as well as a waist circumference less than 35 inches. In addition, obesity is associated with osteoarthritis, cholecystic disease, and urinary incontinence, as well as with cancers such as breast, endometrial, and colorectal (Centers for Disease Control and Prevention, 2012; Obesity Society, 2015). Furthermore, having a BMI greater than 27 kg/m^2 as well as gaining body fat during midlife is associated with a greater frequency of hot flashes, night sweats, and soreness or stiffness in the back, shoulders, and neck (NAMS, 2014; Thurston et al., 2009).

Cardiovascular Disease

The number one cause of mortality for both women and men in the United States is CVD. CVD is an inclusive term that refers to conditions such as hypertension, valvular heart disease, CHD (leading to angina or myocardial infarction), stroke, arrhythmias, congestive heart failure, peripheral arterial disease, aortic disease, arterial and venous thrombosis, pulmonary embolism, and congenital heart defects. In 2010, CVD was the cause of death for approximately 400,000 women in the United States (AHA, 2014). Due to advancements in prevention, diagnosis, and treatment among women in the United States, rates of CVD have declined in recent years; nevertheless, more than one-third of women have some type of CVD, and more women than men will die of CVD. Notably, heart disease disproportionately affects black women, with death rates from CVD being higher among black women when compared to white women (NAMS, 2014).

Women are at a significantly increased risk for developing heart disease following menopause; however, menopause does not appear to independently increase risk for CVD (AHA, 2014; NAMS, 2014). The increased risk is likely a result of changes in cholesterol levels that are found in postmenopausal women: LDL and very-low-density lipoprotein levels (which increase the risk of heart disease) increase, and LDL oxidation is enhanced. Additionally, HDL levels (which are protective against heart disease) may decrease somewhat. However, the HDL changes are far less significant than the LDL changes. Other changes, such as the reduced elasticity in the vascular system and associated hypertension, may be related to decreased levels of estrogen and progesterone. Moreover, production of some procoagulation factors (e.g., fibrinogen, factor VII) and some fibrinolytic factors (e.g., plasminogen, antithrombin III) increase, and they may interact with hormonal and vascular changes to further increase risk.

Major risk factors for CVD include age, cigarette smoking, a sedentary lifestyle, a family history of premature CVD, preexisting hypertension, abnormal serum lipids, and diabetes mellitus. Women who experience premature menopause may have an even greater risk, especially if they smoke, and women with a history of a pregnancy complicated by preeclampsia, hypertension, or gestational diabetes appear to have an increased risk as well (NAMS, 2014; Shifren & Gass, 2014).

Diabetes Mellitus

The likelihood of developing type 2 diabetes mellitus increases with age. This disease disproportionately affects women of minority racial and ethnic groups, such as Native American, Hispanic or Latina, African American, Asian American, and Pacific Islander women. General risk factors for developing diabetes include overweight and obesity (BMI ≥ 25), abdominal adiposity (waist circumference > 35 inches in women), a sedentary lifestyle, insulin resistance, a history of gestational diabetes or polycystic ovary syndrome, and a family history of diabetes. Hypertension and dyslipidemia also predispose an individual to developing diabetes.

Individuals with impaired fasting glucose levels (100–125 mg/dL) or impaired glucose tolerance (2-hour post 75-gm glucose load of 140–199 mg/dL) are identified as having prediabetes. Encouraging lifestyle modifications, such as increasing activity levels, dietary changes and weight loss, is important in this population because such changes have been shown to delay or even prevent the onset of diabetes (ADA, 2010, 2014; Schellenberg, Dryden, Vandemeer, Ha, & Korownyk, 2013). The American Association of Clinical Endocrinologists (2013) recommends weight loss as the primary goal in men and women with prediabetes through therapeutic lifestyle changes, medications, surgery, or a combination of these methods. Insulin resistance is reduced with weight loss and can prevent progression to diabetes as well as improvement in lipids and blood pressure. In addition to significantly increasing the risk for CVD and cerebrovascular disease, diabetes increases the risk for developing infections, foot ulcers, peripheral vascular disease, peripheral neuropathy, nephropathy, and retinopathy (ADA, 2014).

Managing diabetes can be more difficult for women after menopause. This was previously thought to be a result of hormonal changes and their effects on insulin resistance; however, data from the SWAN study suggest that it is more likely the result of weight gain and changes in women's body composition after menopause that further affect insulin resistance. The hormonal changes that occur with menopause appear to have less of an effect on glucose metabolism than was previously thought; aging, weight gain, and changes in body composition are more likely responsible for the increased glucose levels (NAMS, 2014; Wildman et al., 2012). Maintaining optimal glucose control is recommended to reduce the risk of vascular complications associated with diabetes through lifestyle modifications as well as initiating metformin as a first-line therapeutic option. Initiation of statin

therapy in women older than age 40 with diabetes, smoking cessation, and controlling blood pressure are recommended to further reduce the risk of CVD and complications from diabetes (Shifren & Gass, 2014).

Cancer

In 2014, the leading cause of mortality from cancer among women in the United States was estimated to be lung and bronchus cancer (26%), followed by breast (15%) and colon and rectum (9%) cancers (American Cancer Society [ACS], 2014a). These same three types of cancer were expected to be the most frequently diagnosed cancers among women in 2014, with breast cancer being the most commonly diagnosed cancer in the United States. Mortality from cancer has decreased overall among women, with the exception of lung cancer, for which mortality is leveling off.

The risk of developing cancer increases as women age, with approximately 77% of cancers being diagnosed in people 55 years and older. Approximately 12% of women will be diagnosed with breast cancer at some point during their lifetime, and this risk increases as women age. By age 40, the probability of a women developing breast cancer is approximately 1 in 200; by age 60, it increases to 1 in 27 (ACS, 2014a; National Cancer Institute, 2014). Chapter 7 presents cancer screening recommendations, and Chapter 15 provides further information on breast cancer.

Osteoporosis

Osteoporosis is the most common bone disease in humans and is characterized by low bone mass, deterioration of bone tissue, and disruption of bone architecture resulting in reduced bone strength that increases the risk for fracture (National Osteoporosis Foundation [NOF], 2014). Osteoporosis is the most common cause of morbidity among menopausal women, and osteoporotic fractures account for a large portion of morbidity and mortality among postmenopausal women, especially women older than 65 years (NAMS, 2010). **Table 12-3** lists risk factors for osteoporosis.

Osteoporosis is categorized as primary, secondary, or idiopathic. Primary osteoporosis is associated with aging and affects women much more

TABLE **12-3**	Risk Factors for Osteoporosis

Potentially Modifiable Risk Factors	Nonmodifiable Risk Factors
Excessive thinness (BMI < 21 kg/m^2)	Advanced age
Hypogonadal states (e.g., anorexia, athletic amenorrhea, premature menopause, androgen insensitivity, hyperprolactinemia, Turner's and Klinefelter's syndromes)	Female gender
	Race (Caucasian and Asian women at greatest risk, followed by Hispanic and African American women)
Nulliparity	Personal history of fracture during adulthood
Lifestyle factors (e.g., cigarette smoking, excessive alcohol or caffeine intake, sedentary activity level, frequent falling, inadequate calcium or vitamin D intake)	Family history of osteoporosis
	First-degree relative with a history of fracture
Medications (e.g., thyroid hormone, corticosteroids, anticonvulsants, aluminum-containing antacids, lithium, methotrexate, gonadotropin-releasing hormone, cholestyramine, heparin, warfarin, depot medroxyprogesterone acetate [Depo-Provera], premenopausal tamoxifen, selective serotonin reuptake inhibitors, proton-pump inhibitors)	Genetic diseases (e.g., cystic fibrosis, Ehlers-Danlos, osteogenesis imperfecta, porphyria, Gaucher's disease, hemochromatosis, Marfan syndrome, homocystinuria)
	Hematologic disorders (e.g., hemophilia, sickle cell, multiple myeloma, thalassemia, leukemia and lymphomas)
Chronic diseases (e.g., endocrine disorders, gastrointestinal disorders, bone disorders, chronic liver disease, seizure disorders, prolonged immobility, eating disorders, chronic renal failure, frailty)	Rheumatologic and autoimmune disease (e.g., systemic lupus erythematosus, rheumatoid arthritis, ankylosing spondylitis)

Data from National Osteoporosis Foundation (NOF). (2014). *Clinician's guide to prevention and treatment of osteoporosis*. Washington, DC: Author.

significantly than men. Adults achieve peak bone mass in their late 20s to mid-30s, after which time the rates of bone resorption and formation become relatively stable. As women age beyond this point, their bone resorption rate slowly begins to exceed that of bone formation, resulting in a slow decline of bone mass. Because of the loss of estrogen, the rate of bone loss in the first year after menopause is especially rapid, between 1% and 5%, but then slows to approximately 1% per year. In contrast, bone mass is lost in men at a rate of 0.2% to 0.5% per year.

Secondary osteoporosis occurs in response to medication (e.g., corticosteroids, anticonvulsants, or methotrexate) or other disease processes (e.g.,

hyperthyroidism, chronic liver disease, or gastrointestinal diseases, such as malabsorption) that interfere with the normal process of bone formation and can affect women or men at any age. Idiopathic osteoporosis is characterized by low bone density and fracture in young adults when no other cause is identified (NAMS, 2014). Screening recommendations can be found in Chapter 7.

Bone mineral density (BMD) testing by dual-energy x-ray absorptiometry (DXA) is a technique that is used to evaluate central BMD at the spine and hip and is a vital component of the diagnosis and management of osteoporosis. Although DXA can also be used to evaluate the wrist BMD, central testing is much more predictive of overall BMD and fracture risk. Quantitative computed tomography (CT) scan can be used to perform spine measurements and is particularly useful for testing individuals with arthritis, as it is less likely to reflect osteocytes.

BMD results are reported as *T*-scores and *Z*-scores. The *T*-score identifies the number of standard deviations that the patient's BMD is greater or less than that for a young-adult, gender-matched norm. The *Z*-score is compared to the BMD of an age-, sex-, and ethnicity-matched reference population. Low bone mass (osteopenia) is present when the *T*-score is in the range of –1.0 to –2.5. Osteoporosis is present when the *T*-score is –2.5 or less. Severe or established osteoporosis is present when the *T*-score is –2.5 or less and low trauma fractures are present. *T*-scores are used in men older than age 50 and in postmenopausal women, as they are the standard used to determine the risk for fractures. The International Society for Clinical Densitometry recommends the use of *Z*-scores instead of *T*-scores for premenopausal women, children, and men younger than 50 years, with *Z*-scores of –2.0 or less defined as "below the expected range for age" and those greater than –2.0 identified as "within the expected range for age." *Z*-scores are helpful for identifying those individuals who should undergo an evaluation for secondary causes of osteoporosis (NOF, 2014).

Women with osteoporosis are at increased risk for fracture. Although osteoporosis and low bone mass by themselves are painless and not functionally problematic, the risk for fractures puts a patient at significant risk. Following a hip fracture, there is an 8.4% to 36% increase in mortality and 2.5-fold increased risk for a future fracture. Among survivors of such fractures, approximately 20% require long-term nursing home care and only 40% will fully regain their pre-fracture level of independence (NOF, 2014).

Patient Education for Preventing Bone Loss

Prevention is a key component of osteoporosis management. For perimenopausal and postmenopausal women, education should focus on prevention strategies (**Box 12-3**). Exercise is site specific and needs to be continued to maintain bone strength.

Management of Bone Loss

Medication management is recommended for women with *T*-scores of –2.5 or less, and for those with hip or vertebral fractures (NOF, 2014). For women with *T*-scores in the low bone mass range (–1.0 to –2.5), medication is recommended if they also have fractures or are at high risk for fracture (e.g., immobilized, taking glucocorticoids, at high risk for falls).

For women with *T*-scores in the low bone mass range, use of the World Health Organization's (WHO's) Fracture Risk Assessment Tool (FRAX) is recommended to identify those who would realize a cost-effective benefit from initiating medication therapy (Dawson-Hughes et al., 2008; Tosteson et al., 2008; WHO, 2007). The FRAX tool is accessible online (http://www.shef.ac.uk/FRAX) and is applicable to women who have not previously been treated with medications. Information is entered for 11 different risk factors plus the hip raw BMD value (in g/cm^2) to calculate the 10-year probability for a hip fracture and the 10-year probability for any type of major osteoporotic fracture. If the hip fracture probability is equal to or greater than 3%, or if the risk for any major osteoporotic fracture is equal to or greater than 20%, medication therapy is recommended (NOF, 2014).

BOX 12-3 Strategies to Prevent Osteoporosis

- Adequate intake of calcium (1,200 mg/day in postmenopausal women)
- Adequate intake of vitamin D (800–1,000 international units/day for adults 50 and older)
- Weight-bearing and resistance exercise
- Fall prevention
- Avoiding tobacco
- Moderating alcohol intake (fewer than 2 drinks per day for women)

Data from National Osteoporosis Foundation (NOF). (2014). *Clinician's guide to prevention and treatment of osteoporosis.* Washington, DC: Author.

The treatment decision must be weighed against the clinical presentation, with the clinician recognizing the limitations of FRAX. The estimated fracture risk identified by FRAX provides an alert to the clinician that treatment may be useful. The intervention threshold—that is, the point at which treatment should be started for a specific individual—is determined mutually between the clinician and the patient. This threshold is different for different patients and based on multiple factors, including the risks identified previously as well as the FRAX score (Lane & Silverman, 2008). Many of the variables considered in the FRAX instrument are dichotomous (e.g., yes/no) and do not capture the increased risk present with a higher level on a continuous variable scale (e.g., use of higher doses of corticosteroid increases risk for fracture). Additionally, the T-score used in the FRAX calculations is not the same as that obtained with DXA testing; however, a conversion program on the NOF's website can be downloaded to the clinician's computer for use. The converted T-score should then be entered into the FRAX program.

Repeat BMD testing for osteoporosis is recommended every 2 years after treatment is initiated to monitor the effects of therapy (NOF, 2014). **Table 12-4** summarizes the available pharmacologic treatment options for osteoporosis in postmenopausal women. Combination therapy, initiated by an osteoporosis specialist, is also possible; usually a bisphosphonate (alendronate or risedronate) is combined with a drug from another class (e.g., estrogen or raloxifene).

Thyroid Disease

Thyroid disease and depression are other health issues that must be considered at midlife. Thyroid disease affects women more than men, and its incidence increases with age. Thyroid disorders can present with many of the same symptoms that occur during the menopausal transition, such as menstrual cycle changes or irregularities, disruption in sleep, fatigue, mood swings, heat intolerance, and palpitations (NAMS, 2014). Although there is not a general consensus regarding who should be screened for thyroid disorders, the American Association of Clinical Endocrinologists recommends that screening should be considered in older patients, especially women,

and the American Thyroid Association recommends that both women and men older than age 35 be screened every 5 years. Measurement of TSH is the initial step in assessing thyroid function (Garber et al., 2012).

Depression

Despite the fact that most women progress through the menopausal transition without psychological symptoms, many women report symptoms of depression, anxiety, stress, or a decreased sense of well-being. Risk of depression increases during midlife due to symptoms caused by hormonal fluctuations and potential midlife stresses, such as financial concerns, employment issues, relationship problems, family changes, or health issues of self or family members. There appears to be a greater prevalence of depression among perimenopausal women when compared to premenopausal women, and women with a history of clinical depression, postpartum depression, or premenstrual syndrome (PMS) are more likely to experience recurrent depression during perimenopause (NAMS, 2014). Psychological symptoms, thyroid disorders, and other differential diagnoses (**Table 12-2**) must be considered when a woman presents with symptoms that appear to be menopause related.

PATIENT EDUCATION FOR LIFESTYLE APPROACHES TO MANAGE MENOPAUSE-RELATED SYMPTOMS

Several lifestyle approaches have been demonstrated to reduce menopause-related symptoms, and many of these interventions also afford additional health benefits, such as reducing the risk for CVD or osteoporosis. Lifestyle management may encompass dietary changes, exercise, vitamins or supplements, vaginal lubricants and moisturizers, changes in clothing, smoking cessation, stress management techniques, sleep aids, and activities to enhance memory function. Educating women about these approaches to symptom management may reduce symptoms enough to obviate the need for pharmacotherapy or reduce symptoms so that lower doses of pharmacotherapeutics are effective.

TABLE 12-4	Pharmacologic Treatment Options for Postmenopausal Osteoporosis[a]	
Medication	**FDA-Approved Indication**	**Considerations**
Alendronate (Fosamax)	Prevention—5 mg orally daily or 35 mg orally weekly Treatment—10 mg orally daily or 70 mg orally weekly (70-mg dose also available with cholecalciferol/vitamin D_3 as Fosamax Plus D, 70-mg dose also available as an effervescent tablet as Binosto)	Use with caution if the patient has upper gastrointestinal disease, owing to its clinical association with dysphagia, esophagitis, and ulceration Take first thing in the morning on an empty stomach with an 8-oz glass of water; remain upright and take no other food or drink for at least 30 minutes Take 2 hours before antacids/calcium
Risedronate (Actonel)	Prevention—5 mg orally daily or 35 mg orally weekly or 150 mg orally monthly Treatment—5 mg orally daily, 35 mg orally weekly (35-mg dose is also available in a delayed-release formulation as Atelvia 150 mg orally once a month)	Same as alendronate
Ibandronate (Boniva)	Prevention or treatment—150 mg orally once a month Treatment—3 mg intravenously every 3 months	Same as alendronate for tablets but must remain upright and take no other food or drink for at least 60 minutes Intravenous injection is administered over a period of 15–30 seconds
Zoledronic acid (Reclast)	Prevention—5 mg intravenously once every 2 years Treatment—5 mg intravenously once a year	Intravenous infusion is administered over a period of no less than 15 minutes
Calcitonin (Miacalcin, Fortical)	Treatment—200 international units intranasal spray daily or 100 international units subcutaneous injection daily or every other day	Usually administered as nasal spray Has an analgesic effect on osteoporotic fractures

Medication	FDA-Approved Indication	Considerations
Estrogen (i.e., Premarin, Ogen, Alora, Climara, Estrace, Menostar, Vivelle, Vivelle-Dot, Estraderm, Premphase,[b] Prempro,[b] femhrt,[b] Activella,[b] Prefest,[b] Climara Pro[b])	Prevention—Doses and routes vary[c]	Also effective in alleviating most symptoms of menopause. Comes in pills or patch
Raloxifene (Evista)	Prevention or treatment—60 mg orally daily	May cause hot flashes. Not recommended if the patient is taking ET or EPT
Teriparatide (Forteo)	Treatment—20 mcg subcutaneously daily	Reserved for use after failure of first-line agents
Denosumab (Prolia)	Treatment—60 mg subcutaneously every 6 months	Reserved for use after failure of first-line agents

Abbreviations: EPT, estrogen with progestogen therapy; ET, estrogen therapy.
[a] See prescribing reference for full information on doses, side effects, contraindications, and cautions.
[b] Also contains progestogen, which should be used in women with an intact uterus.
[c] Lowest effective dose should be used. The FDA recommends considering nonestrogen osteoporotic agents when ET/EPT use is solely for the purpose of osteoporosis prevention.
Data from ePocrates. (Updated daily). Computerized pharmacology and prescribing reference [Mobile application software]. Retrieved from http://www.epocrates.com; National Osteoporosis Foundation (NOF). (2014). *Clinician's guide to prevention and treatment of osteoporosis.* Washington, DC: Author; North American Menopause Society (NAMS). (2014). *Menopause practice: A clinician's guide* (5th ed.). Mayfield Heights, OH: Author.

Dietary Changes

Many women report perceived hot flash triggers that include hot drinks, spicy foods, caffeine, and alcohol; however, little evidence has been found among large groups of women to support a causative relationship. Avoidance or moderate intake of these substances should be recommended in an attempt to provide some relief from symptoms if women are seeking nonpharmacologic strategies to manage symptoms (NAMS, 2014). Increased water intake is also recommended because of the augmented insensible loss of fluids through sweating. Despite limited data supporting the contention that consuming cool drinks improves menopause-related symptoms, water intake (especially intake of cold water) appears to reduce symptoms such as skin dryness, and may reduce the discomfort associated with hot flashes and sweating (American College of Obstetricians and Gynecologists, 2014).

The usual water intake of 6 to 8 glasses per day should be recommended. However, for women who experience urinary incontinence, water consumption may need to be restricted for social occasions when there is no easy access to a bathroom, or limited to the morning for women who experience nocturia.

Exercise

Lower levels of physical activity have been linked with a higher frequency of menopause-related symptoms (NAMS, 2014). Nevertheless, a recent Cochrane Review of five RCTs found insufficient evidence to state definitively that exercise is an effective treatment for menopause-related vasomotor symptoms (Daley, Stokes-Lampard, Thomas, & MacArthur, 2014). Regular exercise reduces cardiovascular and osteoporosis risks; improves sleep; and assists with maintaining a healthy weight, relieving stress, reducing moodiness, and improving mental function. As a result, the overall benefits of exercise are important even if exercise does not mediate menopause-related vasomotor symptoms for all women (de Villiers, Pines et al., 2013). Women should be encouraged to engage in 30 minutes of moderate exercise on a daily basis; if they are attempting to lose weight, at least 60 minutes of physical activity is recommended (NAMS, 2014).

Vitamins and Supplements

Selected vitamins and supplements may be useful in improving overall health; however, there are limited data on the effectiveness of vitamins and supplements for treating menopause-related vasomotor symptoms (American College of Obstetricians and Gynecologists, 2014). Vitamin E in doses up to 800 international units (IU)/day has been shown to produce either small improvements or no changes in hot flashes in clinical trials (Barton et al., 1998; Blatt, Weisbader, & Kupperman, 1953). A meta-analysis indicated that vitamin E did not provide a reduction in overall mortality, cerebrovascular accident, or cardiovascular death (Vivekananthan, Penn, Sapp, Hsu, & Topol, 2003). As a result, the USPSTF (2014) recommends against the use of vitamin E for prevention of cardiovascular disease or cancer.

In 2011, the Institute of Medicine (IOM) recommended daily intake amounts of calcium (1,200 mg/day) and vitamin D (600 international units (IU)/day) to maintain bone health and prevent fracture in women older than 50 years. In women older than 70 years, 800 IU/day of vitamin D is recommended (Ross et al., 2011). The International Menopause Society recommends 800 to 1,000 IU/day of vitamin D in postmenopausal women, and other professional organizations recommend varying levels of vitamin D intake ranging from 800 to 2,000 IU/day (de Villiers, Pines et al., 2013; NAMS, 2014).

Limited evidence is available to support the use of vitamins and supplements for the prevention of chronic diseases and all-cause mortality. In fact, a potential for harm arises with excessive intake of some nutrients. Limiting dietary supplements and encouraging midlife women to maintain a healthy diet that includes fruits, vegetables, low-fat dairy products, whole grains, chicken, fish, and nuts is recommended, as a healthy diet

appears to have greater health benefits and is associated with reduced rates of diabetes, hypertension, CVD, and colorectal adenoma or cancer (NAMS, 2014).

Vaginal Lubricants and Moisturizers

After menopause, between 25% and 50% of women will experience symptoms of vulvovaginal atrophy (VVA) as a result of decreasing levels of estrogen (de Villiers, Pines et al., 2013). The International Society for the Study of Women's Health and NAMS now recommend the terminology *genitourinary syndrome of menopause (GSM)*, rather than VVA or atrophic vaginitis, to encompass the physiologic genitourinary tract changes and the variety of vulvovaginal (e.g., dryness, burning, irritation), sexual (e.g., inadequate lubrication, pain), and urinary (e.g., urgency, dysuria, urinary tract infections) symptoms associated with decreased estrogen levels (Portman & Gass, 2014). Women with mild symptoms of GSM often respond well to use of vaginal lubricants and moisturizers, and these should be offered as an initial treatment option (NAMS, 2014). Vaginal lubricants can be used to relieve the friction and dyspareunia that results from vaginal dryness during intercourse. Several nonhormonal water-, silicone-, and oil-based lubricants as well as vaginal moisturizers are available as over-the-counter products (**Table 12-5**). Longer-acting vaginal moisturizers may be more appropriate for some women. These products are applied several times weekly, not just at the time of sexual activity. The moisturizers replenish and maintain moisture in the vaginal epithelial cells and provide longer relief. Moisturizers may be particularly beneficial for women who experience daily discomfort, and they can reduce symptoms of vaginitis by supporting a normal pH (American College of Obstetricians and Gynecologists, 2014; NAMS, 2013, 2014).

Women must be cautioned against using petroleum jelly-based products (Vaseline), as these preparations can injure vaginal tissue, are not easily removed, and may increase the incidence of bacterial vaginosis (NAMS, 2013). Use of other products that contain fragrances should also be discouraged, as they often cause vaginitis or irritation. Douching is not effective for moisturizing and will remove normal flora, thereby increasing the risk for infection (NAMS, 2014). Because few tolerability studies

TABLE **12-5**	Nonhormonal Vaginal Lubricants and Moisturizers[a]

Lubricants	Moisturizers
Water Based	Feminease
Astroglide Liquid	K-Y SILK-E
Astroglide Gel Liquid	Luvena
Astroglide	Me Again
Good Clean Love[b,c]	Replens, Rephresh
Just Like Me	Silken Secret
K-Y Jelly	Vagisil
Liquid Silk	
Pre-Seed[b]	
Slippery Stuff[c]	
Sliquid H20[c]	
YES Personal Lubricant	
Silicone Based	
Astroglide X	
ID Millennium	
K-Y Intrigue	
Pink	
Pjur Eros (Bodyglide)[c]	
Oil Based	
Elegance Women's Lubricants	
Coconut oil	
Olive oil	
Vitamin E oil	

[a] Lubricants are applied prior to or during sex. Moisturizers are applied on a regular basis (e.g., daily or two to three times per week).
[b] Osmolality < 380 mOsm/kg, which is the maximum level recommended by the World Health Organization to minimize the risk of epithelial damage. Osmolality is only applicable to water-based lubricants; silicone- and oil-based lubricants do not have an osmolality value because they do not contain water.
[c] Propylene glycol-free. Propylene glycol can cause vaginal irritation for some women.
Data from Edwards, D., & Panay, N. (2015). Treating vulvovaginal atrophy/genitourinary syndrome of menopause: How important is vaginal lubricant and moisturizer composition? Climacteric, 19(2), 151–161; North American Menopause Society (NAMS).(2013). Management of symptomatic vulvovaginal atrophy: 2013 position statement of the North American Menopause Society. *Menopause, 20*(9), 888–902.

are available for over-the-counter products, testing for 24 hours on a small skin area prior to intravaginal use is recommended. If irritation does occur, a silicone-based, iso-osmolar, or propylene glycol-free product (**Table 12-5**) may be better tolerated (NAMS, 2013).

Clothing and Environment

Wearing layered clothes, breathable fabrics (e.g., cotton, linen), or moisture-wicking fabrics (e.g., those worn by runners) is recommended to reduce the discomfort associated with hot flashes and sweats. Avoiding turtlenecks, fabrics that do not allow circulation or absorb sweat (e.g., polyester, silk), and extra layers (e.g., slips, full-length stockings) is also recommended. Keeping the room temperature cool, opening a window or using a fan to circulate air, and using chilling towels and a chilling pillow can help to reduce core body temperature and may be beneficial in reducing the symptoms of menopause (NAMS, 2014).

Smoking Cessation

Smoking is associated with increased morbidity and mortality, especially related to CVD and cancers; earlier age at menopause; increased rate of bone loss; and increased prevalence of vasomotor symptoms (Gold et al., 2000, 2001; NAMS, 2014). Various smoking cessation programs are available, but the most successful programs include one-on-one or group counseling. Ultimately, the best program is the one that is of greatest interest to a specific woman. She needs to be both interested in quitting and motivated to quit. Support from a clinician and use of medications or nicotine replacement therapy (NRT) can significantly improve cessation rates (ACS, 2014b).

Stress Management

Stress and anxiety have been associated with increases in the severity and frequency of hot flashes (Alexander et al., 2003; NAMS, 2014). Additionally, stress can negatively affect quality of life by causing sleep disturbances and decreasing libido as well as aggravating medical conditions such as CVD (NAMS, 2014). At midlife, women may face multiple stressors, such as health changes for themselves or family members, financial concerns, loss of a parent, children leaving home, or relationship struggles with a partner, child, or parent.

Managing stress must be individualized, as each woman may find different tactics helpful. Women are encouraged to identify their own life stressors and find stress-relieving measures that work for them. Some suggestions include regular exercise, meditation, relaxation techniques such as deep breathing, yoga, tai-chi, taking a lukewarm bath, reading, having a massage, seeking support from friends, or activities related to spirituality or religion (NAMS, 2014). Few studies have evaluated the effects of such techniques on menopause-related symptoms, but reports indicate that avoiding and effectively managing stress is associated with less intense and fewer hot flashes (Alexander et al., 2003). While studies have not shown that progressive muscle relaxation and biofeedback

control produce any significant changes in hot flashes, paced respiration has been linked with a significant reduction in hot flashes when initiated with the onset of a hot flash (Freedman & Woodward, 1992; Freedman, Woodward, Brown, Javaid, & Pandy, 1995; Irvin, Domar, Clark, Zuttermeister, & Freidman, 1996). Many women find that yoga breathing—a variation of paced respiration—can enhance relaxation and reduce hot flashes (NAMS, 2014). Yoga breathing consists of a deep inhalation for a count of 4, holding the breath for a count of 7, and slowly exhaling over a count of 8.

Sleep

Evaluating the cause of sleep disruptions is important for developing a plan of management. If sleep disruption is related to hot flashes or other menopausal symptoms, control of those symptoms will usually restore normal sleep patterns. Light blankets, cotton sleepwear or moisture-wicking pajamas, and a well-ventilated room are recommended for reducing nocturnal hot flashes. However, if sleep disruption is unrelated to hot flashes, a more generalized approach is needed.

Developing good sleep hygiene is especially important for perimenopausal and postmenopausal women. Sleep hygiene refers to actions that cue the mind that it is time for sleep and allow the part of the brain that controls the body during sleep to take over. Developing regular routines prior to bedtime, such as brushing the teeth or changing into sleepwear, and doing something relaxing, such as paced respirations, progressive relaxation, guided imagery, taking a warm bath, reading a relaxing book, or drinking a warm beverage without caffeine, can help cue the mind that it is time to sleep. Similarly, activities that tend to stimulate the mind should be avoided just before bed, such as watching television, reading a fast-paced or stimulating book, doing work, or exercise. The bedroom should be reserved for sleep and sexual activities. This consideration is especially important for individuals who have difficulty falling asleep, as doing work or watching television in bed can have a stimulating effect. Establishing regular times for sleep and waking is also important for developing good sleep patterns, as this consistency will facilitate the development of normal daily routines.

Lifestyle changes that can help restore sleep patterns include avoiding caffeine, alcohol, or nicotine. The effects of caffeine can last as long as 20 hours in some individuals, so total elimination is preferable (Landolt, Werth, Borbely, & Dijk, 1995; NAMS, 2014). Although alcohol initially can have a sedative effect, it may cause interruptions in normal sleep patterns after falling asleep, including fragmented sleep and rebound awakening (Landolt, Rioth, Dijk, & Borbely, 1996). Similarly, nicotine can prolong sleep onset and reduces overall sleep duration. Exercise can enhance sleep quality, reduce sleep latency, and increase the amount of time spent in deep sleep. However, timing of exercise is important, as engaging in exercise right before bedtime will increase sleep latency (NAMS, 2014).

Sleep-restriction therapy can be considered to help reestablish a restorative sleep pattern. Use of relaxation techniques prior to bedtime may also benefit women with sleep difficulties. Additionally, yoga and acupuncture have been found to improve sleep among menopausal women with sleep disturbances (Afonso et al., 2012; Hachul et al., 2013).

It is also important to educate women that they may require less sleep as they age. Although the amount of sleep required by adults is very individualized and it is difficult to specify an exact amount of sleep that an individual may need, few postmenopausal women need 8 hours of sleep per night; rather, 6 to 7 hours may be sufficient (National Sleep Foundation, 2015).

Mental Function

Memory and cognitive function tend to decline with advancing age. Difficulty remembering or concentrating commonly occurs among women during the menopausal transition but will often return to premenopause levels when they reach a postmenopausal state. Although poor mental functioning is often associated with lack of sleep or high levels of stress, cognitive impairment can also be related to a myriad of medical problems. Thus the first step in evaluating mental function is to complete a comprehensive assessment to identify potential causes of the cognitive deficit.

Some evidence suggests that women who engage in certain activities or lifestyle changes experience improved memory function and protection against dementia (NAMS, 2014). Maintaining an extensive social network and remaining physically active as well as mentally active by participating in activities that keep the mind engaged (e.g., intellectually stimulating work, puzzles, or other activities) can help to maintain cognitive function. Increasing the intake of omega-3 fatty acids, not smoking, consuming alcohol only in moderation, and adapting lifestyle measures to reduce the risk for hypertension, diabetes, and high cholesterol have the added benefit of protecting against dementia and cognitive decline (NAMS, 2014).

PHARMACOLOGIC OPTIONS FOR MENOPAUSE SYMPTOM MANAGEMENT

The North American Menopause Society (2012, 2014), the International Menopause Society (de Villiers, Pines, et al., 2013), and the Global Consensus (de Villiers, Gass, et al., 2013) identify HT as the most effective therapy for menopause-related moderate to severe vasomotor symptoms. Women with mild vasomotor symptoms will often realize significant benefits from lifestyle changes alone or in combination with nonprescription remedies. In the past, the U.S. Food and Drug Administration (FDA, 2003) defined moderate to severe vasomotor symptoms as 7 to 8 episodes per day or at least 60 episodes per week, but it no longer identifies numbers of episodes as part of defining the severity of vasomotor symptoms (FDA, 2005). NAMS (2014) has also moved to the use of quality of life scales to identify the degree of vasomotor symptom severity on a more individualized basis. In most women, hot flashes will eventually resolve over time without medication.

The Cochrane Group conducted a meta-analysis of 24 randomized, double-blind, placebo-controlled clinical trials that enrolled 3,329 women. The researchers reported that systemic ET/EPT reduced hot flash severity and frequency significantly more than placebos (MacLennan, Broadbent, Lester, & Moore, 2004). Some antidepressant, antihypertensive, and anticonvulsant agents have also been shown to reduce vasomotor symptoms (NAMS, 2014). **Table 12-6** lists currently available HT products. In their review of the efficacy of various preparations, the NAMS researchers concluded that there is no evidence to claim that one product is superior to another in terms of ability to provide symptom relief. **Table 12-7** lists nonhormonal prescription options and **Table 12-8** lists vaginal preparations.

The only FDA-approved prescription therapy for treating hot flashes in women who are at high risk for, or who have been diagnosed with, breast cancer is paroxetine (Noven Therapeutics, 2014). Other nonhormonal agents may also provide hot flash relief for women who have had breast cancer. Herbal alternatives to HT should be used with caution because they can have estrogen-like activity.

Therapy Considerations

Prior to prescribing HT, it is imperative that clinicians and their patients review any cautions or contraindications to hormone use (**Table 12-9**). The clinician must engage the woman in the

TABLE 12-6	Oral and Transdermal Hormone Therapy Options[a]

Type	Product Name	Active Ingredient	Dosage
Estrogens, oral[b]	Cenestin	Conjugated estrogens, A	0.3 mg, 0.45 mg, 0.625 mg, 0.9 mg, or 1.25 mg once daily
	Enjuvia	Conjugated estrogens, B	0.3 mg, 0.45 mg, 0.625 mg, 0.9 mg, or 1.25 mg once daily
	Estrace	17β-estradiol	0.5 mg, 1 mg, or 2 mg once daily
	Menest	Esterified estrogens	0.3 mg, 0.625 mg, 1.25 mg, or 2.5 mg once daily
	Ogen	Estropipate	0.625 mg (0.75 estropipate, calculated as sodium estrone sulfate 0.625), 1.25 (1.5) mg, 2.5 (3) mg, or 5 (6) mg once daily
	Premarin	CEE	0.3 mg, 0.45 mg, 0.625 mg, 0.9 mg, 1.25 mg once daily
Estrogens, transdermal and topical preparations[b]	Minivelle, Vivelle-Dot, Generic	17β-estradiol matrix patch	0.025 mg, 0.0375 mg, 0.05 mg, 0.075 mg, or 0.1 mg patch twice weekly (and 0.06 mg in generic only)
	Alora	17β-estradiol matrix patch	0.025 mg, 0.05 mg, 0.075 mg, or 0.1 mg patch twice weekly
	Climara	17β-estradiol matrix patch	0.025 mg, 0.0375 mg, 0.05 mg, 0.075 mg, or 0.1 mg patch once weekly
	Menostar[c]	17β-estradiol matrix patch	0.014 mg once weekly

Type	Product Name	Active Ingredient	Dosage
	EstroGel	17β-estradiol transdermal gel	0.75 mg/1.25 g gel pump once daily (1 metered pump applied from wrist to shoulder)
	Elestrin	17β-estradiol transdermal gel	0.52 mg/0.87 g gel pump once daily (1–2 metered pumps applied to the upper arm and shoulder)
	Divigel	17β-estradiol transdermal gel	0.25 mg/0.25 g packet, 0.5 mg/0.5 g packet, 1 mg/1 g packet once daily (1 gel packet applied to the upper thigh)
	Estrasorb	17β-estradiol topical emulsion	8.7 mg once daily (2 packets of 1.74 gm of emulsion applied once to each upper leg)
	Evamist	17β-estradiol transdermal spray	1.53 mg/spray once daily (applied as 1–3 sprays to the forearm)
Progestogens, oral	Provera, Generic	MPA	2.5 mg, 5 mg, or 10 mg continuously or on set cycle schedule
	Prometrium, Generic	Micronized progesterone	100 mg or 200 mg continuously or on set cycle schedule
	Micronor,[c] Nor-QD[c]	Norethindrone	0.35 mg continuously or on set cycle schedule
	Aygestin[c]	Norethindrone acetate	5 mg continuously or on set cycle schedule
	Megace[c]	Megestrol acetate	20 mg or 40 mg continuously or on set cycle schedule
Combination estrogen–progestogen products, oral	Premphase	CEE (14 tabs), then CEE + MPA (14 tabs)	0.625 mg E once daily for 14 days, then 0.625 mg E + 5 mg P once daily for 14 days sequentially
	Prempro	CEE + MPA	0.3 mg E + 1.5 mg P once daily, 0.45 mg E + 1.5 mg P once daily, 0.625 mg E + 2.5 mg P once daily, or 0.625 mg E + 5 mg P once daily continuously

(*continues*)

TABLE 12-6	Oral and Transdermal Hormone Therapy Options[a] (*continued*)		

Type	Product Name	Active Ingredient	Dosage
	Femhrt	Ethinyl estradiol + norethindrone acetate	2.5 mcg E + 5 mg P or 5 mcg E + 1 mg P once daily, continuously
	Jinteli	Ethinyl estradiol + norethindrone acetate	5 mcg E + 1 mg P once daily, continuously
	Generic	17β-estradiol + norethindrone acetate	0.5 mg + 0.1 mg P or 1 mg E + 0.5 mg P once daily, continuously
	Mimvey	17β-estradiol + norethindrone acetate	1 mg E + 0.5 mg P once daily
	Angeliq	17β-estradiol + drospirenone	0.25 mg E + 0.5 mg P or 0.5 mg E + 1 mg P once daily, continuously
	Activella	17β-estradiol + norethindrone acetate	0.5 mg E + 0.1 mg P once daily
	Prefest	17β-estradiol (3 tabs) then 17β-estradiol + norgestimate (3 tabs)	1 mg E for 3 days, then 1 mg E + 0.09 mg P for 3 days, once daily sequentially
Combination estrogen–progestogen products, transdermal	Climara Pro	17β-estradiol + levonorgestrel	0.045 mg E + 0.015 mg P once weekly
	CombiPatch	17β-estradiol + norethindrone acetate	0.05 mg E + 0.14 mg P or 0.05 mg E + 0.25 mg P twice weekly
Combination estrogen–BZA product, oral	Duavee	CEE + BZA	0.45 mg E + 20 mg BZA
Combination estrogen–methyltestosterone[b]	Generic	Esterified estrogens + methyltestosterone	0.625 mg E + 1.25 mg MT or 1.25 mg E + 1.25 mg MT cycle 21 days one, 7 days off

Abbreviations: BZA, bazedoxifene; CEE, conjugated equine estrogens; E, estrogen; MPA, medroxyprogesterone acetate P, progestogen.
[a] See prescribing reference for full information on doses, side effects, contraindications, and cautions.
[b] Consider adding progestogen if the woman's uterus is intact.
[c] Evidence-based use; not FDA approved for hormone therapy.
Data from ePocrates. (Updated daily). Computerized pharmacology and prescribing reference [Mobile application software]. Retrieved from http://www.epocrates.com; North American Menopause Society (NAMS). (2014). *Menopause practice: A clinician's guide* (5th ed.). Mayfield Heights, OH: Author.

| TABLE **12-7** | Nonhormonal Pharmacologic Options for Vasomotor Symptoms[a] |

Drug	Dosage	Comments	Side Effects	Contraindications
Antidepressants				
Venlafaxine (Effexor)[b]	37.5–75 mg/day; up-titrate when starting therapy	Response is immediate	Nausea, vomiting, mouth dryness, decreased appetite	Concomitant use of MAO inhibitors; taper when discontinuing
Fluoxetine (Prozac)[b]	20 mg/day; up-titrate when starting therapy	Response is immediate	Asthenia, sweating, nausea, somnolence, anorgasmia, decreased libido	Concomitant use of MAO inhibitors or thioridazine; caution with warfarin; taper when discontinuing
Paroxetine (Paxil,[b] Brisdelle)	10–25 mg/day (Paxil); 7.5 mg/day (Brisdelle)	Response is immediate	See fluoxetine; weight gain, blurred vision	See fluoxetine; taper when discontinuing
Anticonvulsants				
Gabapentin (Neurontin, Gralise)[b]	Initial dose 200–300 mg/day at bedtime, can increase to up to 300 mg 3 times per day at 3- to 4-day intervals		Somnolence, dizziness, ataxia, fatigue, weight gain	Avoid antacids within 2 hours of use; taper when discontinuing
Antihypertensives				
Clonidine (Catapres)[b]	0.05–0.1 mg twice daily	Available as a patch, less effective than antidepressants or gabapentin	Dry mouth, drowsiness, dizziness, weakness, constipation, rash, myalgia, urticaria, insomnia, nausea, agitation, orthostatic hypotension, impotence, arrhythmias	Taper when discontinuing

(continues)

TABLE 12-7	Nonhormonal Pharmacologic Options for Vasomotor Symptoms[a] (*continued*)

Drug	Dosage	Comments	Side Effects	Contraindications
Methyldopa (Aldomet)[b] and belladonna, ergotamine, and phe-nobarbital (Bellergal)[b]		NAMS does not recommend due to limited efficacy data and potential for adverse effects		

Abbreviation: MAO, monoamine oxidase; NAMS, North American Menopause Society.
[a] See prescribing reference for full information on doses, side effects, contraindications, and cautions.
[b] Evidence-based use; not FDA approved for hormone therapy.
Data from ePocrates. (Updated daily). Computerized pharmacology and prescribing reference [Mobile application software]. Retrieved from http://www.epocrates.com; North American Menopause Society (NAMS). (2014). *Menopause practice: A clinician's guide* (5th ed.). Mayfield Heights, OH: Author.

TABLE 12-8	Vaginal and Intrauterine Hormone Therapy Products[a]

Type	Product Name	Active Ingredient	Dose
Estrogen			
Vaginal hormone creams[b]	Estrace	17 β-estradiol	2–4 gm intravaginally daily for 2 weeks, then taper gradually to lowest effective dose; use for shortest effective duration
	Premarin	Conjugated equine estrogens	0.5–2 g intravaginally daily for 2 weeks, then taper gradually to lowest effective dose; use for shortest effective duration
Vaginal tablets[b]	Vagifem	Estradiol hemihydrate	10 mcg intravaginally once daily for 2 weeks; use for shortest effective duration
Ring[b]	Estring	Micronized 17β-estradiol	7.5 mcg/24 hours, 2 mg/90 days ring, replace every 90 days
	Femring	Estradiol acetate	0.05 mg/day or 0.1 mg/day, replace every 3 months; use for shortest effective duration

Type	Product Name	Active Ingredient	Dose
Progestogen			
Gel	Crinone,[c] Prochieve[c]	Progesterone	4% gel—45 mg, 1 applicator every other day, give 6 doses; increase to 8%—90 mg if no response
	Endometrin[c]	Micronized progesterone	100 mg insert
Intrauterine devices	Mirena[c]	Levonorgestrel	20 mcg daily, lasts for 5 years (52 mg over 5 years)
	Skyla[c]	Levonorgestrel	6 mcg/day (13.5 mg over 3 years)

[a] See prescribing reference for full information on doses, side effects, contraindications, and cautions.
[b] Consider adding progestogen if the woman's uterus is intact.
[c] Evidence-based use; not FDA approved for hormone therapy.
Data from ePocrates. (Updated daily). Computerized pharmacology and prescribing reference [Mobile application software]. Retrieved from http://www.epocrates.com; North American Menopause Society (NAMS). (2014). *Menopause practice: A clinician's guide* (5th ed.). Mayfield Heights, OH: Author.

TABLE 12-9 | **Contraindications to Hormone Therapy and Adverse Effects**

Absolute Contraindications to Estrogen Use	Adverse Effects of Estrogen Therapy
Known or suspected cancer of the breast	Uterine bleeding
Known or suspected estrogen-dependent neoplasia	Breast tenderness
History of uterine or ovarian cancer	Nausea
History of coronary heart disease or stroke	Abdominal bloating
History of biliary tract disorder	Fluid retention in extremities
Undiagnosed, abnormal genital bleeding	Headache
History of or active thrombophlebitis or thromboembolic disorders	Dizziness
	Hair loss

Absolute Contraindications to Progestogen Use	Adverse Effects of Estrogen–Progestogen Therapy
Active thrombophlebitis or thromboembolic disorders	Mood changes
Liver dysfunction or disease	Possible increased uterine bleeding than if taking estrogen therapy alone
Known or suspected cancer of the breast	
Undiagnosed abnormal vaginal bleeding	
Pregnancy	

Data from ePocrates. (Updated daily). Computerized pharmacology and prescribing reference [Mobile application software]. Retrieved from http://www.epocrates.com; North American Menopause Society (NAMS). (2014). *Menopause practice: A clinician's guide* (5th ed.). Mayfield Heights, OH: Author.

decision-making process and weigh the risks, benefits, and scientific uncertainty with each woman to individualize her treatment options. The risk of breast cancer increases after 3 to 5 years of EPT (NAMS, 2014; Rossouw et al., 2002). As mentioned earlier, HT should not be used for protection against CVD or dementia. Use of HT within the first 10 years of menopause has not been shown to increase the risk for CVD (NAMS, 2014; Rossouw et al., 2007). Although some data indicate that beginning HT use in early postmenopause may have a cardioprotective effect, the only RCT that tested this hypothesis failed to find any such relationship (Harman, 2012; NAMS, 2014; Salpeter, Walsh, Greyber, & Salpeter, 2006). Recent data do not support a decreased risk of dementia with HT use (NAMS, 2014).

Women considering using HT should have the recommended screening tests for health promotion and disease prevention in addition to a complete history and physical examination. (See Chapter 7 for screening recommendations). Special attention should be paid to any personal or family history of health problems that would contraindicate or increase personal health risks with ET or EPT use. If the woman is considered an appropriate candidate for this therapy, the clinician should explain the various protocols for administering HT: ET alone (for women without a uterus), EPT continuously or sequentially, estrogen with bazedoxifene, or local ET.

Hormone Therapy Protocols and Formulations

Estrogen Therapy
ET has been prescribed exclusively for women who have had a hysterectomy, as the evidence (first reported in 1975) indicates that unopposed estrogen increases the risks for endometrial hyperplasia and cancer. Side effects of ET and strategies to manage them are listed **Table 12-10**.

Estrogen–Progestogen Therapy
Combination estrogen and progestogen therapy can be taken either sequentially (CS-EPT) or continuously (CC-EPT). In the sequential regimen, an estrogen is taken daily with the addition of a progestogen in a cyclic fashion, usually on days 1 to 12 of the month. One side effect often noted with this therapy is that most women will have a withdrawal bleed monthly. To avoid this consequence, the continuous regimen was developed, in which the estrogen and progestogen are taken on a daily basis. Another option includes pulsed combination therapy, wherein the progestogen is taken for 2 days, followed by a day off, in a repeating pattern. The original idea was to reduce potential side effects from the progestogen; however, breakthrough bleeding is usually more problematic with this regimen. A less frequently used regimen is the cyclic regimen, in which estrogen is taken daily for the first 21 days of the cycle and then progestogen is added for days 12 to 21. A withdrawal bleed usually occurs between days 22 and 28, during which neither estrogen nor progestogen is taken. In addition, menopause-related symptoms usually rebound when the estrogen is not taken; therefore, few women opt for the cyclic regimen.

Estrogens
A variety of estrogen compounds exist: estrogens that are bioidentical and transformed into human estrogens, such as 17-beta estradiol, estriol, and estrone; synthetic estrogen analogues, such as ethinyl estradiol; and nonhuman conjugated estrogens, such as CEE, conjugated estrogens, A and B. CEE is the most widely used estrogen and has been the product used in the majority of clinical trials, including the WHI and the Heart and Estrogen/Progestin Replacement Study (HERS).

Estrogens differ in their target tissue response and dose equivalency. They can be administered either systemically or locally. Systemic preparations are available as oral tablets and transdermal patches, creams, sprays, and gels. Local preparations are available as creams, tablets, and rings. The vaginal ring releasing 0.5 mg or 0.1 mg/day of estradiol acetate over 3 months is the only local treatment that has proved effective in treating hot flashes (ePocrates, updated daily; NAMS, 2014). Local treatment with estrogen theoretically avoids systemic absorption; however, in a review of the studies on vaginal preparations, Crandall (2002) found that the ring has slightly more systemic absorption. Women who want to avoid systemic

| TABLE 12-10 | Management of Hormone Therapy Side Effects |

Side Effect	Strategy
Fluid retention	Decrease salt intake; maintain adequate water intake; exercise; use an herbal diuretic or mild prescription diuretic
Bloating	Change to low-dose transdermal estrogen; lower the progestogen dose to a level that still protects the uterus; change the progestogen or try micronized progesterone
Breast tenderness	Lower the estrogen dose; change the estrogen; decrease salt intake; change the progestogen; decrease caffeine and chocolate consumption
Headaches	Change to transdermal estrogen; lower the estrogen and/or progestogen dose; change to a CC-EPT regimen; ensure adequate water intake; decrease salt, caffeine, and alcohol use
Mood changes	Lower the progestogen dose; change to a CC-EPT regimen; ensure adequate water intake; restrict salt, caffeine, and alcohol consumption
Nausea	Take hormones with meals; change the estrogen; change to transdermal estrogen; lower the estrogen or progestogen dose

Abbreviation: CC-EPT, continuous estrogen–progestogen therapy.
Data from ePocrates. (Updated daily). Computerized pharmacology and prescribing reference [Mobile application software]. Retrieved from http://www.epocrates.com; North American Menopause Society (NAMS). (2014). *Menopause practice: A clinician's guide* (5th ed.). Mayfield Heights, OH: Author.

effects, such as breast cancer survivors, should probably use a different preparation until more evidence is available.

Progestogens
Progestogens are hormones that possess progestational properties. The most commonly prescribed progestogen has been MPA, but others are being used with more regularity, such as micronized progesterone (which is bioidentical), norgestimate, and norethindrone acetate. Side effects of adding progestogens to estrogens are listed in **Table 12-9**.

Estrogen–Bazedoxifene Therapy
Therapy combining CEE with bazedoxifene (BZA) is taken daily and continuously. There may be some breakthrough bleeding early during therapy, but this tends to wane over time. This combination formulation is appropriate for women with an intact uterus. No progestogen is needed because the BZA protects against endometrial hypertrophy and malignancy.

Estrogen–Androgen Therapy
Therapy combining androgens and estrogens has been theorized to improve loss of libido in postmenopausal women; however, there is not enough scientific evidence from RCTs to say with certainty that testosterone plus estrogen is more effective than estrogen alone. Known side effects of androgens include alopecia, acne, deepening of the voice, and hirsutism. As of this writing, there are no androgen therapies approved by the FDA for use in women. See Chapter 16 for additional information on use of androgen preparations in women with decreased sexual desire.

Natural Versus Bioidentical Hormones

Many women seek "natural" hormones, believing that they are less likely to cause harmful side effects than pharmaceutically manufactured hormones (Alexander, 2006). The term *natural* actually refers to any product with principal components that originate from plant, animal, or mineral sources. Thus, this definition encompasses pharmaceutically manufactured hormones, which are also derived from animal, plant, or mineral substances. Natural hormones are not necessarily identical to the hormones produced by a woman's body. Hormones that are identical to those made in the human body are available through prescription from both usual and compounding pharmacies.

Several hormones that are pharmaceutically manufactured are available that are bioidentical to the hormones produced in women's bodies. Frequently women requesting "natural hormones" are actually seeking bioidentical formulations (Alexander, 2006). Pharmaceutically manufactured estrogens are available in bioidentical formulations such as estrone, estriol, and 17-beta estradiol. Bioidentical progesterone is also available in micronized form.

"Bioidentical" hormones can also refer to hormones compounded for a specific woman and made in a compounding pharmacy rather than by a commercial pharmaceutical company (NAMS, 2014). It is important to clarify exactly what a women is requesting and to ensure that the source is following FDA regulations. The FDA (2008a) does not recognize the marketing term *bioidentical hormone replacement therapy*. In 2008, the FDA (2008b) took action against compounding pharmacies to stop unwarranted and misleading claims in advertisements that their products are safer than the estrogen products produced by traditional pharmaceutical companies. In reality, all estrogens carry a similar safety and risk profile.

Progesterone Creams

Several different progesterone creams are available as over-the-counter products and from compounding pharmacies. FDA regulations are not currently enforced for these products, again raising concerns about their purity and content. Over-the-counter progesterone creams include products such as PhytoGest, Pro-Gest, Endocreme, and Pro-Dermex; the stated progesterone content varies from less than 2 mg to 700 mg. These creams can also be prepared by compounding pharmacies.

Although some women taking systemic estrogens may want to use progesterone creams for endometrial protection to avoid systemic progesterone effects, there are no data that support this claimed protective effect. One RCT identified some improvement in vasomotor symptoms among women using transdermal progesterone cream as compared with women serving as controls (Leonetti, Longo, & Anasti, 1999). Topical progesterone creams may be a promising option if future research supports these findings.

Plan of Care and Patient Education

NAMS recommends initiating estrogen as ET and EPT at low doses, such as 0.3 mg CEE, 0.25 to 0.5 mg 17-beta estradiol patch, or the equivalent. Studies have shown that these dosages provide adequate vasomotor relief, although the level of endometrial protection afforded by these regimens has not been evaluated in long-term clinical trials. Vasomotor symptoms usually begin to resolve 2 to 6 weeks after initiating HT.

Women should be offered anticipatory guidance about management of side effects, should they occur. Research evidence has absolved HT from contributing to weight gain; however, fluid retention may make women feel as if they are gaining weight. **Table 12-10** lists possible side effects of HT and strategies to manage them.

Women should return for a follow-up visit with the clinician in 6 to 8 weeks to evaluate their progress; if the initial dose of ET/EPT/CEE-BZA does not provide adequate symptom relief, it can be increased or a different combination can be tried. The decision to continue or discontinue HT should be revisited at least annually. On average, vasomotor symptoms last 7.4 years, but some women may experience them for 14 years or more (Avis et al., 2015). The FDA (2005), NAMS (2012, 2014), International Menopause Society (2013), and Global Consensus (2013) all agree that women should take the lowest dose of HT for the shortest period of time. Recommendations for length of time on therapy for women with longer duration of symptoms varies from 3 to 5 years to ongoing if the woman's risk factors are low. Most sources agree that women who experience menopause early should stay on therapy at least until the age when natural menopause usually occurs—age 51 years in North America.

When the woman decides to discontinue therapy, she should be advised there is approximately a 50% chance her symptoms will recur. Rates of recurrence are similar whether HT is tapered or stopped abruptly; therefore, NAMS (2014) recommends individualizing the decision and considering both symptom severity and risks and potential benefits for the individual woman.

COMPLEMENTARY AND ALTERNATIVE MEDICINE OPTIONS FOR MENOPAUSE SYMPTOM MANAGEMENT

The use of complementary and alternative medicine (CAM) is on the rise in the United States (NIH, 2015), especially among women (Smith et al., 2010). Visits to alternative providers now outnumber visits to primary care clinicians, but most patients who use CAM do not report this usage to their primary care clinicians. Furthermore, women are the largest group of CAM users, and the use of CAM to manage menopause-related symptoms is growing (Peng, Adams, Sibbritt, & Frawley, 2014). It is imperative for clinicians to ask patients about the use of CAM and to become knowledgeable about the CAM therapies that women are using.

Herbals

Although many women seek relief of menopause-related symptoms, especially vasomotor symptoms, by using herbal preparations, few studies exist to offer information regarding their efficacy or safety. Because these products are generally identified as diet supplements, rather than as medications, they are not regulated by the FDA in the same way as prescription medications and other over-the-counter products are. Federal regulations for these products do exist, but they are poorly enforced. This lax supervision raises questions about the purity, contents, and consistency from package to package

or tablet to tablet. Various preparations of the same herbal product may contain different amounts of active ingredients (e.g., extract versus tincture), and many products consist of mixtures of many different herbs in a single preparation, making dosing difficult. Furthermore, little is known regarding the interactions between various herbal products and prescription medications or other herbal products.

Despite these concerns, herbal products are widely used for menopause-related symptom relief. Several herbals are commonly included in combination products or in Chinese herb mixtures. **Table 12-11** provides information about some of these preparations.

Isoflavones

Isoflavones are compounds derived from plants that have both estrogenic and nonestrogenic properties. They are present in foods, such as soy (daidzein, genistein, and glycitein) and red clover (*Trifolium pratense*), as well as in commercial preparations. Isoflavones are often referred to as phytoestrogens because of their ability to bind weakly with estrogen receptors, especially the beta receptors, and have been extensively studied as means of reducing vasomotor symptoms.

A systematic review and meta-analysis found that soy isoflavone ingestion (54 mg median aglycone equivalents) from 6 weeks up to 1 year significantly reduced both hot flash severity and frequency compared with placebo (Taku, Melby, Kronenberg, Kurzer, & Messina, 2012). Supplements containing more than 18.8 mg of genistein were more than twice as effective in reducing hot flashes than those with lower levels. Soy isoflavones were also demonstrated to improve quality of life as measured in terms of psychosexual, vasomotor, sexual, and physical scales (Basaria et al., 2009). Studies using red clover isoflavones have not demonstrated beneficial effects from this therapy for vasomotor symptoms or quality of life (Nelson et al., 2006). Studies have not found any effects on vaginal dryness, and results evaluating bone protection and cognitive function have been contradictory (NAMS, 2014). Similarly, soy isoflavones were initially thought to have cardioprotective effects. In 1999, the FDA approved the claim that soy protein (25 gm/day) together with a heart

TABLE 12-11 Herbals Commonly Used for Menopausal Symptom Relief[a]

Product	Usual Dosage[b]	Purpose in Menopause	Comments
Black cohosh (*Cimicifuga racemosa*)	20–40 mg twice daily (proprietary standardized extract)	Vasomotor symptoms	Multiple products and formulations available Research evidence suggests beneficial effect on menopause-related symptoms, benefit similar to estrogen for vasomotor symptom relief Safety for use > 6 months not established Can potentiate antihypertensives Wide variations in product ingredients, extraction processes, and purity Side effects rare, usually intestinal upset, headache, dizziness, hypotension, or painful extremities; more common with higher doses Multiple case reports of liver failure, may be related to contaminants or use of a different cohosh species
Chaste tree berry (*Vitex agnus castus*)	Effective dose unknown, hard to find standardized extract	Menstrual irregularity	More popular in Europe than in the United States; approved in Germany for PMS, mastalgia, and menopause symptoms Often found in combination products Research focuses on PMS symptoms; no data on relief of menopause symptoms Side effects rare, usually headache, intestinal upset
Dong quai (*Angelica sinensis*)	2 capsules 2–3 times per day; usually in combination products	Gynecologic conditions	Widely used in Asia Research found no benefit for menopause symptoms Often found in Chinese herb combination products (*Chinese Materia Medica* advises against giving it alone) A "heating" herb, can cause a red face, hot flashes, sweating, irritability, or insomnia Contains coumarin derivatives; contraindicated in those taking anticoagulants Can cause photosensitivity, hypotension

Product	Usual Dosage[b]	Purpose in Menopause	Comments
Evening primrose oil (Oenothera biennis)	3–4 gm daily in divided doses	Vasomotor symptoms Mastalgia	Data show no benefit in treatment versus controls Potentiates risk for seizure if taken by patients with seizure disorder, with phenothiazines, and with other medications that lower the seizure threshold Side effects include thrombosis, inflammation, immunosuppression, diarrhea and nausea
Ginkgo (Ginkgo biloba)	40–80 mg of standardized extract 3 times daily	Memory changes	Insufficient research on safety and efficacy Memory changes often related to sleep disturbances, menopausal sleep disturbances frequently related to vasomotor symptoms or other life stressors Side effects include gastrointestinal distress, headache, hypotension; chronic use has been linked with subarachnoid hemorrhage, subdural hematoma, and increased bleeding times
Ginseng (Panax ginseng)	1–2 gm root daily in divided doses	General "tonic" Improved mood, fatigue	Heavily adulterated Research showed no benefit on menopause-related symptoms; showed benefits on well-being, general health, and depression Can cause uterine bleeding, mastalgia Contraindicated with breast cancer, and with monoamine oxidase inhibitors, stimulants, or anticoagulants; may potentiate digoxin and others (multiple drug interactions) Side effects include rash, nervousness, dizziness, insomnia, hypertension
Kava (Piper methysticum)	150–300 mg of root extract daily in divided doses	Anxiety Insomnia Vasomotor symptoms	Systematic review indicates effective for anxiety Banned in several countries due to hepatotoxicity; FDA recommends use only after consulting a provider; thus it is not recommended Contraindicated with depression Side effects include gastrointestinal discomfort, impaired reflexes and motor function, weight loss, hepatotoxicity, rash

(continues)

TABLE 12-11 Herbals Commonly Used for Menopausal Symptom Relief[a] (continued)

Product	Usual Dosage[b]	Purpose in Menopause	Comments
Licorice root (Glycyrrhiza glabra)	5–15 mg of root equivalent daily in divided doses; usually in combination products	Expectorant, anti-inflammatory, antiviral, antibacterial Menopause-related symptoms	Found in many Chinese herb mixtures Contains flavonoids, coumarins, and terpenoids No data supporting relief of vasomotor symptoms High doses can lead to primary aldosteronism, cardiac arrhythmias, and cardiac arrest Contraindicated if the woman has hepatic or renal disease, diabetes, hypertension, arrhythmia, hypokalemia, hypertonus, pregnancy, or on diuretics
Passion flower (Passiflora incarnata)	3–10 grains daily in divided doses	Sleep disturbances	Research shows mixed results in sleep improvement Menopausal sleep disturbances frequently related to vasomotor symptoms or other life stressors
St. John's wort (Hypericum perforatum)	300 mg 3 times daily (standardized extract)	Depression Irritability Vasomotor symptoms	Effective for treating depression Some data show efficacy in treating hot flashes Often combined with black cohosh for hot flashes Interferes with metabolism of many medications that are metabolized in the liver (C450) (e.g., estrogen, digoxin, theophylline); reduces INR levels; not to be used concomitantly with antidepressants, monoamine oxidase inhibitors, or immunosuppressants Side effects include gastrointestinal upset (minimized by taking with food), constipation, cramping, photosensitivity, rash, dry mouth, fatigue, dizziness, restlessness, insomnia

Product	Usual Dosage[b]	Purpose in Menopause	Comments
Valerian root (*Valeriana officinalis*)	300–600 mg aqueous extract ½–1 hour before bed (insomnia); 150–300 mg aqueous extract each morning and 300–400 mg each evening (anxiety)	Insomnia Anxiety	Used for insomnia with intermittent dosing, for anxiety with chronic dosing Research showed improvement in sleep and depression/mood scales Side effects are mild; include headache, uneasiness, excitability, arrhythmias, morning sedation, gastrointestinal upset, cardiac function disorders (with long-term use)
Wild yam (*Dioscorea villosa*)	Unknown	Menopause-related symptoms	Products claim that creams are converted to progesterone; however, the human body cannot convert topical or ingested wild yam into progesterone Research showed no benefit on menopausal symptoms

Abbreviations: FDA, U.S. Food and Drug Administration; INR, international normalized ratio; PMS, premenstrual syndrome.

[a] See prescribing reference for full information on doses, side effects, contraindications, and cautions.

[b] Dosages vary and differ according to form (e.g., tincture, liquid extract, drops, essential oil, standardized extract).

Data from Decker, G. M., & Myers, J. (2001). Commonly used herbs: Implications for clinical practice [Insert]. *Clinical Journal of Oncology Nursing, 5*(2); Gaudet, T. W. (2004). CAM approaches to menopause management: Overview of the options. *Menopause Management: Women's Health Through Midlife & Beyond, 13*(Suppl. 1), 48–50; Low Dog, T. (2004). CAM approaches to menopause management: The role for botanicals in menopause. *Menopause Management: Women's Health Through Midlife & Beyond, 13*(Suppl. 1), 51–53; North American Menopause Society. (2014). *Menopause practice: A clinician's guide* (5th ed.). Mayfield Heights, OH: Author.

healthy diet may reduce heart disease risk. More recent research has found that the soy effects are too small to be identified as cardioprotective, with the possible exception of replacing animal protein with soy (NAMS, 2014). NAMS (2014) has concluded that short-term use of soy isoflavones is effective for vasomotor symptoms, does not induce harmful effects on the endometrium or breast, and may be safe for breast cancer survivors.

Other classes of phytoestrogens include flavonoids, lignans, and coumestans. These phytoestrogens have much lower hormonal affinity and are generally not thought to be useful for menopause-related symptom management. They are found in some foods and food products and demonstrate some of the cardioprotective properties of isoflavones. Flavonoids are found in oils, spices, wine, tea, and some vegetables. Lignans are found in flaxseed oil, whole grains, and some fruits and vegetables. Coumestans are found in alfalfa sprouts, red beans, split peas, spinach, and some species of clover. Coumestan phytoestrogens can interfere with bleeding profiles and may interact with anticoagulants.

Acupuncture

Research findings evaluating acupuncture for the relief of menopause-related hot flashes have been contradictory. One concern is that many studies use sham acupuncture as the control, and sham acupuncture is thought to exert some effect. Acupuncture is well known to be an effective and safe treatment for conditions such as headaches and pain. Overall, research suggests that true acupuncture is beneficial for vasomotor symptoms, sleep, and mood among women experiencing menopause-related symptoms (Hachul et al., 2013; NAMS, 2014; Nedeljkovic et al., 2014; Painovich et al., 2012), including breast cancer survivors (Bao et al., 2013; Crew et al., 2010; NAMS, 2014).

CONCLUSION

Menopause is a key landmark in the lives of middle-aged women. This normal developmental stage gives women an opportunity to evaluate their health and risks for diseases of aging, and in turn institute lifestyle changes that can prevent disease and promote health. Although many women will transition through perimenopause to postmenopause without incident, many will also experience mild to severe vasomotor symptoms. Lifestyle modifications, pharmacologic therapies, and use of complementary and alternative medications can often decrease symptoms and improve a woman's quality of life. As the number of postmenopausal women increases, clinicians are in a prime position to counsel their patients about healthy aging.

References

Afonso, R. F., Hachul, H., Kozasa, E. H., Olivera, D. S., Goto, V., Rodrigues, D., . . . Leite, J. R. (2012). Yoga decreases insomnia in postmenopausal women: A randomized clinical trial. *Menopause, 19*(2), 186–193.

Alexander, I. M. (2006). Bioidentical hormones for menopause therapy: Separating the myths from the reality. *Women's Health Care: A Practical Journal for Nurse Practitioners, 5*(1), 7–17.

Alexander, I. M., Ruff, C., Rousseau, M. E., White, K., Motter, S., McKie, C., & Clark, P. (2003). Menopause symptoms and management strategies identified by black women [Abstract]. *Menopause, 10*(6), 601.

American Association of Clinical Endocrinologists (AACE). (2013). American Association of Clinical Endocrinologists' comprehensive diabetes management algorithm 2013 consensus statement. *Endocrine Practice, 19*(Suppl. 2) 1–48.

American Cancer Society (ACS). (2014a). *Cancer facts and figures 2014*. Atlanta, GA: Author.

American Cancer Society (ACS). (2014b). Guide to quitting smoking. Retrieved from http://www.cancer.org/acs/groups/cid/documents/webcontent/002971-pdf.pdf

American College of Obstetricians and Gynecologists. (2014). Practice bulletin: Management of menopausal symptoms. *Obstetrics & Gynecology, 123*(1), 202–216.

American Diabetes Association (ADA). (2010). Position statement: Diagnosis and classification of diabetes mellitus. *Diabetes Care, 33*(Suppl. 1), S62–S69.

American Diabetes Association (ADA). (2014). Standards of medical care in diabetes. *Diabetes Care, 37*(Suppl. 1), S14–S80.

American Heart Association (AHA). (2011). Effectiveness-based guidelines for the prevention of disease in women: 2011 update. *Circulation, 123*, 1243–1262.

American Heart Association (AHA). (2014). Women and cardiovascular disease statistical fact sheet. Retrieved from http://www.heart.org/statistics

Anderson, G. L., Chlebowski, R. T., Aragaki, A. K., Kuller, L. H., Manson, J. E., Gass, M., . . . Wactawski-Wende, J. (2012). Conjugated equine estrogen and breast cancer incidence and mortality in postmenopausal women with hysterectomy: Extended follow-up of the Women's Health Initiative randomised placebo-controlled trial. *Lancet Oncology, 13,* 476–486.

Anderson, G. L., Limacher, M., Assaf, A. R., Bassford, T., Beresford, S. A., Black, H., . . . Wassertheil-Smoller, S. (2004). Effects of conjugated equine estrogen in postmenopausal women with hysterectomy: The Women's Health Initiative randomized controlled trial. *Journal of the American Medical Association, 291*(14), 1701–1712.

Arnold, E. (2005). A voice of their own: Women moving into their fifties. *Health Care for Women International, 26*(8), 630–651.

Avis, N. E., Crawford, S. L., Greendale, G., Bromberger, J. T., Everson-Rose, S. A., Gold, E. B., . . . Thurston, R. C. for the Study of Women's Health Across the Nation (SWAN). (2015). Duration of menopausal vasomotor symptoms over the menopause transition. *JAMA Internal Medicine, 175*(4), 531–539. doi:10.1001/jamainternmed.2014.8063

Avis, N. E., Stellato, R., Crawford, S., Bromberger, J., Ganz, P., Cain, V., & Kagawa-Singer, M. (2001). Is there a menopausal syndrome? Menopausal status and symptoms across racial/ethnic groups. *Social Science and Medicine, 52*(3), 345–356.

Ballard, K. D., Kuh, D. J., & Wadsworth, M. E. J. (2001). The role of the menopause in women's experiences of the "change of life." *Sociology of Health and Illness, 23*(4), 397–424.

Bao, T., Cai, L., Giles, J. T., Gould, J., Tarpinian, K., Betts, K., . . . Stearns, V. (2013). A dual-center randomized controlled double blind trial assessing the effect of acupuncture in reducing musculoskeletal symptoms in breast cancer patients taking aromatase inhibitors. *Breast Cancer Research and Treatment 138*(1), 167–174.

Barton, D. L., Loprinzi, C. L., Quella, S. K., Sloan, J. A., Veeder, M. H., Egner, J. R., . . . Novotny, P. (1998). Prospective evaluation of vitamin E for hot flashes in breast cancer survivors. *Journal of Clinical Oncology, 16*(2), 495–500.

Basaria, S., Wisniewski, A., Dupree, K., Bruno, T., Song M. Y., Yao, F., . . . Dobs, A.B. (2009). Effect of high-dose isoflavones on cognition, quality of life, androgens, and lipoprotein in postmenopausal women. *Journal of Endocrinology Investigation, 32*(2), 150–155.

Blatt, M. H. G., Weisbader, H., & Kupperman, H. S. (1953). Vitamin E and the climacteric syndrome. *Archives of Internal Medicine, 91,* 792–796.

Bromberger, J. T., Matthews, K. A., Kuller, L. H., Wing, R. R., Meilahn, E. N., & Plantinga, P. (1997). Prospective study of the determinants of age at menopause. *American Journal of Epidemiology, 145*(2), 124–133.

Busch, H., Barth-Olofsson, A. S., Rosenhagen, S., & Collins, A. (2003). Menopause transition and psychological development. *Menopause, 10*(2), 179–187.

Centers for Disease Control and Prevention (CDC). (2012, April 27). Adult overweight and obesity. Retrieved from http://www.cdc.gov/obesity/adult

Collins, P. H. (1990). *Black feminist thought: Knowledge, consciousness, and the politics of empowerment.* Boston, MA: Unwin Hyman.

Cooper, G. S., Sandler, D. P., & Bohlig, M. (1999). Active and passive smoking and the occurrence of natural menopause. *Epidemiology, 10*(6), 771–773.

Cramer, G., Xu, H., & Harlow, B. L. (1995). Family history as a predictor of early menopause. *Fertility and Sterility, 64,* 740–745.

Crandall, C. (2002). Vaginal estrogen preparations: A review of safety and efficacy for vaginal atrophy. *Journal of Women's Health, 11*(10), 857–877.

Crew, K. D., Capodice, J. L., Greenlee, H., Brafman, L., Fuentes, D., Awad, D., . . . Hershman, D. L. (2010). Randomized, blinded, sham-controlled trial of acupuncture for the management of aromatase inhibitor–associated joint symptoms in women with early-stage breast cancer. *Journal of Clinical Oncology, 28*(7), 1154–1160.

Daley, A., Stokes-Lampard, H., Thomas, A., & MacArthur, C. (2014). Exercise for vasomotor symptoms. *Cochrane Database of Systematic Reviews, 11,* CD006108. doi:10.1002/14651858.CD006108.pub4

Dawson-Hughes, B., Tosteson, A. N., Melton, L. J., 3rd, Baim, S., Favus, M. J., Khosla, S., & Lindsay, R. L. (2008). Implications of absolute fracture risk assessment for osteoporosis practice guidelines in the USA. *Osteoporosis International, 19*(4), 449–458.

de Bruin, J. P., Bovenhuis, H., van Noord, P. A. H., Pearson, P. L., van Arendonk, J. A. M., te Velde, E. R., . . . Dorland, M. (2001). The role of genetic factors in age at natural menopause. *Human Reproduction, 16*(9), 2014–2018.

Decker, G. M., & Myers, J. (2001). Commonly used herbs: Implications for clinical practice [insert]. *Clinical Journal of Oncology Nursing, 5*(2).

Dennerstein, L., Dudley, E., & Burger, H. (2001). Are changes in sexual functioning during midlife due to aging or menopause? *Fertility & Sterility, 76*(3), 456–460.

de Villiers, T. J., Gass, M. L. S., Haines, C. J., Hall, J. E., Lobo, R. A., Pierroz, D. D., & Rees, M. (2013). Global consensus statement on menopausal hormone therapy. *Climacteric, 16,* 203–204. doi:10.3109/13697137.2013.771520

de Villiers, T. J., Pines, A., Panay, A., Gambacciani, M., Archer, D. F., Baber, R. J., . . . Sturdee, D. W. (2013). Updated 2013 International Menopause Society recommendations on menopausal hormone therapy and preventive strategies for midlife health. *Climacteric, 16,* 316–337.

Duvall, D., & Plourd, D. M. (2014). Update: Management of menopausal and postmenopausal symptoms. *Women's Healthcare, 17–27.* Retrieved from http://npwomenshealthcare.com/wp-content/uploads/2014/01/CE-Meno_F14.pdf

Dvornyk, V., Long, J. R., Liu, P. Y., Zhao, L. J., Shen, H., Recker, R. R., & Deng, H. W. (2006). Predictive factors for age at menopause in Caucasian females. *Maturitas, 54*(1), 19–26.

Edwards, D., & Panay, N. (2015). Treating vulvovaginal atrophy /genitourinary syndrome of menopause: How important is vaginal lubricant and moisturizer composition? *Climacteric, 19*(2), 151–161.

ePocrates. (Updated daily). Computerized pharmacology and prescribing reference [Mobile application software]. Retrieved from http://www.epocrates.com

Freedman, R. R., & Blacker, C. M. (2002). Estrogen raises the sweating threshold in postmenopausal women with hot flashes. *Fertility and Sterility, 77*(3), 487–490.

Freedman, R. R., & Woodward, S. (1992). Behavioral treatment of menopausal hot flashes: Evaluation by ambulatory monitoring. *American Journal of Obstetrics & Gynecology, 167,* 436–439.

Freedman, R. R., Woodward, S., Brown, B., Javaid, J. I., & Pandy, G. N. (1995). Biochemical and thermoregulatory effects of treatment for menopausal hot flashes. *Menopause, 2,* 211–218.

Freeman, E. W., Sammel, M. D., & Sanders, R. J. (2014). Risk of long-term hot flashes after natural menopause: Evidence from the Penn Ovarian Aging Study cohort. *Menopause, 21*(9), 924–932.

Fritz, M. A., & Speroff, L. (2011). *Clinical gynecologic endocrinology and infertility* (8th ed.). Baltimore, MD: Lippincott Williams & Wilkins.

Garber, J. R., Cobin, R. H., Gharib, H., Hennessey, J. V., Klein, I., Mechanik, J. I., . . . Woeber, K. A. (2012). Clinical practice guidelines for hypothyroidism in adults: Cosponsored by the American Association of Clinical Endocrinologists and the American Thyroid Association. *Endocrine Practice, 18*(6), 988–1028.

Garcia, C. R., Sammel, M. D., Freeman, E. W., Lin, H., Langan, E., Kapoor, S., & Nelson, D. B. (2005). Defining menopause status: Creation of a new definition to identify the early changes of the menopausal transition. *Menopause, 12*(2), 128–135.

Gaudet, T. W. (2004). CAM approaches to menopause management: Overview of the options. *Menopause Management: Women's Health Through Midlife & Beyond, 13*(Suppl. 1), 48–50.

Gilligan, C. (1982). *In a different voice: Psychological theory and women's development.* Cambridge, MA: Harvard University Press.

Gold, E. B., Bromberger, J., Crawford, S., Samuels, S., Greendale, G. A., Harlow, S. D., & Skurnick, J. (2001). Factors associated with age at natural menopause in a multiethnic sample of midlife women. *American Journal of Epidemiology, 153*(9), 865–874.

Gold, E. B., Sternfeld, B., Kelsey, J. L., Brown, C., Mouton, C., Reame, N., . . . Stellato, R. (2000). Relation of demographic and lifestyle factors to symptoms in a multi-racial/ethnic population of women 40–55 years of age. *American Journal of Epidemiology, 152*(5), 463–473.

Goodman, M. P. (2012). Are all estrogens created equal? A review of oral vs transdermal therapy. *Journal of Women's Health, 21*(2), 161–169.

Greendale, G. A., Lee, N. P., & Arriola, E. R. (1999). The menopause. *Lancet, 353*(9152), 571–580.

Hachul, H., Garcia, T. K., Maciel, A. L., Yagihara, F., Tufik, S., & Bittencourt, L. (2013). Acupuncture improves sleep in postmenopause in a randomized, double-blind, placebo-controlled study. *Climacteric, 16*(1), 36–40.

Harlow, S. D., Cain, K., Crawford, S., Dennerstein, L., Little, R., Mitchell, E. S., . . . Yosef, M. (2006). Evaluation of four proposed bleeding criteria for the onset of late menopausal transition. *Journal of Clinical Endocrinology and Metabolism, 91*(9), 3432–3438.

Harlow, S. D., Gass, M., Hall, J. E., Lobo, R., Maki, P., Rebar, R. W., . . . de Villiers, T. J. (2012). Executive summary of the Reproductive Aging Workshop + 10: Addressing the unfinished agenda of staging reproductive aging. *Journal of Clinical Endocrinology and Metabolism, 97*(4), 1159–1168.

Harman, S. M. (2012). Effects of oral conjugated estrogen or transdermal estradiol plus oral progesterone treatment on common carotid artery intima media thickness (CIMT) and coronary artery calcium (CAC) in menopausal women: Initial results from the Kronos Early Estrogen Prevention Study (KEEPS) [Abstract]. *Menopause, 19*(12), 1365.

He, C., & Murabito, J. M. (2014). Genome-wide association studies of age at menarche and age at natural menopause. *Molecular and Cellular Endocrinology, 382*(1), 767–779.

Irvin, J. H., Domar, A. D., Clark, C., Zuttermeister, P. C., & Freidman, R. (1996). The effects of relaxation response training on menopausal symptoms. *Journal of Psychosomatic Obstetrics and Gynaecology, 17,* 202–207.

Jacobs Institute on Women's Health. (2003). Expert panel on menopause counseling. Retrieved from http://www.jiwh.org/menodownload.htm

Jordan, J. V., Kaplan, A. G., Miller, J. B., Stiver, I. P., & Surrey, J. L. (1991). *Women's growth in connection.* New York, NY: Guilford Press.

Landolt, H. P., Rioth, C., Dijk, D. J., & Borbely, A. A. (1996). Late-afternoon ethanol intake affects nocturnal sleep and the sleep EEG in middle-aged men. *Journal of Clinical Psychopharmacology, 16,* 428–436.

Landolt, H. P., Werth, E., Borbely, A. A., & Dijk, D. J. (1995). Caffeine intake (200 mg) in the morning affects human sleep and EEG spectra at night. *Brain Research, 675,* 67–74.

Lane, N., & Silverman, S. (2008). Hotline: New NOF guidelines and the WHO Fracture Assessment Tool or FRAX. Retrieved from https://medicalwisdom.wordpress.com/2008/10/18/new-nof-guidelines-and-the-who-fracture-assessment-tool-or-frax

Leonetti, H. B., Longo, S., & Anasti, J. N. (1999). Transdermal progesterone cream for vasomotor symptoms and postmenopausal bone loss. *Obstetrics & Gynecology, 94*(2), 225–228.

Long, M. E., Faubion, S. S., MacLaughlin, K. L., Pruthi, S., & Casey, P. M. (2015). Contraception and hormonal management in the perimenopause. *Journal of Women's Health, 24*(1), 3–10.

Low Dog, T. (2004). CAM approaches to menopause management: The role for botanicals in menopause. *Menopause Management: Women's Health Through Midlife & Beyond, 13*(Suppl. 1), 51–53.

MacLennan, A. H., Broadbent, J. L., Lester, S., & Moore V. (2004). Oral oestrogen and combined oestrogen/progestogen therapy versus placebo for hot flushes. *Cochrane Database of Systematic Reviews, 4,* CD002978. doi:10.1002/14651858.CD002978.pub2

MacPherson, K. I. (1981). Menopause as disease: The social construction of a metaphor. *Advances in Nursing Science, 3,* 95–113.

Manson, J. E. (2014). Current recommendations: What is the clinician to do? *Fertility and Sterility, 101*(4), 916–921.

Manson, J. E., Chlebowski, R. T., Stefanick, M. L., Aragaki, A. K., Rossouw, J. E., Prentice, R. L., . . . Wallace, R. B. (2013). Menopausal hormone therapy and health outcomes during the intervention and extended poststopping of the Women's Health Initiative randomized trials. *Journal of the American Medical Association, 310*(13), 1353–1368.

McKinlay, S. M. (1996). The normal menopause transition: An overview. *Maturitas, 23*(2), 137–145.

Murphy, S. L., Xu, J., & Kochanek, K. D. (2013). Deaths: Final data for 2010. *National Vital Statistics Reports, 61*(4), 1–117.

National Cancer Institute (NCI). (2014, November 25). SEER stat fact sheets: Breast cancer. Retrieved from http://seer.cancer.gov/statfacts/html/breast.html

National Institutes of Health (NIH). (2004). NIH asks participants in Women's Health Initiative Estrogen-Alone Study to stop study pills, begin follow-up phase. Retrieved from http://www.nhlbi.nih.gov/news/press-releases/2004/nih-asks-participants-in-womens-health-initiative-estrogen-alone-study-to-stop-study-pills-begin-follow-up-phase

National Institutes of Health (NIH), National Center for Complementary and Integrative Health. (2015). Use of complementary health approaches in the US. National Health interview survey (NHIS, 2012). Retrieved from https://nccih.nih.gov/research/statistics/NHIS/2012

National Osteoporosis Foundation (NOF). (2014). *Clinician's guide to prevention and treatment of osteoporosis.* Washington, DC: Author.

National Sleep Foundation. (2015). How much sleep do we really need? Retrieved from http://sleepfoundation.org/how-sleep-works/how-much-sleep-do-we-really-need/page/0%2C1

National Women's Health Network. (2000). *Taking hormones and women's health: Choices, risks, and benefits.* Washington, DC: Author.

Nedeljkovic, M., Tian, L., Ji, P., Déglon-Fischer A., Stute P., Ocon E., . . . Ausfeld-Hafter B. (2014). Effects of acupuncture and Chinese herbal medicine (Zhi Mu 14) on hot flushes and quality of life in postmenopausal women: Results of a four-arm randomized controlled pilot trial. *Menopause, 21*(1), 15–24.

Nelson, H. D., Vesco, K. K., Haney, E., Fu, R., Nedrow, A., Miller, J., . . . Humphrey, L. (2006). Nonhormonal therapies for menopausal hot flashes: Systematic review and meta-analysis. *Journal of the American Medical Association, 295*(17), 2057–2071.

North American Menopause Society (NAMS). (2010). Management of osteoporosis in postmenopausal women: 2010 position statement of the North American Menopause Society. *Menopause, 17*(1), 25–54.

North American Menopause Society (NAMS). (2012). The 2012 hormone therapy position statement of the North American Menopause Society. *Menopause,* 19(3), 257–271.

North American Menopause Society (NAMS). (2013). Management of symptomatic vulvovaginal atrophy: 2013 position statement of the North American Menopause Society. *Menopause, 20*(9), 888–902.

North American Menopause Society (NAMS). (2014). *Menopause practice: A clinician's guide* (5th ed.). Mayfield Heights, OH: Author.

North American Menopause Society (NAMS). (2015a). Nonhormonal management of menopause-associated vasomotor symptoms: 2015 position statement of the North American Menopause Society. *Menopause, 22*(11), 1–18.

North American Menopause Society (NAMS). (2015b). The North American Menopause Society statement on continuing use of systemic hormone therapy after 65. *Menopause, 22*(7), 1.

Nosek, M., Kennedy, H. P., Beyene, Y., Taylor, D., Gilliss, C., & Lee, K. (2010). The effects of the perceived stress and attitudes toward menopause and aging on symptoms of menopause. *Journal of Midwifery & Women's Health, 55*(4), 328–334.

Noven Therapeutics. (2014). Brisdell package insert. Retrieved from http://dailymed.nlm.nih.gov/dailymed/drugInfo.cfm?setid =bf208751-e6d8-11e1-aff1-0800200c9a66

Obesity Society. (2015, January). Fact sheets. Retrieved from http:// www.obesity.org/resources/facts-about-obesity/fact-sheets

Painovich, J. M., Shufelt, C. L., Azziz, R., Yang, Y., Goodarzi, M. O., Braunstein, G. D., . . . Merz, C. N. (2012). A pilot randomized, single-blind, placebo-controlled trial of traditional acupuncture for vasomotor symptoms and mechanistic pathways of menopause. *Menopause, 1919*(1), 54–61.

Palmer, J. R., Rosenberg, L., Wise, L. A., Horton, N. J., & Adams-Campbell, L. L. (2003). Onset of natural menopause in African American women. *American Journal of Public Health, 93*(2), 299–306.

Pastore, L. M., Carter, R. A., Hulka, B. S., & Wells, E. (2004). Self-reported urogenital symptoms in postmenopausal women: Women's Health Initiative. *Maturitas, 49*(4), 292–303.

Peng, W., Adams, J., Sibbritt, D. W., & Frawley, J. E. (2014). Critical review of complementary and alternative medicine use in menopause: Focus on prevalence, motivation, decision-making, and communication. *Menopause, 21*(5), 536–548. doi:10.1097/ GME.0b013e3182a46a3e

Portman, D. J., & Gass, M. L. (2014). Genitourinary syndrome of menopause: New terminology for vulvovaginal atrophy from the International Society for the Study of Women's Sexual Health and the North American Menopause Society. *Menopause, 21*(10), 1063–1068.

Quinn, A. A. (1991). A theoretical model of the perimenopausal process. *Journal of Nurse-Midwifery, 36*(1), 25–29.

Ross, C. A., Manson, J. E., Abrams, S. A., Aloia, J. F., Brannon, P. M., Clinton, S. K., . . . Shapses, S. A. (2011) The 2011 report on dietary reference intakes for calcium and vitamin D from the Institute of Medicine: What clinicians need to know. *Journal of Clinical Endocrinology and Metabolism, 96*, 53–58.

Rossouw, J. E., Anderson, G. L., Prentice, R. L., LaCroix, A. Z., Jackson, R. D., Beresford, S. A. A., . . . Ockene, J. (2002). Risks and benefits of estrogen plus progestin in healthy postmenopausal women: Principal results from the Women's Health Initiative Randomized Controlled Trial. *Journal of the American Medical Association, 288*(3), 321–333.

Rossouw, J. E., Prentice, R. L., Manson, J. E., Wy, L., Barad D., Barnabei, V. M., . . . Stefanick, M. L. (2007). Postmenopausal hormone therapy and risk of cardiovascular disease by age and years since menopause. *Journal of the American Medical Association, 287*(13), 1465–1477. Erratum (2008). *Journal of the American Medical Association, 299*(12), 1426.

Salpeter, S. R., Walsh, J. M., Greyber, E., & Salpeter, E. E. (2006). Brief report: Coronary heart disease events associated with hormone therapy in younger and older women: A meta-analysis. *Journal of General Internal Medicine, 21*(4), 363–366. Erratum (2008). *Journal of General Internal Medicine, 23*(10), 1728.

Sampselle, C. M., Harris, V. H., Harlow, S. D., & Sowers, M. (2002). Midlife development and menopause in African American and Caucasian women. *Health Care for Women International, 23*(4), 351–363.

Santen, R. J., Allred, D. C., Ardoin, S. P., Archer, D. F., Boyd, N., Braunstein, G. D., . . . Utian, W. H. (2010). Executive summary: Postmenopausal hormone therapy: An Endocrine Society statement. *Journal of Clinical Endocrinology and Metabolism, 95*(Suppl. 1), S1–S66.

Santoro, N., Brockwell, S., Johnston, J., Crawford, S. L., Gold, E. B., Harlow, S. D., . . . Sutton-Tyrrell, K. (2007). Helping midlife women predict the onset of the final menses: SWAN, the Study of Women's Health Across the Nation. *Menopause, 14*(3, Pt. 1), 415–424.

Santoro, N., Lasley, B., McConnell, D., Allsworth, J., Crawford, S., Gold, E. B., . . . Weiss, G. (2004). Body size and ethnicity are associated with menstrual cycle alterations in women in the early menopausal transition: The Study of Women's Health Across the Nation (SWAN) Daily Hormone Study. *Journal of Clinical Endocrinology & Metabolism, 89*(6), 2622–2631.

Schellenberg, E. S., Dryden, D. M., Vandermeer, B., Ha, C., & Korownyk, C. (2013). Lifestyle interventions for patients with and at risk for type 2 diabetes: A systematic review and meta-analysis. *Annals of Internal Medicine, 159*(8), 543–551.

Sheehy, G. (1976). *Passages: Predictable crises of adult life.* New York, NY: Dutton.

Sheehy, G. (1995). *New passages: Mapping your life across time.* New York, NY: Random House.

Shifren, J. L., & Gass, M. L. S. (2014). The North American Menopause Society recommendations for clinical care of midlife women. *Menopause, 21*(10), 1–25.

Smith, H. A., Matthews, A., Markovic, N., Youk, A., Danielson, M. E., & Talbott, E. O. (2010). A comparative study of complementary and alternative medicine use among heterosexually and lesbian identified women: Data from the ESTHER Project (Pittsburgh, PA, 2003–2006). *Journal of Alternative and Complementary Medicine, 16*(11), 1161–1170. doi:10.1089/acm.2009.0444

Sun, L., Tan, L., Yang, F., Luo, Y., Li, X., Deng, H. W., & Dvornyk, V. (2012). Meta-analysis suggests that smoking is associated with an increased risk of early natural menopause. *Menopause, 19*(2), 126–132.

Taku, K., Melby, M. K., Kronenberg, F., Kurzer, M. S., & Messina, M. (2012). Extracted or synthesized soybean isoflavones reduce menopausal hot flash frequency and severity: Systematic review and meta-analysis of randomized controlled trials. *Menopause, 19*(7), 776–790.

Thurston, R. C., Sowers, M. R., Sternfeld, B., Gold, E. B., Bromberger, J., Chang, Y., . . . Mathews, K. A. (2009). Gains in body fat and vasomotor symptom reporting over the menopausal transition: The Study of Women's Health Across the Nation. *American Journal of Epidemiology, 170*(6), 766–774.

Tosteson, A. N., Melton, L. J. 3rd, Dawson-Hughes, B., Baim, S., Favus, M. J., Khosla, S., & Lindsay, R. L. (2008). Cost-effective osteoporosis treatment thresholds: The United States perspective. *Osteoporosis International.* Retrieved from http://www.ncbi.nlm.nih.gov/entrez/query.fcgi?cmd=Retrieve&db=PubMed&dopt=Citation&list_uids=18292976

U.S. Department of Health, Education, and Welfare, National Institute on Aging. (1979). *Summary of conclusions of the NIH Conference on Estrogen Use and Postmenopausal Women.* Washington, DC: Author.

U.S. Food and Drug Administration (FDA). (2003). Guidance for industry: Estrogen and estrogen/progestin drug products to treat vasomotor symptoms and vulvar and vaginal atrophy symptoms: Recommendations for clinical evaluation. Retrieved from http://www.fda.gov/downloads/Drugs/DrugSafety/InformationbyDrugClass/UCM135338.pdf

U.S. Food and Drug Administration (FDA). (2005). Noncontraceptive estrogen drug products for the treatment of vasomotor symptoms and vulvar and vaginal atrophy symptoms: Recommended prescribing information for health care providers and patient labeling. Retrieved from http://www.fda.gov/downloads/drugs/guidancecomplianceregulatoryinformation/guidances/ucm075090.pdf

U.S. Food and Drug Administration (FDA). (2008a). Bio-identicals: Sorting myths from facts. Retrieved from http://www.fda.gov/downloads/ForConsumers/ConsumerUpdates/ucm049312.pdf

U.S. Food and Drug Administration (FDA). (2008b). FDA takes action against compounded menopause hormone therapy drugs. Retrieved from http://www.fda.gov/NewsEvents/Newsroom/PressAnnouncements/2008/ucm116832.htm

U.S. Preventive Services Task Force (USPSTF). (1996). *Guide to preventive services.* Rockville, MD: Agency for Healthcare Research and Quality.

U.S. Preventive Services Task Force (USPSTF). (2014). Final recommendation statement: Vitamin supplementation to prevent cancer and CVD: Counseling. Retrieved from http://www.uspreventiveservicestaskforce.org/Page/Document/RecommendationStatementFinal/vitamin-supplementation-to-prevent-cancer-and-cvd-counseling

Utian, W. H. (1987). Overview on menopause. *American Journal of Obstetrics & Gynecology, 156,* 1280–1283.

van Noord, P. A., Dubas, J. S., Dorland, M., Boersma, H., & te Velde, E. (1997). Age at natural menopause in a population-based screening cohort: The role of menarche, fecundity, and lifestyle factors. *Fertility & Sterility, 68*(1), 95–102.

Van Voorhis, B. J., Santoro, N., Harlow, S., Crawford, S. L., & Randolph, J. (2008). The relationship of bleeding patterns to daily reproductive hormones in women approaching menopause. *Obstetrics & Gynecology, 112*(1), 101–108.

Vivekananthan, D. P., Penn, M. S., Sapp, S. K., Hsu, A., & Topol, E. J. (2003). Use of antioxidant vitamins for the prevention of cardiovascular disease: Meta-analysis of randomized trials. *Lancet, 361*(9374), 2017–2023.

Waetjen, L. E., Johnson, W. O., Xing, G., Feng, W., Greendale, G. A., & Gold, E. B. (2011). Serum estradiol levels are not associated with urinary incontinence in mid-life women transitioning through menopause. *Menopause, 18*(12), 1283–1290.

Weiss, N. S., Ure, C. L., Ballard, J. H., William, A. R., & Daling, J. R. (1980). Decreased risk of fractures of the hip and lower forearm with postmenopausal use of estrogen. *New England Journal of Medicine, 303,* 1195–1198.

Wildman, R. P., Tepper, P. G., Crawford, S., Finkelstein, J. S., Sutton-Tyrrell, K., Thurston, R. C., . . . Greendale, G. A. (2012). Do changes in sex steroid hormones precede or follow increases in body weight during the menopause transition? Results from the Study of Women's Health Across the Nation. *Journal of Clinical Endocrinology & Metabolism, 97*(9), E1695–E1704.

Wilmoth, M. C. (1996). The middle years: Women, sexuality, and the self. *Journal of Obstetric, Gynecologic, and Neonatal Nursing, 25*(7), 615–621.

Wilson, R. (1966). *Feminine forever.* New York, NY: Evans.

Woods, N. F., & Mitchell, E. S. (2008). Mid-life women's health. In C. I. Fogel & N. F. Woods (Eds.), *Women's health care in advanced practice nursing* (pp. 121–148). New York, NY: Springer.

World Health Organization (WHO). (2007). WHO FRAX technical report. Retrieved from http://www.shef.ac.uk/FRAX

Wysocki, S., Alexander, I., Schnare, S. M., Moore, A., & Freeman, S. B. (2003). Individualized care for menopausal women: Counseling women about hormone therapy. *Women's Health Care: A Practical Journal of Nurse Practitioners, 2*(12), 8–16.

CHAPTER 13

Intimate Partner Violence

Margaret M. Glembocki
Kerri Durnell Schuiling

The editors acknowledge Daniel J. Sheridan, Linda A. Fernandes, Alida D. Wagner, Dawn M. Van Pelt, and Jacquelyn C. Campbell, who were the authors of the previous edition of this chapter.

Intimate partner violence (IPV) is a global issue in which both men and women can be victims; however, statistics reveal that women are more likely to be subjected to violence than men. Perhaps because of that reality, most research and interventions focus on women (Nelson, Bougaatos, & Blazin, 2012). There is no single definition of IPV that is universally accepted. Thus, for the purposes of this chapter, the following definition is used: IPV is the victimization of a person with whom the abuser is currently or has been in an intimate, romantic, or spousal relationship (American College of Obstetricians and Gynecologists, 2014; Burnett & Adler, 2015). Although IPV occurs in both heterosexual and homosexual relationships and the perpetrator can be male or female, it more typically involves violence perpetrated against adolescent and adult women (American College of Obstetricians and Gynecologists, 2014).

Dating violence or adolescent relationship abuse has many aspects that are similar to IPV, but there are also distinct characteristics relative to the age of the victim and/or abuser and the patterns of abuse may differ. To account for these differences, a specific definition of adolescent relationship abuse has been developed (Chamberlain & Levenson, 2013). Adolescent relationship abuse is a pattern of repeated acts in which an individual physically, sexually, or emotionally abuses another person whom the abuser is dating or in a relationship with, regardless whether the relationship is opposite or same sex, and either one or both

parties are minors. The defining characteristic is the abuser's goal to maintain power and control over the victim (American College of Obstetricians and Gynecologists, 2012; Chamberlain & Levenson, 2013).

The term *domestic violence* is sometimes used instead of IPV, although domestic violence can encompass other forms of violence such as elder abuse and child abuse. Both types of abuse include a range of violence, such as physical, psychological, and sexual abuse, as well as sexual coercion and sexual trafficking.

Throughout this chapter, the term *patient* is used more frequently than the terms *victim* and *survivor*. The criminal justice system primarily uses the term *victim* when describing an individual who has experienced a reported assault. Community-based women's advocacy programs often refer to women who have experienced IPV as *survivors* to promote their empowerment. The word *patient* is more often used when discussing or documenting health care provided to individuals who are seeking care due to IPV. Patients experiencing IPV have been criminally victimized and, unless murdered in the process, are survivors of the abuse. Clinicians providing forensic-related care need to keep the boundaries between the criminal justice, advocacy, and the healthcare systems separate. All clinicians need to provide excellent evidence-based patient care that is empathetic and supportive.

This chapter focuses on the prevention of IPV and the screening and treatment of women who live in the United States and who have been victims of violence perpetrated by an intimate partner. Clinicians in primary care settings can be instrumental in providing comprehensive, ongoing assessments and intervention for women experiencing IPV.

EPIDEMIOLOGY

Intimate partner violence in the United States is a serious public health problem that places many women at risk for major injury or death. An estimated 2 million women in the United States are abused by someone whom they know. IPV accounts for approximately 22% of all violent crime experienced by women living in the United States (American College of Obstetricians and Gynecologists, 2014), although the actual number of women assaulted may be higher than the official statistics indicate due to underreporting. Data suggest that between 25% and 33% of all women will be physically assaulted by an intimate partner within their lifetime; 9% will report being raped; 17% will report sexual violence other than rape; and 48% will report psychological aggression (Black et al., 2011).

Research about IPV in same- and opposite-sex relationships suggests that IPV against gay males and lesbian and heterosexual women is more likely than IPV against heterosexual men to be considered illegal (Sorenson & Thomas, 2009). The National Violence Against Women Survey revealed that women respondents who had ever lived with a partner of the same sex had an IPV rate almost twice that of women respondents who had cohabitated only with men (Sorenson & Thomas, 2009).

The National Intimate Partner and Sexual Violence Survey collected data from 16,507 participants, of whom 9,086 were women. Key findings of the survey were that more than 1 in 3 women in the United States have experienced rape, physical violence, and/or stalking by an intimate partner (Black et al., 2011). The study also identified that more than half of women who experienced rape, physical violence, and/or stalking by an intimate partner experienced some type of IPV for the first time before the age of 25 (Black et al., 2011).

Research has shown that women with mental and/or physical disabilities are at higher risk of IPV. In terms of ethnicity, African American and American Indian populations have significantly higher death rates from IPV than other ethnicities (Furlow, 2010; Zolotor, Denham, & Weil, 2009). Risk factors for IPV-related homicide include perpetrators who have access to firearms, previous threats made by the perpetrator using a weapon, recent separation, or use of illicit drugs by the perpetrator and/or the victim (Furlow, 2010; Zolotor et al., 2009).

Violence is associated with a wide range of physical and psychological health needs that compel women victimized by IPV to seek health care. The estimated costs associated with exposure to IPV exceed $5.8 billion annually, with the majority of those costs attributable to direct medical and mental healthcare services (American College of Obstetricians and Gynecologists, 2014).

TYPES OF INTERPERSONAL VIOLENCE

The Centers for Disease Control and Prevention (CDC, 2016) identifies four main types of IPV:

- *Physical violence*: the intentional use of physical force with the potential for causing death, disability, injury, or harm. Examples of physical violence include strangling, slapping, shoving, pushing, biting, shaking, and hitting; burning; use of a weapon; and use of restraints or one's body, size, or strength against another person. Physical violence also includes coercing other people to commit any of these acts.
- *Sexual violence* (five categories): (1) rape or penetration of the victim, (2) victim was made to penetrate someone else, (3) nonphysically pressured unwanted penetration, (4) unwanted sexual contact, and (5) noncontact unwanted sexual experience.
- *Stalking*: a pattern of repeated, unwanted, attention and contact that causes fear or concern for one's own safety or the safety of someone else (e.g., family member or friend).
- *Psychological aggression*: the use of verbal and nonverbal communication with the intent to harm another person mentally or emotionally, and/or to exert control over another person.

Sexual and Reproductive Coercion

Sexual and reproductive coercion is identified as a separate category of IPV (American College of Obstetricians and Gynecologists, 2012; Chamberlain

& Levenson, 2013). Sexual and reproductive coercion involves the use of power and control related to reproductive health. For example, the perpetrator may refuse to allow the partner to use birth control or may refuse to practice safe sex.

Reproductive coercion occurs when a perpetrator exhibits controlling behaviors related to contraception use and pregnancy. The intent of such IPV is for the abuser to maintain power within the relationship; the victim can be either an adult or an adolescent (American College of Obstetricians and Gynecologists, 2012; Chamberlain & Levenson, 2013). Two types of behaviors are most commonly observed among perpetrators of reproductive coercion:

- Sabotage of contraceptive methods: promoting pregnancy by interfering with contraception. Examples include hiding or destroying birth control methods, altering integrity of condoms, and removing condoms during intercourse.
- Pregnancy coercion and pregnancy pressure: acts of violence or threatening behavior if a partner does not observe the perpetrator's wishes about continuing or terminating a pregnancy. Examples include forcing a partner to carry or terminate a pregnancy by use of threats and inflicting injury to the pregnant partner that is intended to cause miscarriage.

In one study approximately 20% of women with a history of abuse who sought care at a family planning clinic reported pregnancy coercion (Miller et al., 2010). Another study analyzing pregnancy-associated homicides between 1993 and 2008 among Maryland residents found that homicides ($n = 110$) were the chief cause of death during pregnancy and the first year postpartum (Cheng & Horan, 2010).

Sexual coercion includes behaviors that pressure a partner to engage in sex without using physical force (Chamberlain & Levenson, 2013). Some of these manipulative behaviors include the following:

- Pressuring the partner to engage in sex
- Threatening to end the relationship if the partner does not engage in sex
- Forcing sexual activity without the use of a condom or other methods of birth control

- Purposefully exposing a partner to a sexually transmitted infection (STI)

All patients who experience sexual and reproductive coercion are at high risk for long-term health issues such as alcohol or drug abuse, sexually transmitted infections, human immunodeficiency virus (HIV) disease, and risky sexual behaviors.

Interventions for Sexual and Pregnancy Coercion

When developing a plan for care, it is important for clinicians to include the differential diagnosis of pregnancy coercion and intimate partner violence when patients present for pregnancy testing, sexually transmitted infection testing, unplanned pregnancy, and any signs or symptoms of violence. When planning interventions and care in patients who are experiencing IPV, it is important to include alternative resources and programs that are available in a setting outside of clinical practice. Treatment and interventions in patients who are victims of reproductive and sexual coercion differ slightly from those in patients who are not subjected to such IPV, as much of the focus is on disease prevention and pregnancy prophylaxis. Interventions may potentially include the following components:

- Education about safety planning and harm reduction
- Education about support services
- Providing discreet and confidential methods of birth control

Concealment of her contraceptive practices by the patient may be needed to protect the woman from further harm. These methods can be discussed and planned by the patient and her clinician. For example, if an intrauterine device (IUD) is used, the pair might consider trimming the string so the abuser is unable to detect and remove the device.

It is important to create a safe environment for patients who are victims of sexual and reproductive coercion and to interview them in an area where the conversation can occur in a confidential manner. It is also essential to inform the patient about mandatory reporting laws. Many times, reporting can place the patient at greater risk.

THEORIES OF INTIMATE PARTNER VIOLENCE

Sociology provides a unique perspective on IPV as a function of social structures versus pathology of the individual; thus the sociological perspective looks at social—rather than individual—causes of violence (Lawson, 2012). When IPV was no longer treated as a private matter (which was the case until the 1970s), the field of sociology split into two bodies of theories on IPV: (1) the general family violence perspective and (2) the feminist perspective (Lawson, 2012).

Family violence theorists view IPV as an aspect of the larger issue of family violence. In this perspective, IPV is not viewed as different from elder violence, child abuse, or sibling violence: They are all expressions of family conflict that could be conceptualized using many different theories (Lawson, 2012). Thus the key to understanding IPV for those using family violence theory is understanding what makes families use violence as a means to resolve their conflict (Lawson, 2012). In this model, the family is viewed as the primary unit of analysis.

Feminist theories, particularly second-wave feminists, treat IPV as fundamentally an issue of gender and specifically the patriarchal domination of men over women (George & Stith, 2014; Lawson, 2012). The fundamental underpinning of such theories is that IPV is an issue of gender and cannot be understood through any lens that does not include gender as the main unit of analysis. Third-wave feminist theories, however, have moved beyond the universalizing view of "sisterhood" to an appreciation that while "we are all women, our experiences within our race, gender, nationality, class and other markers of identity make us different and similar, unequal and equal" (George & Stith, 2014, p. 182.) This line of thinking brought forth the term *intersectionality*—a perspective in which other aspects of identity such as religion, culture, and sexual orientation, are also considered (George & Stith, 2014). Third-wave feminist theories move away from essentializing all men as abusers; they encourage treatment that avoids assumptions and instead addresses violence using an evidence-based method, thereby working toward social justice (George & Stith, 2014).

Lenore Walker (1979) was the first researcher to recognize that repetitive patterns or cycles could be discerned in abusive relationships. She identified three phases in the cycle of abuse; later the third phase (reconciliation and calm) was separated into two different phases. Thus four phases are now identified in the cycle of abuse (see **Appendix 13-A**):

1. *Tension-building phase*: This phase often includes verbal put-downs by the batterer, increased arguing, and, in some cases, the woman trying to appease her batterer.
2. *Acute-battering incident*: This phase can include sexual assault, hitting, kicking, strangulation, and use of weapons.
3. *Reconciliation phase*: During this phase, the abuser will often repent for the abusive actions, will apologize, and may even concede that the abuse occurred.
4. *Calm or loving phase*: During this phase, often referred to as the *honeymoon phase*, the batterer may apologize, promise it will never happen again, or even deny the violence occurred. As time goes on, the calm phase may disappear altogether.

An important aspect of the cycle of abuse theory is the acknowledgment that this cycle is not the same for everyone—some people may experience only some of the stages or even none of the stages.

HEALTH IMPACTS

IPV and domestic abuse represent two of the most pervasive forms of human rights abuse in the United States today (Furlow, 2010). Not only are the victims profoundly affected, but the communities in which they live and work are impacted, as are the social and medical systems that support and treat the victims. The economic costs are extensive. There are significant collateral negative health-related impacts when someone suffers abuse. For example, physical injury, mental health issues, and complications of pregnancy are some of the health consequences that are reported by women who are victims of IPV committed by a current or previous partner (Devries, Mak, & Bacchus, 2013).

Women who survive the abuse are still at a higher risk of developing poor coping skills, and they often suffer a myriad of long-term conditions such as chronic headaches, clinical depression, and suicide ideation (Furlow, 2010). It is also not unusual for a survivor of abuse to suffer from post-traumatic stress syndrome. IPV puts its victims at risk of developing sexually transmitted infections (e.g., HIV), cardiac and circulatory conditions, gastrointestinal disorders (e.g., irritable bowel syndrome), alcohol and drug misuse, anxiety, and insomnia (Trevillion, Agnew-Davis, & Howard, 2013). A need for ongoing health care due to the long-term physical and mental sequelae is common among survivors of IPV (Furlow, 2010).

Anytime a woman presents with one or more of the aforementioned gynecologic conditions, it is crucial that she be screened for IPV. Clinicians should explore the possibility of sexual assault or forced sexual intercourse for all women presenting with gynecologic symptoms. This is especially true for women who present with multiple or persistent gynecologic symptoms. Asking a patient about forced sex from her partner or her partner's sexual practices must be done in a very professional, nonjudgmental, caring, sensitive manner, and in a private and safe environment. Women are often too embarrassed or afraid to volunteer such information, or they may not link their health problems to the abuse in their lives. All women with depression should be screened for IPV; conversely, all women experiencing IPV should be evaluated for depression.

HISTORY AND ASSESSMENT

Risk Factors of IPV

Women who have experienced IPV are more likely to seek healthcare services. In turn, the clinician plays a vital role in identification, intervention, and halting the cycle of abuse through screening, support, and reviewing available prevention and referral programs with the survivor (American College of Obstetricians and Gynecologists, 2012; Feder et al., 2011).

There are multiple risk factors for IPV, which intersect across one's life (**Table 13-1**) (CDC, 2015). A person who has one or more risk factors does not necessarily become an abuser or a victim; rather, the risk factor simply identifies the individual as being *at risk*.

There are also a number of factors that put women at particular risk of being abused:

- History of depression and/or low self-esteem
- Younger age (very high rate in college-aged women)
- History of being raised with violence within the home
- Pregnancy
- Lower educational level
- Unemployment or job instability
- Poverty
- Being in a relationship that involves a dominant or controlling partner
- Living within a community or family with male-dominant norms

Screening and Health History

Guidelines developed by an interdisciplinary team of healthcare experts in IPV recommend that women be screened for IPV in primary care settings during their periodic examinations, especially gynecologic visits, and at all visits for a new concern (American College of Obstetricians and Gynecologists, 2012; Institute of Medicine, 2011). Screening has been shown to increase the identification of IPV; however, there is little evidence to demonstrate that it has an effect on outcomes (Koziol-McLain et al., 2010; Spangaro, Zwi, Poulos, & Mann, 2010; Taft et al., 2015).

Most women who have been battered do not come to healthcare facilities with obvious trauma or injuries, although women who have been battered and who present to an emergency department usually have more injuries to the head, neck, and face than women who have not been physically abused (Campbell, 2002; Furlow, 2010). Clinicians should routinely consider IPV as a possible diagnosis for women who present with gynecologic problems, especially multiple problems, chronic stress-related symptoms, and central nervous system (CNS) symptoms. In addition to the effects of stress and mental distress, patients experiencing IPV usually present with physical health problems. When the question of IPV—either past or present—arises, it is important for the clinician to obtain a focused history and to perform a systematic physical examination to assess the severity and timing

TABLE 13-1 Perpetrator and Victim Risk Factors for Intimate Partner Violence

Individual Risks	Relationship Factors	Community Factors	Societal Factors
Low self-esteem Low income Low academic achievement Young age Aggressive or delinquent behavior as a youth Heavy alcohol and drug use Depression Anger and hostility Antisocial personality traits Borderline personality traits Prior history of being physically abusive Having few friends and being isolated from other people Unemployment Emotional dependence and insecurity Belief in strict gender roles (e.g., male dominance and aggression in relationships) Desire for power and control in relationships Perpetrating psychological aggression Being a victim of physical or psychological abuse (consistently one of the strongest predictors of perpetration) History of experiencing poor parenting as a child History of experiencing physical discipline as a child	Marital conflict—fights, tension, and other struggles Marital instability—divorces or separations Dominance and control of the relationship by one partner over the other Economic stress Unhealthy family relationships and interactions	Poverty and associated factors (e.g., overcrowding) Low social capital—lack of institutions, relationships, and norms that shape a community's social interactions Weak community sanctions against intimate partner violence (e.g., unwillingness of neighbors to intervene in situations where they witness violence)	Traditional gender norms (e.g., women should stay at home, not enter the workforce, and be submissive; men support the family and make the decisions)

Reproduced from Centers for Disease Control and Prevention (CDC). (2015). Intimate partner violence: Risk and protective factors. Retrieved from http://www.cdc.gov/violenceprevention/intimatepartnerviolence/riskprotectivefactors.html.

of trauma, injuries, gynecologic conditions, CNS disorders, and chronic stress-related problems.

With a general understanding of the relationships and patterns associated with partner violence, the clinician can begin to understand the development of stress-related illnesses and mental disorders in women who have been battered. When a woman presents for health care, her symptoms may be very general and vague, including generalized concerns such as unexplained pain or malaise. Clinicians may have misconceived notions that she has some other psychological disorder or is perhaps displaying drug-seeking behaviors. For a variety of reasons, including fear of further abuse and embarrassment, a woman who has been abused is not always forthcoming about her abuse. As a consequence, it is important for clinicians to identify signs of IPV.

Careful questioning during the history can help identify whether the patient is at risk for abuse or has experienced abuse (Agee Shavers, 2013). When obtaining a health history, it is important to be nonjudgmental and supportive. Perform the history in a safe space, and take the time to allow for the therapeutic relationship to develop. If the patient indicates she is experiencing or has experienced IPV, support her in expressing her feelings about the violence and listen without interruption. Research suggests that patients are more likely to respond to universal screening when there is privacy; a nonjudgmental, nonpressured, and supportive environment; and informed consent, especially as to why the screening is being done and who will have access to the information (Todahl & Walters, 2011). Universal screening programs that incorporate numerous screening components at multiple levels and that have institutional support have been shown to yield more successful outcomes. Important components that appear to impact the success rate include ongoing mandatory training for staff so they are comfortable with the screening and referral process; availability of support services that will address the patient's health, social, and safety needs; and a way to facilitate the patient's access to immediate off-site, community-based services (O'Campo, Kirst, Tsamis, Chambers, & Ahmad, 2011).

If the woman's partner has accompanied her, direct her or him to step out of the room during the examination. Do not ask, but rather give a direct request so that there is no option for the partner to remain during the history or physical examination. This practice allows the patient to freely provide information to the clinician without fear of retribution from her partner.

If the patient brings her children to the office visit, it is imperative to ask her if it is acceptable to ask them to step outside. Screening for IPV in the presence of children raises a variety of safety concerns. If the child talks afterward to the perpetrator about the disclosure of IPV to the clinician, the patient may be subjected to retaliation, such as further abuse or prohibiting further contact with the clinician. In addition, the child may be exposed to new information or retraumatized by painful memories (Zink & Jacobson, 2003). Guidelines in the literature indicate that screening in front of children older than 3 years of age should be done only with prior permission from the mother, or with only general IPV screening questions and sensitivity to the mother's nonverbal behaviors and comfort (Zink & Jacobson, 2003). General questions should avoid charged words such as *hit, hurt, harm*, and *afraid*. Clinicians need to be sensitive to the unique privacy, safety, and protection issues of mothers who are survivors of IPV.

Screening Tools

IPV screening remains controversial (Hussain et al., 2015). The U.S. Preventive Services Task Force (USPSTF, 2015) recommends that clinicians screen all women of childbearing age for IPV, such as domestic violence, and provide or refer women who screen positive to intervention services. However, the USPSTF has concluded that the current evidence is insufficient to assess the balance of benefits and harms of screening all elderly or vulnerable adults (physically or mentally dysfunctional) for abuse and neglect (USPSTF, 2015). The American College of Obstetricians and Gynecologists (2012) recommends that IPV screening occur for all women at periodic intervals, including at the first prenatal visit and at least once per trimester and at the postpartum checkup. See Chapter 7 for more on screening for IPV.

IPV screening tools have been evaluated in only a small number of studies and have not been well tested in diverse populations. Thus, while multiple IPV screening tools are available, no single tool has well-established psychometric properties (Hussain et al., 2015; Rabin, Jennings, Campbell, & Bair-Merritt, 2009). The sensitivities and specificities of the tools vary widely (Rabin et al., 2009).

Commonly used IPV screening tools include the nine-question Abuse Assessment Screen (AAS), which was developed by Helton (1987) in an effort to determine if a link exists between IPV health effects on women and fetal health (**Box 13-1**). The number of questions on the AAS has changed over time from nine questions, to six questions (Parker & McFarlane, 1991), to three questions (McFarlane, Parker, Soeken, & Bullock, 1992) to two questions (McFarlane, Greenberg, Weltge, & Watson, 1995). All of these remain widely used today.

During screening for IPV, it is suggested that clinicians avoid the use of stigmatizing words such as *abuse*, *rape*, *battered*, and *violence* (Chamberlain & Levenson, 2013). The American College of Obstetricians and Gynecologists (2012) suggests the following guidelines to facilitate a routine IPV assessment process:

1. Screen for IPV in a private and safe place with the woman alone (no children, partner, or family present).
2. If language is an issue, use professional interpreters instead of family members.
3. Prior to administering a screening tool, it may be helpful to preface its use with a statement that generalizes violence in society and indicates clinicians and many healthcare organizations support the routine screening of all patients for IPV.
4. Incorporate IPV screening into the routine medical history so all patients are screened routinely regardless of whether abuse is suspected.
5. Develop and maintain relationships with community resources for women affectd by IPV.
6. Keep printed take-home resources available, such as locations of shelters and hotline numbers.
7. Ensure that staff have training and regular updates about IPV.

With any "yes" answer on an IPV screen, a recommended interviewer response is "Thank you for sharing. Can you give me an example? When was the last time?"

The three-question AAS (McFarlane et al., 1992) is probably the most widely used IPV screen. However, it does not include questions about being afraid of one's partner or about being emotionally abused or controlled. It is very common to hear from women who have been battered that the pain and scars from being emotionally abused take longer to heal than the pain of physical abuse. Therefore, the clinical pressures to keep IPV screens short must be weighed against the consequences of failure to assess the significant emotional abuse and fear of a partner that could be linked to an increased risk of intimate partner homicide.

Many clinicians are reluctant to screen for IPV because they are uncertain about what to do with a "yes" response (Sheridan, 2003). Patients who give a positive response to being involved in ongoing IPV need to complete Campbell's Danger Assessment (DA; **Box 13-2**) and Sheridan's Harassment in Abusive Relationships: A Self-Report Scale (HARASS; **Box 13-3**). All of the items on these screening instruments have been linked to an increased risk of domestic homicide. The DA is best completed in conjunction with a calendar that serves as a prompt to remind women of abusive events around certain dates. The DA and HARASS take approximately 5 to 10 minutes each to complete; they are self-report scales that can be completed by the patient. Both instruments can be read to patients who are illiterate, have language barriers, or are unable to read secondary to the nature of their injuries.

While studies of the DA instrument have provided some preliminary data to suggest cut-off scores related to risk of homicide, the DA and HARASS instruments are best used as guides to structure safety planning. In general, the more "yes" responses on the DA tool and the more positive responses to some form of harassment, the more dangerous and potentially deadly the relationship.

Screening for Traumatic Brain Injury

Women who have survived IPV or who currently are victims of IPV need to be screened for traumatic brain injury (TBI), particularly if the history suggests she has experienced numerous blows to her face,

BOX 13-1 Original Nine-Question Abuse Assessment Screening Tool

1. Do you know where you would go or who could help you if you were abused or worried about abuse?
   Yes _____ No _____
   If yes, where: _____
   _____

2. Are you in a relationship with a man who physically hurts you?
   Yes _____ No _____ Sometimes _____

3. Does he threaten you with abuse?
   Yes _____ No _____ Sometimes _____

4. Has the man you are with hit, slapped, kicked, or otherwise physically hurt you?
   Yes _____ No _____ Sometimes _____

5. If yes, has he hit you since you've been pregnant?
   Yes _____ No _____ Sometimes _____

6. If yes, did the abuse increase since you've been pregnant?
   Yes _____ No _____ Sometimes _____

7. Have you ever received medical treatment for any abuse injuries?
   Yes _____ No _____ Sometimes _____

8. If you have been abused, remembering the last time he hurt you, mark the places on the body map where he hit you (see body map in **Figure 13-1**).

9. Were you pregnant at the time?
   Yes _____ No _____ Not Applicable _____

Courtesy of March of Dimes National Foundation.

FIGURE 13-1 Body map.

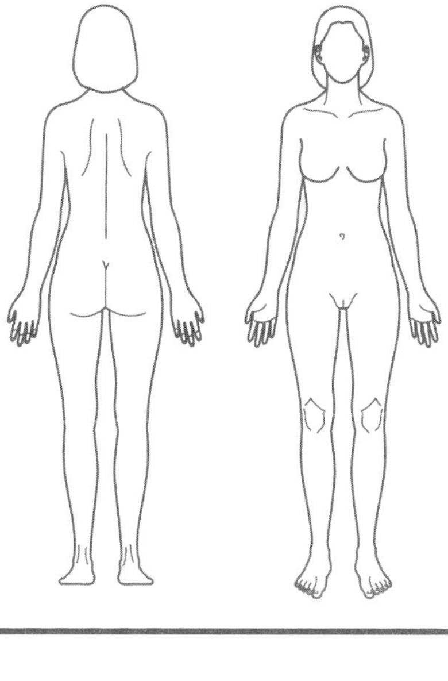

BOX 13-2 Danger Assessment

Several risk factors have been associated with increased risk of homicides (murders) of women and men in violent relationships. We cannot predict what will happen in your case, but we would like you to be aware of the danger of homicide in situations of abuse and for you to see how many of the risk factors apply to your situation.

Using the calendar, please mark the approximate dates during the past year when you were abused by your partner or ex-partner. Write on that date how bad the incident was according to the following scale:

1. Slapping, pushing; no injuries and/or lasting pain
2. Punching, kicking; bruises, cuts, and/or continuing pain
3. "Beating up"; severe contusions, burns, broken bones
4. Threat to use weapon; head injury, internal injury, permanent injury
5. Use of weapon; wounds from weapon

(If any of the descriptions for the higher number apply, use the higher number.)

Mark Yes or No for each of the following. ("He" refers to your husband, partner, ex-husband, ex-partner, or whoever is currently physically hurting you.)

_____ 1. Has the physical violence increased in severity or frequency over the past year?
_____ 2. Does he own a gun?
_____ 3. Have you left him after living together during the past year?
      3a. (If have never lived with him, check here____)
_____ 4. Is he unemployed?
_____ 5. Has he ever used a weapon against you or threatened you with a lethal weapon?
      (If yes, was the weapon a gun?_____)

_____ 6. Does he threaten to kill you?
_____ 7. Has he avoided being arrested for domestic violence?
_____ 8. Do you have a child that is not his?
_____ 9. Has he ever forced you to have sex when you did not wish to do so?
_____ 10. Does he ever try to choke you?
_____ 11. Does he use illegal drugs? By drugs, I mean "uppers" or amphetamines, "meth," speed, angel dust, cocaine, "crack," street drugs or mixtures.
_____ 12. Is he an alcoholic or problem drinker?
_____ 13. Does he control most or all of your daily activities? For instance: does he tell you who you can be friends with, when you can see your family, how much money you can use, or when you can take the car? (If he tries, but you do not let him, check here: ____)
_____ 14. Is he violently and constantly jealous of you? (For instance, does he say "If I can't have you, no one can.")
_____ 15. Have you ever been beaten by him while you were pregnant? (If you have never been pregnant by him, check here: ____)
_____ 16. Has he ever threatened or tried to commit suicide?
_____ 17. Does he threaten to harm your children?
_____ 18. Do you believe he is capable of killing you?
_____ 19. Does he follow or spy on you, leave threatening notes or messages, destroy your property, or call you when you don't want him to?
_____ 20. Have you ever threatened or tried to commit suicide?
_____ Total "Yes" Answers

Thank you. Please talk to your nurse, advocate or counselor about what the Danger Assessment means in terms of your situation.

Reproduced from Campbell, J. C. (2004). Danger assessment. Retrieved from http://www.dangerassessment.org; Campbell, J. C., Webster, D. W., & Glass, N. E. (2009). The danger assessment: Validation of a lethality risk assessment instrument for intimate partner femicide. *Journal of Interpersonal Violence, 24,* 653–674.

BOX 13-3 **HARASS Instrument**

H arassment in

A busive

R elationships:

A

S elf-report

S cale

Many women are harassed in relationships with their abusive partners, especially if the women are trying to end the relationship. You may be experiencing harassment. This instrument is designed to measure harassment of women who are in abusive relationships or who are in the process of leaving abusive relationships. By completing this questionnaire, you may better understand harassment in your life. If you have any questions, please talk with the service provider who gave you this tool.

Harassment is defined as: *a persistent pattern of behavior by an intimate partner that is intended to bother, annoy, trap, emotionally wear down, threaten, frighten, terrify and/or coerce a woman with the overall intent to control her choices and behavior about leaving an abusive relationship.*

There are no right or wrong answers. Do not put your name on the form. The instrument takes about 10 minutes to complete.

For each item, circle the number that best describes how often the behavior occurred. Next, rate how distressing the behavior is to you. If the behavior has never occurred, circle 0 (NEVER) and go to the next question. If the question does not apply to you, circle NA (NOT APPLICABLE). If you are still in the relationship please circle below MY PARTNER. If you have left the relationship, please circle below MY FORMER PARTNER.

THE BEHAVIOR MY PARTNER MY FORMER PARTNER (circle one)	0 = Never 1 = Rarely 2 = Occasionally 3 = Frequently 4 = Very Frequently NA = Not applicable **How often does it occur?**						0 = Not at all distressing 1 = Slightly distressing 2 = Moderately distressing 3 = Very distressing 4 = Extremely distressing NA = Not applicable **How distressing is this behavior to you?**					
1. Frightens people close to me	0	1	2	3	4	NA	0	1	2	3	4	NA
2. Pretends to be someone else in order to get to me	0	1	2	3	4	NA	0	1	2	3	4	NA
3. Comes to my home when I don't want him there	0	1	2	3	4	NA	0	1	2	3	4	NA
4. Threatens to kill me if I leave or stay away from him	0	1	2	3	4	NA	0	1	2	3	4	NA
5. Threatens to harm the kids if I leave or stay away from him	0	1	2	3	4	NA	0	1	2	3	4	NA
6. Takes things that belong to me so I have to see him to get them back	0	1	2	3	4	NA	0	1	2	3	4	NA
7. Tries getting me fired from my job	0	1	2	3	4	NA	0	1	2	3	4	NA
8. Ignores court orders to stay away from me	0	1	2	3	4	NA	0	1	2	3	4	NA
9. Keeps showing up wherever I am	0	1	2	3	4	NA	0	1	2	3	4	NA
10. Bothers me at work when I don't want to talk to him	0	1	2	3	4	NA	0	1	2	3	4	NA
11. Uses the kids as pawns to get me physically close to him	0	1	2	3	4	NA	0	1	2	3	4	NA
12. Shows up without warning	0	1	2	3	4	NA	0	1	2	3	4	NA

THE BEHAVIOR	0 = Never 1 = Rarely 2 = Occasionally 3 = Frequently 4 = Very Frequently NA = Not applicable						0 = Not at all distressing 1 = Slightly distressing 2 = Moderately distressing 3 = Very distressing 4 = Extremely distressing NA = Not applicable					
MY PARTNER MY FORMER PARTNER (circle one)	**How often does it occur?**						**How distressing is this behavior to you?**					
13. Messes with my property (For example: sells my stuff, breaks my furniture, damages my car, steals my things)	0	1	2	3	4	NA	0	1	2	3	4	NA
14. Scares me with a weapon	0	1	2	3	4	NA	0	1	2	3	4	NA
15. Breaks into my home	0	1	2	3	4	NA	0	1	2	3	4	NA
16. Threatens to kill me if I leave or stay away from him	0	1	2	3	4	NA	0	1	2	3	4	NA
17. Makes me feel like he can again force me into sex	0	1	2	3	4	NA	0	1	2	3	4	NA
18. Threatens to snatch or have the kids taken away from me	0	1	2	3	4	NA	0	1	2	3	4	NA
19. Sits in his car outside my home	0	1	2	3	4	NA	0	1	2	3	4	NA
20. Leaves me threatening messages (for example: puts scary notes in the car, sends me threatening letters, sends me threats through family and friends, leaves threatening messages on the telephone answering machine)												
21. Threatens to harm our pet	0	1	2	3	4	NA	0	1	2	3	4	NA
22. Calls me on the telephone and hangs up	0	1	2	3	4	NA	0	1	2	3	4	NA
23. Reports me to the authorities for taking drugs when I don't.	0	1	2	3	4	NA	0	1	2	3	4	NA
Additional harassing behaviors not listed above:												
24. _____	0	1	2	3	4	NA	0	1	2	3	4	NA
25. _____	0	1	2	3	4	NA	0	1	2	3	4	NA

Please answer a few additional questions:

_____ Your age in years

Check the statement that best describes you:

_ Married, living with an abusive partner

_ Single, living with an abusive partner

_ Married, living apart from an abusive partner

_ Single, living apart from an abusive partner.

How long were you in the above relationship? _____

Are you still in the relationship? _ Yes _ No

If you have left the relationship, how long have you been out? _____

What is your approximate annual income? _____

How many years of school have you completed? _____

Check the statement that best describes you:

_ Asian / Pacific Islander

_ Black/African American

_ Caucasian/White

_ Hispanic

_ Native American/American Indian

_ Other _____

head, and neck and recalls losing consciousness or is having a difficult time with her memory. A widely used instrument to screen for TBI is the HELPS screening tool, although it needs validity testing (Furlow, 2010). The acronym HELPS refers to the most important areas of screening around which questions should be asked (Furlow, 2010):

Have you ever:

H = been **H**it in the head or face?

E = had to go to the **E**mergency room treatment for a head injury?

L = had a **L**oss of consciousness?

P = had **P**roblems concentrating or with loss of memory?

S = had **S**ickness or other physical problems following injury?

The HELPS screening instrument cannot be used to diagnose TBI, but affirmative responses suggest further screening and assessment. The Glasgow Coma Scale (GCS) is frequently used to assess the severity of the TBI (Furlow, 2010).

Physical Examination

The physical examination of women suspected of being abused or battered should be conducted just like any other physical assessment of an adult female. Careful attention must be directed to any signs of injury, past and present, with exact measurements taken of even the most insignificant-looking bruises (Campbell, McKenna, Torres, Sheridan, & Landenburger, 1993). Because most injuries affect the face, chest, breasts, and abdomen, special attention should be paid to these areas. If the woman reports sexual violence, a pelvic examination should also be included in the physical examination. If the assault was recent, assessment by a clinician skilled in forensic evidentiary examination is warranted (see Chapter 14 for additional information on evidentiary examinations). The general examination should include observations about the patient's behavior as well as her physical appearance.

When there is a question of IPV, either past or present, it is important for the clinician to obtain a focused history and to perform a systematic physical examination to assess the severity and timing of trauma, illness, or injuries. Although any part of the body can be affected by IPV, special attention should be devoted to those systems that have been found to be most likely to suffer damage.

If there is evidence or suspicion that the patient is involved in an abusive relationship, the clinician should acknowledge the trauma and assess the patient's and her children's (if she has children) immediate safety (Chamberlain & Levenson, 2013). The clinician can help the patient develop a plan for her safety or refer her to a domestic shelter and agencies where she can obtain the help and support she needs to keep herself and her children safe.

Mental Health

The complex relationship between IPV and physical and mental health can be difficult for clinicians to diagnose. Patients may not be forthcoming with pertinent information and may seek to protect the abuser out of fear. Abusive relationships, however, can have a significant impact on a woman's mental health. Mental health problems such as depression, post-traumatic stress disorder (PTSD), anxiety, panic disorder, somatization, attempted suicide, and substance abuse can all result from IPV. Depression and PTSD are the most commonly diagnosed mental health issues among women who have experienced IPV (Agee Shavers, 2013).

Neurologic System

Assessment for traumatic brain injury—as described earlier—is essential for those women who are presenting with injury to the head of neck. Symptoms can include dizziness, memory loss, and difficulty concentrating.

Gastrointestinal System

Women who have experienced IPV often have more gastrointestinal disorders diagnosed than their peers who have not been victims of IPV. These disorders may include irritable bowel syndrome, constipation, diarrhea, stomach ulcers, and frequent indigestion (Wong & Mellor, 2012).

Sexual and Reproductive Health

Women who are victims of IPV are three times more likely to have gynecologic problems than the average woman. Gynecologic problems are considered the most consistent, long-term, and largest physical health difference between women who have and have not experienced IPV (Campbell, 2002). These problems can include sexually transmitted infections, pelvic pain, frequent urinary tract infections, vaginal bleeding, and sexual dysfunction. Pregnancy outcomes can also be impacted by IPV, with worse maternal health behaviors and more medical complications such as hypertension, sexually transmitted infections, and urinary tract infections being noted in victims of IPV.

Strangulation

Strangulation is a common and dangerous form of IPV that causes a variety of health problems and is difficult to detect (Joshi, Thomas, & Sorenson, 2012; Sorenson, Joshi, & Sivitz, 2014). It requires no weapon, causes significant pain and fear in the victim, and is a common cause of homicide death, particularly in women (Sorenson et al., 2014). Strangulation is defined as a reduction of blood flow to and from the brain due to external compression of the blood vessels in the neck (Sorenson et al., 2014). The act of strangulation symbolizes the abuser's power and control over the victim because it often leaves her struggling for air and at the mercy of her abuser (Joshi et al., 2012).

Choking is different from strangulation. Choking is an obstruction in the upper airway that is caused by an external object. The ability to inhale is impeded with choking, whereas the external pressure created during strangulation obstructs oxygen from getting to or from the brain.

Manual strangulation is one of the most common forms of strangulation used in IPV (Sorenson et al., 2014). It takes just 5 to 11 pounds of pressure to occlude the carotid arteries, rendering a woman unconscious within 1 to 15 seconds; death can occur within 3 to 5 minutes (Harle, 2012; Sorenson et al., 2014). If a woman acknowledges that she has been strangled, that admission may indicate the abuse is escalating and she is in grave danger of dying at the hands of her abuser.

Nonfatal strangulation causes immediate symptoms such as loss of consciousness, loss of sphincter control, raspy voice, and symptoms that take a few hours to appear, such as petechiae on the face and eyes (Sorenson et al., 2014; Training Institute on Strangulation Prevention, 2013). Bruising, bleeding from the ear, and other mental or physical health problems (e.g., stroke) may not appear for days after the assault (Sorenson et al., 2014). Women who report any of the following symptoms should be assessed for the possibility of IPV strangulation: loss of consciousness, change in voice (raspy voice), trouble swallowing for no known reason, breathing changes (hyperventilation, shortness of breath, exacerbation of asthma), anxiety, restlessness, and decreased ability to focus or concentrate (which can occur due to the loss of oxygen to the brain).

DOCUMENTATION

It is critical that the clinician accurately document all findings in the patient's record using the correct medical forensic terms. (See Chapter 14 for documenting forensic evidence.) Misuse of common forensic terms in the medical record can lead to questioning of the overall accuracy and competence of the clinician should legal proceedings ensue. The following is a useful summary of the correct usage of common terms:

- *Bruise* can be used interchangeably with *contusion*.
- *Laceration* is related to a partial avulsion.
- *Ecchymosis* is related to (senile) purpura.
- *Petechiae* is related to purpura.
- Rug burn is more accurately described as a *friction abrasion*.
- *Incision* can be used interchangeably with *cut*.
- *Cut* can be used interchangeably with *sharp injury*.
- *Stab wounds* are penetrating, deep, sharp injuries.
- A *hematoma* is a collection of blood that is often, but not always, caused by blunt force trauma (Campbell & Sheridan, 2004, p. 77).

Documentation in the medical record of an IPV history needs to be as thorough and objective as possible. When quoting the patient, the clinician should use such words as *states*, *says*, and *reports*, instead of *claims* or *alleges*, which can be interpreted to mean that the patient is not a credible historian (Sheridan, 2003). If a patient gives an extremely informative and powerful statement concerning the reported abuse, quote it directly in the progress note. Avoid biased documentation by avoiding words or phrases such as *refuses*, *uncooperative*, or *noncompliant*. For example, do not chart this statement: "Patient refused to talk with the police." Instead, make this chart entry: "Patient said she did not want to talk with the police."

Certain principles of medical photography should be followed when using any photographic system. As with any diagnostic procedure, patient consent is required if photographs will be taken. If the patient declines to be photographed (for any reason), this should be documented in her record. All photographs that are taken are part of the patient file and, therefore, are subject to all the rules and regulations related to patient confidentiality.

Photographic evidence of injuries can play a critical role in forensic assessment and subsequent criminal investigation (Verhoff, Kettner, Laszik, & Ramsthaler, 2012). Digital photography offers many advantages, including the ability to check the photographs immediately after they are taken and the ability to easily transfer the photographs to a computer, share them, and print them (Verhoff et al., 2012).

Three components are necessary for documenting injuries: (1) size, (2) location, and (3) a complete description of the wound or injury. Photographs of each injured area need to be taken in a series from farthest away (approximately 6 feet), to a middle distance (4 feet), to close up (2 feet) (Sheridan, 2003). A scale should appear in each photograph to assist in determining the relative size of the injury. If a scale used in the photograph shields any part of the body, an additional photograph is needed of the part of the body without the scale. All photographs should be labeled with the patient's name, date of birth, hospital chart or number, date of photograph, body part location, and photographer's name. The practice of taking a facial image to be used as an identifier is outdated: Many patients felt as if they were having a "mug shot" taken, which suggested they did something wrong.

Using body maps and diagrams is also recommended to accurately portray the patient's physical condition (**Figure 13-1**). Body maps provide pictorial diagrams of all body surfaces, including separate diagrams for external genitalia, vagina, cervix, anus, and rectum. Areas of injury should be drawn on the body maps or diagrams of the corresponding location. A description of the injury should be included with each drawing.

MANAGEMENT

Clinical interventions for patients experiencing IPV should be based on four important principles: empowerment, childbearing cycle-stage specificity, abuse-stage specificity, and cultural competence (Campbell & Campbell, 1996). Abusers take power and control away from their victims by isolating them from the people and information that can help them make thoughtful choices. Therefore, it is crucial that clinicians use an empowerment model of offering information, options, and support. Clinicians must not judge an abused woman's choices, nor should they use any kind of tactics to get her to cooperate.

An empowerment model should include the information given in the following list. Use the mnemonic device of **EMPOWER** to help remember these items:

- **E**mpathic listening
- **M**aking time to properly document findings
- **P**roviding information about domestic violence (including in later life)
- **O**ffering options and choices
- **W**orking with a domestic abuse specialist (including elder domestic abuse)
- **E**ncouraging planning for safety and support
- **R**eferring to local services (Brandl & Raymond, 1997, p. 65)

Women in ongoing abusive relationships may choose to return to the abusive home for many reasons. Prior to leaving the clinician's office, however, all patients need to know where they can find an IPV hotline and shelter information. Wallet-sized referral cards and information posters with tear-off numbers have been effective ways for women who have been abused to access helpful numbers in a manner more easily hidden from perpetrators (Sheridan & Taylor, 1993). Patients who have been abused need to be shown web addresses and pamphlets that list hotline and local shelter-referral numbers. The employees and volunteers who staff the IPV hotlines and women's service programs are experts at safety planning, and they should be called not only by the victims of abuse, but also by clinicians for guidance.

Minimum safety planning by a clinician should include a brief discussion about having the patient pack an emergency bag containing some money, clothing for the patient and her children, copies of bank records, immunization records, birth certificates, and protective legal orders. Patients should be encouraged to call the police before actual abuse occurs, and most definitely after any abusive act. Finally, every abused patient should be encouraged to use any 24-hour health setting as a safety net if she does not have access to any other safe place.

SPECIAL POPULATIONS

Adolescents

All young women should be routinely questioned about IPV during health encounters. Approximately 9% of adolescents report being hit, slapped, or physically hurt by an intimate partner (CDC, 2014; Mitra, Mouradian, & McKenna, 2013). Research suggests that high school girls and boys with disabilities are at an even higher risk for dating violence (Mitra et al., 2013).

Dating violence results in serious and negative health outcomes, with lifelong implications for adolescent victims, including depression, unhealthy weight control behavior, sexually risky behavior, development of sexually transmitted infections, and substance abuse (American College of Obstetricians and Gynecologists, 2012; Lepisto, Astedt-Kurki, Joronen, Luukkaala, & Paavilainen, 2010; Mitra et al., 2013; Silverman et al., 2011).

The simple act of asking adolescents in a private and safe location about dating violence victimization and perpetration may be an important initial step toward effective intervention and prevention strategies. Questioning teenagers in a family planning clinic, emergency department, or pediatric setting about jealous or possessive partners could provide clues to the existence of dating violence. Because many adolescents accept physical and sexual aggression as normal in dating and partner relationships, clinicians can be invaluable in providing an alternative view by talking with them about types of behavior that are appropriate in an intimate relationship. Early identification of dating violence or IPV in adolescents is critical because adolescent IPV is often associated with partner violence in adult life (American College of Obstetricians and Gynecologists, 2012).

Sex Trafficking of Adolescents

Human trafficking is a widespread problem in the United States, with approximately 80% of those exploited being women and young girls (Holland, 2014). Human trafficking is defined as the trade of human beings for the purposes of exploitation, typically in the form of commercial sexual exploitation or forced labor (Androff, 2010). It is a violation of human rights and is largely invisible, although there are probably more than 300,000 victims of sex trafficking at risk in the United States (de Chesnay, 2013). Clearly, it is a gross misunderstanding to suggest that minor sex trafficking is not a problem in the United States; indeed, domestic minor sex trafficking (DMST) is modern-day slavery of children (Kotrla, 2010).

Several factors contribute to adolescents becoming victims of sex trafficking. Adolescents who have been abused (particularly sexual abuse) or come from homes where abuse occurred are at higher risk. Other factors that place adolescents at high risk for becoming victims of sex trafficking include poverty; foster care; parental drug use; identification as lesbian, gay, bisexual, or transgender; and substance abuse (Chaffee & English, 2015). These factors make adolescents easier to recruit through the promise of money, a home, support, and being surrounded by people who care. Often the recruiter is someone the adolescent knows.

A significant number of sex trafficking victims seek health care while they are being trafficked. Unfortunately, they often go unrecognized because many clinicians are not trained to recognize signs and symptoms of such exploitation. Victims themselves often give vague or inconsistent histories; sometimes they do not want anyone to know they are victims and will work hard to avoid disclosure. However, if the victim is younger than age 18, child abuse laws apply.

Clinicians are in a unique position to identify adolescents who are victims of sex trafficking. Medical conditions that may suggest trafficking include a history of multiple partners, frequent visits for reproductive health conditions, and frequent testing for sexually transmitted infections or pregnancy (Chaffee & English, 2015). Patients who are always accompanied by someone who refuses to leave the adolescent alone with the clinician, who have no means of identification and no plausible reason for why they have no documentation, who display signs of physical abuse, and who have signs of fear or anxiety may potentially be victims of trafficking (Hodge, 2014).

Clinicians need to develop an array of effective responses when trafficking is suspected. These responses should address the adolescent's immediate need for safety as well as her immediate health issues. Clinicians need to collaborate with local welfare and law enforcement agencies and establish policies and guidelines for the identification of adolescents at risk or who are in a trafficking situation. Effective responses to victims and survivors should include trauma-informed care education (Chaffee & English, 2015). Due to the hidden nature of this crime, raising awareness and increasing the education of clinicians so they recognize signs of trafficking is essential.

Women Veterans

There is a growing awareness that a significant number of women veterans (WVs) experience IPV. As more women enter the military, it is imperative for clinicians to better understand the impact of IPV on this population and work to make its prevention a priority. It is suspected that the lack of social support for WVs combined with IPV may make for poorer health outcomes (Gerber, Iverson, Dichter, Klap, & Latta, 2014). Research has shown that WVs using the Veterans Health Administration (VA) for health services are more likely to report IPV (Gerber et al., 2014). Many of the risk factors for IPV in WVs are the same as those in women not in the military; however, the fact that they are in

the military may put women at a higher risk for IPV (Dichter, Cerulli, & Bossarte, 2011).

A qualitative study of WVs who were patients in the VA (n = 24) looked at their preferences for IPV screening (Iverson et al., 2014). The findings revealed that WVs support routine IPV screening and comprehensive IPV care within the VA, and that the team-based approach of the VA increases continuity of care and a sense of connectedness.

Women Who Are Pregnant

Many people think of pregnancy as a time of celebration and planning for the unborn child's future. Health professionals, however, have long recognized that pregnancy can be a time of escalating violence in an already troubled relationship (Campbell, 1989; Campbell & Alford, 1989; McFarlane et al., 1992; Wong & Mellor, 2012). Among pregnant women in the United States, homicide is the second most prevalent cause of traumatic death (McMahon & Armstrong, 2012). Bohn and Parker (1993) report that violence during pregnancy affects more women than hypertension, gestational diabetes, or almost any other serious antepartum complication. Additionally, women who are pregnant and experience IPV during their pregnancy are at a significant risk for postpartum depression (Bhandari et al., 2012).

Conversely, pregnancy may provide some measure of protection for some women who suffer the ill effects of IPV (Fagen, Stewart, & Hanson, 1983; Stacey & Schupe, 1983). Despite this period of protection during pregnancy, women need to be aware that the abuse may resume, and they need to understand the implications such abuse can have for both themselves and any children born into the abusive relationship (Campbell, Oliver, & Bullock, 1993). Even if the violence does not escalate, but simply continues at the rate prior to pregnancy, there are negative health effects associated with the violence for both the woman and her unborn fetus.

Complications associated with abuse during pregnancy can be the result of trauma or side effects of the psychological or controlling effects of the abuse. Mechanisms of injury are related to direct trauma to the pregnant abdomen, leading to premature labor due to rupture of membranes, placental abruption, and uterine rupture. In addition, abusive environments are associated with indirect mechanisms leading to low-birth-weight infants. Women in abusive situations are more likely than women not in abusive relationships to use alcohol, nicotine, and prescription, over-the-counter, and illicit drugs to help them deal with their stress (Curry, 1998). Low birth weight may also be due to poor maternal weight gain, anemia, an unhealthy diet, STIs, and lack of social support—all potential problems stemming from the effects of stress related to an abusive relationship. As a consequence of these mechanisms, Murphy and colleagues (2001) state that abuse should be recognized as a factor contributing to low-birth-weight infants.

Women with Disabilities

Women with disabilities may be at particular risk of IPV due to their disabilities. They may not be able to care for themselves and may be reliant upon an abusive partner, which sets up a dangerous dynamic because the power resides with the caregiver. It is important for clinicians to ask their patients who have disabilities if they are experiencing IPV. Also, many shelters are unprepared to provide the necessities needed by women with disabilities and are not trained or equipped to respond adequately to women with disabilities (American College of Obstetricians and Gynecologists, 2012). Clinicians need to identify shelters or community agencies that can support women with disabilities who are in abusive relationships.

Women Who Are Elderly

Family violence involving the elderly has been addressed by laws in all 50 states requiring the reporting of elder or vulnerable person abuse (Fulmer & Wetle, 1986). Clinicians are mandated by law to report a case if there is reasonable cause to suspect that an elderly patient has been the victim of abuse, neglect, or mistreatment. Estimates suggest that 500,000 to 1.5 million older adults are subjected to abuse and neglect each year in the United States (Brandl, 1997; Jogerst et al., 2003; Spivak et al., 2014). Accurate detection and assessment of elder patients subjected to abuse are critical duties of all clinicians, but especially those in ambulatory care settings.

Although IPV affects women of all ages, often the literature focuses on women in their childbearing years, ignoring the unique problems of aging women who are experiencing IPV. All too frequently, elder abuse and mistreatment is viewed from an inadequate care perspective—a view that obscures important issues. Some forms of elder abuse and mistreatment derive from inadequate care and are rooted in the dynamics of caregiving. Other forms of elder abuse and mistreatment, especially physical assaults, are, in fact, domestic violence. Also, the notion that elder abuse is equivalent to inadequate care obfuscates the gender issues and power dynamics inherent in IPV as they apply to older women. Serious physical and emotional harm, and even death, may result from wife or partner abuse at any age, but among older women, because of their physical vulnerability that increases with age, even "low-severity violence" can cause serious injury or death (Phillips, 2000; Roberto, McCann, & Brossoie, 2013). In an analysis of national news reports, researchers identified a higher rate of murder–suicide among older adults; most reported cases of IPV in this population involved murder in which men were the perpetrators and women were the victims (Roberto et al., 2013).

Although injury may be the reason an older woman seeks health care, it is important to remember that the physical and mental sequelae of IPV could be more subtle, including depression, sleeplessness, chronic pain, atypical chest pain, and other kinds of somatic symptoms (Phillips, 2000). Interactions with cognitively impaired or unresponsive elderly women require that the clinician assess for nonverbal cues and focus assessment on the caregiver. Characteristics of batterers that might trigger suspicion include showing possessiveness toward and jealousy of the victim, denying or minimizing the seriousness of the violence, refusing to take responsibility for the violence, and holding a rigid view of sex roles or negative attitudes toward women.

Influences of Culture

Cultural awareness is the process that allows the clinician to interact sensitively with persons from other cultures. It requires self-examination for biases and prejudices toward other cultures, and assists the clinician in avoiding cultural imposition—that is, the tendency to impose his or her own beliefs, values, and patterns of behavior on persons from other cultures (Campbell & Campbell, 1996). Cultural skill is a process in which the clinician learns how to assess the woman's cultural values, beliefs, and practices without solely relying on written "facts" about a specific cultural group. It enables the clinician to learn systematically from the woman her perception of her situation and what she believes can be done about it (Campbell & Campbell, 1996).

Women from different cultures may have a different sense or perception of what constitutes IPV. They also may not be aware of support services that are available to them and their children. Some cultures support rigid sex roles, with the male partner holding all of the power. For example, many migrant and seasonal farm workers believe a good wife is one who supports her husband, does not question his actions, and stays at home to care for the children (Wilson, Rappleyea, Hodgson, Hall, & White, 2014). Additionally, women who are immigrants may be fearful of reporting IPV because they fear deportation (American College of Obstetricians & Gynecologists, 2012).

The patient experiencing IPV may assume that a clinician from a majority ethnic group will perceive either her or her whole cultural group as stigmatized if the clinician learns of the family violence. Women of color who have been battered may be particularly afraid that a clinician who is a member of another ethnic group will call the police because, historically, police have physically assaulted men of minority ethnic groups (Campbell & Campbell, 1996). Further, women of color who have been battered may consider IPV to be a relatively unimportant issue in comparison to a serious health problem or issues of economic survival (Campbell & Campbell, 1996). Minority cultural groups often perceive IPV to be merely an outgrowth of other community problems, such as joblessness, prejudice, or substance abuse. They may consider IPV not a particularly important problem in comparison to others, or one not to be addressed in isolation (Campbell & Campbell, 1996). Thus the patient experiencing IPV may not see the healthcare clinician as a person who understands the complexities of family violence in her cultural context and, therefore, may prefer that the clinician concentrate on other areas of care (Campbell & Campbell, 1996).

When the clinician does not speak the primary language of the patient, assessing and intervening in the area of IPV may become very difficult. To prevent a breakdown in communication, clinicians should ask the meaning of unfamiliar words. Such requests for clarification demonstrate a willingness to learn and appreciate cultural nuances rather than pretending such differences do not exist or are related to a lack of education (Campbell & Campbell, 1996). The clinician must learn to listen with a sensitive ear and must accept the challenges and rewards inherent in effective cultural communications as the patient from a different ethnic group discloses her experiences.

To practice culturally competent care, clinicians need culturally competent risk assessment instruments (Messing, Amanor-Boadu, Cavanaugh, Glass, & Campbell, 2013). Even though women who are immigrants have been identified as being at increased risk for IPV, culturally competent risk assessment instruments are not always available for such populations. Messing et al. (2013) adapted the original 20-item Danger Assessment Instrument to test its effectiveness in predicting re-assault and severe IPV among immigrant women of diverse backgrounds— the first test of an adapted risk assessment tool for use with immigrant women. The findings revealed that the adapted instrument predicted risk with a much greater accuracy than the original instrument, which provides further support for attempts to adapt other instruments because the risk for this population may be different than for nonimmigrant women.

PREVENTION

Many factors are involved in the prevention of IPV. The most difficult, yet most effective, method of prevention is encouraging a societal culture change that no longer accepts or tolerates violence toward women. Clinicians can promote this change by becoming involved in making laws and policies at both the state and federal levels that encourage cessation of violence against women (Modi, Palmer, & Armstrong, 2014). The World Health Organization (2013) has stated that all forms and types of IPV are preventable with appropriate intervention by individuals, families, communities, and society in general. Clinicians play a significant role in early detection and identification of women at risk for IPV by screening and obtaining a detailed history at each and every visit.

Raising awareness and encouraging the development and implementation of evidence-based programs and practice to prevent IPV are essential in preventing violent behavior. Priority needs to be placed on the development of healthy relationships across the life span, with special focus on children and adolescents. The best hope for prevention is early education in fostering a society without IPV (Spivak et al., 2014).

VIOLENCE AGAINST WOMEN ACT

The Violence Against Women Act (VAWA) was introduced in the United States in 1994. VAWA addresses domestic violence, dating violence, sexual assault, stalking, and human trafficking. It is reauthorized every 5 years and helps shape the federal response to violence against women (Modi et al., 2014). VAWA was revised most recently in 2013 and contains many needed guidelines for Native Americans; lesbian, gay, bisexual, transgender, and queer (LGBTQ) individuals; and victims of human trafficking. Unfortunately, it stops short of providing guidelines for the growing immigrant population (Modi et al., 2014). All clinicians who provide care to women should be aware of and understand the provisions of VAWA.

References

Agee Shavers, C. (2013). Intimate partner violence. *Nurse Practitioner, 38*(12), 39–46.

American College of Obstetricians and Gynecologists (2012). Committee Opinion No. 518: Intimate partner violence. *Obstetrics & Gynecology, 119,* 412–7. Retrieved from https://www.acog.org/-/media/Committee-Opinions/Committee-on-Health-Care-for-Underserved-Women/co518.pdf?dmc=1&ts=20160219T0918473135

American College of Obstetricians and Gynecologists. (2014). Intimate partner and domestic violence: Guidelines for Women's Health Care Part III. Retrieved from http://www.acog.org

Androff, D. K. (2010). The problem of contemporary slavery: An international human rights challenge for social work. *International Social Work, 54,* 2009–2222.

Bhandari, S., Bullock, L. E., Bair-Merritt, M., Rose, L., Marcantonio, K., Campbell, J. C., & Sharps, P. (2012). Pregnant women experiencing IPV: Impact of supportive and non-supportive relationships with their mothers and other supportive adults on perinatal depression: A mixed methods analysis. *Issues in Mental Health Nursing, 22,* 827–837.

Black, M. C., Basile, K. C., Breiding, M. J., Smith, S. G., Walters, M. L., Merrick, M. T., . . . Stevens, M. R. (2011). The National Intimate Partner and Sexual Violence Survey (NISVS): 2010 summary report. Centers for Disease Control and Prevention, National Center for Injury Prevention and Control. Retrieved from http://www.cdc.gov/violenceprevention/pdf/nisvs_executive_summary-a.pdf

Bohn, D. K., & Parker, B. (1993). Domestic violence and pregnancy: Health effects and implications for nursing practice. In J. C. Campbell & J. Humphreys (Eds.), *Nursing care of survivors of family violence* (pp. 156–172). St. Louis, MO: Mosby.

Brandl, B. (1997). *Developing services for older abused women.* Madison, WI: Wisconsin Coalition Against Domestic Violence.

Brandl, B., & Raymond, J. (1997). Unrecognized elder abuse victims: Older abused women. *Journal of Case Management, 6*(2), 62–68.

Burnett, L. B., & Adler, J. (2015). Domestic violence. *Medscape.* Retrieved from http://emedicine.medscape.com/article/805546-overview

Campbell, J. C. (1989). Women's response to sexual abuse in intimate relationships. *Women's Healthcare International, 38,* 335–347.

Campbell, J. C. (2002). Health consequences of intimate partner violence. *Lancet, 359*(9314), 1331–1336.

Campbell, J. C. (2004). Danger assessment. Retrieved from http://www.dangerassessment.org

Campbell, J. C., & Alford, P. (1989). The dark consequences of marital rape. *American Journal of Nursing, 89,* 946–949.

Campbell, J. C., & Campbell, D. W. (1996). Cultural competence in the care of abused women. *Journal of Nurse-Midwifery, 41*(6), 457–462.

Campbell, J. C., McKenna, L. S., Torres, S., Sheridan, D., & Landenburger, K. (1993). Nursing care of abused women. In J. C. Campbell & J. Humphreys (Eds.), *Nursing care of survivors of family violence* (pp. 248–289). St. Louis, MO: Mosby.

Campbell, J. C., Oliver, C., & Bullock, L. (1993). Why battering during pregnancy? In J. C. Campbell & J. A. Lewis (Eds.), *Clinical issues in perinatal and women's health nursing* (pp. 343–349). Philadelphia, PA: Lippincott.

Campbell, J. C., & Sheridan, D. J. (2004). Domestic violence assessments. In C. Jarvis (Ed.), *Physical examination and health assessment* (4th ed., pp. 73–82). St. Louis, MO: Saunders.

Campbell, J. C., Webster, D. W., & Glass, N. E. (2009). The danger assessment: Validation of a lethality risk assessment instrument for intimate partner femicide. *Journal of Interpersonal Violence, 24,* 653–674.

Centers for Disease Control and Prevention (CDC). (2014). Understanding teen dating violence: Fact sheet. Retrieved from http://www.cdc.gov/violenceprevention/pdf/teen-dating-violence-factsheet-a.pdf

Centers for Disease Control and Prevention (CDC). (2015). Intimate partner violence: Risk and protective factors. Retrieved from http://www.cdc.gov/violenceprevention/intimatepartnerviolence/riskprotectivefactors.html

Centers for Disease Control and Prevention (CDC). (2016). Intimate partner violence: Definitions. Retrieved from http://www.cdc.gov/ViolencePrevention/intimatepartnerviolence/definitions.html

Chaffee, T., & English, A. (2015). Sex trafficking of adolescents and young adults in the United States: Healthcare provider's role. *Adolescent and Pediatric Gynecology, 27*(5), 339–344.

Chamberlain, .L., & Levenson, R. (2013). Addressing intimate partner violence reproductive and sexual coercion: A guide for obstetric, gynecologic and reproductive health settings (3rd ed.). American College of Obstetricians and Gynecologists and Futures Without

Violence. Retrieved from http://www.futureswithoutviolence.org/addressing-intimate-partner-violence

Cheng, D., & Horan, I. L. (2010). Intimate-partner homicide among pregnant and postpartum women. *Obstetrics & Gynecology, 115,* 1181–1186.

Curry, M. A. (1998). The interrelationships between abuse, substance use, and psychosocial stress during pregnancy. *Journal of Obstetric, Gynecologic, and Neonatal Nursing, 27*(6), 692–699.

de Chesnay, M. (2013). Psychiatric–mental health nurses and the sex trafficking pandemic. *Issues in Mental Health Nursing, 34,* 901–907.

Devries, K. M., Mak, J. Y., & Bacchus, L. J. (2013). Intimate partner violence and incident depressive symptoms and suicide attempts: A systematic review of longitudinal studies. *PLOS Medicine, 10*(5). Retrieved from http://www.plosmedicine.org/article/fetchObject.action?uri=info:doi/10.1371/journal.pmed.1001439&representation=PDF

Dichter, M. E., Cerulli, C., & Bossarte, R. M. (2011). Intimate partner violence victimization among women veterans and associated heart health risks. *Women's Health Issues, 24*(4 suppl), 190–194.

Fagen, J., Stewart, D., & Hanson, K. (1983). Violent men or violent husbands? In D. Finkelhor, R. Gelles, G. Hotaling, & M. Straus (Eds.), *The dark side of families* (pp. 49–67). Beverly Hills, CA: Sage.

Feder, G., Davies, R. A., Baird, K., Dunne, D., Eldridge, S., Griffiths, C., . . . Sharp, D. (2011). Identification and referral to improve safety (IRIS) of women experiencing domestic violence with a primary care training and support program: A cluster randomized controlled trial. *Lancet, 378*(9805), 1788–1795.

Fulmer, T., & Wetle, T. (1986). Elder abuse screening and intervention. *Nurse Practitioner, 11*(5), 33–38.

Furlow, B. (2010). Domestic violence. *Radiologic Technology, 82*(2), 133–153.

George, J., & Stith, S. M. (2014). An updated feminist view of intimate partner violence. *Family Process, 53*(2), 179–193.

Gerber, M. R., Iverson, K. M., Dichter, M. E., Klap, R., & Latta, R. E. (2014). Women veterans and intimate partner violence: Current state of knowledge and future directions. *Journal of Women's Health, 23*(4), 302–309.

Harle, L. (2012). Forensics: Asphyxia. Retrieved from http://www.pathologyoutlines.com/topic/forensicsasphyxia.html

Helton, A. (1987). *A protocol of care for battered women.* White Plains, NY: March of Dimes Birth Defects Foundation.

Hodge, D. R. (2014). Assisting victims of human trafficking: Strategies to facilitate identification, exit from trafficking, and the restoration of wellness. *Social Work, 59*(2), 111–118.

Holland, A. C. (2014). The role of the healthcare professional in human trafficking. *Journal of Obstetric, Gynecologic & Neonatal Nursing, 43*(suppl 1), S98.

Hussain, N., Sprague, S., Madden, K., Hussain, F.N., Pindiproul, B. & Bhandari, M. (2015). A comparison of the types of screening tool administration methods used for the detection of intimate partner violence: A systematic review and meta-analysis. *Trauma, Violence & Abuse, 16*(1), 60–69.

Institute of Medicine. (2011). Recommendations. In *Clinical preventive services for women: Closing the gaps* (pp. 71–141). Washington, DC: National Academies Press.

Iverson, K. M., Huang, K., Wells, S. Y., Wright, J. D., Gerber, M. R., & Wiltsey-Stirman, S. (2014). Women veterans' preferences for intimate partner violence screening and response procedures within the Veterans Health Administration. *Research in Nursing and Health, 37,* 302–311.

Jogerst, G. J., Daly, J. M., Brinig, M. F., Dawson, J. D., Schmuch, G. A., & Ingran, J. G. (2003). Domestic elder abuse and the law. *American Journal of Public Health, 93*(12), 2131–2137.

Joshi, M., Thomas, K. A., & Sorenson, S. B. (2012). "I didn't know I could turn colors": Health problems and health care experiences of women strangled by an intimate partner. *Social Work in Health Care, 51,* 798–814.

Kotrla, K. (2010). Domestic minor sex trafficking in the United States. *Social Work, 55*(2), 181–187.

Koziol-McLain, J., Garrett, N., Fanslow, J., Hassall, I., Dobbs, T., Hanare-Toka, T. A., & Lovell, V. (2010). A randomized controlled trial of a brief emergency department intimate partner violence screening intervention. *Annals of Emergency Medicine, 56*(4), 413–423.

Lawson, J. (2012). Sociological theories of intimate partner violence. *Journal of Human Behavior in the Social Environment, 22*(5), 572–590.

Lepisto, S., Astedt-Kurki, P., Joronen, K., Luukkaala, T., & Paavilainen, E. (2010). Adolescents' experiences of coping with domestic violence. *Journal of Advanced Nursing, 66*(6), 1232–1245.

McFarlane, J., Greenberg, L., Weltge, A., & Watson, M. (1995). Identification of abuse in emergency departments: Effectiveness of a two-question screening tool. *Journal of Emergency Nursing, 21*(5), 391–394.

McFarlane, J., Parker, B., Soeken, K., & Bullock, L. (1992). Assessing for abuse during pregnancy: Severity and frequency of injuries and associated entry into prenatal care. *Journal of the American Medical Association, 267*(23), 3176–3178.

McMahon, S., & Armstrong, D.Y. (2012). Intimate partner violence during pregnancy: Best practices for social workers. *Health and Social Work, 37*(1), 9–17.

Messing, J. T., Amanor-Boadu, Y., Cavanaugh, C. E., Glass, N. E., & Campbell, J. C. (2013). Culturally competent intimate partner violence risk assessment: Adapting the danger assessment for immigrant women. *Social Work Research, 37*(3), 263–275.

Miller, E., Decker, MR, McCauley, HL, Tancredi, DJ, Levenson, RR, Waldman, J.,...Silverman, JG. (2010). Pregnancy, coercion, intimate partner violence and unintended pregnancy. *Contraception, 81:* 316–322.

Mitra, M., Mouradian, V. E., & McKenna, M. (2013). Dating violence and associated health risks among high school students with disabilities. *Maternal Child Health, 17,* 1088–1094.

Modi, M. N., Palmer, S., & Armstrong, A. (2014). The role of Violence Against Women Act in addressing intimate partner violence: A public health issue. *Journal of Women's Health, 23*(3), 253–259.

Murphy, C. C., Schei, B., Myhr, T. L., & Du Mont, J. (2001). Abuse: A risk factor for low birth weight? A systematic review and meta-analysis. *Canadian Medical Association Journal, 164,* 1567–1572.

Nelson, H. D., Bougaatos, C., & Blazin, I. (2012). Screening women for intimate partner violence: A systematic review to update the U.S. Prevention Services Task Force recommendation. *Annals of Internal Medicine, 156,* 796–808.

O'Campo, P., Kirst, M., Tsamis, C., Chambers, C., & Ahmad, F. (2011). Implementing successful intimate partner violence screening programs in health care settings: Evidence generated from a realist-informed systematic review. *Social Science & Medicine, 72,* 855–866.

Parker, B., & McFarlane, J. (1991). Identifying and helping battered pregnant women. *Maternal Child Nursing, 16*(3), 161–164.

Phillips, L. R. (2000). Domestic violence and aging women. *Geriatric Nursing, 21*(4), 188–193.

Rabin, R. F., Jennings, J. M., Campbell, J. C., & Bair-Merritt, M. H. (2009). Intimate partner violence screening tools. *American Journal of Preventive Medicine, 36*(5), 439–445.

Roberto, K. A., McCann, B. R., & Brossoie, N. (2013). Intimate partner violence in late life: An analysis of national news reports. *Journal of Elder Abuse and Neglect, 25*(3), 230–241.

Sheridan, D. J. (2003). Forensic identification and documentation of patients experiencing intimate partner violence. *Clinics in Family Practice, 5*(1), 113–143.

Sheridan, D. J., & Taylor, W. K. (1993). Developing hospital-based domestic violence programs, protocols, policies, and procedures. *Association of Women's Health, Obstetrics and Neonatal Nurses Clinical Issues in Perinatal and Women's Health Nursing, 4*(3), 471–482.

Silverman, J. G., McCauley, H. L., Decker, M. R., Miller, E., Reed, E., & Raj, A. (2011). Coercive forms of sexual risk and associated violence perpetrated by male partners of female adolescents. *Perspectives on Sexual and Reproductive Health, 43*(1), 60–65.

Sorenson, S. B., & Thomas, K. A. (2009). Views of intimate partner violence in same- and opposite-sex relationships. *Journal of Marriage and Family, 71*(2), 337–352.

Sorenson, S. B., Joshi, M., & Sivitz, E. (2014). A systematic review of the epidemiology of nonfatal strangulation, a human rights and health concern. *American Journal of Public Health, 104*(11), 54–61.

Spangaro, J. M., Zwi, A. B., Poulos, R. G., & Mann, W. Y. N. (2010). Six months after routine screening for intimate partner violence: Attitude change, useful and adverse effects. *Women & Health, 50*(2), 125–143.

Spivak, H. R., Jenkins, E. L., VanAudenove, K., Lee, D., Kelly, M., & Iskander, J. (2014). CDC grand rounds: A public health approach to prevention of intimate partner violence. *Morbidity and Mortality Weekly Report, 63*(2), 38–41.

Stacey, W., & Schupe, A. (1983). *The family secret: Domestic violence in America.* Boston, MA: Beacon Press.

Taft, A., O'Doherty, L., Hegarty, K., Ramsay, J., Davidson, L., & Feder, G. (2015). Screening women for intimate partner violence in healthcare settings. *Cochrane Database of Systematic Reviews, 7,* CD007007. doi:10.1002/14651858.CD007007.pub3

Todahl, J., & Walters, E. (2011). Universal screening for intimate partner violence: A systematic review. *Journal of Marital & Family Therapy, 37*(3), 355–369.

Training Institute on Strangulation Prevention, California District Attorneys Association. (2013). *The investigation and prosecution of strangulation cases.* San Diego, CA: Training Institute on Strangulation Prevention.

Trevillion, K., Agnew-Davis, R., & Howard, R. (2013). Healthcare professionals' response to domestic violence. *Primary Health Care, 23*(9), 34–42.

U.S. Preventive Services Task Force (USPSTF). (2015). Final update summary: Intimate partner violence and abuse of elderly and vulnerable adults. Retrieved from http://www.uspreventiveservicestaskforce.org/Page/Document/UpdateSummaryFinal/intimate-partner-violence-and-abuse-of-elderly-and-vulnerable-adults-screening

Verhoff, M. A., Kettner, M., Laszik, A., & Ramsthaler, F. (2012). Digital photo documentation of forensically relevant injuries as part of the clinical first response protocol. *Medicine, 109*(39), 638–642.

Walker, L. E. (1979). *The battered woman.* New York, NY: Harper & Row.

Wilson, J. B., Rappleyea, D. L., Hodgson, J. L., Hall, T. L., & White, M. B. (2014). Intimate partner violence screening among migrant/seasonal farmworker women and healthcare: A policy brief. *Journal of Community Health, 39,* 372–377.

Wong, J., & Mellor, D. (2012). Intimate partner violence and women's health and wellbeing: Impacts, risk factors and responses. *Contemporary Nurse, 46*(2), 170–179.

World Health Organization. (2013). Responding to intimate partner violence and sexual violence against women: WHO clinical and policy guidelines. Retrieved from http://apps.who.int/iris/bitstream/10665/85240/1/9789241548595_eng.pdf

Zink, T. M., & Jacobson, J. (2003). Screening for intimate partner violence when children are present. *Journal of Interpersonal Violence, 18*(8), 872–890.

Zolotor, A. J., Denham, A. C., & Weil, A. (2009). Intimate partner violence. *Obstetrics & Gynecology Clinics of North America, 36*(4), 847–860.

The Four Phases in the Cycle of Abuse

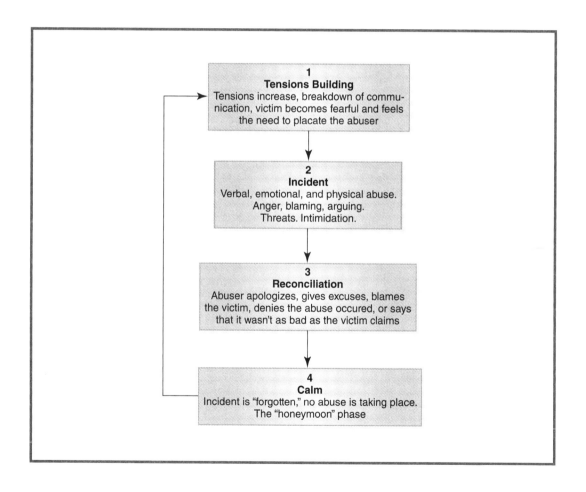

1
Tensions Building
Tensions increase, breakdown of communication, victim becomes fearful and feels the need to placate the abuser

2
Incident
Verbal, emotional, and physical abuse.
Anger, blaming, arguing.
Threats. Intimidation.

3
Reconciliation
Abuser apologizes, gives excuses, blames the victim, denies the abuse occured, or says that it wasn't as bad as the victim claims

4
Calm
Incident is "forgotten," no abuse is taking place.
The "honeymoon" phase

CHAPTER 14

Sexual Assault

Kelly A. Berishaj

The editors acknowledge Linda E. Ledray, who was the author of the previous edition of this chapter.

Sexual assault is a violent act committed in the name of power and control. It is a significant global societal problem and often leads to both acute and chronic physical and mental health consequences in victims who survive the assault (Black et al., 2011). Sexual assault and other forms of sexual violence are serious issues, and it is imperative that clinicians providing health care for women be properly educated to care for and treat a woman who is a victim of sexual violence.

Although men, women, and children can all be victims of sexual violence, this chapter focuses primarily on the care and treatment of women who have been victims of sexual violence and the management of their healthcare needs related to the assault. The chapter presents information pertaining to the health care of adolescent and adult women who have been victims of sexual assault. Care of the pediatric sexual assault patient is beyond the scope of this chapter. Children who are victims of sexual violence should receive care from clinicians who have additional specialty education and training in how to care for this vulnerable population.

The physical and psychological effects of sexual violence are presented here, along with information to assist clinicians in providing treatment according to the current standard of care. Throughout this chapter, the term *victim* is used when referring to a woman who has recently been sexually assaulted, and the term *survivor* is used when the woman has begun to heal from the traumatic event. The term *patient* is used to describe and document the health care provided to a woman who has been sexually assaulted.

DEFINITIONS

Sexual violence is an umbrella term used to refer to any sexual act, attempted or committed, against a woman who has not freely given her consent (Basile, Smith, Breiding, Black, & Mahendra, 2014). Types of sexual violence, as described in **Box 14-1**, include completed sex acts, attempted sex acts, abusive sexual contact, and noncontact sexual abuse (Basile et al., 2014).

Sexual assault is a subcategory of sexual violence that refers to a range of nonconsensual sexual acts or behavior, including rape, sexual abuse, and sexual misconduct (American College of Emergency Physicians [ACEP], 2013; Office on Violence Against Women [OVAW], 2014). *Rape* is defined as "penetration, no matter how slight, of the vagina or anus with any body part or object, or oral penetration by a sex organ of another person, without the consent of the victim" (Federal Bureau of Investigation [FBI], 2013, para. 2). The terms *sexual assault* and *rape* are often used interchangeably.

All acts of sexual violence involve a lack of freely given consent and may include situations in which the woman is unable to consent or refuse the sexual act (Basile et al., 2014). Inability to consent may occur as a result of alcohol or drug intoxication, whether the substances are consumed voluntarily or involuntarily. The woman may also be unable to consent if she is younger than the legal age of consent, has certain disabilities, or is unconscious. Inability to refuse a sexual act occurs when the victim is forced to comply under the threat of physical harm or psychological coercion (Basile et al., 2014).

BOX 14-1   Types of Sexual Violence

- A completed sex act—contact between the penis and the vulva or the penis and the anus involving penetration, however slight; contact between the mouth and penis, vulva, or anus; or penetration of the anal or genital opening of another person by a hand, finger, or an object.
- An attempted (but not completed) sex act.
- Abusive sexual contact—intentional touching, either directly or through the clothing, of the genitalia, anus, groin, breast, inner thigh, or buttocks of any person.
- Noncontact sexual abuse—abuse that does not involve physical contact. Examples include voyeurism, intentional exposure of an individual to exhibitionism, pornography, verbal or behavioral sexual harassment, threats of sexual violence, and taking nude photographs of a sexual nature of another person.

Data from Basile, K. C., Smith, S. G., Breiding, M. J., Black, M. C., & Mahendra, R. R. (2014). *Sexual violence surveillance: Uniform definitions and recommended data elements, version 2.0.* Atlanta, GA: National Center for Injury Prevention and Control, Centers for Disease Control and Prevention. Retrieved from http://www.cdc.gov/violenceprevention/pdf/sv_surveillance_definitionsl-2009-a.pdf.

No clinical definition of sexual assault or rape has gained widespread acceptance as yet (Basile et al., 2014). This lack of a consistent definition impedes the ability to accurately monitor the incidence of sexual violence and makes measuring risk and identifying preventive measures more difficult (Basile et al., 2014). It is important for clinicians to be familiar with their state's definitions of terms and corresponding sexual assault laws to ensure they follow legal dictates in their state of practice.

EPIDEMIOLOGY AND INCIDENCE

In 2010, an estimated 270,000 women were victims of sexual assault or rape in the United States (U.S. Department of Justice [DOJ], 2013b). Globally, more than one-third of the world's women have reported experiencing physical and/or sexual violence (World Health Organization [WHO], 2013b).

In the National Intimate Partner and Sexual Violence Survey (NISVS), data on sexual violence were collected from participants who were English and/or Spanish speaking and older than age 18 in all 50 states and the District of Columbia from January to December 2010. A total of 18,049 telephone interviews were conducted, with 9,970 women and 8,079 men participating in the survey; this equates to a 27.5% to 33.6% overall weighted response rate (Black et al., 2011). According to the NISVS, nearly 1 in 5 women in the United States has been raped at some point in her life (Black et al., 2011). This equates to almost 22 million women, with approximately 1.2 million of these women also reporting a victimization in the previous year. In almost 80% of cases where women experienced completed rape, the assault occurred before the age of 25, with more than 42% of victims being raped prior to age 18. Approximately 45% of the women participating in the survey also reported experiencing some form of sexual violence other than rape during their lifetime (Black et al., 2011).

The findings of the NISVS also revealed that American Indian/Native Alaskan and multiracial women had a significantly higher incidence of rape—26.9% and 33.5%, respectively (Black et al., 2011)—compared to women of other races. In this survey, 22% of black women reported that they had experienced rape, compared to 18.8% of white women and 14.6% of women of Hispanic origin.

The National Crime Victimization Survey (NCVS), conducted by the U.S. Census Bureau, collects data annually on reported and nonreported nonfatal personal and household property crime. "In 2010, about 81,950 households and 146,570 individuals age 12 or older were interviewed for the NCVS. The response rate was 92.3% of households and 87.5% of eligible individuals" (DOJ, 2013b, p. 9). Results from the NCVS for the years 1994 to 2010 (DOJ, 2013b) showed that sexual assault or rape victimization in women age 12 and older declined by 58% over this time span—from 5.0 victimizations per 1,000 females in 1994 to 2.1 per 1,000 in 2010. Despite this encouraging trend, between 2005 and 2010, women aged 34 and younger who were living in low-income, rural areas experienced some of the highest rates of sexual violence. During this same period, almost 80% of the incidents of sexual violence were perpetrated by a known individual (family member, intimate partner, friend, or acquaintance). Of women injured during a sexual assault or rape, 35% received treatment for their injuries, with 80% of the injured receiving care in a hospital, physician's office, or emergency department (DOJ, 2013b).

These statistics do not account for the probable underreporting by victims of rape and other forms of sexual violence. According to the DOJ (2013b), 65% of women who are victims of sexual assault or rape do not report the assault to police. Women ages 18 to 24 years have the highest incidence of rape and sexual assault in the nation, yet only 20% of student victims and 32% of nonstudent victims in this age group report the incident to the police (DOJ, 2014b).

CLINICAL PRESENTATION AND CONCERNS FOLLOWING SEXUAL ASSAULT

A woman who has been sexually assaulted may delay seeking treatment following the assault (ACEP, 2013). She may wait days or even weeks, if treatment is sought at all. Zinzow and colleagues (2012) conducted a study to examine the prevalence and factors associated with seeking medical care following rape. In their national sample of 3,001 adult women in the United States, 15% ($n = 445$) of the women met the criteria for the category of most-recent/only rape and of those women in that category only 21% ($n = 93$) received medical attention following their assault. Even when they suffered physical injury, only 27% ($n = 201$) of the women sought medical treatment for their injuries.

A woman may choose to delay or avoid treatment because she feels ashamed or embarrassed, or blames herself for playing a role in her own vulnerability and victimization (DOJ, 2013a). She may fear that others will not believe her story, particularly if drugs or alcohol were voluntarily consumed (Aronowitz, Lambert, & Davidoff, 2012; Carr et al., 2014). Women are also less likely to report this crime to law enforcement, seek treatment, or disclose the assault if the perpetrator was a current or former intimate partner, friend, family member, or acquaintance (Deming, Covan, Swan, & Billings, 2013; Heath, Lynch, Fritch, & Wong, 2013), which is the case in almost 80% of sexual assaults (DOJ, 2013b). A woman may avoid treatment if she is uninsured, lacks the means to pay for medical expenses, or does not have transportation. Other deterrents may include fear of retaliation from the assailant or the woman's desire to just move on from the event and avoid having to recount the assault (DOJ, 2013a).

Women who do seek treatment following sexual assault may present with a variety of acute and chronic health concerns that may be of a physical or psychological nature (Basile & Smith, 2011; WHO, 2013a). Common reasons for seeking acute or initial treatment include concern over sexually transmitted infections (STIs), human immunodeficiency virus (HIV), pregnancy, and physical health (ACEP, 2013; Zinzow et al., 2012).

Women who are survivors of sexual assault may also present with chronic health concerns, making more visits to clinicians during their lifetime compared to nonvictims (Basile & Smith, 2011; Black et al., 2011). Women who have survived sexual assault tend to have significantly higher rates of chronic pain, headaches, difficulty sleeping, activity limitations, asthma, irritable bowel syndrome, and overall poor physical and mental health (Black et al., 2011). Clinicians must be familiar with these potential variations in health to provide competent, quality care to women who are victims of sexual violence.

Acute Traumatic Injury

Immediately following a sexual assault, a woman may present with a variety of physical injuries as well as anogenital injuries, or she may have no injuries at all (Carr et al., 2014). Carr and colleagues conducted a cross-sectional descriptive study to examine time to report, resistance during the assault, and presence of injury following the assault. Their sample consisted of 317 female sexual assault victims who were examined by a Sexual

Assault Nurse Examiner (SANE) in an emergency department (ED). The largest percentage of patients presented to the ED in 4 hours or less 26% ($n = 78$) and between 1 to 5 days after the assault 28% ($n = 84$). In this study, 59% ($n = 185$) of women who were sexually assaulted sustained physical (non-anogenital) injury, 43% ($n = 134$) had anogenital injury, and 30% ($n = 95$) sustained no identifiable injury.

Injuries that are sustained during a sexual assault are generally categorized by a clinician as mild, with moderate and severe injuries occurring only rarely (ACEP, 2013). Even though the categorization may be *mild*, it in no way reflects the impact of the assault and accompanying injury on the woman's psyche—this damage is more often severe and can cause myriad related sequelae during the woman's lifetime. Injuries from sexual assault can occur anywhere on the body, including the head, neck, oral cavity, torso, extremities, and anogenital region. Mild injuries may include abrasions, bruises, tenderness, or sore muscles and generally do not require clinical intervention; however, this does not mean the woman should not be seen by a clinician for treatment and follow-up. Moderate injuries often require intervention and include superficial tears or lacerations, bites, and chipped or broken teeth. Severe injuries that require extensive clinical intervention may include deep lacerations, broken bones, and traumatic brain injury (Carr et al., 2014).

No matter which type of injury is incurred, a woman who is a victim of a sexual assault should seek health care from a clinician who is capable of caring for her and educating her about follow-up options, including counseling. Additionally, reporting options should be made clear.

Genital Injury

Statistics regarding the presence of genital injury in women post sexual assault vary greatly, with such injury occurring in 20% to 81% of cases (Anderson & Sheridan, 2012). Lacerations or tears, abrasions, and bruising or ecchymosis are the most common genital injuries found in women who are victims of sexual assault (Lincoln, Perera, Jacobs, & Ward, 2013; McLean, Roberts, White, & Paul, 2010). While any structure in the genital region may suffer trauma, the most common sites for injury include the labia minora, posterior fourchette, and fossa navicularis (Lincoln et al., 2013; Linden, 2011; McLean et al., 2010). Injury may also occur to the labia majora, hymen, vaginal wall, cervix, and other genital structures (McLean et al., 2010).

The presence of injury may depend on the time from the assault to the time of examination. Women examined within 24 hours of an assault may be more likely to have injury visualized (Lincoln et al., 2013; Linden, 2011) than women who wait a longer time, because anogenital tissue can heal in as little as 36 to 48 hours (Markowitz & Scalzo, 2011).

Astrup, Ravn, Lauritsen, and Thomsen (2012) examined 98 women following consensual sexual intercourse within 48 hours of the contact using the naked eye, colposcopy, and toluidine blue dye. They found that 34% of the women examined had an injury detected by the naked eye, 49% had an injury detected by colposcopy, and 52% had an injury detected with toluidine blue dye. "The median survival time for lesions is 24 [hours] ([confidence interval] 19–42 [hours]) using the naked eye, 40 [hours] ([confidence interval] 20–83 [hours]) using the colposcope, and 80 [hours] ([confidence interval] 21–108 [hours]) using toluidine blue dye" (Astrup et al., 2012, p. 53). The use of technology, such as the colposcope and toluidine blue dye, can increase the ability to detect anogenital injury and at longer intervals compared to the naked eye alone.

It is important to recognize that genital injury can be found in women after both consensual and nonconsensual intercourse (Anderson & Sheridan, 2012; Lincoln et al., 2013; McLean et al., 2010). While studies have attempted to link injury type, pattern, and location so as to distinguish consensual from nonconsensual sex, no definitive data on the topic currently exist (Anderson & Sheridan, 2012). Thus, genital trauma does not prove that sexual assault occurred, nor does the absence of trauma exclude the possibility of sexual assault (ACEP, 2013). A lack of anogenital injury could signify that a colposcope or toluidine blue dye was not used to detect injury, or that the injury healed prior to examination (Markowitz & Scalzo, 2011).

Sexually Transmitted Infections

The most frequently diagnosed STIs among women who have been sexually assaulted are chlamydia, gonorrhea, trichomoniasis, and bacterial vaginosis

(Centers for Disease Control and Prevention [CDC], 2010). However, because the incidence of these particular infections is also high in sexually active women, it is not always feasible to determine whether the infection was a direct result of the assault (CDC, 2010). Improperly treated chlamydia and gonorrhea can lead to pelvic inflammatory disease, ectopic pregnancy, and infertility in woman (CDC, 2010). Given these risks, it is crucial for clinicians to consider prophylactic treatment for these common infections in women following sexual assault.

Human Immunodeficiency Virus

Transmission of the human immunodeficiency virus (HIV) is also a concern of women who have been sexually assaulted. The risk of contracting HIV through receptive penile–vaginal intercourse is estimated at 8 infections for every 10,000 exposures, or 0.08% risk (CDC, 2014; Patel et al., 2014). Receptive penile–anal intercourse has a higher risk, estimated to be 138 infections for every 10,000 exposures or 1.38% risk. Receptive penile–oral intercourse has a minuscule transmission risk, much lower than other forms of HIV transmission; nevertheless, it is not a zero risk (Patel et al., 2014). Sexual assault may potentially increase the likelihood of HIV transmission if the woman suffers trauma and bleeding. Other factors that increase transmission risk are the site of ejaculation, viral load in the ejaculate, and presence of genital lesions or current STIs in the woman or assailant (CDC, 2010). All women who have been sexually assaulted should be counseled on the importance of follow-up STI and HIV testing and adherence to prescribed treatment regimens to prevent these infections.

Pregnancy

Women who are victims of sexual assault and who are of reproductive age often fear becoming pregnant. The incidence of an unintended pregnancy as a result of a rape is difficult to identify because of limited research on this topic, but is estimated to be approximately 2% to 5%, which is similar to the risk of pregnancy from a one-time sexual encounter (DOJ, 2013a). Most notably, Holmes, Resnick, Kilpatrick, and Best (1996) conducted a study to determine the prevalence of rape-related pregnancy. Of the 3,031 adult women in their

sample, 413 had experienced 616 completed rapes in their lives. Of these women, 19 became pregnant once and 1 woman became pregnant twice from two separate rapes. In this study, there was a 5% rape-related pregnancy rate in women ages 12 to 45. Prompt care for female patients following a sexual assault is critical for preventing unintended or unwanted pregnancy.

Psychological Health

Behavioral reactions following assault vary from woman to woman. Some may present with evident signs of distress such as crying, trembling, or expressions of anger. Conversely, a woman's reaction may be more composed and controlled, with minimal to no outward sign that she is in distress (Linden, 2011; Mason & Lodrick, 2013). A woman may be in shock or denial, and she may feel embarrassed or guilty, and even blame herself for the assault (Mason & Lodrick, 2013).

A woman who has been sexually assaulted may have problems providing accurate details and recalling the assault secondary to the trauma of the event and the impairment that this has on brain functioning (Campbell, 2012; Mason & Lodrick, 2013). Dr. Rebecca Campbell, who is well recognized for her research on the neurobiology of trauma, has reported extensively about how the brain responds to a traumatic event such as a sexual assault. Her work identifies that the hormonal responses mediated by the hypothalamus, pituitary gland, and adrenal glands mount a "fight, flight, or freeze" response during the assault. In contrast, the hippocampus and amygdala play crucial roles in the processing, storing, and recollection of memories. If the information is emotionally charged, such as with an assault, it becomes much harder to encode that information into retrievable memories (Campbell, 2012). Additionally, the hormones released during the stress response make recalling the details of the event even more difficult, which in turn further fragments the memories. Collectively, these effects explain why it is difficult for assault victims to recall the trauma in an orderly or organized manner. Their memory is disorganized and in pieces, and time may need to pass before they can recall the trauma, if they ever do. If alcohol was involved, there may have been no encoding of the memory so there may be nothing left to retrieve (Campbell, 2012). Educating clinicians and members of the legal and criminal justice system about the effects of trauma on memory is crucial to help support women who have been victims of sexual assault as they attempt to navigate the criminal justice system and heal from the effects of their trauma.

Psychological symptoms may become more visible and severe in the weeks and months following the sexual assault. These responses can include fear, anger, anxiety, depression, substance use or abuse, and post-traumatic stress disorder (Mason & Lodrick, 2013; Zinzow et al., 2012). Women who have been sexually assaulted are prone to more severe trauma responses when (1) the assault is completed rather than attempted, (2) the assailant is known to the woman, (3) the woman experiences a freeze reaction or is restrained and unable to move during the assault, or (4) the woman has experienced previous psychological trauma or has a history of mental illness (Mason & Lodrick, 2013).

The greatest influence on the psychological health of the woman is the response that she receives from those surrounding and supporting her. Women who are subject to victim blaming, lack of belief or support, and continued violence have more severe and long-lasting psychological impact from the assault (Mason & Lodrick, 2013).

Post-Traumatic Stress Disorder

Women who are victims of sexual violence are at an extremely high risk for developing post-traumatic stress disorder (PTSD) (Mason & Lodrick, 2013; WHO, 2013b; Zinzow et al., 2012). As many as one-third to more than half of all survivors are diagnosed with PTSD (American Psychiatric Association [APA], 2013).

In a study of 119 women who had been sexually assaulted in the previous month, a majority demonstrated high levels of probable PTSD: 78% (n = 93) at 1 month, 67% (n = 79) at 2 months, 48% (n = 57) at 3 months, and 41% (n = 48) at 4 months (Steenkamp, Dickstein, Salters-Pedneault, Hofmann, & Litz, 2012). Symptoms of PTSD generally develop within 3 months of the trauma and may fluctuate over time. As many as 50% of those with PTSD will experience recovery from symptoms within 3 months; however, some will experience symptoms for as long as 12 months to several years after the trauma (APA, 2013). The diagnostic criteria for PTSD defined by the

American Psychiatric Association in the *Diagnostic and Statistical Manual of Mental Disorders, Fifth Edition* (*DSM-5*) is in **Box 14-2**.

As many as 30% of female assault survivors who experience PTSD will use substances such as alcohol and drugs as coping mechanisms (Mason & Lodrick, 2013). These women may also engage in self-harm behaviors and injure themselves (Mason & Lodrick, 2013). More specifically, younger survivors who are from a racial minority or are bisexual report increased suicidal ideation. Additionally, women who disclose their assault have been reported to have more traumas, tend to engage in drug use, and report increased suicide attempts (Ullman & Najdowski, 2009). PTSD in general has been found to be a risk factor for completed suicide (Gradus et al., 2010). For this reason, it is essential that a clinician treating a woman who is a victim of sexual assault assess her suicide risk during the initial and all follow-up visits.

Substance Abuse

The use of alcohol, marijuana, and other illicit drugs may be factors that increase a woman's vulnerability to sexual assault, as the effects of these substances prevent the woman from being able to legally give consent (McCauley, Kilpatrick, Walsh, & Resnick, 2013; Turchik & Hassija, 2014). McCauley and colleagues surveyed 104 women, aged 18 to 61, who reported seeking medical treatment following sexual assault, regarding their substance use surrounding their assault. One-third of these women reported consuming alcohol and/or drugs at the time of their sexual assault, with alcohol being the most commonly used substance (71%). Almost 40% of these women reported passing out from the consumption, and more than 65% were too incapacitated to be in control.

Conversely, sexual assault can lead to increased substance use and abuse in women as a means to attempt to cope with the trauma (Johnson & Johnson, 2013; Turchik & Hassija, 2014). The more severe the sexual trauma (e.g., completed rape), the more likely the woman is to develop problematic substance use. Further, the substance use may lead to an increase in risky sexual behavior, which in turn puts the woman at risk for STIs and possible sexual dysfunction (Johnson & Johnson, 2013; Turchik & Hassija, 2014).

BOX 14-2 Diagnostic Criteria of Post-Traumatic Stress Disorder

Note: The following criteria apply to adults, adolescents, and children older than 6 years.

A. Exposure to actual or threatened death, serious injury, or sexual violence in one (or more) of the following ways:
   1. Directly experiencing the traumatic event(s).
   2. Witnessing, in person, the event(s) as it occurred to others.
   3. Learning that the traumatic event(s) occurred to a close family member or close friend. In cases of actual or threatened death of a family member or friend, the event(s) must have been violent or accidental.
   4. Experiencing repeated or extreme exposure to aversive details of the traumatic event(s) (e.g., first responders collecting human remains; police officers repeatedly exposed to details of child abuse).

Note: Criterion A4 does not apply to exposure through electronic media, television, movies, or pictures, unless this exposure is work related.

B. Presence of one (or more) of the following intrusion symptoms associated with the traumatic event(s), beginning after the traumatic event(s) occurred:
   1. Recurrent, involuntary, and intrusive distressing memories of the traumatic event(s).

Note: In children older than 6 years, repetitive play may occur in which themes or aspects of the traumatic event(s) are expressed.

   2. Recurrent distressing dreams in which the content and/or affect of the dream are related to the traumatic event(s).

Note: In children, there may be frightening dreams without recognizable content.

   3. Dissociative reactions (e.g., flashbacks) in which the individual feels or acts as if the traumatic event(s) were recurring. (Such reactions may occur on a continuum, with the most extreme expression being a complete loss of awareness of present surroundings).

Note: In children, trauma-specific reenactment may occur in play.

   4. Intense or prolonged psychological distress at exposure to internal or external cues that symbolize or resemble an aspect of the traumatic event(s).
   5. Marked physiological reactions to internal or external cues that symbolize or resemble an aspect of the traumatic event(s).

C. Persistent avoidance of stimuli associated with the traumatic event(s), beginning after the traumatic event(s) occurred, as evidenced by one or both of the following:
   1. Avoidance of or efforts to avoid distressing memories, thoughts, or feelings about or closely associated with the traumatic event(s).
   2. Avoidance of or efforts to avoid external reminders (people, places, conversations, activities, objects, situations) that arouse distressing memories, thoughts, or feelings about or closely associated with the traumatic event(s).

D. Negative alterations in cognitions and mood associated with the traumatic event(s), beginning or worsening after the traumatic event(s) occurred, as evidenced by two (or more) of the following:
   1. Inability to remember an important aspect of the traumatic event(s) (typically due to dissociative amnesia and not to other factors such as head injury, alcohol, or drugs).
   2. Persistent and exaggerated negative beliefs or expectations about oneself, others, or the world (e.g., "I am bad," "No one can be trusted," "The world is completely dangerous," "My whole nervous system is permanently ruined").
   3. Persistent, distorted cognitions about the cause or consequences of the traumatic

(continues)

BOX 14-2 Diagnostic Criteria of Post-Traumatic Stress Disorder (*continued*)

event(s) that lead the individual to blame himself/herself or others.

4. Persistent negative emotional state (e.g., fear, horror, anger, guilt, or shame).

5. Markedly diminished interest or participation in significant activities.

6. Feelings of detachment or estrangement from others.

7. Persistent inability to experience positive emotions (e.g., inability to experience happiness, satisfaction, or loving feelings).

E. Marked alterations in arousal and reactivity associated with the traumatic event(s), beginning or worsening after the traumatic event(s) occurred, as evidenced by two (or more) of the following:

1. Irritable behavior and angry outbursts (with little or no provocation) typically expressed as verbal or physical aggression toward people or objects.

2. Reckless or self-destructive behavior.

3. Hypervigilance.

4. Exaggerated startle response.

5. Problems with concentration.

6. Sleep disturbances (e.g., difficulty falling or staying asleep or restless sleep).

F. Duration of the disturbance (Criteria B, C, D, and E) is more than 1 month.

G. The distrubrance causes clinically significant distress or impairment in social, occupational, or other important areas of functioning.

H. The disturbance is not attributable to the physiological effects of a substance (e.g., medication, alcohol) or another medical condition.

Specify whether:

With dissociative symptoms: The individual's symptoms meet the criteria for post-traumatic stress disorder, and in addition, in response to the stressor, the individual experiences persistent or recurrent symptoms of either of the following:

1. **Depersonalization:** Persistent or recurrent experiences of feeling detached from, and as if one were an outside observer of, one's mental processes or body (e.g., feeling as though one were in a dream; feeling a sense of unreality of self or body or of time moving slowly).

2. **Derealization:** Persistent or recurrent experiences of unreality of surroundings (e.g., the world around the individual is experienced as unreal, dreamlike, distant, or distorted).

Note: To use this subtype, the dissociative symptoms must not be attributable to the physiological effects of a substance (e.g., blackouts, behavior during alcohol intoxication) or another medical condition (e.g., complex partial seizures).

Specify if:

With delayed expression: If the full diagnostic criteria are not met until at least 6 months after the event (although the onset and expression of some symptoms may be immediate).

Sexual Dysfunction

Sexual dysfunction is a common and sometimes chronic problem after sexual assault—particularly loss of sexual desire and lack of ability to orgasm (Turchik & Hassija, 2014). Sexual dysfunction may also include an inability to become sexually aroused, slow arousal, pelvic pain associated with sexual activity, a lack of sexual enjoyment, fear of sex, avoidance of sex, intrusive thoughts of the assault during sex,

vaginismus, or abstinence (Turchik & Hassija, 2014). Chapter 10 provides a thorough discussion of sexuality and the impact of stress on sexual functioning.

EVALUATION OF THE SEXUAL ASSAULT PATIENT

Evaluation of a woman who has been sexually assaulted is often referred to as the medical forensic or clinical forensic examination. Sexual assault victims are entitled to a prompt, high-quality medical forensic examination to promote healing, minimize trauma, and increase the likelihood of recovering evidence from the assault (DOJ, 2013a). The medical forensic examination should include a complete history, general physical examination, anogenital examination, and evidentiary collection.

The STOP Violence Against Women (VAWA) Formula Grant Program provides support to each state for the costs associated with the medical forensic examination. Thus the victim does not incur the cost of the forensic examination regardless of whether she has healthcare insurance. Further, VAWA, which was renewed by the federal government in 2013, ensures that women receive this examination free of charge even if they choose not to report the crime to law enforcement or participate in the criminal justice system (ACEP, 2013; DOJ, 2013a).

A National Protocol for Sexual Assault Medical Forensic Examinations—Adults/Adolescents, published by the DOJ (2013a), provides recommendations on the proper evaluation and treatment of women who have been sexually assaulted. Sexual Assault Forensic Examiners and SANE are clinicians who are specially educated and clinically trained to evaluate and treat sexual assault patients; they are recommended to conduct the forensic examination to ensure competent, quality care (ACEP, 2013; DOJ, 2013a). Clinicians treating women who experience sexual violence must be able to not only treat women's injuries and address health-related concerns, but also coordinate crisis intervention, collect evidence and maintain the appropriate chain of custody, follow jurisdictional reporting procedures, and testify in legal proceedings if necessary (DOJ, 2013a).

The clinician should ensure that a safe and private setting is provided for a woman when she is waiting for the medical forensic examination, undergoing the examination, and participating in law enforcement reporting. The woman should be asked if she would like the victim services organization to be contacted so that an advocate can be made available to offer crisis intervention, advocacy, and support to the patient before, during, and after the medical forensic examination (ACEP, 2013; DOJ, 2013a). The clinician should also help the woman to contact a support person such as a family member or friend if desired (ACEP, 2013; DOJ, 2013a). It is important that the clinician inform the woman and support person that information obtained during the history may be used to prosecute a crime; thus, support persons could be subpoenaed to testify in court. It is important that persons who are present during the evaluation do not participate in answering questions or influence the woman's answers in anyway (DOJ, 2013a).

Consent

Prior to engaging in care of the sexual assault victim, the clinician must obtain two types of informed consent. The first type is a general consent that signifies the woman has agreed to receive medical evaluation and treatment. The second type grants the clinician permission to collect evidence and gives the woman the option to release the evidence to the appropriate law enforcement and criminal justice agencies (DOJ, 2013a). The process of obtaining consent from the woman should follow agency policy, with consent usually obtained verbally and in writing in the presence of a witness.

In cases of reversible incapacitation (e.g., medication, drug, or alcohol ingestion and intoxication), the sexual assault medical forensic examination should be deferred until the patient is legally able to consent. In cases where the patient is younger than the age of consent, is comatose, or is suffering from a permanent cognitive or developmental disability, consent should be obtained from the person legally responsible for making healthcare decisions for the patient (DeVore & Sachs, 2011). It is important for the clinician to follow state statutes regarding age of consent for medical forensic examinations as well as treatment for pregnancy and STIs, as the age limit for consent for each situation varies by state.

Confidentiality and Reporting

Clinicians are required to maintain the privacy and confidentially of patient health information as outlined in the federal privacy law, the Health Insurance Portability and Accountability Act (HIPAA), unless legally mandated to report to law enforcement officials. In some states, clinicians are required to report all incidents of sexual assault; in others, reporting is required only if a weapon, such as a gun or knife, was used during the crime (ACEP, 2013). In still other states, the competent, adult victim is the sole decision maker regarding whether she will file a police report (ACEP, 2013; National District Attorneys Association, 2010).

In many states, statutory rape (sexual contact between a minor and an adult), although against the law, is not a crime that clinicians are mandated to report unless the patient is younger than the age of sexual consent and the perpetrator was a relative, caregiver, someone in a position of authority over the patient (e.g., teacher, coach, babysitter), or someone living in the same household (U.S. Department of Health and Human Services, 2006). Clinicians may also be mandated to report the sexual assault, or suspected assault, of vulnerable adults, such as the elderly or those with physical and/or mental disability.

If a clinician is unsure about the duty to report, he or she should contact the local prosecutor's office or protective services agency to find out the rules for mandated reporting. The Rape, Abuse, and Incest National Network (RAINN, 2013) has compiled a summary of relevant state sexual assault laws, which can be found on RAINN's website: https://www.rainn.org/public-policy/laws-in-your-state. Clinicians can also obtain information about state sexual assault laws from their local law enforcement agency, prosecutor's office, or State Attorney General's office.

If the patient desires to report the assault, or a report is mandated, the clinician should explain the reporting process and the clinician's responsibilities to the patient. The police should be notified and requested to come to the facility and take the report. A quiet and private area should be provided during the report, and the clinician should be available to provide support to the woman throughout the visit. Importantly, the woman should be made aware that law enforcement agencies are not bound by the same privacy and confidentially standards as clinicians. Once the patient's health information is released to law enforcement agencies, they may share that information with other members of the criminal justice system who will prosecute the case (DOJ, 2013a).

It is important for the woman to understand that she has the right to receive medical evaluation and treatment even if she declines to report the assault to law enforcement or participate in the criminal justice process. Further, she may receive this medical treatment without having evidence collected (DOJ, 2013a). The woman should also be informed that costs associated with the medical forensic examination will be covered with monies each state receives from the STOP Violence Against Women Formula Grant, no matter what her level of participation with law enforcement (DOJ, 2013a). Some women may need more time to process their options before reporting to law enforcement. The woman should be informed about the agency's policy on storing collected evidence and the process by which she may contact the agency if she decides to release the material to law enforcement at a later date.

Patient History

During the patient history or medical forensic history, the clinician should collect information related to the chief complaint, including information about the sexual assault as well as general medical information pertinent to the assault. The purpose of the history is to help guide the clinician during the physical examination, to help formulate diagnoses, and to determine a plan of care appropriate for the patient. The history further assists the clinician in deciding whether to collect evidentiary samples (DeVore & Sachs, 2011), which the crime lab may subsequently analyze.

Communication with the patient should be supportive and nonjudgmental. Avoid using language that is derogatory, is accusatory, or could be considered victim-blaming, such as "How drunk were you?" or "Why were you in that area by yourself?" It is imperative to carefully document the details provided by the patient, even those that may seem insignificant. Importantly, the clinician should use the patient's exact words placed in quotation marks when documenting the history.

Although specific questions asked in the history may vary between agencies, **Box 14-3** provides an example of the type of information that should be requested from patients who are victims of sexual assault. Such information includes pertinent medical–surgical history, medications, allergies, disabilities, immunizations, menstrual history, and recent consensual sexual contact (ACEP, 2013; DOJ, 2013a). It is important to ask the woman about her gynecologic health and variances so that the clinician can determine baseline abnormalities versus injury that could be a result of the assault (DeVore &

BOX 14-3   Information to Obtain During the Medical Forensic History

General Medical Information

- Pertinent medical–surgical history (e.g., previous anogenital injury/surgery, hysterectomy)
- History of disability
- Current medications
- Immunization history
- Allergies
- Date of last menstrual period; usual duration of menses; length of time between menses (cycle)
- Current contraception use and type
- Whether the patient had consensual intercourse within the past 72 to 120 hours; if yes, how many hours since the last consensual intercourse and was a condom used

Sexual Assault History

- Time, date, and location of the assault
- General appearance and emotional status of the patient
- Use of drugs or alcohol prior to the assault; if these substances were used, the amount of substance used
- Use of force, threat, weapon, coercion, or suspected drug or alcohol facilitation? Describe.

- Ask questions to determine if strangulation occurred. Was pressure, restraint, or force applied to the neck or upper chest with the assailant's hands, arms, or another object?
- Ask the patient about her level of consciousness during the attack. If she indicates she was unconscious, ask her to explain and document the response carefully using her words.
- Number and gender of assailants
- Ask the patient if she was kissed, bitten, or licked, and if so, on which locations
- Document orifices (mouth, vagina, anus, rectum, other) involved and attempted or completed acts
- Were objects used during the attack and if so, in which body part were they used?
- Did the assailant(s) use a condom?
- Did the assailant(s) ejaculate and if yes, where (e.g., in vagina, on clothes)?
- Has the patient bathed, showered, urinated, or defecated since the attack?
- Has the patient changed clothes since the attack? If not, document the status (condition) of her clothes.
- Ask her if there is any other information she would like to provide at this time.

Data from American College of Emergency Physicians (ACEP). (2013). *Evaluation and management of the sexually assaulted or sexually abused patient* (2nd ed.). Retrieved from http://www.acep.org/resources; U.S. Department of Justice (DOJ). (2013a). *A national protocol for sexual assault medical forensic examinations: Adults/adolescents* (2nd ed.). Retrieved from https://www.ncjrs.gov/pdffiles1/ovw/241903.pdf.

Sachs, 2011). The clinician should ask about recent consensual intercourse to rule out DNA that would be expected to be found on the woman.

Questions specific to the assault should also be explored. The purpose of these questions is not to obtain an exhaustive account of the event, but rather to collect enough information to guide the physical examination and evidence collection, and provide appropriate treatment for the patient (DeVore & Sachs, 2011). The clinician should ask the patient to identify the time, date, and location of the assault (ACEP, 2013; DOJ, 2013a). Time and date

are important because they dictate whether certain medications should be given and whether evidence is to be collected as directed by the jurisdiction of practice (DOJ, 2013a). Identifying the location of the assault may help to determine the origin of debris found on the woman. Questions regarding postassault activities, such as if the woman showered, douched, used intravaginal products, ate, drank, smoked, brushed teeth, changed clothes, or had consensual intercourse, should be asked to help explain the amount or type of evidence found on the woman (ACEP, 2013; DOJ, 2013a).

The clinician should ask about all orifices invaded and by which means; this information suggests where to look for injury and identify the possibility and presence of evidentiary material (ACEP, 2013; DOJ, 2013a). It is also important to ask about drug or alcohol consumption immediately prior to the assault to determine if the woman's ability to consent was compromised (ACEP, 2013; DOJ, 2013a). The clinician should specifically ask about loss of memory or consciousness, as the woman may be a victim of drug-facilitated rape and the testing for the presence of these substances is extremely time sensitive (DeVore & Sachs, 2011). The woman should also be asked about force or restraint used during the assault, particularly if strangulation occurred.

Psychological Assessment

The clinician should assess the woman's psychological health throughout the evaluation. This part of the evaluation can be completed by asking the woman about her thoughts and feelings and by observing the woman's behavior. Each woman copes differently with psychological trauma; thus women may present with a variety of behaviors, including anger, indifference, humor, emotional distress, or hostility (DOJ, 2013a). It is important for the woman to be given as much control as possible throughout the examination, meaning that she has the right to decline any part of the evaluation, to take breaks as needed, and to have her questions answered throughout the process.

General Physical Examination

The clinician should begin with a general head-to-toe physical examination to assess the woman's appearance, maturational stage, and general health. The body surface should be systematically examined to identify acute injury that may be a result of the sexual assault. Evidentiary collection is completed in conjunction with the physical examination and is discussed in more detail later in this chapter.

Prior to beginning the examination, the woman's clothing and undergarments should be collected if they are the same items worn during the assault, and she should be provided with an examination gown. When removing her clothes, the woman should stand on a clean sheet so that foreign material and debris that fall on the sheet can be collected as evidence (ACEP, 2013; DOJ, 2013a). Each article of clothing should be packaged separately in a paper bag and marked with her name, date, time of collection and name of the person collecting the evidence (ACEP, 2013).

The clinician should examine the woman's entire body, including her head, neck, oropharynx, extremities, and torso, looking for injury as well as foreign debris or biological fluids that could be collected as evidence (ACEP, 2013). All instances of acute injury should be documented on a body diagram (DOJ, 2013a) (see **Appendix 14-B**). Documentation should include the injury type, location, measurement, color, and if pain or tenderness is present.

Assessing the woman for signs, symptoms, and complications associated with strangulation, which has life-threatening consequences, should be included as part of the evaluation, particularly if the woman recounts that physical or mechanical force was applied to her face, neck, or upper chest. The patient who has been strangled may lose consciousness as a result of blocking of the carotid arteries or jugular veins, or closing off of the trachea, which prevents breathing (Alliance for Hope International [AHI], n.d.). The patient may present with signs such as scratches, abrasions, or bruises around the head, neck, face, eyes, ears, or shoulders. These injuries may be a result of the strangulation, or they may be defensive injuries that occurred when the patient attempted to remove the force restricting her oxygenation or breathing (AHI, n.d.). The clinician should specifically assess for the presence of petechiae on the scalp, eyes, eyelids, ears, and soft palate (AHI, n.d.).

The patient may also present with symptoms such as sore throat, difficulty speaking or swallowing, breathing problems, mental status changes, or behavioral changes (ACEP, 2013; AHI, n.d.). The clinician should inquire about memory loss, agitation, dizziness, headaches, and loss of bowel or bladder control (AHI, n.d.). Strangulation is a felonious assault and can constitute attempted homicide (AHI, n.d.). The use of an approved strangulation screening tool is recommended to ensure that appropriate and thorough documentation of the injuries is completed. **Appendix 14-C** provides the Alliance for HOPE International's Documentation Chart for Strangulation Cases.

Photographic Documentation

In addition to the history and documentation using the body diagram, the clinician may take photographs to further document the woman's injuries. Photographs may be taken with a variety of cameras dependent upon agency resources. The clinician may use a digital camera to capture images on the body surface. If available, a colposcope may be used to take photographs of the anogenital structures and/or injury.

Three photographs should be taken of each injury (DeVore & Sachs, 2011). First, a reference photograph is taken at a distance so that the body structure being photographed is identifiable. The second photograph is a close-up image of the injury, allowing characteristics of the injury to be identified. The third photograph is another close-up image, this time with a measuring device next to the injury so that its size can be documented.

Anogenital Examination

Examination of the anogenital structures should be consistent with the woman's history of the sexual assault. **Box 14-4** outlines the steps of the anogenital examination. As with the entire evaluation process, the clinician should reconfirm verbal consent with the woman prior to moving on to the anogenital examination, as it may be psychologically traumatizing and physically painful, particularly if injury is present.

Perianal Tissue

The clinician should begin the anogenital examination by visually inspecting the perianal area for signs of injury and foreign material. The woman should be put in a knee–chest position while lying in a supine, prone, or side-lying position to assist with relaxation of the anal sphincter. Several minutes may be needed until relaxation occurs.

BOX 14-4 Steps of the Anogenital Examination

1. Visually inspect the perianal tissue for injury and the presence of foreign material.
2. Photograph the perianal tissue.
3. Collect evidentiary samples from the perianal tissue.
4. Palpate the perianal tissue for pain or tenderness.
5. Apply manual traction to the perianal tissue to examine perianal folds and the anal canal.
6. Collect evidentiary samples from the anal canal.
7. Visually inspect the external genitalia for injury and the presence of foreign material.
8. Photograph the external genitalia.
9. Collect evidentiary samples from the external genitalia.
10. Palpate the external genitalia for pain or tenderness.
11. Separate the labial folds to further examine external genital structures.
12. Apply manual traction to the labia minora to further examine external genital structures.
13. Apply toluidine blue dye (to external genital structures only) to assist with identification of external genital injury that is not visible by the unassisted eye.
14. With patient consent, complete a speculum examination to assess the internal genitalia (vaginal wall and cervix). Speculum examinations are completed on post-pubescent females only.
15. Collect evidentiary samples from the internal genitalia.
16. Reinspect the external genitalia for injury that may have been caused by the speculum examination; document this finding if present.
17. Use a Foley catheter or other related technique to inspect the hymen for injury. The Foley technique is completed on post-pubescent females only.

Evidentiary swabs should be collected prior to palpating the perianal tissue, as the clinician may need to use manual traction to examine the perianal folds and visualize the anal canal. Prolonged separation of the perianal tissue may result in venous congestion or pooling, which may give the illusion that there is bruising when, in fact, there is no injury. Releasing the pressure and allowing the woman to change position will alleviate the discoloration in this area (Wieczorek, 2013). Injury occurring to any part of the anogenital anatomy should be documented on a body diagram (**Figure 14-1**) according to the times on a clock (DeVore & Sachs, 2011), with 12:00 always being closest to the urethra.

External Genitalia

The clinician should begin by visually inspecting the external genitalia for signs of trauma and the presence of foreign material. The external genitalia, or vulva, includes the mons pubis, labia majora, labia minora, clitoris, vestibule, and perineum. The vestibule, bordered by the clitoris, inner aspects of the labia minora, and the posterior fourchette, is composed of the urethral os,

hymen, vaginal introitus, fossa navicularis, and Bartholin and Skene glands (Wieczorek, 2013). Special attention should be paid to the posterior fourchette, as this is a common site for injury following sexual assault, consensual intercourse, anogenital inspection using labial separation, or speculum insertion. The labia minora, hymen, and fossa navicularis are also areas frequently injured following sexual assault (Wieczorek, 2013). See Chapter 5 for illustrations of the normal female anatomy.

The clinician should pay special attention when examining the hymen, as it may contain many folds that can mask injury. There is a myth that the hymen completely covers the vaginal introitus and once ruptured—for example, after sexual intercourse—is no longer found in women. Barring congenital defect or prior injury, all women have a hymen. The shape and presentation will differ from woman to woman and may change throughout the woman's life, particularly with hormonal fluctuations (Wieczorek, 2013).

After visual inspection of the external genitalia, evidentiary samples should be collected prior to palpation, separation, and traction of the genital tissue. When examining the hymen, the clinician may use a moistened swab or a 14 French Foley catheter, in which the balloon has been inflated with air, to better visualize the hymen and its edges (ACEP, 2013; DeVore & Sachs, 2011). It is critical that the clinician accurately document the exact anatomic location from which evidentiary samples are collected. Criminal sexual conduct laws can vary from state to state, and depending on the extent of the sexual assault (i.e., contact versus penetration) different criminal charges may apply. Finding DNA on the hymen versus the labia majora may constitute more serious criminal sexual conduct charges.

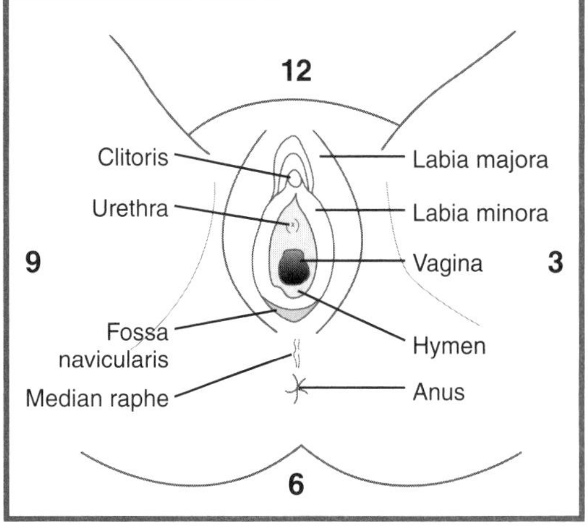

Internal Genitalia

If the woman consents, the vagina and cervix should be assessed by speculum examination. So as to not alter evidence that may be present within the vaginal vault, only warm water should be used to lubricate the speculum; lubricating gel should not be used (DeVore & Sachs, 2011). Speculum insertion should be attempted only in post-pubescent females, as pre-pubescent females

FIGURE 14-1 **Documenting anogenital injuries.**

12

Clitoris
Urethra

9

Fossa navicularis
Median raphe

Labia majora
Labia minora
Vagina
Hymen
Anus

3

6

lack a fully estrogenized hymen and contact with this area can be extremely painful (DeVore & Sachs, 2011).

Special Equipment

If available, a colposcope—a digital camera with magnifying capability—may be used during the anogenital examination to identify injury that would otherwise go undetected by the unassisted eye. The colposcope (**Figure 14-2**) can also be used to take pictures of injury or foreign material (ACEP, 2013; Rossman, Jones, & Dunnuck, 2013). Documentation of all findings should be completed on the body diagram.

Clinicians may apply toluidine blue dye, a nuclear stain, to the external genitalia and the perianal tissue as a means to highlight areas of injury not detected with the unassisted eye (ACEP, 2013). The dye is taken up by de-epithelialized tissue with exposed nucleated cells, occurring as a result of injury (ACEP, 2013; DeVore & Sachs, 2011). Areas of injury will appear deep, royal blue (Rossman et al., 2013). The toluidine blue dye should be applied to external structures only, and prior to the insertion of a speculum. The dye can be removed with lubricating jelly or a 1% acetic acid solution. The dye and acetic acid solution may be irritating to the woman's skin, particularly on areas of injury (DeVore & Sachs, 2011).

Evidentiary Collection

Evidentiary samples are collected if indicated by the patient's history in conjunction with the physical and anogenital examinations. Evidence should be collected following inspection of the area and prior to palpation or physical manipulation of the tissue. The clinician should use an evidentiary collection kit (**Figure 14-3**) and follow the provided instructions, which detail how evidence should be collected, preserved, sealed, and stored. At a minimum, the kit should contain an instruction sheet, documentation forms, and materials for collecting evidence such as clothing, hair, oral/anogenital swabs/smears, body swabs, urine/blood samples for toxicology or alcohol testing, and blood or saliva samples for DNA testing (DOJ, 2013a).

It is important for clinicians to know their agency's policy on evaluation of sexual assault victims, as institutions may differ on how long evidence should be collected after the time of the assault. Some jurisdictions may request evidence collection up to 72 hours after the assault; however, with advances in DNA technology, other areas are collecting evidence as long as 120 hours post assault (ACEP, 2013; DOJ, 2013a). Whether or not evidence is collected, all women who seek treatment following sexual assault should be evaluated and treated according to their specific healthcare needs (DOJ, 2013a).

This discussion provides general guidelines for evidentiary collection; however, clinicians should follow the policies, protocols, and procedures established in their jurisdiction of practice. The clinician should always wear gloves when examining the patient and collecting samples, and should change gloves when moving to different body sites to limit the transfer of DNA (ACEP, 2013). All wet samples should be air-dried before being packaged. Evidence should be placed in paper bags or containers, as packaging in plastic can facilitate mold and bacterial growth, which could then degrade biological material (DeVore & Sachs, 2011; DOJ, 2013a).

It is the responsibility of the clinician to maintain the chain of custody—that is, control over the evidence—during collection and when sealing and storing the evidence kit (Devore & Sachs, 2011; DOJ, 2013a). The chain of custody is the

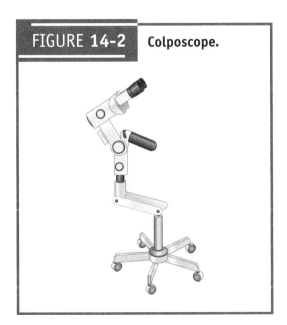

FIGURE **14-2** **Colposcope.**

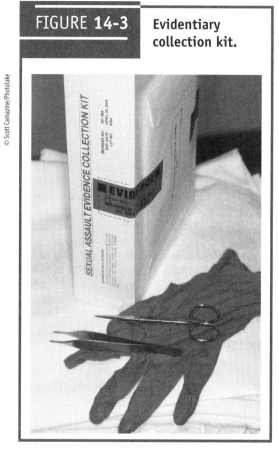

FIGURE 14-3   Evidentiary collection kit.

© Scott Camazine/Phototake

chronological documentation that describes the seizure, custody, control, transfer, analysis, and disposition of evidence collected. Such evidence can be used in court to convict persons of crimes, so it must be handled in a specific and careful manner. The chain of custody is intended to establish that the evidence collected is related to the crime and was not put there by someone else to make a person appear guilty (DOJ, 2013a). Clinicians should know their agency's policy regarding safely storing evidence if the kit will not be immediately turned over to law enforcement.

Known Sample

A known sample from the woman should be collected so that the woman's DNA can be compared

to non-self DNA found on her body. The clinician may be required to collect a buccal swab or a blood sample for this purpose. If there is a history of oral penetration, a blood sample may be recommended, as the buccal sample could be contaminated with the assailant's DNA (DOJ, 2013a).

Hair Samples

The evidentiary kit may contain a paper towel, comb, and envelope to collect head hair and pubic hair combings. Hair should be combed over a towel or paper so that loose hair or foreign material may be collected as evidence. The clinician may consider allowing the woman to complete these acts while supervising.

Reference hair samples are sometimes collected; these samples are compared to samples taken from the hair combings. As many as 15 to 30 hairs must be pulled from various areas of the scalp or pubic region as reference samples. The patient should be given the option to decline collection of reference hair, as this can be collected at a later time if needed to prosecute a criminal case (DOJ, 2013a).

Body Samples

While completing the physical examination, the clinician may find cause to collect evidentiary samples from the woman's body surface. The clinician should collect any material from the woman's body that may have originated from another person or from the scene of the assault, such as fibers, hair, or dried secretions (DOJ, 2013a).

The use of an alternative light source may be helpful in detecting evidence, as body fluids will notably fluoresce under ultraviolet (UV) light (ACEP, 2013). Dried secretions may include saliva, seminal fluid, blood, vomit, urine, or fecal matter. To collect dried secretions, the clinician should moisten a swab with sterile water or saline and then roll the swab over the area, completely covering the swab surface. This process should be repeated with a second dry swab. Swabs may also be used to remove material from under the woman's fingernails.

Oral and Anogenital Swabs and Smears

Samples from the oral cavity, external and internal genitalia, and perianal area may be taken with either an oral swab or a smear based on the woman's history of sexual assault. If the woman is unable to provide a history of the assault as a result of incapacitation or memory loss, all orifices should be swabbed (DOJ, 2013a).

The number of swabs used will depend on the recommendations in the jurisdiction of practice. The clinician should swab the identified orifice and then may be required to prepare a slide by swiping the swabs in a circular manner around the target area on the slide. Both the swabs and the slide should be allowed to at least partially air-dry, while avoiding contact or contamination from other objects or substances (DOJ, 2013a). Once dry, the slide should be housed in the slide holder and closed, and the swabs should be placed in the swab box. The swab box is then placed in the appropriate envelope and sealed according to jurisdictional policy.

Documentation

Thorough documentation by the clinician is crucial. The clinician may be responsible for documenting the results of the examination in both the patient's medical record and the evidence collection kit report. The medical record includes all information from the patient's admission, whereas the evidence kit report includes only the evidence collection consent form, a history of the assault, and information pertaining to evidence collection to assist the crime lab in analyzing samples. Only medical information that could affect evidentiary findings should be included in the kit report. If the sexual assault is reported to law enforcement, the evidence collection kit and report will be provided to the law enforcement agency as well as the state crime laboratory. The patient's medical record is not part of the evidence kit and should not be released to the aforementioned agencies (DOJ, 2013a).

Diagnostic Testing

Sexually Transmitted Infections

Treating patients prophylactically is often preferable to performing STI testing unless the woman presents with signs and symptoms consistent with an STI. Women who are evaluated soon after the sexual assault may not test positive for an STI, as the infectious agent may not be present in significant quantity to illicit a positive result (CDC, 2010). Testing at this time would more than likely detect STIs the woman had prior to the assault; thus

testing is often deferred and prophylactic treatment is provided with follow-up recommendations (CDC, 2010).

The CDC (2010) recommends that women who are tested for STIs have nucleic acid amplification testing (NAAT), which can detect the presence of *Chlamydia trachomatis* and *Neisseria gonorrhoeae*—the organisms responsible for chlamydia and gonorrhea, respectively. The sample can be collected via vaginal swab. A wet mount and culture of the swab can also be tested for *Trichomonas vaginalis* and examined for bacterial vaginosis and candidiasis (CDC, 2010).

Based on the exposure risk, a baseline serum sample for HIV, hepatitis B virus (HBV), and syphilis may be indicated (CDC, 2010). In women who have previously received the HBV vaccine, titers should be drawn to determine immunization status. Those who receive initial STI testing should receive follow-up testing 1 to 2 weeks after the assault. Follow-up testing for HIV and syphilis is recommended at 6 weeks, 3 months, and 6 months (CDC, 2010).

Pregnancy

A baseline pregnancy test should be performed on all women of childbearing age prior to the administration of oral contraceptives and antibiotics, as the results may impact treatment options.

Drug-Facilitated Sexual Assault

Alcohol and other drugs, such as benzodiazepines and gamma-hydroxybutyrate (GHB), may be used to incapacitate a woman and facilitate sexual assault. Toxicology is not routinely performed unless indicated by the woman's history and when drug-facilitated sexual assault (DFSA) is suspected (DOJ, 2013a). Testing for DFSA should be conducted in cases where the woman is unable to recall details of the assault or state whether an assault even occurred even though she has missing clothing, is experiencing genital pain, or suspects that she may have been victimized (DeVore & Sachs, 2011). The woman who has been subjected to DFSA may also be lethargic, light-headed, or confused; have motor impairment; or be hemodynamically unstable (DOJ, 2013a).

Drugs used to facilitate sexual assault are typically cleared from the body quickly; therefore, samples should be taken as soon as possible from the urine and blood as indicated (DOJ, 2013a). Most drugs clear more quickly from the bloodstream, so the first available urine sample is preferred as evidence: The drug is more concentrated and readily detected in the first sample. Clinicians should collect 30 to 100 mL of urine if DFSA is suspected within the last 96 hours and 20 mL of blood if DFSA is suspected within the last 24 hours (DOJ, 2013a). Toxicology samples are collected separately from the evidence collection kit, as the samples may be tested in different labs. If not immediately tested, the toxicology samples should be refrigerated. Similar to the discussion about evidence collection, the chain of custody should be maintained for toxicology samples that may be related to a crime (DOJ, 2013a).

MANAGEMENT

Psychological Health

During the initial evaluation, the clinician must make an assessment of the woman's psychological health sufficient to determine the level of orientation, possible suicidal ideation, and need for referral for follow-up support, evaluation, or treatment. During this evaluation, the woman may or may not present with outward signs of psychological distress. The clinician should inform the woman that any type of psychological response is normal and that her thoughts, feelings, and behavior may fluctuate or change over time (Mason & Lodrick, 2013).

A referral to a community-based agency that specializes in long-term management and care of the psychological needs of sexual assault victims should be offered. A "watchful waiting" approach may be implemented over several months, in which the woman engages in follow-up appointments with the referred agency (WHO, 2013a). If during these appointments it is determined that the woman is suffering from alcohol or drug abuse, depression, psychotic symptoms, or suicidal ideation; is self-harming; or is unable to participate in day-to-day activities, referral to a qualified mental health clinician is recommended (WHO, 2013a).

Pharmacologic Management

Sexually Transmitted Infection Prevention

The Centers for Disease Control and Prevention (2010) recommends administration of the HBV vaccine at the time of initial evaluation in the woman who has not been previously vaccinated. Follow-up vaccination should be provided at 1 to 2 months and 4 to 6 months to complete the series of three vaccinations. Hepatitis B immune globulin (HBIG) may be recommended to the woman who is not fully vaccinated at the time of the assault after a high-risk exposure involving an assailant known to have hepatitis B (CDC, 2010).

Antibiotic therapy should be administered to prevent chlamydia, gonorrhea, and trichomoniasis infections. Recommendations include (1) a single dose of ceftriaxone 250 mg IM or cefixime 400 mg orally for gonorrhea; (2) a single dose of azithromycin 1 g or doxycycline 100 mg twice daily for 7 days orally for chlamydia and gonorrhea; and (3) a single dose of metronidazole 2 g orally for trichomoniasis (CDC, 2010). Metronidazole should not be given to women who have consumed alcohol within the past 24 hours.

Importantly, *N. gonorrhoeae* has become increasingly resistant to antibiotics, specifically fluoroquinolones. Cephalosporins are the only class of antibiotics that currently meet the efficacy standards set by the CDC to treat gonorrhea (CDC, 2010). *N. gonorrhoeae* is also becoming less susceptible to cephalosporins; thus the CDC recommends dual therapy with ceftriaxone and either azithromycin or doxycycline to prevent and treat gonorrhea.

Women need to be educated on the importance of refraining from sexual contact until the prescribed treatment regimen is completed. They should also be educated on identification of the signs and symptoms of STIs so that evaluation and treatment can be sought if they develop.

HIV Prevention

The clinician should consider several factors when deciding whether to recommend HIV nonoccupational post-exposure prophylaxis (nPEP) to a woman who has been sexually assaulted. Factors that increase the likelihood of HIV transmission include risk behaviors in the assailant (e.g., IV drug use, men who have sex with men) and high-risk characteristics of the assault (e.g., vaginal or anal penetration, ejaculation on mucous membranes) (CDC, 2010). An assault by multiple assailants or the presence of genital lesions or ulcers on the assailant or woman also increases the possibility of transmission. It is important for the clinician to inform the woman of the known toxicity of antiretroviral drugs and that close follow-up while taking the nPEP regimen is recommended. This information enables the patient to make an educated decision on whether she would like to begin nPEP therapy (CDC, 2010).

To be effective, the nPEP regimen should be initiated as soon as possible; it may be given up to 72 hours after the sexual assault (CDC, 2010). A 28-day course of antiretroviral medications is generally prescribed. Clinicians should refer to the local infectious disease guidelines in their agency of practice for medication selection and dosing; however, the U.S. Public Health Service Working Group recommends prescription of a combination of three or more antiretroviral agents (Kuhar et al., 2013). Currently, the preferred standard regimen includes the use of Truvada (combination of tenofovir 300 mg and emtricitabine 200mg) once daily plus Isentress (raltegravir 400mg) twice daily *or* Truvada once daily plus Tivicay (dolutegravir 50 mg) once daily (Kuhar et al., 2013). If the clinician and woman decide to initiate nPEP therapy, the woman should be given a 3- to 5-day supply of medication—enough to last until her follow-up appointment, preferably with an infectious disease specialist (CDC, 2010).

Pregnancy Prevention

All women who have been sexually assaulted need to be informed of the risk of conception and the availability of emergency contraception. Emergency contraceptive (EC) therapy is highly effective if administered to the woman who seeks treatment immediately following sexual assault; it may be given within 120 hours of the assault, although its efficacy decreases with time (WHO, 2013a). A single, oral dose of 1.5 mg of levonorgestrel (Plan B, Next Choice), a progestogen-only EC, is recommended if available (WHO, 2013a), as it has a higher efficacy rate, greater ease of use, and less nausea and vomiting compared with other medications (DOJ, 2013a). Levonorgestrel may also be given in two doses of 0.75 mg 12 to 24 hours apart (WHO, 2013a). If levonorgestrel is unavailable, the clinician may offer a combined estrogen–progestogen regimen (WHO, 2013a), such as ethinyl estradiol and norgestrel in 2 tablets (0.05 mg ethinyl estradiol and 0.5 mg norgestrel) orally at the time of examination,

with a repeat dose of 2 tablets given 12 hours later (DeVore & Sachs, 2011). An antiemetic agent may be offered given that nausea and vomiting may occur, although this is more commonly observed with estrogen–progestogen ECs (WHO, 2013a).

Other Medications

Pain medication should be offered if indicated. The type of medication will depend on the severity of the woman's injury, but a nonsteroidal anti-inflammatory drug (NSAID) or acetaminophen is often sufficient for minor injury. The woman may be given an antiemetic agent, as a common side of effect of antibiotics, emergency contraceptives, and antiretrovirals is gastrointestinal distress. If the woman vomits within 3 hours of receiving emergency contraception, it may be suggested that she take an additional dose of EC to ensure its efficacy. If the woman sustained a bite or injury from a foreign object, a tetanus shot may also be recommended.

Referral to Sexual Assault Forensic Examiners

Recommendations by the Department of Justice (2013a) are that clinicians serving as examiners of sexual assault victims should have advanced knowledge and skill, as well as certification, in this specialty area of practice. If the clinician has not received the appropriate education and clinical training, referral to a Sexual Assault Forensic Examiner (SAFE) should be initiated if available. A SAFE may be any clinician who has completed the required didactic and clinical training to care for sexual assault patients. Oftentimes this role is assumed by a registered nurse, referred to as a Sexual Assault Nurse Examiner (SANE). The SANE performs all of the components of the medical forensic examination, psychological and physical management of the patient, and relevant patient education. The International Association of Forensic Nurses (IAFN) provides education guidelines and certification requirements for SANEs. For more information about the education, certification, and role of the SANE, refer to the IAFN's website (http://www.iafn.org).

It is recommended that a clinician trained in sexual assault evaluation and treatment should be available at all times, either on call or on location, in facilities that evaluate patients who have experienced sexual assault (WHO, 2013a). The major benefit of having a SAFE/SANE is that a standardized approach to evaluation, treatment, and evidence collection is employed, assuring patients receive quality, competent healthcare services (ACEP, 2013).

Patient Education

Prior to discharge, the woman should receive oral and written instructions regarding the care she received during her evaluation. Education should be provided regarding the importance of medical follow-up and the availability of victims' advocacy services. The clinician should also ask about safety concerns and, if necessary, facilitate referral to the appropriate agencies to assist with developing a safety plan for the woman.

MEDICAL FOLLOW-UP

The clinician must impress upon the woman the importance of routine follow-up after the initial examination. Medical follow-up should occur within 1 to 2 weeks after the assault (CDC, 2010). During this follow-up, the woman is assessed for the presence of STIs acquired during the assault, completes treatment for other STIs, completes hepatitis B immunization if indicated, and is assessed for side effects and adherence to the prescribed treatment regimen (CDC, 2010; DOJ, 2013a). The clinician should offer information to the woman on how to obtain these follow-up services if she does not have a primary care provider, does not have health insurance, or is afraid to disclose the assault to her usual clinician. It is recommended that the clinician or healthcare agency contact the woman by phone or text message within 24 to 48 hours following the initial evaluation, as this step may increase compliance with the prescribed treatment regimen and follow-up services (DOJ, 2013a).

ADVOCACY SERVICES

The woman should be made aware of the various services that the victims' advocacy agency can provide to help her deal with the acute and chronic sequelae of sexual violence (DOJ, 2013a). Advocates can serve as a support person, offer crisis intervention, provide information and referrals, and help ensure the woman's rights and wishes are respected. Long-term resources such as counseling, support groups, and legal advocacy may also be offered (DOJ, 2013a).

SAFETY PLANNING

The clinician should assist the woman with contacting local law enforcement to file a report of the assault if she desires. The clinician may also partner with law enforcement officials and advocacy agencies to develop a plan to help ensure the woman's safety following sexual assault. Making sure the woman has a safe place to stay and a support system in place is important for both the physical and psychological health of the woman. If necessary, the victim services' agency may be able to assist with finding emergency shelter or an alternative living arrangement if it is unsafe for the woman to return home. It may also be able to provide legal advocacy services, including assisting the woman with obtaining a personal protection order and providing information and support while she is participating in legal proceedings (DOJ, 2013a).

SPECIAL CONSIDERATIONS

Certain populations of sexual assault victims deserve special consideration because they may have higher levels of vulnerability than other victim groups. In particular, special consideration should be given to the age of the victim (children, adolescents, elderly), any disability (physical and cognitive), the gender and sexual orientation of the victim, and relevant cultural issues.

Age

The age of the victim is important for many reasons. The very young and the very old may not have opportunities to report sexual violence if they are in a situation in which they are living with the perpetrator. They may exhibit a sense of loyalty to the abuser if they rely on the abuser for food, shelter, and basic needs. Such victims may also be physically unable to leave the situation and find someone to whom they can report the sexual assault. The abuse in such cases may have occurred over an extended period of time—months or even years; as a result, the collection of forensic evidence may not be possible at the time of the examination.

Sexual assault of the elderly occurs more frequently in an institutional setting than in the home (ACEP, 2013). Elderly women tend to experience more genital injuries as a result of their decreased estrogen levels (ACEP, 2013). The elderly in general are more likely to have bruising related to the effects of aging and medication use. Further, impairments in memory may prohibit accurate retelling of the assault, and physical decline can make the actual examination process more difficult (ACEP, 2013).

Most states have mandatory reporting laws that apply to children and elderly victims of abuse. Clinicians should ensure that they are familiar with the laws in their state of practice.

Disability

People with disabilities are almost three times as likely to experience violent victimization (60 per 1,000) compared to those without disability (22 per 1,000) (DOJ, 2014a). Persons with cognitive disability suffer the highest incidence of violent victimization. In individuals with cognitive or developmental disability, there may be issues with obtaining informed consent to perform a forensic examination. It is best if the clinician is experienced in interviewing individuals with disabilities; alternatively, individuals with specialized interviewing skills may be called upon to obtain consent and assist with collection of the medical forensic history.

In persons with communication or physical disabilities, the clinician should ensure that the patient has access to adaptive devices. If caretakers or family are requested by the patient to be present during the examination, it is crucial to minimize the influence of these individuals over the patient when relating the history of the assault. In the case of communication deficits, the use of an independent interpreter with no personal relationship to the patient may be required (DOJ, 2013a).

Reporting the sexual abuse of disabled persons is mandated in every state.

Persons Who Are Lesbian, Gay, Bisexual, or Transgender

Similar to other victims, many lesbian, gay, bisexual, and transgender (LGBT) persons who are sexually assaulted do not report the assault. This failure or resistance to reporting may result from a fear of possible homophobic response or "outing" of their sexual orientation or gender identity (ACEP, 2013). To provide quality care to the LGBT population, forms that ask for gender or sex should be left open so that patients can fill in the term that best represents them. Forms should also provide for differentiation between gender identity and sex of the patient, which may not always coincide (DOJ, 2013a). The patient's preferred name and pronoun should always be used.

It is critical to maintain professionalism and to avoid outward demonstrations of surprise, shock, or disapproval if a patient reveals that she is transgender (DOJ, 2013a). Patients who are transgender may demonstrate increased shame or disassociation with their body parts. Vaginas that have been surgically created or that have been exposed to testosterone may be more fragile and, therefore, may demonstrate increased injury from a sexual assault (DOJ, 2013a). Male patients who are transgender and who still have ovaries and a uterus may become pregnant after the assault, so emergency contraceptive should be offered. There may also be higher rates of self-harm in the transgender population as a means to cope (DOJ, 2013a).

When providing referrals for after-care, it is important to recommend agencies that are skilled in providing care to the LGBT population. It is also critical for clinicians to appreciate the diversity of LGBT individuals so that care focuses on the needs of the person. See Chapter 9 for further discussion on health care for patients who identify as LGBT.

Culture

Cultural values and beliefs vary greatly and may play a role in whether a woman reports the assault and how she deals with the psychological and physical aftermath of the assault. Clinicians must be cognizant that these differences exist and be willing to adapt care to address the cultural needs of women during the provision of services.

Women of different racial or ethnic backgrounds may fear or distrust the healthcare system or may worry about confidentiality and receiving fair, unbiased treatment (DOJ, 2013a). Immigrants, for example, may worry about the assault being reported to law enforcement and the impact that this would have on their presence in the country.

Clinicians should educate their patients on the process of applying for a U-Visa. The U-Visa allows immigrants who are victims of serious crime, including sexual assault, and who work with law enforcement, to obtain temporary, legal status to reside and work in the United States (U.S. Citizenship and Immigration Services, 2014). The U-Visa is intended to encourage victims of crimes to speak up and participate in legal proceedings without fear of repercussion.

In some cultures, it is considered taboo to be touched or seen by opposite-sex clinicians. In such a case, it may beneficial to have a same-sex clinician or someone of the same culture provide care for the woman. For some, the loss of virginity prior to marriage—even as a result of an assault—could lead to the woman being shunned by her family or even prevent her from marrying (DOJ, 2013a). Sexual assault in these instances may be a source of significant shame and embarrassment.

Women of different ethnicities may have the added barrier of limited English language proficiency. Any such difficulty in communicating may be exacerbated by the stress of the assault. It is important to make necessary accommodations for the woman's communication needs by offering a clinician who speaks the woman's language or utilizing interpreter services (DOJ, 2013a).

Prevention

Clinicians will most often provide medical services to women who are victims of sexual violence. Nevertheless, clinicians should be expected to begin their involvement at the primary prevention level, so as to stop sexual violence from occurring. Clinicians can participate in primary sexual violence prevention by applying individual prevention skills, such as challenging behaviors in others that promote violence, engaging in healthy professional and personal relationships, and learning to identify risk factors for sexually abusive behaviors (IAFN, n.d.). At an organizational level, the clinician can participate in efforts to make the workplace an environment of zero tolerance for violence and harassment (IAFN, n.d.). The clinician may also assist in the education of facility administration and staff regarding sexual violence by presenting in-service programs on primary prevention strategies.

To have an impact on the incidence of sexual violence and effectively participate in prevention efforts, clinicians must receive proper education and training (Academy on Violence and Abuse [AVA], 2007). Unfortunately, the academic curriculum, particularly in medicine, is deficient in providing content addressing sexual violence. Because violence is an overarching issue that does not belong to a single practice specialty, the topic of violence must be covered throughout program curriculum (AVA, 2007). Oftentimes, the care of patients who have been exposed to violence falls under forensics, but forensic education may not be part of an undergraduate academic curriculum and is more often offered at the graduate or continuing education level.

To provide the necessary education, experts in the field of sexual violence must lend their knowledge to those educating new clinicians (AVA, 2007). It will also be up to clinicians to independently seek out educational opportunities to expand their practice expertise. Education should include bystander intervention strategies and methods to facilitate the development of sexual violence prevention strategies across the healthcare community (IAFN, n.d.).

CONCLUSION

Sexual violence perpetrated against women continues to be a significant public health concern in the United States and globally. Clinicians must be properly educated and trained to address the physical and psychological needs of women who have been sexually assaulted and have the courage to seek treatment in a healthcare setting. It is recommended that clinicians advocate for and follow a written policy in their place of practice when caring for women in all cases involving suspected or known sexual assault. This may include the completion of a medical forensic examination and possible evidence collection if the woman desires this type of evaluation. The clinician must also consider the need for STI, HIV, and pregnancy testing and treatment. Clinicians should also be familiar with mandatory reporting requirements and laws pertaining to consent for treatment to ensure they are following the legal mandates in their state of practice.

Clinicians should seek out formal education and clinical training that prepares them to best care for patients who have been sexually assaulted. If available, clinicians may consider referral of the patient to a SAFE/SANE to ensure the woman receives appropriate treatment and services that follow the current standard of care. Education should also be provided to the patient regarding the importance of medical follow-up, the availability and resources provided by victims' advocacy services, and the importance of a safety plan. The care that the clinician provides can make a significant positive difference for the woman who has suffered a sexual assault.

References

Academy on Violence and Abuse (AVA). (2007). Building academic capacity and expertise in the health effects of violence and abuse: A blueprint for advancing professional health education. Retrieved from http://www.avahealth.org/resources/ava_publications

Alliance for Hope International (n.d.). Training institute on strangulation prevention. Retrieved from http://www.allianceforhope.com

American College of Emergency Physicians (ACEP). (2013). *Evaluation and management of the sexually assaulted or sexually abused patient* (2nd ed.). Retrieved from http://www.acep.org/resources

American Psychiatric Association (APA). (2013). *Diagnostic and statistical manual of mental disorders* (5th ed.). Washington, DC: Author.

Anderson, J. C., & Sheridan, D. J. (2012). Female genital injury following consensual and nonconsensual sex: State of the science. *Journal of Emergency Nursing, 12*(38), 518–522.

Aronowitz, T., Lambert, C. A., & Davidoff, S. (2012). The role of rape myth acceptance in the social norms regarding sexual behavior among college students. *Journal of Community Health Nursing, 29*, 173–182.

Astrup, B. S., Ravn, P., Lauritsen, J., & Thomsen, J. L. (2012). Nature, frequency, and duration of genital lesions after consensual sexual intercourse: Implications for legal proceedings. *Forensic Science International, 219*(1), 50–56.

Basile, K. C., & Smith, S. G. (2011). Sexual violence victimization of women: Prevalence, characteristics, and the role of public health and prevention. *American Journal of Lifestyle Medicine, 5*(5), 407–417.

Basile, K. C., Smith, S. G., Breiding, M. J., Black, M. C., & Mahendra, R. R. (2014). *Sexual violence surveillance: Uniform definitions and recommended data elements, version 2.0.* Atlanta, GA: National Center for Injury Prevention and Control, Centers for Disease Control and Prevention. Retrieved from http://www.cdc.gov/violenceprevention/pdf/sv_surveillance_definitionsl-2009-a.pdf

Black, M. C., Basile, K. C., Breiding, M. J., Smith, S. G., Walters, M. L., Merrick, M. T., . . . Stevens, M. R. (2011). *The National Intimate Partner and Sexual Violence Survey (NISVS): 2010 summary report.* Atlanta, GA: National Center for Injury Prevention and Control, Centers for Disease Control and Prevention.

Campbell, R. (2012). National Institute of Justice: Transcript "the neurobiology of sexual assault." Retrieved from http://www.nij.gov/multimedia/presenter/presenter-campbell/pages/presenter-campbell-transcript.aspx

Carr, M., Thomas, A. J., Atwood, D., Muhar, A., Jarvis, K., & Wewerka, S. S. (2014). Debunking three rape myths. *Journal of Forensic Nursing, 10*(4), 217–225.

Centers for Disease Control and Prevention (CDC). (2010). Sexually transmitted diseases treatment guidelines. Retrieved from http://www.cdc.gov/std/treatment/2010/std-treatment-2010-rr5912.pdf

Centers for Disease Control and Prevention (CDC). (2014). HIV transmission risk. Retrieved from http://www.cdc.gov/hiv/policies/law/risk.html

Deming, M. E., Covan, E. K., Swan, S. C., & Billings, D. L. (2013). Exploring rape myths, gendered norms, group processing, and the social context of rape among college women: A qualitative analysis. *Violence Against Women, 19*(4), 465–485.

DeVore, H. K., & Sachs, C. J. (2011). Sexual assault. *Emergency Medicine Clinics of North America, 29*, 605–620.

Federal Bureau of Investigation (FBI). (2013). Uniform crime reports: Rape addendum. Retrieved from http://www.fbi.gov/about-us/cjis/ucr/crime-in-the-u.s/2013/crime-in-the-u.s.-2013/rape-addendum/rape_addendum_final

Gradus, J. L., Qin, P., Lincoln, A. K., Miller, M., Lawler, E., Sørensen, H. T., & Lash, T. L. (2010). Posttraumatic stress disorder and completed suicide. *American Journal of Epidemiology, 171*, 721–727.

Heath, N. M., Lynch, S. M., Fritch, A. M., & Wong, M. M. (2013). Rape myth acceptance impacts the reporting of rape to the police: A study of incarcerated women. *Violence Against Women, 19*(9), 1065–1078.

Holmes, M., Resnick, H., Kilpatrick, D., & Best, C. (1996). Rape related pregnancy: Estimates and descriptive characteristics from a national sample of women. *American Journal of Obstetrics & Gynecology, 175*, 320–324.

International Association of Forensic Nurses (IAFN). (n.d.). Primary sexual violence prevention project. Retrieved from http://c.ymcdn.com/sites/www.forensicnurses.org/resource/resmgr/imported/Primary%20Prevention%20Brochure.pdf

Johnson, N. L., & Johnson, D. M. (2013). Factors influencing the relationship between sexual trauma and risky sexual behavior in college students. *Journal of Interpersonal Violence, 28*(11), 2315–2331.

Kuhar, D. T., Henderson, D. K., Struble, K. A., Heneine, W., Thomas, V., Cheever, L. W., . . . Panlilio, A. L. (2013). US Public Health Service guidelines for the management of occupational exposures to human immunodeficiency virus and recommendations for postexposure prophylaxis. *Infection Control and Hospital Epidemiology, 34*(9), 875–892.

Lincoln, C., Perera, R., Jacobs, I., & Ward, A. (2013). Macroscopically detected female genital injury after consensual and non-consensual vaginal penetration: A prospective comparison study. *Journal of Forensic and Legal Medicine, 20*, 884–901.

Linden, J. A. (2011). Care of the adult patient after sexual assault. *New England Journal of Medicine, 365*(9), 834–841.

Markowitz, J., & Scalzo, T. (2011). Understanding anogenital injury in adult sexual assault cases. *Strategies in Brief, 5,* 1–3.

Mason, F., & Lodrick, Z. (2013). Psychological consequences of sexual assault. *Best Practice & Research Clinical Obstetrics and Gynaecology, 27*(2013), 27–37.

McCauley, J. L., Kilpatrick, D. G., Walsh, K., & Resnick, H. S. (2013). Substance use among women receiving post-rape medical care, associated post-assault concerns and current substance abuse: Results from a national telephone household probability sample. *Addictive Behaviors, 38,* 1952–1957.

McLean, I., Roberts, S. A., White, C., & Paul, S. (2010). Female genital injuries resulting from consensual and non-consensual vaginal intercourse. *Forensic Science International, 204*(2011), 27–33.

National District Attorneys Association. (2010). Mandatory reporting of domestic violence and sexual assault statutes. Retrieved from http://www.evawintl.org/PAGEID8/Forensic-Compliance/Resources/Mandated-Reporting

Office on Violence Against Women (OVAW). (2014). What is sexual assault? Retrieved from http://www.justice.gov/ovw/sexual-assault#sa

Patel, P., Borkowf, C. B., Brooks, J. T., Lasry, A., Lansky, A., & Mermin, J. (2014). Estimating per-act HIV transmission risk: A systematic review. *AIDS, 28*(10), 1509–1519.

Rape, Abuse, and Incest National Network (RAINN). (2013). The laws in your state. Retrieved from https://www.rainn.org/public-policy/laws-in-your-state

Rossman, L., Jones, J., & Dunnuck, C. K. (2013). Anogenital injury. In T. Henry (Ed.), *Atlas of sexual violence* (pp. 93–112). St. Louis, MO: Elsevier.

Steenkamp, M. M., Dickstein, B. D., Salters-Pedneault, K., Hofmann, S. G., & Litz, B. T. (2012). Trajectories of PTSD symptoms following sexual assault: Is resilience the modal outcome? *Journal of Traumatic Stress, 25,* 469–474.

Turchik, J. A., & Hassija, C. M. (2014). Female sexual victimization among college students: Assault severity, health risk behaviors, and sexual functioning. *Journal of Interpersonal Violence, 29*(13) 2439–2457.

Ullman, S. E., & Najdowski, C. J. (2009). Correlates of serious suicidal ideation and attempts in female adult sexual assault survivors. *Suicide and Life-Threatening Behavior, 39*(1), 47–56.

U.S. Citizenship and Immigration Services. (2014). Victims of criminal activity: U nonimmigrant status. Retrieved from http://www.uscis.gov/humanitarian/victims-human-trafficking-other-crimes/victims-criminal-activity-u-nonimmigrant-status/victims-criminal-activity-u-nonimmigrant-status

U.S. Department of Health and Human Services. (2006). Exploring community responses to statutory rape: Final report. Retrieved from http://aspe.hhs.gov/hsp/08/sr/commresp/index.shtml

U.S. Department of Justice (DOJ). (2013a). *A national protocol for sexual assault medical forensic examinations: Adults/adolescents* (2nd ed.). Retrieved from https://www.ncjrs.gov/pdffiles1/ovw/241903.pdf

U.S. Department of Justice (DOJ). (2013b). Special report: Female victims of sexual violence, 1994–2010. Retrieved from http://www.bjs.gov/content/pub/pdf/fvsv9410.pdf

U.S. Department of Justice (DOJ). (2014a, February). Crime against persons with disabilities, 2009–2012: Statistical tables. Retrieved from http://www.bjs.gov/content/pub/pdf/capd0912st.pdf

U.S. Department of Justice (DOJ). (2014b, December). Rape and sexual assault victimization among college-age females, 1995–2013. Retrieved from http://www.bjs.gov/content/pub/pdf/rsavcaf9513.pdf

Wieczorek, K. (2013). Anatomy and physiology. In T. Henry (Ed.), *Atlas of sexual violence* (pp. 45–63). St. Louis, MO: Elsevier.

World Health Organization (WHO). (2013a). Responding to intimate partner violence and sexual violence against women: WHO clinical and policy guidelines. Retrieved from http://apps.who.int/iris/bitstream/10665/85240/1/9789241548595_eng.pdf?ua=1

World Health Organization (WHO). (2013b). Global and regional estimates of violence against women: prevalence and health effects of intimate partner violence and nonpartner sexual violence. Retrieved from http://apps.who.int/iris/bitstream/10665/85239/1/9789241564625_eng.pdf?ua=1

Zinzow, H. M., Resnick, H. S., McCauley, J. L., Amstadter, A. B., Ruggiero, K. J., & Kilpatrick, D. G. (2012). Prevalence and risk of psychiatric disorders as a function of variant rape histories: Results from a national survey of women. *Social Psychiatry; Psychiatric Epidemiology, 47,* 893–902.

Clinician Resources

American College of Emergency Physicians (ACEP)

1125 Executive Circle

Irving, TX 75038 2522

1-972-550-0911

1-800-798-1822

1-972-580-2816 (Fax)

http://www.acep.org

Centers for Disease Control and Prevention (CDC)

1600 Clifton Road NE

Atlanta, GA 30333

1-800-CDC-INFO

http://www.cdc.gov

CDC Treatment Guidelines 2010: http://www.cdc.gov/std/treatment/2010

International Association of Forensic Nurses (IAFN)

6755 Business Parkway, Suite 303

Elkridge, MD 21075

1-410-626-7804

http://www.iafn.org

National Alliance to End Sexual Violence (NAESV)

1130 Connecticut Avenue, NW

Suite 300

Washington, DC 20036

http://endsexualviolence.org

National Center for the Prosecution of Violence Against Women (NCPVAW)

National District Attorneys Association

99 Canal Center Plaza, Suite 330

Alexandria, VA 22314

http://www.ndaajustice.org/ncpvaw_home.html

National Sexual Violence Resource Center (NSVRC)

123 North Enola Drive

Enola, PA 17025

1-717-909-0710

1-877-739-3895

http://www.nsvrc.org

Rape, Abuse, and Incest National Network (RAINN)

2000 L Street, NW

Suite 406

Washington, DC 20036

1-202-544-3064

http://www.rainn.org

Body Diagram

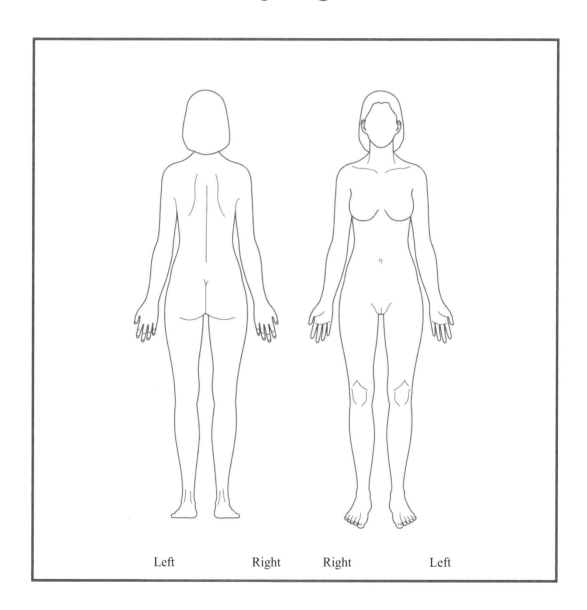

Left   Right   Right   Left

Documentation Chart for Strangulation Cases

Documentation Chart for Strangulation Cases

Symptoms and/or Internal Injury:

Breathing Changes	Voice Changes	Swallowing Changes	Behavioral Changes	OTHER
☐ Difficulty breathing ☐ Hyperventilation ☐ Unable to breathe Other:	☐ Raspy voice ☐ Hoarse voice ☐ Coughing ☐ Unable to speak	☐ Trouble swallowing ☐ Painful to swallow ☐ Neck pain ☐ Nausea/vomiting ☐ Drooling	☐ Agitation ☐ Amnesia ☐ PTSD ☐ Hallucinations ☐ Combativeness	☐ Dizzy ☐ Headaches ☐ Fainted ☐ Urination ☐ Defecation

Use face & neck diagrams to mark visible injuries:

Face	Eyes & Eyelids	Nose	Ear	Mouth
☐ Red or flushed ☐ Pinpoint red spots (petechiae) ☐ Scratch marks	☐ Petechiae to R and/or L eyeball (circle one) ☐ Petechiae to R and/or L eyelid (circle one) ☐ Bloody red eyeball(s)	☐ Bloody nose ☐ Broken nose (ancillary finding) ☐ Petechiae	☐ Petechiae (external and/or ear canal) ☐ Bleeding from ear canal	☐ Bruising ☐ Swollen tongue ☐ Swollen lips ☐ Cuts/abrasions (ancillary finding)

Under Chin	Chest	Shoulders	Neck	Head
☐ Redness ☐ Scratch marks ☐ Bruise(s) ☐ Abrasions	☐ Redness ☐ Scratch marks ☐ Bruise(s) ☐ Abrasions	☐ Redness ☐ Scratch marks ☐ Bruise(s) ☐ Abrasions	☐ Redness ☐ Scratch marks ☐ Finger nail impressions ☐ Bruise(s) ☐ Swelling ☐ Ligature mark	☐ Petechiae (on scalp) Ancillary findings: ☐ Hair pulled ☐ Bump ☐ Skull fracture ☐ Concussion

Jones & Bartlett Learning gratefully acknowledges Alliance for HOPE International for allowing us to reproduce, in part or in whole, the Documentation Chart for Strangulation Cases. The documents were accessed through the online Resource Library hosted by the Training Institute on Strangulation Prevention.

Women's Gynecologic Healthcare Management

CHAPTER 15

Breast Conditions

Kathryn J. Trotter

The editors acknowledge Heather M. Aliotta and Nancy J. Schaeffer, who were the authors of the previous edition of this chapter.

Breasts remain innate to the feminine image, sexuality, and reproductive function; in turn, they are the subject of much attention, especially in Western society. Breasts are admired and even worshipped in depictions of women in the media and art. Some women place great importance on the appearance of their breasts and will seek surgeries to enhance their appearance. As with most human features, breasts have basic similarities but unique features, including different sizes, shapes, and asymmetries, which can be normal variants. Like any organ, the mammary gland deserves particular attention to symptomology, even if benign, and due diligence is required to verify any abnormalities or any needed treatment. The clinician should be respectful, deliberate, and conscientious in the history, examination, and plan of care for breast concerns.

The presence of symptoms in the breasts that may be associated with pathology causes understandable concern for women. A woman may have an underlying fear, which may not be articulated or even conscious, that she has breast cancer. The meaning of her breasts to a woman will greatly influence how she reacts to having a breast condition. Providing adequate emotional support when a woman presents with a breast condition is as important as ensuring accurate assessment, diagnosis, and management of the condition. The breast conditions that are the focus of this chapter are mastalgia, nipple discharge, benign breast masses, and breast cancer. Online resources for caring for women with breast conditions can be found in **Appendix 15-A**.

MASTALGIA

Mastalgia, also called mastodynia or breast pain, is one of the most commonly reported symptoms in women with breast concerns. Breast pain is a significant cause of anxiety, even though mastalgia is benign in 90% of cases (Iddon & Dixon, 2013; Yildirim, Yildiz, Yildiz, Kahramanca, & Kargici, 2015).

Mastalgia is classified as cyclic or noncyclic, depending on whether its presence is related to the menstrual cycle. The majority of breast pain is cyclic, occurring 1 to 2 weeks prior to menses. As many as 70% of women experience cyclic mastalgia, and 10% to 22% of women have moderate to severe breast pain (Kataria, Dhar, Srivastava, Kumar, & Goyal, 2014; Scurr, Hedger, Morris, & Brown, 2014). Noncyclic mastalgia is less common, with approximately 25% of women reporting this symptom (Iddon & Dixon, 2013).

Etiology and Pathophysiology

Mild cyclic mastalgia is considered a normal, physiologic condition caused by the hormonal changes of the menstrual cycle (Klimberg, Kass, Beenken, & Bland, 2009). It is clearly linked to the reproductive cycle, with onset at menarche, monthly cycling, and cessation at menopause. Three hormonally oriented theories have emerged to explain moderate or severe breast pain: increased estrogen secretion from the ovary, deficient progesterone production, and hyperprolactinemia. One study found similar serum hormone levels in women with breast pain and a control group (Malarkey, Schroeder, Stevens, James, & Lanese, 1977), although two other studies found that women with breast pain had a significantly greater elevation in prolactin levels compared with women in a control group (Kumar et al., 1984; Peters, Pickardt, Zimmermann, & Breckwoldt, 1981). The effects of stress on the hypothalamic–pituitary axis and prolactin levels are difficult to prove, but seem a reasonable explanation for at least some cases of mastalgia (Cole, Sellwood, England, & Griffiths, 1977; Parker, Menzies, & Douglas, 2011).

Mastalgia can also be caused by certain medications, including combined estrogen and progestin contraceptives (i.e., pills, vaginal ring, and transdermal patch), hormone therapy (HT), antidepressants, digoxin, methyldopa, cimetidine, spironolactone, oxymetholone, and chlorpromazine (King & Brucker, 2011). Interestingly, some women may obtain relief from their breast pain with combined contraceptives or HT (Kataria et al., 2014) or selective serotonin reuptake inhibitors (SSRIs; Iddon & Dixon, 2013).

Fibrocystic breast changes are common among women with mastalgia, although not all women with fibrocystic breast changes experience pain, and not all women with mastalgia have fibrocystic breast changes (Amin, Purdy, Mattingly, Kong, & Termuhlen, 2013). Fibrocystic breast changes were originally called fibrocystic breast disease, but the associated constellation of symptoms has become increasingly recognized as common to many women; thus, these symptoms are no longer considered to constitute a disease. Such changes include tender, nodular, and swollen breast tissue.

Clinical Presentation

Three classifications are commonly used to distinguish the various types of breast pain: cyclic mastalgia, noncyclic mastalgia, and chest wall pain.

Cyclic mastalgia typically begins in the luteal phase of the menstrual cycle and subsides with menses. This pain is usually bilateral; can be poorly localized, but is most frequently associated with the outer quadrants; and described as soreness or aching. Cyclic mastalgia most commonly occurs in women who are 30 to 50 years old and accounts for two-thirds of mastalgia cases (Klimberg et al., 2009). It seems to be equally distributed in smaller- and larger-breasted women.

In contrast, noncyclic mastalgia may be constant or intermittent, and is unrelated to the menstrual cycle. Approximately 25% of all women with breast pain have this variant, and its incidence peaks in the fourth decade of life. Noncyclic mastalgia is more likely to cause unilateral, localized pain that is sharp or burning in nature (Ferrara, 2011). Women with macromastia (very large breasts) may report shoulder grooving, neck pain, and back pain in addition to breast pain.

Chest wall pain is usually quite localized, becomes worse with movement, and affects approximately 5% to 10% of women with mastalgia symptoms (Amin et al., 2013).

Assessment

History

The clinician must determine whether the mastalgia is cyclic or noncyclic, diffuse or focal, and must eliminate nonbreast causes of the discomfort, such as chest wall pain. When taking the history, ask the woman about the timing (especially in relation to the menstrual cycle), frequency, location, nature, severity, and mitigating factors of the pain as well as its effects on her functioning (Amin et al., 2013). The use of an instrument such as a visual analog scale to rate pain may be helpful in evaluating mastalgia and monitoring the response to treatment. Prospective evaluation of pain with a daily diary can be useful in differentiating cyclic and noncyclic mastalgia (Kataria et al., 2014). In addition, the clinician should ask the woman about other breast symptoms, such as nipple discharge or breast mass, and whether there is a previous history of any type of breast disease or surgery.

Menstrual, pregnancy, lactation, and general medical histories are all necessary as part of a comprehensive assessment for mastalgia. Note current medications, including exogenous hormones. Although this factor has not been definitively established as a causal factor, ask about the amount of caffeine in case a pattern exists. Caffeine contains the chemical methylxanthine, which causes dilation of blood vessels and overstimulation of breast cells that could theoretically result in mastalgia. However, randomized trials have failed to demonstrate a benefit of caffeine restriction in relieving the discomfort (Ernster et al., 1982).

Also obtain a family history, particularly regarding breast and ovarian cancer. A complete review of systems is helpful in eliminating nonbreast causes (see the discussion of differential diagnoses).

Physical Examination

Perform a comprehensive breast examination, including inspection and palpation of the breasts with the unclothed woman in both the upright and supine positions, and evaluate the lymph nodes (see Chapter 6). Assess for skin changes, nipple discharge, and breast masses. If the pain can be reproduced with examination, note its location. The chest wall structures should also be examined for nonbreast causes of pain.

Diagnostic Testing

Pregnancy testing should be performed if indicated by the woman's history, because mastalgia can be a sign of pregnancy. Diagnostic imaging is frequently used in the evaluation of breast conditions; information about these tests is provided in **Table 15-1**. A mammogram with ultrasound can be performed for women older than 30 years; a targeted ultrasound is recommended for women younger than age 30. Such diagnostic imaging is helpful only to rule out the unlikely diagnosis of cancer, because there are no radiologic findings associated with mastalgia (Yildirim et al., 2015). Mammography or other appropriate imaging should also be considered for women with focal breast pain who have a family history of early breast cancer or other breast cancer risk factors (Yildirim et al., 2015). If a breast mass is discovered during the evaluation of mastalgia, it needs to be evaluated appropriately, as described later in this chapter

Differential Diagnoses

Breast pain can originate from the breast with conditions such as pregnancy, mastitis, cysts, abscess, and cancer. Extramammary or nonbreast causes of pain are also important differential diagnoses. If the pain is reproducible with palpation of the chest wall, costochondritis or Tietze syndrome should be suspected (Kataria et al., 2014). Costochondritis is characterized by

TABLE **15-1**	Diagnostic Imaging Tests		
Test	**Source of Images**	**Best for Detecting**	**Limitations of Test**
Mammogram	X-rays	Calcifications, masses, and architectural distortion	Cannot show if mass is solid or cystic; has lower sensitivity in women with dense breast tissue
Ultrasound (US)	Sound waves	Differentiation of solid and cystic masses	Typically cannot show calcifications
Magnetic resonance imaging (MRI)	Magnetic fields, must be enhanced with gadolinium contrast	Tissue with increased blood flow such as tumors; high sensitivity and negative predictive value	Expensive; limited to specific indications; high rate of false-positive results (lack of specificity)
Tomosynthesis	X-rays (provide 3-D digital images); use with a standard mammogram	Architectural distortion, masses, and calcifications, in dense breast tissue	Slight increase in radiation exposure versus standard mammogram, takes twice as long to read

inflammation of the costochondral or chondro-sternal joints; the second through fifth costochondral junctions are most likely to be affected. Tietze syndrome is differentiated from costochondritis by the presence of swelling with or without erythema. Nonsteroidal anti-inflammatory drugs (NSAIDs) can be helpful in relieving the symptoms of both conditions. Other potential etiologies of breast pain include medications (see the section on etiology), arthritis, pleuritis, cervical spondylitis, herpes zoster, cholecystitis, and myocardial ischemia (Amin et al., 2013).

Mastalgia is rarely the principal sign of a developing breast cancer, but the possibility of cancer increases when breast pain occurs postmenopausally in the absence of HT or is accompanied by skin changes or a palpable abnormality (Ahmed et al., 2014; American Cancer Society, 2015; Klimberg et al., 2009). Mastalgia related to breast cancer usually occurs in only one area of one breast and does not follow a cyclic pattern (Yildirim et al., 2015).

Management

Once a clinician has ruled out malignancy and non-breast causes of mastalgia, attention turns to reassuring the woman that she does not have a serious illness and relieving her symptoms. Nonpharmacologic, complementary, and alternative therapies are often successful in the treatment of mastalgia. Severe breast pain can be chronic and relapsing, and may require pharmacologic treatment.

Nonpharmacologic Therapies

Reassurance is the first-line treatment for mastalgia and has been found to be effective for as many as 85% of women, with more success in women with mild or moderate symptoms than in those with severe mastalgia (Kataria et al., 2014). Wearing a supportive and well-fitting bra is frequently recommended, especially for women with large, heavy breasts (Hadi, 2000; Salzman, Fleegle, & Tully, 2012). Reductions in caffeine and dietary fat have shown limited effectiveness in diminishing breast pain; however, neither of these dietary recommendations is likely to be harmful. Supplementation with vitamins A, B, or E has not consistently demonstrated effectiveness in relieving mastalgia (Amin et al., 2013).

Pharmacologic Therapies

Modifying the dose or route of HT may be helpful in reducing breast pain in a postmenopausal woman. Some women report increased mastalgia with use of hormonal contraception. Trying a different contraceptive method or delivery system, such as changing from combined oral contraceptives to a nonoral combined method (i.e., the ring or patch), may sometimes prove helpful in reducing pain. Conversely, some women report an improvement in mastalgia with use of hormonal contraception.

Danazol, tamoxifen, and bromocriptine are the primary pharmacologic therapies for mastalgia, and a meta-analysis of randomized trials found that all three of these medications offer significant relief (Srivastava et al., 2007). These medications can produce significant side effects, however, and relapses after discontinuation of therapy are common (Colak, Ipek, Kanik, Ogetman, & Aydin, 2003; Iddon & Dixon, 2013; Kataria et al., 2014). Tamoxifen has the least problematic side effects, but danazol is the only medication approved by the U.S. Food and Drug Administration (FDA) for the treatment of mastalgia. In a randomized trial that compared cabergoline with bromocriptine in 140 women with premenstrual mastalgia, researchers found that two-thirds of participants responded positively to treatment (66.6% in the bromocriptine group and 68.4% in the cabergoline group), but women in the cabergoline group had significantly less vomiting, nausea, and headache (Aydin, Atis, Kaleli, Uludag, & Goker, 2010).

Localized therapies have also been evaluated for the treatment of mastalgia. Topical use of di-clofenac diethyl ammonium gel (an NSAID), three times daily for 6 months, was found to be superior to a placebo for relieving the pain of both cyclical and noncyclical mastalgia in one study (Colak et al., 2003). In another study, women with non-cyclical mastalgia were offered injection of 1 mL of 2% lidocaine and 40 mg of methyl prednisone at the area of maximum tenderness. Participants who were given an injection experienced greater relief of symptoms than those who were treated with either reassurance or oral or topical NSAIDs. Recurrence of symptoms occurred in 16% of the women who had an injection, and all elected to receive a second injection (Khan, Rampaul, & Blamey, 2004). A more recent study comparing oral versus topical diclofenac for mastalgia treatment, however, failed to show any difference in efficacy based on the route of NSAID administration (Zafar & Rehman, 2013).

Complementary and Alternative Therapies

The herbal product evening primrose oil (EPO) is frequently recommended for the treatment of mastalgia; however, a systematic review refuted its effectiveness (Edwards, da Costa Rocha, Williamson, & Heinrich, 2015), and a meta-analysis of four randomized controlled trials found EPO to be ineffective compared to placebo (Srivastava et al., 2007). The herbal treatment *Agnus castus* (also called vitex, chaste tree, or chaste berry) is used for cyclic mastalgia and is well tolerated, but there is not sufficient evidence to rate it as effective ("Vitex agnus-castus," 2015). Isoflavones, which are naturally occurring phytoestrogens, have also been proposed as a treatment for mastalgia. A small, randomized, controlled trial found that women taking isoflavones had a greater reduction in pain than women taking a placebo (Ingram, Hickling, West, Mahe, & Dunbar, 2002). In a small short-term study, a flaxseed bread diet was more effective than omega-3 fatty acid supplementation in reducing cyclical mastalgia (Vaziri et al., 2014).

Surgical Therapies

Surgery is rarely indicated in the treatment of mastalgia and runs the risk of replacing a painful area with a painful scar. Potential surgical candidates include women with macromastia whose symptoms warrant reduction mammoplasty and women with refractory mastalgia who resort to mastectomy after nonsurgical options have proved unsuccessful in providing pain relief. Mastectomy should be reserved for refractory cases and may not be curative (Klimberg et al., 2009). As with any surgery, the risks and benefits of this procedure must be considered.

Special Considerations

Mastalgia is common during pregnancy and lactation. The pain in such cases is attributed to the proliferation of breast tissue and hormonal influences on that tissue. Mastitis is the most likely diagnosis when breast pain in a lactating woman is accompanied by inflammation, erythema, chills, myalgia, and, in more advanced cases, fever. Mastitis is estimated to occur in approximately 10% of breastfeeding mothers (Bergmann et al., 2014). Abscesses can also develop and should be suspected when mastitis is unresponsive to antibiotic therapy and the breast pain is worsening.

NIPPLE DISCHARGE

Nipple discharge is another breast symptom that often causes women to seek care—it is the third most common presenting symptom to a breast clinic (Amin et al., 2013). The level of a woman's concern can range from minor embarrassment to fear and anxiety about underlying pathology. Nipple discharge can be classified as normal lactation; galactorrhea unrelated to childbearing; and nonmilky discharge, which is sometimes referred to as pathologic discharge (Pearlman & Griffin, 2010). Nonmilky discharge that is spontaneous, unilateral, from a single duct (uniductal), and clear or bloody in color is more likely to be associated with cancer than the physiologic discharge that can occur in approximately 50% of women with nipple manipulation (squeezing the nipple) (Isaacs, 1994). Physiologic discharge is often bilateral, comes from multiple ducts (multiductal), and is white, clear, yellow, green, or brown in color (Patel, Falcon, & Drukteinis, 2015). See **Color Plate 11** for an example of nipple discharge. Nipple discharge is usually the result of a benign process, but malignancy must always be considered in its evaluation.

Etiology, Pathophysiology, and Clinical Presentation

Numerous etiologies of nipple discharge exist. Among the most common are pregnancy and lactation, galactorrhea, intraductal papilloma, mammary duct ectasia, and cancer. During pregnancy, women begin having bilateral, milky discharge that can continue as long as one year after birth or stopping breastfeeding. Clear nipple discharge during pregnancy, particularly in the third trimester, usually consists of colostrum. Bloody nipple discharge during pregnancy or lactation can occur as well, as a result of the increased vascularity of the breasts and changes in the epithelium (Sabate et al, 2007); however, evaluation is warranted if bloody discharge occurs at any point (Patel et al., 2015; Pearlman & Griffin, 2010).

Galactorrhea is milky nipple discharge in a woman who has not been pregnant or lactated in the last 12 months. This type of discharge is usually bilateral and multiductal, and it may occur spontaneously or only with nipple or breast manipulation. Galactorrhea is not caused by breast pathology (Hussain, Policarpio, & Vincent, 2006; Pearlman & Griffin, 2010). Instead, it results from hyperprolactinemia, which may be caused by pituitary prolactin-secreting tumors, medications, hypothyroidism, stress, trauma, chronic renal failure, hypothalamic lesions, previous thoracotomy, and herpes zoster. In addition to galactorrhea, pituitary tumors can cause headaches and visual disturbances. Numerous medications can cause galactorrhea, including combined contraceptives containing estrogen and progestin, phenothiazines and other antipsychotics, tricyclic antidepressants, SSRIs, monoamine oxidase inhibitors (MAOIs), metoclopramide, domperidone, methadone, methyldopa, reserpine, verapamil, cimetidine, calcium-channel blockers, and amphetamines (Morgan, 2015). Most of these medications inhibit dopamine, which can lead to hyperprolactinemia. Hyperprolactinemia can also interfere with the normal menstrual cycle, resulting in anovulation, oligomenorrhea or amenorrhea, and infertility (Fritz & Speroff, 2011). Marijuana use has also been implicated in nipple discharge (Rizvi, 2006).

Intraductal papilloma and mammary duct ectasia are the most common causes of nonmilky nipple discharge. Intraductal papilloma typically occurs in women aged 40 to 50 and results from a small, benign growth in the duct. The discharge with intraductal papilloma is typically bloody, unilateral, and uniductal (Klimberg et al., 2009). Mammary duct ectasia, in contrast, usually occurs in women older than age 50 and results from dilation of the ducts with surrounding inflammation and fibrosis. Nipple discharge with mammary duct ectasia is typically bilateral; multiductal; sticky; and green, brown, or black in color (Morgan, 2015). Both intraductal papilloma and mammary duct ectasia may be accompanied by a palpable mass.

While women with nipple discharge are often concerned that they have cancer—and indeed, it is the presenting symptom in 5% to 12% of breast cancers (Patel et al., 2015)—such pathology is the least likely etiology, although it certainly must be considered carefully during assessment. Cancer is more likely if the nipple discharge is accompanied by a palpable mass or abnormal mammogram, and the woman is older than age 50 (Morgan, 2015; Patel et al., 2015).

Assessment

History
Ask the woman about the duration and color of her nipple discharge, as well as whether it occurs spontaneously or only with manipulation of the nipple or breast, whether it is unilateral or bilateral, and whether it comes from one or more ducts/points on the nipple. Review the medications she is taking and determine whether any of them could cause galactorrhea. Note other breast symptoms, such as mastalgia or breast mass, and identify any history of any type of breast disease or surgery. Ask about symptoms of hypothyroidism (e.g., fatigue, weight gain, cold intolerance), hyperthyroidism (e.g., nervousness, weight loss despite increased appetite, heat intolerance), pituitary tumor (e.g., headaches, visual problems), and hyperprolactinemia (e.g., irregular menses, infertility, decreased libido) (Morgan, 2015; Patel et al., 2015). Menstrual, pregnancy, lactation, general medical, and family histories should be obtained as well. Any family history of breast and ovarian cancer should be noted.

Physical Examination
Perform a comprehensive breast examination, including inspection and palpation with the woman in both the upright and supine positions, and palpation of the lymph nodes (see Chapter 6). If the nipple discharge can be reproduced, note the color, consistency, unilateral versus bilateral locations, and the number of ducts involved, using the clock method for documentation. Assess for skin changes, breast masses, and tenderness. Additional examination may be warranted based on the woman's history, such as thyroid palpation if symptoms of a thyroid disorder are present or examination of the visual fields for women with galactorrhea who are not pregnant or breastfeeding.

Diagnostic Testing
If the woman has bilateral, milky discharge, perform a pregnancy test. If this test is negative, obtain

a serum prolactin level and thyroid-stimulating hormone (TSH) measurement (Patel et al., 2015). If hyperprolactinemia is present, imaging of the sella turcica with magnetic resonance imaging (MRI) should be performed to rule out a pituitary prolactin-secreting tumor (Fritz & Speroff, 2011).

Evaluation of the woman with a nonmilky discharge depends on the presence or absence of a mass and the characteristics of the discharge (Pearlman & Griffin, 2010). When a palpable mass is present, it should be evaluated as described later in this chapter. If the discharge is spontaneous, unilateral, uniductal, and reproducible on examination, a mammogram and ultrasound should be performed if the woman is 30 years or older (Morgan, 2015; Patel et al., 2015; Pearlman & Griffin, 2010). If she is younger than age 30, an ultrasound of the affected breast is recommended and possibly a diagnostic mammogram (National Comprehensive Cancer Network [NCCN], 2015a). Additional evaluation is based on imaging findings. For mammogram results classified as Breast Imaging Reporting and Data System (BI-RADS) categories 1 to 3, an option of MRI may be considered (NCCN, 2015a). Referral to a surgeon for evaluation for duct incision may be offered.

If the discharge occurs only with manipulation, is multiductal, and is yellow, green, brown, or gray in color, the woman can be observed and advised to avoid nipple stimulation, with a follow-up examination occurring in 3 to 4 months. Guaiac testing is used if the color of the discharge is black and concern for bleeding exists. Women fitting this description should have diagnostic mammography if they are 40 years or older and have not had a mammogram in the preceding 6 months (Pearlman & Griffin, 2010). Avoiding nipple stimulation via compression is ideal, and all women should report any spontaneous discharge (NCCN, 2015a).

Cytology testing is generally not recommended as part of assessment of nipple discharge because it has a low sensitivity for cancer detection and does not change the management of galactorrhea (Pearlman & Griffin, 2010). Additional diagnostic modalities that assist in ruling out malignancy include duct excision, ductoscopy, and ductography. Excision of the affected duct or ducts allows for definitive evaluation, remains the gold standard, and may also be therapeutic. Ductography is rarely used because it has low sensitivity and is painful to women. A fiber-optic ductoscope can be used to visualize the ducts and may prove helpful both in the diagnosis and as a guide for duct excision, particularly sparing excessive duct removal in young women, thereby allowing them to retain the ability to lactate (Amin et al., 2013). The limited availability of ductoscopy may preclude its use.

Differential Diagnoses

In addition to the conditions already described, sexual stimulation, infection or abscess, and Paget's disease (described in the section on breast cancer later in this chapter) can cause nipple discharge.

Management

Women who express colostrum during pregnancy should be reassured that the discharge is benign and advised that avoiding nipple stimulation will generally lead to resolution of the discharge. Physiologic discharge has a similar management plan.

The treatment of galactorrhea unrelated to pregnancy or lactation depends on the etiology. Pituitary tumors may be treated surgically, with medications, or expectantly in certain circumstances (Fritz & Speroff, 2011). Discontinuing a medication that causes galactorrhea or treating hypothyroidism if it is present may resolve the discharge. Bromocriptine and cabergoline can be used to treat galactorrhea, but symptoms often recur upon discontinuation of these medications; thus, long-term therapy is usually required (Fritz & Speroff, 2011).

Intraductal papillomas without atypia that are solitary and less than 1 cm in size are generally not removed, but women who have multiple papillomas or a single papilloma 1 cm or larger are treated with duct excision (Cuneo, Dash, Wilke, Horton, & Koontz, 2012). Mammary duct ectasia can be managed expectantly (because it is associated with a benign process), or it can be surgically treated with removal of the subareolar duct system if imaging shows focal thickening of the duct wall (Ferris-James, Iuanow, Mehta, Shaheen, & Slanetz, 2012) or if symptoms are severe.

If breast cancer is diagnosed, appropriate management should be initiated according to the disease stage, as is discussed in the breast cancer section later in this chapter.

BENIGN BREAST MASSES

A breast mass can be alarming for the woman as well as her clinician. Fortunately, most breast masses are benign; however, malignancy must always be considered in the evaluation of a breast mass. The likelihood of malignancy increases with age and risk factors for breast cancer, which are detailed in the breast cancer section later in this chapter.

Incidence, Etiology, and Clinical Presentation

The most common benign breast masses are fibroadenomas and cysts. Lipomas, fat necroses, phyllodes tumors, hamartomas, and galactoceles may also be encountered.

Fibroadenomas, which are composed of dense epithelial and fibroblastic tissue, are usually nontender, encapsulated, round, movable, and firm. They are the most common type of breast mass in adolescents and young women. Their incidence decreases with increasing age, but they still account for 12% of masses in menopausal women (Pearlman & Griffin, 2010). Multiple fibroadenomas occur in 10% to 15% of cases (Vashi, Hooley, Butler, Geisel, & Philpotts, 2013). A proposed etiology for formation of these masses is the effect of estrogen on susceptible tissue (Vashi et al., 2013).

Cysts are fluid-filled masses that are most commonly found in women aged 35 to 50 years (Berg, Sechtin, Marques, & Zhang, 2010). They are thought to result from cystic lobular involution. Although many of these lesions can be dismissed as benign simple cysts requiring intervention only for symptomatic relief, complex cystic and solid masses require biopsy.

A lipoma is an area of fatty tissue that may occur in the breast or other areas of the body, including the arms, legs, and abdomen. Lipomas typically occur in the later reproductive years (Grobmeyer, Copeland, Simpson, & Page, 2009). Fat necrosis is usually the result of trauma to the breast, whether as a result of external force against the tissue (e.g., a seat belt in a motor vehicle accident) or subsequent to surgical manipulation of tissue (Grobmeyer et al., 2009)

Phyllodes tumors form from periductal stromal cells of the breast and present as a firm, palpable mass. These typically large and fast-growing masses account for fewer than 1% of all breast neoplasms. Phyllodes tumors, which can range from a benign mass to a sarcoma, are usually seen in women aged 30 to 50 years (Pearlman & Griffin, 2010). Hamartomas are composed of glandular tissue, fat, and fibrous connective tissue; the average age at presentation for these masses is 45 years (Sevim et al., 2014).

Galactoceles are milk-filled cysts that usually occur during or after lactation. They result from duct dilation and often have an inflammatory component (Vashi et al., 2013). See **Color Plate 12** for an example of a breast mass.

Assessment

A woman may present with a breast mass found on self-examination, or a mass may be discovered on clinical breast examination.

History

If the woman found the mass, determine when she first noticed it and any changes she has observed since that time. Ask about other breast symptoms, such as mastalgia or nipple discharge, and determine whether the woman has a history of any type of breast disease or surgery. Menstrual, pregnancy, lactation, and general medical histories should be taken. A family history of breast and ovarian cancer is particularly important.

Physical Examination

Perform a comprehensive breast examination, including inspection and palpation with the woman in both the upright and supine positions, and evaluation of the lymph nodes. If a mass is palpable, identify the size (in centimeters), the shape, and the consistency or texture. Determine whether the mass is discrete (well-delineated, distinct edges) or poorly differentiated, tender to palpation, and mobile or fixed. Assess for skin changes, nipple discharge, and lymphadenopathy. When documenting the location of a mass, it may be helpful to draw a sketch of the breast with the site of the mass marked, or more importantly to describe the position of the mass on the breast relative to a clock face, such as "at seven o'clock." Typical physical examination findings for benign breast masses are described in **Table 15-2**.

TABLE 15-2	Features of Benign Breast Masses	

Type of Mass	Typical Physical Examination Findings	Tissue Sampling Findings
Fibroadenoma	Discrete, smooth, round or oval, nontender, mobile	Ductal epithelium, dense stroma, numerous elongated nuclei without fat
Cyst	Discrete, tender, mobile; size may fluctuate with the menstrual cycle	Cyst fluid and inflammation
Lipoma	Discrete, soft, nontender; may or may not be mobile	Fatty tissue
Fat necrosis	Ill defined, firm, nontender, nonmobile	Necrotic fat with inflammation
Phyllodes tumor	Discrete, firm, round, mobile, findings similar to a fibroadenoma, but mass is usually larger; may observe stretching of skin due to rapid tumor growth	Stromal hypercellularity with glandular and ductal elements
Hamartoma	Discrete, nontender, nonmobile; may be nonpalpable with incidental diagnosis on imaging studies	Glandular tissue, fat, and fibrous connective tissue
Galactocele	Discrete, firm, sometimes tender	Fat globules

Diagnostic Testing

If the physical examination suggests a palpable area of concern, order an ultrasound if the woman is younger than age 30, and a diagnostic mammogram with or without an ultrasound if she is 30 years or older. If the mass is suspicious for malignancy on physical examination and the woman is least 30 years of age, order a mammogram and ultrasound (NCCN, 2015a; Salzman et al., 2012). Ultrasound helps to distinguish a cystic mass from a solid mass, but is not as accurate as tissue sampling. Mammography can be used to detect nonpalpable abnormalities if a woman is of appropriate screening age or has a solid mass. Palpable breast masses may not be visible with diagnostic imaging tests, however, so these tests cannot rule out malignancy.

Biopsy is required to definitively ascertain whether a mass is solid versus cystic, and benign versus malignant. A fine-needle aspiration (FNA) biopsy is a minimally invasive way to differentiate solid and cystic masses, and provides for cytologic evaluation of a palpable mass. FNA biopsy may also be therapeutic if the mass is filled with fluid. Tissue sample findings for benign breast masses are described in **Table 15-2**. If cytologic evaluation does not yield definitive findings, a more invasive method of tissue sampling (**Table 15-3**) is required to rule out breast cancer or determine the type of tumor if the mass is benign (Kerlikowske, Smith-Bindman, Ljung, & Grady, 2003).

Differential Diagnoses

In addition to the types of breast masses already discussed, differential diagnoses for breast masses include fibrocystic changes, infection or abscess, and malignancy. Women with fibrocystic breast tissue may present with a perceived mass, although these changes are typically associated with nodularity or thickening rather than formation of a discrete mass. Intradermal cysts, such as epidermal inclusion cysts and periareolar sebaceous cysts, occur in 3% to 5% of women and are benign

TABLE 15-3	Breast Tissue Sampling Procedures

Procedure	Description	Breast Target
Fine-needle aspiration biopsy	Tissue for cytologic evaluation aspirated with a small needle Differentiates solid and cystic masses	Palpable breast mass or thickening
Stereotactic-guided core-needle biopsy	Large-bore needle used to obtain cores of tissue for histologic examination Stereotactic mammography used for localization and targeting	Calcification seen on mammogram, masses or other abnormalities visible only by mammography (i.e. not visible with ultrasound)
Ultrasound-guided core-needle biopsy	Large-bore needle used to obtain cores of tissue for histologic examination Ultrasound used for localization and targeting	Solid or indeterminate lesion (most commonly a mass) seen on ultrasound
Magnetic resonance imaging (MRI)–guided needle biopsy	MRI with intravenous contrast material used for localization and targeting	Lesions visible only with MRI
Needle-localized breast biopsy	Use of a wire (or radioactive seed) to localize an occult mammographic, sonographic, or MRI-detected abnormality prior to excisional biopsy	Mass or calcification seen on imaging in a location that cannot be effectively assessed with core biopsy
Excisional breast biopsy	Surgical procedure that requires a skin excision Mass is removed with a surrounding margin of normal-appearing tissue	Palpable breast mass, thickening or skin change; used for initial diagnosis only when needle biopsy is not feasible

findings (Giess, Raza, & Birdwell, 2011); however, they can cause discomfort when inflamed, especially if on the bra line. These cysts seem to be more prevalent in cigarette smokers and can be intermittently chronic.

Management

Management of benign breast masses depends on the type of mass. A fibroadenoma that has been definitively diagnosed by cytologic or histologic analysis does not need to be removed. Instead, it can be expectantly managed and removed only if the mass becomes enlarged, such as doubling in size

or becoming 4 cm or larger (Hubbard, Cagle, Davis, Kaups, & Kodama, 2015). Fibroadenomas usually decrease in size postmenopausally, and many resolve completely (Hubbard et al., 2015).

Management of cysts is based on symptoms, with these sac-like structures sometimes requiring incision and drainage. Asymptomatic simple cysts do not require intervention. Aspiration can be used to treat large or painful cysts (Berg et al., 2010). Complicated cysts will need biopsy of the debris to rule out atypia or malignancy.

Excision of a lipoma is not required if a breast mass is consistent with lipoma on clinical examination and tissue sampling, and there are no suspicious findings at the site on mammography and ultrasound. Otherwise, excision should be performed. Fat necroses typically resolve spontaneously (Grobmeyer et al., 2009).

Excisional biopsy is recommended for suspected phyllodes tumor, and typically a wide margin of normal surrounding tissue is also removed due to the tendency for such masses to recur (Pearlman & Griffin, 2010). Hamartomas may require excision for diagnosis, but otherwise do not have to be removed and may be expectantly managed. Aspiration of a galactocele allows for diagnosis and appropriate treatment (Vashi et al., 2013).

When benign breast masses are managed expectantly, the woman should be advised to report any new symptoms and encouraged to follow up with her clinician for examinations and diagnostic testing as recommended.

Special Considerations

Adolescents

In approximately two-thirds of adolescents presenting with a breast mass, the diagnosis is a fibroadenoma. Ultrasound is the best diagnostic imaging test for this age group. Mammography is not indicated, and aspiration for diagnostic purposes can be avoided (Giess et al., 2011). Breast cancer in women younger than age 20 is very rare (American Cancer Society, 2015).

Pregnant or Breastfeeding Women

Evaluation of palpable findings in pregnant and lactating women is complicated by the complex breast parenchyma. Nevertheless, appropriate diagnostic imaging and breast tissue sampling should not be deferred, with the exception of mammography—this modality is not generally used during pregnancy because physiologic changes in the breast result in poor sensitivity for such imaging (Vashi et al., 2013). Fibroadenomas may increase in size and become symptomatic during pregnancy (Amin et al., 2013).

Older Women

The likelihood of malignancy increases with age. Among women aged 55 years and older, 85% of breast masses are malignant. Masses in postmenopausal women are presumed to be malignant until proven otherwise (Vaidya & Joseph, 2014).

BREAST CANCER

Breast cancer is one of the most feared diseases among women, even though treatment of this condition has become increasingly successful in prolonging women's lives after diagnosis. From the Halsted radical mastectomy of the 1890s to breast-sparing surgery in conjunction with other treatment modalities, the management of breast cancer has changed dramatically over time. With increased public awareness and earlier detection, comprehensive treatment can be initiated promptly for this disease process.

Incidence

Breast cancer is the most prevalent cancer diagnosed among U.S. women after skin cancer, with an incidence rate of more than 220,000 new invasive cases annually (American Cancer Society, 2013). One out of every eight U.S. women (12%) will be diagnosed with breast cancer during her lifetime (American Cancer Society, 2013). The risk increases gradually with age, from 1 in 227 for women ages 30 to 39 to 1 in 28 for women ages 60 to 69 (National Cancer Institute, 2012). Breast cancer is the second leading cause of cancer deaths in women, after lung cancer (Centers for Disease Control and Prevention, 2014).

Etiology

Two aspects of breast cancer are especially challenging: Many of the risk factors are nonmodifiable, and most women with breast cancer (85%) have no identifiable risk factors other than age (Fritz & Speroff, 2011). In fact, fewer than 10% of women with breast cancer have an identified germline mutation that puts them at known risk for this disease (Petrucelli, Daly, & Feldman, 2013). Known risk factors for developing breast cancer are listed in **Box 15-1**.

The discovery of the *BRCA1* and *BRCA2* genetic mutations was a monumental step in the understanding of breast cancer, because mutations of these genes account for 5% to 10% of breast cancer cases (American Cancer Society, 2015; Petrucelli et al., 2013). In normal cells, these genes help prevent cancer by making proteins that keep the cells from growing abnormally. If a woman inherits a mutated copy of either gene from a parent, she has

BOX 15-1 Risk Factors for Breast Cancer

- Female
- Advancing age
- Personal history of invasive breast cancer, ductal carcinoma in situ, or lobular carcinoma in situ
- Family history of invasive breast cancer, ductal carcinoma in situ, or lobular carcinoma in situ, especially in first-degree relatives
- Inherited detrimental genetic mutations
- Biopsy-confirmed proliferative breast lesions with atypia
- Dense breast tissue on mammogram
- High-dose radiation to chest, especially during puberty or young adulthood
- Menarche before age 12 years
- Menopause at age 55 years or older
- Nulliparity
- First full-term pregnancy after age 30 years
- Current use of combined oral contraceptives (likely due to detection bias of regular screening)
- Use of combined estrogen– progestogen hormone therapy after menopause
- Weight gain leading to overweight or obese status after age 18 years
- Physical inactivity
- Consumption of one or more alcoholic beverages per day
- Jewish ancestry (Ashkenazi)
- Place of birth (North America and Northern Europe versus Asia and Africa)

Data from American Cancer Society. (2015). Cancer facts & figures 2015. Retrieved from http://www.cancer.org/research/cancerfactsstatistics/cancerfactsfigures2015; Vaidya, J. S., & Joseph, D. (2014). Fast facts: Breast cancer (5th ed.). Oxford, UK: Health Press Limited.

a high risk of developing breast cancer during her lifetime. These mutations are also associated with an increased risk of developing ovarian cancer. In two meta-analyses, the estimated cumulative risks of breast cancer by age 70 years were found to be 55% to 65% for BRCA1 mutation carriers and 45% to 47% for BRCA2 mutation carriers. Ovarian cancer risks were 39% for BRCA1 mutation carriers and 11% to 17% for BRCA2 mutation carriers (National Cancer Institute, 2015d). Expanded panel testing is now available that can detect additional genetic mutations (BRACAnalysis Large Rearrangement Test [BART] panel), which may warrant management for increased risk (NCCN, 2015b). Given the growing knowledge base about genetic influences on the development of breast cancer, the genetic counselor has a significant role working in collaboration with the healthcare team in the care of women with breast cancer (Moyer & U.S. Preventive Services Task Force, 2014).

Other potential risk factors for breast cancer include cigarette smoking and shift work, particularly at night (American Cancer Society, 2015). The 2014 U.S. Surgeon General's report on smoking concluded that there is "suggestive but not sufficient" evidence that smoking increases the risk of breast cancer (U.S. Department of Health and Human Services, 2014). Studies have yielded conflicting results about other putative risk factors, such as diet, vitamin intake, and chemicals in the environment (American Cancer Society, 2015), and research in this area is ongoing.

Conversely, breastfeeding is a protective factor against developing breast cancer. A woman's relative risk of breast cancer decreases by 4.3% for every 12 months of breastfeeding, in addition to 7% for each birth (National Cancer Institute, 2015a). This effect increases with longer duration of lactation, especially at least 1 year (Collaborative Group on Hormonal Factors in Breast Cancer, 2002).

Moderate or vigorous physical activity for at least 4 hours per week is also associated with reduced breast cancer risk, with the average relative risk reduction being 30% to 40% (National Cancer Institute, 2015a). Maintaining a normal weight protects against breast cancer as well (American Cancer Society, 2015).

Pathophysiology

Breast cancer develops when erratic cell growth and proliferation occur in the breast tissue. Which hormones are most critical in the development of breast cancer and why a large percentage of women who develop breast cancer have no identified risk factors remain unclear (National Cancer Institute, 2015a). While the discovery of pertinent genetic factors has clarified the predisposition toward developing breast cancer in some women, a significant amount of ongoing research is dedicated to further elucidating the development of this disease.

Clinical Presentation and Types of Breast Cancer

Breast cancer may be detected by identification of a palpable lesion or by screening mammography. It is important to note that pain (or lack thereof) does not indicate the presence or the absence of breast cancer (American Cancer Society, 2015); nevertheless, pain is not usually a sign of breast cancer (Vaidya & Joseph, 2014). Skin changes can also be the initial manifestation of breast cancer. Types of breast cancer include carcinoma in situ, invasive breast cancer, Paget's disease, and inflammatory carcinoma. Breast cancer is further classified based on whether it originated in the ducts or lobules. See Chapter 5 for a discussion of breast anatomy and physiology.

Carcinoma in Situ

Ductal carcinoma in situ (DCIS), or intraductal carcinoma, is the earliest manifestation of breast cancer and involves abnormal cells that are confined to the ducts. This condition is usually diagnosed in association with microcalcifications seen on mammography; it is rare to find a palpable mass in such cases. DCIS is sometimes referred to as a precancerous condition, although the likelihood of DCIS progressing to invasive cancer is unknown. Currently, researchers are evaluating a 12-gene assay (the DCIS Score) that has the potential to assess recurrence risk based on the individual woman's tumor biology and, therefore, guide treatment decisions (Wood et al., 2014).

With lobular carcinoma in situ (LCIS), the abnormal cells are limited to the breast lobules. LCIS is a noninvasive lesion that differs from DCIS in that it does not always progress to invasive cancer; thus, the term *lobular neoplasia* is often used to describe this condition. LCIS may be bilateral and is often an incidental finding noted during biopsy for another lesion (Simpson, Reis-Filho, & Lakhani, 2010).

Invasive Breast Cancer

Invasive or infiltrating ductal carcinoma is the most common malignancy of the breast. Invasive ductal carcinoma usually presents as a discrete, solid mass, with malignant cells escaping the confines of the ducts and infiltrating the breast parenchyma. The most common sites of metastatic spread of such cancer are the lymph nodes, bones, liver, and lungs (Price, 2009).

Invasive or infiltrating lobular carcinoma is less common and may also present as a discrete mass. The mass may be characterized only by thickening or induration, with margins that are diffuse and ill defined, both on physical examination and on mammogram. Invasive lobular carcinoma is more frequently characterized by bilateral involvement than other types of breast cancer; it is associated with unusual spread of metastases, including carcinomatous meningitis, intra-abdominal metastases with intestinal and ureteral obstruction, and metastases to the uterus and ovaries (Dillon, Guidi, & Schnitt, 2010).

Paget's Disease

Paget's disease is a rare form of breast cancer (1% of all cases) that causes eczematous nipple changes as well as ulceration, itching, erythema, and nipple discharge. As many as half of all women with Paget's disease present with a palpable mass that is usually an underlying DCIS or invasive ductal carcinoma. Controversy exists regarding whether the nipple involvement arises from infiltration from an underlying breast tumor or is a separate process involving the nipple epidermis. Nevertheless, women with Paget's disease demonstrating nipple change should be assumed to have underlying breast cancer (Helme, Harvey, & Agrawal, 2015).

Inflammatory Carcinoma

Inflammatory breast carcinoma is a rapidly progressive type of breast cancer, with more than half of all cases already demonstrating lymphovascular invasion at the time of diagnosis (Matro et al., 2015). This type of carcinoma causes diffuse inflammatory changes of the breast skin with erythema, edema, warmth, skin thickening, and peau d'orange (fine dimpling that makes the breast skin appear similar to the skin of an orange). Thus, it can be mistaken for mastitis. Often there is not a distinct palpable mass (Matro et al., 2015).

Assessment

History

The initial history for a woman with a breast mass is the same as that described in the earlier section on benign breast masses. If the cancer is already diagnosed and classified as a T3 or T4 lesion (**Table 15-4**), the woman should be asked

---

TABLE 15-4	TNM Classification of Breast Cancers

Primary Tumor (T)

TX	Primary tumor cannot be assessed
T0	No evidence of primary tumor
Tis	Carcinoma in situ: ductal carcinoma in situ, lobular carcinoma in situ, or Paget's disease of the nipple with no associated invasive carcinoma or carcinoma in situ (Paget's disease with a tumor is classified according to tumor size)
T1	Tumor 2 cm or smaller in greatest dimension (may be subdivided into T1mi, T1a, T1b, and T1c, depending on the exact size of the tumor)
T2	Tumor larger than 2 cm but not larger than 5 cm in greatest dimension
T3	Tumor larger than 5 cm in greatest dimension
T4	Tumor of any size with direct extension to the chest wall (T4a), skin (T4b), or both (T4c); inflammatory carcinoma (T4d)

Regional Lymph Nodes (N)

NX	Regional lymph nodes cannot be assessed (e.g., previously removed)
N0	No regional lymph node metastases
N1	Metastases in movable ipsilateral axillary node(s)
N2	Metastases in ipsilateral axillary lymph nodes that are clinically fixed or matted (N2a), or in clinically detected (by imaging studies or clinical examination) ipsilateral internal mammary nodes in the absence of clinically evident axillary lymph node metastases (N2b)
N3	Metastases in ipsilateral infraclavicular lymph node(s) with or without axillary lymph node involvement (N3a), or in clinically detected (by imaging studies or clinical examination) apparent ipsilateral internal mammary lymph node(s) with clinically evident axillary lymph node metastasis (N3b), or metastases in ipsilateral supraclavicular lymph node(s) with or without axillary or internal mammary lymph node involvement (N3c)

Distant Metastases (M)

M0	No clinical or radiographic evidence of distant metastases
M1	Distant detectable metastases

Data from Edge, S. B., Byrd, D. R., Compton, C. C., Fritz, A. G., Greene, F. L., & Trotti, A. (2010). *AJCC cancer staging manual* (7th ed.). New York, NY: Springer.

about symptoms of metastases such as bone pain, arthralgias, cough, jaundice, abdominal pain, headaches, visual disturbances, malaise, loss of appetite, weight loss, fever, and fatigue. Clinicians should remain vigilant for symptoms of metastasis in any woman with a history of breast cancer.

Physical Examination

The clinician should perform a comprehensive breast examination when breast cancer is suspected. Note any skin changes, palpable masses, and nipple discharge. A suspicious lesion is usually hard, is painless, and has irregular borders that may be immobile and fixed to the skin or surrounding breast tissue. Palpate for the axillary, cervical, and supraclavicular lymph nodes—enlargement of any of these nodes is suspicious. Examination of the lungs, abdomen, and neurologic system should also be performed to detect signs of metastasis. See Chapter 6 for further information on breast examination.

Diagnostic Testing

Diagnostic testing for breast cancer includes both imaging studies and tissue sampling. The diagnostic imaging tests most frequently used in the evaluation of breast cancers are mammography, ultrasound, and sometimes MRI (**Table 15-1**).

Mammography can identify breast cancers that are too small to palpate on physical examination, and can detect both benign and malignant calcifications. Benign calcifications are typically characterized by their large, coarse, and scattered appearance. Malignant-appearing calcifications tend to be fainter, resembling grains of sand. With digital mammography as well as tomosynthesis, a wider range of tissue contrast can be seen; subtle contrast differences can be amplified with these technologies, and the images are immediately available. Mammography can also identify masses that ultrasound can then further characterize as solid or fluid filled. Solid masses require further intervention or follow-up, whereas simple fluid-filled cysts generally do not.

MRI is recommended for screening women at high risk for breast cancer (20% or greater lifetime risk), but evidence does not support the use of this modality for screening women at average risk (Griffin & Pearlman, 2010; NCCN, 2015c). MRI is helpful in identifying occult breast cancer when there are axillary node metastases but no visible carcinoma on mammogram or ultrasound. This imaging technology can also assist with staging and therapy evaluation (NCCN, 2015c). MRI should be used judiciously due to its expense and high false-positive rate (lack of specificity); moreover, it may be unnecessary depending on findings of other imaging studies.

Breast tissue sampling procedures are described in **Table 15-3**.

Further Assessment When Breast Cancer Is Diagnosed

Several factors guide appropriate treatment options and serve as prognostic indicators when breast cancer is diagnosed. Malignancies are staged using the TNM system, which incorporates information on the size of tumor, lymph node involvement, and metastatic spread (**Table 15-4**). Tumors can also be graded; grading indicates the tumor's extent of differentiation, or how closely the cells resemble normal tissue. A well-differentiated tumor has a more favorable prognosis than a poorly differentiated lesion (Chang & Hilsenbeck, 2010; Yamamoto et al., 2014).

Tumors are also assessed for estrogen and progesterone receptor (ER/PR) and *HER2/neu* status. ER/PR-positive tumors are more likely to respond to hormonal manipulation, whereas ER/PR-negative tumors have a less favorable prognosis (Chang & Hilsenbeck, 2010; Yamamoto et al., 2014). The *HER2/neu* oncogene is closely related to human epidermal growth factor. Overexpression of *HER2*, which occurs in 20% to 25% of breast cancers, is associated with more aggressive tumor cells and a poorer prognosis (Niikura et al., 2012). Other biomarkers in breast cancers, such as radiosensitivity index and MRE11, vascular endothelial growth factor (VEGF), and proliferating cellular nuclear antigen (PCNA), are also being studied as means to help predict individual recurrence risk and develop personalized treatment plans.

The status of the axillary lymph nodes is critical in determining treatment options for women with invasive breast cancer. For women who have early-stage tumors less than 5 cm in size and no palpable axillary lymph nodes, sentinel node biopsy provides necessary staging information without the associated morbidities of a full dissection (e.g., lymphedema, immobility of the upper extremity, and accompanying diminished quality of life). With this technique, dye is injected into the region surrounding the tumor to identify the first node draining the breast. This node, which is termed the sentinel axillary node, is then removed (Cowher et al., 2014). If the sentinel node is positive, dissection of the Level I and II axillary lymph nodes is needed, although FNA or core biopsy should be considered first to confirm malignancy and the need for dissection (Lyman et al., 2014).

Additional tests are performed if there is evidence of advanced cancer (stage 3 or 4) to detect metastases. These tests routinely include a complete blood count, liver function tests, and a chest radiograph. Brain imaging, a bone scan, and abdominal imaging (computed tomography [CT], MRI, or ultrasound) are not routine, but may be warranted if metastases are suspected due to the tumor's clinical stage or signs and symptoms (NCCN, 2015c). Positron emission tomography (PET) scan may also be indicated when considering metastatic disease, but it is no longer routinely used in women with clinical stage 1 or 2 disease (Schnipper et al., 2012).

Differential Diagnoses

A palpable breast mass can be caused by any of the benign conditions discussed earlier in this chapter. Differential diagnoses for Paget's disease include eczema, psoriasis, contact dermatitis, and, rarely, squamous cell carcinoma in situ arising in the skin (Bowen's disease). Differential diagnoses for inflammatory carcinoma include breast abscess, infection, and mastitis. The presence of any of these conditions in a woman who is not lactating is highly suspicious for malignancy.

Prevention

Two selective estrogen receptor modulators (SERMs), tamoxifen (Nolvadex) and raloxifene (Evista), as well as aromatase inhibitors, such as anastrazole (Arimidex), exemestane (Aromasin), and letrozole (Femara), are used to prevent breast cancer in women who are at high risk for developing this disease; this indication is known as preventive therapy or chemoprevention (Bambhroliya, Chavez-MacGregor, & Brewster, 2015; Visvanathan et al., 2013). To date, FDA approval for breast cancer prevention has been granted to only tamoxifen and raloxifene (Bambhroliya et al., 2015). All of these medications have potentially serious side effects. For example, SERMs are associated with thromboembolic events and endometrial cancer; aromatase inhibitors have been linked to decreased bone mineral density, which can increase fracture risk (National Cancer Institute, 2015a). Evidence supporting the use of particular agents is emerging rapidly, and the choice of agent should be made by an expert after careful consideration of patient factors and current data.

Those women who are at very high risk for breast cancer may elect to undergo prophylactic mastectomy, particularly after childbearing is complete. Salpingo-oophorectomy may also be performed in women with BRCA1 or BRCA2 mutations (NCCN, 2015b). In premenopausal women who are BRCA positive, salpingo-oophorectomy reduces the risk of developing breast cancer by 50% (NCCN, 2015b). The benefits of risk reduction and decreased anxiety about the possibility of developing cancer must be weighed against the risks of the surgeries themselves. Although such disease is uncommon, women must be advised that breast cancer can develop in the chest wall after prophylactic mastectomy (Ho et al., 2012).

Management

Suspected or diagnosed breast cancer requires collaborative care with breast cancer specialists, such as a surgeon or medical oncologist. The primary treatment strategies for breast cancer include surgery, chemotherapy, radiation, hormone therapies, bisphosphonates, and monoclonal antibodies. A combination of these modalities is often used, and the specific therapies employed must be individualized based on a variety of clinicopathologic factors (e.g., cancer stage; age and menopausal status; ER, PR, and HER2 results; and genetic assays).

Breast-conserving surgery—lumpectomy or partial mastectomy—removes the cancer but not the breast itself. In addition to removal of breast tissue alone (total or simple mastectomy), mastectomy may include removal of the breast and Level I and II lymph nodes (modified radical mastectomy). Radical mastectomy, which includes removal of the breast, pectoralis major and minor muscles, and Level I to III lymph nodes, is no longer performed, as it is associated with severe morbidities and does not offer any survival advantage over less radical surgery. Breast-conserving surgery may be performed instead of mastectomy depending on the disease stage. Studies examining surgical treatment outcomes in women for 20 years after the procedures indicate that breast-conserving surgeries do not increase the future risk of death from recurrent disease when compared to mastectomy (Goldhirsch et al., 2013; Ye, Yan, Christos, Nori, & Ravi, 2015). When mastectomy is performed, breast reconstruction is an option.

Chemotherapy may be administered after surgery (adjuvant therapy) or preoperatively (neoadjuvant therapy) to decrease the size of a large tumor prior to surgery. Radiation therapy is used regularly following breast-sparing surgery and may also be administered after mastectomy. In addition, radiation is useful for treatment of locally advanced disease of the chest wall or breast, for palliation for bone pain from bone metastases, and to strengthen a region that contains bony disease that is at risk for pathologic fracture.

The SERM tamoxifen and the aromatase inhibitors letrozole, exemestane, and anastrazole are the hormonal therapies used in breast cancer treatment when ER/PR receptors are positive. The optimal duration of tamoxifen therapy appears to be 10 years, rather than 5 years as was previously recommended (Burstein et al., 2014).

Ductal Carcinoma in Situ

Historically, DCIS was treated with mastectomy, but this can be more radical surgery than is necessary for a carcinoma that may not progress to invasive carcinoma (Bleicher, 2013). Current options for DCIS treatment include breast-conserving surgery, with or without radiation, and if women have large or high-grade tumors, total mastectomy. Tamoxifen therapy after surgery may be recommended, especially for women who are ER positive. The most appropriate treatment strategy depends on patient characteristics, the extent of disease, and patient preferences (Bleicher, 2013;

Morrow & Harris, 2010; National Cancer Institute, 2015b; NCCN, 2015c).

Lobular Carcinoma in Situ

Optimal management of LCIS must balance the fact that this condition is a risk factor for cancer with the fact that it is not malignant per se. Risk of cancer is increased when LCIS is present in both breasts (King & Reis-Filho, 2014). Treatment options include surgical excision, careful observation with clinical examination and mammography, preventive therapy/chemoprevention with tamoxifen, participation in breast cancer prevention trials, and bilateral prophylactic mastectomy for those women deemed to be at high risk for developing breast cancer (King & Reis-Filho, 2014; National Cancer Institute, 2015b).

Invasive Breast Cancer

Treatment of invasive carcinoma depends on multiple factors, including the size and grade of the tumor, the involvement of lymph nodes, the presence of metastases, first-time diagnosis versus recurrent disease, and the results of ER/PR and *HER2* testing. A combination of treatments, including surgery, chemotherapy, radiation, hormonal therapies, bisphosphonates (e.g., zoledronic acid [Reclast, Zometa] and pamidronate [Aredia]), and monoclonal antibodies, may be used. FDA-approved monoclonal antibodies for use in treatment of invasive cancer include bevacizumab (Avastin), cetuximab (Erbitux), panitumumab (Vectibix), and trastuzumab (Herceptin). Poly (ADP-ribose) polymerase (PARP) inhibitors are currently being evaluated in clinical trials for women with *BRCA* mutations and triple-negative (i.e., no estrogen, progesterone, or *HER2* receptors) breast cancer (National Cancer Institute, 2015b). When cancer has metastasized, the goal of treatment is control or palliative, rather than curative (National Cancer Institute, 2015b; NCCN, 2015c).

Paget's Disease

Suspicion for Paget's disease should be high in any woman with nipple symptoms, as diagnosis of this disease is often delayed. Breast-conserving surgery with complete excision of the nipple and areola to clear margins, followed by radiation, is recommended if the margins are negative. Mastectomy should be considered if the margins are positive or if the disease is multicentric or extends beyond the central portion of the breast. Tamoxifen therapy after surgery may be recommended as well (NCCN, 2015c).

Inflammatory Carcinoma

Women with signs and symptoms of inflammatory breast carcinoma may initially be treated with antibiotics because inflammatory carcinoma can be mistaken for mastitis. If a 7- to 10-day course of antibiotics does not result in complete resolution of symptoms, or if the cutaneous findings are highly suspicious, immediate mammography and referral for skin biopsy are indicated. Treatment of inflammatory carcinoma involves multiple modalities, including surgery, chemotherapy, radiation, hormonal therapy, aromatase inhibitors, and monoclonal antibodies (NCCN, 2015c).

Emerging Evidence That May Change Practice

Recommendations regarding breast cancer screening, diagnostic techniques, and management are constantly evolving. A December 2015 search of the National Cancer Institute's website (National Cancer Institute, 2015c) identified more than 340 ongoing clinical trials related to breast cancer treatment alone. These trials will inevitably change clinical practice related to breast cancer, and clinicians must keep up-to-date with new developments. In addition, women at high risk for breast cancer, or who already have breast cancer, should be encouraged to participate in clinical trials, as these interventions are considered the best management (NCCN, 2015c).

Special Considerations

Pregnant Women

The incidence of breast cancer in pregnancy is difficult to estimate. When this disease is defined as breast cancer diagnosed either during pregnancy or within 1 year postpartum, the incidence has been reported as 0.2% to 3.8% of all breast cancers or 2.4 cases per 100,000 births (Guidroz, Scott-Conner, & Weigel, 2011). The incidence of breast cancer in pregnant and postpartum women is likely to increase with the trend toward delayed childbearing (Azim et al., 2012; National Cancer Institute, 2015a).

Delays in diagnosis in this population are common because breast abnormalities can be difficult to detect in the presence of the normal breast changes that occur during pregnancy and lactation. Mammography, with appropriate abdominal shielding during pregnancy, and ultrasound can be used to evaluate a mass or other abnormality on clinical examination (Litton & Theriault, 2010). Any palpable mass should be biopsied regardless of the imaging results (Litton & Theriault, 2010; National Cancer Institute, 2015b).

Management of breast cancer during pregnancy must take into account the benefits and risks for both the woman and the fetus, and can involve making complex decisions. Surgery—either mastectomy or lumpectomy—can be performed during pregnancy. Chemotherapy can be used during the second and third trimesters, but is stopped at 35 weeks' gestation or 3 weeks prior to planned birth. Radiation is contraindicated during pregnancy (Colfry, 2013; Litton & Theriault, 2010; NCCN, 2015c).

References

Ahmed, A., Malone, C., Sweeney, K., Barry, K., Kerin, M., & McLaughlin, R. (2014). Symptomatic breast: How does breast cancer present? Symptoms and clues to diagnosis. *Research*, 1087. http://dx.doi.org/10.13070/rs.en.1.1087

American Cancer Society. (2013). Breast cancer facts & figures 2013–2014. Retrieved from http://www.cancer.org/acs/groups/content/@research/documents/document/acspc-042725.pdf

American Cancer Society. (2015). Cancer facts & figures 2015. Retrieved from http://www.cancer.org/research/cancerfactsstatistics/cancerfactsfigures2015

Amin, A. L., Purdy, A. C., Mattingly, J. D., Kong, A. L., & Termuhlen, P. M. (2013). Benign breast disease. *Surgical Clinics of North America*, 93(2), 299–308. doi:10.1016/j.suc.2013.01.001

Aydin, Y., Atis, A., Kaleli, S., Uludag, S., & Goker, N. (2010). Cabergoline versus bromocriptine for symptomatic treatment of premenstrual mastalgia: A randomised, open-label study. *European Journal of Obstetrics, Gynecology, and Reproductive Biology*, 150(2), 203–206. doi:10.1016/j.ejogrb.2010.02.024

Azim, H. A., Jr., Santoro, L., Russell-Edu, W., Pentheroudakis, G., Pavlidis, N., & Peccatori, F. A. (2012). Prognosis of pregnancy-associated breast cancer: A meta-analysis of 30 studies. *Cancer Treatment Reviews*, 38(7), 834–842. doi:10.1016/j.ctrv.2012.06.004

Bambhroliya, A., Chavez-MacGregor, M., & Brewster, A. M. (2015). Barriers to the use of breast cancer risk reduction therapies. *Journal of the National Comprehensive Cancer Network*, 13(7), 927–935.

Berg, W. A., Sechtin, A. G., Marques, H., & Zhang, Z. (2010). Cystic breast masses and the ACRIN 6666 experience. *Radiologic Clinics of North America, 48*(5), 931–987. doi:10.1016/j.rcl.2010.06.007

Bergmann, R. L., Bergmann, K. E., von Weizsäcker, K., Berns, M., Henrich, W., & Dudenhausen, J. W. (2014). Breastfeeding is natural but not always easy: Intervention for common medical problems of breastfeeding mothers: A review of the scientific evidence. *Journal of Perinatal Medicine, 42*(1), 9–18. doi:10.1515/jpm-2013-0095

Bleicher, R. J. (2013). Ductal carcinoma in situ. *Surgical Clinics of North America, 93*(2), 393–410. doi:10.1016/j.suc.2012.12.001

Burstein, H. J., Temin, S., Anderson, H., Buchholz, T. A., Davidson, N. E., Gelmon, K. E., . . . Griggs, J. J. (2014). Adjuvant endocrine therapy for women with hormone receptor–positive breast cancer: American Society of Clinical Oncology clinical practice guideline focused update. *Journal of Clinical Oncology, 32*(21), 2255–2269. doi:10.1200/jco.2013.54.2258

Centers for Disease Control and Prevention. (2014, September 2). Cancer among women. Retrieved from http://www.cdc.gov/cancer/dcpc/data/women.htm

Chang, J. C., & Hilsenbeck, S. G. (2010). Prognostic and predictive markers. In J. R. Harris, M. E. Lippman, M. Morrow, & C. K. Osborne (Eds.), *Diseases of the breast* (4th ed., pp. 443–457). Philadelphia, PA: Lippincott Williams & Wilkins.

Colak, T., Ipek, T., Kanik, A., Ogetman, Z., & Aydin, S. (2003). Efficacy of topical nonsteroidal antiinflammatory drugs in mastalgia treatment. *Journal of the American College of Surgeons, 196*(4), 525–530. doi:10.1016/s1072-7515(02)01893-8

Cole, E. N., Sellwood, R. A., England, P. C., & Griffiths, K. (1977). Serum prolactin concentrations in benign breast disease throughout the menstrual cycle. *European Journal of Cancer, 13*(6), 597–603.

Colfry, A. J., 3rd. (2013). Miscellaneous syndromes and their management: Occult breast cancer, breast cancer in pregnancy, male breast cancer, surgery in stage IV disease. *Surgical Clinics of North America, 93*(2), 519–531. doi:10.1016/j.suc.2012.12.003

Collaborative Group on Hormonal Factors in Breast Cancer. (2002). Breast cancer and breastfeeding: Collaborative reanalysis of individual data from 47 epidemiological studies in 30 countries, including 50302 women with breast cancer and 96973 women without the disease. *Lancet, 360*(9328), 187–195. doi:10.1016/s0140-6736(02)09454-0

Cowher, M. S., Grobmyer, S. R., Lyons, J., O'Rourke, C., Baynes, D., & Crowe, J. P. (2014). Conservative axillary surgery in breast cancer patients undergoing mastectomy: Long-term results. *Journal of the American College of Surgeons, 218*(4), 819–824. doi:10.1016/j.jamcollsurg.2013.12.041

Cuneo, K. C., Dash, R. C., Wilke, L. G., Horton, J. K., & Koontz, B. F. (2012). Risk of invasive breast cancer and ductal carcinoma in situ in women with atypical papillary lesions of the breast. *Breast J, 18*(5), 475–478. doi: 10.1111/j.1524-4741.2012.01276.x

Dillon, D. A., Guidi, A. J., & Schnitt, S. J. (2010). Pathology of invasive breast cancer. In J. R. Harris, M. E. Lippman, M. Morrow, & C. K. Osborne (Eds.), *Diseases of the breast* (4th ed., pp. 374–407). Philadelphia, PA: Lippincott Williams & Wilkins.

Edge, S. B., Byrd, D. R., Compton, C. C., Fritz, A. G., Greene, F. L., & Trotti, A. (2010). *AJCC cancer staging manual* (7th ed.). New York: Springer.

Edwards, S. E., da Costa Rocha, I., Williamson, E. M., & Heinrich, M. (2015). Evening primrose (oil) *Oenothera biennis L.* In *Phytopharmacy: An evidence-based guide to herbal medicinal products* (pp. 144–148). Chichester, UK: John Wiley & Sons.

Ernster, V. L., Mason, L., Goodson, W. H., 3rd, Sickles, E. A., Sacks, S. T., Selvin, S., . . . Hunt, T. K. (1982). Effects of caffeine-free diet on benign breast disease: A randomized trial. *Surgery, 91*(3), 263–267.

Ferrara, A. (2011). Benign breast disease. *Radiologic Technology, 82*(5), 447M–462M.

Ferris-James, D. M., Iuanow, E., Mehta, T. S., Shaheen, R. M., & Slanetz, P. J. (2012). Imaging approaches to diagnosis and management of common ductal abnormalities. *Radiographics, 32*(4), 1009–1030. doi:10.1148/rg.324115150

Fritz, M. A., & Speroff, L. (2011). *Clinical gynecologic endocrinology and infertility* (8th ed.). Philadelphia, PA: Lippincott Williams & Wilkins.

Giess, C. S., Raza, S., & Birdwell, R. L. (2011). Distinguishing breast skin lesions from superficial breast parenchymal lesions: Diagnostic criteria, imaging characteristics, and pitfalls. *Radiographics, 31*(7), 1959–1972. doi:10.1148/rg.317115116

Goldhirsch, A., Winer, E. P., Coates, A. S., Gelber, R. D., Piccart-Gebhart, M., Thurlimann, B., & Senn, H. J. (2013). Personalizing the treatment of women with early breast cancer: Highlights of the St Gallen International Expert Consensus on the Primary Therapy of Early Breast Cancer 2013. *Annals of Oncology, 24*(9), 2206–2223. doi:10.1093/annonc/mdt303

Griffin, J. L., & Pearlman, M. D. (2010). Breast cancer screening in women at average risk and high risk. *Obstetrics & Gynecology, 116*(6), 1410–1421. doi:10.1097/AOG.0b013e3181fe714e

Grobmeyer, S. R., Copeland, E. M., Simpson, J. F., & Page, D. L. (2009). High-risk and premalignant lesions of the breast. In A. I. Bland & E. M. Copeland (Eds.), *The breast: Comprehensive managment of benign and malignant disease* (4th ed., pp. 169–188). Phildelphia, PA: Saunders.

Guidroz, J. A., Scott-Conner, C. E., & Weigel, R. J. (2011). Management of pregnant women with breast cancer. *Journal of Surgical Oncology, 103*(4), 337–340. doi:10.1002/jso.21673

Hadi, M. S. (2000). Sports brassiere: Is it a solution for mastalgia? *Breast J, 6*(6), 407–409.

Helme, S., Harvey, K., & Agrawal, A. (2015). Breast-conserving surgery in patients with Paget's disease. *British Journal of Surgery, 102*(10), 1167–1174. doi:10.1002/bjs.9863

Ho, A., Cordeiro, P., Disa, J., Mehrara, B., Wright, J., Van Zee, K. J., . . . McCormick, B. (2012). Long-term outcomes in breast cancer patients undergoing immediate 2-stage expander/implant reconstruction and postmastectomy radiation. *Cancer, 118*(9), 2552–2559. doi:10.1002/cncr.26521

Hubbard, J. L., Cagle, K., Davis, J. W., Kaups, K. L., & Kodama, M. (2015). Criteria for excision of suspected fibroadenomas of the breast. *American Journal of Surgery, 209*(2), 297–301. doi:10.1016/j.amjsurg.2013.12.037

Hussain, A. N., Policarpio, C., & Vincent, M. T. (2006). Evaluating nipple discharge. *Obstetrics and Gynecological Survey, 61*(4), 278–283. doi:10.1097/01.ogx.0000210242.44171.f6

Iddon, J., & Dixon, J. M. (2013). Mastalgia. *BMJ, 347*, f3288. doi:10.1136/bmj.f3288

Ingram, D. M., Hickling, C., West, L., Mahe, L. J., & Dunbar, P. M. (2002). A double-blind randomized controlled trial of isoflavones in the treatment of cyclical mastalgia. *Breast, 11*(2), 170–174. doi:10.1054/brst.2001.0353

Isaacs, J. H. (1994). Other nipple discharge. *Clinical Obstetrics and Gynecology, 37*(4), 898–902.

Kataria, K., Dhar, A., Srivastava, A., Kumar, S., & Goyal, A. (2014). A systematic review of current understanding and management of mastalgia. *Indian Journal of Surgery, 76*(3), 217–222. doi:10.1007/s12262-013-0813-8

Kerlikowske, K., Smith-Bindman, R., Ljung, B. M., & Grady, D. (2003). Evaluation of abnormal mammography results and palpable breast abnormalities. *Annals of Internal Medicine, 139*(4), 274–284.

Khan, H. N., Rampaul, R., & Blamey, R. W. (2004). Local anaesthetic and steroid combined injection therapy in the management of non-cyclical mastalgia. *Breast, 13*(2), 129–132. doi:10.1016/j.breast.2003.09.010

King, T. A., & Reis-Filho, J. S. (2014). Lobular neoplasia. *Surgical Oncology Clinics of North America, 23*(3), 487–503. doi:10.1016/j.soc.2014.03.002

King, T. L., & Brucker, M. C. (2011). *Pharmacology for women's health.* Sudbury, MA: Jones and Bartlett.

Klimberg, V. S., Kass, R. B., Beenken, S. W., & Bland, K. I. (2009). Etiology and management of benign breast disease. In K. I. Bland & E. M. Copeland (Eds.), *The breast: Comprehensive management of benign and malignant diseases* (4th ed., Vol. 1, pp. 87–106). Philadelphia, PA: Saunders Elsevier.

Kumar, S., Mansel, R. E., Scanlon, M. F., Hughes, L. E., Edwards, C. A., Woodhead, J. S., & Newcombe, R. G. (1984). Altered responses of prolactin, luteinizing hormone and follicle stimulating hormone secretion to thyrotrophin releasing hormone/gonadotrophin releasing hormone stimulation in cyclical mastalgia. *British Journal of Surgery, 71*(11), 870–873.

Litton, J. K., & Theriault, R. L. (2010). Breast cancer during pregnancy and subsequent pregnancy in breast cancer survivors. In J. R. Harris, M. E. Lippman, M. Morrow, & C. K. Osborne (Eds.), *Diseases of the breast* (4th ed., pp. 808–816). Philadelphia, PA: Lippincott Williams & Wilkins.

Lyman, G. H., Temin, S., Edge, S. B., Newman, L. A., Turner, R. R., Weaver, D. L., . . . Giuliano, A. E. (2014). Sentinel lymph node biopsy for patients with early-stage breast cancer: American Society of Clinical Oncology clinical practice guideline update. *Journal of Clinical Oncology, 32*(13), 1365–1383. doi:10.1200/jco.2013.54.1177

Malarkey, W. B., Schroeder, L. L., Stevens, V. C., James, A. G., & Lanese, R. R. (1977). Twenty-four-hour preoperative endocrine profiles in women with benign and malignant breast disease. *Cancer Research, 37*(12), 4655–4659.

Matro, J. M., Li, T., Cristofanilli, M., Hughes, M. E., Ottesen, R. A., Weeks, J. C., & Wong, Y. N. (2015). Inflammatory breast cancer management in the National Comprehensive Cancer Network: The disease, recurrence pattern, and outcome. *Clinical Breast Cancer, 15*(1), 1–7. doi:10.1016/j.clbc.2014.05.005

Morgan, H. S. (2015). Primary care management of the female patient presenting with nipple discharge. *Nurse Practitioner, 40*(3), 1–6. doi:10.1097/01.npr.0000460856.83105.61

Morrow, M., & Harris, J. R. (2010). Ductal carcinoma in situ and microinvasive carcinoma. In J. R. Harris, M. E. Lippman, M. Morrow, & C. K. Osborne (Eds.), *Diseases of the breast* (4th ed. pp. 349–362). Philadelphia, PA: Lippincott Williams & Wilkins.

Moyer, V. A., & U.S. Preventive Services Task Force. (2014). Risk assessment, genetic counseling, and genetic testing for *BRCA*-related cancer in women: U.S. Preventive Services Task Force recommendation statement. *Annals of Internal Medicine, 160*(4), 271–281. doi:10.7326/m13-2747

National Cancer Institute. (2012, September 24). Breast cancer risk in women. Retrieved from http://www.cancer.gov/types/breast/risk-fact-sheet

National Cancer Institute. (2015a, May 28). Breast cancer prevention (PDQ): Health professional version. Retrieved from http://www.ncbi.nlm.nih.gov/pubmedhealth/PMH0032634

National Cancer Institute. (2015b, July 24). Breast cancer treatment (PDQ): Health professional version. Retrieved from http://www.ncbi.nlm.nih.gov/pubmedhealth/PMH0032676

National Cancer Institute. (2015c). Find a clinical trial. Retrieved from http://www.cancer.gov/about-cancer/treatment/clinical-trials/search

National Cancer Institute. (2015d, June 5). Genetics of breast and gynecologic cancers (PDQ). Retrieved from http://www.cancer.gov/types/breast/hp/breast-ovarian-genetics-pdq

National Comprehensive Cancer Network (NCCN). (2015a). NCCN clinical practice guidelines in oncology: Breast cancer screening and diagnosis, version 1.2015. Retrieved from http://www.nccn.org/professionals/physician_gls/pdf/breast-screening.pdf

National Comprehensive Cancer Network (NCCN). (2015b). NCCN clinical practice guidelines in oncology: Genetic/familial high-risk assessment: Breast and ovarian, version 2.2015. Retrieved from http://www.nccn.org/professionals/physician_gls/pdf/genetics_screening.pdf

National Comprehensive Cancer Network (NCCN). (2015c). NCCN clinical practice guidelines in oncology: Breast cancer, version 2.2015. Retrieved from http://www.nccn.org/professionals/physician_gls/pdf/breast.pdf

Niikura, N., Liu, J., Hayashi, N., Mittendorf, E. A., Gong, Y., Palla, S. L., . . . Ueno, N. T. (2012). Loss of human epidermal growth factor receptor 2 (*HER2*) expression in metastatic sites of *HER2*-overexpressing primary breast tumors. *Journal of Clinical Oncology, 30*(6), 593–599. doi:10.1200/jco.2010.33.8889

Parker, V. J., Menzies, J. R., & Douglas, A. J. (2011). Differential changes in the hypothalamic–pituitary–adrenal axis and prolactin responses to stress in early pregnant mice. *Journal of Neuroendocrinology, 23*(11), 1066–1078. doi:10.1111/j.1365-2826.2011.02204.x

Patel, B. K., Falcon, S., & Drukteinis, J. (2015). Management of nipple discharge and the associated imaging findings. *American Journal of Medicine, 128*(4), 353–360. doi:10.1016/j.amjmed.2014.09.031

Pearlman, M. D., & Griffin, J. L. (2010). Benign breast disease. *Obstetrics & Gynecology, 116*(3), 747–758. doi:10.1097/AOG.0b013e3181ee9fc7

Peters, F., Pickardt, C. R., Zimmermann, G., & Breckwoldt, M. (1981). PRL, TSH, and thyroid hormones in benign breast diseases. *Klinische Wochenschrift, 59*(8), 403–407.

Petrucelli, N., Daly, M. B., & Feldman, G. L. (2013). *BRCA1* and *BRCA2* hereditary breast and ovarian cancer. In R. A. Pagon, M. P. Adam, H. H. Ardinger, S. E. Wallace, A. Amemiya, L. J. H. Bean, . . . K. Stephens (Eds.), *GeneReviews* [Internet]. Seattle, WA: University of Washington, Seattle.

Price, J. E. (2009). Concepts and mechanisms of breast cancer metastasis. In K. I. Bland & E. M. Copeland (Eds.), *The breast: Comprehensive management of benign and malignant disease* (4th ed., pp. 549–564). Philadelphia, PA: Saunders/Elsevier.

Rizvi, A. A. (2006). Hyperprolactinemia and galactorrhea associated with marijuana use. *Endocrinologist, 16*(6), 308–310. doi:10.1097/01.ten.0000250184.10041.9d

Sabate, J. M., Clotet, M., Torrubia, S., Gomez, A., Guerrero, R., de las Heras, P., & Lerma, E. (2007). Radiologic evaluation of breast disorders related to pregnancy and lactation. *Radiographics, 27*(Suppl. 1), S101–124. doi:10.1148/rg.27si075505

Salzman, B., Fleegle, S., & Tully, A. S. (2012). Common breast problems. *American Family Physician, 86*(4), 343–349.

Schnipper, L. E., Smith, T. J., Raghavan, D., Blayney, D. W., Ganz, P. A., Mulvey, T. M., & Wollins, D. S. (2012). American Society of Clinical Oncology identifies five key opportunities to improve care and reduce costs: The top five list for oncology. *Journal of Clinical Oncology, 30*(14), 1715–1724. doi:10.1200/jco.2012.42.8375

Scurr, J., Hedger, W., Morris, P., & Brown, N. (2014). The prevalence, severity, and impact of breast pain in the general population. *Breast J, 20*(5), 508–513. doi:10.1111/tbj.12305

Sevim, Y., Kocaay, A. F., Eker, T., Celasin, H., Karabork, A., Erden, E., & Genc, V. (2014). Breast hamartoma: A clinicopathologic analysis of 27 cases and a literature review. *Clinics (Sao Paulo), 69*(8), 515–523.

Simpson, P. T., Reis-Filho, J. S., & Lakhani, S. R. (2010). Lobular carcinoma in situ: Biology and pathology. In J. R. Harris, M. E. Lippman, M. Morrow, C. K. Osborne. (Eds.), *Diseases of the breast* (4th ed., pp. 333–340). Philadelphia, PA: Lippincott Williams & Wilkins.

Srivastava, A., Mansel, R. E., Arvind, N., Prasad, K., Dhar, A., & Chabra, A. (2007). Evidence-based management of mastalgia: A meta-analysis of randomised trials. *Breast, 16*(5), 503–512. doi:10.1016/j.breast.2007.03.003

U.S. Department of Health and Human Services. (2014, January). The health consequences of smoking—50 years of progress: A report of the Surgeon General. Retrieved from http://www.surgeongeneral.gov/library/reports/50-years-of-progress/full-report.pdf

Vaidya, J. S., & Joseph, D. (2014). *Fast facts: Breast cancer* (5th ed.). Oxford, UK: Health Press.

Vashi, R., Hooley, R., Butler, R., Geisel, J., & Philpotts, L. (2013). Breast imaging of the pregnant and lactating patient: physiologic changes and common benign entities. *American Journal of Roentgenology, 200*(2), 329–336. doi:10.2214/ajr.12.9845

Vaziri, F., Lari, M. Z., Dehaghani, A. S., Salehi, M., Sadeghpour, H., Akbarzadeh, M., & Zare, N. (2014). Comparing the effects of dietary flaxseed and omega-3 fatty acids supplement on cyclical mastalgia in Iranian women: A randomized clinical trial. *International Journal of Family Medicine, 2014*(Article ID 174532), 1–7. doi:10.1155/2014/174532

Visvanathan, K., Hurley, P., Bantug, E., Brown, P., Col, N. F., Cuzick, J., . . . Lippman, S. M. (2013). Use of pharmacologic interventions for breast cancer risk reduction: American Society of Clinical Oncology clinical practice guideline. *Journal of Clinical Oncology, 31*(23), 2942–2962. doi:10.1200/jco.2013.49.3122

Vitex agnus-castus. (2015). *Natural Medicines Professional Database*. Retrieved from https://naturalmedicines.therapeuticresearch.com/databases/food,-herbs-supplements/professional.aspx?productid=968#effectiveness

Wood, W. C., Alvarado, M., Buchholz, D. J., Hyams, D., Hwang, S., Manders, J., . . . Willey, S. (2014). The current clinical value of the DCIS Score. *Oncology (Williston Park, NY), 28*(Suppl. 2), C2, 1–8, C3.

Yamamoto, M., Hosoda, M., Nakano, K., Jia, S., Hatanaka, K. C., Takakuwa, E., . . . Yamashita, H. (2014). p53 accumulation is a strong predictor of recurrence in estrogen receptor–positive breast cancer patients treated with aromatase inhibitors. *Cancer Science, 105*(1), 81–88. doi:10.1111/cas.12302

Ye, J. C., Yan, W., Christos, P. J., Nori, D., & Ravi, A. (2015). Equivalent survival with mastectomy or breast-conserving surgery plus radiation in young women aged < 40 years with early-stage breast cancer: A national registry–based stage-by-stage comparison. *Clinical Breast Cancer*. doi:10.1016/j.clbc.2015.03.012

Yildirim, A. C., Yıldız, P., Yıldız, M., Kahramanca, Ş., & Kargıcı, H. (2015). Mastalgia–cancer relationship: A prospective study. *Journal of Breast Health, 11*, 88–91. doi:10.5152/tjbh.2015.2492

Zafar, A., & Rehman, A. (2013). Topical diclofenac versus oral diclofenac in the treatment of mastalgia: A randomized clinical trial. *Rawal Medical Journal, 38*(4), 371–377.

Online Resources

The *CRICO/RMF Breast Care Management Algorithm: Improving Breast Patient Safety* includes risk assessment and screening recommendations; algorithms for management of screening mammogram results, nipple discharge, palpable mass, and breast pain; and discussion points for providing breast care.

http://www.rmf.harvard.edu/files/documents/cricormf_bca.pdf

The California Department of Public Health, Cancer Detection Section, has a website that offers multiple clinician resources, including forms for recording the results of a breast-related history and physical examination as well as diagnostic algorithms for management of a palpable mass, abnormal screening mammogram results, nipple discharge, breast skin changes, breast pain, and breast biopsy results.

http://qap.sdsu.edu/resources/tools/index.html

The National Cancer Institute's Breast Cancer page includes information about screening and testing, prevention, genetics, causes, treatment, clinical trials, cancer literature, research, and statistics. Materials for health professionals and patients are available.

http://www.cancer.gov/cancertopics/types/breast

The National Comprehensive Cancer Network provides detailed evidence-based guidelines and algorithms for breast cancer screening, diagnosis, risk reduction, and treatment.

http://www.nccn.org/professionals/physician_gls/f_guidelines.asp

CHAPTER 16

Alterations in Sexual Function

Brooke Faught
The editors acknowledge Susan Chasson, who was the author of the previous edition of this chapter.

Over the past century, human sexuality has evolved from a risqué topic to a more commonplace subject in media and among the general public. As a result, clinicians regularly encounter women seeking care for sexual concerns as well as women who disclose sexual concerns in the course of a visit for another purpose. These sexual concerns may reflect a normal variation of sexuality; indicate the need for education (e.g., inadequate knowledge about the sexual stimulation needed for arousal and/or orgasm); result from a medical or mental health condition, medication, or substance; or lead to a diagnosis of sexual dysfunction.

This chapter is entitled "Alterations in Sexual Function," rather than "Female Sexual Dysfunction" as it was titled in previous editions of this text, because sexual function varies widely among women, and alterations in sexual function are not necessarily sexual dysfunction. A diagnosis of sexual dysfunction requires that the woman perceive her symptoms as distressing. For example, a woman who is unable to achieve orgasm but is satisfied by her sexual relationship with her partner and is not distressed by her lack of orgasm is not considered to have a sexual dysfunction. While not all alterations in sexual function are dysfunctional, that statement does not discount the right of women and clinicians to consider and implement safe and effective therapies when appropriate to improve sexual function. Each woman should be considered as the unique individual that she is; she should be evaluated from a holistic, unbiased, and nonjudgmental perspective, and provided with multimodal treatment options.

From a feminist perspective, it is important to appreciate the history of gender imbalance in treatment for sexual dysfunction. In 1998, the U.S. Food and Drug Administration (FDA) approved sildenafil (Viagra) for erectile dysfunction in men. In 1999, Laumann et al. published findings from the landmark National Health and Social Life Survey, which found that more women report sexual dysfunction than their male counterparts—43% versus 31%, respectively. Yet, there were no FDA-approved medications for libido, arousal, or orgasm in women until 2015, when flibanserin (Addyi) became the first medication to win FDA approval for the indication of hypoactive sexual desire disorder in women. At the time when flibanserin was approved, there were already nearly 30 FDA-approved medications to directly or indirectly enhance sexual functioning in men. The issue is not whether a "magic pill" exists to cure a medical problem, but rather how gender equality is perceived by researchers, clinicians, and the government. Although the focus of sexual health research was on men in the immediate post-sildenafil era, women are now demanding more gender-specific research and treatment options for sexual dysfunction.

This chapter begins with an overview of models of sexual response and evolving definitions of female sexual dysfunction. This is followed by a description of the scope and etiology of sexual concerns in women and a discussion of the elements to include in a general assessment of sexual concerns. The remainder of the chapter focuses on the assessment and management of the three specific types of female sexual dysfunction: female sexual interest/arousal disorder, female orgasmic disorder, and genito-pelvic pain/penetration disorder.

MODELS OF SEXUAL RESPONSE

Many models of sexual response have been proposed over the years. Alfred Kinsey (1953) is deemed the original researcher of human sexuality and began his research in the 1950s. Approximately a decade later, Masters and Johnson (1966) published a linear model of sexual response, which included a progressive occurrence of excitement, plateau, orgasm, and resolution. This model was believed to describe sexual response in both men and women. Another linear model proposed by Helen Singer Kaplan (1979) in the late 1970s was narrowed down to three phases: desire, arousal, and orgasm. Unlike the aforementioned models, a biopsychosocial model takes into account multiple etiologic factors and determinants that include biological, psychological, sociocultural, and interpersonal influences (Althof et. al., 2005; Rosen & Barsky, 2006).

In 2000, Dr. Rosemary Basson proposed a new model for female sexual response based on a changed perspective of female sexual dysfunction and desire disorders. Instead of the traditional model of excitement, desire, orgasm, and resolution, Basson (2000) describes many women as moving from a state of sexual neutrality to a state where they become motivated to seek stimuli that will cause sexual arousal. Orgasm is not always a necessary component to satisfying sexual encounters, according to Basson's model; other factors—such as emotional intimacy and relationship status—are of just as much importance as physiologic and biochemical changes. A diagram of Basson's model can be found in Chapter 10.

DEFINITIONS OF FEMALE SEXUAL DYSFUNCTION

Various definitions of female sexual dysfunction have been proposed, and they remain inconsistent among different organizations and committees due to advancing research. To further complicate the situation, most well-known sexual health research relied on older terminology, which therefore perpetuates the use of certain outdated terms. Although many clinicians remain familiar with the terminology developed in 1998 by the American Foundation for Urologic Disease (AFUD) Consensus Panel (Basson et al., 2000), these definitions are actually outdated and inconsistent with current diagnostic terms.

In 2003, an international committee sponsored by the American Urological Association Foundation developed definitions for female sexual dysfunction that expanded upon definitions presented by the AFUD Consensus Panel. These definitions attempted to incorporate the evolving conceptualization of women's sexual response cycle, which was not reflected in earlier diagnostic criteria (Basson et al., 2003).

The *Diagnostic and Statistical Manual of Mental Disorders, Fourth Edition, Text Revision* (*DSM-IV-TR*) (American Psychiatric Association, 2000) included six categories of female sexual dysfunction. These six categories were narrowed down to three with the release of the *Diagnostic and Statistical Manual of Mental Disorders, Fifth Edition* (*DSM-5*) in 2013: female sexual interest/arousal disorder, female orgasmic disorder, and genito-pelvic pain/penetration disorder (American Psychiatric Association, 2013). These three *DSM-5* categories are used as the organizational structure for assessment and management of female sexual dysfunction in this chapter.

Table 16-1 reviews the evolution of female sexual dysfunction terms and definitions, noting their requirement of patient distress for a diagnosis of sexual dysfunction. An important part of the evaluation of sexual concerns is determining whether the patient perceives the sexual dysfunction as distressing (American Psychiatric Association, 2013).

SCOPE OF THE PROBLEM

Many women have concerns about sexual issues. In the National Health and Social Life Survey, which was one of the first national U.S. surveys to address sexual concerns, 43% of women reported sexual dysfunction. Of the 1,486 women responding, 27% to 32% reported a lack of interest in sex, 22% to 28% were unable to achieve orgasm, 17% to 27%

TABLE 16-1	Female Sexual Dysfunction Definitions

Type of Dysfunction	*Diagnostic and Statistical Manual of Mental Disorders, Fourth Edition, Text Revision (DSM-IV-TR), 2000*[a]	**American Foundation for Urologic Disease Consensus Panel, 2000**[b]	**American Urological Association Foundation Committee, 2003**	*Diagnostic and Statistical Manual of Mental Disorders, Fifth Edition (DSM-5), 2013*[c]
Desire	Hypoactive sexual desire disorder Sexual aversion disorder	Hypoactive sexual desire disorder Sexual aversion disorder	Women's sexual interest/desire disorder Sexual aversion disorder	Female sexual interest/ arousal disorder
Arousal	Female sexual arousal disorder	Sexual arousal disorder	Subjective sexual arousal disorder Genital sexual arousal disorder Combined genital and subjective arousal disorder Persistent sexual arousal disorder	
Orgasm	Female orgasmic disorder	Orgasmic disorder	Women's orgasmic disorder	Female orgasmic disorder
Sexual pain	Dyspareunia Vaginismus	Dyspareunia Vaginismus Other sexual pain disorders	Dyspareunia Vaginismus	Genito-pelvic pain/ penetration disorder

[a] Diagnosis requires that the disturbance causes marked distress or interpersonal difficulty.
[b] Diagnosis requires that the symptoms cause personal distress.
[c] Diagnosis requires that the symptoms cause clinically significant distress.

Data from American Psychiatric Association. (2000). *Diagnostic and statistical manual of mental disorders* (4th ed., text revision). Washington, DC: Author; American Psychiatric Association. (2013). *Diagnostic and statistical manual of mental disorders* (5th ed.). Washington, DC: Author. Basson, R., Berman, J., Burnett, A., Derogatis, L., Ferguson, D., Fourcroy, J., . . . Whipple, B. (2000). Report of the international consensus development conference on female sexual dysfunction: Definitions and classifications. *Journal of Urology, 163,* 888–893; Basson, R., Leiblum, S. L., Brotto, L., Derogatis, L., Fourcroy, J., Fugl-Myer, K., . . . Schultz, W. W. (2003). Definitions of women's sexual dysfunctions reconsidered: Advocating expansion and revision. *Journal of Psychosomatic Obstetrics & Gynecology, 24,* 221–229.

reported sex was not pleasurable, 18% to 27% described trouble lubricating, 8% to 21% experienced pain during sex, and 6% to 16% were anxious about performance (the ranges reflect variations among age groups) (Laumann et al., 1999). More recent national estimates are available from the Prevalence of Female Sexual Problems Associated with Distress and Determinants of Treatment Seeking (PRESIDE) study, which had 31,581 respondents. Nearly half of women (44%) reported having some type of sexual problem. Prevalence of specific problems was 39% for low desire, 26% for low arousal, and 21% for orgasm difficulties. Sexually related personal distress, as measured by the Female Sexual Distress Scale, was present in 23% of women, and 12% reported both a sexual problem and sexually related personal distress (Shifren, Monz, Russo, Segreti, & Johannes, 2008). These surveys indicate that sexual concerns in women are relatively common.

ETIOLOGY

Developmental, health-related, partner, and relationship factors as well as sociocultural influences may all contribute to female sexual dysfunction. Etiologies may stem from environmental and genetic origins, and oftentimes overlap (Clayton & Groth, 2013). The number and complexity of potential contributing factors highlights the importance of a comprehensive assessment and evaluation for women reporting sexual concerns. Although many women presenting with issues related to their sexual health may have biologic etiologies, there is frequently a push to medicalize nonmedical symptoms by both clinicians and women seeking health care for sexual concerns (Bellamy, Gott, & Hinchliff, 2013). Women with sexual concerns may actually be experiencing normal variations of sexuality—a possibility that must be considered in the assessment. In this circumstance, referral to a sexuality educator or sex therapist can frequently prove beneficial.

GENERAL ASSESSMENT FOR SEXUAL CONCERNS

This section describes the general assessment of any woman presenting with sexual concerns. Sexual health assessment and screening for sexual concerns is discussed in Chapters 6 and 10. Additional assessments specific to the different types of sexual dysfunction are detailed later in this chapter. The purpose of the general assessment is to identify all potential biological and psychosocial sources of the concern(s). When assessing a woman for sexual dysfunction, it is necessary to determine whether the concerns have been lifelong (primary) or emerged more recently after a period of normal sexual function (secondary), and whether they are situational (specific to certain circumstances) or generalized (occur across all circumstances—masturbation, intercourse, manual stimulation, and so on).

Relationship stressors also need to be evaluated as a possible source of sexual dysfunction. For example, if a woman is experiencing intimate partner violence, changing the time and location of sex is not an appropriate recommendation to help increase her sexual desire. In addition, using an intervention in such circumstances may lead to further deterioration of the woman's sexual health and possibly even aggravate the violent episodes.

History

Assessment of the woman with sexual concerns requires a comprehensive health history that includes physical and psychosocial history questions as well as assessment of her general and sexual health. Investigation of physical concerns should include surgeries, injuries, chronic illnesses, medications, and allergies. Reports of surgeries that could affect vascular or neurologic function of the genital tract and other erogenous areas, such as the breasts, indicate a need for further investigation. Past injuries to the pelvis, the genital structures, the spine, and even the brain can affect sexual response in women. Chronic illnesses of relevance include, but are not limited to, thyroid disease, diabetes, hypertension, certain cancers, chronic pain, hyperprolactinemia, cognitive disorders, and heart disease. In addition, pregnancy history is important to review, because pregnancy, birth, and lactation can pose unique challenges to sexual functioning. A review of medications is important as well, because several drugs are known to cause or exacerbate sexual dysfunction (**Box 16-1**). Screening for latex allergies should be a standard part of any

---

BOX 16-1 Drugs Known to Cause or Exacerbate Female Sexual Dysfunction

- Amphetamines
- Anticonvulsants
- Antidepressants
- Antihypertensives and other cardiovascular agents
- Antiulcer drugs
- Benzodiazepines
- Combined estrogen and progestin contraceptives
- Digoxin
- Gonadotropin-releasing hormone (GnRH) agonists
- Histamine receptor blockers
- Hormone therapy (estrogen and/or progestogen)
- Lipid-lowering agents
- Nonsteroidal anti-inflammatory drugs
- Opioid pain medications
- Psychotropic medications
- Substances: alcohol, amphetamines, cocaine, heroin, marijuana

Data from Kingsberg, S., & Woodard, T. (2015). Female sexual dysfunction: Focus on low desire. *Obstetrics & Gynecology, 125*(2), 477–486.

---

gynecologic examination, because latex products used for contraception and during pelvic examinations may be a source of sexually related pain.

The psychosocial history should include information about the woman's sexual orientation as well as her past and present partner(s) and relationship(s). Never assume sexual orientation or monogamous relationship status based on marital status, background, religious beliefs, or other sociodemographic factors. Some women may be uncomfortable answering sexual history questions in a face-to-face interview, so providing patient-completed history forms may yield more information about sensitive topics than only asking questions verbally. Providing such forms prior to the appointment date allows the woman to answer intimate questions in the privacy of her own home.

Ask the woman if she has a prior or present history of physical, emotional, or sexual abuse, or if she has ever been sexually assaulted. Assess for signs and symptoms of major depression and other mental health conditions, such as post-traumatic stress disorder and obsessive–compulsive disorder, as well as cognitive conditions that might affect memory and attention.

Diet and exercise habits, life stressors, coping mechanisms, and body image should also be evaluated. In addition, it is important to inquire about the use of alcohol, cigarettes, and illegal drugs, because these habits may be factors in sexual dysfunction. Screen the woman for risk factors associated with sexual activity, including multiple sexual partners and use of contraception. Sexually transmitted infections can be a source of sexual pain, and use of hormonal contraceptives may cause decreased desire in some women (Burrows, Basha, & Goldstein, 2012).

The cultural and religious beliefs of the woman should be considered when evaluating and recommending treatment for sexual dysfunction as well. For example, if a woman is unable to achieve orgasm through intercourse, encouraging self-stimulation may not be an option if that practice conflicts with her religious or cultural beliefs.

Box 16-2 lists some open-ended questions that can be used to begin a discussion of a patient's sexual concerns. The Female Sexual Function Index (FSFI) can be helpful in assessment but should not replace a thorough sexual history. The FSFI is a validated questionnaire that assesses six domains: desire, arousal, lubrication, orgasm, satisfaction, and pain (Rosen et al., 2000). The FSFI questionnaire contains 19 items and is available online at http://www.fsfi-questionnaire.com. Additionally, the Female Sexual Distress Scale-Revised (FSDS-R) is a validated 13-item questionnaire that can determine whether distress accompanies the sexual concern(s) (DeRogatis, Clayton, Lewis-D'Agostino, Wunderlich, & Fu, 2008).

When evaluating the woman with a sexual concern, reviewing normal sexual response may be all that is needed to reassure her that what she is experiencing is normal. The clinician may also need

---

BOX 16-2 **Initial Questions for Assessment of Sexual Concerns**

- Do you have any concerns related to your sexual health?
- Are you sexually active?
- Which sexual concerns, problems, or issues are you experiencing?
- How does this concern affect your sexual function, relationship(s), and life?
- What is the most distressing part of this concern?
- Which treatments have you used?
- What kind of conversations have you had with your partner(s) so far, and how have they gone?
- What do you think is the source of your sexual concern?

Data from Association of Reproductive Health Professionals. (2010). Sexual health fundamentals for patient care: A report on 2010 consensus outcomes and guidance for women's health professionals. Retrieved from http://www.arhp.org /uploadDocs/SHF_meetingreport.pdf; Steege, J. F., & Zolnoun, D. A. (2009). Evaluation and treatment of dyspareunia. *Obstetrics & Gynecology, 113*, 1124–1136; van Lankveld, J. J. D. M., Granot, M., Weijmar Schultz, W. C. M., Binik, Y. M., Wesselmann, U., Pukall, C. F., . . . Achtrari, C. (2010). Women's sexual pain disorders. *Journal of Sexual Medicine, 7*, 615–631.

---

to evaluate the woman's understanding of normal sexual anatomy and function. One technique is to use a diagram to discuss genital anatomy and physiology. Women's sexual response cycle is often not well understood. For example, many people do not realize that the majority of women cannot achieve orgasm without direct or indirect stimulation of the clitoris. As a consequence, women who cannot achieve orgasm through intercourse often believe they have a problem. Discussing and describing sexual anatomy may give the woman enough information to allow her to understand and improve her sexual response.

Physical Examination

The physical examination should specifically look for potential health conditions that could affect sexual function, such as undiagnosed diabetes or hypertension. Height, weight, and vital signs should be recorded. Women with sexual dysfunction who are overweight or obese tend to have worse symptoms (Mozafari et al., 2015). Neurologic and vascular systems should be examined as well. A pelvic examination should be incorporated into an assessment for sexual dysfunction, including inspection and palpation of both external and internal genital and pelvic structures. See Chapter 6 for pelvic examination techniques.

Diagnostic Testing

Laboratory tests should be performed only when there is a clinical indication for them. Although a comprehensive battery of laboratory tests in every woman reporting sexual concerns is unnecessary, appropriate screening based on history and specific symptoms can facilitate individualized care. General tests to consider based on individual history and symptomatology include fasting glucose, a lipid profile, thyroid-stimulating hormone (TSH), and prolactin (Brotto, Bitzer, Laan, Leiblum, & Luria, 2010; Hatzichristou et al., 2010). Testing for women presenting with sexual pain should include vaginal pH and microscopy of vaginal secretions with normal saline and 10% potassium hydroxide. See Chapter 6 for microscopic examination techniques.

Measurement of androgen levels, such as free and total testosterone, androstenedione, dihydrotestosterone, and dehydroepiandrosterone sulfate (DHEA-S), as well sex hormone–binding globulin (SHBG) and albumin is considered controversial because assay methods vary in terms of their accuracy, precision, and reliability, and because a consistent correlation between androgen levels and sexual dysfunction has not been found in past studies. Despite the inconsistency, a recent correlation has been made among free testosterone levels, androstenedione levels, and sexual desire in women between the ages of 19 and 65 (Wåhlin-Jacobsen et al., 2015).

Clinicians who obtain androgen levels must be well versed in the latest research on the topic so that they can use this information appropriately. Additionally, there is the issue of how to manage a women who is believed to have insufficient levels of endogenous testosterone. As of November 2015, there was no FDA-approved testosterone replacement product for women in the United States; however, testosterone products, including compounded testosterone, are widely used on an off-label basis (Snabes & Simes, 2009). This issue is discussed in more detail in the section on women's sexual interest/arousal disorder.

For women who are on combined hormonal contraceptives (i.e., estrogen and progestin pills, patch, or ring) and present with sexual pain, some evidence suggests a correlation between low free testosterone levels and an increase in cytosine–adenine–guanine (CAG) trinucleotide repeat length, which results in an inefficient androgen receptor on the X chromosome with vestibulodynia (Goldstein et al., 2014). Testing for CAG repeat length is not yet appropriate for clinical use, but this information is certainly of relevance in understanding why some women develop pain while using these contraceptive methods and other women do not.

Differential Diagnoses

The clinician should begin by categorizing the type of sexual dysfunction as sexual interest/arousal disorder, orgasmic disorder, or genito-pelvic pain/penetration disorder (**Table 16-1**), keeping in mind that overlap among the types is frequent and common. Using the information obtained in the history, physical examination, and possibly laboratory testing, the clinician should then determine whether the source of the dysfunction is psychological, physical, or a combination of the two. The rest of this chapter presents specific assessment and management recommendations for each type of sexual dysfunction.

FURTHER ASSESSMENT AND MANAGEMENT OF SPECIFIC TYPES OF SEXUAL DYSFUNCTION

Female Sexual Interest/Arousal Disorder

Female sexual interest/arousal disorder is the complete lack of or significant reduction in sexual interest or sexual arousal, associated with three or more of the following six symptoms: (1) the absence or reduction of interest in sex; (2) an absence of or reduction in fantasies and erotic thoughts; (3) absent or decreased desire to initiate sexual encounters with her partner and usually unreceptiveness when the partner attempts to initiate such encounters; (4) absent or reduced sense of excitement/pleasure during sex; (5) absent or reduced response to sexual cues (e.g., verbal, visual); and (6) absent or reduced sensations in the genitals or elsewhere during sex. These symptoms must be distressing to the woman and must have persisted for a minimum of 6 months. The symptoms may be either lifelong or acquired after previously normal sexual function, and either situational (occurring only in certain circumstances, such as intercourse) or generalized (occurring in all circumstances, such as intercourse, digital and manual stimulation, and masturbation). Severity may fall on a continuum from mild to moderate to severe distress over the symptoms. Lastly, there must be no other known mental health, physical, or substance-induced cause of the condition (American Psychiatric Association, 2013).

Assessment of Sexual Interest Disorder

Assessment of issues related to sexual interest should start with determining the duration of the concern and factors surrounding the symptoms. Has the woman always felt this way, or does her current state represent a change in her level of desire? It is important to look for any negative factors, either psychological or physical, that may affect desire. Does the woman have a history of sexual abuse? Are there conflicts about other issues in the woman's relationship with her partner? Is the woman experiencing pain with intercourse? Other social factors that may influence desire include financial stress, small children who continue to require care at night, or work schedules that make it difficult for couples to find the time or energy to plan for sexual intimacy.

Frequency of sexual activity is another important factor to evaluate. Instead of experiencing a lack of sexual interest caused by a physical or psychological source, there may be a difference in expectations between the woman and her partner. In a national study, married women aged 25 to 69 years reported the following frequencies of sexual activity: not at all in the past year, 3.5% to 37.9%; a few times per year to monthly, 11.6% to 23.7%; a few times per month to weekly, 35.9% to 50.2%; two to three times per week, 6.2% to 35.2%; and four or more times per week, 0 to 5.1% (ranges reflect variations among age groups) (Herbenick et al., 2010). These statistics demonstrate a wide variation in the frequency of sexual activity.

It is also important to inquire about whether the change in desire has resulted in a change in sexual frequency. Does the woman continue to have sex even when the encounters are unwanted? A woman who believes she does not have a choice about frequency of sex may first need to deal with issues of power and control in the relationship before it can be determined whether her sexual concern has a physical basis.

Basson (2000) believes that many women are motivated to initiate sexual activity for reasons other than a desire for sexual gratification. These motivating factors for sexual relations may include "emotional closeness, increased commitment, bonding, and tolerance of imperfections in the relationship" (p. 53). If a woman achieves these nonsexual goals, she will view her sexual experience as positive, whether or not she personally experiences sexual gratification. Therefore, when assessing a woman for a sexual interest disorder, it is important to consider what motivates her desire for sexual relations.

When using Basson's (2000) model, if a woman does not initiate sex, it is necessary to find out if she is willing to participate in and able to enjoy sex if the encounter is initiated by her partner. If so, the woman can be told that her pattern of response is normal for many women. Working with the woman, explore any changes that may have altered her satisfaction with her sexual relationship. Does the woman experience orgasm with her partner? Although many anorgasmic women report satisfying sexual relationships, over time the lack of physical pleasure may decrease motivation to engage in sexual activity.

Do the negatives that result from sex outweigh the positive rewards? If a woman's need for intimacy is not being met during the sexual encounter, because of either lack of time or fatigue, then she may lose her motivation for future sexual encounters. Although the hormonal changes associated with menopause can affect desire, a woman's inability to achieve pregnancy—a previous motivating factor for sex—may act as a factor in decreasing desire for sex after menopause or sterilization. In addition, infertility and the associated testing, medications, interventions, and other therapies can medicalize sex and eliminate spontaneity.

Do associated physical symptoms indicate that a woman's lack of interest is the result of underlying illness? Fatigue may be related to thyroid dysfunction or sleep disorders. Does the woman have a chronic medical condition, such as arthritis or back pain, that makes sex painful or uncomfortable? Sexual interest disorder is also associated with thyroid disease, epilepsy, and renal disease. Screen the woman for use of medications (see **Box 16-1**) or a history of surgeries that could alter desire by changing hormone levels, particularly combined contraceptives, gonadotropin-releasing hormone (GnRH) agonists, antiestrogens, and hysterectomy or oophorectomy.

Menopause may be a time of decreased desire, and the reasons for this change may go beyond alterations in hormone levels, such as hot flashes, night sweats, fatigue, weight gain, vaginal dryness, and painful intercourse. Despite these changes, distressing low desire does not progressively increase in the postmenopausal years (Kingsberg, 2014). The highest prevalence of distressing sexual arousal disorder occurs in the 45- to 64-year-old age range, with a decline in the 65 and older population (Shifren et al., 2008).

Although there is no clear consensus on the usefulness of androgen testing and replacement in women, there is some understanding of androgens' relevance and use in women with sexual dysfunction. Androgens are produced both by the ovaries and the adrenal glands. The ovaries produce testosterone and androstenedione, which are converted to dihydrotestosterone by way of 5-alpha-reductase enzyme (Cohen, Catherine, & Goldstein, 2014), and the adrenal glands produce dehydroepiandrosterone (DHEA and DHEA-S). Testosterone levels decrease approximately 50% between the ages of 30 and 50 years, then decline another 15% after menopause—although the latter decrease is thought to be related to age rather than menopause (Mathur & Braunstein, 2010). Androgen levels can vary significantly from one woman to another, and the two main factors that can decrease androgen levels (other than age) are oophorectomy and oral estrogen therapy. Oophorectomy can result in a 50% loss of testosterone production, whereas oral estrogen therapy can increase SHBG, triggering a relative decrease in free testosterone levels. Androgen insufficiency can be diagnosed by history and exclusion of other causes of symptoms. Measurement of androgen levels is not required to initiate testosterone therapy or to monitor this treatment's effectiveness (American College of Obstetricians and Gynecologists, 2011, reaffirmed 2015; Mathur & Braunstein, 2010), although such testing can help to correlate objective changes with subjective perceptions of improvement.

Management of Sexual Interest Disorder

The appropriate treatment for decreased sexual interest in women depends on the etiology of this condition. If relationship discord is affecting intimacy, the clinician should avoid suggesting a medical intervention and instead provide a referral to an appropriate therapist. Patients with undiagnosed or untreated physical or mental health conditions require applicable interventions to remedy the underlying illness. Consider changing any medications that may be affecting sexual desire (**Box 16-1**). If decreased desire is related to pain with intercourse, the source of the pain should be diagnosed and treated. If sexual dysfunction already exists, be aware of how medical interventions may cause the sexual symptoms to increase in severity. For example, decreased libido has been reported by as many as 80% to 90% of patients with depression (Clayton & Balon, 2009). At the same time, use of most antidepressants can lead to sexual side effects. Selective serotonin reuptake inhibitors (SSRIs) tend to carry the highest potential for sexual side effects, which are dose dependent (Waldinger, 2015).

Women should be educated about normal alterations in desire that result from the aging process, longer duration of a relationship, and life changes such as those resulting from pregnancy, lactation, and menopause. For instance, all domains of sexual function in women decrease throughout each trimester of pregnancy, including desire, arousal, orgasm, and lubrication, resulting in decreased sexual activity over the course of pregnancy

(Galazka, Drosdzol-Cop, Naworska, Czajkowska, & Skrzypulec-Plinta, 2015). Women who are postpartum are believed to have decreased sexual desire due to a generalized decrease in amygdala response to arousing stimuli compared to nulliparous women (Rupp et al., 2013). The rise in prolactin levels that occurs during lactation can certainly have a negative impact on sexual desire. Finally, distressing sexual concerns peak in the perimenopausal and early postmenopausal age group (ages 45 to 64), indicating another possible hormonal connection (Shifren et al., 2008).

Individual or couples counseling may help patients whose decreased desire is the result of life stressors or relationship problems. Some strategies to promote healthy sexuality among couples include planning time for intimacy, writing a "to-do" list of tasks that a woman may worry about during a sexual encounter and placing it outside the door prior to intimacy, and encouraging honest communication between partners. While sex therapy tends to benefit women with sexual pain disorders more than women with desire, arousal, and orgasmic dysfunction, it is still the most widely used therapy for any form of sexual dysfunction (Pereira, Arias-Carrion, Machado, Nardi, & Silva, 2013)—likely due to the longstanding lack of FDA-approved treatment for sexual dysfunction in women.

In August 2015, flibanserin was approved for use in the United States as the first ever medication indicated for hypoactive sexual desire disorder (HSDD) in premenopausal women. Flibanserin is a $5\text{-}HT_{1A}$ receptor agonist and $5\text{-}HT_2$ receptor antagonist. In nine studies, it was found to improve women's sexual desire, increase satisfying sexual events, and decrease distress. Five long-term safety studies demonstrated the drug's safety and verified that the benefits outweigh the risks of this medication; such risks include dizziness, somnolence, nausea, fatigue, insomnia, and dry mouth. Night-time dosing is recommended to avoid many of these potential side effects. Hypotension and syncope are additional potential adverse reactions in a small subset of flibanserin users (FDA, 2015).

Women who have sexual side effects from SSRIs may be helped by taking bupropion SR (Wellbutrin) 150 mg twice daily (Safarinejad, 2011) or sildenafil 50 mg to 100 mg before sexual activity (Nurnberg et al., 2008). Switching the woman to an antidepressant that is associated with fewer sexual side effects, such as mirtazapine (Remeron), nefazodone (Serzone), or bupropion, is another option (Clayton & Balon, 2009). In addition, off-label use of bupropion SR (150 mg once daily) in women without a history of depression can often improve desire and decrease distress (Safarinejad, Hosseini, Asgari, Dadkhah, & Taghva, 2010).

Transdermal estrogen therapy may be beneficial for the woman experiencing decreased desire after menopause. If symptoms persist and all other causes of low desire have been excluded, testosterone therapy can be considered, although its use for this indication remains controversial (Mathur & Braunstein, 2010). Testosterone plays a vital role in production of estrogen in women, and it also directly acts on testosterone receptor sites throughout the female body (Davis & Braunstein, 2012). As of November 2015, there were no androgen therapies approved by the FDA for use in women; in contrast, the agency has approved oral, injectable, and transdermal androgen preparations for men. Transdermal preparations are frequently used in symptomatic postmenopausal women (Snabes & Simes, 2009), but achieving proper dosing can be difficult because products are packaged in a dose appropriate for male replacement. Compounded androgen preparations are available but are considered controversial due to their lack of standardization. The most common potency of testosterone used in women is 1%, with varying application amounts based on individual patient need.

Known adverse effects from excessive androgen supplementation include hirsutism, acne, deepening of the voice, liver damage, hair loss, mood changes, and enlargement of the clitoris. Lowering of high-density lipoprotein (HDL) cholesterol—that is, "good" cholesterol—levels can be avoided by using transdermal testosterone versus oral formulations (Davis, 2011). These potential risks must be discussed with the patient prior to prescribing androgen therapy. To date, little evidence has been published to support the efficacy and safety of androgen supplementation in premenopausal women and long-term (more than 6 months) androgen supplementation in menopausal women (American College of Obstetricians and Gynecologists, 2011, reaffirmed 2015; Mathur & Braunstein, 2010). Moreover, no causal relationship has been identified between exogenous testosterone use

in women and cardiovascular disease and breast cancer (Brand & van der Schouw, 2010; Laughlin, Goodell, & Barrett-Connor, 2010).

Additional medications on the horizon to treat low sexual desire in women include bremelanotide, a melanocortin receptor 4 agonist (Portman, Edelson, Jordan, Clayton, & Krychman, 2014); Lybrido, a phosphodiesterase inhibitor (PDE) combined with a sublingual testosterone (Poels et al., 2013); and Lybridos, a 5-HT$_{1A}$ receptor agonist combined with a sublingual testosterone (van Rooij et al., 2013). Lybrido and Lybridos are believed to also enhance vascular sexual response, which may have a dual benefit in treating arousal disorders in women (Kingsberg & Woodard, 2015).

Assessment of Sexual Arousal Disorder

Women should be asked whether they are experiencing vaginal lubrication or feelings of genital engorgement with sex play. It is important to determine whether the woman is having stimulation adequate to achieve arousal prior to her partner attempting intercourse and whether difficulty with arousal exists with all forms of sexual stimulation. Women with difficulties in achieving arousal should be assessed for physiologic conditions causing vascular or neurologic changes to the body. Diabetes, hypertension, and coronary artery disease can affect genital vasculature, for example. The woman should also be questioned about exercise or physical activities such as bicycle riding, horseback riding, and motorcycle riding where there is prolonged compression of the nerves and blood vessels leading to the genitals. Atrophic vaginitis and use of certain medications, particularly SSRIs, can also cause arousal disorders (American College of Obstetricians and Gynecologists, 2011, reaffirmed 2015). Other medications associated with arousal disorder include anticholinergics, antihistamines, monoamine oxidase inhibitors (MAOIs), tricyclic antidepressants, and antihypertensives. Smoking and alcohol use can also affect a woman's ability to achieve sexual arousal, which may provide a more enticing reason to stop smoking and limit alcohol use than simply citing the general health benefits from smoking cessation and limited alcohol use.

Management of Sexual Arousal Disorder

If arousal disorder is the result of inadequate stimulation of the clitoris, instructing the woman on the use of artificial lubricants and clitoral stimulation may allow for adequate arousal to achieve orgasm. Vaginal moisturizers, lubricants, and topical arousal products may help increase stimulation, although caution should be urged given the potential for contact irritation. Many lubricants and arousal gels contain chemicals and vulvar irritants to which some women may be sensitive. Natural moisturizing products, such as coconut oil and Emu oil, are often used as alternatives to traditional lubricants. Other glycerin-free lubricants include Slippery Stuff, Wet, Pjur, and Sliquid.

Treatments for medical conditions associated with arousal disorder are usually based on trying to restore blood flow to the genital tissues. For perimenopausal and postmenopausal women with atrophic vaginitis, localized estrogen therapy may be beneficial (see Chapter 12). Women who are breastfeeding may benefit from localized estrogen therapy. Some vulvar skin conditions such as lichen sclerosus can result in scarring and clitoral phimosis, thereby decreasing clitoral sensitivity and increasing potential for irritation and pain (see Chapter 26).

Sexual aids and toys can facilitate and enhance the sexual experience in some women. Vibrators are commonly used to enhance genital arousal and increase the potential for orgasm. Such devices can be used for masturbation or with partnered sexual activity. If women have no personal experience purchasing or using sexual aids and toys, some counseling may be required to identify safe distributors and provide directions on proper use at home. For women who may be hesitant to consider sexual aids and toys, normalizing their use can help them feel comfortable incorporating this into their sexual practice. In some circumstances, referral to a sexuality educator or sex therapist can be helpful. See Chapter 10 for additional information about vibrator use.

In 2000, the FDA cleared the Eros-CTD to treat sexual arousal and orgasmic disorders. Eros-CTD is a clitoral therapy device that fits over the clitoris and increases blood flow to the area by creating gentle suction (Feldhaus-Dahir, 2010). While this device is no longer manufactured by the original distributor, it can still be obtained through third-party vendors. More recently, the Fiera device was developed to serve as a sexual primer. Fiera is a hands-free device that works by providing concurrent suction and vibration to the clitoris.

Complementary and alternative treatments for sexual arousal include yohimbine, L-arginine, and Zestra. Yohimbine, an extract from the bark of an African tree, is available as an over-the-counter (OTC) bark extract (yohimbe) and a prescription pure extract (yohimbine). Yohimbine is FDA approved for use in men but has also been used on an off-label basis in women. It must be taken consistently for at least 14 days and can cause tachycardia and hypertension (Feldhaus-Dahir, 2010). L-Arginine, which is one of the ingredients in the nutritional supplements ArginMax and Vesele, has been shown to increase sexual desire, intercourse frequency, and sexual satisfaction (Ito, Polan, Whipple, & Trant, 2006). Topical products with L-arginine are also available on an over-the-counter basis. Zestra, a topical formulation, contains a blend of botanical oils and extracts. In a randomized controlled trial, women who used Zestra had significantly greater mean improvement in the desire and arousal domains of the FSFI compared to women who used placebo. Mean improvements were also greater with Zestra than with placebo in the lubrication, pain, orgasm, and satisfaction domains of the FSFI, but these results were not statistically significant (Ferguson, Hosmane, & Heiman, 2010). In women with a recent history of cancer and concurrent vaginal atrophy, application of Zestra resulted in improved orgasmic response and decreased latency of time to orgasms. Additionally, all patients in the study reported improved sexual satisfaction at the 4-week follow-up visit (Krychman, Kellogg, Damaj, & Hachicha, 2014).

Although not approved for use in women, sildenafil has been tested in clinical trials. The outcomes of these trials have produced mixed results, but sildenafil may be beneficial for women whose arousal disorder is associated with a neurodegenerative disease (Brown, Kyle, & Ferrill, 2009). Sildenafil should not be used in women with cardiovascular disease and should never be used in conjunction with nitroglycerin.

Compounding offers the option to utilize some of the aforementioned off-label treatments into a topical preparation. For instance, ingredients such as sildenafil, arginine, aminophylline, and testosterone may be mixed into a cream at various potencies, with the final product frequently referred to as "scream cream" or "O cream."

Female Orgasmic Disorder

Female orgasmic disorder is present when there is a marked delay in, marked infrequency of, or absence of orgasm or reduced intensity of orgasm sensations lasting more than 6 months. To warrant this diagnosis, the anorgasmia cannot be related to other physical or mental health conditions or relational problem(s) and must involve some degree of distress. Symptoms may have been present lifelong or be more recent, and they may be generalized to all types of sexual encounters or more situational based on the type of stimulation. For example, some women may be able to attain orgasm with use of a vibrator but be unable to achieve orgasm during coitus (situational), whereas other women cannot achieve orgasm with any modality (generalized). In addition, some women who were previously orgasmic may not be able to achieve orgasm after menopause with any mode of stimulation (secondary), whereas other women may have never been able to achieve orgasm (primary). As the name states, this diagnosis is gender specific (American Psychiatric Association, 2013).

Assessment of Women's Orgasmic Disorder

Assessment of orgasmic disorder begins with determining the duration and extent of the problem. Has the woman ever experienced an orgasm? If so, did she reach orgasm through self-stimulation or with a partner? Which sexual activities led to orgasm in the past? Inability to achieve orgasm is often related to lack of sufficient stimulation. As noted previously, many people are unaware that most women need clitoral stimulation to reach orgasm. Other causes of orgasmic disorders may include trauma and abuse, particularly for women who have never had an orgasm; chronic illness, such as multiple sclerosis, chronic kidney disease, or fibromyalgia; pelvic disorders or surgery; use of medications—most notably SSRIs but also other antidepressants, antipsychotics, and mood stabilizers; alcohol and illegal drug use; relationship issues; inadequate communication between partners; and cultural, religious, or familial beliefs or inhibitions (American College of Obstetricians and Gynecologists 2011, reaffirmed 2015; IsHak, Bokarius, Jeffrey, Davis, & Bakhta, 2010). Inhibition of the orgasmic reflex may also occur for psychological reasons or as a response to genital pain.

Management of Women's Orgasmic Disorder

As part of the management process, it is critical to address any underlying cause of the orgasmic disorder. For example, consider referring women who have been abused for counseling, and consider switching medications for women whose orgasmic disorder seems to be drug related.

There is no specific method for a woman to achieve orgasm. For the woman who has never experienced orgasm, the clinician should begin by using a diagram to demonstrate genital anatomy to the woman. During this education, it is important to explain to the woman that most women can achieve orgasm only through direct or indirect stimulation of the clitoris. Women should be encouraged to try self-exploration of their genital area to determine which type of touching achieves the best response, if they are comfortable with this exercise. Practicing Kegel exercises allows the woman to control her muscular tension, which may decrease inhibition of her orgasmic response. For some women, the use of a vibrator will produce the required stimulation to achieve orgasm. Women who are uncomfortable with self-stimulation may be able to instruct their partners to provide direct clitoral stimulation either manually or with a vibrator to achieve orgasm. Although dated by age, *Becoming Orgasmic* (Heiman & Lopiccolo, 1988) is an excellent self-help guide for women who need more coaching to achieve orgasm. Cognitive-behavioral therapy or sexual therapy may be useful for women with orgasmic disorder that does not resolve with self-help measures.

Pharmaceutical options for female orgasmic disorder are also limited, as there are no FDA-approved medications for arousal and orgasmic dysfunction in women. As mentioned previously in the discussion of female sexual interest/arousal disorder, off-label use of PDE5 inhibitors can occasionally benefit the woman battling anorgasmia related to insufficient arousal. Oxytocin is also used on an off-label basis in some women with orgasmic dysfunction. In one study, intranasal oxytocin increased the intensity of orgasm and contentment after sexual intercourse, although these effects were more pronounced in men (Behnia et al., 2013).

Genito-Pelvic Pain/Penetration Disorder

Genito-pelvic pain/penetration disorder is present when a woman experiences one or more of the following: difficulty with vaginal penetration during intercourse; vulvovaginal or pelvic pain during intercourse or attempted penetration; fear or anxiety about pain before, during, or after vaginal penetration; and the pelvic floor muscles tensing or tightening when vaginal penetration is attempted. To make this diagnosis, symptoms must be present for a minimum of 6 months, must cause significant distress, and cannot be better explained by another physical or mental condition (American Psychiatric Association, 2013).

Assessment of Sexual Pain

In the evaluation of sexual pain (also called dyspareunia), it is important to determine the exact location and experience of the pain. Ask about the pain onset, duration, quality, and severity as well as any factors that cause the pain to improve or worsen. The timing of the pain in relation to the menstrual cycle should be assessed as well, especially if endometriosis is suspected. Determine whether painful sexual encounters occur with penetrative sexual activity only or with all internal and external stimulation. Ask if direct contact is required for pain or if arousal and orgasm result in pain independent from contact.

Causes of external pain may include vaginal infections, dermatologic disorders, atrophic vaginitis, trauma, allergy, and vulvodynia (persistent vulvar pain without a clear identifiable cause). Vaginal infections to consider include vulvovaginal candidiasis, trichomoniasis, bacterial vaginosis, herpes simplex virus, and human papillomavirus (see Chapters 19 and 20). Dermatologic disorders that can cause pain with intercourse include lichen sclerosus, lichen planus, and lichen simplex chronicus (Seehusen, Baird, & Bode, 2014). Vulvar colposcopy and a punch biopsy should be performed to properly diagnose any chronic skin conditions (see Chapter 26).

Women who are perimenopausal, postmenopausal, on long-term hormonal contraceptives, or lactating should be evaluated for atrophic changes to the vulvovaginal tissue (see Chapters 12 and 19). Genitourinary syndrome of menopause (GSM) is the term endorsed by the International Society for the Study of Women's Sexual Health (ISSWSH) and the North American Menopause Society (NAMS) to replace the terms vulvovaginal atrophy and atrophic vaginitis in premenopausal and postmenopausal women (Portman & Gass, 2014). This term more appropriately describes the condition as a syndrome and acknowledges that it affects the entire urogenital tract. Use of certain medications, including tamoxifen, danazol, medroxyprogesterone acetate, and GnRH agonists, can result in GSM-like changes. Physical examination may demonstrate pale and dry vaginal walls with decreased rugae, vulvar fissures, petechiae, and loss of vulvar architecture. In addition, vaginal pH is typically greater than 5.0 in women with GSM/atrophic vaginitis (Reimer & Johnson, 2011).

If the woman is using a latex barrier method for contraception, it is important to consider a latex allergy as the source of the pain. Although the condition is fairly rare, some women are sensitive to human semen. A woman with semen hypersensitivity can demonstrate localized symptoms of vaginal pain after intercourse as well as systemic symptoms of diffuse urticaria, angioedema, and malaise (Bernstein, 2011). If the clinician suspects a woman has a seminal fluid allergy, and use of latex condoms does not alleviate symptoms, the woman should be assessed for a concurrent latex allergy.

Women who report persistent pain at the vaginal introitus or inability to achieve penetration secondary to pain should be evaluated for vestibulodynia (also known as localized provoked vulvodynia, vulvar vestibular syndrome, and vestibulitis). Many of these women will describe experiencing pain while attempting to insert tampons prior to their first intercourse, but this condition can also develop in women with no previous vulvar pain. To evaluate a woman for vestibulodynia, gently palpate the vestibule (see Chapter 5 for location) with a moist cotton swab or Q-tip. The woman will often describe a sharp or burning sensation when this area is lightly touched with the swab. Pain is most often elicited at the six o'clock region of the vulvar vestibule but can occur at any area of the vestibule. Erythema may or may not be present. The etiology of vestibulodynia is not well understood but is thought to be multifactorial (Bonham, 2015; Edwards, 2015). Women with chronic vulvar pain should also be assessed for musculoskeletal dysfunction, anxiety, and comorbid pain conditions (Lamvu et al., 2015).

The woman with vaginal pain or pain after intercourse should be evaluated for chronic vaginitis, atrophic vaginitis, and allergy. Trauma related to episiotomy or birth-related perineal lacerations may also be a source of sexual pain, with pressure during intercourse placed on the perineum or the outer third of the vagina. Deep pelvic pain or pain with thrusting may be caused by adenomyosis, endometriosis, pelvic adhesions, or adnexal pain (see Chapters 26 and 28). Nongynecologic etiologies (e.g., Crohn's disease, irritable bowel syndrome, painful bladder syndrome, and interstitial cystitis) can also cause deep pelvic pain (Seehusen et al., 2014). Trying to duplicate the pain during pelvic examination may give an indication of the source of the pain.

Management of Sexual Pain

Treatment of sexual pain depends on the etiology of the pain. Vaginal infections should be treated with appropriate antibiotic or antifungal medication. Dermatologic disorders of the genital area are often treated with topical corticosteroids (see Chapter 27). A variety of vaginal estrogen preparations are available to treat perimenopausal and postmenopausal women with GSM (see Chapter 12); these products can also be used for short-term therapy in postpartum women with atrophic urogenital changes. Women who dislike the discharge associated with vaginal estrogen creams often prefer to use the vaginal tablets or ring. Women who prefer to avoid hormonal medications or who are not candidates for vaginal estrogen can consider ospemifene, an FDA-approved, nonhormonal, selective estrogen receptor modulator (SERM) for atrophic vaginitis. In addition, the Monalisa Touch fractional CO_2 vaginal laser treatment helps to stimulate healthy collagen production and may improve symptoms of GSM including vaginal dryness, itching, burning and pain. This device was approved by the FDA in 2014.

Women with vulvodynia, including vestibulodynia, should wear cotton underwear and avoid common irritants to the vulvar area such as glycerin-based lubricants, scented panty liners, and harsh soaps (Bonham, 2015; Edwards, 2015). In addition, women with vulvar sensitivities should be encouraged to avoid self-treatment for perceived, undiagnosed infections. Multidisciplinary care can be particularly valuable for women with vulvodynia (Brotto, Yong, Smith, & Sadownik, 2015). Nonpharmacologic treatment modalities include pelvic floor physical therapy, pelvic floor muscle desensitization with vaginal dilators, biofeedback, transcutaneous electrical nerve stimulation (TENS), and cognitive-behavioral therapy (Bonham, 2015; Edwards, 2015; Landry, Bergeron, Dupuis, & Desrochers, 2008; Vallinga, Spoelstra, Hemel, van de Wiel, & Weijmar Schultz, 2015). Likewise, acupuncture can be helpful for some women afflicted with vulvodynia (Schlager, Xu, Park, & Wilkie, 2015). Pharmacologic therapy options include topical lidocaine, oral antidepressants (e.g., tricyclics, venlafaxine, duloxetine), and oral anticonvulsants (e.g., gabapentin, pregabalin); a variety of topical compounded therapies are used as well (Bonham, 2015; De Andres et al., 2015; Edwards, 2015). For women who do not obtain relief with nonpharmacologic, pharmacologic, or complementary and alternative therapies, surgical removal of the vestibule (modified vestibulectomy) can provide long-term pain relief (Swanson, Rueter, Olson, Weaver, & Stanhope, 2014).

Treatment for pelvic pain with intercourse will depend on the source of the pain. Many women report feeling periodic sharp pain when their partner thrusts during intercourse. This pain is often the result of the penis brushing against an ovary or the cervix. Teaching the woman to shift the position of her hips to change the angle of the uterus and ovaries should eliminate this type of pelvic pain. Women with pelvic infections or endometriosis should receive appropriate treatment to remedy these conditions. Physical therapy that teaches the woman to relax her pelvic muscles may also be beneficial in reducing pelvic pain. In some circumstances, compounded diazepam vaginal suppositories can serve as an adjunctive treatment for high-tone pelvic floor dysfunction (Rogalski, Kellogg-Spadt, Hoffmann, Fariello, & Whitmore, 2010).

REFERRAL TO A THERAPIST SPECIALIZING IN SEXUAL DYSFUNCTION

Clinicians who see women with sexual dysfunction should be aware of the counseling resources available in their communities. Circumstances that warrant referral to a therapist include, but are not limited to, longstanding dysfunction, multiple dysfunctions, history of sexual abuse, a psychological disorder or acute psychological event, dysfunction with an unknown etiology, dysfunction that does not respond to therapy, poor relationship status, and negative portrayal of sex from parents as a child.

The American Association of Sex Educators, Counselors, and Therapists (AASECT) is a national organization that provides certification for sex counselors and sex therapists. Sex therapists are mental health professionals with specialized training in psychotherapy for sexual health and dysfunction. The AASECT website (http://www.aasect.org) can help clinicians locate a certified sex therapist in their community.

In addition to mental health services, physical therapy should be frequently considered for patients reporting sexual pain. The American Physical Therapy Association (APTA) website (http://www.apta.org) can direct providers to local physical therapists who specialize in pelvic floor physical therapy.

References

Althof, S. E., Leiblum, S. R., Chevret-Measson, M., Hartmann, U., Levine, S. B., McCabe, M., . . . Wylie, K. (2005). Psychological and interpersonal dimensions of sexual function and dysfunction. *Journal of Sexual Medicine, 2*(6), 793–800.

American College of Obstetricians and Gynecologists. (2011, reaffirmed 2015). Female sexual dysfunction. ACOG Practice Bulletin No. 119. *Obstetrics & Gynecology, 117*, 996–1007.

American Psychiatric Association. (2000). *Diagnostic and statistical manual of mental disorders* (4th ed., text revision). Washington, DC: Author.

American Psychiatric Association. (2013). *Diagnostic and statistical manual of mental disorders* (5th ed.). Washington, DC: Author.

Association of Reproductive Health Professionals. (2010). Sexual health fundamentals for patient care: A report on 2010 consensus outcomes and guidance for women's health professionals. Retrieved from http://www.arhp.org/uploadDocs/SHF_meetingreport.pdf.

Basson, R. (2000). The female sexual response: A different model. *Journal of Sex and Marital Therapy, 26*, 51–65.

Basson, R., Berman, J., Burnett, A., Derogatis, L., Ferguson, D., Fourcroy, J., . . . Whipple, B. (2000). Report of the international consensus development conference on female sexual dysfunction: Definitions and classifications. *Journal of Urology, 163*, 888–893.

Basson, R., Leiblum, S. L., Brotto, L., Derogatis, L., Fourcroy, J., Fugl-Myer, K., . . . Schultz, W. W. (2003). Definitions of women's sexual dysfunctions reconsidered: Advocating expansion and revision. *Journal of Psychosomatic Obstetrics & Gynecology, 24*, 221–229.

Behnia, B., Heinrichs, M., Bergmann, W., Jung, S., Germann, J., Schedlowski, M., . . . Kruger, T. H. (2013). Differential effects of intranasal oxytocin on sexual experiences and partner interactions in couples. *Hormones and Behavior, 65*(3), 308–318.

Bellamy, G., Gott, M., & Hinchliff, S. (2013). Women's understandings of sexual problems: Findings from an in-depth interview study. *Journal of Clinical Nursing, 22*, 3240–3248.

Bernstein, J. A. (2011). Human seminal plasma hypersensitivity: An under-recognized women's health issue. *Postgraduate Medicine, 123*, 120–125.

Bonham, A. (2015). Vulvar vestibulodynia: Strategies to meet the challenge. *Obstetrical and Gynecological Survey, 70*(4), 274–283.

Brand, J. S., & van der Schouw, Y. T. (2010). Testosterone, SHBG and cardiovascular health in postmenopausal women. *International Journal of Impotence Research, 22*, 91–104.

Brotto, L. A., Bitzer, J., Laan, E., Leiblum, S., & Luria, M. (2010). Women's sexual desire and arousal disorders. *Journal of Sexual Medicine, 7*, 586–614.

Brotto, L. A., Yong, P., Smith, K. B., & Sadownik, L. A. (2015). Impact of a multidisciplinary vulvodynia program on sexual functioning and dyspareunia. *Journal of Sexual Medicine, 12*(1), 238–247.

Brown, D. A., Kyle, J. A., & Ferrill, M. J. (2009). Assessing the clinical efficacy of sildenafil for the treatment of female sexual dysfunction. *Annals of Pharmacotherapy, 43*, 1275–1285.

Burrows, L. J., Basha, M., & Goldstein, A. T. (2012). The effects of hormonal contraceptives on female sexuality: A review. *Journal of Sexual Medicine, 9*, 2213–2223.

Clayton, A. H., & Balon, R. (2009). The impact of mental illness and psychotropic medications on sexual functioning: The evidence and management. *Journal of Sexual Medicine, 6*, 1200–1211.

Clayton, A. H., & Groth, J. (2013). Etiology of female sexual dysfunction. *Women's Health (London), 9*(2), 135–137.

Cohen, S., Catherine, J., & Goldstein, I. (2014, April). *5 Alpha-reductase enzyme deficiency in women: A new syndrome of "female androgen insufficiency."* Poster session presented at the 13th Annual Meeting of the International Society for the Study of Women's Sexual Health, San Diego, CA.

Davis, S. R. (2011). Cardiovascular and cancer safety of testosterone in women. *Current Opinions in Endocrinology, Diabetes and Obesity, 18*, 198–203.

Davis, S. R., & Braunstein, G. D. (2012). Efficacy and safety of testosterone in the management of hypoactive sexual desire disorder in postmenopausal women. *Journal of Sexual Medicine, 9*, 1134–1148.

De Andres, J., Sanchis-Lopez, N., Asensio-Samper, J. M., Fabregat-Cid, G., Villanueva-Perez, V. L., Monsalve Dolz, V., & Minguez, A. (2015). Vulvodynia: An evidence-based literature review and proposed treatment algorithm. *Pain Practice, 16*, 204–236.

DeRogatis, L., Clayton, A., Lewis-D'Agostino, D., Wunderlich, G., & Fu, Y. (2008). Validation of the Female Sexual Distress Scale—Revised for assessing distress in women with hypoactive sexual desire disorders. *Journal of Sexual Medicine, 5*(2), 357–364.

Edwards, L. (2015). Vulvodynia. *Clinical Obstetrics and Gynecology, 58*(1), 143–152.

Feldhaus-Dahir, M. (2010). Treatment options for female sexual arousal disorder: Part II. *Urologic Nursing, 30,* 247–251.

Ferguson, D. M., Hosmane, B., & Heiman, J. R. (2010). Randomized, placebo-controlled, double-blind, parallel design trial of the efficacy and safety of Zestra in women with mixed desire/interest/arousal/orgasm disorders. *Journal of Sex and Marital Therapy, 36,* 66–86.

Food and Drug Administration (FDA), Center for Drug Evaluation and Research (CDER). (2015, June 4). *Joint Meeting of the Bone, Reproductive and Urologic Drugs Advisory Committee and the Drug Safety and Risk Management Advisory Committee.* Silver Spring, MD: Author.

Galazka, I., Drosdzol-Cop, A., Naworska, B., Czajkowska, M., & Skrzypulec-Plinta, V. (2015). Changes in the sexual function during pregnancy. *Journal of Sexual Medicine, 12*(2), 445–54.

Goldstein, A. T., Belkin, Z. R., Krapf, J. M., Song, W., Khera, M., Jutrzonka, S. L., . . . Goldstein, I. (2014). Polymorphisms of the androgen receptor gene and hormonal contraceptive-induced provoked vestibulodynia. *Journal of Sexual Medicine, 11,* 2764–2771.

Hatzichristou, D., Rosen, R. C., Derogatis, L., Low, W. Y., Meuleman, E. J. H., Sadovsky, R., & Symonds, T. (2010). Recommendations for the clinical evaluation of men and women with sexual dysfunction. *Journal of Sexual Medicine, 7,* 337–348.

Heiman, J. R., & Lopiccolo, J. (1988). *Becoming orgasmic.* New York, NY: Simon & Schuster.

Herbenick, D., Reece, M., Schick, V., Sanders, S. A., Dodge, B., & Fortenberry, J. D. (2010). Sexual behaviors, relationships, and perceived health status among adult women in the United States: Results from a national probability sample. *Journal of Sexual Medicine, 7*(Suppl. 5), 277–290.

IsHak, W. W., Bokarius, A., Jeffrey, J. K., Davis, M. C., & Bakhta, Y. (2010). Disorders of orgasm in women: A literature review of etiology and current treatments. *Journal of Sexual Medicine, 7,* 3254–3268.

Ito, T. Y., Polan, M. L., Whipple, B., & Trant, A. S. (2006). The enhancement of female sexual function with ArginMax, a nutritional supplement, among women differing in menopausal status. *Journal of Sex & Marital Therapy, 32*(5), 369–378.

Kaplan, H. (1979). *Disorders of sexual desire.* New York, NY: Brunner/Mazel.

Kingsberg, S. (2014). Attitudinal survey of women living with low sexual desire. *Journal of Women's Health, 10,* 817–823.

Kingsberg, S., & Woodard, T. (2015). Female sexual dysfunction: Focus on low desire. *Obstetrics & Gynecology, 125*(2), 477–486.

Kinsey, A. (1953). *Sexual behavior in the human female.* Philadelphia, PA: W.B. Saunders.

Krychman, M., Kellogg, S., Damaj, B., & Hachicha, M. (2014, October). *Female arousal and orgasmic complaints in a diverse cancer population treated with Zestra: A topical applied blend of botanical oils.* Paper presented at the 16th World Meeting on Sexual Medicine, Sao Paulo, Brazil.

Lamvu, G., Nguyen, R. H., Burrows, L. J., Rapkin, A., Witseman, K., Marvel, R. P., . . . Zolnoun, D. (2015). The Evidence-based Vulvodynia Assessment Project: A national registry for the study of vulvodynia. *Journal of Reproductive Medicine, 60*(5–6), 223–235.

Landry, T., Bergeron, S., Dupuis, M-J., & Desrochers, G. (2008). The treatment of provoked vestibulodynia: A critical review. *Clinical Journal of Pain, 24,* 155–171.

Laughlin, G. A., Goodell, V., & Barrett-Connor, E. (2010). Extremes of endogenous testosterone are associated with increased risk of incident coronary events in older women. *Journal of Clinical Endocrinology and Metabolism, 95,* 740–747.

Laumann, E. O., Paik, A., & Rosen, R. C. (1999). Sexual dysfunction in the United States: Prevalence and predictors. *Journal of the American Medical Association, 281,* 537–544.

Masters, W., & Johnson, V. (1966). *Human sexual response.* Boston: Little, Brown.

Mathur, R., & Braunstein, G. D. (2010). Androgen deficiency and therapy in women. *Current Opinion in Endocrinology, Diabetes, & Obesity, 17,* 342–349.

Mozafari, M., Khajavikhan, J., Jaafarpour, M., Khani, A., Direkvand-Moghadam, A., & Najafi, F (2015). Association of body weight and female sexual dysfunction: A case control study. *Iranian Red Crescent Medical Journal, 17*(1), 23.

Nurnberg, H., Hensley, P., Heiman, J., Croft, H., Debattista, C., & Paine, S. (2008). Sildenafil treatment of women with antidepressant-associated sexual dysfunction: A randomized controlled trial. *Journal of the American Medical Association, 300*(4), 395–404.

Pereira, V. M., Arias-Carrion, O., Machado, S., Nardi, A. E., & Silva, A. C. (2013), Sex therapy for female sexual dysfunction. *International Archives of Medicine, 6*(1), 37.

Poels, S., Bloemers, J., van Rooij, K., Goldstein, I., Gerritsen, J., van Ham D, . . . Tuiten, A. (2013). Toward personalized sexual medicine (part 2): Testosterone combined with a PDE5 inhibitor increases sexual satisfaction in women with HSDD and FSAD, and a low sensitive system for sexual cues. *Journal of Sexual Medicine, 10,* 810–823.

Portman, D. J., Edelson, J., Jordan, R., Clayton, A., & Krychman, M. L. (2014). Bremelanotide for hypoactive sexual desire disorder: Analyses from a phase 2B dose-ranging study. *Obstetrics and Gynecology, 123*(Suppl. 1), 31S.

Portman, D. J., & Gass, M. L. (2014). Genitourinary syndrome of menopause: New terminology for vulvovaginal atrophy from the International Society for the Study of Women's Sexual Health and the North American Menopause Society. *Menopause, 21*(10), 1063–1068.

Reimer, A., & Johnson, L. (2011). Atrophic vaginitis: Signs, symptoms, and better outcomes. *Nurse Practitioner, 36,* 22–28.

Rogalski, M. J., Kellogg-Spadt, S., Hoffmann, A. R., Fariello, J. Y., & Whitmore, K. E. (2010). Retrospective chart review of vaginal diazepam suppository use in high-tone pelvic floor dysfunction. *International Urogynecology Journal, 21*(7), 895–899.

Rosen, R. C., & Barsky J. L. (2006). Normal sexual response in women. *Obstetrics and Gynecology Clinics of North America, 33*(4), 515–526.

Rosen, R., Brown, C., Heiman, J., Leiblum, S., Meston, C., Shabsigh, R., . . . D'Agostino, R., Jr. (2000). The Female Sexual Function Index (FSFI): A multidimensional self-report instrument for the assessment of sexual function. *Journal of Sex & Marital Therapy, 26,* 191–208.

Rupp, H., James, T., Ketterson, E., Sengelaub, D., Ditzen, B., & Heiman, J. (2013). Lower sexual interest in postpartum women: Relationship to amygdala activation and intranasal oxytocin. *Hormones and Behavior, 63*(1), 114–121.

Safarinejad, M. R. (2011). Reversal of SSRI-induced female sexual dysfunction by adjunctive bupropion in menstruating women: A double-blind, placebo-controlled and randomized study. *Journal of Psychopharmacology, 25,* 370–378.

Safarinejad, M. R., Hosseini, S.Y., Asgari, M. A., Dadkhah, F., & Taghva, A. (2010). A randomized, double-blind, placebo-controlled study of the efficacy and safety of bupropion for treating hypoactive sexual desire disorder in ovulating women. *British Journal of Urology International, 106,* 832–839.

Schlager, J. M., Xu, N., Park, C. G., & Wilkie, D. J. (2015). Acupuncture for the treatment of vulvodynia: A randomized wait-list controlled pilot study. *Journal of Sexual Medicine, 12*(4), 1019–1027.

Seehusen, D. A., Baird, D. C., & Bode, D. V. (2014). Dyspareunia in women. *American Family Physician, 90*(7), 465–470.

Shifren, J. L., Monz, B. U., Russo, P. A., Segreti, A., & Johannes, C. B. (2008). Sexual problems and distress in United States women: Prevalence and correlates. *Obstetrics & Gynecology, 112,* 970–978.

Snabes, M. C., & Simes, S. M. (2009). Approved hormonal treatments for HSDD: An unmet medical need. *Journal of Sexual Medicine, 6,* 1846–1849.

Steege, J. F., & Zolnoun, D. A. (2009). Evaluation and treatment of dyspareunia. *Obstetrics & Gynecology, 113,* 1124–1136.

Swanson, C. L., Rueter, J. A., Olson, J. E., Weaver, A. L., & Stanhope, C. R. (2014). Localized provoked vestibulodynia: Outcomes after modified vestibulectomy. *Journal of Reproductive Medicine, 59*(3–4), 121–126.

Vallinga, M. S., Spoelstra, S. K., Hemel, I. L., van de Wiel, H. B., & Weijmar Schultz, W. C. (2015). Transcutaneous electrical nerve stimulation as an additional treatment for women suffering from therapy-resistant provoked vestibulodynia: A feasibility study. *Journal of Sexual Medicine, 12*(1), 228–237.

van Lankveld, J. J. D. M., Granot, M., Weijmar Schultz, W. C. M., Binik, Y. M., Wesselmann, U., Pukall, C. F., . . . Achtrari, C. (2010). Women's sexual pain disorders. *Journal of Sexual Medicine, 7,* 615–631.

van Rooij, K., Poels, S., Bloemers, J., Goldstein, I., Gerritsen, J., van Ham, D., . . . Tuiten, A. (2013). Toward personalized sexual medicine (part 3): Testosterone combined with a serotonin 1A receptor agonist increases sexual satisfaction in women with HSDD and FSAD, and dysfunctional activation of sexual inhibitory mechanisms. *Journal of Sexual Medicine, 10,* 824–837.

Wåhlin-Jacobsen, S., Pedersen, A. T., Kristensen, E., Læssøe, N. C., Lundqvist, M., Cohen, A. S., . . . Giraldi, M. (2015). Is there a correlation between androgens and sexual desire in women? *Journal of Sexual Medicine, 12,* 358–373.

Waldinger, M. D. (2015). Psychiatric disorders and sexual dysfunction. *Handbook of Clinical Neurology, 130,* 469–489.

CHAPTER 17

Unintended Pregnancy

Katherine Simmonds

Frances E. Likis

Evelyn Angel Aztlan-James

Nearly 6.6 million pregnancies occur in the United States each year, and slightly more than half are reported as unintended at the time of conception (Finer & Zolna, 2014). Although the binary classification of pregnancy as intended or unintended has been criticized for failing to reflect the complexity of women's reproductive experiences (Borrero et al., 2015; Higgins, Popkin, & Santelli, 2012; Petersen & Moos, 1997), the concept of pregnancy intendedness continues to be widely embraced by demographers and within public health. Santelli and colleagues (2003) highlight the tension between women's lived experiences and the need for population-level data for planning purposes: "Although current measures of unintended pregnancy seem reasonable, reliable, and predictive at a population level, they were not designed to be used at an individual level" (p. 99). Although this chapter presents population-level data on unintended pregnancy, the main focus is on providing sensitive, quality, patient-centered care to those in the process of pregnancy discovery, decision making, and resolution.

SCOPE OF THE PROBLEM

According to the National Survey of Family Growth (NSFG), an estimated 51% of pregnancies in the United States are unintended, occurring among women of all ages and socioeconomic groups (Finer & Zolna, 2014). This widely referenced survey defines and categorizes pregnancies as *intended* if they occurred at the time or later than they were desired (Guzzo & Hayford, 2014; Klerman, 2000).

Unintended pregnancies are further subcategorized as either mistimed or unwanted according to the definitions in **Box 17-1** (Santelli, Lindberg, Orr, Finer, & Speizer, 2009). Evidence suggests that such dichotomous categorization of pregnancy is excessively simplistic (Borrero et al., 2015; Higgins et al., 2012; Petersen & Moos, 1997); nevertheless, because the NSFG is a well-established, nationally representative survey, it continues to provide the most readily available epidemiologic data on pregnancy in the United States and is the main source in this section. Criticisms of this survey are discussed later in this chapter.

Unintended pregnancy is most frequent among women who are between the ages of 18 and 24, are unmarried, have incomes less than 200% of the federal poverty level, are members of minority groups, or have not finished high school—all characteristics that signal significant socioeconomic disparities (Finer & Zolna, 2014). Approximately 40% of unintended pregnancies end in abortion (Finer & Zolna, 2014). An estimated 1.1 million abortions took place in the United States in 2011, continuing a general trend of decline in the abortion rate since its peak in the early 1980s (Jones & Jerman, 2014). Placing an infant for adoption is an alternative to parenting for a woman who chooses to carry an unintended pregnancy to term. Comprehensive adoption statistics have not been collected in the United States for many years; thus current information about how frequently adoption is the outcome of unintended pregnancy is limited. Estimates from the 2002 NSFG indicate that 1% of infants born to never-married women

Data from Santelli, J. S., Lindberg, L. D., Orr, M. G., Finer, L. B., & Speizer, I. (2009). Toward a multidimensional measure of pregnancy intentions: Evidence from the United States. *Studies in Family Planning, 40*(2), 87–100.

BOX 17-1   Commonly Used Pregnancy Intention Categorizations

- Intended pregnancy: Occurring at or about the right time; occurring later than desired (subfertility and infertility).
- Unintended pregnancy, mistimed: Occurring earlier than desired. Subcategorized as moderately mistimed (less than 2 years earlier than desired) or seriously mistimed (more than 2 years earlier than desired).
- Unintended pregnancy, unwanted: Occurring when a woman wanted no children or no more children.

---

younger than age 45 were relinquished for adoption between 1996 and 2002 (Jones, 2008). More recent data focus on the annual number of adoptions (Child Welfare Information Gateway, 2011), but they include older children and intercountry adoptions, which makes it difficult to identify the number of U.S. women who relinquish newborns.

Studies on the consequences of the decision to continue an unintended pregnancy and parent the child have suggested that there may be potentially adverse effects for both women and their children (Brown & Eisenberg, 1995; Dibaba, Fantahun, & Hindin, 2013; Gipson, Koenig, & Hindin, 2008; Logan, Holcombe, Manlove, & Ryan, 2007). Unintended pregnancy precludes the opportunity to receive preconception care that might improve pregnancy outcomes. Unintended pregnancy has been associated with later entry into prenatal care, low birth weight, and decreased likelihood of breastfeeding. In addition, children born as a result of an unintended pregnancy have been found to have poorer mental and physical health as well as poorer educational and behavioral outcomes. Women who experience unintended births are at

greater risk of negative mental health outcomes during and after pregnancy, and at greater risk of physical abuse while pregnant. These findings must be interpreted with caution, however, because newer research suggests associations between unintended pregnancy and adverse outcomes may vary by whether the pregnancy was unwanted or mistimed and the extent of mistiming (Kost & Lindberg, 2015; Lindberg, Maddow-Zimet, Kost, & Lincoln, 2015). Unintended pregnancy must not be assumed to cause or predict adverse outcomes for individual women.

Challenges in Measuring Pregnancy Intention

The framework of pregnancy intention described in the previous section has existed essentially unchanged in the United States for more than 50 years (Klerman, 2000). Recently, however, its validity—both on an individual level and on a population level—has come under criticism. As it is most commonly measured, pregnancy intention assesses a woman's feelings at the time of conception (Guzzo & Hayford, 2014). This is problematic for two reasons. First, it is difficult to accurately measure intention at conception when women are most often asked this question retrospectively. Second, the usefulness to women of a measure at conception may be limited (Petersen & Moos, 2007). Women answer questions related to pregnancy intention differently at different stages of a pregnancy, and the intendedness they report may not be static (Poole, Flowers, Goldenberg, Cliver, & McNeal, 2000). Additionally, time may affect how a woman views a pregnancy: She may think of it in the context of her life situation and with regard to her happiness at the time of confirmation of the pregnancy, rather than around the time of conception. The perception of whether a pregnancy is unacceptable or unwanted in a woman's *current* situation may not be the same as her perception of the pregnancy prior to conception.

The NSFG measure uses a few questions to categorize pregnancies, and these questions may not fully reflect the complex realities in which women live their reproductive lives. This is especially important when acknowledging that unintended pregnancies account for more than half of all U.S. pregnancies (51%) as determined by the current measures. Additionally, these measures may not fully capture the commonly reported experience of ambivalence around pregnancy. Women in clinical settings often report "not, not trying to get pregnant" instead of explicitly planning a pregnancy. While the importance of preventing unwanted pregnancies and the benefits of preconception folic acid supplementation are certain, we must ask ourselves, If more than half of women experience a life event, is it really abnormal? How accurate are our measurements? And how can we help women achieve the healthiest pregnancies with optimal maternal and neonatal outcomes possible in ways that are consistent with their lived experiences?

ETIOLOGY

Given the complexity of women's lived sexual, contraceptive, pregnancy, and parenting experiences as well as the variation in meaning and value placed on pregnancy planning for different women, a wide range of causes can be identified for pregnancies that are classified as unintended. Ayoola, Nettleman, and Brewer (2007) performed a comprehensive literature search to develop a summary of women's reasons for engaging in unprotected intercourse, which they organized into categories of individual/personal reasons, interpersonal reasons, and societal reasons. Individual/personal reasons women have unprotected intercourse include contraceptive side effects and health concerns; procedural reasons (e.g., contraceptive method is difficult to use or inconvenient, did not have method on hand, unexpected/unplanned sex); perceived low risk of getting pregnant; knowledge and attitudes (e.g., lack of understanding about where or how to obtain contraception, dislike contraception, didn't think or care about contraception, ambivalence about pregnancy); and personal beliefs or values (e.g., religious objection to contraceptive use). Interpersonal reasons can be divided between those related to partners (e.g., partner opposed to use of contraception, uncomfortable discussing contraception with partner) and the influence of family and friends (e.g., family members oppose contraception use, woman's parents want a grandchild, friends don't use contraception). Societal reasons include access to contraception, which includes access to a provider and the preferred method;

quality of contraceptive care (e.g., woman has unanswered questions or was given incomplete or incorrect information about contraception); cost of contraception and health insurance coverage; and forced or unwanted sex (Ayoola et al., 2007).

In addition, ambivalence about pregnancy and motherhood, pleasure-seeking during sex, and the irrelevance of a planned behavior framework with respect to pregnancy have been identified as reasons women experience so-called unintended pregnancies (Borrero et al., 2015; Higgins, Hirsch, & Trussell, 2008; Higgins et al., 2012). For clinicians who provide care to individual reproductive-aged women, understanding that there are numerous reasons—both personal and structural—why a given pregnancy may have occurred can help with maintaining a patient-centered focus.

PREGNANCY DISCOVERY, DECISION MAKING, AND RESOLUTION

For women, the discovery of a pregnancy

can be a complex and sometimes protracted process that begins with assessing pregnancy risk, perceiving and correctly interpreting pregnancy signs and symptoms, seeking confirmation, accepting (or denying) the pregnancy, disclosure to others, and deciding actively or by default to continue with the pregnancy. (Peacock et al., 2001, p. 110)

A woman may present to the health system for care at any point during this process, including for pregnancy confirmation, options counseling, and/or decision-making support, or to obtain health services related to her pregnant state (prenatal care, abortion, or miscarriage management). In some cases, a woman may present for care completely unaware that she is pregnant, and its discovery may take place during the clinical visit.

Given the frequency of pregnancy, clinicians who provide care to reproductive-aged women—particularly in primary, urgent, or emergency care settings—are likely to be called on to confirm or diagnose pregnancy, provide options counseling and decision-making support, and deliver pregnancy-related clinical services or referrals. These professional responsibilities require clinicians to have adequate knowledge and skills to deliver safe, quality care to women at any point during this pregnancy discovery-resolution process. In addition, when providing care to women and their partners, clinicians need to be aware of any potential conflicts between their personal beliefs and these professional responsibilities so that patients' rights to autonomy and dignity will be respected.

CONFLICTS IN CARING FOR WOMEN IN THE PREGNANCY DISCOVERY-RESOLUTION PROCESS

When providing care to women who have just discovered they are pregnant, are in the process of pregnancy decision making, or are seeking pregnancy-related care (prenatal care, abortion, or miscarriage management), clinicians may experience complex personal responses. Professional organizations have established ethical codes to guide health professionals in providing sound clinical care to patients, including in morally complex circumstances. For example, the American Nurses Association (ANA, 2011) mandates that all nurses, including advanced practice registered nurses, "practice with compassion and respect for the inherent dignity, worth and uniqueness of every individual, unrestricted by considerations of social or economic status, personal attributes, or the nature of health problems." This code of ethics applies to all clinical care, including the care of those women who present during the pregnancy discovery-resolution process. Values clarification is a process that can help clinicians explore the intersection of their personal beliefs and professional responsibilities, so that ultimately patients' rights are upheld (Simmonds & Likis, 2011).

Professional Responsibilities

Clinicians have professional responsibilities to uphold patient rights and autonomy, and to treat patients with respect and compassion. These responsibilities related to care for women experiencing unintended pregnancy have been codified by a number of professional organizations, including the American Academy of Physician Assistants (2008, reaffirmed 2013), the American College of Nurse-Midwives (1997, reviewed 2011), the American College of Obstetricians and Gynecologists (2014a, 2014b), and the National Organization of Nurse Practitioner Faculties (2013). These organizational statements (**Box 17-2**) provide an ethical and legal mandate for clinicians to ensure patient access to comprehensive reproductive health services, including pregnancy options counseling.

Applying these principles in the clinical setting means that women must be given the opportunity to express their concerns, desires, and need for additional information in a supportive environment. Creating such conditions can sometimes be challenging, however. Opinions about what patients "should" do may subtly or overtly influence the therapeutic relationship, particularly for clinicians who are not fully aware of the boundaries between their personal beliefs and their professional responsibilities. Although a woman may make a decision that is different from what a clinician wishes or believes is best, upholding patient autonomy is paramount (Simmonds & Likis, 2011).

Values Clarification

Because unintended pregnancy and its outcomes—including such possibilities as adolescent pregnancy, single parenthood, and abortion—are socially and politically controversial and may stir up personal sentiments, it is important for clinicians who provide care to women of reproductive age to clarify their own values regarding these issues. Ideally, self-assessment should take place before having a clinical encounter with a woman who is seeking pregnancy confirmation, decision-making support, or other pregnancy-related health services. In addition, because personal beliefs and professional work environments are dynamic, engaging in a process of ongoing values clarification may benefit clinicians and the women they care for (Simmonds & Likis, 2005).

Several resources have been developed to assist clinicians with clarifying their personal beliefs about pregnancy options and helping them examine the intersection of their beliefs with their professional responsibilities. These materials include books, articles, and exercises that may be used individually or in groups (**Table 17-1**). Given the heightened controversy surrounding abortion in the United States, many of these resources focus

BOX 17-2 Statements of Professional Organizations

American Academy of Physician Assistants (2008, reaffirmed 2013)

"Reproductive decision making: Patients have a right to access the full range of reproductive healthcare services, including fertility treatments, contraception, sterilization, and abortion. Physician assistants (PAs) have an ethical obligation to provide balanced and unbiased clinical information about reproductive health care.

When the PA's personal values conflict with providing full disclosure or providing certain services such as sterilization or abortion, the PA need not become involved in that aspect of the patient's care. By referring the patient to a qualified provider who is willing to discuss and facilitate all treatment options, the PA fulfills their ethical obligation to ensure the patient's access to all legal options."[a]

American College of Nurse-Midwives (1997, reviewed 2011)

"The American College of Nurse-Midwives (ACNM) affirms the following:

- Every woman has the right to make reproductive health choices that meet her individual needs.
- Every woman has the right to access to factual, evidence-based, unbiased information about available reproductive health choices, in order to make an informed decision.
- Women with limited means should have available financial resources to support access to services to meet their reproductive health care needs.

Certified nurse-midwives (CNMs) and certified midwives (CMs) believe that every individual has the right to safe, satisfying health care with respect for human dignity and cultural variations. The philosophy of the ACNM supports each person's right to self-determination, access to comprehensive health information, and to active participation in all aspects of their health care. We acknowledge the wide range of cultural, religious, and ethnic diversity of CNMs and CMs and their clients allowing for a variety of personal and professional choices related to reproductive health care."

American College of Obstetricians and Gynecologists (2014)

In its abortion policy, the American College of Obstetricians and Gynecologists (2014a) recognizes that individual healthcare providers may hold personal beliefs about abortion but asserts that such beliefs should not compromise patient health, access to care, or informed consent in any way. Furthermore, the American College of Obstetricians and Gynecologists states that healthcare providers have an ethical obligation to provide pregnant women with accurate information about all options—including parenting, adoption, and abortion—that is free of personal bias so patients can make fully informed decisions. In addition, an American College of Obstetricians and Gynecologists (2014b) Committee Opinion authored by the Committee on Health Care for Underserved Women endorses appropriately trained and credentialed advanced practice clinicians as providers of medication and first trimester aspiration abortion services as a means to increase access to abortion.

National Organization of Nurse Practitioner Faculties (2013)

"Women's health/gender-related nurse practitioner competencies:

- Supports a woman's right to make her own decisions regarding her health and reproductive choices within the context of her belief system."

[a]Courtesy of APAOG Association of Physician Assistants in Obstetrics & Gynecology.

TABLE 17-1   Resources for Values Clarification

Title	Type of Resource	Where to Obtain the Resource
Abortion and Options Counseling: A Comprehensive Reference	Book	The Hope Clinic for Women, Ltd.: https://www.hopeclinic.com/publications.html
The Abortion Option: A Values Clarification Guide for Health Professionals	Workbook	National Abortion Federation (NAF): http://prochoice.org/?s=abortion+option
"Induced Abortion: An Ethical Conundrum for Counselors"	Article	Millner, V. S., & Hanks, R. B. (2002). Induced abortion: An ethical conundrum for counselors. *Journal of Counseling & Development, 80*, 57–63.
"Options Counseling: Techniques for Caring for Women with Unintended Pregnancies"	Article	Singer, J. (2004). Options counseling: Techniques for caring for women with unintended pregnancies. *Journal of Midwifery & Women's Health, 49*, 235–242.
Values Clarification for Providing Abortion Care Self-Assessment for Providing Abortion Care Exploring Attitudes Towards Abortion	Group exercises that include some components for individuals to do independently	The Association for Reproductive Health Professionals Curricula Organizer for Reproductive Health Education: http://core.arhp.org
Values Clarification Workshop	Curriculum for workshop including exercises for participants	The Reproductive Health Access Project: http://www.reproductiveaccess.org/wp-content/uploads/2014/12/values_clarification-workshop.pdf

largely or exclusively on that option. Although this attention may be warranted, exploring beliefs about women's decisions to parent or place a child for adoption are equally important. Unexamined personal beliefs about these options may also inadvertently affect clinical encounters. For example, a clinician may have strong personal feelings about an adolescent who reports she has decided to parent a child or about a woman who has no hesitation about placing an infant for adoption. During the values clarification process, attention to all pregnancy options is warranted.

By engaging in values clarification, clinicians can identify areas of potential conflict between their personal beliefs and professional responsibilities. If this process reveals these conflicts are irreconcilable, the clinician is obligated to ensure that patients will not be denied their right to comprehensive, respectful pregnancy options counseling. Upholding this professional responsibility may require referring patients to a colleague or a different setting entirely. When alternative arrangements are necessary, these should not result in undue hardship for women, such as necessitating long-distance travel, paying out of pocket for services rendered, or creating significant delays in delivery of care. In addition, if patients are referred to another facility, it is the referring clinician's responsibility to ensure that the counseling offered in that site includes factual information about all available options and is nondirective. In particular, referral to "crisis pregnancy centers"—agencies known to provide biased counseling that tries to dissuade women from having abortions—is not an acceptable alternative (Rosen, 2012). In general, clinicians who identify a high level of personal conflict with providing comprehensive pregnancy options counseling are advised not to work in settings where such counseling is frequently one of their job responsibilities (Higginbotham, 2002).

ASSESSMENT

A qualitative, urine pregnancy test is performed to diagnose or confirm previous testing. If pregnancy is confirmed, gestational age should be calculated by ascertaining the last menstrual period (LMP) and applying Nägele's rule or using a pregnancy calculator. If the LMP is unknown or unsure, a bimanual examination to size the uterus or ultrasound is warranted to determine gestational age (see Chapter 30). Assessment of a woman's thoughts about whether she will continue the pregnancy or have an abortion is more complex and is discussed in the next section.

MANAGEMENT

Prevention

Healthy People 2020 objectives include increasing the percentage of pregnancies that are intended to 56% of all pregnancies (HealthyPeople.gov, 2011). When providing reproductive health care, clinicians should adhere to professional codes of ethics with regard to respect for the dignity of the individual, and not confuse this responsibility with national efforts to meet population-level pregnancy prevention goals.

Levi, Simmonds, and Taylor (2009) suggest a framework for unintended pregnancy prevention using a public health approach. In this model, primary prevention strategies include contraceptive and emergency contraceptive counseling, dispensing, and prescribing. Secondary strategies include pregnancy diagnostics; options counseling, referrals, and support; and abortion counseling. Tertiary prevention strategies involve care provided to women with pregnancies that are more complicated, due to advanced gestational age or other psychosocial or medical factors. Depending on the clinical setting, scope of practice, and state laws and regulations, a clinician may provide all or some

of women's desired services (prenatal care, abortion, and/or miscarriage management).

Moos (2003) suggests that eliminating practice routines that impede obtaining timely services (e.g., long waits for appointments for contraceptive services, requiring a pelvic examination prior to prescribing hormonal contraception) and removing financial barriers to contraceptive access are important strategies for supporting women who do not want to become pregnant. Elements of these suggested strategies are discussed in more detail here and elsewhere in this book. See Chapter 11 for contraception and Chapter 30 for pregnancy diagnosis.

Pregnancy Options Counseling

While many women know what they will do immediately or shortly after they discover they are pregnant, some may want or benefit from exploring their options with a healthcare provider. Pregnancy options counseling is appropriate for a woman who knows she is pregnant and needs to clarify her thoughts and feelings about how she will resolve the pregnancy, whereas abortion counseling is provided when a woman needs additional information or emotional support specifically related to her decision to have an abortion (Baker & Beresford, 2009). To provide quality pregnancy options counseling, clinicians need current, accurate knowledge about all of the available options, including continuing the pregnancy and parenting the child, placing an infant for adoption, or having an abortion, as well as about the fundamental principles of pregnancy options counseling.

It is essential for clinicians who provide pregnancy options counseling to be nondirective, and to withhold personal judgment about a woman's situation and decision. Equally important is ensuring patient confidentiality, as some women may avoid or forgo counseling because of fear that parents, a partner, or other members of their social network will find out about the pregnancy. Other essentials of pregnancy options counseling include establishing rapport, using neutral language, and asking open-ended questions—all of which should be part of the established communication skills of clinicians. Baker (1995) describes options counseling as a form of crisis intervention that usually takes place during one clinician–patient interaction. As such, it is short term, addresses an immediate problem, and involves a major life crisis requiring a time-limited decision.

Although every patient encounter is unique—necessitating variations in approach—four general steps are suggested for clinicians when providing pregnancy options counseling:

- Explore how the woman feels about the pregnancy and her options
- Help identify support systems and assess risks
- Provide decision-making support or discuss a timetable for decision making
- Provide or refer the woman to the desired services (Simmonds & Likis, 2011)

Explore How the Woman Feels About the Pregnancy and Her Options

When delivering pregnancy test results or initiating pregnancy options counseling, begin by asking neutral, open-ended questions that encourage a woman to share her thoughts and emotions about the pregnancy. **Table 17-2** suggests questions or statements to use and to avoid during this conversation. Questions that allow a clinician to ascertain a woman's level of understanding and her feelings about continuing a pregnancy, parenting, adoption, and abortion can help guide subsequent education and counseling. Having the woman list the pros and cons of each option may also help her clarify her situation and make an informed decision.

Help Identify Support Systems and Assess Risks

Asking a woman whether she has told anyone that she is pregnant can help a clinician determine if there is need for additional support.

Asking specifically about partner's and parents' (with adolescents in particular) possible reactions to the news of the pregnancy can identify situations where coercion or abuse is present or may arise. If abuse, neglect, or statutory rape is suspected or confirmed, clinicians are bound by state laws regarding mandatory reporting. Assessing for interpersonal violence (IPV) and reproductive coercion should be a standard component of pregnancy options counseling, as women experiencing unintended pregnancy have been found to be at increased risk for both (Miller & McCauley, 2013; Miller et al., 2014; Saltzman, Johnson, Gilbert, & Goodwin, 2003). Sexual and reproductive coercion includes "explicit attempts to impregnate a partner against her will, control outcomes of a pregnancy, coerce a partner to have unprotected sex, and interfere with contraceptive methods" (American College of Obstetricians and Gynecologists, 2013). Engaging the assistance of other members of the healthcare team, including social work, IPV specialists, and/or legal advisors, is advised when such situations are identified. Futures Without Violence has created resources for clinicians and others who work in health-related settings to support efforts to screen and appropriately manage women experiencing IPV and reproductive coercion (Chamberlain & Levenson, 2013).

Encouraging a woman to talk with someone (or people) whom she trusts and feels will be supportive of her decision, as well as helping her explore how to tell someone who might not be supportive, can be valuable aspects of the counseling session. Clinicians should arrange additional follow-up for women who report they are unable to tell anyone

---

TABLE **17-2**	Examples of Statements or Questions to Use or Avoid When Delivering Pregnancy Test Results or Initiating Pregnancy Options Counseling
Recommended	**Avoid**
<ul><li>How do you feel about being pregnant?</li><li>Do you know what your choices are?</li><li>What are your thoughts about becoming a parent? About adoption? About abortion?</li></ul>	<ul><li>Are you happy about the pregnancy?</li><li>Congratulations!</li></ul>

about the pregnancy, which may include referral to a professional counselor in some cases.

Provide Decision-Making Support or Discuss a Timetable for Decision Making

Depending on how recently a woman discovered she was pregnant, she may need time to accept her situation or discuss it with others. Determining with her whether to proceed immediately with pregnancy options counseling, postpone it until a later time, or forgo it altogether is appropriate. If a woman reports that she already knows how she wants to proceed, a clinician may simply assess whether she needs any additional information or would like to discuss any of the options further. Some women may benefit from being directed to additional resources to further explore their options on their own (**Table 17-3**).

Resources that facilitate understanding of fetal development may be helpful to some as part of the decision-making process, whereas such resources may not be welcomed or desired by other women. For those who express interest, accurate patient education resources should be made available. The National Library of Medicine (2013) has developed one such resource, a free app called "Embryo."

Another important component of pregnancy options counseling is ensuring that a woman is aware of the estimated gestational age of the pregnancy and the clinical and legal implications of this fact. With regard to abortion, postponing the decision may render a woman ineligible to use a preferred method (medication), increase cost, or—in cases where gestational age extends beyond services that are locally available or legal (e.g., within a

TABLE 17-3	Patient Resources for Exploring Pregnancy Options		
Title	**Type**	**Where to Obtain the Resource**	**Description**
Are You Pregnant and Thinking About Adoption?	Factsheet	https://www.child welfare.gov /pubPDFs /f_pregna.pdf	Provides information about adoption, including community resources and considerations for fathers and relatives.
Pregnancy Options Workbook Abortion: Which Method Is Right for Me?	Web and print-based	http://www .pregnancyoptions .info	Resource includes exercises for individuals undecided about what to do about a pregnancy as well as information on all three pregnancy options. Addresses topics such as decision making, getting support, male partners, fetal development, and spiritual and religious concerns.
Talking with Your Parents About Your Pregnancy	Online resource	https://www.abortion carenetwork.org /exceptional-care /get-help/talking-with -your-parents-about -your-pregnancy	Resource created to assist young people explore their options and tell parents about a pregnancy.

(continues)

TABLE 17-3	Patient Resources for Exploring Pregnancy Options (*continued*)		
Title	**Type**	**Where to Obtain the Resource**	**Description**
Talkline	Telephone	1-888-493-0092	Peer-based counseling and support for people making decisions about a current pregnancy, as well as other pregnancy-related concerns (parenting, abortion, infertility, miscarriage). Free, confidential, nonjudgmental.
Unsure About Your Pregnancy? A Guide to Making the Right Decision for You	Brochure	https://www.prochoice.org/pubs_research/publications/downloads/are_you_pregnant/pregnancy_guide_english.pdf	Provides exercises for pregnant women who are undecided about their pregnancy. Website also provides links to information about all three options.

particular state)—eliminate this option altogether. For those women who ultimately continue a pregnancy, a delay in decision making can result in later entry into prenatal care, which may be associated with poorer pregnancy outcomes as well as missed opportunities for early fetal risk assessment.

Provide or Refer the Woman to the Desired Services

Depending on a woman's decision, she may be able to receive services within that setting or, alternatively, she may need to be referred elsewhere. It is essential for clinicians to know which services are available and accessible for each option in the area. The Child Welfare Information Gateway and the National Abortion Federation offer information about adoption and abortion services in specific geographic areas. Backline also maintains current lists of service providers, resources, and support networks for all pregnancy options (**Box 17-3**).

It can be worthwhile to consult colleagues and others in the community to determine the reputation and practices of any agency or clinic prior to referring patients there. Following up with women after they have received services at another site can also help clinicians develop a deeper knowledge of the quality of these services. Finally, when providing referrals, verify with the woman that she knows how to access them and is able to make contact. Additional assistance should be provided to any woman who has difficulty arranging desired services due to linguistic barriers, developmental limitations, fear, or other psychosocial or economic factors.

OPTIONS FOR WOMEN EXPERIENCING UNINTENDED PREGNANCIES

Continuing the Pregnancy: Parenting or Adoption

The decision about whether to parent or place a child for adoption can be made at any point during a pregnancy. Optimally, those who decide to parent would have adequate support, time, ability, and financial resources to care for a child. Clinicians can provide women who are pregnant with information about state and local programs that offer social and financial support to pregnant women and their children. Such information may prove critical in their decision-making process.

BOX **17-3** **Resources on Reproductive Options, Legislation, and Policies**

Abortion Care Network

http://www.abortioncarenetwork.org

Advancing New Standards in Reproductive Health (ANSIRH)

http://www.ansirh.org/research/pci/access.php

Backline

http://yourbackline.org/resources

Child Welfare Information Gateway

http://www.childwelfare.gov (click on "Adoption" under "Topics")

Clinicians for Choice

http://prochoice.org/health-care-professionals /clinicians-for-choice/resource-center

Guttmacher Institute

http://www.guttmacher.org
Research and analysis for individual states:
http://www.guttmacher.org/statecenter

Kaiser Family Foundation

http://www.kff.org
Specifics regarding state policies and legislation:
http://www.statehealthfacts.kff.org (click on "Women's Health")

NARAL Prochoice America

http://www.naral.org
State-by-state guide to legislative bills:
http://www.prochoiceamerica.org /government-and-you/state-governments

National Abortion Federation

http://www.prochoice.org

National Network of Abortion Funds (NNAF)

http://www.fundabortionnow.org

Unintended Pregnancy Prevention and Care Modules

http://provideaccess.org/nursingcurriculum

Women who decide to continue a pregnancy should be encouraged to follow recommendations for promoting a healthy pregnancy, including early initiation of prenatal care, taking folic acid supplements, and addressing other maternal and fetal health threats, such as chronic disease management and avoidance of teratogens. If a clinician is not a provider of prenatal care or other needed services (e.g., management of medical or psychological conditions relevant to maternal or fetal well-being), referrals should be provided. For more information on guidelines for promoting health in early pregnancy, see Chapter 30.

Arrangements for adoption vary according to state law. Children may be placed for adoption through public or private agencies, independently with assistance from an adoption lawyer or facilitator, directly between the birth and adoptive parents, or formally or informally through kinship networks. Adoptions may be closed or open. Parents in a confidential or closed adoption do not

know each other or have contact, but the adoptive parents are given relevant information about the birth parents such as medical histories. Open adoption encompasses options along a broad continuum that may range from birth parents reading about families and selecting one, to ongoing contact between the families (American College of Obstetricians and Gynecologists, 2012; Smith & Brandon, 2008).

Abortion

There are four general approaches for inducing an abortion: aspiration, medication, labor induction, and surgery (i.e., hysterectomy or hysterotomy). Of these, aspiration is the most frequently used method in the United States (Pazol, Creanga, Burley, & Jamieson, 2014). Since the U.S. Food and Drug Administration's (FDA) approval of mifepristone in 2000, medication abortion has become increasingly common; it accounted for 18.3% of all abortions in 2011 (Pazol et al., 2014). Induction and surgical methods of abortion are now relatively rare in this country (Pazol et al., 2014). The most recent data on timing of abortions indicates that 91.4% were performed prior to 13 weeks' gestation, 7.1% between 14 and 20 weeks' gestation, and 1.4% after 20 weeks' gestation (Pazol et al., 2014). Because the vast majority of abortions in the United States are performed by either aspiration or medication administration, these methods will be the main focus of this section. **Table 17-4** compares these options.

Abortion can be performed as early as pregnancy is detected, although some clinicians prefer to wait until a gestational sac can be visualized by ultrasound or directly as part of routine tissue examination immediately following completion of the procedure, which is usually by 4 to 6 weeks' gestation. Aspiration abortion prior to 6 weeks' gestation has been shown to be safe and effective, particularly if protocols that guard against missed ectopic or continuing pregnancies are followed (Edwards & Carson, 1997). Upper limits beyond which therapeutic abortion may be performed are based on

legal (rather than medical) restrictions, and vary from state to state. **Box 17-3** lists resources for locating information on specific state laws.

The decision about which method will be used in an individual case depends on a number of factors, including gestational age of the pregnancy, patient preference, and provider training and availability. Depending on state laws and regulations, nurse practitioners, nurse-midwives, and physician assistants may be able to provide medical and/or aspiration abortion (Taylor, Safriet, Dempsey, Kruse, & Jackson, 2009). State-specific information about the current status of such laws and regulations and considerations for clinicians interested in offering abortion is available from Advancing New Standards in Reproductive Health (ANSIRH) and Clinicians for Choice (**Box 17-3**).

In addition to providing education and answering patients' questions about the various abortion methods, clinicians who do not or are not able to provide abortion services must be able to relay pertinent information about specific referral sites, including the type(s) of abortion available and their

TABLE 17-4   Comparison of Aspiration and Medication Abortion

Consideration	Aspiration Abortion	Medication Abortion
Invasive procedure	Yes	No, except when medication fails (5% or less)
Anesthesia	If desired	Usually avoids
Time to complete	Predictable: typically a few minutes, can be longer with advancing gestation	Somewhat unpredictable: typically 4–6 hours after misoprostol use, 80% within 24 hours
Available during early pregnancy	Yes	Yes
Success rate	High, 99%	High, approximately 95%
Women's common perception of bleeding	Light	Not light
Follow-up	Not required in most cases	Required to ensure completion of abortion
Required visits to provider	One for procedure; may be more depending on state laws about required waiting period after counseling	Generally minimum of one to two; may be more depending on state laws about required waiting period after counseling

limits based on gestational age, cost, type of insurance accepted, language(s) spoken, and likelihood of encountering protestors at a particular site. Both state and federal legislation that may affect a patient's abortion experience, such as parental consent laws, state-mandated counseling, or waiting periods, should also be discussed. Resources for identifying abortion services in a particular state or region are listed in **Table 17-5**. Clinicians can also deepen their knowledge about the local services by communicating directly with providers and staff from clinics and hospitals where abortions are performed, talking to colleagues, and asking patients about their abortion experiences.

The Abortion Care Network has created a set of guidelines that both women and clinicians can use to find high-quality service delivery sites. The National Abortion Federation also has suggestions for determining if a clinic delivers safe, quality care. Links to these resources can be found in **Table 17-5**. Given the illicit history of abortion in the United States prior to the Supreme Court's 1973 *Roe v. Wade* ruling, and its continued illegality in many parts of the world, safety and quality are prominent concerns for many women that should be addressed as part of pregnancy options and abortion counseling.

Paying for an Abortion

The majority of women in the United States pay out of pocket for their abortions, regardless of their insurance status (Jones, Finer, & Singh, 2010). In recent years, increasing restrictions on insurance coverage for abortions have forced even more

TABLE **17-5**	Resources for Women Seeking Abortion Services	
Organization	**Where to Obtain the Resource**	**Description**
Abortion Care Network	https://www.abortioncarenetwork.org /abortion-care-providers	List of independent abortion care providers who belong to the Abortion Care Network, organized by state
Abortion Clinics Online	http://abortionclinics.com	List of sites that offer abortion services, searchable by city and state
Full Spectrum Doulas	http://www.fullspectrumdoulas.org	Information about doulas who provide abortion support
National Abortion Federation	1-877-257-0012	Provides referrals to quality abortion providers in the caller's area
	http://prochoice.org/think-youre -pregnant/find-a-provider	State-by-state map with information about state legislation that impacts abortion service delivery (e.g., waiting periods, mandated counseling) and contact information of National Abortion Federation member providers
	http://prochoice.org/think-youre -pregnant/i-want-an-abortion -what-should-i-expect	Includes questions to help determine if an abortion provider is safe

(continues)

TABLE **17-5**	Resources for Women Seeking Abortion Services (*continued*)	
Organization	**Where to Obtain the Resource**	**Description**
Planned Parenthood	1-800-230-PLAN (7526)	Helps the caller find the nearest Planned Parenthood health center
	https://www.plannedparenthood.org/health-center	Search for Planned Parenthood health centers by state or zip code
Radical Doula	http://radicaldoula.com	Includes profiles of doulas that provide full-spectrum care, including abortion support

women to draw on their personal resources to cover their abortions (Roberts, Gould, Kimport, Weitz, & Foster, 2014). Because of the Hyde Amendment, which prohibits the use of federal funds to pay for abortion services, in 33 states and the District of Columbia, women who are Medicaid recipients must also use alternative sources to pay when they have an abortion. Given that the average cost of a first-trimester abortion in the United States is approximately $500 (Jones & Jerman, 2014), this may represent a prohibitive expense for many women. In some cases, this cost has been linked to delays in obtaining services (Roberts et al., 2014). Nationally, a number of independent state and national funds have been established to assist women who are seeking but are unable to afford an abortion. For information on these funds, refer to the National Network of Abortion Funds (**Box 17-3**).

Aspiration Abortion

All aspiration abortion methods involve removing the products of conception (POC) by introducing a cannula through the cervical os into the uterine cavity. The cannula is attached to a source of suction, generated by either a manual or electric vacuum aspirator (MVA or EVA, respectively). MVA is generally used only for abortions before 14 weeks' gestation (Meckstroth & Paul, 2009). The decision to use MVA or EVA depends on the clinician's preference and training as well as equipment availability.

In early abortions, evacuation of the uterus can be completed in a few minutes and through the use

of suction alone. Some clinicians choose to curette the walls of the uterus after suctioning (a process referred to as dilation and curettage [D & C]) to ensure that the procedure is complete. However, because D & C has been associated with increased rates of complications and has no demonstrable benefits, the World Health Organization has recommended that this technique be replaced by suction alone for first-trimester abortions (Meckstroth & Paul, 2009).

In abortions after the first trimester, forceps may be used in conjunction with suction to remove the POC. This technique is termed dilation and evacuation (D & E). Research has shown D & E to be at least as safe and less physically and emotionally stressful for patients as labor induction (Hammond & Chasen, 2009; Henshaw, 2009). However, because second-trimester D & E requires more advanced training, the decision to employ labor induction instead of D & E may be based on clinician availability rather than patient preference or other medical considerations (Hammond & Chasen, 2009; Jerman & Jones, 2014).

Dilation of the cervix is usually necessary to remove the POC, except in very early aspiration abortions. The degree of dilation required depends on the gestational age of the pregnancy. It may be accomplished either by inserting dilating rods of increasing diameter into the cervical os immediately prior to inserting the cannula or by placing osmotic dilators into the cervix several hours to a day before the procedure. In general, osmotic dilators are used in later abortions, although clinician training and experience may guide this decision as well. Oral or vaginal pharmacologic agents, such as misoprostol, are also used in some settings to promote cervical softening and subsequent dilation (Meckstroth & Paul, 2009).

In the United States, women are offered various options for pain relief during and following aspiration and D & E abortions. In most settings, a paracervical block is routinely administered prior to cervical dilation and is promoted as a standard of care (National Abortion Federation, 2015). In addition, many sites offer women options of intravenous or oral pain medications; in some facilities, general anesthesia is available. Studies suggest that the use of intravenous and general anesthesia increases patient satisfaction, contributes to faster recovery and improved physiologic benefits for patients, and may positively influence operative conditions for clinicians (Nichols, Halvorson-Boyd, Goldstein, Gevirtz, & Healow, 2009); however, these benefits must be weighed against the risks associated with the use of anesthesia. Nonpharmacologic approaches, including positive suggestion, relaxation, and guided imagery, have also been used successfully to decrease pain, including for women undergoing abortion (Nichols et al., 2009). There is a growing movement of "full-spectrum" and abortion-specific doula care providers in the United States. While no studies to date have been conducted that prove their presence reduces pain, intuitively such support would seem likely to help ameliorate the overall stressful experience that many women have when undergoing an abortion, possibly including with respect to pain. **Table 17-5** provides more information on this option and ways to find a doula to support a woman who is having an abortion.

Recovery after an abortion depends on the type of procedure and anesthesia used, the gestational age of the pregnancy, and whether the woman has any preexisting medical or psychosocial conditions or experienced any complications during the procedure. After an uncomplicated early abortion in which only local anesthesia was used, a woman may be able to leave the facility as soon as 20 minutes after the procedure. Greater levels of anesthesia generally require longer periods of stabilization and monitoring. Before discharge, women are instructed that they may resume regular activity as

soon as they feel ready, although they are usually advised to not engage in sexual intercourse, rigorous exercise, or lifting heavy objects for a few days to a week after the procedure. Evidence to support these recommendations is limited (Espey & MacIsaac, 2009).

Some abortion services providers advise women to return to the facility where the abortion was performed or to their primary care provider for a routine examination 2 to 3 weeks after the procedure to ensure a complete and uncomplicated recovery, assess emotional well-being, and initiate or follow up on any newly established contraceptive method. There is also little evidence to support this practice, which is costly for both women and the healthcare system. Alternative approaches for follow-up care have been suggested, including better patient education regarding self-monitoring for post-abortion complications and improved delivery of contraceptive services at the time of the abortion (Grossman, Ellertson, Grimes, & Walker, 2004; Kapp, Whyte, Tang, Jackson, & Brahmi, 2013).

Medication Abortion

Since the approval of mifepristone by the FDA in 2000, use of medication as a method for inducing early abortion has grown steadily. Currently, nearly one-fifth of all abortions performed in the United States are achieved through the administration of mifepristone in conjunction with misoprostol (Pazol et al., 2014). Alternative medications that can be used for an early abortion include methotrexate in conjunction with misoprostol, and misoprostol alone. Because of the greater frequency of mifepristone–misoprostol abortions in the United States, this method is the primary focus of this section. All methods of medication abortion are currently used only for early abortions.

Mifepristone works by binding to progesterone receptors more effectively than progesterone itself, thereby blocking the hormone's effects. As a result, the endometrium sloughs and the cervix softens, both of which promote expulsion of pregnancy tissue. Adding misoprostol (a prostaglandin) increases the efficacy of this regimen (Creinin & Danielsson, 2009; Creinin & Grossman, 2014). Multiple studies have shown mifepristone to be highly effective (95–99%) when given in combination with vaginal or buccal misoprostol up to 63 days' gestation (Creinin & Grossman, 2014; Gatter, Cleland, & Nucatola, 2015). Recent research has demonstrated comparable efficacy in abortions up to 70 days' gestation (Winikoff et al., 2012). Methotrexate, when given with misoprostol, has been found to have similar efficacy rates in gestations of 49 days or less. Misoprostol alone has also been investigated for use as an abortifacient; however, it has been found to be significantly less effective than the other options (Creinin & Grossman, 2014).

In March 2016, the FDA approved a number of changes to the label of mifepristone; **Table 17-6** compares the old and new labeling. While some clinicians may continue to recommend approaches that differ from the new label when prescribing mifepristone, overall these changes bring the FDA-approved regimen into greater alignment with the evidence that has been gathered over the past 2 decades about the medication's efficacy, safety, and acceptability. One particularly pertinent change is the label's new language about who can prescribe mifepristone, which is now stated as any "healthcare provider who prescribes," thereby expanding the ability of clinicians other than physicians (i.e., advanced practice registered nurses and physician assistants) to provide medication abortions to their patients.

Currently in most settings in the United States, mifepristone (200 mg) is taken orally by the patient at the clinical site. She is then instructed to self-administer misoprostol (400–800 mcg) vaginally, buccally, or orally at home, which—depending on the guideline being followed—may be specified to occur between several hours and several days later (Creinin & Grossman, 2014). For most women, bleeding and passage of the POC ensues within 2 to 4 hours after misoprostol administration, but it can take up to 24 hours or longer (Creinin & Danielsson, 2009).

It is common for women to continue to bleed for several weeks after a medication abortion; however, subsequent bleeding is usually much lighter than during pregnancy expulsion. Having the woman return for follow-up several days to weeks later to ensure that the POC have been successfully expelled is generally the standard of care in the United States (Creinin & Grossman, 2014). Transvaginal ultrasound is commonly performed at this visit; however, clinical examination, pregnancy testing, and patient symptomatology have also been found to be acceptable alternatives for verifying the abortion is complete (Creinin & Grossman, 2014).

TABLE 17-6 Mifepristone Abortion Regimens

	Old FDA Labeling	New FDA Labeling (2016)
Recommended gestational age	Up to 49 days from last menstrual period	Up to 70 days from last menstrual period
Mifepristone dose	600 mg orally	200 mg orally
Misoprostol dose, route, and patient location at administration	400 mcg orally; administered on site at the second office visit	800 mcg via buccal administration; no specification as to location (i.e., office vs. home)
Misoprostol timing	72 hours after mifepristone	24–48 hours after mifepristone
Misoprostol repeat dose	Not optional	Optional
Follow-up visit	Day 14	About 1–2 weeks post treatment
Prescriber	By or under the supervision of a physician	By or under the supervision of a healthcare provider who prescribes

Data from Danco Laboratories. (2016). Mifeprex labeling and medication guide. Retrieved from http://earlyabortionpill.com/wp-content/uploads/2016/03/MIFEPREX-Labeling-and-MG-FINAL_March2016.pdf; U.S. Food and Drug Administration. (2016). Questions and answers on Mifeprex. Retrieved from http://www.fda.gov/Drugs/DrugSafety/PostmarketDrugSafetyInformationforPatientsandProviders/ucm492705.htm.

Only a few medical contraindications to medication abortion with mifepristone–misoprostol exist; they include known allergies to either of the medications; ectopic pregnancy; presence of an intrauterine device (IUD); severe hypertension or liver, adrenal, renal, or cardiovascular disease; or long-term corticosteroid use. In addition, because of the expected bleeding, caution should be used when providing any type of medication abortion to women with severe anemia or coagulopathies, or who use anticoagulants. Other psychosocial conditions may also render some women inappropriate candidates for medication abortion (Creinin & Grossman, 2014). Careful counseling and screening that addresses a woman's expectations of the experience, her ability to communicate with the clinical facility in case of complications, and the need to return for follow-up are important considerations prior to providing a medication abortion. In addition, because of the potential teratogenicity of misoprostol, in the small number of cases when medication abortion fails, uterine aspiration is necessary. Therefore, prior to medication administration, all candidates are required to consent to a uterine aspiration in case the method fails (Creinin & Grossman, 2014). Although research has demonstrated comparable levels of satisfaction among women following aspiration and medication abortion (Creinin & Danielsson, 2009), it is important for women to understand that medication abortion is not the optimal choice for every individual.

Medication abortion with methotrexate is similar to mifepristone in the manner of service delivery, but it does have several distinguishing clinical features. The most important clinical difference lies in the timing of bleeding and expulsion of pregnancy tissue, which may take longer (up to several weeks following medication administration) for 20% to 30% of women. For some women, this unpredictability renders methotrexate less desirable than mifepristone (Wiebe, Dunn, Guilbert, Jacot, & Lugtig, 2002). In addition, methotrexate is administered via intramuscular injection rather than orally, which may lead some women to prefer mifepristone. Nevertheless, methotrexate does offer some advantages relative to mifepristone: It can be used when ectopic pregnancy cannot be ruled out, offers a lower-cost alternative to mifepristone, and may be available in countries where mifepristone is not available or abortion is legally restricted (Creinin & Grossman, 2014).

Labor Induction Abortion

After the first trimester of pregnancy, medication can also be used to induce labor as a method of abortion; however, this method is not typically referred to as a medication abortion but rather as labor induction abortion. Current approaches involve administering prostaglandins, with or without the addition of misoprostol, to stimulate uterine contractions that eventually lead to expulsion of the fetus. Less commonly, oxytocin may be used for this purpose. In the United States, labor induction has become a less common method (used in fewer than 2% of all abortions) than D & E for abortions in later pregnancy (Borgatta & Kapp, 2011). Because D & E requires advanced training, it is not readily available in some areas (Jerman & Jones, 2014). In-depth discussion of labor induction abortion is beyond the scope of this chapter.

Safety of Abortion

Risks associated with early abortion, including death, are relatively low when procedures are carried out under modern medical conditions. Legality is an important prerequisite for such conditions to be present. In places where abortion is illegal or restricted, associated morbidity and mortality rates remain high. According to the World Health Organization (WHO, 2011), nearly half of all abortions that take place around the world are unsafe, leading to significant health and economic consequences for women, their families, and the countries in which they reside. In the United States, abortion mortality rates have decreased considerably since the 1970s, largely as a result of advances in technique and elimination of many legal restrictions (Shah & Ahman, 2009). The current mortality rate for legal, reported abortions in the United States is 0.6 deaths per 100,000 abortions (WHO, 2011). Risk of death increases with advancing gestational age (Bartlett et al., 2004). Nevertheless, given the limited number of abortions that occur after the first trimester and particularly after 20 weeks' gestation, death from abortion is relatively rare in the United States. Compared to abortion, the risk of death associated with live birth has been found to be approximately 14 times higher (Raymond & Grimes, 2012).

Serious and minor complications following legal aspiration or D & E abortion are also infrequent. Possible complications (from most to least likely) include infection, missed or incomplete abortion, cervical tear, uterine perforation, hemorrhage requiring transfusion, and hematometra. Overall, minor complications are estimated to occur in fewer than 2.5% of abortions, and serious complications requiring hospitalization in fewer than 0.5% (Henshaw, 2009; Weitz et al., 2013; White, Carroll, & Grossman, 2015). In a systematic review, other major complications requiring intervention, including hemorrhage requiring transfusion and uterine perforation needing repair, occurred in fewer than 0.1% of cases (White et al., 2015). In general, these conditions are treatable and rarely lead to long-term morbidity or death.

Strong evidence shows that first-trimester abortion, when performed safely, does not increase a woman's risks of subsequent infertility, miscarriage, ectopic pregnancy, birth defects, preterm birth, or birth of a low-birth-weight infant (Boonstra, Gold, Richards, & Finer, 2006). When abortions are performed under conditions that are not safe, or with other methods (e.g., dilation and sharp curettage), certain reproductive risks, such as midtrimester spontaneous abortions and low birth weight, may increase (Hogue, Boardman, & Stotland, 2009). To reduce potential risks, it is important for clinicians to encourage women to seek abortion services as early as possible and from experienced providers.

Overall, the risk associated with medication abortion is comparable to that associated with aspiration and D & E abortions (Creinin & Grossman, 2014). With medication abortion, complications attributable to instrumentation (i.e., cervical tear and uterine perforation) are avoided; however, other complications are possible, including incomplete abortion, hemorrhage, and infection. From 2004 to 2008, six unusual, sepsis-related deaths occurred among women in the United States following the use of the mifepristone-misoprostol regimen, leading to an overall increase in the risk of death associated with this method. These infections are being followed by the Centers for Disease Control and Prevention (CDC, 2010). At the present time, mifepristone–misoprostol abortion remains available in the United States and is generally believed to be safe for use.

SPECIAL CONSIDERATIONS

When providing care to reproductive-aged women, clinicians need to be aware that both personal characteristics and structural forces influence individuals' experiences and decisions about a given pregnancy. In this section, we discuss some of the considerations relevant to one special population, pregnant adolescents. For any particular woman, however, multiple "identities"—including those related to her age, race, gender identity, cultural membership(s), class, immigrant status, language, and mental and developmental ability—intersect to shape her unique reality, including with regard to reproductive acts and decisions about sex, contraception, pregnancy, abortion, adoption, and childrearing. This is true for all women, and clinicians are advised to keep this point in mind as they strive to provide patient-centered reproductive health care.

Adolescents

In the United States, 615,000 women between the ages of 15 and 19 became pregnant in 2010 (Kost & Henshaw, 2014). Most (82%) adolescent pregnancies have been found to be unintended (Finer & Zolna, 2014). Recently, the U.S. adolescent pregnancy rate has dropped to an all-time low (Boonstra, 2014); however, compared to other countries with similar levels of economic development, the adolescent pregnancy rate in the United States still ranks among the highest (Kearney & Levine, 2015). Most adolescent pregnancies in the United States end in birth (60%), and approximately one-fourth end in abortion (Kost & Henshaw, 2014).

Laws and statutes regarding adolescents' rights to access confidential health services for reproductive and sexual concerns vary by state, and recently this has been an area of shifting practice. Clinicians should familiarize themselves with the relevant laws and statutes in the state where they practice. In 38 states, minors must involve at least one of their parents or seek a judicial bypass to obtain an abortion, except in cases of medical emergency or where there is evidence of abuse or neglect (Guttmacher Institute, 2015b). In addition to awareness about abortion laws and regulations, clinicians who work with young women need to be familiar with current legislation regarding adolescents' rights to confidential reproductive health services in the state where they practice. These rights are an area of great controversy in the United States, as reflected by legislative battles at both the federal and state levels. As of late 2015, 26 states and the District of Columbia allowed minors to seek contraceptive services without the consent of a parent; the other 24 states either placed restrictions on minors (20) or had no relevant policy or case law (4) regarding this issue. Thirty-two states explicitly allowed minors to consent to prenatal care without their parents' involvement, although 12 of those allowed a clinician to inform parents that their daughter was seeking these services if deemed "in the minor's interest." Four other states allowed minors to consent when they were "mature." The remaining states had no policy or case law on this subject (Guttmacher Institute, 2015a). Pregnancy options counseling falls between these three aspects of reproductive health care (i.e., prenatal care and contraceptive and abortion services).

Where legislative conditions allow, reassuring adolescent patients that all counseling and follow-up related to pregnancy will be kept confidential is an important aspect of providing pregnancy options counseling. Before delivering services, it is also essential to inform adolescents about clinical situations when parents or guardians may or must be informed. A full discussion of the reproductive health rights of adolescents is beyond the scope of this chapter, and readers are referred to the references cited and to the resource listing (**Box 17-3**) regarding laws specifically pertaining to adolescents in their practice location.

Influences of Sociodemographic Characteristics and Cultural Heritage

As previously noted, significant disparities in rates of unintended pregnancy and abortion in the United States have been identified. Women who are between the ages of 18 and 24, unmarried, Latina or black, with incomes less than 200% of the federal poverty level, or without a high school

diploma experience both of these reproductive health events at disproportionate levels relative to older, married, white, more affluent, or more educated women. However, a closer review of these data reveals a complex picture. Recent research has demonstrated that how pregnancy is viewed once it is discovered, including unintended pregnancy, may differ among black and Latina women when compared to white women (Aiken & Potter, 2013; Borrero et al., 2015; Rocca, Harper, & Raine-Bennett, 2013). While women who are black and Latina experience more unintended pregnancies, it is important to remember that race/ethnicity may simply be a visible and measurable proxy for such complicated factors as increased life stress related to experiencing daily racism, poverty, and structural and institutional racial barriers (Nuru-Jeter et al., 2009), and even differing cultural beliefs about one's ability to control childbearing or the benefits of childbearing (Borrero et al., 2015; Rocca et al., 2013).

Subtleties in relation to other sociodemographic characteristics also exist. Although most women who have abortions in the United States are not married, 31% of married women report that their pregnancies are unintended (Finer & Zolna, 2014). Among married women with unintended pregnancies, 20% have an abortion (Finer & Zolna, 2014). The majority of women (61%) who have abortions have had one or more previous births (Jones & Kavanaugh, 2011). Three-fourths of women who have an abortion report a religious affiliation. Many of these women identify themselves with religions that typically prohibit abortion: 28% of women who have abortions are Catholic, and 15% are Born-Again, Evangelical, or Fundamentalist Christians (Jones & Kavanaugh, 2011). Women who have not graduated from high school have a rate of unintended pregnancy three times higher than that of college graduates, but are far less likely to have abortions (Finer & Zolna, 2014). Regardless of an individual's demographic characteristics and cultural heritage, for the clinician providing care to a woman who is in the process of pregnancy discovery, decision making, and/or resolution, it is important *not* to make assumptions based on population-level trends, but rather to keep the woman's unique needs, situation, and wishes at the center of her care.

References

Aiken, A. R., & Potter, J. E. (2013). Are Latina women ambivalent about pregnancies they are trying to prevent? Evidence from the Border Contraceptive Access Study. *Perspectives on Sexual and Reproductive Health, 45*(4), 196–203. doi:10.1363/4519613

American Academy of Physician Assistants. (2008, reaffirmed 2013). *Guidelines for ethical conduct for the physician assistant profession.* Alexandria, VA: Author.

American College of Nurse-Midwives. (1997, reviewed 2011). *Reproductive choices* [Position statement]. Silver Spring, MD: Author.

American College of Obstetricians and Gynecologists. (2012). ACOG Committee Opinion No. 528: Adoption. *Obstetrics & Gynecology, 119*(6), 1320–1324.

American College of Obstetricians and Gynecologists. (2013). ACOG Committee Opinion No. 554: Reproductive and sexual coercion. *Obstetrics & Gynecology, 121*(2), 411–415.

American College of Obstetricians and Gynecologists. (2014a). *Abortion policy* [Policy statement]. Washington, DC: Author.

American College of Obstetricians and Gynecologists. (2014b). ACOG Committee Opinion no. 613: Increasing access to abortion. *Obstetrics & Gynecology, 124*(5), 1060–1065.

American Nurses Association (2011). Code of ethics for nurses with interpretive statements. Retrieved from http://www.nursingworld.org/MainMenuCategories/EthicsStandards/CodeofEthicsforNurses/Code-of-Ethics-For-Nurses.html

Ayoola, A. B., Nettleman, M., & Brewer, J. (2007). Reasons for unprotected intercourse in adult women. *Journal of Women's Health, 16*, 302–310.

Baker, A. (1995). *Abortion and options counseling: A comprehensive reference.* Granite City, IL: Hope Clinic for Women.

Baker, A., & Beresford, T. (2009). Informed consent, patient education and counseling. In M. Paul, E. S. Lichtenberg, L. Borgatta, D. Grimes, P. Stubblefield, & M. Creinin (Eds.), *Management of unintended pregnancy and abnormal pregnancy: Comprehensive abortion care* (pp. 48–62). Chichester, UK: Wiley-Blackwell.

Bartlett, L., Berg, C., Shulman, H., Zane, S., Green, C., Whitehead, S., & Atrash, H. K. (2004). Risk factors for legal induced abortion-related mortality in the United States. *Obstetrics & Gynecology, 103*(4), 729–737.

Boonstra, H. (2014). What is behind the decline in teenage pregnancy rates? *Guttmacher Policy Review, 17*(3), 15–21.

Boonstra, H., Gold, R., Richards, C., & Finer, L. (2006). *Abortion in women's lives.* New York, NY: Guttmacher Institute, 2006.

Borgatta, L., & Kapp, N. (2011). Labor induction abortion in the second trimester. *Contraception, 84*(1), 4–18. doi:10.1016/j.contraception.2011.02.005

Borrero, S., Nikolajski, C., Steinberg, J. R., Freedman, L., Akers, A. Y., Ibrahim, S., & Schwarz, E. B. (2015). "It just happens": A qualitative study exploring low-income women's perspectives on pregnancy intention and planning. *Contraception, 91*(2), 150–156. doi:10.1016/j.contraception.2014.09.014

Brown, S. S., & Eisenberg, L. (Eds.). (1995). *The best intentions: Unintended pregnancy and the well-being of children and families.* Washington, DC: National Academy Press.

Centers for Disease Control and Prevention. (2010). *Clostridium sordelli.* Retrieved from http://www.cdc.gov/HAI/organisms/cSordellii.html

Chamberlain, L., & Levenson, R. (2013). *Addressing intimate partner violence, reproductive and sexual coercion: A guide for obstetric, gynecologic, and reproductive health care settings.* San Francisco,

CA: Futures Without Violence and the American College of Obstetricians & Gynecologists. Retrieved from http://www.futureswithoutviolence.org/addressing-intimate-partner-violence

Child Welfare Information Gateway. (2011). *How many children were adopted in 2007 and 2008?* Washington, DC: U.S. Department of Health and Human Services, Children's Bureau.

Creinin, M. D., & Danielsson, K. (2009). Medical abortion in early pregnancy. In M. Paul, E. S. Lichtenberg, L. Borgatta, D. Grimes, P. Stubblefield, & M. Creinin (Eds.), *Management of unintended pregnancy and abnormal pregnancy: Comprehensive abortion care* (pp. 208–223). Chichester, UK: Wiley-Blackwell.

Creinin, M., & Grossman, D. (2014). Medical management of first-trimester abortion. Society of Family Planning Clinical Guideline #2014-1. American College of Obstetricians and Gynecologists Practice Bulletin No. 143. *Contraception, 89*(3), 148–161.

Danco Laboratories. (2016). Mifeprex labeling and medication guide. Retrieved from http://earlyabortionpill.com/wp-content/uploads/2016/03/MIFEPREX-Labeling-and-MG-FINAL_March2016.pdf

Dibaba Y., Fantahun, M., & Hindin, M. J. (2013). The effects of pregnancy intention on the use of antenatal care services: Systematic review and meta-analysis. *Reproductive Health, 10.* doi:10.1186/1742-4755-10-50

Edwards, J., & Carson, S. A. (1997). New technologies permit safe abortion at less than six weeks' gestation and provide timely detection of ectopic gestation. *American Journal of Obstetrics & Gynecology, 176*(5), 1101–1106.

Espey, E., & MacIsaac, L. (2009). Contraception and surgical abortion aftercare. In M. Paul, E. S. Lichtenberg, L. Borgatta, D. Grimes, P. Stubblefield, & M. Creinin (Eds.), *Management of unintended pregnancy and abnormal pregnancy: Comprehensive abortion care* (pp. 157–177). Chichester, UK: Wiley-Blackwell.

Finer, L., & Zolna, M. (2014). Shifts in intended and unintended pregnancies in the United States, 2001–2008. *American Journal of Public Health, 104*(Suppl. 1), S43–S48. doi:10.2105/AJPH.2013.301416

Gatter, M., Cleland, K., & Nucatola, D. L. (2015). Efficacy and safety of medical abortion using mifepristone and buccal misoprostol through 63 days. *Contraception, 91*(4), 269–273. http://dx.doi.org/10.1016/j.contraception.2015.01.005

Gipson, J. D., Koenig, M. A., & Hindin, M. J. (2008). The effects of unintended pregnancy on infant, child, and parental health: A review of the literature. *Studies in Family Planning, 39*(1), 18–38.

Grossman, D., Ellertson, C., Grimes, D. A., & Walker, D. (2004). Routine follow-up visits after first trimester induced abortion. *Obstetrics & Gynecology, 103*, 738–745.

Guttmacher Institute. (2015a). An overview of minors' consent laws. *State Policies in Brief.* Retrieved from http://www.guttmacher.org/statecenter/spibs/spib_OMCL.pdf

Guttmacher Institute. (2015b). Parental involvement in minors' abortions. *State Policies in Brief.* Retrieved from http://www.guttmacher.org/statecenter/spibs/spib_PIMA.pdf

Guzzo, K. B., & Hayford, S. R. (2014). Revisiting retrospective reporting of first-birth intendedness. *Maternal and Child Health Journal, 18*(9), 2141–2147. doi:10.1007/s10995-014-1462-7

Hammond, C., & Chasen, S. (2009). Dilation and evacuation. In M. Paul, E. S. Lichtenberg, L. Borgatta, D. Grimes, P. Stubblefield, & M. Creinin (Eds.), *Management of unintended pregnancy and abnormal pregnancy: Comprehensive abortion care* (pp. 157–177). Chichester, UK: Wiley-Blackwell.

HealthyPeople.gov. (2011). 2020 topics and objectives. Retrieved from http://www.healthypeople.gov/2020/topicsobjectives2020/default.aspx

Henshaw, S. K. (2009). Unintended pregnancy and abortion in the USA: Epidemiology and public health impact. In M. Paul, E. S. Lichtenberg, L. Borgatta, D. Grimes, P. Stubblefield, & M. Creinin (Eds.), *Management of unintended pregnancy and abnormal pregnancy: Comprehensive abortion care* (pp. 24–35). Chichester, UK: Wiley-Blackwell.

Higginbotham, E. (2002). When your beliefs run counter to care. *RN, 65*(11), 69–72.

Higgins, J. A., Hirsch, J. S., & Trussell, J. (2008). Pleasure, prophylaxis and procreation: A qualitative analysis of intermittent contraceptive use and unintended pregnancy. *Perspectives on Sexual and Reproductive Health, 40*(3), 130–137. doi:10.1363/4013008

Higgins, J. A., Popkin, R. A., & Santelli, J. S. (2012). Pregnancy ambivalence and contraceptive use among young adults in the United States. *Perspectives on Sexual and Reproductive Health 44*(4), 236–243.

Hogue, C. J., Boardman, L. A., & Stotland, N. (2009). Answering questions about long-term outcomes. In M. Paul, E. S. Lichtenberg, L. Borgatta, D. Grimes, P. Stubblefield, & M. Creinin (Eds.), *Management of unintended pregnancy and abnormal pregnancy: Comprehensive abortion care* (pp. 252–263). Chichester, UK: Wiley-Blackwell.

Jerman, J., & Jones, R. K. (2014). Secondary measures of access to abortion services in the United States, 2011 and 2012: Gestational age limits, cost, and harassment. *Women's Health Issues, 24*(4), e419–e424. doi:10.1016/j.whi.2014.05.002

Jones, J. (2008). Adoption experiences of women and men and demand for children to adopt by women 18–44 years of age in the United States, 2002. *Vital and Health Statistics, 23*(27), 1–36.

Jones, R. K., Finer, L. B., & Singh, S. (2010) *Characteristics of U.S. abortion patients, 2008.* New York, NY: Guttmacher Institute.

Jones, R. K., & Jerman, J. (2014). Abortion incidence and service availability in the United States, 2011. *Perspectives on Sexual and Reproductive Health, 46*(1), 3–14. doi:10.1363/46e0414

Jones, R. K., & Kavanaugh, M. L. (2011). Changes in abortion rates between 2000 and 2008 and lifetime incidence of abortion. *Obstetrics & Gynecology, 117*, 1358–1366.

Kapp, N., Whyte, P., Tang, J., Jackson, E., & Brahmi, D. (2013). A review of evidence for safe abortion care. *Contraception, 88*(3), 350–363. doi:10.1016/j.contraception.2012.10.027

Kearney, M. S., & Levine, P. B. (2015). Investigating recent trends in the US teen birth rate. *Journal of Health Economics, 41*, 15–29. doi:10.1016/j.jhealeco.2015.01.003

Klerman, L. K. (2000). The intendedness of pregnancy: A concept in transition. *Maternal and Child Health Journal 4*(3), 155–162.

Kost, K., & Henshaw, S. (2014). U.S. teenage pregnancies, births and abortions, 2010: National and state trends and trends by age, race and ethnicity. Retrieved from http://www.guttmacher.org/pubs/USTPtrends10.pdf

Kost, K., & Lindberg, L. (2015). Pregnancy intentions, maternal behaviors, and infant health: Investigating relationships with new measures and propensity score analysis. *Demography, 52*(1), 83–111. doi:10.1007/s13524-014-0359-9

Levi, A. J., Simmonds, K. E., & Taylor, D. (2009). The role of nursing in the management of unintended pregnancy. *Nursing Clinics of North America, 44*, 301–314.

Lindberg, L., Maddow-Zimet, I., Kost, K., & Lincoln, A. (2015). Pregnancy intentions and maternal and child health: An analysis of longitudinal data in Oklahoma. *Maternal and Child Health Journal, 19*(5), 1087–1096. doi:10.1007/s10995-014-1609-6

Logan, C., Holcombe, E., Manlove, J., & Ryan, S. (2007). *The consequences of unintended childbearing* [White paper]. Washington, DC: Child Trends.

Meckstroth, K., & Paul, M. (2009). First-trimester aspiration abortion. In M. Paul, E. S. Lichtenberg, L. Borgatta, D. Grimes, P. Stubblefield, & M. Creinin (Eds.), *Management of unintended pregnancy and abnormal pregnancy: Comprehensive abortion care* (pp. 135–156). Chichester, UK: Wiley-Blackwell.

Miller, E., & McCauley, H. L. (2013). Adolescent relationship abuse and reproductive and sexual coercion among teens. *Current Opinion in Obstetrics and Gynecology, 25,* 364–369.

Miller, E., McCauley, H. L., Tancredi, D. J., Decker, M. R., Anderson, H., & Silverman, J. G. (2014). Recent reproductive coercion and unintended pregnancy among female family planning clients. *Contraception, 89*(2), 122–128. doi:10.1016/j.contraception.2013.10.011

Moos, M.-K. (2003). Unintended pregnancies: A call for nursing action. *MCN: The American Journal of Maternal/Child Nursing, 28*, 24–30.

National Abortion Federation. (2015). *Clinical policy guidelines.* Washington, DC: Author.

National Library of Medicine. (2013). National Library of Medicine announces release of "Embryo" app. Retrieved from https://www.nlm.nih.gov/news/apps_embryo.html

National Organization of Nurse Practitioner Faculties. (2013). *Population-focused nurse practitioner competencies: Family, neonatal, pediatric acute care, pediatric primary care, psychiatric-mental health, and women's health/gender-related.* Washington, DC: Author.

Nichols, M., Halvorson-Boyd, G., Goldstein, R., Gevirtz, C., & Healow, D. (2009). Pain management. In M. Paul, E. S. Lichtenberg, L. Borgatta, D. Grimes, P. Stubblefield, & M. Creinin (Eds.), *Management of unintended pregnancy and abnormal pregnancy: Comprehensive abortion care* (pp. 90–110). Chichester, UK: Wiley-Blackwell.

Nuru-Jeter, A., Dominguez, T. P., Hammond, W. P., Leu, J., Skaff, M., Egerter, S., . . . Braveman, P. (2009). "It's the skin you're in": African-American women talk about their experiences of racism. An exploratory study to develop measures of racism for birth outcome studies. *Maternal and Child Health Journal, 13*(1), 29–39. doi:10.1007/s10995-008-0357-x

Pazol, K., Creanga, A., Burley, K., & Jamieson, D. (2014). Abortion surveillance—United States, 2011. *MMWR Surveillance Summaries, 63*(SS11), 1–41.

Peacock, N. R., Kelley, M. A., Carpenter, C., Davis, M., Burnett, G., Chavez, N., . . . Chicago Social Networks Project. (2001). Pregnancy discovery and acceptance among low-income primiparous women: A multicultural exploration. *Maternal and Child Health Journal, 5*(2), 109–118.

Petersen, R., & Moos, M. (1997). Defining and measuring unintended pregnancy: Issues and concerns. *Women's Health Issues, 7*(4), 234–240. doi:10.1016/S1049-3867(97)00009-1

Poole, V. L., Flowers, J. S., Goldenberg, R. L., Cliver, S. P., & McNeal, S. (2000). Changes in intendedness during pregnancy in a high-risk multiparous population. *Maternal and Child Health Journal, 4*(3), 179–182.

Raymond, E., & Grimes, D. (2012). The comparative safety of legal induced abortion and childbirth in the United States. *Obstetrics & Gynecology, 119*(2 Pt 1), 215–219.

Roberts, S. C., Gould, H., Kimport, K., Weitz, T. A., & Foster, D. G. (2014). Out-of-pocket costs and insurance coverage for abortion in the United States. *Women's Health Issues, 24*, e211–e218.

Rocca, C. H., Harper, C. C., & Raine-Bennett, T. R. (2013). Young women's perceptions of the benefits of childbearing: Associations with contraceptive use and pregnancy. *Perspectives on Sexual and Reproductive Health, 45*(1), 23–32. doi:10.1363/4502313

Rosen, J. D. (2012). The public health risks of crisis pregnancy centers. *Perspectives on Sexual and Reproductive Health, 44*(3), 201–205. doi:10.1363/4420112

Saltzman, L. E., Johnson, C. H., Gilbert, B. C., & Goodwin, M. M. (2003). Physical abuse around the time of pregnancy: An examination of prevalence and risk factors in 16 states. *Maternal and Child Health Journal, 7*, 31–43.

Santelli, J. S., Lindberg, L. D., Orr, M. G., Finer, L. B., & Speizer, I. (2009). Toward a multidimensional measure of pregnancy intentions: Evidence from the United States. *Studies in Family Planning, 40*(2), 87–100.

Santelli, J., Rochat, R., Hatfield-Timajchy, K., Gilbert, B., Curtis, K., Cabral, R., . . . Unintended Pregnancy Working Group. (2003). The measurement and meaning of unintended pregnancy. *Perspectives on Sexual and Reproductive Health, 35*(2), 94–101. doi:10.1111/j.1931-2393.2003.tb00111.x

Shah, I., & Ahman, E. (2009). Unsafe abortion: The global public health challenge. In M. Paul, E. S. Lichtenberg, L. Borgatta, D. Grimes, P. Stubblefield, & M. Creinin (Eds.), *Management of unintended pregnancy and abnormal pregnancy: Comprehensive abortion care* (pp. 10–23). Chichester, UK: Wiley-Blackwell.

Simmonds, K., & Likis, F. E. (2005). Providing options counseling for women with unintended pregnancies. *Journal of Obstetric, Gynecologic, and Neonatal Nursing, 34*, 373–379.

Simmonds, K., & Likis, F. E. (2011). Caring for women with unintended pregnancies. *Journal of Obstetric, Gynecologic, and Neonatal Nursing, 40*, 794–807.

Smith, K. J., & Brandon, D. (2008). The hospital-based adoption process: A primer for perinatal nurses. *MCN, 33*(6), 382–388.

Taylor, D., Safriet, B., Dempsey, G., Kruse, B., & Jackson, C. (2009). Providing abortion care: A professional toolkit for nurse–midwives, nurse practitioners, and physician assistants. Retrieved from http://www.apctoolkit.org

U.S. Food and Drug Administration. (2016). Questions and answers on Mifeprex. Retrieved from http://www.fda.gov/Drugs/DrugSafety/PostmarketDrugSafetyInformationforPatientsandProviders/ucm492705.htm

Weitz, T., Taylor, D., Desai, S., Upadhyay, U., Waldman, J., Battistelli, M., & Drey, E. (2013). Safety of aspiration abortion performed by nurse practitioners, certified nurse midwives, and physician assistants under a California legal waiver. *American Journal of Public Health, 103*(3), 454–461. doi:10.2105/AJPH.2012.301159

White, K., Carroll, E., & Grossman, D. (2015). Complications from first-trimester aspiration abortion: A systematic review of the literature. *Contraception, 92*, 422–438.

Wiebe, E., Dunn, S., Guilbert, E., Jacot, F., & Lugtig, L. (2002). Comparison of abortions induced by methotrexate or mifepristone followed by misoprostol. *Obstetrics & Gynecology, 99*(5), 813–819. doi:10.1016/S0029-7844(02)01944-0

Winikoff, B., Dzuba, I. G., Chong, E., Goldberg, A., Lichtenberg, E., Ball, C., . . . Swica, Y. (2012). Extending outpatient medical abortion services through 70 days of gestational age. *Obstetrics & Gynecology, 120*(5), 1070–1076.

World Health Organization (WHO). (2011). *Unsafe abortion: Global and regional estimates of the incidence of unsafe abortion and associated mortality in 2008* (6th ed.). Geneva, Switzerland: Author.

CHAPTER 18

Infertility

Lucy Koroma

The editors acknowledge Ellen Olshansky, who was the author of the previous edition of this chapter.

Infertility is a condition that generates a variety of meanings among those experiencing it, including those who care for people with infertility, family members and friends of people with infertility, and the society in which infertility occurs. Infertility is a complex, multifactorial disorder that significantly affects physical, psychosocial, and economic aspects of women's and men's lives (Koroma & Stewart, 2012). The inability to become a mother or a father due to a diagnosis of infertility is a profound and difficult challenge for a significant portion of the population. People who desire to conceive and bear a child but are unable to do so often suffer immensely.

We live in a pronatalist society, which adds to the emotionally charged nature of infertility. Definitions of femininity are socially constructed and interlaced with the ability to give birth. Historically, infertility has been viewed as a woman's problem. This view is now changing, because of enhanced abilities to diagnose various etiologies of infertility, which have led to the recognition that both male and female factors cause infertility. Nevertheless, matters of reproduction, childbearing, and childrearing continue to be viewed primarily as women's issues. Many women have grown up rehearsing to be mothers, believing that their femininity and identity are interrelated with childbearing. Finding that they are unable to conceive can be both shocking and devastating to these individuals. Some women may be able to deconstruct such ideas through involvement in organizations and groups that support greater choices of lifestyles for women. Yet even women who may not feel that it is their duty to bear children may continue to desire children.

Clinicians may find it difficult to provide care for women with infertility due to the amount of suffering they may endure in their quest to have a child. Women often define themselves by their infertility; consequently, it is essential for the clinician to recognize that providing care for women with infertility involves more than just physical treatment. The psychological effects of infertility must be dealt with when treating women with this condition (Koroma & Stewart, 2012).

Advances in the technologies used to treat infertility have raised some new issues and created some new opportunities. For example, treatments for cancer, such as chemotherapy and radiation, may cause individuals to become infertile. Today, these individuals may preserve their fertility through cryopreservation of oocytes or spermatozoa. Some technological advances, however, have led to ethical dilemmas, including issues of who has the right to use a frozen embryo, who is the real parent, and who is considered eligible for certain treatments.

This chapter describes the incidence and causes of infertility, the assessment of individuals experiencing infertility, and treatments for infertility. It also highlights the various options available beyond trying to conceive, including adoption and child-free living. The chapter concludes with a discussion of psychosocial, controversial, and ethical issues related to infertility.

SCOPE OF THE CONDITION

The medical definition of infertility is the inability "to achieve a successful pregnancy after 12 months or more of regular unprotected intercourse" (Practice

Committee of the American Society for Reproductive Medicine [ASRM], 2015b, p. e44). Infertility is classified as primary or secondary according to the pregnancy history. A woman who has never been pregnant has primary infertility. Secondary infertility is "the inability to become pregnant, or to carry a pregnancy to term, following the birth of one or more biological children" (Resolve, 2015). Estimates of infertility in the United States range from 6% to 15% (Chandra, Copen, & Stephen, 2013; Practice Committee of the ASRM, 2015b, 2015c). However, only 43% of women who meet the criteria for infertility and want to become pregnant have spoken to a clinician about their condition, and only 19% have received medical treatment for infertility (Greil, Slauson-Blevins, Tiemeyer, McQuillan, & Shreffler, 2015).

For women older than age 35, evaluation and treatment of infertility are considered after 6 months of attempting pregnancy, instead of 1 year, because fertility declines gradually beginning at age 32 and more rapidly after age 37, and because the incidence of spontaneous abortion and conditions that may impair fertility (e.g., endometriosis, tubal disease) increases with age (American College of Obstetricians and Gynecologists & Practice Committee of the ASRM, 2014; Practice Committee of the ASRM, 2015b). Both the mean age at first birth and the birth rates of women aged 35 years and older continue to increase in the United States (Martin, Hamilton, Osterman, Curtin, & Mathews, 2015). Immediate infertility evaluation is warranted for women who are older than age 40 or have medical conditions that may impair fertility, should those women desire to become pregnant (**Box 18-1**).

Male fertility takes a different trajectory than female fertility, in that men are usually able to father children throughout their lives. Men have little or no overall measurable decline in fertility before age 45 to 50. Pregnancy rates for men older than age 50 are 23% to 38% lower than those for their counterparts who are younger than age 30, however, and time to conception is 5 times longer for men older than age 45 compared with men younger than age 25 (Fritz & Speroff, 2011).

From a personal perspective, an individual often constructs his or her own definition of infertility, which is influenced by the social context in

---

> ## BOX 18-1 Indications for Early Infertility Evaluation
>
> - Age > 35 years[a]
> - Age > 40 years[b]
> - History of oligomenorrhea or amenorrhea[b]
> - Known or suspected uterine, tubal, or peritoneal disease[b]
> - Known or suspected stage 3 or 4 endometriosis[b]
> - Other condition known to limit fertility[b]
> - Known or suspected male subfertility[b]
>
> [a] Evaluate for infertility if the woman has not conceived after 6 months of unprotected intercourse.
> [b] Immediate diagnostic evaluation for infertility when the woman desires pregnancy.
> Data from American College of Obstetricians and Gynecologists & Practice Committee of the American Society for Reproductive Medicine (ASRM). (2014). Committee Opinion No. 589. Female age-related fertility decline. *Obstetrics & Gynecology, 123*, 719–721; Practice Committee of the American Society for Reproductive Medicine (ASRM). (2015b). Diagnostic evaluation of the infertile female: A committee opinion. *Fertility and Sterility, 103*(6), e44–e50.

---

which that person lives. For example, a couple who has been trying to conceive for 3 months and has many friends who have recently become pregnant with no apparent difficulty may begin to see themselves as infertile even though they are not considered infertile according to the medical definition. Such a couple may become very anxious and seek health care, but be turned away because they do not fit the medical definition of infertility. The clinician can validate the couple's concerns by taking a thorough history, acknowledging their fears, and scheduling a follow-up visit in 9 months. If they are pregnant, the visit can be canceled. If they are not pregnant, that visit is scheduled and their anxiety is not heightened by hearing their clinician's first available visit is not for several weeks or months.

Conversely, a clinician may warn a 40-year-old nulligravida woman seeking a routine gynecologic examination that she should consider conceiving very soon because her childbearing years are almost over. There may be an assumption that this woman—and all women, for that matter—choose to be mothers. For this particular woman, her life goals may not include parenting. Although it would be correct to provide her with information about childbearing, it would be even more appropriate to ask her, in a nonjudgmental manner, about her goals related to childbearing with the recognition that not all women choose to become mothers.

OVERVIEW OF ANATOMY AND PHYSIOLOGY RELATED TO INFERTILITY

An understanding of the anatomy and physiology of the female and male reproductive systems as well as the processes of fertilization and implantation is crucial to understanding the etiology of infertility. The discussion in this chapter is limited to an overview of men's reproductive anatomy and physiology, fertilization, and implantation, as women's reproductive anatomy and physiology are discussed elsewhere in this text. See Chapter 5 for further information.

Anatomy and Physiology of the Male Reproductive System

The anatomic components of the male reproductive system include the penis, urethra, seminal vesicles, prostate gland, vas deferens, epididymis, and testes (testicles); see **Figure 18-1**, **Color Plate 13**, and **Table 18-1**. Sperm production relies on a functioning hypothalamic–pituitary–testicular axis that has many similarities to the hypothalamic–pituitary–ovarian axis in women. The pituitary produces follicle-stimulating hormone (FSH) and luteinizing hormone (LH) in response to secretion of gonadotropin-releasing hormone (GnRH) by the hypothalamus. FSH and LH initiate testicular production of sperm and testosterone, which are also necessary for spermatogenesis. The process of spermatogenesis takes approximately 72 days, after which sperm mature in the epididymis and then travel out of the vas deferens during ejaculation (Fritz & Speroff, 2011).

Fertilization and Implantation

The processes of fertilization (also known as conception) and implantation involve several steps.

Sperm must be produced and deposited in the vagina, and then transported through the vagina, cervix, and fallopian tubes. In the fallopian tubes, the sperm are transformed by a process called capacitation, which changes the surface characteristics of sperm. Capacitation is essential to the sperm's ability to fertilize an ovum and enables the sperm to undergo acrosome reaction, to bind to the zona pellucida, and to acquire hypermotility—all of which help to increase the sperm's ability to penetrate the ovum. The ovaries must produce a mature ovum (oocyte), which requires integrated functioning along the hypothalamic–pituitary–ovarian axis. The ovum is transported from the ovary into the fallopian tube, where it is fertilized by the sperm. The fertilized ovum then travels down the fallopian tube into the uterus. Implantation is the process by which the fertilized ovum attaches to the uterine wall and penetrates the uterine epithelium and the maternal circulatory system. Implantation can occur only if there is destruction of the zona pellucida, which is the surface of the fertilized ovum.

ETIOLOGIES OF INFERTILITY

Approximately 55% of infertility cases are due to female factors, and 35% of cases are due to male factors (Fritz & Speroff, 2011). In some cases, no apparent cause can be found; the diagnosis of unexplained infertility is then made. The incidence of unexplained infertility ranges from 8% to 28% in couples, depending on their ages and other individual characteristics (Gelbaya, Potdar, Jeve, & Nardo, 2014).

When presenting or discussing the pathophysiology of infertility, attention should be given to avoiding the use of terms that reflect negatively upon women. Clinicians should be mindful that women with infertility are often listening closely to every word that clinicians utter and may internalize subtle nuances in wording. For example, cervical mucus that is not receptive to sperm is commonly referred to as "hostile cervical mucus," and a cervix that prematurely dilates is commonly called an "incompetent cervix." Although some may view such adjectives as innocuous from a medical perspective, this negative terminology can connote blame on the woman's part for the infertility. Clinicians should use alternative terms (e.g., cervical insufficiency) that have a less negative connotation

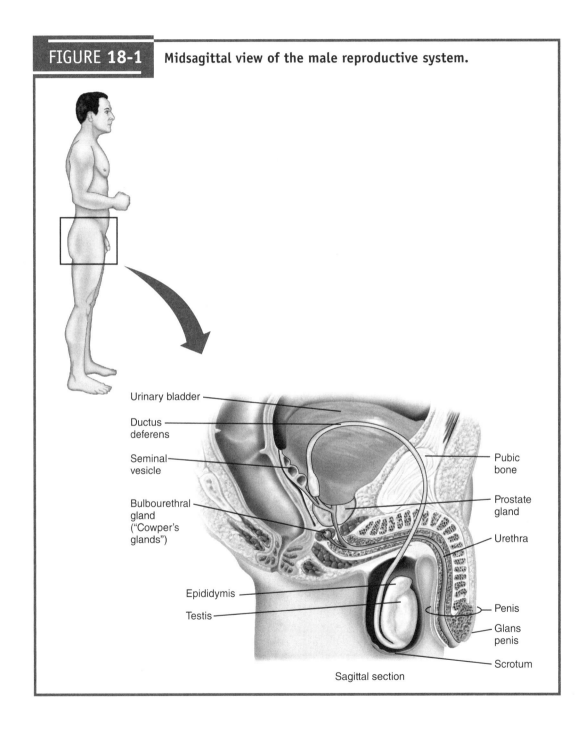

FIGURE 18-1 Midsagittal view of the male reproductive system.

Urinary bladder

Ductus deferens

Seminal vesicle

Bulbourethral gland ("Cowper's glands")

Epididymis

Testis

Pubic bone

Prostate gland

Urethra

Penis

Glans penis

Scrotum

Sagittal section

TABLE 18-1	Functions of the Male Reproductive Anatomy

Organs	Functions
Penis	External organ through which semen and urine are expelled
Urethra	Tube that carries semen and urine through the penis; its external opening is at the tip of the penis
Seminal vesicles	Two internal saclike structures that secrete fructose and other substances into the seminal fluid to promote viability of the semen
Prostate gland	Internal gland that secretes substances into the seminal fluid to nourish and increase the motility of the sperm
Vas deferens	Bilateral tubes through which sperm are propelled from each epididymis to the urethra for ejaculation
Epididymis	Stores sperm while they mature and connects the testicles to the vas deferens; each testicle has an adjacent epididymis
Testes	Produce testosterone and immature sperm; suspended externally in the scrotum
Bulbourethral gland	Two internal glands that produce an alkaline mucoid secretion that coats and lubricates the urethra

to avoid exacerbating women's guilt and distress about their infertility.

Female Etiologies

The majority of female infertility is due to ovulatory dysfunction (20–40%) and tubal and peritoneal pathology (30–40%); uterine pathology is relatively uncommon. Unexplained infertility and combined (interactional) infertility, which are discussed separately in this chapter, account for most other cases of infertility among women.

Ovulatory dysfunction may involve either a total lack of ovulation or the occurrence of irregular ovulation. Anovulation is usually—but not always—evidenced by irregular menstrual bleeding patterns or amenorrhea. Numerous causes of ovulatory dysfunction are possible, stemming from any interruption of the hypothalamic–pituitary–ovarian axis. Etiologies of ovarian dysfunction include hyperandrogenic disorders, physiologic anovulation at either end of the reproductive spectrum, hyperprolactinemia, pituitary tumors, thyroid disorders, eating disorders, low or high body mass index (BMI), medications, and possibly stress. Further

information about etiologies of anovulation can be found in Chapters 24 and 25.

A short duration of the luteal phase may also contribute to female infertility. This condition is commonly referred to as *luteal phase insufficiency*, *luteal phase deficiency*, or *inadequate luteal phase*, because it is associated with abnormally low levels of progesterone production by the corpus luteum. The term *luteal phase defect* is no longer used because it may reflect negatively upon women, as previously explained. The luteal phase is important for establishing a healthy normal pregnancy, and luteal phase insufficiency occurs when endogenous progesterone is not sufficient to maintain the endometrium adequately to allow an embryo to implant and develop. The corpus luteum must produce sufficient amounts of progesterone to support the endometrium until the placenta develops and takes over progesterone production. The luteal phase is considered short when fewer than 13 days elapse between the mid-cycle LH surge and the onset of menses (Fritz & Speroff, 2011). Nevertheless, luteal phase insufficiency has not been proven as a cause of infertility, and its management is controversial, as noted later in this chapter (Practice Committee of the ASRM, 2015a).

The primary cause of tubal disease and tubal blockage is pelvic inflammatory disease (PID, see Chapter 20). The sexually transmitted infections (STIs) chlamydia and gonorrhea can also cause tubal scarring. The STI may have been asymptomatic and, therefore, gone unrecognized and untreated, resulting in tubal scarring; however, tubal scarring may result even when STIs are treated. Other tubal factors that can impact fertility are stage 3 and 4 endometriosis, which can cause severe adhesive disease, making oocyte and spermatozoa transport through the fallopian tube very difficult; adhesions or blockage from uterine fibroids; and blockage from previous ectopic pregnancy or tubal surgery (Practice Committee of the ASRM, 2015d).

Other pelvic conditions to consider when assessing women for causes of infertility include endometriosis, Asherman syndrome, and other uterine factors. Endometriosis is a condition in which endometrial tissue retrogrades back through the fallopian tubes and attaches to other organs, typically near the uterus and within the pelvis. Endometriosis may or may not cause pain; paradoxically, pain may not correlate with the extent of the disease process. For example, slight pain may be present with severe endometriosis, and severe pain may occur in conjunction with very minimal disease. This disease process can be elusive to diagnose and treat. See Chapter 26 for further information about endometriosis.

With Asherman syndrome, women have intrauterine adhesions as a result of trauma to the uterine cavity (Conforti, Alviggi, Mollo, De Placido, & Magos, 2013). The adhesions can be located within the uterus or go down inside the cervical canal, causing the cervix to become completely agglutinated. The lower uterine segment can have bands of adhesions crossing from the anterior endometrium to the posterior endometrium. Over time, and as white blood cells continually attack the adhesions, inflammation begins in the uterus, and the bands of adhesions become increasingly thicker. The most common causes of Asherman syndrome are curettage after spontaneous abortion, postpartum curettage, myomectomy, and endometrial ablation (Conforti et al., 2013).

Other potential uterine causes of infertility include submucosal fibroids and chronic endometritis. Fibroids not only can cause infertility, but also may lower the success rates of assisted reproductive technology (ART) to treat infertility (Owen & Armstrong, 2015; Practice Committee of the ASRM, 2008b). Chronic endometritis appears to cause inhibition of embryo implantation during an in vitro fertilization (IVF) cycle if untreated (Cicinelli et al., 2015). Congenital anomalies of the uterus, such as a bicornuate uterus or septate uterus, are typically associated with pregnancy loss and complications but not infertility (Fritz & Speroff, 2011).

Male Etiologies

A male factor is the sole cause of the inability to conceive in 20% of couples with infertility. In another 30% to 40% of couples, a male factor contributes to infertility (Practice Committee of the ASRM, 2015c). Four categories of causes of male infertility are distinguished: idiopathic (40–50%), primary gonadal disorders (30–40%), disorders of sperm transport (10–20%), and hypothalamic–pituitary disorders (1–2%) (Fritz & Speroff, 2011).

Gonadal failure can result from chromosomal disorders (e.g., Klinefelter syndrome, Y chromosome deletions), cryptorchidism (undescended testes), varicoceles, infections, medications, radiation, environmental exposures, and chronic illness. A varicocele is caused by a dilation of the pampiniform plexus of spermatic veins and occurs in 15% to 20% of postpubertal males. It is more common to diagnose men with a varicocele on the left than on the right, because the left spermatic vein is longer and enters the left renal vein at a perpendicular angle (Fritz & Speroff, 2011). A varicocele can range from minimal fullness to a bulge or large scrotal mass that when palpated feels like a "sac of worms." Varicocele repair can improve semen parameters and male fertility, with such improvement occurring 3 to 6 months after the procedure (Practice Committee of the ASRM, 2014).

Men who contract mumps later in life, particularly after adolescence, may become infertile due to orchitis (testicular inflammation). Symptoms of orchitis include high fever; unilateral, swollen, warm testicle; inflamed scrotum; and severe testicular pain. Not all men who have mumps orchitis will become sterile (Davis et al., 2010). Gonorrhea and chlamydia infections can also cause orchitis (Fritz & Speroff, 2011).

Environmental factors may negatively affect sperm production in some men, although more research is needed to elucidate these associations. In addition, febrile illness and increased scrotal temperature can cause sperm abnormalities. Thus, men who are trying to get their partners pregnant should avoid the use of hot tubs or saunas and minimize the practice of resting their laptop computers on their laps. Sperm transport may be impaired by congenital or acquired (e.g., infection, vasectomy) obstruction of the vas deferens.

Combined Causes

Combined or interactional causes of infertility include the inability of sperm to survive in the woman's cervical mucus because of the presence of antisperm antibodies. These antibodies can be present in either the male or the female, and their presence causes the sperm to agglutinate or clump, which decreases their motility. Testing for antisperm antibodies is no longer performed routinely; therefore, this condition may go undetected. Other interactional causes of infertility include simultaneous female and male causes of infertility that together increase the risk for infertility and sexual difficulties. Psychological distress in one or both partners may contribute to infertility and can also occur as a result of infertility.

Unexplained Infertility

Unexplained infertility refers to situations in which no specific cause for the infertility can be found. Unexplained infertility is a diagnosis of exclusion, meaning that all other possible causes for the infertility must be ruled out. Interestingly, before the application of various technological means to diagnose specific etiologies of infertility, the rate of unexplained infertility was much higher. As scientific advances have enhanced clinicians' ability to identify an increasing number of causes of infertility, fewer people are being diagnosed with unexplained infertility. Having a diagnosis can give individuals a sense of relief, as they know there is a cause for their difficulty conceiving. In contrast, a diagnosis of unexplained infertility can be especially distressing because individuals have no etiology to blame for their condition.

ASSESSMENT OF INFERTILITY

A diagnosis of infertility is not made until a couple has attempted pregnancy for 12 months; therefore, evaluation is not initiated until this amount of time has elapsed. Earlier assessment is warranted in women who are older than age 35 or have medical conditions that may impair fertility (**Box 18-1**).

Evaluation of infertility begins with a thorough history and physical examination. Clinicians who provide gynecologic care often perform limited assessment of male partners (e.g., obtaining relevant history and ordering semen analysis) and then refer men to a urologist or other specialist in male reproduction if additional evaluation is needed. Diagnostic tests for infertility are most useful and cost-effective if they proceed sequentially in a logical order.

History

Initially, it is essential that the clinician obtain an accurate and detailed history from the woman and her partner. This history will inform which diagnostic tests are ordered, how urgently these tests are performed, and how quickly the woman should return for a follow-up visit. Ideally, the woman and her partner should be interviewed separately and then together to encourage the most complete evaluation. Given the large number of patients that clinicians must provide care for, however, obtaining a thorough infertility history in a timely manner while also providing compassionate care is a skill that should be honed over time.

The information to be gathered in history taking includes general medical, mental health, family health, social, occupational, and personal habits (including exercise) histories. If the woman is a previous patient of the clinician, her history should be reviewed in detail. The clinician should identify the duration of infertility and any previous evaluation or treatment. A detailed gynecologic history, with particular attention to the menstrual and pregnancy histories as well as any previous surgeries or procedures, is crucial to the infertility evaluation. When obtaining the history of the woman's previous surgeries, make certain to identify the specific type of procedure (e.g., laparoscopic versus open), the indication for the procedure, and any complications. The clinician should also ascertain which type of contraception the woman was previously using. This information can clarify whether there have been other periods of unprotected intercourse without pregnancy and identify whether infertility might be related to contraception (e.g., the expected delayed return to fertility after discontinuation of the depot medroxyprogesterone acetate injection [Depo-Provera]). The frequency of coitus, any sexual dysfunction, and history of STIs in either partner are other important pieces of information to collect.

When asking about previous pregnancies, clarify whether the woman and her partner have ever become pregnant together or with other partners. If so, obtain a pregnancy history, including whether the woman had a vaginal or cesarean birth. Cesarean births can cause adhesion formation, which can potentially make it difficult for the oocyte to move through the fallopian tube.

Ask if the woman has had any abnormal Pap tests and if so, what treatment she had. Clinicians should also ask about family history of birth defects, developmental delay, early menopause, or reproductive problems. Note the woman's occupation, exposure to environmental hazards, and substance use (Practice Committee of the ASRM, 2015b).

During the review of systems, ask the woman specifically about nipple discharge, hirsutism, pelvic and abdominal pain, and dyspareunia. Also ask about symptoms of thyroid disorders such as fatigue, heat or cold intolerance, hair loss, and weight gain or loss (Practice Committee of the ASRM, 2015b).

When taking a male infertility history, ask about general medical history, previous surgeries, current medications, and family genetic disorders that could interfere with conceiving. The reproductive history should include duration of infertility, frequency and timing of sex, and history of STIs. Ask if the man has ever attempted to conceive with his current partner or a previous partner. Note exposure to environmental or chemical toxins in the home or workplace as well as exposure to heat that could raise scrotal temperature. Ask how much alcohol, tobacco, cannabis, illegal drugs, and anabolic steroids the man is using, as these substances can affect fertility (Practice Committee of the ASRM, 2015c).

Physical Examination

A complete physical examination of the woman, including a pelvic examination, should be performed (Practice Committee of the ASRM, 2015b). During the general examination, it is particularly important to note weight, BMI, blood pressure, and pulse; the presence of thyroid enlargement, nodules, or tenderness; acne, hirsutism, male pattern baldness, or alopecia that could indicate a hyperandrogenic disorder (see Chapter 25); and nipple discharge or visual changes that could indicate a pituitary mass. The pelvic examination should focus on identifying any abnormalities of the genitalia, such as enlargement of the clitoris, tenderness, masses, and organ enlargement. Assess uterine size and shape, and determine whether there is evidence of gynecologic infections or STIs. If infection is suspected, microscopic examination of vaginal secretions and chlamydia and gonorrhea testing should be performed (see Chapter 6).

The male partner should also have a complete physical examination, by either the primary care physician or a urologist, with attention to the reproductive organs to rule out structural problems.

Diagnostic Testing and Procedures

The basic and simple diagnostic procedures that should be performed in an initial evaluation include documentation of ovulation detection and obtaining a semen analysis from the male partner or donor. More specific tests that may be warranted include laboratory testing, sonohysterosalpingography, hysterosalpingography, transvaginal ultrasound, hysteroscopy, laparoscopy, postcoital testing, endometrial biopsy, and sperm penetration assay. The history should guide the clinician's decisions as to which testing is needed and in which order so that time and money are not wasted. Evaluation generally proceeds from least invasive to most invasive testing. If a woman is ovulatory, it is preferable to organize the infertility evaluation according to the menstrual cycle. With this approach, many of the tests can be performed within the same month without disturbing her ability to conceive.

Ovulation Detection

Women can detect ovulation by monitoring and recording their basal body temperature (BBT) each day upon awakening. A BBT thermometer is different from a fever thermometer, in that the BBT thermometer is calibrated in tenths of degrees, allowing for the detection of smaller changes in temperature. The woman should measure her temperature before eating or drinking; this measurement is most accurate if taken before rising from bed. The temperature can be taken orally, vaginally, or rectally, but should be taken the same way each time.

If a woman ovulates, the biphasic cycle is indicated by consistently lower temperatures during the follicular phase and consistently higher temperatures during the luteal phase. A temperature increase of at least 0.4°F is expected after ovulation. Although fluctuations inevitably occur within each of the phases, plotting the temperatures on a graph makes a biphasic pattern evident. Usually a slight drop in temperature occurs just prior to ovulation, and a surge in temperature accompanies ovulation (**Figure 18-2**).

Recording the BBT is helpful because it provides useful data for confirmation of ovulation. The BBT should be recorded for at least 3 months. One menstrual cycle does not provide enough information; rather, it is best to have a record of at least three menstrual cycles to assess whether the cycles follow a pattern. BBT charting is an inexpensive, noninvasive testing methodology that is controlled by the woman. The only caveat to BBT charting is that by the time a woman's temperature has risen, she has already ovulated. This information must be communicated effectively to the woman, or she may be frustrated that she has missed the correct window of peak fertility to time coitus and feel that she has wasted a cycle.

Although keeping a record of the woman's BBT provides useful information, an alternative and more accurate method of ovulation detection is available in the form of over-the-counter urine tests for LH. Women can perform these tests in their home. Identification of an LH surge indicates that ovulation will likely occur within the next 24 to 36 hours. Some women may consider urine LH testing cost-prohibitive if used for an extended period. However, ovulation predictor kits are much less expensive and invasive than serial ultrasounds to look for follicular maturation.

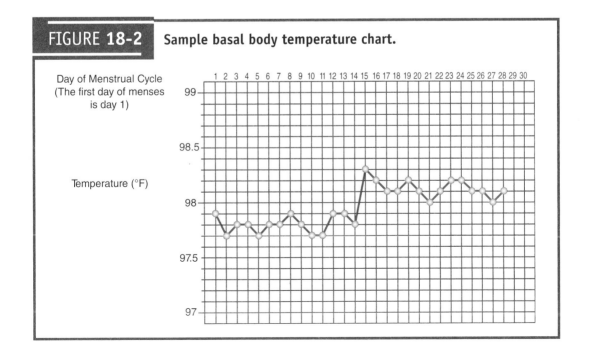

FIGURE 18-2 **Sample basal body temperature chart.**

Semen Analysis

A semen analysis is the cornerstone of the male infertility assessment and can detect most male factor infertility. A complete male evaluation usually includes at least two semen analyses, performed a month apart. It is important that semen analysis be performed early in the infertility evaluation so that male factor infertility can be diagnosed before the woman undergoes extensive, invasive diagnostic procedures.

Male partners should be provided with specific, standardized instructions before collecting a semen sample (Practice Committee of the ASRM, 2015c). Semen can be collected by masturbation with ejaculation into a sterile container or by intercourse with ejaculation into a special collection condom that contains no toxins to sperm (if a man is uncomfortable with masturbation). Instructions should also include a defined period of abstinence of 2 to 5 days prior to sample collection. Men with severe oligospermia should be instructed to adhere to a shorter duration of abstinence and may need to provide several sperm samples (Practice Committee of the ASRM, 2015c). While semen collection in

the office or laboratory is ideal, some men prefer to collect their semen sample at home. In this case, no more than 1 hour should elapse between collection and microscopic examination of the semen sample, and the sample should be kept at room or body temperature during transport (Practice Committee of the ASRM, 2015c). If a woman presents with her partner and his semen analysis is older than 6 months, the clinician should repeat the semen analysis, as sperm counts and morphology change over time.

The World Health Organization (WHO) reference values (Cooper et al., 2010) are widely used to determine if a semen sample falls within normal ranges for semen volume and sperm concentration, motility, and morphology (Practice Committee of the ASRM, 2015c). The 2010 WHO reference limits (**Table 18-2**) help to differentiate a male specimen as fertile or subfertile. It is important to appreciate that these values are reference ranges—they are *not* the minimum values needed for fertilization. Thus, a man whose semen falls outside the ranges can be fertile, whereas a man whose semen is within the ranges can be infertile (Practice

---

TABLE 18-2   World Health Organization Lower Reference Limits for Semen Characteristics

Characteristic	Lower Reference Limit	
	5th Centile	**95% CI**
Semen volume per mL	1.5	1.4–1.7
Total sperm number (10^6 per ejaculate)	39	33–46
Sperm concentration (10^6 per mL)	15	12–16
Total motility (PR + NP, %)	40	38–42
Progressive motility (PR, %)	32	31–34
Vitality (live spermatozoa, %)	58	55–63
Sperm morphology (normal forms, %)	4	3.0–4.0
pH	≥ 7.2	NA

Abbreviations: CI, confidence interval; mL, milliliter; NA, not applicable; NP, nonprogressive motility; PR, progressive motility.
Data from Cooper, T. G., Noonan, E., von Eckardstein, S., Auger, J., Baker, H. W. G., Behre, H., . . . Vogelson, K. (2010). World Health Organization reference values for human semen characteristics. *Human Reproduction Update, 16*(3), 231–245. doi:10.1093/humupd /dmp048; World Health Organization (WHO). (2010). *WHO laboratory manual for the examination and processing of human semen* (5th ed.). Retrieved from http://www.who.int/reproductivehealth/publications/infertility/9789241547789/en/index.html.

Committee of the ASRM, 2015c). If the male partner's semen analysis indicates subfertility, the clinician should repeat the semen analysis a month from the first test prior to referring the man to a specialist.

The semen analysis helps determine treatment options for male factor infertility, including intrauterine insemination (IUI), which may be accompanied by ovulation induction; IVF; and intracytoplasmic sperm injection (ICSI, discussed later in this chapter). Both IVF and ICSI are performed by reproductive endocrinology and infertility (REI) specialists.

Laboratory Testing

Evaluation for infertility usually includes serum tests to identify the cause and guide treatment. Important hormones in conception are produced by the hypothalamus, pituitary gland, thyroid gland, and ovaries. Tests during initial evaluation most often include thyroid-stimulating hormone (TSH), free thyroxine (T4), and prolactin levels, as women can have asymptomatic thyroid disease or hyperprolactinemia. If thyroid or pituitary abnormalities are detected, these conditions will need to be treated prior to infertility treatment commencing, or it is quite possible that the infertility treatment may not be successful (Practice Committee of the ASRM, 2015b).

A repeatedly elevated serum prolactin level in the absence of lactation requires magnetic resonance imaging (MRI) of the pituitary and sella turcica, with and without contrast, to rule out a pituitary mass. Of women who have hyperprolactinemia, 50% to 60% have a pituitary tumor, regardless of the numeric value of their prolactin level (Practice Committee of the ASRM, 2008a). The poor correlation between tumor presence and prolactin level indicates that the clinician should have a low threshold for ordering a pituitary MRI.

If hysterosalpingography cannot be obtained for financial or other reasons, chlamydia antibody testing can be performed as a screen for tubal blockage. If the chlamydia antibody test is negative, the likelihood of tubal pathology is less than 20% (Practice Committee of the ASRM, 2015b).

If BBT charting or LH urine testing does not demonstrate a biphasic curve, measuring serum progesterone levels midway through the luteal phase, on cycle day 21, can be helpful in confirming whether a woman is ovulating (Practice Committee of the ASRM, 2015b). A progesterone level greater than 3 ng indicates the woman has ovulated. Additional laboratory serum tests may be warranted if the woman has oligomenorrhea, amenorrhea, or signs and symptoms of a hyperandrogenic disorder. These tests may include FSH, LH, estradiol, free testosterone, total testosterone, and dehydroepiandrosterone sulfate (DHEA-S) measurements (Practice Committee of the ASRM, 2015b).

Ovarian reserve testing assesses a woman's reproductive potential by measuring the quality and quantity of her remaining oocytes (Practice Committee of the ASRM, 2015f). Ovarian reserve testing can be used to guide the choice of infertility treatment options and predict the likelihood of success of treatment. Routine ovarian reserve testing is not recommended, but such testing can be useful for women at risk of decreased or diminished ovarian reserve (**Box 18-2**) or those who are planning treatment with ART (Practice Committee of the ASRM, 2015b). A common method for measuring ovarian reserve is to obtain serum FSH and estradiol levels on cycle day 3; however, the reliability of a single FSH measurement is very limited due to variations in FSH levels between and within cycles (Practice Committee of the ASRM, 2015f).

BOX 18-2 **Risk Factors for Decreased or Diminished Ovarian Reserve**

- Age > 35 years
- Family history of early menopause
- Poor response to gonadotropin stimulation
- Single ovary or history of previous ovarian surgery, chemotherapy, or pelvic radiation therapy
- Unexplained infertility

Data from Practice Committee of the American Society for Reproductive Medicine (ASRM). (2015b). Diagnostic evaluation of the infertile female: A committee opinion. *Fertility and Sterility, 103*(6), e44–e50.

Another measurement of ovarian reserve is the clomiphene citrate challenge test, which entails measuring serum FSH and estradiol levels on cycle day 3, administering clomiphene citrate (100 mg/day) from cycle days 5 to 9, and repeating serum FSH and estradiol levels on cycle day 10. Use of the clomiphene citrate challenge test has declined due to newer, simpler, highly predictive tests of ovarian reserve, such as the serum anti-Müllerian hormone (AMH) and antral follicle count (Practice Committee of the ASRM, 2015b). As the primordial follicle pool declines with age, AMH levels gradually decline until they become undetectable by menopause. AMH testing is reliable and can be performed at any time in the menstrual cycle because levels remain consistent within and between cycles. The antral follicle count measures the number of antral follicles in both ovaries during the early follicular phase using transvaginal ultrasound. Both the AMH level and antral follicle count appear to have high specificity (78–92% and 73–100%, respectively) for screening for poor ovarian response to gonadotropin stimulation; however, neither test has sufficient evidence as a screening test for failure to conceive (Practice Committee of the ASRM, 2015f).

Sonohysterosalpingography and Hysterosalpingography

Sonohysterosalpingography is an inexpensive, minimally invasive test that uses transvaginal ultrasound to confirm the shape of the uterine cavity, measure the thickness of the endometrium, and assess the patency of the fallopian tubes. During a sonohysterosalpingogram (SHG), sterile saline and air are injected into the uterus through the cervix.

Hysterosalpingography is a procedure in which radiopaque contrast is injected through the woman's cervix into her uterus. During a hysterosalpingogram (HSG), the transport of the contrast through the uterus and into the fallopian tubes is observed by x-ray. In a normal HSG, the contrast travels unobstructed; therefore, this test indicates whether the fallopian tubes are patent or whether a structural abnormality is present in the uterus or tubes (Fritz & Speroff, 2011).

An SHG or HSG is ideally performed on cycle days 6 through 9 and after menstruation ends to avoid interference from menstrual tissue and disruption of potential fertilization and implantation; however, these tests can be performed through cycle day 12. The SHG has better sensitivity and specificity for detecting anomalies of the uterine cavity than the HSG and allows the clinician to examine the ovaries for abnormalities. In addition, the woman does not have not to be exposed to the radiation hazards and risk of iodine allergy that occur with an HSG (Maheux-Lacroix et al., 2014). Both an SHG and an HSG are excellent screening tools for diagnosing tubal factor infertility, and one of these tests should be obtained prior to consideration of laparoscopy, which is the gold standard for diagnosing tubal occlusion but is an invasive procedure.

Transvaginal Ultrasound and Hysteroscopy

Transvaginal ultrasound can help identify uterine factors associated with infertility, such as fibroids and endometrial polyps. It is not a necessary test to obtain during the initial infertility evaluation, however, and it may not be needed at all now that hysteroscopy can be performed as an outpatient procedure in the clinician's office.

Hysteroscopy can be used for definitive diagnosis and treatment of intrauterine conditions causing infertility. This procedure allows the clinician to assess the uterine cavity and endometrium. A hysteroscopy is performed early in the follicular phase, typically between cycle days 7 through 11, and preferably after cessation of menses, for optimal visualization of the cavity (Makled, Farghali, & Shenouda, 2014).

Laparoscopy

The outside surfaces of the uterus, tubes, and ovaries can be observed via a laparoscope, which is inserted into the abdomen through the umbilicus. In this procedure, the pelvic organs are examined for any abnormalities, including structural alterations, endometriosis, or pelvic adhesions. Laparoscopy can be used not only for diagnosis of endometriosis and pelvic adhesions, but also for treatment by excision of endometriosis. Hysteroscopy may be performed at the time of laparoscopy to evaluate the uterine cavity as well. Laparoscopy should be considered when advanced stage endometriosis, tubal occlusive disease, or peritoneal factors are strongly suspected, but is not recommended for routine evaluation without a specific indication (Practice Committee of the ASRM, 2015b). Given that laparoscopy is an invasive diagnostic tool and other tests are available to assess tubal patency (i.e., SHG and HSG), laparoscopy is not used as a first-line assessment of tubal patency (Maheux-Lacroix et al., 2014).

Diagnostic Testing and Procedures That Are No Longer Recommended Routinely

Three diagnostic tests and procedures previously used in infertility assessment are no longer recommended during the initial infertility evaluation: the postcoital test, endometrial biopsy, and the sperm penetration assay.

A postcoital test evaluates the interaction between the sperm and the cervical mucus around the time of ovulation. After a couple has sexual intercourse, a sample of the woman's cervical mucus is obtained by the clinician for microscopic examination. Normally, live, motile sperm will be seen. If there are fertility-related problems, such as the cervical mucus being too acidic or the man having an abnormally low sperm count, the clinician might see predominantly immotile sperm or no sperm at all in the sample. Due to the subjectivity of postcoital test results and the availability of treatments that avoid cervical factors (e.g., IUI and IVF), the postcoital test is no longer routinely recommended (Practice Committee of the ASRM, 2015b).

In the past, cells from endometrial biopsy were microscopically examined to assess the phase of the menstrual cycle. The day of the woman's menstrual cycle was compared with the phase of the endometrial tissue to determine if the two were consistent. Endometrial biopsy was considered the gold standard for the diagnosis of short luteal phase for many years, but research has shown that it is not a valid diagnostic method. Consequently, endometrial biopsy is no longer recommended for routine infertility evaluation and should be used as an assessment only in women strongly suspected to have endometrial pathology (e.g., cancer, chronic endometritis) (Practice Committee of the ASRM, 2015b). However, a form of endometrial biopsy called an *endometrial scratch*, in which the endometrium is not scraped three times as it is in a typical endometrial biopsy, is now used as part of the infertility treatment for women with recurrent implantation failure (RIF). Women with RIF do not conceive during ART despite having good-quality embryos, satisfactory endometrial development, and good hormonal response. Women who have their endometrium scratched in the cycle prior to having IVF are 70% more likely to have a clinical pregnancy in the following month (Potdar, Gelbaya, & Nardo, 2012).

Sometimes the cause of infertility is the inability of the sperm to penetrate the ovum. In the sperm penetration assay, sperm are exposed to hamster ova to determine their ability to penetrate, because there is a correlation between the ability of sperm to penetrate human ova and hamster ova. This test is mentioned because it highlights the fact that sperm abnormalities are sometimes better understood in interaction with the ova. It is no longer performed, however, because ICSI is routinely used during IVF for couples who have male factor infertility (Practice Committee of the ASRM, 2015c).

DIFFERENTIAL DIAGNOSIS

The differential diagnosis of infertility includes the etiologies detailed previously. It is important to recognize that several causes may exist simultaneously.

PREVENTION OF INFERTILITY

The focus in infertility has traditionally been on diagnosis and treatment, but recently more attention has been paid to prevention. Young women can be taught to prevent STIs, or if they have symptoms or suspect they may have been exposed to infection, to seek care early to prevent PID and subsequent infertility. Paradoxically, certain contraceptive methods may protect future fertility by decreasing the risk of PID and ectopic pregnancies (see Chapter 11). It is important for clinicians to ask women about cigarette smoking and alcohol and caffeine intake at annual visits, not only for their general health, but also because these habits are associated with reduced fertility (Sharma, Biedenharm, Felor, & Agarwal, 2013). Simple health promotion education can greatly impact women's future fertility.

MANAGEMENT OF INFERTILITY

Treatments for infertility are usually specific to the cause. Sometimes treatments are general because a specific cause of infertility cannot be determined (unexplained infertility). Approaches to treatment in these instances raise complex issues about risks and benefits. Usually the least invasive, least costly option is offered as first-line treatment. If that is unsuccessful, treatment proceeds to more invasive and costly procedures. Throughout the treatment process, clinicians must take into account the physical and mental health, financial resources, and overall well-being of the woman and her partner.

Patient Education

Education about when a woman is fertile during the menstrual cycle and coital timing is extremely important for women who are trying to conceive. The "fertile window" is the 6-day interval that ends on the day of ovulation. Couples who have intercourse every 1 to 2 days during this time have the highest pregnancy rates, but pregnancy rates are similar with intercourse two to three times a week (Practice Committee of the ASRM, 2013a). Education about how to time intercourse with ovulation is all the information needed to improve conception rates for some women.

The infertility evaluation is also an opportune time to suggest health-promoting behaviors. Behaviors that may specifically improve fertility include achieving a BMI in the range of 20 to 25 if the woman is underweight or overweight, smoking cessation for both partners, and reducing alcohol and caffeine consumption (to 4 or fewer drinks per week and less than 250 mg per day, respectively) (Fritz & Speroff, 2011).

Subclinical Hypothyroidism

Management of subclinical hypothyroidism (SCH) in women with infertility is controversial due to disagreement about the thresholds for diagnosis as well as conflicting findings regarding the association of SCH with infertility and the ability of treatment to improve outcomes. The ASRM defines SCH as a TSH level greater than the upper limit of normal (4 mIU/L for women who are not pregnant) with normal free T4 levels (Practice Committee of the ASRM, 2015e). **Table 18-3** summarizes the recent ASRM guidelines regarding management of SCH in women with infertility.

Ovulation Induction

The oral ovulation induction agents used in infertility treatment are clomiphene citrate (Clomid) and letrozole (Femara).

Clomiphene Citrate

The first-line medication for ovulation induction in women who do not have polycystic ovary syndrome (PCOS) is clomiphene citrate, which is indicated for women who are anovulatory or have unexplained infertility. For those with unexplained infertility, clomiphene citrate should be used in conjunction with IUI; empiric treatment with clomiphene citrate with intercourse is no more effective than expectant management for unexplained infertility and, therefore, is discouraged (Practice Committee of the ASRM, 2013b).

Clomiphene citrate works by binding to estrogen receptors in the hypothalamus, thereby

---

TABLE 18-3 Preconception Management of Subclinical Hypothyroidism in Women with Infertility

Thyroid-Stimulating Hormone Level	Management
>4 mIU/L	Treat with levothyroxine to maintain levels < 2.5 mIU/L
2.5–4 mIU/L	Monitor TSH and treat when > 4 mIU/L or Treat with levothyroxine to maintain levels < 2.5 mIU/L

Data from Practice Committee of the American Society for Reproductive Medicine (ASRM). (2015e). Subclinical hypothyroidism in the infertile female population: A guideline. *Fertility and Sterility*, *104*(3), 545–553.

blocking those receptors from detecting circulating estrogen. As a result, the hypothalamus increases its secretion of GnRH, which stimulates the pituitary to secrete FSH and LH. These hormones, in turn, stimulate and initiate an ovulatory menstrual cycle (Practice Committee of the ASRM, 2013b).

Clomiphene citrate is taken orally once a day at the same time of day for 5 consecutive days. Women are instructed to start Clomid on cycle days 3 to 5 after the start of a spontaneous menses or menses induced with progestin withdrawal. The initial dose is 50 mg (Practice Committee of the ASRM, 2013b). Ovulation usually occurs 14 days after the first dose, and it is typical for ovulation to occur a couple of days later with clomiphene citrate use than it does in the woman's natural cycle. The dose can be increased in increments of 50 mg if ovulation does not occur, up to a maximum dose of 250 mg. Women with greater BMI may require higher doses than women with lower BMI (Practice Committee of the ASRM, 2013b). If ovulation occurs at a specific dose, the woman should remain on that dose each month, because an increased dose provides no advantage.

Pregnancy is most likely to occur in the first three to six cycles. The maximum number of cycles for which a woman should take clomiphene citrate before moving to other interventions (e.g., letrozole, IVF) is usually three for women with unexplained infertility and six for women who are anovulatory; however, the number of cycles varies depending on multiple factors, including age and laboratory results, and should be individualized for each woman.

The combination of insulin-sensitizing agents, such as metformin, with clomiphene citrate may be beneficial in women with polycystic ovary syndrome (see Chapter 25) who have not responded to either medication by itself. Metformin should be added only if the women has a diagnosis of insulin resistance. In addition, clomiphene citrate is sometimes combined with glucocorticoids, if the women has a diagnosis of hyperandrogenemia and her serum DHEA-S is elevated.

Appropriate monitoring of women using clomiphene citrate includes ovulation detection with BBT charting, urine LH testing, or follicular ultrasound monitoring. A serum progesterone level is obtained on cycle day 21, or 7 days after a positive LH test or follicular ultrasound monitoring, to determine effectiveness of the treatment. Close follow-up for ovarian enlargement is also warranted, although monthly pelvic or ultrasound examinations are no longer routinely required.

Common side effects of clomiphene citrate include hot flashes, headaches, ovarian enlargement, ovarian cyst, multiple gestation, and, less frequently, nausea and visual disturbances. Women may also report pelvic pain due to the formation of an ovarian cyst. In pregnancies that occur among women taking clomiphene citrate, 8% are multiple gestations. Almost all of those pregnancies (99% or more) are twin gestations; triplet and higher-order gestations are rare but possible (Practice Committee of the ASRM, 2013b).

Letrozole

The first-line medication for ovulation induction in women who have PCOS is letrozole, now that a landmark randomized controlled trial has demonstrated it is more effective than clomiphene citrate for this population (Legro et al., 2014). Letrozole is also used as a second-line treatment for women who do not become pregnant with clomiphene citrate.

Letrozole is an aromatase inhibitor that decreases the amounts of estrogen produced by the brain, the ovaries, and conversion of androgens to estrogens. This decreased estrogen production increases FSH secretion, which stimulates follicular development (Pavone & Bulun, 2013). Letrozole was first developed to suppress estrogen production in women with breast cancer, but has been used on an off-label basis in the last decade to induce ovulation (Koroma & Stewart, 2012).

Women start taking letrozole on cycle day 3 and continue its use for 5 consecutive days. The initial dose can be 2.5 mg or 5 mg. If the woman does not ovulate, the dose can be titrated up to 7.5 mg. Women should begin urine LH testing on cycle day 9, as they tend to ovulate sooner than in a natural cycle. Letrozole's label carries a "black box" warning stating that this agent is a category X drug, which women who are trying to get pregnant should not take without discussing such use with their clinician. The half-life of letrozole is 2 days, so by the time a woman ovulates, the drug is completely out of her system and will not interfere with a developing ova.

The most common side effects of letrozole are fatigue, hot flashes, and dizziness (Legro et al., 2014). If a woman does not conceive after three to five cycles of letrozole, she should be referred to a REI physician.

Exogenous Gonadotropins

More potent ovulation induction with injectable exogenous gonadotropins can be tried for women who do not respond to clomiphene citrate or letrozole. Recombinant or purified FSH (Follistim, Gonal-F) or human menopausal gonadotropins containing FSH and LH (Pergonal, Repronex) are most commonly used for this purpose. These medications work by directly stimulating development of the ovarian follicles and are used in conjunction with human chorionic gonadotropin (hCG), recombinant LH, or a GnRH agonist, which is administered in the final stages of follicle maturation to induce oocyte release.

Administration of exogenous gonadotropins increases the risk of ovarian hyperstimulation and tends to result in multiple gestations—even more so than with clomiphene citrate or letrozole. Careful timing of the medication used to induce oocyte release is necessary to limit this risk (Practice Committee of the ASRM, 2008c). The complex protocols and potential serious side effects of exogenous gonadotropins require careful treatment and extensive monitoring that is best performed by REI physicians who are experienced in their use.

Clinicians must use ovulation induction methods judiciously and provide women with education about these medications, including their risks and benefits, so they can make an informed decision about their use. Exogenous gonadotropins can be very expensive, which is a consideration for many people. Some studies in the 1990s found an association between the use of ovulation induction medications and ovarian cancer later in life. More recent studies and a Cochrane review (Rizzuto, Behrens, & Smith, 2013) have found that when confounding variables are controlled for, there is no evidence of an increased risk of ovarian cancer with fertility drug treatment.

Insemination Procedures

Insemination procedures may be used to treat infertility or by women who wish to conceive but do not have a male partner (e.g., women who are single or lesbians). Depending on the circumstances, sperm may be obtained from a heterosexual couple's male partner, a known donor, or an unknown donor, and insemination may be used with natural cycles or in conjunction with ovulation induction. Insemination must be performed in a precisely timed manner based on the woman's menstrual cycle

Insemination procedures begin with a man masturbating to collect semen, which is placed in the vagina, in the cervix (intracervical insemination [ICI]), or directly into the uterus (IUI), bypassing the cervix. Women who are having vaginal insemination may choose to use fresh, unprocessed semen from a known donor. For ICI and IUI, the semen is washed in a centrifuge to remove the seminal plasma, creating a more highly concentrated specimen of motile sperm.

Performing insemination is a simple office procedure. A needleless syringe is used for vaginal insemination. For ICI and IUI, the sperm are inserted into the cervix or uterus, respectively, via a flexible catheter attached to a syringe that contains the sperm. The training and supplies needed for insemination procedures are minimal; therefore, all women's healthcare providers—not just REI specialists—can easily provide these services and in doing so offer increased continuity of care for women and their families (Markus, Weingarten, Duplessi, & Jones, 2010).

Tubal Blockage

Distal tubal disease can sometimes be repaired with a fimbrioplasty, a procedure in which the fimbrial adhesions are lysed. If a fimbrial stricture at the distal portion of the tube can be released surgically to alleviate the distal tubal blockage, then the woman can attempt natural conception. Because there is a high rate of ectopic pregnancy after fimbrioplasty (58%), the clinician should have a very low suspicion for ectopic pregnancy if a woman reports pelvic pain or severe dysmenorrhea during early gestation after fimbrioplasty.

If the woman's fallopian tubes are blocked at the proximal end, she can have a cannulation procedure. If the woman has tubal blockage that cannot be repaired surgically and can afford it, she may be referred for IVF treatment after undergoing a bilateral salpingectomy. The salpingectomy improves the likelihood of IVF success. Otherwise, if the woman has bilateral hydrosalpinges, the fluid in the tubes will create an inhospitable uterine environment and compromise the ability to achieve successful embryo implantation (Practice Committee of the ASRM, 2015d).

Luteal Phase Insufficiency

Management of short luteal phase is controversial. The Practice Committee of the ASRM (2015a) does not recommend treating luteal phase insufficiency unless the woman has ovulatory dysfunction. Fritz and Speroff (2011) also do not recommend treating luteal phase insufficiency, noting that such therapy simply gets women's hopes up, delays menses if they are not pregnant, and causes women stress. A serum progesterone level can be drawn in the luteal phase of a woman's cycle, which would be 7 days after a positive ovulation predictor kit or positive follicular monitoring ultrasound, or on cycle day 21 (Practice Committee of the ASRM, 2015a). A serum progesterone level greater than 3 ng/mL means a woman has ovulated, and a serum progesterone level greater than 10 ng/mL is high enough to support a pregnancy (Fritz & Speroff, 2011).

Some clinicians treat luteal phase insufficiency with progesterone supplementation starting 2 to 3 days after a positive LH surge predictor kit. In naturally conceived cycles, women can discontinue their exogenous progesterone between 7 and 9 weeks' gestation based on either their last menstrual period (LMP), providing they are accurate with their dating, or a first-trimester ultrasound to confirm dating. In ovulation induction, women take exogenous progesterone starting 2 to 3 days after they ovulate and continue this treatment until approximately 5 to 7 weeks' gestation. Women using ART must take progesterone supplementation at least for 7 weeks and up to 10 weeks' gestation (Fritz & Speroff, 2011). The placental–luteal transition typically occurs somewhere between 7 and 9 weeks' gestation.

While progesterone intramuscular injection (IM) of 50 to 100 mg/1 cc in each gluteus maximus has been considered superior in its ability to quickly raise progesterone levels, this treatment is often used as a last resort. The injections are difficult to administer, as they must be injected into the gluteus maximus due to the progesterone being compounded in peanut, olive, or sesame oil. Progesterone vaginal suppositories (100 or 200 mg twice a day) work just as well and actually support the endometrium more quickly than the injection. Women may find the suppositories to be messy, in which case they can try using a suppository once a day at bedtime. Oral progesterone does not work well because this formulation is cleared from the body too rapidly. The half-life of oral progesterone is 4 hours; therefore, it must be given 3 times a day to even possibly be somewhat effective on the endometrium.

Treatment for Male Factor Infertility

Treatment for male factor infertility depends on the specific etiology. For example, certain hormonal conditions respond to medical therapy, and surgical repair of a varicocele can be beneficial. Unfortunately, many causes of male factor infertility are not amenable to treatment. In such cases, pregnancy may still be achieved with IUI, IVF, or ICSI.

The precise timing in the menstrual cycle that is required for insemination and ART procedures can lead to increased stress. A man may feel greater pressure to perform by producing the semen on a schedule, and a woman may feel more anxious about having intercourse at "appropriate" times and abstaining at "inappropriate" times.

Assisted Reproductive Technology

The first IVF birth in the United States occurred in 1981, and today IVF is the most widely used ART procedure. More than 99% of the ART cycles in the United States are IVF (Centers for Disease Control and Prevention [CDC], ASRM, & Society for Assisted Reproductive Technology, 2015). In this technique, the ovaries are hyperstimulated with gonadotropin medication; several mature ova are then surgically retrieved, placed in a laboratory dish, and mixed with sperm. Fertilization takes place in vitro, after which one or more embryos are transferred directly into the woman's uterus for implantation. The number of embryos transferred into the women's uterus is based on a variety of factors, including age, quality of embryos, previous success with infertility treatment, and whether this will be her only IVF cycle (Practice Committee of the ASRM & Practice Committee of the Society for

Assisted Reproductive Technology, 2013). Because IVF bypasses the fallopian tubes, it is commonly used in women who have tubal blockage from structural conditions or secondary to pelvic infection or scar tissue. It is also used for women who have not gotten pregnant with ovulation induction and IUI, and when the etiology of infertility remains unknown.

Gamete intrafallopian transfer (GIFT) is another form of ART. In this case, however, fertilization occurs in vivo rather than in vitro. With GIFT, the ooycte and the sperm are both placed directly into the fallopian tube via laparoscopy so that fertilization can occur. The woman must have at least one patent fallopian tube for GIFT to be successful. Women and men who are Catholic may choose this method over IVF because the Catholic Church condones GIFT, but not IVF.

Zygote intrafallopian transfer (ZIFT) is a process in which the ovaries are hyperstimulated and the ova are surgically retrieved. They are then fertilized in vitro, as with IVF. The zygotes are placed in the fallopian tube laparoscopically the day after fertilization.

ICSI is a newer technique, used in conjunction with IVF or ZIFT, in which an oocyte is directly injected with one sperm. This procedure is indicated when the man has a low sperm count or another form of male factor infertility, and it is increasingly being used with IVF procedures even when there is not a diagnosis of male factor infertility. In 2013, ICSI was used in 69% of all IVF cycles in the United States (CDC, ASRM, & Society for Assisted Reproductive Technology, 2015).

The likelihood that ART will be successful varies depending on a number of factors, most notably the woman's age. For U.S. women using fresh embryos from nondonor eggs, the percentage of ART cycles resulting in live births is 39.9% in women younger than 35 years, 31.6% in women ages 35 to 37, 21.1% in women ages 38 to 40, 11.1% in women ages 41 to 42, 5.2% in women ages 43 to 44, and 1.6% in women older than 44 years (CDC, ASRM, & Society for Assisted Reproductive Medicine, 2015). All U.S. clinics that perform ART must report procedural characteristics and outcomes to the CDC, which publishes national and clinic-specific ART success rates (http://www.cdc.gov/art/reports/index.html).

Collaborative Reproduction

Collaborative or third-party assisted reproduction refers to the involvement of a person who will not be raising the child, such as a sperm or egg donor or a surrogate mother. When this approach is used, one person may donate sperm or oocytes (genetic parent) and/or carry the pregnancy (gestational mother) for another person or couple who will raise the child (rearing parents). Collaborative reproduction may involve insemination procedures or ART. Collaborative reproduction may be chosen when infertility treatment or ART has been unsuccessful or is not possible because of individual factors. Individuals who are situationally infertile (e.g., have a chronic illness or take a medication for which pregnancy would be unadvisable) or those who are unable to conceive because they are not in a heterosexual relationship (e.g., individuals who are single, lesbian women, gay men), may also seek collaborative reproduction.

Use of donor sperm is the most common type of collaborative reproduction, but women may also become pregnant with donor oocytes. For example, a known or anonymous woman may donate her oocytes to an individual or couple. The oocytes are fertilized in vitro with sperm, most likely from the male partner in a couple with infertility (rearing father), and then transferred to the female partner with infertility for gestation. In this instance, the oocyte donor is the genetic mother and the woman who becomes pregnant is the gestational and rearing mother. Surrogate mothers can be genetic and gestational mothers if they carry a fetus who is conceived from their own oocyte, or solely gestational mothers if they carry a fetus conceived from another woman's oocyte.

Complementary and Alternative Therapies

In the United States, 29% to 91% of individuals seeking infertility treatment use complementary and alternative therapies; however, only one-fourth of patients report use of these modalities to their clinicians (Clark, Will, Moravek, Xu, & Fisseha, 2013; Smith, Eisenberg, Millstein et al., 2011). The most commonly used complementary and alternative therapies are exercise, vitamins and supplements, prayer, massage, chiropractic, and meditation (Clark, Will, Moravek, Xu, & Fisseha, 2013). A recent systematic review (Clark, Will, Moravek, & Fisseha, 2013) examined complementary and alternative therapies for infertility and found four modalities had three or more studies demonstrating their beneficial effects:

- Acupuncture: improves anxiety levels but has mixed results regarding improvement of pregnancy rates
- Selenium supplementation: improves semen parameters but data are lacking regarding pregnancy rates
- Weight loss: consider for women with PCOS
- Psychotherapy: improves psychological well-being but has mixed results regarding improvement of pregnancy rates

The two most recent systematic reviews and meta-analyses of use of acupuncture with IVF had conflicting results. One review found higher pregnancy rates, but not higher birth rates, in women who had acupuncture compared with women who did not; however, birth rates were higher when studies using a specific control needle that may not be inactive were excluded from the analysis (Zheng, Huang, Zhang, & Wang, 2012). The other review did not find improved pregnancy and live birth rates with acupuncture (Cheong, Dix, Hung Yu Ng, Ledger, & Farquhar, 2013). Studies of the use of acupuncture in women who are not undergoing ART are lacking. In a systematic review of acupuncture for men with infertility, there was improvement in some parameters of semen quality but not in pregnancy rates with acupuncture; however, the number of studies was small, and the studies were heterogeneous, with a high risk of bias and poor quality of reporting (Jerng, Jo, Lee, Lee, & Kwon, 2014).

Two Cochrane reviews have examined the use of antioxidants for infertility. Antioxidant use by women with infertility does not increase pregnancy and live birth rates (Showell, Brown, Clarke, & Hart, 2013); however, antioxidant use in men with infertility may improve pregnancy and live birth rates (Showell et al., 2014).

OTHER OPTIONS FOR WOMEN AND MEN WITH INFERTILITY

Despite the array of infertility treatment, ART, and third-party assisted reproduction options now available, some women and men will not be able to have children via any of these methods. These individuals may choose adoption or child-free living.

Adoption

Adoption is often an ideal option for individuals who are able to separate pregnancy from parenting. Those who choose to adopt can go through a public or private adoption agency, or they may work with an attorney and have an independent or private adoption. International adoption has become common as more people have begun to go outside of the United States to adopt children.

Child-Free Living

Some individuals or couples eventually come to a decision to live their lives without children. The term *child-free* connotes that this state has now become a choice rather than something occurring against their will. People without children may be referred to as *childless*, but this term can connote a loss or absence. Granted, this situation was initially childlessness for those who hoped to conceive, but through the process of reconciling their loss, some people are able to come to a conclusion of their own volition to remain child-free.

EVIDENCE FOR BEST PRACTICES RELATED TO INFERTILITY CARE

The Practice Committee of the ASRM regularly publishes updated evidence-based guidelines for infertility care (https://www.asrm.org/Guidelines). Practices that offer ART are urged to follow the guidelines developed by the Practice Committee of the ASRM, Practice Committee of the Society for Assisted Reproductive Technology, and Practice Committee of the Society of Reproductive Biology and Technology (2014). These guidelines address necessary personnel, the specialized training and experience required for personnel, ethical and experimental procedures, recordkeeping, and informed consent. The guidelines are updated periodically and are considered the standard for the delivery of ART care.

SPECIAL CONSIDERATIONS

This section presents some of the controversial issues related to infertility and its treatment. Infertility can have psychosocial effects on the individuals and couples involved as well as on their larger families. The use of oocyte cryopreservation for both medical and nonmedical reasons is increasing, and new technologies have made it possible for women to have children at later ages. The new technologies that are now used to both diagnose and treat infertility have created many ethical issues.

Psychological, Family, Relationship, and Social Issues

Extensive research suggests that many psychological issues are related to infertility, as either causes or consequences of this condition. Historically, women were viewed as psychogenically infertile—a very negative term implying that women who were unable to conceive were psychologically unstable, had unresolved relationship issues with their mothers, or were hysterical or neurotic (Boivin & Gameiro, 2015). Psychoanalytic theory in the 1950s and 1960s explained infertility as solely a woman's problem, to the exclusion of any involvement by men. A few decades later, the scientific literature developed an increasing focus on psychological problems in both women and men that occurred as a consequence of infertility rather than as a cause, mitigating the negative labels placed on women. A better understanding was developed about the difficulties and stresses that both women and men experienced as a result of their inability to conceive or bear a child. Recently, the scientific literature has taken a more complex view, indicating that infertility has both psychological causes and consequences for women and men.

Infertility is profoundly distressing for those experiencing it, and some studies have shown that stress, anxiety, and depression can reduce chances of pregnancy with ART (Matthiesen, Frederiksen, Ingerslev, & Zachariae, 2011; Reis, Xavier, Coelho, & Montenegro, 2013). Infertility is directly intertwined with family issues, because it represents the inability to expand a family. Some people even view it as an inability to have a family, implying that two people in a couple are not a family by virtue of not having children and further emphasizing a societal bent toward pronatalism. Family gatherings can be extremely difficult for persons dealing with infertility because they may be directly confronted with their inability to conceive, especially if young children are present. Family issues may also extend to other people beyond the couple themselves, such as the parents of people with infertility who are experiencing the loss related to not being grandparents. Family members may pressure couples with infertility with comments such as "Why are they taking so long to have a baby?"

As stated earlier, women and men experience infertility within a socially pronatalist context. As a result, women and men experiencing infertility are often viewed as abnormal or as not fulfilling their responsibilities to continue the human race. Women, by virtue of the general social approach to and view of women's roles, may experience feeling even more "aberrant" than do men.

Complicated psychological issues can come to the fore surrounding a decision or inability to make a decision to stop infertility treatment. The introduction of new treatments may raise hopes and make it difficult to stop treatment for fear that there will be a feeling of not having done everything possible to conceive, which could then make it difficult to resolve infertility later. In this situation, the clinician should advise patients about their options, including the pros and cons of continuing treatment.

Some evidence indicates that providing psychosocial interventions—particularly cognitive-behavioral therapy—to women and men being treated for infertility can be beneficial in terms of both decreasing psychological distress and improving clinical pregnancy rates (Frederiksen, Farver-Vestergaard, Skovgård, Ingerslev, & Zachariae, 2015). Some infertility treatment centers now have a mental health professional on site (Domar, 2015). This type of specialist can be helpful not only for the patients, but also for the center's clinicians and staff because caring for women and men with infertility can be difficult.

Fertility Preservation

Advances in ART have created the opportunity for individuals to cryopreserve spermatozoa, oocytes, and embryos for future use. Initially this technology was used by patients facing disease- or treatment-related infertility, such as patients having chemotherapy and radiation for cancer or women undergoing oophorectomy for chemoprophylaxis. Today, increased awareness of the age-related decline in fertility has led to interest in oocyte cryopreservation among women who want to delay childbearing due to a variety of life circumstances, such as not yet having a partner or wanting to accomplish specific life goals before having children. The Ethics Committee of the ASRM (2013b) recommends that clinicians counsel patients about fertility preservation options and future reproduction prior to any gonadotoxic treatments. Fertility preservation for nonmedical reasons remains controversial, although the European Society of Human Reproduction and Embryology (ESHRE) says it should be available (ESHRE Task Force on Ethics and Law including Dondorp et al., 2012). Individuals considering cryopreservation must be informed this is an emerging technology, and long-term follow-up data are not yet available (Ethics Committee of the ASRM, 2013b; ESHRE Task Force on Ethics and Law including Dondorp et al., 2012). Cryopreservation has complex ethical and legal considerations (Shah, Goldman, & Fisseha, 2011). As one example, individuals must give instructions about what should be done with their cryopreserved spermatozoa, oocytes, or embryos should they die, divorce, or experience other life changes.

Infertility and Women in the Later Years of Childbearing

With the increased use of technology to treat infertility, more options have been developed for women at the end of their childbearing years. Thus women in their mid-40s to 50s may conceive and carry a pregnancy to term. Although this flexibility provides more opportunities for women, it also creates more complex decisions for women and their families. Certain genetic risks to the fetus, such as Down syndrome, and obstetric risks are known to be higher when women become pregnant at later ages. At the same time, some women have circumstances that make them want to have children at older ages. More research is needed in this area.

Ethical Issues

Many of the ethical issues related to infertility occur as a result of the increasing use of technology; however, it is important to note that ethical issues existed prior to and may be independent of advances in infertility treatment. Access to infertility treatment has always been an issue, but it has been particularly compounded by the never-ending stream of technology that has been introduced within the healthcare realm. The expense of infertility treatment raises the question of whether these therapies will be limited to those with the financial means to afford them, as the costs for such treatment are frequently not covered by insurance (Ethics Committee of the ASRM, 2015b; Smith, Eisenberg, Glidden et al., 2011). The ability to conceive with technology but without a partner also leads to questions regarding whether single, lesbian, gay, and transgender individuals will be treated (Ethics Committee of the ASRM, 2013a, 2015a).

Other ethical issues concern who the parents are in situations where extra embryos have been frozen and a couple subsequently divorces, or when a surrogate mother decides she no longer wants to relinquish the newborn. In fact, the larger issue is how the "real parent" is defined. Parties involved in various third-party assisted reproduction conflicts may include the genetic mother, the genetic father, the surrogate mother, the gestational mother, and the rearing mother and/or father.

Another ethical dilemma can occur when several embryos are transferred into the woman's uterus and multiple embryos survive. The presence of multiple embryos may create a high-risk situation for all of them, and the woman may choose to selectively abort one or more embryos to reduce this risk. This situation creates complex ethical as well as emotional issues. Limiting the number of embryos transferred is advisable (Practice Committee of the ASRM & Practice Committee of the Society for Assisted Reproductive Technology, 2013).

Ethical concerns have also arisen in relation to the ability to perform preimplantation genetic screening and diagnosis with ART. After IVF, a cell is removed from the embryo for genetic testing. This evaluation allows individuals with known inherited disorders to select nonaffected embryos for transfer, but leads to questions about genetic engineering. The sex of the embryo can also be predetermined, which is useful for sex-linked disorders, but is controversial when sex selection is performed for nonmedical reasons (Ethics Committee of the ASRM, 2015c).

These are just a few of the many ethical issues that arise in relation to infertility care and treatment. There are no simple answers to these conflicts, but they warrant consideration both from a societal perspective and on the level of caring for individual patients. The Ethics Committee of the ASRM regularly publishes reports that address ethical issues in infertility treatment (https://www.asrm.org/EthicsReports).

References

American College of Obstetricians and Gynecologists & Practice Committee of the American Society for Reproductive Medicine (ASRM). (2014). Committee Opinion No. 589. Female age-related fertility decline. *Obstetrics & Gynecology, 123,* 719–721.

Boivin, J., & Gameiro, S. (2015). Evolution of psychology and counseling in infertility. *Fertility and Sterility, 104*(2), 251–259.

Centers for Disease Control and Prevention (CDC), American Society for Reproductive Medicine (ASRM), & Society for Assisted Reproductive Technology. (2015). *2013 Assisted Reproductive Technology National Summary Report.* Atlanta, GA: U.S. Department of Health and Human Services.

Chandra, A., Copen, C. E., & Stephen, E. H. (2013). Infertility and impaired fecundity in the United States, 1982–2010: Data from the National Survey of Family Growth. *National Health Statistics Reports, 67,* 1–18.

Cheong, Y. C., Dix, S., Hung Yu Ng, E., Ledger, W. L., & Farquhar, C. (2013). Acupuncture and assisted reproductive technology. *Cochrane Database of Systematic Reviews, 7,* CD006920.

Cicinelli, E., Matteo, M., Tinelli, R., Lepara, A., Alfonso, R., Indracolo, U., . . . Resta, L. (2015). Prevalence of chronic endometritis in repeated unexplained implantation failure and the IVF success rate after antibiotic therapy. *Human Reproduction, 30*(2), 323–330.

Clark, N. A., Will, M. A., Moravek, M. B., & Fisseha, S. (2013). A systematic review of the evidence for complementary and alternative medicine in infertility. *International Journal of Gynecology & Obstetrics, 122,* 202–206.

Clark, N. A., Will, M. A., Moravek, M. B., Xu, X., & Fisseha, S. (2013). Physician and patient use of and attitudes toward complementary and alternative medicine in the treatment of infertility. *International Journal of Gynecology & Obstetrics, 122,* 253–257.

Conforti, A., Alviggi, C., Mollo, A., De Placido, G., & Magos, A. (2013). The management of Asherman syndrome: A review of literature. *Reproductive Biology and Endocrinology, 11,* 118

Cooper, T. G., Noonan, E., von Eckardstein, S., Auger, J., Baker, H. W. G., Behre, H., . . . Vogelson, K. (2010). World Health Organization reference values for human semen characteristics. *Human Reproduction Update, 16*(3), 231–245. doi:10.1093/humupd/dmp048

Davis, N. F., McGuire, B. B., Mahon, J. A., Smyth, A. E., O'Malley, K. J., & Fitzpatrick, J. M. (2010). The increasing incidence of mumps orchitis: A comprehensive review. *British Journal of Urology, 105,* 1060–1065.

Domar, A. D. (2015). Creating a collaborative model of mental health counseling for the future. *Fertility and Sterility, 104*(2), 277–280.

ESHRE Task Force on Ethics and Law, including Dondorp, W., de Wert, G., Pennings, G., Shenfield, F., Devroey, P., Tarlatzis, B., . . . Diedrich, K. (2012). Oocyte cryopreservation for age-related fertility loss. *Human Reproduction, 27*(5), 1231–1237.

Ethics Committee of the American Society for Reproductive Medicine (ASRM). (2013a). Access to fertility treatment by gays, lesbians, and unmarried persons: A committee opinion. *Fertility and Sterility, 100*(6), 1524–1527.

Ethics Committee of the American Society for Reproductive Medicine (ASRM). (2013b). Fertility preservation and reproduction in patients facing gonadotoxic therapies: A committee opinion. *Fertility and Sterility, 100*(5), 1224–1231.

Ethics Committee of the American Society for Reproductive Medicine (ASRM). (2015a). Access to fertility treatment by transgender persons: An ethics committee opinion. *Fertility and Sterility, 104*(5), 1111–1115.

Ethics Committee of the American Society for Reproductive Medicine (ASRM). (2015b). Disparities in access to effective treatment for infertility in the United States: An ethics committee opinion. *Fertility and Sterility, 104*(5), 1104–1110.

Ethics Committee of the American Society for Reproductive Medicine (ASRM). (2015c).Use of reproductive technology for sex selection for nonmedical reasons. *Fertility and Sterility, 103*(6), 1418–1422.

Frederiksen, Y., Farver-Vestergaard, I., Skovgård, N. G., Ingerslev, H. J., & Zachariae, R. (2015). Efficacy of psychosocial interventions for psychological and pregnancy outcomes in infertile women and men: A systematic review and meta-analysis. *BMJ Open, 5,* e006592. doi:10.1136/bmjopen-2014-006592

Fritz, M., & Speroff, L. (2011). *Clinical gynecologic endocrinology and infertility* (8th ed.). Baltimore, MD: Lippincott Williams & Wilkins.

Gelbaya, T. A., Potdar, N., Jeve, Y. B., & Nardo, L. G. (2014). Definition and epidemiology of unexplained infertility. *Obstetrical & Gynecological Survey, 69*(2), 109–115.

Greil, A. L., Slauson-Blevins, K. S., Tiemeyer, S., McQuillan, J., & Shreffler, K. M. (2015). A new way to estimate the potential unmet need for infertility services among women in the United States. *Journal of Women's Health, 25*(2),133–138. doi:10.1089/jwh.2015.5390

Jerng, U. M., Jo, J. Y., Lee, S., Lee, J. M., & Kwon, O. (2014). The effectiveness and safety of acupuncture for poor semen quality in infertile males: A systematic review and meta-analysis. *Asian Journal of Andrology, 16*(6), 884–891.

Koroma, L., & Stewart, L. (2012). Infertility: Evaluation and initial management. *Journal of Midwifery & Women's Health, 57*(6), 614–621.

Legro, R. S., Brzyski, R. G., Diamond, M. P., Coutifaris, C., Schlaff, W. D., Casson, P., . . . Zhang, H. (2014). Letrozole versus clomiphene for infertility in the polycystic ovary syndrome. *New England Journal of Medicine, 371*(2), 119–129.

Maheux-Lacroix, S., Boutin, A., Moore, L., Bergeron, M., Bujold, E., Laberge, P., . . . Dodin, S. (2014). Hysterosalpingosonography for diagnosing tubal occlusion in subfertile women: A systematic review with meta-analysis. *Human Reproduction, 29*(5), 953–963.

Makled, A. K., Farghali, M. M., & Shenouda, D. S. (2014). Role of hysteroscopy and endometrial biopsy in women with unexplained infertility. *Archives of Gynecology and Obstetrics, 289,* 187–192.

Markus, E., Weingarten, A., Duplessi, Y., & Jones, J. (2010). Lesbian couples seeking pregnancy with donor insemination. *Journal of Midwifery&Women's Health, 55*(2), 124– 132.

Martin, J. A., Hamilton, B. E., Osterman, M. J. K., Curtin, S. C., & Mathews, T. J. (2015). Births: Final data for 2013. *National Vital Statistics Reports, 64*(1), 1–65.

Matthiesen, Sm. M. S., Frederiksen, Y., Ingerslev, H. J., & Zachariae, R. (2011). Stress, distress and outcomes of assisted reproductiv technology (ART): A meta-analysis. *Human Reproduction, 26*(10), 2764–2776.

Owen, C., & Armstrong, A. Y. (2015). Clinical management of leiomyoma. *Obstetrics and Gynecology Clinics of North America, 42*(1), 67–85.

Pavone, M. W., & Bulun, S. E. (2013). The use of aromatase inhibitors for ovulation induction and superovulation. *Journal of Clinical Endocrinology & Metabolism, 98*(5), 1838–1844.

Potdar, N., Gelbaya, T., & Nardo, L. G. (2012). Endometrial injury to overcome recurrent embryo implantation failure: A systematic review and meta-analysis. *Reproductive BioMedicine, 25*(6), 561–571.

Practice Committee of the American Society for Reproductive Medicine (ASRM). (2008a). Current evaluation of amenorrhea. *Fertility and Sterility, 90*(Suppl. 5), S219–S225.

Practice Committee of the American Society for Reproductive Medicine (ASRM). (2008b). Myomas and reproductive function. *Fertility and Sterility, 90*(Suppl. 3), S125–S130.

Practice Committee of the American Society for Reproductive Medicine (ASRM). (2008c). Use of exogenous gonadotropins in anovulatory women: A technical bulletin. *Fertility and Sterility, 90*(Suppl. 1), S7–S12.

Practice Committee of the American Society for Reproductive Medicine (ASRM). (2013a). Optimizing natural fertility: A committee opinion. *Fertility and Sterility, 100*(3), 631–637.

Practice Committee of the American Society for Reproductive Medicine (ASRM). (2013b). Use of clomiphene citrate in infertile women: A committee opinion. *Fertility and Sterility, 100*(2), 341–348.

Practice Committee of the American Society for Reproductive Medicine (ASRM). (2014). Report on varicocele and infertility: A committee opinion. *Fertility and Sterility, 102*(6), 1556–1560.

Practice Committee of the American Society for Reproductive Medicine (ASRM). (2015a). Current clinical irrevance of luteal phase deficiency: A committee opinion. *Fertility and Sterility, 103*(4), e27–e32.

Practice Committee of the American Society for Reproductive Medicine (ASRM). (2015b). Diagnostic evaluation of the infertile female: A committee opinion. *Fertility and Sterility, 103*(6), e44–e50.

Practice Committee of the American Society for Reproductive Medicine (ASRM). (2015c). Diagnostic evaluation of the infertile male: A committee opinion. *Fertility and Sterility, 103*(3), e18–e25.

Practice Committee of the American Society for Reproductive Medicine (ASRM). (2015d). Role of tubal surgery in the era of assisted reproductive technology: A committee opinion. *Fertility and Sterility, 103* (6), e37–e45.

Practice Committee of the American Society for Reproductive Medicine (ASRM). (2015e). Subclinical hypothyroidism in the infertile female population: A guideline. *Fertility and Sterility, 104*(3), 545–553.

Practice Committee of the American Society for Reproductive Medicine (ASRM). (2015f). Testing and interpreting mesausres of ovarian reserve: A committee opinion. *Fertility and Sterility, 103*(3), e9–e17.

Practice Committee of the American Society for Reproductive Medicine (ASRM) & Practice Committee of the Society for Assisted Reproductive Technology. (2013). Criteria for number of embryos to transfer: A committee opinion. *Fertility and Sterility, 99*(1), 44–46.

Practice Committee of the American Society for Reproductive Medicine (ASRM), Practice Committee of the Society for Assisted Reproductive Technology, & Practice Committee of the Society of Reproductive Biology and Technology. (2014). Revised minimum standards for practices offering assisted reproductive technologies: A committee opinion. *Fertility and Sterility, 102*(3), 682–686.

Reis, S., Xavier, M. R., Coelho, R., & Montenegro, N. (2013). Psychological impact of single and multiple courses of assisted reproductive treatments in couples: A comparative study. *European Journal of Obstetrics & Gynecology and Reproductive Biology, 171*(1), 61–66.

Resolve. (2015). Secondary infertility. Retrieved from http://www.resolve.org/about-infertility/medical-conditions/secondary-infertility.html

Rizzuto, I., Behrens, R. F., & Smith, L. A. (2013). Risk of ovarian cancer in women treated with ovarian stimulating drugs for infertility. *Cochrane Database of Systematic Reviews, 8,* CD008215.

Shah, D. K., Goldman, E., Fisseha, S. (2011). Medical, ethical, and legal considerations in fertility preservation. *International Journal of Gynecology & Obstetrics, 115,* 11–15.

Sharma, R., Biedenharn, K. R., Felor, J. M., & Agarwal, A. (2013). Lifestyle factors and reproductive health: Taking control of your fertility. *Reproductive Biology and Endocrinology, 11,* 66. doi:10.1186/1477-7827-11-66

Showell, M. G., Brown, J., Clarke, J., & Hart, R. J. (2013). Antioxidants for female subfertility. *Cochrane Database of Systematic Reviews, 8,* CD007807.

Showell, M. G., Mackenzie-Proctor, R., Brown, J., Yazdani, A., Stankiewicz, M. T., & Hart, R. J. (2014). Antioxidants for male subfertility. *Cochrane Database of Systematic Reviews, 12,* CD007411.

Smith, J., Eisenberg, M., Glidden, D., Millstein, S., Cedars, M., Walsh, T., . . . Katz, P. P. (2011). Socioeconomic disparities in the use and success of fertility treatments: Analysis of data from a prospective cohort in the United States. *Fertility and Sterility, 96*(1), 95–101.

Smith, J., Eisenberg, M., Millstein, S., Nachtigall, R. D., Shindel, A. W., . . . Katz, P. P. (2011). The use of complementary and alternative fertility treatment in couples seeking fertility care: Data from a prospective cohort in the United States. *Fertility and Sterility, 93*(7), 2169–2174.

World Health Organization (WHO). (2010). *WHO laboratory manual for the examination and processing of human semen* (5th ed.). Retrieved from http://www.who.int/reproductivehealth/publications/infertility/9789241547789/en/index.html

Zheng, C. H., Huang, G. Y., Zhang, M. M., & Wang, W. (2012). Effects of acupuncture on pregnancy rates in women undergoing in vitro fertilization: A systematic review and meta-analysis. *Fertility and Sterility, 97*(3), 599–611.

Gynecologic Infections

Sharon M. Bond

The editors acknowledge Catherine Ingram Fogel, who was the author of the previous edition of this chapter.

Vulvovaginal symptoms are among the most frequent reasons why a woman seeks care from a clinician. Women perceive vulvovaginal symptoms such as discharge, odor, pain, and itching in unique ways. One woman may be extremely uncomfortable with these symptoms, another may feel only minor distress, a third may be very anxious, and a fourth may be mildly concerned. Women's reactions depend on many factors, including their previous experiences or knowledge; concurrent or chronic medical conditions; societal, religious, and cultural beliefs; and the number and severity of symptoms.

This chapter begins with an overview of vaginal secretions, vaginitis and vaginosis, and prevention measures. The remaining sections address bacterial vaginosis, vulvovaginal candidiasis, atrophic vaginitis, desquamative inflammatory vaginitis, toxic shock syndrome, Bartholin gland duct cysts and abscesses, and genital piercing. Atrophic vaginitis and genital piercing are included in this chapter because they are associated with an increased risk of infection. In addition, atrophic vaginitis can mimic the symptoms of some gynecologic infections and should be considered in the differential diagnosis of women with vulvovaginal symptoms.

VAGINAL SECRETIONS

Normal Characteristics

During reproductive years, vaginal secretions are a normal, regularly occurring experience. The numerous variations in the amount and characteristics of vaginal secretions are determined by physiology, timing in relation to the menstrual cycle, use of local or systemic medications, sexual practices, and pathology. Women who have adequate endogenous or exogenous estrogen will have vaginal secretions. The major source of these secretions is the cervical mucosa, although small amounts are also secreted by the Bartholin, sebaceous, sweat, and apocrine glands of the vulva. Unique combinations of organisms in the vagina are believed to protect a woman by providing an initial line of defense against infection through production of lactic acid by *Lactobacillus* species, which maintain the vaginal pH between 3.5 and 4.5. Conversely, the growth of opportunistic and pathogenic organisms is facilitated when the woman uses antibiotics, vaginal lubricants, hormonal contraceptives, or douching, and is affected by other behavioral and intrinsic factors (Ma, Forney, & Ravel, 2012). However, at least some women with minimal lactobacilli populations are otherwise healthy and do not report vaginal symptoms.

Vaginal secretions provide physiologic lubrication and represent a response to the hormonal milieu. These secretions vary throughout the menstrual cycle and increase in amount around ovulation, during the premenstrual period, during pregnancy, and when sexual arousal occurs. Normal vaginal secretions are usually clear or cloudy and nonirritating in nature, although they may leave a yellow cast on clothing after drying. An increase in the amount of vaginal secretion is known as *leukorrhea* and is classically described as a thin or thick white discharge resulting from congestion of the vaginal mucosa and an increase in polymorphonuclear leukocytes (white blood cells) that is visible under microscopy (Lazenby,

Soper, & Nolte, 2013). Leukorrhea may be seen under normal circumstances, such as pregnancy or menstruation, or in the presence of vaginal infection. Normal vaginal discharge is slightly slimy, is non-irritating, and has a mild inoffensive odor. The alkaline, shiny mucoid substance secreted by the cervix, by comparison, is more abundant than vaginal secretions and less viscous at ovulation. The amount of vaginal discharge a woman experiences is not, in itself, an indication of infection.

Life-Cycle Changes

The female newborn may have a mucous discharge for 1 to 10 days following birth as a result of in utero stimulation of the uterus and vagina by maternal estrogen. A similar mucoid discharge may be seen a few years before and after menarche as a result of increased estrogen production by the maturing ovaries. Pregnant women often report substantially increased mucus production, with a resulting profuse discharge, particularly during the last few weeks before childbirth.

Throughout the reproductive years, vaginal secretions and cervical mucus vary during the menstrual cycle. Typically around day 9 of the menstrual cycle, rising levels of estradiol will increase the amount of cervical mucus, making it thin and watery to enable penetration of sperm immediately prior to ovulation. Once ovulation occurs, progesterone secreted from the corpus luteum converts the cervical mucus into a thickened, tenacious substance, making penetration by sperm unlikely (Steward, Melamed, Granat, & Mishell, 2012).

During two phases of a woman's life—before menarche and following menopause—estrogen levels are low and, consequently, vaginal secretions are minimal. The vaginal epithelium is inactive and thin, the cells contain very little glycogen, lactobacilli are absent, and the vaginal pH is between 6 and 7. Such inactive mucosa is particularly susceptible to infection, whereas the estrogen-stimulated vaginal mucosa during the reproductive years is less vulnerable to such disease.

VAGINITIS AND VAGINOSIS

Vaginitis is an inflammation of the vagina characterized by an increased vaginal discharge containing numerous white blood cells. In contrast,

vaginosis is not associated with an increase in white blood cells. Vaginitis and vaginosis occur when the vaginal environment is altered, either by microorganisms (**Table 19-1**) or by a disturbance allowing pathogens normally found in the vagina to proliferate.

Vulvovaginitis, which is inflammation of the vulva and vagina, may be caused by vaginal infection or copious amounts of leukorrhea. In addition, chemical irritants, allergens, and foreign bodies may produce inflammatory reactions. Bacterial vaginosis (BV), vulvovaginal candidiasis (VVC), and trichomoniasis are the most common causes of abnormal vaginal discharge. See Chapter 20 for a discussion of trichomoniasis and **Color Plate 14** for an example of vaginal discharge.

Prevention Measures

Clinicians can help women alleviate the discomfort associated with abnormal vaginal discharge by teaching preventive measures, providing information to assist in recognizing symptoms, and suggesting self-care activities to prevent and treat vaginitis. Preventive measures are important for all types of vaginal infections, but particularly for women with recurrent episodes of vaginitis. General health promotion, including adequate rest, reduction of life stressors, and a healthy diet low in refined sugars, may help to decrease the likelihood of infection. Good personal hygiene is essential for preventing vaginal infections. Regular, gentle cleansing and drying of the perineal area removes perspiration and smegma accumulations. Towels, washcloths, sponges, douching equipment, vaginal diaphragms, cervical caps, sexual devices, and underwear should be cleaned following each use and never shared.

Critical to prevention efforts is teaching women the proper way to wipe after voiding and defecation. One should always wipe from front to back to avoid introducing bacteria into the vagina or urethra. Sprays, powders, soaps, and deodorants that are perfumed or irritating should be avoided. Chemicals that irritate the skin or vaginal mucosa, or alter the vaginal environment, are best avoided. Avoid clothing that is restrictive or tight in the crotch area, does not allow free air flow to the perineum, or traps moisture. Discourage daily use

TABLE **19-1**	Vaginal Discharge		
	Normal Discharge	**Bacterial Vaginosis**	**Vulvovaginal Candidiasis**
Vaginal pH	3.5–4.5	> 4.5	< 4.5 (usually)
Wet prep	Normal flora	With saline solution: positive for clue cells, decreased lactobacilli	With KOH: pseudohyphae with yeast buds
Discharge	White/clear Thin/mucoid	Thin, homogenous, grayish-white, adherent	Thick or thin, white, curd-like ("cottage cheese"), adherent
Amine odor (KOH "whiff" test)	Absent	Present (fishy)	Absent
Vulvar pruritus	No	Mild, if present at all	Yes, swelling, excoriation, redness
Genital ulceration	No	No	Skin may crack with severe cases
Pelvic pain	No	No	No
Dysuria	No	Occasionally	Severe cases
Dyspareunia	No	Occasionally	Occasionally
Main patient concern	None or variable	May be asymptomatic; vaginal discharge, vaginal odor that is often worse after intercourse	Vaginal itching, burning, and/or discharge
Risk of pelvic inflammatory disease	No	Yes	No

Abbreviation: KOH, potassium hydroxide
Data from Centers for Disease Control and Prevention (CDC). (2015). Sexually transmitted diseases treatment guidelines 2015. *Morbidity and Mortality Weekly Report, 64*(3), 1–138; Eckert, L. O. (2006). Acute vulvovaginitis. *New England Journal of Medicine, 355*(12), 1244–1252.

of panty liners that trap moisture and irritate vulvar skin. Counsel women to change tampons, sanitary pads, and panty liners frequently. Advise women not to wear tampons to bed and not to use them when flow is scanty, as the tampon may adhere to the vaginal wall or cervix and cause trauma when removed. In addition, advise women to avoid perfumed sanitary products because they may cause allergic or irritating skin reactions.

Recommend against vulvar shaving, waxing, and use of depilatories, as these practices strip the vulva—and, therefore, the vagina—of protective hair, expose the skin to bacteria, and may lead to severe inflammatory reactions. Excessive vulvar hair can be clipped with scissors rather than shaved or waxed. Cotton crotches are advisable in underwear and pantyhose. Except when recommended by a clinician to treat a vaginal problem, women should avoid douching, because it can remove normal, protective vaginal flora, introduce bacteria, and aggravate inflammation.

Bacterial Vaginosis

Bacterial vaginosis (see **Color Plate 15**) is a highly prevalent cause of vaginal discharge, accounting for 22% to 50% of women who present with vaginitis symptoms (Fethers, Fairley, Hocking, Gurrin, & Bradshaw, 2008; Verstraelen & Verhelst, 2009). Among reproductive-age women in the United States, the prevalence of BV has been reported to be approximately 29% (Koumans et al., 2007). BV has long been associated with multiple gynecologic and obstetric sequelae, such as spontaneous abortion, upper genital tract infection, preterm birth, and postpartum endometritis (Fethers et al., 2008).

Normally, the vagina of a reproductive-age woman is colonized with lactobacilli that produce hydrogen peroxide, lactic acid, and bacteriocins to maintain the pH of the vagina in an acidic range, between 3.5 and 4.5. An acidic pH creates a hostile environment for bacteria other than the lactobacilli. If the vaginal pH becomes more alkaline, an overgrowth of anaerobic and facultative organisms may occur, producing the characteristic symptoms of BV. Although these organisms, such as *Gardnerella*, *Corynebacterium*, and *Escherichia coli*, may be part of the normal vaginal flora, their growth is typically suppressed in the acidic vaginal environment.

Although the majority of women with BV are asymptomatic, a significant number experience recurring and chronic symptoms. The scientific literature has not settled the controversy regarding whether and when to screen women with chronic recurrence and how to treat them.

Risk factors for BV include the presence of menstrual bleeding, douching, a new sexual partner, smoking, lack of condom use, and race/ethnicity (Fettweis et al., 2014; Secor & Coughlin, 2013; Srinivasan et al., 2012). Hensel, Randis, Gelber, and Ratner (2011) investigated low vitamin D levels as a possible risk factor for BV; their findings may help explain the disparate rates of BV in women who are pregnant, black, or of Mexican American ethnicity. Marrazzo et al. (2002) found BV is common among women who have sex with women, suggesting BV may be acquired via sexual exchange of vaginal secretions.

The most common symptom of BV is a malodorous discharge. The woman or her partner may notice a fishy odor after heterosexual intercourse because semen releases the vaginal amines. When present, the vaginal discharge associated with BV is usually increased, thin, white or gray, and milky in appearance. Some women also may experience mild irritation, vulvar pruritus, postcoital spotting, irregular bleeding episodes, vaginal burning after intercourse, and urinary discomfort.

Assessment

A careful history may help distinguish BV from other causes of vaginitis if the woman is symptomatic. Reports of fishy odor, vaginal irritation, and increased thin vaginal discharge are considered the most significant findings. Reports of increased odor after intercourse are also suggestive of BV. Previous occurrences of similar symptoms, diagnoses, and treatments should be investigated, because recurrence is common.

A speculum examination is performed to inspect the vaginal walls and cervix. A microscopic examination of vaginal secretions is performed with both 10% potassium hydroxide (KOH) and normal saline (see Chapter 6). The KOH solution is used to test for amine odor; amines are produced as a by-product of anaerobic metabolism. The fishy odor released when KOH is added to vaginal secretions on a slide or on the lip of the withdrawn speculum results in a positive KOH or whiff test. The presence of clue cells (vaginal epithelial cells coated with bacteria that obscure cell borders) in the sample with normal saline is a characteristic sign because this phenomenon is specific to BV (**Figure 19-1**). In addition, a reduction in lactobacilli and typically very few white blood cells are noted. Increased numbers of white blood cells in addition to the presence of clue cells suggest a concurrent vaginitis or coinfection with trichomoniasis, chlamydia, or candidiasis.

Vaginal secretions can also be tested for pH. Nitrazine paper is sensitive enough to detect a pH of 4.5 or greater. Normal vaginal secretions have a pH in the range of 3.5 to 4.5. An elevated pH (4.5 or higher) is more commonly seen in the presence of BV or trichomoniasis. A sample for pH testing is best collected from the lateral walls of the vagina to ensure an accurate pH assessment; pH is more variable in the cervix, reflecting the current point in the woman's hormonal cycle. While vaginal pH can be a useful

FIGURE **19-1**   Wet mount findings with bacterial vaginosis.

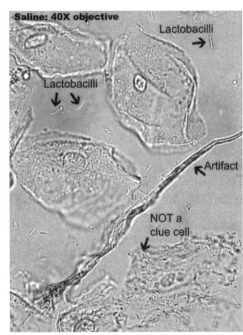

A No bacterial vaginosis: presence of normal epithelial cells and *Lactobacillus*.

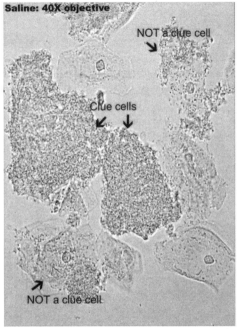

B Bacterial vaginosis: clue cells and absence of *Lactobacillus*.

adjunct test, it is nonspecific and its results may be altered by the presence of blood in the vagina.

While a clinical diagnosis of BV can be reliably made using the Amsel criteria (Amsel et al., 1983; **Box 19-1**), the gold standard for BV diagnosis remains the Gram stain. Although cytology reports may include comments such as "predominance of coccobacilli consistent with shift in vaginal flora," Pap testing is both nonspecific and nonsensitive for diagnosing BV. Furthermore, vaginal cultures are not useful because BV is multibacterial in origin and cultures are nonspecific.

Differential Diagnoses
The differential diagnoses for BV include trichomoniasis, VVC, presence of a foreign body,

chemical vaginitis, contact vaginitis, desquamative inflammatory vaginitis (DIV), atrophic vaginitis, lactational vaginitis, chlamydia, gonorrhea, genital herpes, cervicitis, and normal physiologic discharge (Girerd, 2014).

Management
Table 19-2 outlines treatment guidelines for BV. The Centers for Disease Control and Prevention (CDC) recommends treatment for symptomatic women. Vaginal metronidazole is not recommended for women with a known allergy to oral metronidazole; however, it can be used in women who do not tolerate oral metronidazole (CDC, 2015). Clindamycin cream is preferred in case of allergy or intolerance to metronidazole or tinidazole; however, women

---

BOX **19-1** Criteria for Clinical Diagnosis of Bacterial Vaginosis

Clinical diagnosis of bacterial vaginosis is based on the presence of three out of four of the following Amsel criteria:

- White, thin adherent vaginal discharge
- pH ≥ 4.5
- Positive whiff/KOH test
- Clue cells on microscopic examination (more than 20% of epithelial cells are clue cells)

Reproduced from Amsel, R., Totten, P. A., Spiegel, C. A., Chen, K. C., Eschenbach, D., & Holmes, K. K. (1983). Nonspecific vaginitis: Diagnostic criteria and microbial and epidemiologic associations. *American Journal of Medicine*, *74*(1), 14–22. Reprinted with permission of Elsevier.

---

should be advised that clindamycin may weaken latex condoms or contraceptive diaphragms. Treatment of sexual partners of women who have BV is not recommended because it does not affect the woman's response to treatment or the likelihood of relapse or recurrence. The CDC recommends that all women with BV be tested for HIV and other sexually transmitted infections (STIs).

Table 19-3 lists alternative therapies for BV. Nearly 65% of women have used alternative therapies to treat chronic vaginitis (Nyirjesy et al., 2011). The most commonly used alternative therapies for vaginitis include probiotics, boric acid, douching, tea tree oil, and garlic (Van Kessel, Assefi, Marrazzo, & Eckert, 2003).

Patient Education

The importance of completing the course of medication and avoiding alcohol while taking metronidazole or tinidazole and after completing the treatment (24 hours after treatment with metronidazole, 72 hours after treatment with tinidazole) must be emphasized. Inform women that nitroimidazole antibiotics can cause a metallic taste, nausea, vomiting, and cramps even if they do not consume alcohol. In addition, women should be

counseled to avoid intercourse until treatment is complete and to consistently use condoms. Instruct women to refrain from douching, both in general and during treatment. Many women develop VVC symptoms following treatment with nitroimidazole; therefore, providers often co-prescribe an antifungal, such as fluconazole.

When considering the use of alternative therapies for treatment of BV or vaginitis, inform women that while research in this area is actively under way, including investigations being carried out by the National Institutes of Health National Center for Complementary and Alternative Medicine, few existing studies adequately demonstrate the safety, effectiveness, and long-term outcomes of alternative therapies. Some herbal preparations may lead to adverse interactions when used with prescribed or over-the-counter (OTC) medications. Encourage women considering alternative therapies to consult reliable sources (e.g., healthcare providers, Lexicomp, MedlinePlus Herbs and Supplements, National Center for Complementary and Integrative Health) and to be wary of Internet blogs and unsubstantiated websites.

Special Considerations

Pregnant Women BV is associated with chorioamnionitis, premature rupture of fetal membranes, preterm labor and birth, and postpartum endometritis (CDC, 2015). However, conflicting evidence exists about whether treatment of asymptomatic pregnant women reduces the likelihood of adverse outcomes of pregnancy. Treatment is recommended for pregnant women with BV who have symptoms, and guidelines for treatment can be found in **Table 19-2**. Clindamycin vaginal cream is not recommended in pregnancy because it is associated with low birth weight and neonatal infections in newborns whose mothers were treated with this medication (CDC, 2015).

Recurrent Bacterial Vaginosis As many as 70% of women who have experienced an episode of BV report a recurrence within 3 to 6 months (Johnson, 2014; Sobel, 2015). The CDC has considered the problem of recurrent BV and suggests retreating women with this condition with the original

---

TABLE **19-2** | Bacterial Vaginosis and Vulvovaginal Candidiasis Treatment

---

Vaginitis	Recommended Regimens	Alternative Regimens
BV	Metronidazole 500 mg orally twice a day for 7 days OR Metronidazole gel 0.75%, one full applicator (5 g) intravaginally, daily for 5 days OR Clindamycin cream 2%, one full applicator (5 g) intravaginally, at bedtime for 7 days **Pregnant Women** Metronidazole 500 mg orally twice a day for 7 days OR Metronidazole 250 mg orally three times a day for 7 days OR Clindamycin 300 mg orally twice a day for 7 days	Tinidazole 2 g orally once daily for 2 days OR Tinidazole 1 g orally once daily for 5 days OR Clindamycin 300 mg orally twice a day for 7 days OR Clindamycin ovules 100 g intravaginally once at bedtime for 3 days **Pregnant Women** None
Recurrent BV	Retreat with original therapy	Metronidazole 0.75% intravaginally once weekly for 4–6 months OR Metronidazole 2 g orally and fluconazole 150 mg orally in a single dose once monthly
Uncomplicated VVC	**Over-the-Counter Intravaginal Agents** Clotrimazole 1% cream 5 g intravaginally for 7–14 days OR Clotrimazole 2% cream 5 g intravaginally for 3 days OR Miconazole 2% cream 5 g intravaginally for 7 days OR Miconazole 4% cream 5 g intravaginally for 3 days OR Miconazole 100 mg vaginal suppository, one suppository daily for 7 days OR Miconazole 200 mg vaginal suppository, one suppository daily for 3 days OR Miconazole 1,200 mg vaginal suppository, one suppository for 1 day OR Tioconazole 6.5% ointment 5 g intravaginally in a single application **Prescription Intravaginal Agents** Butoconazole 2% cream (single-dose bioadhesive product), 5 g intravaginally for a single application OR Terconazole 0.4% cream 5 g intravaginally for 7 days OR Terconazole 0.8% cream 5 g intravaginally for 3 days OR Terconazole 80 mg vaginal suppository, one suppository for 3 days **Oral Agent** Fluconazole 150 mg oral tablet, one tablet in single dose **Pregnant Women**[a] Topical azole therapy, applied for 7 days	

(continues)

TABLE 19-2   Bacterial Vaginosis and Vulvovaginal Candidiasis Treatment (*continued*)

Vaginitis	Recommended Regimens	Alternative Regimens
Complicated VVC	**Recurrent VVC Initial Therapy** Longer duration of initial therapy, such as topical azole for 7–14 days OR Fluconazole 150 mg orally every third day for a total of 3 doses (days 1, 4, and 7) OR Itraconazole 200 mg orally twice daily for 3 days **Recurrent VVC Maintenance Therapy** Fluconazole 150 mg orally weekly for 6 months OR Itraconazole 100–200 mg daily for 6 months OR Miconazole 1,200 mg vaginal suppository, one suppository weekly for 6 months OR Intermittent use of topical treatments **Severe VVC** Topical azole for 7–14 days OR Fluconazole 150 mg in 2 sequential doses, second dose 72 hours after initial dose **Non-*albicans* VVC Initial Therapy** Optimal treatment unknown; options include nonfluconazole azole drug (oral or topical) for 7–14 days **Recurrent Non-*albicans* VVC** Boric acid 600 mg in gelatin capsule vaginally once daily for 14 days **HIV Infection** Should not differ from that of seronegative women	

Abbreviations: BV, bacterial vaginosis; HIV, human immunodeficiency virus; VVC, vulvovaginal candidiasis.

[a] Some experts categorize VVC in pregnant women as complicated (American College of Obstetricians & Gynecologists, 2006, reaffirmed 2013; Sobel, 2007).

Data from Centers for Disease Control and Prevention (CDC). (2015). Sexually transmitted diseases treatment guidelines 2015. *Morbidity and Mortality Weekly Report, 64*(3), 1–138; Sobel, J. D. (2016). Recurrent vulvovaginal candidiasis. *American Journal of Obstetrics & Gynecology, 214*(1), 15–21.

TABLE 19-3	Alternative Therapies for Bacterial Vaginosis, Vulvovaginal Candidiasis, or Vulvovaginal Symptoms

Intervention	Dosage	Administration	Use
Gentian violet	Few drops in water, 0.25–2%	Douche or local application	VVC
Vinegar (white)	1 teaspoon per quart of water 1–2 tablespoons per quart of water	Douche every 5–7 days or twice a day for 2 days Douche 1–2 times/week	VVC or BV
Acidophilus culture	2 tablespoons per pint of water	Douche twice a day	VVC
Vitamin C	500 mg 2–4 times daily	Orally	VVC
Acidophilus tablet	40 million–1 billion units (1 tab) daily	Orally	VVC
Yogurt	1 application to labia or in vagina	Hourly as needed	VVC
Goldenseal	1 teaspoon in 3 cups warm water, strain and cool	Douche	BV (not safe for use in pregnancy)
Garlic clove	1 peeled clove wrapped in cloth dipped in olive oil	Overnight in vagina, change daily	BV
Boric acid powder	600 mg in gelatin capsule	Every day in vagina for 14 days (toxic if ingested orally)	BV
Sassafras bark	Steep in warm water Compress	Wash affected area	VVC
Cold milk, cottage cheese, yogurt	Compress or insert in vagina	Apply to affected area	Pruritus
Calendula	Steep in boiling water than cool	Douche	Vulvovaginal inflammation
Tea tree oil	Soaked tampon or 1 suppository	Douche or 1 suppository daily	Vulvovaginal inflammation

Abbreviations: BV, bacterial vaginosis; VVC, vulvovaginal candidiasis.
Data from The Gale Group, Inc. (2016). Vaginitis. Retrieved from http://www.altmd.com/Articles/Vaginitis--Encyclopedia-of -Alternative-Medicine; University of Maryland Medical Center. (2012). Vaginitis. Retrieved from http://umm.edu/health/medical /altmed/condition/vaginitis; Van Kessel, K., Assefi, N., Marrazzo, J., & Eckert, L. (2003). Common complementary and alternative therapies for yeast vaginitis and bacterial vaginosis: A systematic review. *Obstetrical & Gynecological Survey, 58*(5), 351–358.

therapy, using metronidazole gel intravaginally weekly for 4 to 6 months, or monthly oral metronidazole with fluconazole (see **Table 19-2**). No studies have found a regimen effective enough to be recommended for treatment of recurrent BV. Indeed, recurrent BV remains a clinical enigma and a source of distress among affected women. Studies showing direct evidence of etiology, treatments demonstrating better cure rates, and prevention of recurrence are needed (Marazzo et al., 2010).

Vulvovaginal Candidiasis

Worldwide, vulvovaginal candidiasis (VVC) is one of the most common infections of the lower genital tract in women; however, information on its exact incidence is incomplete because it is not a reportable condition. Furthermore, accurate collection of data on VVC is impeded by the imprecise diagnostic methods and the availability of OTC treatments. As many as 75% of women will have VVC at least once during their lifetime (Sobel, 2007).

The most common cause of VVC is infection with *Candida albicans*. Indeed, 90% or more of VVC episodes in women are believed to be caused by this organism. However, VVC can also be caused by non-*albicans* species such as *Candida glabrata*, *Candida tropicalis*, *Candida parapsilosis*, and *Candida krusei*. These non-*albicans* species may be more resistant to commonly used azole antifungal therapies, whether OTC or prescribed products (American College of Obstetricians and Gynecologists, 2006, reaffirmed 2013). New research is shifting the understanding of the pathogenesis of VVC toward a more complex set of circumstances working synchronously to facilitate infection. These etiologic factors involve host immune function, availability of estrogen, virulence of the specific organism, and an increase in vaginal pH as reflected by diminished levels of lactobacilli (Peters, Yano, Noverr, & Fidel, 2014). Numerous factors have been identified as predisposing a woman to development of VVC (**Box 19-2**). Clinical observations and research have also suggested that wearing tight-fitting clothing and underwear or pantyhose made of nonabsorbent materials creates an environment in which *Candida* can grow.

VVC is classified as either uncomplicated or complicated according to four features: clinical

---

BOX **19-2** **Risk Factors for Vulvovaginal Candidiasis**

- Repeated courses of systemic or topical antibiotic therapy, particularly broad-spectrum antibiotics
- Diabetes, especially when uncontrolled
- Pregnancy
- Obesity
- Consumption of a diet high in refined sugars or artificial sweeteners
- Use of corticosteroids and exogenous hormones
- Immunosuppressed states, including HIV seropositivity
- Local allergic or hypersensitivity reactions
- Postmenopausal hormone therapy, especially vaginal topical use

---

presentation, microbiology, host factors, and response to therapy (CDC, 2015). Most (80–90%) women who have VVC will have uncomplicated disease. Those with complicated VVC will need special diagnostic testing and treatment regimens (**Table 19-4**).

Candida albicans is a normal inhabitant of the vagina and the most common cause of VVC (see **Color Plate 16**). The most common symptom of VVC is vulvar and possibly vaginal pruritus (**Table 19-1**). This itching may be mild or intense, interfere with rest and activities, and occur during or after intercourse. Some women report a feeling of dryness. Others may experience painful urination as the urine flows over the vulva; this symptom usually occurs in women who have excoriation resulting from scratching. Most often the discharge is thick, white, and lumpy with the consistency of cottage cheese. Often the discharge is found in patches on the vaginal walls, cervix, and labia. The vulva is commonly red and swollen, as are the labial folds, vagina, and cervix. Although no characteristic odor is associated with VVC, sometimes a yeasty or musty smell occurs.

TABLE 19-4	Classification of Vulvovaginal Candidiasis

Uncomplicated VVC	Complicated VVC	RVVC
Sporadic or infrequent VVC AND Mild to moderate VVC AND Likely to be *C. albicans* AND Immunocompetent women	RVVC OR Severe VVC OR Non-*albicans* candidiasis OR Women with diabetes, immunocompromising conditions (e.g., HIV infection), debilitation, or immunosuppressive therapy	4 or more episodes of symptomatic VVC in 1 year Pathogenesis of RVVC is poorly understood, and most women with RVVC have no apparent predisposing or underlying conditions Obtain vaginal cultures to confirm the clinical diagnosis and identify unusual species

Abbreviations: RVVC, recurrent vulvovaginal candidiasis; VVC, vulvovaginal candidiasis.
Data from Centers for Disease Control and Prevention (CDC). (2015). Sexually transmitted diseases treatment guidelines 2015. *Morbidity and Mortality Weekly Report, 64*(3), 1–138.

Assessment

In addition to obtaining a thorough history of the woman's symptoms (their onset and course), it is valuable to identify predisposing risk factors. The physical examination includes a thorough inspection of the vulva and vagina. A speculum examination and microscopic examination of vaginal secretions with saline and KOH are performed. The characteristic pseudohyphae may be seen on a wet smear done with normal saline, although these organisms may sometimes be confused with other cells and artifacts. Pseudohyphae are best seen on the KOH wet smear (**Figure 19-2**). Vaginal pH can be tested and is normal with VVC (3.5–4.5). If the pH is greater than 4.5, the clinician should suspect coinfection with trichomoniasis or BV. In recurrent or resistant cases, vaginal cultures for *Candida* can confirm the diagnosis, identify less common species, and redirect treatment when candidiasis is suspected but the KOH prep is negative (CDC, 2015).

Given the wide availability of OTC therapies, many symptomatic women presume their symptoms are VVC related and choose to self-treat rather than see a healthcare provider. When self-treatment is ineffective and women seek professional advice, accurate identification of the offending organism(s) is sometimes obscured by intravaginal OTC preparations.

Differential Diagnoses

The differential diagnoses for VVC include BV, trichomoniasis, chemical vaginitis, contact vaginitis, chlamydia, gonorrhea, genital herpes, atrophic vaginitis, desquamative inflammatory vaginitis, and normal physiologic discharge. Clinicians should also consider candidiasis secondary to diabetes, pregnancy, HIV seropositivity, and infection with non-*albicans* species such as *Candida glabrata* or *Candida tropicalis.*

Management

A number of antifungal preparations are available for the treatment of VVC (**Table 19-2**), and no single brand is significantly more effective than another. Vaginal creams and suppositories recommended for treatment of this condition are oil based, so they may weaken latex condoms and diaphragms. Many effective topical azole drugs are available as OTC products; they have cure rates ranging from 80% to 90% (Sobel, 2007). Only women who have been previously diagnosed with

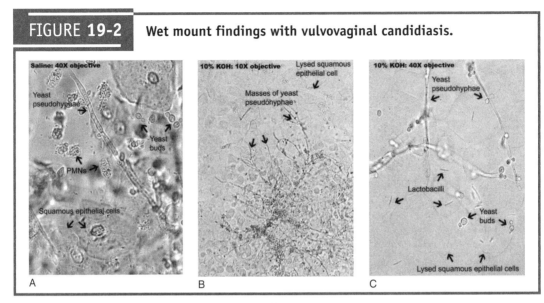

FIGURE **19-2**   **Wet mount findings with vulvovaginal candidiasis.**

Abbreviation: PMNs, polymorphonuclear leukocytes/white blood cells.
Used with permission from Washington State Department of Health STD/TB Program, Seattle STD/HIV Prevention Training Center, and Cindy Fennell, MS, MT, ASCP.

VVC and who are experiencing the same symptoms should attempt self-treatment with OTC medications. Any woman whose symptoms persist or who develops a recurrence of symptoms within 2 months of treatment should be evaluated by a clinician (CDC, 2015). Unnecessary or inappropriate use of OTC preparations is common and can lead to delays in treating other causes of vulvovaginitis.

If vaginal discharge is extremely thick and copious, vaginal debridement with a cotton swab followed by application of vaginal medication may be useful. Alternative therapies for VVC can be found in **Table 19-3**. Women who have extensive irritation, swelling, and discomfort of the labia and vulva may find sitz baths helpful in decreasing inflammation and discomfort. Adding colloidal oatmeal to the bath may also decrease vulvar itching and inflammation.

Diabetes screening should be considered for women with recurrent infections and comorbidities such as obesity or family history of diabetes. Testing for chlamydia, gonorrhea, and HIV is recommended if the history indicates the presence of risk factors for STIs. For more information, see Chapter 20.

Patient Education
Bathing daily with lots of water and minimal, unscented soap may help prevent recurrent infections. Additional health measures include not wearing underpants to bed, wearing loose-fitting slacks and jeans, wearing cotton-crotched underwear or pantyhose, and not sitting in wet bathing suits or clothing for long periods. Completing the full course of treatment prescribed is essential; instruct women to continue applying the medication even during menstruation. Advise against tampon use during treatment, as tampons will absorb the vaginal medication. If possible, avoid intercourse during treatment. If this is not feasible, use of a nonlatex condom during intercourse may decrease introduction of more organisms. Counsel women to avoid feminine hygiene sprays, deodorants, scented tampons or pads, perfumed or colored toilet paper, and fabric softeners—all of which may cause irritation and allergies. Ingesting vitamin C (500 mg two to four times per day), oral acidophilus (40 million to 1 billion units daily), or plain yogurt containing live cultures (several times a week) may be helpful in preventing recurrences. Decreasing use of unnecessary antibiotics and reducing

intake of refined sugars in the diet may diminish *Candida* colonization. Advise women that no randomized controlled trials have been published that have evaluated these common interventions. Other studies continue to explore host genetic and microbiome factors, probiotic therapy, anti-*Candida* defense mechanisms, and genetic yeast factors that facilitate persistence of VVC (Sobel, 2007, 2016).

Special Considerations

Pregnant and Breastfeeding Women VVC frequently occurs during pregnancy. In 2006, the CDC categorized VVC during pregnancy as complicated; however, pregnancy was not specified in this classification in the 2010 and 2015 updates. The American Congress of Obstetricians and Gynecologists (2006, reaffirmed 2013) and Sobel (2007) consider VVC in pregnancy to be complicated.

Pregnant women who suspect they have VVC should be counseled not to self-treat their symptoms, but instead to contact their healthcare provider. Currently, topical azoles are the only forms of treatment for VVC recommended for use by pregnant women (CDC, 2015). Oral medication for VVC (fluconazole) is not recommended in pregnancy. Fluconazole is an FDA Pregnancy Category C drug due to teratogenicity found in animal studies when high doses were used. A recent study found an increased risk of spontaneous abortion in women who used fluconazole during pregnancy (Mølgaard-Nielsen, Svanström, Melbye, Hviid, & Pasternak, 2016). Fluconazole is found in breastmilk; therefore caution is recommended in breastfeeding women. Boric acid should not be used during pregnancy (Sobel, 2007).

Complicated VVC Complicated VVC cases affect a relatively small number of women and are generally caused by *C. albicans* or *C. glabrata*. These infections respond favorably to the azole medications but may require longer than the 1- to 3-day period of therapy recommended for uncomplicated VVC. The optimal treatment for non-*albicans* VVC is unknown. Boric acid has been shown to be an effective treatment for non-*albicans* species, in the form of a 600-mg suppository or capsule administered per vagina once daily for 14 days (American College of Obstetricians and Gynecologists, 2006, reaffirmed 2013; Pappas et al., 2009). One review of 14 studies, including 2 randomized controlled trials, concluded that use of intravaginal boric acid capsules for recurrent and chronic VVC symptoms is a safe, alternative option when conventional therapies fail and where non-*albicans* or azole-resistant strains have been identified (Iavuzzo, Gkegkes, Zarkada, & Falagas, 2011). The long-term safety of intravaginal boric acid has not been established (Sobel, 2016). An observational study by Powell, Gracely, and Nyirjesy (2015) found most non-*albicans* infections can be effectively cured using either boric acid or fluconazole. At all times, when using intravaginal boric acid, counsel women to keep capsules away from children and pets because oral ingestion of this medication can be fatal.

Atrophic Vaginitis

Atrophic vaginitis (AV) is a symptomatic condition seen frequently among women experiencing decreased estrogen production as a result of perimenopause, postmenopausal status, or lactation. Cancer treatments such as surgical therapy and radiation can damage the vaginal epithelium, lead to vaginal stenosis, induce AV, and increase the risk of other vaginal infections. Pharmacologic therapies used as a component of breast cancer treatment—specifically aromatase inhibitors such as anastrazole, letrozole, and exemestane—produce a symptomatic estrogen-deficiency state. Aromatase inhibitors prevent the conversion of androgens to estrogens, thereby causing vaginal dryness and dyspareunia (North American Menopause Society [NAMS], 2013). Other conditions leading to a reduced estrogen state include surgical menopause (bilateral oophorectomy with or without removal of the uterus), use of medications used to treat endometriosis or uterine fibroids such as gonadotropin-releasing hormone (GnRH) agonists, and hypothalamic amenorrhea caused by excessive physical activity seen in athletes or by eating disorders such as anorexia (NAMS, 2013). In summary, a state of decreased estrogen, attributable to any cause, may result in AV.

Atrophic vaginitis develops as a consequence of vulvovaginal atrophy (VVA); although these terms are often used interchangeably, they are not necessarily the same. Some authors distinguish between an atrophic vagina, resulting from urogenital atrophy, and AV, also resulting from urogenital atrophy but additionally accompanied by inflammation (Edwards & Goldbaum, 2014; NAMS, 2013). In premenopausal and postmenopausal women, VVA and AV may collectively be referred to as genitourinary syndrome of menopause (GSM), which is an encompassing term for the range of vulvar, vaginal, and urinary tract symptoms and physical changes associated with estrogen deficiency (Portman & Gass, 2014).

Untreated VVA is a progressive condition that can significantly interfere with women's quality of life. An estimated 10% to 40% of women have symptoms of AV after menopause, but few will discuss these symptoms with their providers due to embarrassment (Bond & Horton, 2010; NAMS, 2013).

Very little has been published specifically about lactational AV. A case study published in 2003 noted only three articles found in a MEDLINE search dating back to 1966 (Palmer & Likis, 2003); more recent articles on lactational AV were not found in PubMed as of November 2015.

Assessment

A thorough history is key when AV is suspected. Because women often do not report symptoms of AV or VVA, it is important for providers to routinely address these issues with women who are of reproductive age, perimenopausal, or postmenopausal. Symptoms include vulvovaginal itching and burning as well as urinary frequency and pain. Some women experience nocturia and urge incontinence, although these symptoms may not be directly attributable to AV or VVA. A sensation of lack of lubrication and dryness during intercourse, which can be associated with dyspareunia, is commonly reported. Women may have symptoms of AV whether or not they are sexually active.

AV is characterized by scant vaginal secretions, immature epithelial cells, elevated vaginal pH, and an increase in white blood cells. On examination, the vaginal epithelium is pale, with diminished rugae. Petechiae may or may not be seen on the cervix. Vaginal pH is typically greater than 5.0. On microscopy, parabasal cells with large nuclei are seen. When compared with mature epithelial cells, parabasal cells are typically smaller in size, have a rounded appearance, and have denser nuclei (**Figure 19-3**). The nuclear to cytoplasmic ratio is increased; the size of the nuclei is large relative to the amount of cytoplasm in the cells. White blood cells are often increased, while lactobacilli are diminished or absent. Consequently, the atrophic vagina is frequently repopulated with enteric organisms previously kept in check by the healthy, acidic vagina (NAMS, 2013).

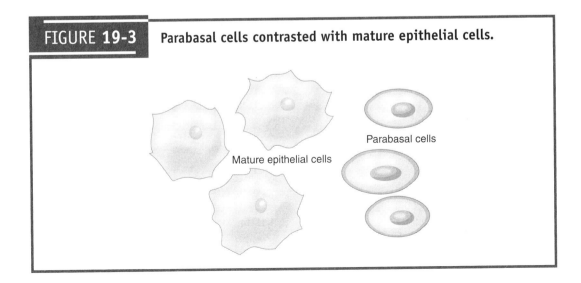

FIGURE **19-3**   **Parabasal cells contrasted with mature epithelial cells.**

Parabasal cells

Mature epithelial cells

The diagnosis of AV is often made based on the woman's history and clinical findings. While there are no specific diagnostic tests for this condition, testing vaginal pH and calculating a vaginal maturation index (VMI) can be helpful. Unfortunately, many laboratories no longer perform VMI testing, which measures relative proportions of parabasal, intermediate, and superficial vaginal epithelium cell types (Mac Bride, Rhodes, & Shuster, 2010). The proportion of superficial cells in women with VVA is less than 5% (Mac Bride et al., 2010).

Differential Diagnoses

The differential diagnoses for AV include BV, VVC, desquamative inflammatory vaginitis, trichomoniasis, presence of a foreign body, chemical vaginitis, contact vaginitis, lactational vaginitis, chlamydia, gonorrhea, genital herpes, cervicitis, and normal physiologic discharge (Girerd, 2014). Vulvovaginal dermatoses may be considered as differential diagnoses; these include lichen sclerosis, lichen planus, and lichen simplex chronicus. Symptoms similar to AV may also arise in conjunction with cancer, precancerous lesions, or extramammary Paget disease. If the diagnosis is unclear or therapy has been ineffective, consider vaginal or vulvar biopsy (Mac Bride et al., 2010).

Management

The treatment for AV will depend on the woman's preference, severity of symptoms, effectiveness, and safety of treatments (NAMS, 2013). Nonprescriptive therapies include regular use of lubricants and moisturizing agents to decrease symptoms and discomfort, especially in women who do not desire to, or are unable to, use estrogen therapy. These agents may be water, silicone, or oil based. A combination of a vaginal preparation of vitamin E and phytoestrogen has been shown to improve symptoms in some women (Morali et al., 2006). In the Herbal Alternatives for Menopause (HALT) study—a randomized placebo-controlled, double-blind trial of 351 women using herbal products to treat VVA—the authors concluded there were no improvements in symptoms as measured by VMI (Reed et al., 2008).

In general, OTC products, such as moisturizers and lubricants, have few clinical trials supporting their efficacy, though at least one study found they reduce or eliminate symptoms for many women (Bygdeman & Swahn, 1996). Another study examining the safety of OTC lubricants and moisturizers found several to have hyperosmolar properties, which could be damaging to vaginal tissues (Dezzutti et al., 2012). In summary, adequate well-controlled trials of complementary and alternative methods for treating AV are lacking.

Low-dose vaginal estrogen therapy can replace the loss of estrogen in women with AV and is administered either locally (vaginal), orally, or transdermally. Estrogen therapy promotes revascularization of the vaginal epithelium and restores the normal pH of the vagina. Vaginal preparations include creams, suppositories, and ring. Prescription vaginal estrogens are available as either estradiol or conjugated estrogen formulations. While systemic or transdermal methods can be used, vaginal application is the preferred mode of delivery and is generally more effective than other routes when vaginal symptoms are the primary concern (NAMS, 2013). Systemic therapy (e.g., patch, pill) is helpful when women also report vasomotor symptoms; however, 10% to 20% of women describe continued symptoms of VVA when using systemic preparations, often leading to an additional prescription for a local therapy (Mac Bride et al., 2010). Nonoral routes are also more advantageous than oral routes because local therapy avoids the first-pass effect through the liver, helps to maintain steadier blood levels, and decreases gastrointestinal side effects. Low-dose vaginal therapy has a less severe risk profile than oral therapy because serum levels are lower, yet results are effective. Most investigations show that the risk of endometrial cancer in women using low-dose vaginal estrogen is low, but long-term studies in this area are lacking. See Chapter 12 for more detailed information about prescribing estrogen therapy including formulations, dosages, and contraindications.

A study of 21 postmenopausal women with breast cancer on aromatase inhibitors found that a 4-week course of vaginal testosterone improved symptoms, vaginal pH, and maturation of vaginal epithelial cells without increasing serum estradiol or testosterone levels (Witherby et al., 2011). Currently, there are no FDA-approved uses for testosterone in women, and additional studies are needed to examine its safety and efficacy for topical use.

Tamoxifen, a selective estrogen receptor modulator (SERM), demonstrates an estrogenic effect on the uterus. Its use has been associated with endometrial hyperplasia and increased vaginal discharge (Conzen, 2013).

Ospemifene is a SERM with specific vaginal effects, which is approved by the FDA for treatment of moderate to severe dyspareunia. This agent has been shown to improve vaginal maturation, vaginal pH, and most symptoms associated with dyspareunia caused by vaginal dryness. In a multicenter study of 605 women, ages 40 to 80, with self-reported dyspareunia and a diagnosis of VVA, participants were randomized to ospemifene or placebo for 12 weeks. The researchers found that treatment with ospemifene was highly effective compared with placebo, and no serious adverse events were reported (Portman, Bachmann, Simon, & Ospemifene Study Group, 2013). The recommended dose of ospemifene is 60 mg orally daily.

Patient Education

Healthcare providers can discuss preserving and protecting women's sexual health and the availability of treatment for AV and VVA, which can occur not only in response to the menopause transition, but also in conjunction with other circumstances leading to an estrogen-deficient state. Regular, safe, sexual activity can help maintain vaginal health and delay atrophic symptoms. For symptomatic, sexually abstinent women, information on use of dilators, vibrators, and lubricants can minimize symptoms. Currently, there are few, if any, data on the prevention of AV or VVA, and the value of educating women proactively that symptoms may occur in response to a low-estrogen state has not been determined. Theoretically, it may be possible that regular use of low-dose vaginal estrogen may avert symptoms associated with AV and VVA; however, current studies focus on treatment rather than prevention (NAMS, 2013).

Desquamative Inflammatory Vaginitis

Desquamative inflammatory vaginitis (DIV) is an uncommon syndrome characterized by a profuse, noninfectious, vaginal discharge, accompanied by vaginal irritation, burning, and dyspareunia. DIV is found in both premenopausal and postmenopausal women. In this condition, the predominant lactobacilli flora of the vagina is replaced with gram-positive coccobacilli, usually group B *Streptococcus*. Often the diagnosis of DIV occurs only after more common conditions have been ruled out.

Assessment

Women with DIV may present with burning, dyspareunia, and yellow discharge with a green tinge. Vaginal examination often reveals a profuse, purulent-appearing discharge with or without vaginal and vestibular erythema. An amine test will be negative, and a pH test will be elevated toward the basic end of the scale (> 5). Microscopic examination of vaginal secretions shows large numbers of polymorphonuclear cells and parabasal cells. DIV can appear very similar to trichomoniasis; however, no motile trichomonads will be seen and cultures for *Candida*, trichomoniasis, chlamydia, and gonorrhea will be negative (American College of Obstetricians and Gynecologists, 2006, reaffirmed 2013).

Differential Diagnoses

The differential diagnoses for DIV include BV, VVC, trichomoniasis, presence of a foreign body, chemical vaginitis, contact vaginitis, atrophic vaginitis, lactational vaginitis, chlamydia, gonorrhea, genital herpes, cervicitis, and normal physiologic discharge (Girerd, 2014).

Management

Clindamycin cream 2% is used intravaginally for both its anti-inflammatory and antimicrobial activities for 2 to 4 weeks; women are then reevaluated. Sobel (2011) reported results of a study examining 98 women diagnosed with DIV who used 2% clindamycin suppositories (54%) or 10% hydrocortisone cream (46%). Improvement was reported in 86% of women by 3 weeks. However, relapse is common, lending support to the perception of DIV as a chronic inflammatory process. If women are concurrently diagnosed with vaginal estrogen deficiency, local estrogen therapy may aid in maintaining remission (Sobel, 2011). The most noticeable difference between DIV and AV is that DIV does not respond to estrogen therapy alone. Prescribers may consider the addition of weekly oral fluconazole in conjunction with intravaginal azole to minimize the occurrence of secondary VVC when women are using intravaginal antimicrobials or corticosteroids as therapies (Edwards, 2010).

TOXIC SHOCK SYNDROME

Toxic shock syndrome (TSS) was first named in 1978 by two pediatricians and their colleagues who described a set of symptoms that included high fever, rash, headache, vomiting, and acute renal failure in young boys and girls ages 8 to 17 between 1975 and 1977 (Todd, Fishaut, Kapral, & Welch, 1978). *Staphylococcus aureus* was identified as the primary pathogenic agent, with *Streptococcal pyogenes* subsequently, but less frequently, implicated (Smit, Nyquist, & Todd, 2013). *S. aureus* is a common bacteria that is responsible for several diseases and conditions, including skin boils, acne, and some severe forms of food poisoning. Approximately 20% of the adult population carries *S. aureus* on the skin and in mucous membranes such as the nose and the vagina (Vostral, 2011). Some strains of *S. aureus* and *S. pyogenes* produce powerful toxins that result in massive immune cell activation and cytokine release, leading to shock and organ failure (McDermott & Sheridan, 2015).

In 1980, it became apparent that young menstruating women using highly absorbent tampons were at high risk for this type of infection. Subsequently, the incidence of TSS declined from a high of 13.7 cases per 100,000 persons in 1980 to between 1 and 0.3 case per 100,000 persons in 1986 (DeVries et al., 2011). This decline in incidence directly followed public health messages regarding safe tampon use in conjunction with removal from the market of a highly absorbent tampon brand that contributed to risk. While TSS incidence is monitored by the National Notifiable Diseases Surveillance System, an arm of the CDC, there has not been population-based active surveillance of this disease since 1986 (DeVries et al., 2011).

There is no definitive test to diagnose TSS. Symptoms include fever, rash, hypotension, myalgia, and vomiting (CDC, 2015) (**Table 19-5**).

Assessment

In addition to a careful history of the woman's symptoms, their onset, and the course of the infection, the history is a valuable screening tool for identifying predisposing risk factors such as menses with tampon use (usually within 5 days of onset of symptoms), history of TSS, and history of recent surgery or wound. Upon physical examination, dermatologic findings may differ depending on the stage of the illness. Early signs may include generalized erythematous and macular rash; generalized, nonpitting edema; and erythema of the palms and soles. After the acute phase, findings may include generalized maculopapular rash and desquamation of the fingers, palms, toes, and soles. Pelvic examination may reveal hyperemic vaginal mucosa and vulvar and vaginal tenderness (CDC, 2015). The diagnosis of TSS is made on the basis of clinical manifestations meeting the 2011 CDC case definition (**Table 19-5**).

Differential Diagnoses

Numerous conditions can cause fever and/or rash. TSS should be considered in any woman with unexplained fever and a rash during or immediately following menses or use of intravaginal menstrual products (McDermott & Sheridan, 2015).

Management

Toxic shock syndrome can constitute an acute, life-threatening emergency. Women with a suspected case of TSS need emergency evaluation and medical care. Although TSS is rare, all women and others at risk for TSS should be educated about the signs and symptoms of this condition and steps to prevent its occurrence, such as using low-absorbency tampons, changing tampons frequently, alternating pad and tampon use, avoiding overnight use of tampons, and removing barrier contraception within 24 hours. Host factors also play a role in susceptibility to TSS. Instruct women who have had TSS not to use barrier contraceptive methods or tampons.

BARTHOLIN GLAND DUCT CYSTS AND ABSCESSES

The Bartholin glands are two mucus-secreting, nonpalpable glandular structures with duct openings within the posterolateral vulvar vestibule that provide minimal lubrication. Obstruction of the

TABLE 19-5	Centers for Disease Control and Prevention's 2011 Case Definition for Toxic Shock Syndrome

Clinical Criteria	An illness with the following clinical manifestations:
	• Fever: temperature greater than or equal to 102.0°F (greater than or equal to 38.9°C)
	• Rash: diffuse macular erythroderma
	• Desquamation: 1–2 weeks after onset of rash
	• Hypotension: systolic blood pressure less than or equal to 90 mm Hg for adults or less than the fifth percentile by age for children younger than 16 years
	• Multisystem involvement (three or more of the following organ systems):
	  • Gastrointestinal: vomiting or diarrhea at onset of illness
	  • Muscular: severe myalgia or creatine phosphokinase level at least twice the upper limit of normal
	  • Mucous membranes: vaginal, oropharyngeal, or conjunctival hyperemia
	  • Renal: blood urea nitrogen or creatinine at least twice the upper limit of normal for laboratory or urinary sediment with pyuria (greater than or equal to 5 leukocytes per high-power field) in the absence of urinary tract infection
	  • Hepatic: total bilirubin, alanine aminotransferase enzyme, or aspartate aminotransferase enzyme levels at least twice the upper limit of normal for laboratory
	  • Hematologic: platelets less than 100,000/mm^3
	  • Central nervous system: disorientation or alterations in consciousness without focal neurologic signs when fever and hypotension are absent

Laboratory Criteria for Diagnosis	Negative results on the following tests, if obtained: • Blood or cerebrospinal fluid cultures (blood culture may be positive for *Staphylococcus aureus*) • Negative serologies for Rocky Mountain spotted fever, leptospirosis, or measles
Case Classification	• Probable: a case that meets the laboratory criteria and in which four of the five clinical criteria described above are present • Confirmed: a case that meets the laboratory criteria and in which all five of the clinical criteria described above are present, including desquamation, unless the patient dies before desquamation occurs

narrow ducts results in a nontender mass approximately 1 to 8 cm in size. Obstruction may occur as a result of either nonspecific inflammation or trauma. Continued fluid secretion after obstruction results in cyst formation (Kessous et al., 2013). Abscess formation occurs when the cystic fluid becomes infected.

Studies from the 1960s and 1970s identified *Neisseria gonorrhea* and other sexually transmitted pathogens in Bartholin gland abscess development; however, the more recent literature reports that most cases are not caused by sexually transmitted organisms, but rather by opportunistic bacteria (Mattila, Miettinen, & Heinonen, 1994). Positive cultures for Bartholin gland abscesses typically contain multiple bacteria, many of which are normal vaginal flora (Kessous et al., 2013). Between 2006 and 2011, Kessous et al. found *Escherichia coli* to be the most common pathogen among women with Bartholin gland abscesses.

Approximately 2% of all reproductive-age women will develop a Bartholin gland cyst (Quinn & Schraga, 2014). Most women with such a cyst are asymptomatic. An abscess usually develops rapidly over 2 to 4 days, and most will spontaneously rupture within 3 to 4 days. Symptoms include varying amounts of pain or tenderness, difficulty sitting or walking, and dyspareunia. Extensive inflammation may cause systemic symptoms.

Assessment

A Bartholin gland cyst may be an incidental finding during a routine pelvic examination (see **Color Plate 17**). The cyst appears as a visible round or oval mass causing a crescent-shaped vestibular entrance. It is nontender but tense, and palpable swelling—usually unilateral and without erythema or inflammation—is apparent.

A Bartholin gland abscess is a very tender, edematous fluctuant mass with erythema of the overlying skin (see **Color Plate 18**). Labial edema and distortion are observed on the affected area. The affected area is rarely larger than 5 cm in size. An area of softening or pointing suggests an impending rupture. Routine culture of draining fluid is not recommended, as the results are rarely useful in treatment (Quinn & Schraga, 2014).

Differential Diagnoses

Differential diagnoses include Skene duct cyst, Bartholin gland malignancy, vulvar malignancy, endometriosis, Gartner duct cyst, hematoma, hidradenoma, abscess, neoplasm, STI, mesonephric cyst of the vagina, and epithelial inclusion cyst (Quinn & Schraga, 2014).

Management

Small asymptomatic cysts do not require treatment. In contrast, treatment is indicated for a symptomatic cyst or abscess. The aim of abscess treatment is to permit drainage of cyst contents and prevent reaccumulation of fluid. One option is incision and drainage (I&D), irrigation, and packing; these procedures are often performed in an office setting. However, I&D with packing is associated with a higher rate of recurrence (Quinn & Schraga, 2014).

A Word catheter is a device with a balloon tip that allows drainage and fistula formation to occur. It can be placed in the office setting following a small incision using a local anesthetic. Use of a Word catheter is generally considered tolerable by patients.

Marsupialization is a surgical procedure consisting of a wide excision of the mass and is reserved for recurrent abscesses. A gynecologist or urologist performs marsupialization in the operating room.

Other newer techniques under investigation for treatment of Bartholin gland abscesses include carbon dioxide laser therapy, alcohol sclerotherapy, and silver nitrate gland ablation (Quinn & Schraga, 2014).

Referral is indicated for marsupialization, recurrent cyst or abscess formation, any solid mass, and cyst or abscess in women older than 40 years of age to rule out neoplasm.

Patient Education

Other than routine bathing and hygienic practices, avoidance of STIs, and seeking prompt evaluation for pain, there are no special steps that women need to take to avoid Bartholin gland cysts.

GENITAL PIERCING

The practice of genital piercing, especially among young adults and adolescents, has increased substantially in recent years. In many early studies, individuals with various forms of body art were presumed to be involved with questionable or criminal behaviors, perhaps contributing to a sense of disapproval of these persons among healthcare professionals (Schmidt & Armstrong, 2014). Today, various forms of body art and piercing have become mainstream for a variety of reasons. Among individuals ages 15 to 25 years, estimates of body piercing rates range from 25% to 35%, excluding earlobe piercing in males and females (Kohut, Parker, Keeter, Doherty, & Dimock, 2007). While generally safe when practiced by authorized, licensed practitioners, genital piercing in women is associated with potentially serious health risks about which women and their healthcare providers should be informed. Body piercing services are most often regulated by state regulations or local ordinances, and there are no national guidelines (Holbrook, Minocha, & Lauman, 2012). Unless a body piercing practitioner is also a licensed healthcare professional, local anesthesia is not used for procedures (Schmidt & Armstrong, 2014).

Assessment

The most common complications associated with genital piercing are allergic reactions, compromise of barrier contraceptive methods, infection, and keloid formation (Meltzer, 2005). Women with any increased vulnerability to infection (e.g., diabetes, HIV, use of steroid medications, anticoagulants) may be more likely to experience infection after a piercing procedure (Meltzer, 2005). Genital piercings may require 2 to 6 weeks for adequate

healing. The locations of body piercings and condition of the surrounding tissues can be documented in the woman's health record in the event that injury or infection develops later (Schmidt & Armstrong, 2014).

Management

Millner et al. (2005) do not recommend routinely counseling against genital piercing. Pregnant women with existing piercings on any body part are recommended to remove them (Holbrook et al., 2012). Women considering pregnancy within a year are recommended to defer genital piercing, as piercing tracts may lead to infection and blood-borne diseases, such as hepatitis, or cause fetal effects as a consequence of medications used to treat infection (Holbrook et al., 2012).

Patient Education

It is important to avoid projecting judgmental or dismissive attitudes when counseling women considering genital piercing. This is especially true when educating adolescents, so as to avoid missing teachable moments for providing accurate health information about the process and its potential health risks (Schmidt & Armstrong, 2014). Barrier methods of contraception—specifically condoms and diaphragms—are more likely to tear during sexual activity when genital piercings are present (Meltzer, 2005). Women considering genital piercing are advised to select authorized, licensed practitioners in established business settings and thoroughly understand the risks of infection, allergic responses, poor healing, scarring, and possible disfigurement. The importance of informed decision making should be reviewed. Adolescents younger than age 18 considering body piercing may need parental permission.

References

American College of Obstetricians and Gynecologists. (2006, reaffirmed 2013). ACOG Clinical Practice Bulletin, No. 72: Vaginitis. *Obstetrics & Gynecology*, 107(5), 1195.

Amsel, R., Totten, P. A., Spiegel, C. A., Chen, K. C., Eschenbach, D., & Holmes, K. K. (1983). Nonspecific vaginitis: Diagnostic criteria and microbial and epidemiologic associations. *American Journal of Medicine*, 74(1), 14–22.

Bond, S. M., & Horton, L. S. (2010). Management of postmenopausal vaginal symptoms in women. *Journal of Gerontological Nursing*, 36(7), 3–7.

Bygdeman, M., & Swahn, M. L. (1996). Replens versus dienoestrol cream in the symptomatic treatment of vaginal atrophy in postmenopausal women. *Maturitas, 23*, 259–263.

Centers for Disease Control and Prevention (CDC). (n.d.). Toxic shock syndrome (other than Streptococcal) (TSS). 2011. case definition. Retrieved from https://wwwn.cdc.gov/nndss/conditions/toxic-shock-syndrome-other-than-streptococcal/case-definition/2011

Centers for Disease Control and Prevention (CDC). (2015). Sexually transmitted diseases treatment guidelines 2015. *Morbidity and Mortality Weekly Report, 64*(3), 1–138.

Conzen, S. (2013, November 26). Managing the side effects of tamoxifen. *Up To Date.* Retrieved from http://www.uptodate.com/contents/managing-the-side-effects-of-tamoxifen

DeVries, A. S., Lesher, L., Schlievert, P. M., Rogers, T., Villaume, L. G., Danila, R., & Lynfield, R. (2011). Staphylococcal toxic shock syndrome 2000–2006: Epidemiology, clinical features, and molecular characteristics. *PLoS ONE, 6*(8), e22997. doi:10.1371/journal.pone.0022997

Dezzutti, C. S., Brown, E. R., Moncla, B., Russo, J., Cost, M., Wang, L., . . . Rohan, L. C. (2012). Is wetter better? An evaluation of over-the-counter personal lubricants for safety and anti-HIV-1 activity. *PLoS ONE, 7*(11), e48328. doi:10.1371/journal.pone.0048328

Eckert, L. O. (2006). Acute vulvovaginitis. *New England Journal of Medicine, 355*(12), 1244–1252.

Edwards, L. (2010). Dermatologic causes of vaginitis: A clinical review. *Dermatologic Clinics, 28,* 727–735.

Edwards, L., & Goldbaum, B. E. (2014). Chronic vulvar irritation, itching, and pain: What is the diagnosis? *OBG Management, 26*(6), 30–37.

Fethers, K. A., Fairley, C. K., Hocking, J. S., Gurrin, L. C., & Bradshaw, C. S. (2008). Sexual risk factors and bacterial vaginosis: A systematic review and meta-analysis. *Clinical Infectious Diseases, 47,* 1426–1435.

Fettweis, J. M., Brooks, J. P., Serrano, M. G., Sheth, N. U., Girerd, P. H., Edwards, D. J., . . . Buck, G. A. (2014). Differences in vaginal microbiome in African American women versus women of European ancestry. *Microbiology, 160,* 2272–2282.

Girerd, P. H. (2014, March 27). Bacterial vaginosis differential diagnoses. Retrieved from http://emedicine.medscape.com/article/254342-differential

Hensel, K. J., Randis, T. M., Gelber, S. E., & Ratner, A. J. (2011). Pregnancy-specific association of vitamin D deficiency and bacterial vaginosis. *American Journal of Obstetrics & Gynecology, 204,* 41.e1–41.e9.

Holbrook, J., Minocha, J., & Lauman, A. (2012). Body piercing: Complications and prevention of health risks. *American Journal of Clinical Dermatology, 13*(1), 1–17.

Iavuzzo, C., Gkegkes, I. D., Zarkada, I. M., & Falagas, M.E. (2011). Boric acid for recurrent vulvovaginal candidiasis: The clinical evidence. *Journal of Women's Health, 20*(8), 1245–1255.

Johnson, M. (2014, December 25). Metronidazole: An overview. Retrieved from http://www.uptodate.com/contents/metronidazole-an-overview

Kessous, R., Aricha-Tamir, B., Sheizaf, B., Steiner, N., Moran-Gilad, J., & Weintraub, A. Y. (2013). Clinical and microbiological characteristics of Bartholin gland abscesses. *Obstetrics & Gynecology, 122*(4), 794–799.

Kohut, A., Parker, K., Keeter, S., Doherty, C., & Dimock, M. (2007, January 9). How young people view their lives, futures, and politics: A portrait of "generation next." Washington, DC: Pew Research Center. Retrieved from http://www.people-press.org/files/legacy-pdf/300.pdf

Koumans, E. H., Sternberg, M., Bruce, C., McQuillan, G., Kendrick, J., Sutton, M., & Markowitz, L E. (2007). The prevalence of bacterial vaginosis in the United States, 2001–2004: Associations with symptoms, sexual behaviors, and reproductive health. *Sexually Transmitted Diseases, 34*(11), 864–869.

Lazenby, G. B., Soper, D. E., & Nolte, F. S. (2013). Correlation of leukorrhea and *Trichomonas vaginalis* infection. *Journal of Clinical Microbiology, 51*(7), 2323–2327.

Ma, B., Forney, L. J., & Ravel, J. (2012). Vaginal microbiome: Rethinking health and disease. *Annual Review of Microbiology, 66,* 731–789.

Mac Bride, M. B., Rhodes, D. J., & Shuster, L. T. (2010). Vulvovaginal atrophy. *Mayo Clinic Proceedings, 85*(1), 87–94.

Marrazzo, J. M., Koutsky, L. A., Eschenbach, D. A., Agnew, K., Stine, K., & Hillier, S. L. (2002). Characterization of vaginal flora and bacterial vaginosis in women who have sex with women. *Journal of Infectious Diseases, 185*(9), 1307–1313.

Marrazzo, J. M., Martin, D. H., Watts, D. H., Schulte, J., Sobel, J. D., Hillier, S. L., . . . Fredricks, D. N. (2010). Bacterial vaginosis: Identifying research gaps: Proceedings of a workshop sponsored by DHHS/NIH/NIAD. *Sexually Transmitted Diseases, 37*(12), 732–744.

Mattila, A., Miettinen, A., & Heinonen, P. K. (1994). Microbiology of Bartholin's duct abscess. *Infectious Diseases in Obstetrics and Gynecology, 1,* 265–268.

McDermott, C., & Sheridan, M. (2015). Case report: Staphylococcal toxic shock syndrome caused by tampon use. *Case Reports in Critical Care,* 640373. http://dx.doi.org/10.1155/2015/640373

Meltzer, D. I. (2005). Complications of body piercing. *American Family Physician, 72*(10), 2029–2034.

Millner, V. S., Eichold, B. H., Sharpe, T. H., & Sherwood, S. C. (2005). First glimpse of the functional benefits of clitoral hood piercings. *American Journal of Obstetrics & Gynecology, 193*(3), 675–676.

Mølgaard-Nielsen, D., Svanström, , H., Melbye, M., Hviid, A., & Pasternak, B. (2016). Association between use of oral fluconazole during pregnancy and risk of spontaneous abortion and stillbirth. *Journal of the American Medical Association, 315*(1), 58–67.

Morali, G., Polatti, F., Metelitsa, E. N., Mascarucci, P., Magnani, P., & Marrè, G. B. (2006). Open, non-controlled clinical studies to assess the efficacy and safety of a medical device in form of gel topically and intravaginally used in postmenopausal women with genital atrophy. *Arzneimittelforschung, 56*(3), 230–238.

North American Menopause Society (NAMS). (2013). Symptomatic Vaginal Atrophy Advisory Panel. Management of symptomatic vulvovaginal atrophy: 2013 position statement of the North American Menopause Society. *Menopause, 20*(9), 888–902.

Nyirjesy, P., Robinson, J., Mathew, L., Lev-Sagie, A., Reyes, I., & Culhane, J. F. (2011). Alternative therapies in women with chronic vaginitis. *Obstetrics & Gynecology, 117*(4), 856–861.

Palmer, A. E., & Likis, F. E. (2003). Lactational atrophic vaginitis. *Journal of Midwifery & Women's Health, 48*(4), 282–284.

Pappas, P. G., Kauffman, C. A., Andes, D., Benjamin, D. K., Calandra, T. F., Edwards, J. E., . . . Sobel, J. D. (2009). Clinical practice guidelines for the management of candidiasis: 2009 update by the Infectious Diseases Society of America, *Clinical Infectious Diseases, 48,* 503–535.

Peters, B. M., Yano, J., Noverr, M. C., & Fidel, P. L. (2014). Candida vaginitis: When opportunism knocks, the host responds. *PLoS Pathogens, 10*(4), e1003965.

Portman, D. J., Bachmann, G. A., Simon, J. A., & Ospemifene Study Group. (2013). Ospemifene, a novel selective estrogen receptor modulator for treating dyspareunia associated with postmenopausal vulvar and vaginal atrophy. *Menopause, 20*(6), 623–630.

Portman, D. J., & Gass, M. L. S. (2014). Genitourinary syndrome of menopause: New terminology for vulvovaginal atrophy from the International Society for the Study of Women's Sexual Health and the North American Menopause Society. *Menopause, 21*(10), 1063–1068.

Powell, A. M., Gracely, E., & Nyirjesy, P. (2015). Non-*albicans* candida vulvovaginitis: Treatment experience at a tertiary care vaginitis center. *Journal of Lower Genital Tract Disease, 20,* 85–89. doi:10.1097/LGT.0000000000000126

Quinn, A., & Schraga, E. D. (2014, August 8). Bartholin gland diseases. Retrieved from http://emedicine.medscape.com /article/777112-overview

Reed, S. D., Newton, K. M., LaCroix, A. Z., Grothaus, L. C., Grieco, V. S., & Erlich, K. (2008). Vaginal, endometrial, and reproductive hormone findings: Randomized placebo-controlled trial of black cohosh, multibotanical herbs, and dietary soy for vasomotor symptoms: The Herbal Alternatives for Menopause (HALT) Study. *Menopause, 15,* 51–58.

Schmidt, R. M., & Armstrong, M. L. (2014). Body piercing in adolescents and young adults. *UpToDate.* Retrieved from http://www.uptodate .com/contents/body-piercing-in-adolescents-and-young -adults

Secor, M., & Coughlin, G. (2013). Advances in the diagnosis and treatment of acute and recurrent infections: Bacterial vaginosis update. *Advance for NPs and PAs, 4*(7), 23.

Smit, M. A., Nyquist, A., & Todd, J. K. (2013). Infectious shock and toxic shock syndrome diagnoses in hospitals, Colorado, USA. *Emerging Infectious Diseases, 19*(11), 1855–1858.

Sobel, J. D. (2007). Vulvovaginal candidiasis. *Lancet, 369,* 1961–1971.

Sobel, J. D. (2011). Prognosis and treatment of desquamative inflammatory vaginitis. *Obstetrics & Gynecology, 117*(4), 850–855.

Sobel, J. D. (2015, August 28). Bacterial vaginosis. Retrieved from http://www.uptodate.com/contents/bacterial-vaginosis

Sobel, J. D. (2016). Recurrent vulvovaginal candidiasis. *American Journal of Obstetrics & Gynecology, 214*(1), 15–21.

Srinivasan, S., Hoffman, N. G., Morgan, M. T., Matsen, F. A., Fiedler, T. L., Hall, R. W., . . . Fredericks, D. N. (2012). Bacterial communities in women with bacterial vaginosis: High resolution phylogenetic analyses reveal relationships of microbiota to clinical criteria. *PLoS One, 7*(6), e37818. doi:10.1371/journal. pone.0037818

Steward, R., Melamed, A., Granat, A., & Mishell, D. R. (2012). Comparison of cervical mucus of 24/4 vs. 24/7 combined oral contraceptives. *Contraception, 86,* 710–715.

The Gale Group, Inc. (2016). Vaginitis. Retrieved from http://www .altmd.com/Articles/Vaginitis--Encyclopedia-of-Alternative -Medicine

Todd, J., Fishaut, M., Kapral, F., & Welch, T. (1978). Toxic-shock syndrome associated with phage-group-I staphylococci. *Lancet, 312*(8100), 1116–1118.

University of Maryland Medical Center. (2012). Vaginitis. Retrieved from http://umm.edu/health/medical/altmed/condition/vaginitis

Van Kessel, K., Assefi, N., Marrazzo, J., & Eckert, L. (2003). Common complementary and alternative therapies for yeast vaginitis and bacterial vaginosis: A systematic review. *Obstetrical & Gynecological Survey, 58*(5), 351–358.

Verstraelen, H., & Verhelst, R. (2009). Bacterial vaginosis: An update on diagnosis and treatment. *Expert Review of Anti-infective Therapy, 7*(9), 1109–1124.

Vostral, S. L. (2011). Rely and toxic shock syndrome: A technological health crisis. *Yale Journal of Biology and Medicine, 84,* 447–459.

Witherby, S., Johnson, J., Demers, L., Mount, S., Littenberg, B., Maclean, C. D., . . . Muss, H. (2011). Topical testosterone for breast cancer patients with vaginal atrophy related to aromatase inhibitors: A Phase I/II study. *Oncologist, 16*(4), 424–431.

CHAPTER 20

Sexually Transmitted Infections

Heidi Collins Fantasia

The editors acknowledge Catherine Ingram Fogel, who was the author of the previous edition of this chapter.

INTRODUCTION

Sexually transmitted infections (STIs) are a major public health issue in the United States, with approximately 20 million new STIs occurring every year (Centers for Disease Control and Prevention [CDC], 2014a). As many as 50% of Americans will contract one or more reportable STIs during their lifetime, and as many as 80% will be infected with a nonreportable STI such as genital herpes or the human papillomavirus (HPV) (CDC, 2014a, 2014c, 2015d). STIs are a direct cause of tremendous human suffering, place heavy demands on healthcare services, and cost the U.S. healthcare system as much as $16 billion each year (CDC, 2013a).

The term *sexually transmitted infection* does not refer to any one specific disease, but rather refers to "a variety of clinical syndromes caused by pathogens that can be acquired and transmitted through sexual activity" (CDC, 2015d, p. 1). This term has replaced the older designation of *venereal disease*, which primarily described gonorrhea and syphilis. STIs may be caused by a wide spectrum of bacteria, viruses, protozoa, and ectoparasites (organisms that live on the outside of the body, such as a louse). Historically, many STIs were considered to be symptomatic illnesses usually afflicting men; however, women and children can have more severe symptoms and sequelae from these infections than do men. Common STIs are listed in **Table 20-1**.

Preventing, identifying, and managing STIs are essential components of women's health care.

Clinicians can assume an important role in promoting women's reproductive and sexual health by counseling women about the risks of STIs, including human immunodeficiency virus (HIV); encouraging sexual and other risk-reduction measures; and being familiar with assessment and management strategies related to STIs. Through screening, early detection, treatment, and education, clinicians can assist women in reducing their risk for STIs and in living better lives with the sequelae and chronic infections of STIs.

This chapter begins with an overview of STI transmission, screening, and detection. Topics that need to be addressed when talking with a woman who has been diagnosed with an STI are presented as well. The remaining sections address specific STIs, including HPV, genital herpes, chancroid, pediculosis pubis, trichomoniasis, chlamydia, gonorrhea, pelvic inflammatory disease (PID), syphilis, hepatitis B virus (HBV), hepatitis C virus (HCV), and HIV infection.

TRANSMISSION OF SEXUALLY TRANSMITTED INFECTIONS

The chance of contracting, transmitting, or suffering complications from STIs depends on multiple biologic, behavioral, social, and relationship risk factors (**Box 20-1**). That is, a myriad of microbiologic, hormonal, and immunologic factors influence individual susceptibility and transmission potential

TABLE 20-1	Common Sexually Transmitted Infections

Infection	Causative Organism
Chancroid	*Haemophilus ducreyi*
Chlamydia	*Chlamydia trachomatis*
Genital herpes	Herpes simplex virus
Genital warts	Human papillomavirus (HPV)
Gonorrhea	*Neisseria gonorrhoeae*
Hepatitis	Hepatitis B virus (HBV), hepatitis C virus (HCV)
Human immunodeficiency virus (HIV) infection and acquired immunodeficiency syndrome (AIDS)	Human immunodeficiency virus (HIV)
Molluscum contagiosum	Molluscum contagiosum virus
Pubic lice	*Phthirus pubis*
Syphilis	*Treponema pallidum*
Trichomoniasis	*Trichomonas vaginalis*

BOX 20-1 Risk Factors for Sexually Transmitted Infections and HIV

- Previous or current sexually transmitted infection
- Sex with multiple or new partners
- Initiating sex at a young age
- Unprotected sex
- Sex with high-risk partners
- Sex with an partner who has HIV
- Sex in exchange for money or drugs
- Sex while intoxicated
- Illegal drug use
- Injection drug use
- Mental illness
- Age < 25 years
- Living in an area with high sexually transmitted infection/HIV prevalence
- Residing in a detention or correctional facility

Abbreviation: HIV, human immunodeficiency virus.
Data from Centers for Disease Control and Prevention (CDC). (2015d). Sexually transmitted diseases treatment guidelines, 2015. *Morbidity and Mortality Weekly Report*, *64*(3), 1–137; Vasilenko, S. A., Kugler, K. C., Butera, N. M., & Lanza, S. T. (2015). Patterns of adolescent sexual behavior predicting young adult sexually transmitted infections: A latent class analysis approach. *Archives of Sexual Behavior, 44*, 705–714. doi:10.1007/s10508-014-0258-6

for STIs. These factors are partially influenced by a woman's sexual practices, substance use, and other health behaviors. Health behaviors, in turn, are influenced by socioeconomic factors and other social influences (Senie, 2014).

Biologic Factors

Women are biologically more likely to become infected with STIs than men. Women are also more likely than men to acquire an STI from a single heterosexual sexual encounter. For example, the risk of a woman contracting gonorrhea from a single act of intercourse is 50% or greater, whereas the corresponding risk for a man is 20% to 30%. In addition, men are 2 to 3 times more likely to transmit HIV to women than the reverse (Marrazzo & Cates, 2011). This difference arises because the vagina has a larger amount of genital mucous membranes exposed and is an environment more conducive to development of infections than the penis. Further, risk for trauma is greater during vaginal intercourse for women than for men (Fogel, 2008; Marrazzo & Cates, 2011; Youngkin, Davis, Schadewald, & Juve, 2013).

STIs are frequently asymptomatic in women and, therefore, are more likely to go undetected than the same infections in men (Marrazzo & Cates, 2011). Additionally, when or if symptoms develop, they are often confused with those of other conditions that are not transmitted sexually, such as bacterial vaginosis, vulvovaginal candidiasis, and urinary tract infections. The relative frequency of asymptomatic and unrecognized infections in women often results in delayed diagnosis and treatment, chronic untreated infections, and complications. Further, it can be more difficult to diagnose STIs in a woman because the anatomy of her genital tract makes clinical examination more difficult. Lesions that occur inside the vagina and on the cervix are not readily visible, for example, and the normal vaginal environment (a warm, moist, enriched medium) is ideal for nurturing an infection.

The prevalence rates of many STIs are highest among adolescents, whose lack of immunity and biologic susceptibility are contributing factors to their vulnerability to such infections (CDC, 2015d). An estimated 70% of all adolescent girls have had vaginal sex by age 19 years, with the end result being that many young women are at risk for STIs

(Alan Guttmacher Institute, 2011). The earlier a woman begins to have sexual intercourse, the longer her period of sexual activity is, the greater her number of partners, and the less apt she is to use barrier contraception (Fogel, 2008; Youngkin et al., 2013). Compared to older women prior to menopause, female adolescents and young women are more susceptible to cervical infections, such as chlamydial infections, gonorrhea, and HIV, because of the ectropion of the immature cervix and resulting larger exposed surface area of cells unprotected by cervical mucus. As women age, these cells eventually recede into the inner cervix. Nevertheless, women who are postmenopausal also are at increased risk because of the thin vaginal and cervical mucosa that occurs as estrogen levels decline. Further, women who are pregnant have a higher cervical ectropion area due to the influence of estrogen levels in pregnancy (Cunningham et al., 2010).

Other biologic factors that may increase a woman's risk of acquiring, transmitting, or developing complications of certain STIs include vaginal douching, risky sexual practices, use of hormonal contraceptives, and bacterial vaginosis (Marrazzo & Cates, 2011). The risk for contracting infections that can lead to PID may be increased with vaginal douching, and risk for PID may also increase with greater frequency of douching (CDC, 2015d). Certain sexual practices—for example, anal intercourse, sex during menses, and vaginal intercourse without sufficient lubrication (dry sex)—may also predispose a woman to acquiring an STI; the bleeding and tissue trauma that can result from these practices facilitate invasion by pathogens (CDC, 2015d; Marrarzzo & Cates, 2011).

The role of contraceptive choice in the acquisition and transmission of STIs is not fully understood, however. Some researchers have reported an increased risk of HPV, chlamydia, and herpes simplex virus (HSV) among high-risk female sex workers who use oral contraceptive pills (OCPs) (Henneke et al., 2015), and others have reported an increased rate of chlamydia infection in the general population of women who use OCPs (Nelson & Cwiak, 2011). It has been postulated that women who use OCPs have a greater area of cervical ectropion, which may make them more susceptible to STIs, especially when they do not use condoms (Nelson & Cwiak, 2011).

Social Factors

Preventing the spread of STIs, including HIV, is difficult without addressing community and individual issues that have a tremendous influence on prevention, transmission, and treatment of these infections. Societal factors such as poverty, lack of education, social inequity, immigration status, and inadequate access to health care may all indirectly increase the prevalence of STIs in at-risk populations. Persons with the highest rates of many STIs are often those with the least access to health care, and health insurance coverage influences whether and where a woman obtains STI treatment and preventive services (CDC, 2015d; Marrazzo & Cates, 2011; Senie, 2014).

Social Interactions and Relationships

Sexual behavior within the context of relationships is a critical risk factor for preventing and acquiring STIs, because intimate human contact is the most common vehicle of these infections' transmission. Notably, many researchers have reported on gender-related power imbalances and cultural proscriptions associated with sexual relationships that may lead to difficulty in negotiating condom use and other behaviors that protect against STIs (Teitelman, Calhoun, Duncan, Washio, & McDougall, 2015; Ulibarri et al., 2014; Woolf-King & Maisto, 2015). Women may perceive that they have less control than men over when and under which circumstances intercourse occurs. Young women are particularly at risk in this context, as they may lack the negotiating skills, self-efficacy, and self-confidence needed to successfully negotiate for safer sex practices. Premarital and extramarital sexual activity are common practices among many women, yet because of the secrecy and cultural proscriptions surrounding such activities, women may engage in them without preparation, leading to increased risks for both themselves and their partners.

Some women may be dependent upon an abusive male partner or a partner who places a woman at risk through his own risky behaviors. The risk of acquiring STIs is high among women who are physically and sexually abused (Fontenot, Fantasia, Sutherland, & Lee-St. John, 2014). Past and current experiences with violence—particularly sexual abuse—may erode women's sense of self-efficacy that enables them to exercise control over sexual behaviors, engender feelings of anxiety and depression, and increase the likelihood of risky sexual behaviors. Additionally, fear of physical harm and loss of economic support may hamper women's efforts to enact protective practices. Past and current abuse is also strongly associated with substance abuse, which also increases the risk of contracting an STI (Fantasia, Sutherland, Fontenot, & Lee-St. John, 2012; Fontenot et al., 2014; Sutherland, Fantasia, Fontenot, & Harris, 2012).

Risk of acquiring an STI is determined not only by a woman's actions, but also by her partner's behaviors. Although prevention counseling customarily recommends that women identify any partner who is at high risk and the nature of their sexual practices, this advice may be unrealistic or culturally inappropriate in many relationships.

Women who engage in sexual activities only with other women may also be at risk for infection. Many women who identify themselves as women who have sex with women (WSW) or lesbian have had intercourse with a man by choice, by force, or by necessity. Their female partners may also have other STI risk factors, such as injection drug use.

Dating and relationship patterns can also influence the acquisition and transmission of STIs. Concurrent partnership (i.e., having two or more partnerships at the same time) among men and women in established relationships can vary widely but has been reported by 20% to 45% of individuals and has been identified as a significant risk factor for STIs (Hamilton & Morris, 2015; Kogan, Cho, Barnum, & Brown, 2015; Lilleston et al., 2015). In addition to partner concurrency, sexual mixing patterns are a significant determinant of STIs. Sex partner mixing can occur among people of similar and different sexual risk categories and can include differing characteristics such as age differences and alcohol and substance use. Mixing between partners with higher-risk behaviors and lower-risk behaviors is a key factor in the spread of STIs within geographic areas (Prah, Copas, Mercer, Nardone, & Johnson, 2015).

Societal Norms

Relationships and sexual behavior are regulated by cultural norms that influence sexual expression in interpersonal relationships. Women are often socialized to please their partners and to place men's needs and desires first; as a consequence, they may find it difficult to insist on safer sex behaviors. Traditional cultural values associated with passivity and subordination may also diminish the ability of many women to adequately protect themselves (Edwards & Collins, 2014).

Power imbalances in relationships are the product of, and contribute to, the maintenance of traditional gender roles that identify men as the initiators and decision makers of sexual activities and women as passive gatekeepers. As long as traditional gender norms define the roles in sexual relationships such that men have the dominant role in sexual decision making, women will find it difficult to negotiate with their partners about condom use. Additionally, cultural norms may define talking about condoms as implying that women do not trust their male partner, which in turn may conflict with traditional gender norm expectations for women. Women may not request condom use because of a need to establish and maintain intimacy with partners. Urging women to insist on condom use may be unrealistic if their cultural norm includes traditional gender roles that do not encourage women to talk about sex, initiate sexual practices, or control intimate encounters (Minnis et al., 2015; Sastre et al., 2015).

Substance Use

Use of alcohol and drugs is associated with increased risk of HIV and STIs. This association may arise for several reasons, including social factors such as poverty, lack of access to health care, lack of treatment options, and lack of educational or economic opportunities, as well as individual factors such as high risk-taking propensity, survival sex, exchange of sex for money or drugs, and low self-esteem (Marrazzo & Cates, 2011). In addition to the risk from needle sharing, use of drugs and alcohol may contribute to risk of HIV infection by undermining cognitive and social skills, thereby making it more difficult for users to engage in HIV-protective actions. Further, depression and other psychological problems as well as history of sexual abuse are associated with substance abuse, which in turn contributes to risky behaviors (Jackson, Seth, DiClemente, & Lin, 2015). Being high and unable to clean drug paraphernalia can be a pervasive barrier to protective practice. Further, drug use

may take place in settings where persons participate in sexual activities while using drugs (Blankenship, Reinhard, Sherman, & El-Bassel, 2015).

Past and current physical, emotional, and sexual abuse characterize the lives of many, if not most, women using drugs (Sutherland, Fantasia, & McClain, 2013). For women who have experienced violence, use of alcohol and drugs can evolve into a coping mechanism by which they self-medicate to relieve feelings of anxiety, guilt, fear, and anger stemming from the violence. Women's drug use is strongly linked to relationship inequities and the ability of some men to mandate women's sexual behavior (Fontenot et al., 2014; Wechsberg et al., 2015).

SEXUALLY TRANSMITTED INFECTION SCREENING AND DETECTION

Prompt diagnosis and treatment are predicated on the assumption that any person who believes he or she may have contracted an STI, has symptoms of an STI, has had sexual relations with someone who has symptoms of an STI, or has a partner who has been diagnosed with an STI will seek care. To obtain prompt diagnosis and treatment, women and men must know how to recognize the major signs and symptoms of all STIs and must be willing and able to obtain health care if they experience symptoms or have sexual contact with someone who has an STI. Clinicians have a responsibility to educate their patients regarding the signs and symptoms of STIs. This education may be provided when a woman comes in for her annual health examination or episodic care, seeks contraception, or obtains preconception or prenatal care.

Clinicians must also ensure that their patients know where and how to obtain care if they suspect they might have contracted an STI. Many local health departments have clinics specifically designed to treat STIs, with services often available for free or at a reduced cost.

Screening

All women who are sexually active should be screened for STIs regularly through history, physical examination, and laboratory studies based on risk factors. To identify those women at increased risk, specific questions should be asked during the collection of a health history (**Box 20-2** and **Box 20-3**). The accuracy of risk assessment, however, depends on a woman's willingness to self-identify risk factors that may be seen as socially unacceptable or stigmatizing. Some women may not reveal such risk factors directly to clinicians, but might be willing to do so if asked to fill out a questionnaire using questions similar to those

---

BOX 20-2 The Five P's of Sexual Health

Partners

- Do you have sex with men, women, or both?
- In the past 2 months, how many partners have you had sex with?
- In the past 12 months, how many partners have you had sex with?
- Is it possible that any of your sex partners in the past 12 months had sex with someone else while they were still in a sexual relationship with you?

Practices

- To understand your risks for sexually transmitted infections, I need to understand the kind of sex you have had recently.
- Have you had vaginal sex, meaning "penis-in-vagina sex?" If yes, do you use condoms never, sometimes, or always?
- Have you had anal sex, meaning "penis-in-rectum/anus sex?" If yes, do you use condoms never, sometimes, or always?
- Have you had oral sex, meaning "mouth-on-penis/vagina?"

For condom answers:
- If "never": Why don't you use condoms?
- If "sometimes": In which situations (or with whom) do you use condoms?

Prevention of Pregnancy

- What are you doing to prevent pregnancy?

Protection from Sexually Transmitted Infections

- What do you do to protect yourself from sexually transmitted infections and HIV?

Past History of Sexually Transmitted Infections

- Have you ever had a sexually transmitted infections?
- Have any of your partners had a sexually transmitted infections?

Additional questions to identify HIV and viral hepatitis risk:
- Have you or any of your partners ever injected drugs?
- Have your or any of your partners exchanged money or drugs for sex?
- Is there anything else about your sexual practices that I need to know about?

Reproduced from Centers for Disease Control and Prevention (CDC). (2015d). Sexually transmitted diseases treatment guidelines, 2015. *Morbidity and Mortality Weekly Report, 64*(3), 1–137.

BOX 20-3 Gynecologic History Questions to Assess Risk of Sexually Transmitted Infections

Do you experience now or have you ever experienced:

- Frequent vaginal infections
- Unusual vaginal discharge or odor
- Vaginal itching, burning, sores, or warts
- Sexually transmitted infections (ask about individual infections)
- Abdominal pain
- Pelvic inflammatory disease/infection of the uterus, tubes, ovaries
- Sexual assault/rape
- Physical, emotional, sexual abuse
- Abnormal Pap test
- Pain or bleeding with intercourse
- Severe menstrual cramps occurring at end of period
- Ectopic pregnancy

Data from Carcio, H. A., & Secor, M. C. (2015). *Advanced health assessment of women* (3rd ed.). New York, NY: Springer; Hawkins, J. W., Roberto-Nichols, D. M., & Stanley-Haney, J. L. (2016). *Guidelines for nurse practitioners in gynecologic settings* (11th ed.). New York, NY: Springer.

given in the Five P's (**Box 20-2**). The Five P's—an instrument developed by the CDC—is one way to gather sexual history information in an organized and nonjudgmental way. Any woman who has been diagnosed with an STI should also be screened for other STIs, because comorbidity of such infections is high and many STIs can be asymptomatic (CDC, 2015d).

ASSESSMENT

The diagnosis of an STI is based on the integration of relevant history, physical examination, and laboratory data. A history that is accurate, comprehensive, and specific is essential for accurate diagnosis.

Generally the history should be taken first, with the woman dressed. Information should be collected in a nonjudgmental manner, avoiding assumptions about sexual preference. All partners should be referred to as "partners," rather than by gender. It is helpful to begin with open-ended questions because they often elicit information that might otherwise be missed. These queries can be followed with symptom-specific questions and relevant history. Specific areas to address include the reason why the woman has sought care and any symptoms she has noticed; a sexual history, including a description of the date and type of sexual activity; number of partners; whether she has had contact with someone who recently had an STI; and potential sites of infection (e.g., mouth, cervix, urethra, and rectum). Pertinent medical history includes anything that will influence the management plan, such as history of drug allergies, previously diagnosed chronic illnesses, and general health status. A menstrual and contraceptive history, including the date of the woman's last menstrual period, must always be obtained to determine if the woman might be pregnant. When indicated, a systems review should be conducted that may assist in diagnosis of specific STIs. Any positive answers regarding symptoms should be followed up to elicit information about systemic and local onset, duration, and characteristics.

Before the actual physical examination is performed, the clinician should discuss the procedure to be followed with the woman so that she is prepared. The physical examination begins with careful visualization of the external genitalia, including the perineum. Erythema, edema, distortions, lesions, trauma, and any other abnormalities are noted. Palpation can locate areas of tenderness. During the speculum examination, the vagina and cervix are inspected for edema, thinning, lesions, abnormal coloration, trauma, discharge, and bleeding. Thorough palpation of inguinal area and pelvic organs through bimanual examination, milking of the urethra for discharge, and assessment of vaginal secretion odors is essential.

Appropriate laboratory studies will be suggested, in part, by the history and physical examination results. These tests include microscopic examination of vaginal secretions (wet mount), chlamydia and gonorrhea testing, treponemal tests with reflex to Venereal Disease Research Laboratory (VDRL) or rapid plasma reagin (RPR) testing for syphilis, and a hepatitis B/C panel. When an STI is diagnosed, testing for other STIs is essential. The woman should be notified that HIV testing will be performed unless she specifically declines such testing (see the section on HIV testing later in this chapter). Other laboratory tests, such as a complete blood count, urinalysis, and urine culture and sensitivity, should be obtained only if indicated. If the history or physical examination indicates pregnancy is possible, a urine human chorionic gonadotropin (hCG) test should also be performed because treatment for STIs can differ in pregnant and nonpregnant women, and because certain antibiotics are contraindicated in pregnancy (CDC, 2015d).

EDUCATION AND PREVENTION

Counseling is an essential part of caring for a patient with an STI (**Box 20-4** and **Table 20-2**). The woman with an STI will need support in seeking care at the earliest possible stage of symptoms. Counseling women about STIs is essential for the following reasons:

- Preventing new infections or reinfection
- Increasing adherence to treatment and follow-up
- Providing support during treatment
- Assisting women in discussions and disclosure with their partners
- Increasing awareness of the serious potential consequences of untreated STIs

The clinician must make sure that the woman understands which infection she has, how it is transmitted, and why it must be treated. Women should be given a brief description of the infection in language they can understand. This description should include modes of transmission, incubation period, symptoms, infectious period, and potential complications.

Effective treatment of STIs necessitates a careful, thorough explanation of the treatment regimen and follow-up procedures. Comprehensive and precise instructions about medications must be provided, both verbally and in writing. Side effects, benefits, and risks of medications should be discussed. Unpleasant side effects or early relief of symptoms may sometimes discourage women from completing their medication course. All patients should be strongly urged to continue taking their medication until the full regimen is finished, regardless of whether their symptoms diminish or disappear a few days after they begin the therapeutic regimen. Comfort measures that decrease symptoms such as pain, itching, or nausea should be suggested. Providing written information is a useful strategy because diagnosis of an STI is a time of high anxiety for many women, and they may not be able to hear or remember what they were told. A number of booklets on STIs are available, or the clinician may wish to develop literature specific to the practice setting and patient population.

In general, women should be advised to refrain from intercourse until all treatment is finished. After treatment, women should be urged to continue using condoms to prevent recurring infections. Women may wish to avoid having sex with partners who have many other sexual partners. All women who have contracted an STI should be taught safer sex practices, if this education has not been provided already. Follow-up appointments should be made as needed (CDC, 2015d; Hawkins, Roberto-Nichols, & Stanley-Haney, 2016).

Addressing the psychosocial component of STIs is essential. Be aware that a woman may be afraid or embarrassed to tell her partner and ask him or her to seek treatment, or she may be concerned about confidentiality. The effect of a diagnosis of an STI on a committed relationship for the woman, who is now faced with the necessity of dealing with uncertain monogamy, can be significant. In other instances, the woman may be afraid that telling her partner about the STI may place her in danger of escalating abuse. The potential consequences of talking with her partner must be discussed with each woman.

In most situations involving STIs, sexual partners should be examined; thus the woman is asked to identify and notify all partners who might have been exposed (partner notification). Empathizing with the woman's feelings and suggesting specific ways

BOX 20-4 Patient Information About Sexually Transmitted Infections

The only certain way to prevent STIs is to avoid sexual contact with others. If you choose to be sexually active, there are things you can do to decrease your risk of developing an STI:

- Have sex with only one person who does not have sex with anyone else and who has no infections.
- Always use a condom and use it correctly.
- Use clean needles if you inject any drugs.
- Prevent and control other STIs to decrease your susceptibility to HIV infection and to reduce your infectiousness if you are HIV positive.
- Wait to have sex for as long as possible. The younger you are when you have sex for the first time, the more likely you are to get an STI. The risk of acquiring an STI also increases with the number of partners you have over a lifetime.

Anyone who is sexually active should do the following:

- Always use protection unless you are having sex with only one person who does not have sex with anyone else and who has no infections.
- Have regular checkups for STIs even if you have no symptoms, and especially when having sex with a new partner.
- Learn the common symptoms of STIs. Seek health care immediately if any suspicious symptoms develop, even if they are mild.
- Avoid having sex during menstruation. Women with HIV are probably more infectious during menstruation, and women without HIV are probably more susceptible to becoming infected during that time.
- Avoid anal intercourse, but if practiced, use a condom.
- Avoid douching. It removes some of the normal protective bacteria in the vagina and increases the risk of getting some STIs.

Anyone diagnosed as having an STI should do the following:

- Be treated to reduce the risk of transmitting an STI to another person.
- Notify all recent and current sex partners and urge them to get tested and treated as soon as possible to reduce the risk of reinfection from an untreated partner.
- Follow the clinician's recommendations and complete the full course of medication prescribed. Have a follow-up test if necessary.
- Avoid all sexual activity while being treated.

Abbreviations: HIV, human immunodeficiency virus; STI, sexually transmitted infection.
Data from Centers for Disease Control and Prevention (CDC). (2015d). Sexually transmitted diseases treatment guidelines, 2015. *Morbidity and Mortality Weekly Report, 64*(3), 1–137; Hawkins, J. W., Roberto-Nichols, D. M., & Stanley-Haney, J. L. (2016). *Guidelines for nurse practitioners in gynecologic settings* (11th ed.). New York, NY: Springer; Marrazzo, J. M., & Cates, W. (2011). Reproductive tract infections, including HIV and other sexually transmitted infections. In R. A. Hatcher, J. Trussell, A. L. Nelson, W. Cates, D. Kowal, & M. S. Policar (Eds.), *Contraceptive technology* (20th ed., pp. 571–620). New York, NY: Ardent Media.

TABLE 20-2	Sexual Risk Practices		
Safest	**Lower Risk**	**Possibly Risky (Possible Exposure)**	**High Risk (Unsafe)**
Behavior			
Abstinence	Wet kissing	Cunnilingus	Unprotected anal intercourse
Self-masturbation	Urine contact with intact skin	Fellatio	Unprotected vaginal intercourse
Monogamous (both partners and no high-risk activities)		Mutual masturbation with skin breaks	Oral–anal contact
Hugging,[a] massage,[a] touching[a]		Vaginal intercourse with condom	Fisting
Dry kissing		Anal intercourse with condom	Multiple sexual partners
Mutual masturbation		Vaginal intercourse after anal contact without new condom	Sharing uncleaned sex toys, douche equipment
Drug abstinence			Sharing needles
Prevention			
Avoid high-risk behaviors	Avoid exposure to potentially infected body fluids	Dental dam or female condom with cunnilingus	Avoid exposure to potentially infected body fluids
	Consistently use condom and spermicide	Use condom with fellatio	Consistently use condom and spermicide
	Avoid anal intercourse	Use latex gloves for digital/hand penetration	Avoid anal intercourse
			If having anal penetration, use condom with intercourse, latex glove with digital/hand penetration
			Avoid oral–anal contact
			Do not share sex toys, needles, douching equipment
			If sharing needles, clean with bleach before and after use

[a] Assumes no breaks in skin.
Modified from Fogel, C. I. (2008). Sexually transmitted infections. In C. I. Fogel & N. F. Woods (Eds.), *Women's health care in advanced practice nursing* (pp. 475–526). New York, NY: Springer.

of talking with partners will help decrease her anxiety and assist in efforts to control infection. For example, the clinician might suggest that the woman say, "I care about you and I'm concerned about you. That's why I'm calling to tell you that I have a sexually transmitted infection. My clinician is _____ and she will be happy to talk with you if you would like." Offering literature and role-playing situations with the woman may also be of assistance. It is often helpful to remind the woman that, although this may be a potentially embarrassing situation, most persons would rather know than not know they have been exposed to an STI. Clinicians who take the time to counsel their patients on how to talk with their partners can improve adherence and case finding (Marrazzo & Cates, 2011).

In situations when patient referral may not be effective or possible, clinicians and local health departments should be prepared to assist the woman. Women can notify their partners themselves or can seek assistance through local health departments that can attempt to contact partners. With the woman's permission, clinicians can also attempt to contact partners. In some areas, this contact can be made through Internet services, although this ability is not consistently available. More information on Internet-based notification can be found at http://www.ncsddc.org/Internet_Guidelines (CDC, 2015d).

SPECIAL CONSIDERATIONS

Reporting

Accurate identification and timely reporting of STIs are integral components of successful infection control efforts. Clinicians are required to report certain STIs to their state public health officials, who in turn report these infection rates to the CDC. Nationally notifiable STIs include chancroid, chlamydia, gonorrhea, hepatitis, HIV, and syphilis (CDC, 2015d). A full list of all nationally notifiable STIs can be found at the National Notifiable Diseases Surveillance System (NNDSS) website: http://www.cdc.gov/nndss/default.aspx. The requirements for reporting other STIs differ from state to state, and clinicians need to be aware of reporting laws in their practice area. Clinicians are legally responsible for reporting all cases of those infections identified as

reportable. Additionally, individuals with STIs should be asked to identify and notify all partners who might have been exposed to the infection.

Confidentiality is a crucial issue for many patients. When an STI is reportable, the woman must be informed her case will be reported and told why. Failure to inform a woman that her case will be reported is considered a serious breach of professional ethics. Women need to be told that the diagnosis will be reported to the state health department and they may be contacted by a health department representative. They should be assured that the information reported to and collected by health authorities is maintained in strictest confidence. Reports are protected by statute from subpoena in most jurisdictions (CDC, 2015d). Every effort, within the limits of the clinician's public health responsibilities, should be made to reassure patients that their confidentiality will be protected.

Sexual Assault

Woman who have experienced sexual assault and sexual violence are a vulnerable group at risk for STIs. To the extent possible, all examinations should be conducted as soon as feasible after the assault, by a clinician trained in sexual assault care and evidence collection. Care must be taken to avoid secondary trauma. Among women who have been sexually assaulted, the most commonly diagnosed STIs are gonorrhea, chlamydia, and trichomoniasis (CDC, 2015d). Broad-spectrum antibiotic treatment is offered to sexual assault victims to cover these infections. As HPV is prevalent in the general population, women younger than age 26 who have not been vaccinated for HPV should be offered the vaccine (CDC, 2015d). More detailed care and specific treatment for sexual assault victims can be found in the *CDC Sexually Transmitted Disease Treatment Guidelines* (CDC, 2015d). See also Chapter 14.

Older Women

Perimenopausal and postmenopausal women have historically been neglected in both STI screening and assessment, most likely due to the fact that statistically this age group has the lowest rates for all STIs. Clinicians may also make assumptions that aging women are not sexually active. To counteract this bias, all women, regardless of age, should be asked about sexual activity and sexual function.

In older women, the dry, friable vaginal tissue that results from vulvovaginal atrophy associated with declining estrogen levels in menopause may increase microabrasions with intercourse and increase the risk for STI transmission (Archer, 2015). This factor must be considered in conjunction with the knowledge that with age, the columnar epithelium regresses into the cervical canal, which can result in decreased exposure to infected seminal fluids and may be protective against STI acquisition (Jackson, McNair, & Coleman, 2015). As natural fertility ends with menopause, however, condoms may not be seen as necessary. Screening for STIs in older women should be based on their various risk factors as identified via a thorough sexual health history (Fantasia, Fontenot, Sutherland, & Harris, 2011).

Women Who Have Sex with Women

Women who have sex with women (WSW) represent a diverse group who vary in their sexual identity and sexual practices (see Chapter 9). Therefore, information on sexual risk and the transmission of most STIs between female partners is extremely limited (Marrazzo & Gorgos, 2012). Additionally, many WSW also have either a past or present history of male partners and other risk behaviors such as transactional sex and substance use that may contribute to an increased risk of STIs (Tat, Marrazzo, & Graham, 2015).

Some bacterial STIs, such as gonorrhea and chlamydia, may potentially be spread between women via oral sex or shared penetrative sex items (CDC, 2015d). Additionally, viral STIs, such as HSV and HPV, can be spread via skin-to-skin mucosal contact without penetrative sex. Women who report sexual activity with other women should be asked about their specific sexual practices and relationship characteristics to assess their actual STI risk (CDC, 2015d).

Pregnancy

Considerations for woman who are pregnant are discussed individually within each STI section in this chapter.

HUMAN PAPILLOMAVIRUS AND GENITAL WARTS

HPV infection is now the most common STI in the United States (CDC, 2014c, 2015d). Its exact incidence is not known, because clinicians are not required to report these cases. Nevertheless, as many as 6 million people are believed to become newly infected with HPV each year, and nearly all sexually active men and women will have HPV at some point in their lives but may not be aware of the infection (CDC, 2014c, 2015d).

HPV comprises a group of double-stranded DNA viruses with more than 100 known serotypes, of which more than 40 can infect the genital tract, including the external genitalia, vagina, urethra, and anus (CDC, 2015d). Most HPV infections are asymptomatic, subclinical, or unrecognized, and clear spontaneously (CDC, 2014c, 2015d). HPV can cause genital warts, and persistent infection with high-risk, oncogenic strains can cause cervical, penile, vulvar, vaginal, anal, and oropharyngeal cancers. Most (90%) genital warts are caused by HPV types 6 and 11, which carry a low risk for triggering invasive cancer. Some other types (i.e., 16, 18, 31, 33, and 35) that are occasionally found in genital warts are associated with cervical intraepithelial neoplasia. Two high-risk HPV types, 16 and 18, cause 70% of all cervical cancers (CDC, 2015d).

Although the period of communicability is unknown, the transmission rate of HPV is high. More than 60% of individuals with a partner who has HPV will acquire the virus (Giuliano et al., 2015).

Genital warts in women are most frequently seen around the vaginal introitus, but can also occur on the cervix, vagina, perineum, and anus/perianal area. Typically the lesions present as small, soft, papillary swellings, occurring singularly or in clusters on the genital and anal–rectal region (see **Color Plate 19**). Growths can be flat, papular, or pedunculated (Fantasia, 2012). Warts are usually flesh-colored or slightly darker on Caucasian women, black on African American women, and brownish on Asian women. Infections of long duration may appear as a cauliflower-like mass. In moist areas such as the vaginal introitus, the lesions may appear to have multiple, fine, fingerlike projections. Vaginal lesions can appear as multiple warts. Flat-topped papules are sometimes seen on the cervix, but often these lesions are visualized only under magnification with a colposcope (Carcio & Secor, 2015). Although they are usually painless and often asymptomatic, the lesions may sometimes be uncomfortable, particularly when very large, inflamed, or ulcerated. Chronic vaginal discharge, pruritus, or dyspareunia can occur as well.

Assessment

A woman with HPV lesions may be asymptomatic or present with "bumps" on her vaginal introitus, vulva, labia, or anus. Symptoms such as vaginal discharge, itching, dyspareunia, and postcoital bleeding are possible but less common (Carcio & Secor, 2015; Hawkins et al., 2016). History of known exposure to the virus is important because of the potentially long latency period for HPV infection and the possibility of subclinical infections in men and women. Nevertheless, the lack of a history of known exposure cannot be used to exclude a diagnosis of HPV infection, as viral transmission can occur between asymptomatic partners (CDC, 2015d).

Physical inspection of the vulva, perineum, anus, vagina, and cervix is essential whenever HPV lesions are suspected or seen. Gloves should be changed between vaginal and rectal examinations to prevent the potential spread of vulvar or vaginal lesions to the anus (Hawkins et al., 2016). Because speculum examination of the vagina may block some lesions, it is important to rotate the speculum blades until all areas are visualized. When lesions are visible, the characteristic appearance previously described is considered diagnostic (CDC, 2015d). In many instances, however, cervical lesions are not visible; moreover, some vaginal or vulvar lesions may be unobservable to the naked eye. Diagnosis is made by careful, thorough clinical examination of visible genital warts or by biopsy of cervical lesions and (rarely) of lesions at other sites if the diagnosis is not clear (CDC, 2015d). Perform testing for other STIs when genital warts are present.

Women with genital warts should have cervical cancer screening according to the standard recommendations (see Chapter 7); more frequent screening is not recommended (CDC, 2015d). HPV DNA testing should be performed only in women aged 21 years and older with a Pap test result indicating atypical squamous cells of undetermined significance (ASC-US) or for women aged 30 years and older in conjunction with Pap testing for cervical cancer screening. HPV DNA testing is inappropriate for STI screening, in adolescents (women 20 years and younger), for women with abnormal Pap results other than ASC-US (e.g., atypical squamous cells cannot rule out a high-grade lesion [ASC-H], low-grade squamous intraepithelial lesion [LSIL], and high-grade squamous intraepithelial lesion [HSIL]), and as routine screening in women younger than age 30. Women considering vaccination against HPV should not be tested for HPV prior to vaccination (CDC, 2015d; Saslow et al., 2012).

Differential Diagnoses

HPV lesions must be differentiated from molluscum contagiosum, condylomata lata, and carcinoma. Molluscum contagiosum lesions are half-domed, smooth, and flesh-colored to pearly white papules with depressed centers. Condylomata lata—a form of secondary syphilis—are generally flatter and wider than genital warts. Cancers to be ruled out include squamous cell carcinoma, carcinoma in situ, and malignant melanoma. An extensive list of other differential diagnoses for vulvar lesions can be found in Chapter 26.

Prevention

The most clinically significant HPV types can now be prevented with vaccination. The bivalent vaccine (HPV2, Cervarix), the quadrivalent vaccine (HPV4, Gardasil), and the 9-valent vaccine (HPV9, Gardasil 9) all protect against HPV types 16 and 18, which cause the majority of cervical cancers. In addition, the quadrivalent and 9-valent vaccines protect against HPV types 6 and 11, which cause the majority of genital warts, and provide some protection against vulvar and vaginal cancers and precancers. The 9-valent HPV vaccine protects against another 5 strains of HPV (31, 33, 45, 52, and 58) that are responsible for an additional 15% of cervical cancers (CDC, 2015d).

Routine HPV vaccination is recommended for girls aged 11 to 12 years. HPV vaccines can be given to girls as young as age 9, and are also recommended for adolescents and women aged 13 to 26 years who were not vaccinated or did not complete the series earlier (CDC, 2015d). Ideally, vaccination should occur before the adolescent or woman becomes sexually active and, therefore, has the potential for HPV exposure; nevertheless, previous sexual activity does not preclude women from receiving any of the available HPV vaccines. Vaccination is recommended for women who have evidence of existing HPV infection, such as Pap test abnormalities or genital warts, to provide protection against HPV types that they have not yet acquired (CDC, 2015d). Vaccination will not treat existing HPV infection, cervical cytologic abnormalities, or genital warts (American College of Obstetricians and Gynecologists, 2010b; CDC, 2015d).

All three HPV vaccines are given as a series of three intramuscular injections over a 6-month period. The second dose is given 1 to 2 months (and at least 4 weeks) after the first dose. The third dose is given 6 months (and at least 12 weeks) after the second dose. The series does not need to be restarted if the second and third doses are delayed. When possible, the same vaccine (bivalent, quadrivalent, or 9-valent) should be given for all three doses. HPV testing prior to vaccination is not recommended (CDC, 2015d).

The HPV vaccines are not recommended during pregnancy but can be given during lactation (GlaxoSmithKline, 2015). Routine pregnancy testing prior to vaccination is not recommended. If a woman is found to be pregnant after the vaccine is given, the remaining vaccines in the series should be delayed until after she gives birth, and the clinician should report the exposure to the vaccine manufacturer (Merck [800-986-8999] for the quadrivalent and 9-valent vaccines and Glaxo-SmithKline [888-452-9622] for the bivalent vaccine); no intervention is needed.

All three vaccines are contraindicated for women with hypersensitivity to any vaccine component. The quadrivalent and 9-valent vaccines are also contraindicated for women with yeast hypersensitivity. Women with anaphylactic latex allergy who are receiving the bivalent vaccine should be given the vaccine from a single-dose vial rather than using a prefilled syringe, as the latter contains latex (GlaxoSmithKline, 2015).

Syncope has been reported after administration of all three HPV vaccines. Given this risk, it is advisable to observe patients for 15 minutes after each injection (GlaxoSmithKline, 2015).

Management

The primary goals of treatment of visible genital warts are removal or reduction of warts and relief of signs and symptoms, not the eradication of HPV. If left untreated, genital warts may resolve, remain unchanged, or increase in size and number (CDC, 2015d). Treatment of genital warts can be difficult. A woman often must make multiple office visits if clinician-administered regimens are used. Patient-applied treatments need to be repeated for months, and even with treatment recurrence is common (CDC, 2015d).

Treatment of genital warts should be guided by the woman's preferences, available resources, cost considerations, ability to return for multiple visits if needed, size and location of warts, and experience of the clinician. None of the treatments is superior to any of the others, and no one treatment is ideal for all women or all warts (CDC, 2015d). Available treatments are outlined in **Table 20-3**. Any concurrent vaginal infections or STIs should also be treated along with the genital warts.

Patient Education

Women who are experiencing discomfort associated with genital warts may find that bathing with an oatmeal solution and drying the area with a hair dryer on a lower setting may provide some relief. Keeping the area clean and dry may also decrease discomfort. Cotton underwear and loose-fitting clothes that decrease friction and irritation may be helpful as well (Hawkins et al., 2016). Women should be advised to maintain a healthy lifestyle to aid the immune system. Women can also be counseled regarding diet, rest, stress reduction, and exercise. All women who smoke should be counseled in smoking-cessation techniques.

Counseling messages for women with HPV infection and genital warts are outlined in **Box 20-5**. The partners of women with genital warts should be evaluated and treated if lesions are present. Condoms should be used until both partners are lesion free and for as long as 9 months after the appearance of lesions, as subclinical HPV may remain infectious (CDC, 2015d). All sexually active women with multiple partners or a history of HPV should be encouraged to use latex condoms during intercourse to decrease HPV acquisition or transmission, although HPV transmission may still occur

TABLE 20-3	Treatment of External Genital Warts

Patient-Applied Regimens	Clinician-Administered Regimens	Alternative Regimens
Podofilox 0.5% solution or gel **or** Imiquimod 3.75% or 5% cream **or** Sinecatechins 15% ointment	Cryotherapy with liquid nitrogen or cryoprobe, repeat applications every 1–2 weeks **or** Trichloroacetic acid or bichloracetic acid 80–90% **or** Surgical removal by tangential scissor excision, tangential shave excision, curettage, or electrosurgery	Intralesional interferon **or** Photodynamic therapy **or** Topical cidofovir **or** Podophyllin resin 10–25% in a compound tincture of benzoin[a]

[a] Consider only if strict adherence to application guidelines is followed to avoid systemic toxicity.
Modified from Centers for Disease Control and Prevention (CDC). (2015d). Sexually transmitted diseases treatment guidelines, 2015. *Morbidity and Mortality Weekly Report, 64*(3), 1–137.

BOX 20-5 Counseling Messages for Women with Human Papillomavirus and Genital Warts

The CDC recommends that the following key counseling points be conveyed to all persons with HPV:

- Genital HPV infection is very common and can be passed through vaginal, anal, or oral sexual contact.
- Most sexually active adults will get HPV at some point in their lives, although most will never know it because HPV infection usually has no signs or symptoms.
- HPV infection usually clears spontaneously without causing health problems, but some infections progress to genital warts, precancerous conditions, and cancers. The types of HPV that cause genital warts are not the same as the types that can cause cancer.
- A diagnosis of HPV in one sex partner is not indicative of sexual infidelity in the other partner.
- Treatments are available for genital warts but cannot eradicate the actual virus.
- HPV does not affect female fertility or the ability to carry a pregnancy to term.
- Correct and consistent condom use might lower the chances of giving or getting genital HPV, but condom use is not fully protective because HPV can infect areas that are not covered by a condom. The only way to definitively avoid giving and getting HPV is to abstain from sexual activity.
- Tests for HPV are available to screen for cervical cancer in certain women.
- Three HPV vaccines are available, which protect against the HPV types that cause 70% to 85% of cancers. Two of the vaccines also protect against the HPV types that cause 90% of genital warts. All three vaccines are most effective when all doses are administered before sexual contact.

The following key counseling points are for persons diagnosed with genital warts and their partners:

- Genital warts are not life threatening. If they are not treated, genital warts might go away, stay the same, or increase in size or number. It is very unusual for genital warts to turn into cancer.

(continues)

BOX 20-5 Counseling Messages for Women with Human Papillomavirus and Genital Warts (*continued*)

- It is difficult to determine how or when a person became infected with HPV. Genital warts can be transmitted even when no visible signs of warts are present and even after warts are treated.
- It is not known how long a person remains contagious after warts are treated or whether informing subsequent sexual partners about a history of genital warts is beneficial to their health.
- Genital warts commonly recur after treatment, especially in the first 3 months.
- Women with HPV do not need more frequent Pap tests.
- HPV testing is unnecessary in sexual partners of persons with genital warts. In contrast, STI screening for both sex partners is beneficial if one partner has genital warts.
- Persons with genital warts should inform their current sex partner(s) because warts can be transmitted to other partners. They should refrain from sexual activity until the warts are gone or removed.

Abbreviations: CDC, Centers for Disease Control and Prevention; HPV, human papillomavirus.
Data from Centers for Disease Control and Prevention (CDC). (2015d). Sexually transmitted diseases treatment guidelines, 2015. *Morbidity and Mortality Weekly Report, 64*(3), 1–137.

---

from areas not covered by a condom. Women with HPV infection may radically alter their sexual practices both out of fear of transmission of the virus to or from a partner, and owing to genital discomfort associated with treatment, which may have a negative effect on their sexual relationships. Unless the partner accepts and understands the necessary precautions, it may be difficult for the woman to follow the treatment regimen. The clinician can offer to discuss feelings that the woman may have and, when indicated, joint counseling can be suggested.

Special Considerations

Pregnancy
Although various options exist for treating genital warts, not all are safe during pregnancy. Specifically, podophyllin, sinecatechins, and imiquimod should be avoided in pregnant women.

External genital warts can multiply during pregnancy and become friable. Unless the vaginal opening is obstructed by large warts, a cesarean birth is not warranted. The risk of HPV transmission to the newborn and subsequent development of respiratory papillomatosis is low, and the presence of small warts that do not block the vaginal opening does not preclude a vaginal birth (CDC, 2015d).

GENITAL HERPES

Genital herpes is a recurrent, incurable viral infection characterized by painful vesicular eruptions of the skin and mucosa of the genitals. Two types of herpes simplex virus have been identified as causing genital herpes: HSV-1 and HSV-2. HSV-2 is usually transmitted sexually, whereas HSV-1 is transmitted either nonsexually or through oral–genital contact. Although HSV-1 is more commonly associated with gingivostomatitis and oral ulcers (fever blisters) and HSV-2 with genital lesions, both types are not exclusively associated with those sites, and an increasing number of genital infections are being attributed to HSV-1 (CDC, 2015d). HSV-2 infection significantly increases the risk of women acquiring HIV, most likely related to inflammatory processes, but HSV-1 infection does not appear to carry the same risk (Masson et al., 2015).

Genital herpes is one of the most common STIs in the United States, but its exact prevalence is unknown because HSV is not a reportable infection. It is the primary cause of genital ulcer disease in the United States. According to CDC surveillance data, the overall prevalence rate of genital HSV in non-Hispanic Caucasian women is approximately 15%. Non-Hispanic women of African descent have the highest reported rates among all females—approximately 50%, more than 3 times higher than the rates in Caucasian women (CDC, 2014b). HSV prevalence also increases with a higher number of lifetime sex partners: Seroprevalence has been reported as 5.4% in women with one lifetime sex partner, 18.8% in women with two to four lifetime partners, 21.8% in women with five to nine lifetime partners, and 37.1% in women with 10 or more lifetime partners.

Although HSV rates are high, more than 85% of individuals who are positive for HSV-2 antibodies report that they have never had a clinician tell them they had genital herpes (CDC, 2014b). In fact, most people with HSV-2 antibodies have never been diagnosed with genital herpes. Despite their mild or unrecognized infections, they intermittently shed the HSV-2 virus in the genital tract. As a result, most genital herpes infections are transmitted by individuals who do not know they have HSV-2 or who do not have symptoms at the time of transmission (CDC, 2015d).

An initial or primary genital herpes infection characteristically has both systemic and local symptoms and lasts approximately 3 weeks. Flu-like symptoms with fever, malaise, and myalgia first appear about a week after exposure, peak within 4 days, and subside over the next week. Multiple genital lesions develop at the site of infection, which is usually the vulva, but may be present anywhere in the anogenital area. Other commonly affected sites are the perianal area, vagina, and cervix. The lesions begin as small painful blisters or vesicles that become "unroofed," leaving behind ulcerated lesions (see **Color Plate 20**). Individuals with a primary herpes infection often develop bilateral, tender, inguinal lymphadenopathy; vulvar edema; vaginal discharge; and severe dysuria (Hawkins et al., 2016).

Ulcerative lesions last 4 to 15 days before crusting over, and new lesions may develop over a period of 10 days during the course of the infection. Cervicitis is also common with initial HSV-2 infections. The cervix may appear normal, or it may be friable, reddened, ulcerated, or necrotic if cervical lesions are present. A heavy, watery to purulent vaginal discharge is possible. Extragenital lesions may be present because of autoinoculation. Urinary retention and dysuria may occur secondary to autonomic involvement of the sacral nerve root (Hawkins et al., 2016).

Women experiencing recurrent episodes of genital herpes typically develop only local symptoms that are less severe than those associated with the initial infection due to the initial immune response. Systemic symptoms are usually absent with recurrences, although the characteristic prodromal genital tingling is common. Recurrent lesions are unilateral, are less extensive than the original lesions, and usually last 7 to 10 days without prolonged viral shedding. Lesions begin as vesicles and progress rapidly to ulcers (Hawkins et al., 2016). Very few women with recurrent infection have cervicitis.

Assessment

Establishing a diagnosis of genital HSV can be challenging. Many individuals with HSV do not have overt symptoms. Thus, in making the diagnosis of genital herpes, a history of exposure to a person with HSV infection is important, although infection from an asymptomatic individual is common. A history of viral symptoms, such as malaise, headache, fever, or myalgia, is suggestive of HSV infection. Likewise, local symptoms such as vulvar pain, dysuria, itching, or burning at the site of infection, and painful genital lesions that heal spontaneously are very suggestive of HSV infection. The clinician should also ask about prior history of a primary infection, prodromal symptoms, vaginal discharge, dysuria, and dyspareunia.

During the physical examination, the clinician should assess for inguinal and generalized lymphadenopathy and elevated temperature. Carefully inspect the entire vulvar, perineal, vaginal, and cervical areas for vesicles, ulcers, or crusted areas. A speculum examination may be very difficult for the patient because of the extreme tenderness often associated with genital herpes. Any genital lesion that is extremely tender should be tested for HSV even if the appearance is not consistent with the classic herpes lesions.

Although a diagnosis of HSV infection may be suspected from the woman's history and physical examination, it can be confirmed only by laboratory studies. Isolation of HSV in cell culture or by polymerase chain reaction (PCR) is the preferred test in women who have genital ulcers or other mucocutaneous lesions. Viral culture is less sensitive than PCR, with the best culture yield being found during a primary infection or if the specimen is taken during the vesicular stage of the infection—the sensitivity of a culture declines rapidly as lesions begin to heal. Both culture and PCR can be negative in a person with HSV infection because the virus is shed only intermittently (CDC, 2015d).

Type-specific serologic tests are useful in confirming a clinical diagnosis given the frequency of false-negative HSV cultures, especially in women with healing lesions or recurrent infection. Antibodies are present within the first several weeks after infection and persist indefinitely. Clinicians should be certain to specifically request serologic type-specific glycoprotein G (IgG)–based assays. Serologic test options include laboratory-based assays and point-of-care tests using capillary blood or serum during a clinic visit. The sensitivity of these tests varies from 80% to 98%, and false-negative results can occur, especially in early-stage infection when antibodies are still developing. If there is a strong clinical suspicion of HSV in the presence of a negative result, testing can be repeated within a few months. The specificity of these assays is 96% or greater, and false-positive results can occur in individuals with a low likelihood of HSV infection.

Serologic screening for HSV is not recommended for the general population, but should be considered in women who experience recurrent or atypical genital symptoms with negative HSV cultures, have a clinical diagnosis of genital herpes without laboratory confirmation, present for STI evaluation (especially if they have multiple sexual partners), or have HIV. Testing should also be considered for asymptomatic partners of women with HSV infection (CDC, 2015d). All women with genital herpes should be tested for other STIs, including chlamydia, gonorrhea, syphilis, and HIV.

Differential Diagnoses

Differential diagnoses for HSV infection include syphilis, chancroid, lymphogranuloma venereum, and granuloma inguinale, as well as non-STI vulvar lesions such as those caused by Crohn's disease or Behcet's syndrome (Youngkin et al., 2013).

Prevention

There is currently no vaccine available to prevent HSV infection, so changes in sexual behavior are the only way to protect against this infection. Safer sexual practices are detailed in **Box 20-4** and **Table 20-2**. Although condoms provide some protection against HSV, they cover only a portion of the genital skin. Transmission of HSV via skin-to-skin contact can still occur among partners, even in the absence of symptoms (CDC, 2015d).

Management

Genital herpes is a chronic and recurring condition for which there is no known cure. Systemic antiviral drugs may partially control the symptoms and signs of HSV infections when used for primary or recurrent episodes, and they may completely control symptoms when used as daily suppressive therapy. These drugs do not cure the infection, however, nor do they alter the subsequent risk, frequency, or rate of recurrence after discontinuation. Three antiviral medications provide clinical benefits for genital herpes: acyclovir, valacyclovir, and famciclovir (**Table 20-4**). Topical antiviral therapy is not recommended due to its minimal benefits (CDC, 2015d).

Systemic antiviral therapy should be given to all individuals experiencing their first genital herpes episode. Most people with a symptomatic first episode of genital HSV-2 infection will experience recurrent episodes of genital lesions; by comparison, recurrence is less common among individuals with genital HSV-1 infection. Lifelong, intermittent, asymptomatic, genital shedding occurs in those persons who have HSV-2 infection. Recurrent genital herpes can be treated with daily suppressive therapy, which decreases the frequency of recurrences and the risk of transmitting HSV, or episodic therapy may be implemented when lesions occur to help them heal more quickly. Episodic therapy should be started within one day of when the lesion begins or during the prodromal symptoms if present. Individuals using episodic therapy should be provided with a prescription or medication in advance to facilitate immediate treatment of outbreaks. All women who have a history of HSV and desire suppressive therapy should be offered treatment if they do not have any contraindications to antiviral medications (CDC, 2015d).

Oral analgesics, such as aspirin or ibuprofen, may be used to relieve pain and systemic symptoms associated with initial infections. Any topical

TABLE 20-4	Treatment of Genital Herpes

Primary Infection[a]	Recurrent Infection	Suppressive Therapy
Acyclovir 400 mg orally 3 times a day for 7–10 days	Acyclovir 400 mg orally 3 times a day for 5 days	Acyclovir 400 mg orally 2 times a day
or	or	or
Acyclovir 200 mg orally 5 times a day for 7–10 days	Acyclovir 800 mg orally 2 times a day for 5 days	Famciclovir 250 mg orally 2 times a day
or	or	or
Famciclovir 250 mg orally 3 times a day for 7–10 days	Acyclovir 800 mg orally 3 times a day for 2 days	Valacyclovir 500 mg orally once a day (may be less effective than other valacyclovir or acyclovir dosing regiments in patients who have 10 or more episodes per year)
or	or	
Valacyclovir 1 gm orally 2 times a day for 7–10 days	Famciclovir 125 mg orally 2 times a day for 5 days	
	or	or
	Famciclovir 1,000 mg orally 2 times a day for 1 day	Valacyclovir 1 gm orally once a day
	or	
	Famciclovir 500 mg orally once, followed by 250 mg 2 times a day for 2 days	
	or	
	Valacyclovir 500 mg orally 2 times a day for 3 days	
	or	
	Valacyclovir 1 gm orally once a day for 5 days	

[a] Treatment can be extended if healing is incomplete after 10 days of therapy.
Modified from Centers for Disease Control and Prevention (CDC). (2015d). Sexually transmitted diseases treatment guidelines, 2015. *Morbidity and Mortality Weekly Report, 64*(3), 1–137.

agents should be used with caution, because the mucous membranes affected by herpes are very sensitive. Ointments containing cortisone should be avoided. Women should be informed that occlusive ointments may prolong the course of infections.

Complementary measures that may increase comfort for women when lesions are active include warm sitz baths; keeping lesions warm and dry by using a hair dryer set on cool or patting dry the area with a soft towel; wearing cotton underwear and loose clothing; applying cold milk or witch hazel compresses followed by aloe vera gel or Burrow's solution (Domeboro) to lesions four times a day for 30 minutes; oatmeal baths; applying cool, wet, black tea bags to lesions; and applying compresses with an infusion of cloves or peppermint oil and clove oil to lesions (Hawkins et al., 2016; Youngkin et al., 2013).

Many complementary and alternative products are used for genital herpes, although no or only limited evidence supports the effectiveness of most of these products. The amino acid L-lysine has been used for active lesions and suppression. It is thought that L-lysine has an inhibitory effect on the amino acid L-arginine, which supports HSV infection. Minimizing consumption of the foods that contain arginine may help as well; these foods include coffee, grains, chicken, chocolate, corn, dairy products, meat, peanut butter, nuts, and seeds. Avoiding citrus foods may also be helpful (Gaby, 2006; Hassan,

Masarcikova, & Berchova, 2015; Heslop, Jordan, Trivella, Papastamopoulos, & Roberts, 2013).

A number of herbal remedies may also help diminish the discomforts of herpes infections and possibly expedite healing of lesions. Zinc has been tested as an oral treatment and as applied via a topical solution or intravaginal sponges, but results have been conflicting and there is no recommended dose. Vitamin C, in doses up to 10,000 mg/day (or to bowel tolerance), can be considered during outbreaks (Gaby, 2006). Although data are limited, individuals using honey, propolis, lemon balm, and aloe vera as creams or ointments have reported improvement in symptoms in small studies (Gaby, 2006; Perfect, Bourne, Ebel, & Rosenthal, 2005). Echinacea extract has antiviral properties, stimulates the body's immune system, and may be taken orally or applied locally to reduce inflammation and pain. Data from studies examining echinacea for the treatment of HSV are limited and/or contradictory, and currently there is no clinical evidence to support its use for genital herpes.

Patient Education

Women should be advised that viral shedding—and, therefore, transmission of HSV to a partner—is most likely with active lesions, but can occur even when they are asymptomatic. Therefore, all current and future sex partners should be informed that the woman has genital HSV infection. Women whose partners do not have HSV infection should refrain from sexual contact from the onset of the prodrome until the complete healing of lesions. During asymptomatic periods, condoms and suppressive therapy can be used to reduce the risk of transmission to partners who do not have HSV infection.

Researchers have established the effectiveness of antiviral suppressive therapy among discordant couples (Lebrun-Vignes et al., 2007; Le Cleach et al., 2014). All women who are diagnosed with genital HSV should be informed of the availability of suppressive therapy that can help prevent transmission of the virus to partners.

Women should be taught how to examine themselves for herpetic lesions using a mirror and good light source. The clinician should ensure that women understand that when lesions are active, they should avoid sharing intimate articles (e.g., washcloths, wet towels, sex toys) that come into contact with the lesions.

Special Considerations

Pregnancy

HSV infection has significant implications for women and their neonates. Women should be educated about the risk of neonatal HSV infection and advised that if they become pregnant, they need to be certain to disclose their history of genital herpes to the clinicians providing their prenatal care and the care for their newborn (CDC, 2015d). Preventing neonatal herpes depends on preventing a primary infection in pregnant women during late pregnancy and avoiding exposure of the neonate to the HSV virus via shedding or exposure to active lesions during birth. Rates of HSV transmission to neonates are as high as 50% among women who first acquire HSV close to birth, but much lower in women with recurrent HSV or a more remote history of primary infection (CDC, 2015d).

Women who have not have genital HSV should be counseled to abstain from vaginal intercourse and receptive oral sex if their partner is known or suspected to have oral or genital HSV. Women with a known history of HSV should be questioned during labor about active lesions or prodromal symptoms. Women without lesions can give birth vaginally. Women who have active lesions at the time of labor should have a cesarean birth to decrease the possibility of transmission to their newborn. Women with a history of HSV can take suppressive acyclovir during the third trimester to reduce the risk of an outbreak during labor and subsequent need for cesarean birth (CDC, 2015d).

CHANCROID

Chancroid is a bacterial infection of the genitourinary tract caused by the gram-negative bacteria *Haemophilus ducreyi*. Chancroid is uncommon in the United States, with only 10 cases being reported in the country in 2013. This number may be an underestimate, however, reflecting the fact that the causative organism of chancroid is difficult to culture (CDC, 2014b, 2015d). Chancroid is a genital ulcer and, therefore, is a risk factor for HIV transmission. The major way chancroid is acquired is through sexual contact and trauma (CDC, 2015d), although infection through autoinoculation of fingers or other sites occasionally occurs. The incubation period for the infection, though not well established, usually ranges from 4 to 7 days but may be as long as 3 weeks (CDC, 2015d).

Most women with chancroid present with a history of a painful macule on the external genitalia that rapidly changes to a pustule and then to an ulcerated lesion (see **Color Plate 21**). They may also develop enlarged unilateral or bilateral inguinal nodes known as buboes. After 1 to 2 weeks, the skin overlying the lymph node becomes erythematous, the center necroses, and the node becomes ulcerated (Hawkins et al., 2016).

Assessment

A probable diagnosis of chancroid can be made when one or more painful genital ulcers are present; there is no evidence of syphilis (per dark-field examination of ulcer exudate or serologic testing at least 7 days after ulcer onset); the clinical presentation, ulcer appearance, and regional lymphadenopathy (if present) are typical for chancroid; and HSV testing of the exudate is negative (CDC, 2015d). Because chancroid is more prevalent in certain geographic areas and less common in the United States, women should be asked about recent travel to or sexual activity with a partner from Africa or the Caribbean, where chancroid outbreaks are more common (Hawkins et al., 2016). Definitive diagnosis of chancroid is difficult because the organism can be identified only by culture on a special medium that is not used routinely; even when this technique is used, the test's sensitivity is less than 80% (CDC, 2015d). Testing for HIV and syphilis should be performed at the time of diagnosis and repeated in 3 months if initial testing was negative.

Differential Diagnoses

Differential diagnoses include syphilis, HSV, lymphogranuloma venereum, folliculitis, metastatic genital cancer (cervical, vagina, vulvar), and other vulvar lesions (Hawkins et al., 2016; Youngkin et al., 2013).

Prevention

There is no vaccine to prevent chancroid. General STI prevention strategies are detailed in **Box 20-4** and **Table 20-2**.

Management

The recommended treatments for chancroid are azithromycin 1 gm orally in a single dose, ceftriaxone 250 mg IM in a single dose, ciprofloxacin 500 mg orally twice a day for 3 days, or erythromycin base 500 mg orally 4 times a day for 7 days (CDC, 2015d). Women with comorbid HIV infection may require repeated or longer therapy (CDC, 2015d).

Women should be reexamined 3 to 7 days after beginning therapy. If treatment is successful, symptomatic improvement should be apparent within 3 days of starting therapy. Objective clinical improvement should be noticeable on examination 7 days after treatment, although it may take more than 2 weeks for complete healing of large ulcers.

Patient Education

All sexual partners who have had sexual contact with a person diagnosed with chancroid within 10 days preceding the onset of that individual's symptoms should be evaluated and treated, regardless of whether symptoms are present (CDC, 2015d). Complete symptom resolution could take weeks and permanent scarring is possible, even with successful treatment.

Special Considerations

Pregnancy
Although ciprofloxacin is generally considered to be safe during pregnancy, toxicity has been reported among infants who are breastfeeding. Consequently, one of the other antibiotics recommended for chancroid should be used in women who are pregnant or breastfeeding (CDC, 2015d).

PEDICULOSIS PUBIS

Pediculosis is a parasitic infection caused by any of three species of lice: *Pediculosis humanus capitis* (head louse infecting the scalp), *Pediculosis humanus corporus* (body or clothing louse infecting the trunk), and *Phthirus pubis* (pubic lice or "crabs"). *P. pubis* inhabits the genital area but may also be found in other hair-bearing areas of the body, including the axillae, chest, thighs, eyelashes, and head. A woman may be infected through sexual transmission or contact with infected clothing or bedding (Hawkins et al., 2016).

Assessment

Individuals with pediculosis usually present with pruritus, caused by the lice ingesting saliva and then depositing digestive juices and feces into the skin. Women may report seeing the lice or known exposure to a household member or sexual partner with head, body, or pubic lice. A history of shared clothing, bathing equipment, or bedding may also be given. Diagnosis is made by direct examination of the egg cases (nits) in the involved area (see **Color Plate 22**). Although the nits are usually visible to the naked eye, a hand lens and light can be helpful in identifying them. Black dots (excreta) may be visible on the surrounding skin and underclothing, and crusts or scabs may be seen in the pubic area. Women with pediculosis pubis should be tested for other STIs (Hawkins et al., 2016).

Differential Diagnoses

Differential diagnoses include anogenital eczema and pruritus, seborrheic dermatitis, pruritus vulvae, folliculitis, tinea cruris, and scabies. Other concomitant STIs should be ruled out as well (Hawkins et al., 2016).

Prevention

General STI prevention strategies are detailed in **Box 20-4** and **Table 20-2**. Some evidence suggests that pubic hair removal is associated with a decreased rate of pubic lice, but there is no current recommendation to use this as a mechanism to reduce the risk of infection (Dholakia et al., 2014).

Management

Recommended treatments for pediculosis pubis include permethrin 1% cream rinse and pyrethrins with piperonyl butoxide. These medications are applied to the affected areas and washed off after 10 minutes. If symptoms do not resolve within a week and treatment failure is thought to be due to drug resistance, an alternative regimen consists of Malathion 0.5% lotion applied for 8 to 12 hours and washed off. Oral ivermectin (250 mcg/kg) taken initially and repeated in 2 weeks is another alternative regimen, although this medication has limited ovicidal activity. Taking ivermectin with food increases this medication's bioavailability (CDC, 2015d).

Patient Education

Advise women with pediculosis to wash all clothing, bed linens, and towels in hot water and to dry these items thoroughly on the hot cycle to destroy lice and nits. During treatment with topical agents, care should be taken to avoid contact with the eyes. Sexual partners within the past month should be evaluated and treated if necessary. Sexual contact should be avoided until the woman and her partner(s) have been successfully treated and all linens and clothing have been decontaminated (CDC, 2015d; Hawkins et al., 2016).

Special Considerations

Pregnancy

Pregnant women with pubic lice should be treated. Permethrin or pyrethrins with piperonyl butoxide are recommended. Additionally, ivermectin is considered to be compatible with pregnancy and lactation and can be used as an additional or alternative treatment. In contrast, topical lindane has been shown to cause fetal harm and should not be used during pregnancy (CDC, 2015d).

TRICHOMONIASIS

Trichomoniasis is caused by *Trichomonas vaginalis*, an anaerobic one-celled protozoan with characteristic flagellae. This organism most commonly lives in the vagina in women, and in the urethra in men. Among women presenting with vaginitis symptoms, 4% to 35% will have trichomoniasis. The prevalence of *T. vaginalis* has been reported by researchers as approximately 4.1% for white women and 16.1% for black women (Rogers et al., 2014). Higher rates have been seen in specific populations of women, including those who are incarcerated and women who seek care at STI clinics (Alcaide et al., 2015). Trichomoniasis is sexually transmitted during vaginal–penile intercourse or vulva-to-vulva contact. Nonsexual transmission is possible but rare. Trichomoniasis is strongly associated with an increased risk of HIV transmission (Rogers et al., 2014; Van Der Pol et al., 2008).

Although trichomoniasis is often asymptomatic, women can experience a characteristically yellow to greenish, frothy, mucopurulent, copious, malodorous discharge. Inflammation of the vulva, vagina, or both may be present, and the woman may have irritation, pruritus, dysuria, or dyspareunia. Typically, the discharge worsens during and after menstruation (CDC, 2015d).

Assessment

In addition to the history of current symptoms, a careful sexual history, including information on last intercourse and last sexual contract, should be obtained from the woman with suspected trichomoniasis. Any history of similar symptoms in the past and treatment used should be noted. The clinician should determine whether the woman's partners were treated and whether she has engaged in subsequent relations with new partners. Additional important information includes the last menstrual period, method of contraception, condom use, and use of other medications (Hawkins et al., 2016).

Inspect the external genitalia for excoriation, erythema, edema, ulceration, and lesions. On speculum examination, note the quantity, color, consistency, and any odor of the vaginal discharge. In women with trichomoniasis, the cervix and vaginal walls may demonstrate characteristic "strawberry spots," or tiny petechiae, especially after prolonged infection (see **Color Plate 23**), and the cervix may bleed on contact. In severe infections, the vaginal walls, the cervix, and occasionally the vulva may be acutely inflamed. The pH of vaginal discharge is elevated (Carcio & Secor, 2015; Hawkins et al., 2016).

Diagnosis is usually made by visualization of the typical one-celled flagellate trichomonads on microscopic examination of vaginal discharge (**Figure 20-1**), although this method has a sensitivity of only approximately 51% to 65%. The slide must be viewed immediately to ensure optimal results. Nonmotile trichomonads are more challenging to recognize. Microscopic examination of the wet mount may also reveal increased numbers of white blood cells, and a strong amine odor will be produced with the addition of potassium hydroxide (KOH) to the specimen. Point-of-care tests are also available that typically have higher sensitivity (more than 82%) and specificity (more than 95%) (CDC, 2015d).

Culture is a sensitive and highly specific method of diagnosis, but is no longer routinely performed because of the availability of nucleic acid amplification tests (NAATs). Culture should be performed when trichomoniasis is suspected but cannot be confirmed with microscopy or NAAT is not available. Although *T. vaginalis* may be an incidental finding on a Pap test, this test is not considered diagnostic (even with liquid-based specimens), and confirmatory testing is still needed. All patients with trichomoniasis should be tested for other STIs, including chlamydia, gonorrhea, syphilis, and HIV (CDC, 2015d).

Differential Diagnoses

Differential diagnoses for trichomoniasis include other conditions that cause vaginal discharge (see Chapter 19), such as vulvovaginal candidiasis, bacterial vaginosis, chlamydia, and gonorrhea (Youngkin et al., 2013).

Prevention

General STI prevention strategies are detailed in **Box 20-4** and **Table 20-2**.

Management

The nitroimidazoles are the only antimicrobial medications that are effective against *T. vaginalis*. The recommended treatment for trichomoniasis is metronidazole 2 gm orally in a single dose or tinidazole 2 gm orally in a single dose. Tinidazole is equivalent or superior to metronidazole in terms of cure and symptom resolution, and has fewer gastrointestinal side effects, but is more expensive than metronidazole. Topical metronidazole is less effective and not recommended.

Most reoccurrences of trichomoniasis are thought to be due to reinfection. If single-dose metronidazole treatment fails and reinfection is excluded, metronidazole 500 mg orally twice a day for 7 days should be prescribed. If infection persists, consider metronidazole or tinidazole 2 gm orally for 7 days. If infection persists, consultation with a specialist is warranted (CDC, 2015d).

Patient Education

When taking metronidazole or tinidazole, women should be educated not to drink alcoholic beverages due to the high likelihood of experiencing a disulfiram-like reaction, including severe abdominal

| FIGURE 20-1 | Wet mount findings with trichomoniasis. |

Note: Trichomonads must be motile for conclusive diagnosis.
Abbreviation: PMNs, polymorphonuclear leukocytes/white blood cells.
Used with permission from Washington State Department of Health STD/TB Program, Seattle STD/HIV Prevention Training Center, and Cindy Fennell, MS, MT, ASCP.

distress, nausea, vomiting, and headache. Abstinence from alcohol should continue 24 hours after completing metronidazole treatment and 72 hours after completing tinidazole treatment.

Sex partners of women with trichomoniasis should be treated as well as the women themselves, and all individuals should abstain from sex until both partners have been treated and are asymptomatic. Because rates of reinfection have been documented as high as 17% within the first 3 months after treatment, women should be evaluated within this time frame even if they and their partners have completed treatment (CDC, 2015d).

Special Considerations

Pregnancy

Pregnant women with trichomoniasis are at risk for pregnancy complications, including premature rupture of membranes (PROM), preterm labor and birth, and low-birth-weight infants (Silver, Guy, Kaldor, Jamil, & Rumbold, 2014). Treatment during pregnancy has not been shown to reduce perinatal morbidity. Recommended treatment for pregnant women with trichomoniasis is metronidazole 2 gm orally as a single dose.

Routine screening for asymptomatic pregnant women is currently not recommended unless the woman has HIV. Trichomoniasis infection is a risk for vertical HIV transmission, and all pregnant women who have HIV should be promptly treated for trichomoniasis if infection is suspected or diagnosed (CDC, 2015d).

Women with HIV Infection
Women with HIV are at increased risk for infection with *T. vaginalis.* It is estimated that more than 50% of women with HIV may also be infected with *T. vaginalis* at some point in time, and this coinfection significantly increases their risk for PID. Recommended screening for *T. vaginalis* among women with HIV includes screening upon entry to care and at least annually; more frequent screening can occur based on the woman's specific history and symptoms.

The recommended treatment for trichomoniasis in women with HIV infection is metronidazole 500 mg orally twice daily for 7 days. Treatment with a single 2 mg dose is less effective among women with HIV (CDC, 2015d).

CHLAMYDIA

Chlamydia, which is caused by the bacterium *Chlamydia trachomatis*, is the most commonly reported nationally notifiable infection in the United States and the most common bacterial STI. More than 1.45 million cases were reported to the CDC in 2013, with at least that many more estimated to have gone undetected (CDC, 2014b). Sexually active adolescents and women aged 15 to 24 years of age have nearly three times the prevalence of chlamydia as women aged 25 and 39 years, and women are infected at a rate of two times that of men. The prevalence of chlamydia is six times higher in black women than in white women (CDC, 2014b). Risk factors for this infection include multiple sexual partners and failure to use barrier methods of contraception. The most serious complication of chlamydial infections for women is PID (see the section on PID later in this chapter).

Assessment

When assessing patients for chlamydia, in addition to obtaining information about any risk factors, inquire about the presence of any symptoms, while recognizing that chlamydia is usually asymptomatic. Women experiencing symptoms may report vaginal spotting or postcoital bleeding, mucoid or purulent cervical discharge, urinary frequency, dysuria, lower abdominal pain, or dyspareunia. Bleeding results from inflammation and erosion of the cervical columnar epithelium. Symptoms of chlamydia infection in women may mimic those of a urinary tract infection (UTI). In sexually active women who present with urinary symptoms only, it may be prudent to test a urine sample for chlamydia if urine is already being collected for dipstick analysis or culture (Hawkins et al., 2016).

Physical examination findings of abdominal guarding, referred pain, or rebound tenderness upon abdominal examination should raise the level of suspicion for PID. Cervical friability may be detected with the speculum examination. Discharge, if present, is characteristically mucopurulent (see **Color Plate 24**). During the bimanual examination, a woman may report cervical motion tenderness (pain with cervical movement), and the examiner may detect adnexal fullness and uterine tenderness. These findings are also suggestive of PID (Hawkins et al., 2016).

In recent years, the CDC has expanded recommendations for chlamydia screening among asymptomatic women. All sexually active women younger than 25 years should be screened for chlamydia annually (CDC, 2014b, 2015d). Women 25 years and older with risk factors (e.g., new or multiple partners, partner with an STI, partner with other partners) should also be screened.

Chlamydia testing can be performed using first-catch urine or swab specimens from the endocervix or vagina. Screening procedures for chlamydial infection include NAATs, cell culture, direct immunofluorescence, enzyme immunoassay (EIA), and nucleic acid hybridization tests. NAATs are the preferred technique because they provide the highest sensitivity (see Chapter 6). Although less sensitive than urine or cervical/vaginal swabs, NAATs can also be used with liquid-based Pap tests. All patients with chlamydia should be tested for other STIs, including gonorrhea, syphilis, and HIV (CDC, 2015d).

Differential Diagnoses

Differential diagnoses for chlamydia include gonorrhea, trichomoniasis, PID, appendicitis, and cystitis (Hawkins et al., 2016; Youngkin et al., 2013).

TABLE 20-5 — Treatment of Chlamydial Infections

Recommended Regimens	Alternative Regimens
Azithromycin 1 gm orally in a single dose **or** Doxycycline 100 mg orally 2 times a day for 7 days	Erythromycin base 500 mg orally 4 times a day for 7 days **or** Erythromycin ethylsuccinate 800 mg orally 4 times a day for 7 days **or** Levofloxacin 500 mg orally once daily for 7 days **or** Ofloxacin 300 mg orally 2 times a day for 7 days

Modified from Centers for Disease Control and Prevention (CDC). (2015d). Sexually transmitted diseases treatment guidelines, 2015. *Morbidity and Mortality Weekly Report, 64*(3), 1–137.

Prevention

General STI prevention strategies are detailed in **Box 20-4** and **Table 20-2**.

Management

Recommendations for treatment of chlamydial infections are found in **Table 20-5**. Treatment of current and recent sexual partners is imperative. A test of cure (3–4 weeks after treatment) is not necessary unless a woman is pregnant, has persistent symptoms, was unable to complete treatment, or may have been re-exposed or reinfected. A high prevalence of reinfection is observed in women who have had chlamydial infections in the preceding several months, usually from reinfection by an untreated partner. Clinicians should advise all individuals with chlamydia to be rescreened 3 months after treatment to assess for reinfection (CDC, 2015d).

Treatment should be given as soon as possible after diagnosis, as a delay may increase a woman's chances of developing PID.

Patient Education

All of the woman's sexual partners in the past 60 days should be referred for testing and possible treatment. If partners are unable or unwilling to be evaluated by a healthcare provider, expedited partner therapy (EPT) should be considered if permitted by state law. EPT is the practice of treating sexual partners of individuals who have been diagnosed with chlamydia by providing medication or prescriptions for medication to the individual to provide to

the partner. Examination of the partner is not necessary (CDC, 2015d). Women should be advised to abstain from sex until their sexual partners are treated and to wait 7 days after single-dose treatment or until completion of a 7-day regimen before resuming sexual activity.

Special Considerations

Pregnancy

All pregnant women younger than 25 years should be screened for chlamydia at their first prenatal visit. Women aged 25 and older should be screened based upon risk factors (see the "Assessment" section). Asymptomatic screening in pregnancy may also be considered for women living in communities with high rates of documented chlamydia infections.

Pregnant women who are diagnosed with chlamydia should have a test of cure 3 to 4 weeks after the completion of treatment and again in 3 months to reduce the risk of neonatal transmission and infection. Chlamydia infection can cause conjunctivitis and pneumonia in newborns. Pregnant women should be treated with a macrolide antibiotic (i.e., azithromycin or erythromycin). Doxycycline is known to discolor teeth and should be avoided in the second and third trimesters.

GONORRHEA

Gonorrhea, which is caused by the aerobic, gram-negative diplococcus *Neisseria gonorrhoeae*, is the second most commonly reported bacterial STI in the United States, after chlamydia. In 2013, 333,004 cases of gonorrhea were reported in the United States, although it is estimated that more than twice this number occurred but were not diagnosed or reported. The rate of infection was slightly higher in men than in women (109.5/100,000 versus 102.4/100,000, respectively). Gonorrhea rates are highest among adolescents and young adult women aged 15 to 24 years. The rate of gonorrhea in black women is more than 12 times the rate in white women (CDC, 2014b).

Gonorrhea is almost exclusively transmitted by sexual activity, primarily through genital-to-genital contact; however, it is also spread by oral-to-genital and anal-to-genital contact. Sites of infection in females include the cervix, urethra, oropharynx, Skene's glands, and Bartholin's glands. In addition to age, other risk factors for this infection include early onset of sexual activity and multiple sexual partners.

The main complication of gonorrheal infections is PID. Women may also develop a pelvic abscess or Bartholin's abscess. Disseminated gonococcal infection (DGI) is a rare (0.5–3%) complication of untreated gonorrhea. DGI occurs in two stages: The first stage is characterized by bacteremia with chills, fever, and skin lesions; it is followed by the second stage during which the patient experiences acute septic arthritis with characteristic effusions, most commonly in the wrists, knees, and ankles (CDC, 2015d; Hawkins et al., 2016).

Assessment

Women with gonorrhea often remain asymptomatic, with as many as 80% of women having no symptoms from this infection (Hawkins et al., 2016). When symptoms are present, they are often less specific than the symptoms in men. Women may report dyspareunia, a change in vaginal discharge, unilateral labial pain and swelling, or lower abdominal discomfort. Later in the infection's course, women may describe a history of purulent, irritating vaginal discharge, or rectal pain and discharge. Menstrual irregularities may be the presenting symptom, with longer, more painful menses being noted. Women may also report chronic or acute lower abdominal pain. Unilateral labial pain and swelling may indicate Bartholin's gland infection (see Chapter 19), whereas periurethral pain and swelling may indicate inflamed Skene's glands.

Infrequently, dysuria, vague abdominal pain, or low backache prompts women to seek care. Later symptoms may include fever (possibly high), nausea, vomiting, joint pain and swelling, or upper abdominal pain (liver involvement) (Hawkins et al., 2016; Marrazzo & Cates, 2011).

Women may develop a gonococcal rectal infection following anal intercourse, in which case they may report symptoms of profuse purulent anal discharge, rectal pain, and blood in the stool. Rectal itching, fullness, pressure, and pain are also commonly noted symptoms. Women with gonococcal pharyngitis may appear to have viral pharyngitis, as some individuals will have a red, swollen uvula and pustule vesicles on the soft palate and tonsils similar to streptococcal infections (Hawkins et al., 2016).

Physical examination is individualized based on the woman's presenting symptoms. The clinician should obtain vital signs and perform a general skin inspection for signs of classic DGI lesions, which are painful necrotic pustules on an erythematous base, approximately 1 mm to 2 cm in diameter. Inspect the pharynx and oral cavity for erythema, edema, and lesions. Assess for cervical lymphadenopathy. Palpate the abdomen for masses, tenderness, and rebound tenderness. During the speculum examination, inspect the vaginal walls for discharge and redness, and examine the cervix for mucopurulent discharge, ectopy, and friability (see **Color Plate 25**). During the bimanual examination, observe for cervical motion tenderness, uterine tenderness, adnexal tenderness, and adnexal masses—all of these findings are associated with PID (Hawkins et al., 2016).

Annual screening for gonorrhea is recommended for all sexually active women younger than 25 years. Women who are 25 or older should be screened based on risk factors such as inconsistent or absent condom use, new or multiple partners, partner with an STI or other partners, and exchange of sex for drugs or money. Clinicians should also inquire about recent travel that included sexual partners outside the United States (CDC, 2015d).

Gonorrhea testing can be performed by culture and NAATs. NAATs can be performed using urine or swab specimens from the endocervix or vagina. Although the U.S. Food and Drug Administration (FDA) has not formally approved NAATs for use in the rectum or pharynx, some laboratories have established performance specifications for using these tests with specimens from these sites. NAAT products vary, however, and clinicians must be certain that the test they are using is appropriate for the specimen type (CDC, 2015d). Culture is also available for the detection of gonorrhea infection of the rectum and pharynx. All patients with gonorrhea should be offered testing for other STIs, including chlamydia, syphilis, and HIV.

Differential Diagnoses

Differential diagnoses for gonorrhea include chlamydia, trichomoniasis, PID, appendicitis, and cystitis (Hawkins et al., 2016; Youngkin et al., 2013).

Prevention

General STI prevention strategies are detailed in **Box 20-4** and **Table 20-2**.

Management

Recommended therapies for gonorrhea are listed in **Box 20-6**. Treatment of current and recent sexual partners is imperative. Patients who are treated for gonorrhea should be concomitantly treated for chlamydia because coinfection rates are high, and dual therapy may help hinder the development of antimicrobial-resistant *N. gonorrhoeae*. Quinolones are no longer used to treat gonorrhea because of the high prevalence of quinolone-resistant strains of the organism (CDC, 2015d).

A test of cure (typically performed 3–4 weeks after treatment) is not necessary (CDC, 2015d). Decreased susceptibility of the infectious organism to cefixime has been reported, which has raised concerns about the potential for development of cephalosporin-resistant strains of *N. gonorrhoeae*. Additionally, cefixime has decreased efficacy against pharyngeal gonorrhea. Treatment with cefixime should be considered only if ceftriaxone is not available. It should not be prescribed based on the patient's preference for an oral medication instead of an injection or the patient not wanting to return to the office for treatment.

Clinicians must be vigilant for treatment failures (CDC, 2015d). Individuals whose symptoms do not resolve after treatment should have a culture, with

---

BOX 20-6 **Treatment of Uncomplicated Gonococcal Infections of the Cervix, Urethra, and Rectum**

Ceftriaxone 250 mg IM in a single dose

or

Cefixime 400 mg orally in a single dose[a]

or

Other single-dose injectable cephalosporin regimens[b] (ceftizoxime 500 mg IM, cefoxitin 2g IM with probenecid 1 gm orally, or cefotaxime 500 mg IM)

plus

Azithromycin 1 gm orally in a single dose (preferred)

or

Doxycycline 100 mg orally 2 times a day for 7 days

Abbreviation: IM, intramuscularly.
[a] Consider only as an alternative due to its decreased efficacy and increasing resistance.
[b] Do not offer any advantage over ceftriaxone for urogenital infection, and efficacy for pharyngeal infection is less certain.
Data from Centers for Disease Control and Prevention (CDC). (2015d). Sexually transmitted diseases treatment guidelines, 2015. *Morbidity and Mortality Weekly Report, 64*(3), 1–137.

---

any gonococci that are isolated being tested for antimicrobial susceptibility. All individuals with gonorrhea should be retested 3 months after treatment due to the high rate of reinfection (CDC, 2015d).

Patient Education

If a woman has gonorrhea, all of her partners within the past 60 days or the last partner outside of that time period should be tested and treated. Women and their partners should abstain from sexual activity for 7 days after single-dose injection treatment or during oral therapy to avoid reinfection (CDC, 2015d). The rationale for cotreatment for chlamydia should be explained. Safer sexual practices and strategies to prevent future infections need to be discussed in a nonjudgmental conversation.

Special Considerations

Pregnancy

All pregnant women younger than 25 years should be screened for gonorrhea at their first prenatal visit. Women aged 25 and older should be screened based upon risk factors. Asymptomatic screening in pregnancy may also be considered for women living in communities with high rates of documented gonococcal infections. Women who were diagnosed with gonorrhea in the first trimester and women who remain at high risk for gonorrhea throughout their pregnancies should be retested in the third trimester prior to birth to prevent maternal complications and neonatal infection. Gonorrhea can cause conjunctivitis in newborns. Pregnant women should be treated with dual therapy consisting of ceftriaxone 250 mg IM and azithromycin 1gm orally as a single dose. If a woman is allergic to these medications, consultation with an infectious disease specialist is indicated (CDC, 2015d).

PELVIC INFLAMMATORY DISEASE

PID occurs in the upper female genital tract and includes any combination of endometritis, salpingitis, tubo-ovarian abscess, and pelvic peritonitis (CDC, 2015d). Each year, more than 750,000 women in the United States will have an episode of acute PID (Brunham, Gottleib, & Paavonen, 2015; Goyal et al., 2013). This estimate does not include women who have PID that is undiagnosed because it is asymptomatic or presents atypically (Soper, 2010). Adolescents have the highest risk of developing PID because of their decreased immunity to infectious organisms and increased risk of contracting gonorrhea and chlamydia (Goyal et al., 2013; Youngkin et al., 2013).

Multiple organisms have been found to cause PID, and most cases are associated with infection by more than one organism. Common causative agents include *N. gonorrhoeae* and *C. trachomatis*. In addition to the pathogens that cause gonorrhea and chlamydia, a wide variety of anaerobic and aerobic microorganisms, including some found in the vaginal flora, are associated with PID (Brunham et al., 2015; CDC, 2015d)—for example, *Gardnerella vaginalis, Haemophilus influenzae,* and *Mycoplasma genitalium*. Bacterial vaginosis is common in women with PID and may facilitate the ascent of microorganisms into the upper genital tract, but it remains unclear whether treating bacterial vaginosis can reduce the incidence of PID (CDC, 2015d; Soper, 2010).

Major health complications are associated with PID. Acute and chronic reproductive sequelae include tubo-ovarian abscess, ectopic pregnancy, infertility, chronic pelvic and abdominal pain, dyspareunia, and recurring PID. Although rare, inflammation of the liver capsule (Fitz-Hugh-Curtis syndrome) can also occur with PID (Brunham et al., 2015; Soper, 2010).

As noted earlier, PID may be caused by a variety of infectious agents, and it encompasses a wide variety of pathologic processes; therefore, the infection can be acute, subacute, or chronic, and may be associated with a wide range of symptoms. Diagnosis of PID is difficult because almost all of the most common signs and symptoms could accompany other urinary, gastrointestinal, or gynecologic tract problems. Accurate and prompt diagnosis is crucial to minimize long-term sequelae; thus, clinicians should maintain a high suspicion for PID and a low threshold for its diagnosis and treatment (Brunham et al., 2015; CDC, 2015d).

Assessment

When PID is suspected, the history taking must be comprehensive. Relevant history includes recent pelvic surgery, abortion, childbirth, dilation of the cervix, and insertion of an intrauterine device (IUD) within the last month. A thorough sexual risk history should be obtained, including the current or most recent sexual activity, number of partners, and method of contraception; this information will assist the clinician in identifying possible increased risk for STI exposure.

The severity and extent of symptoms that women with PID experience vary widely. Historically, the abrupt onset of acute lower abdominal pain following menses has been considered the characteristic presenting symptom of PID. More recently, it has been recognized that symptoms of this infection can be very mild and nonspecific. Commonly reported symptoms include abdominal, pelvic, and low back pain; abnormal vaginal discharge; intermenstrual or postcoital bleeding; fever; nausea and vomiting; and urinary frequency (Brunham et al., 2015). Women may report levels of pain ranging from minimal discomfort to dull, cramping, and intermittent pain to severe, persistent, and incapacitating pain. Pelvic pain is usually exacerbated by the Valsalva maneuver, intercourse, or movement. Symptoms of STIs in a woman's partners also should be noted.

As part of the assessment for PID, the clinician should obtain vital signs and perform a complete physical examination. While fever may be present, the majority of women with PID are afebrile when they present for evaluation (Brunham et al., 2015). Thus, absence of fever does not rule out PID. Physical examination may reveal adnexal tenderness, abdominal tenderness, uterine tenderness, and tenderness with cervical movement. Pelvic tenderness is usually bilateral. There may or may not be a palpable adnexal swelling or thickening. A pelvic mass suggests tubo-ovarian abscess.

A clinical diagnosis of PID is often made based on findings of pelvic organ tenderness and signs of lower genital tract infection, including mucopurulent cervicitis and cervical friability (Brunham et al., 2015). There is no single laboratory test that can be used to detect upper genital tract infections. Instead, a pH test and wet mount of the vaginal secretions should be performed, along with tests for chlamydia and gonorrhea, although negative results do not rule out these infections' presence in the upper genital tract. Other laboratory tests that are not needed for diagnosis but are recommended for women with clinically severe PID are a complete blood count (CBC) and erythrocyte sedimentation rate (ESR), which, if positive, increase the specificity of the PID diagnosis (Brunham et al., 2015). All women with PID should be offered testing for syphilis and HIV as well. Laboratory data are useful only when considered in conjunction with the history and physical examination findings. Pelvic ultrasound should be performed in women requiring hospitalization and those with a pelvic mass found on examination (Brunham et al., 2015).

Clinical diagnosis of PID is imprecise; nevertheless, most diagnoses of PID are made clinically because laparoscopy and biopsy are too expensive and invasive to be practical screening tools. In 2002 (reaffirmed in 2015), the CDC established new minimum criteria for beginning treatment of PID (**Box 20-7**), in recognition of the fact that delay in diagnosis and treatment of PID is associated with severe sequelae. In addition, a diagnosis of PID should be considered in a woman with any of the common symptoms of PID (CDC, 2015d).

Differential Diagnoses

Symptoms of PID may mimic those associated with other conditions such as ectopic pregnancy, endometriosis, ovarian cyst with torsion, pelvic adhesions, inflammatory bowel disease, and acute appendicitis (Hawkins et al., 2016; Youngkin et al., 2013).

Prevention

Perhaps the most important action a clinician can take to prevent PID in women is counseling. Primary prevention consists of education about avoiding STIs, whereas secondary prevention involves prompt treatment of lower genital tract infections to prevent ascension to the upper genital tract. Instructing women in self-protective behaviors such as practicing safer sex and using barrier contraceptive methods is critical (see **Box 20-4** and **Table 20-2**). Also important is the detection of asymptomatic gonorrheal and chlamydial infections through routine screening of women with risk factors. Partner notification when an STI is diagnosed is essential to prevent reinfection (Brunham et al., 2015).

Management

In the past, the majority of women with PID were hospitalized so that bed rest and parenteral therapy could be started. Today, most women with PID receive outpatient treatment, especially for mild PID, and do not experience any adverse reproductive outcomes (Savaris, Ross, Fuhrich, Rodriguez-Malagon, & Duarte, 2013). The decision of whether to hospitalize a woman should be based on each woman's individual circumstances. To guide clinicians' decisions regarding hospitalization, the CDC (2015d) has developed specific criteria for hospitalization, including the need to rule out surgical emergencies (e.g., appendicitis); pregnancy; no

BOX 20-7 Diagnosing Pelvic Inflammatory Disease

Empiric treatment of PID should be initiated in sexually active young women and other women at risk for STIs if they are experiencing pelvic or lower abdominal pain, if no cause for the illness other than PID can be found, and if one or more of the following minimum criteria are present on pelvic examination:

- Cervical motion tenderness
- Uterine tenderness
- Adnexal tenderness

One or more of the following additional criteria can be used to enhance the specificity of the minimum criteria and support a diagnosis of PID:

- Oral temperature $>$ 101°F (38.3°C)
- Abnormal cervical or vaginal mucopurulent discharge
- Presence of abundant numbers of white blood cells on saline microscopy of vaginal fluid
- Elevated erythrocyte sedimentation rate
- Elevated C-reactive protein level
- Laboratory documentation of cervical infection with *N. gonorrhoeae* or *C. trachomatis*

The most specific criteria for diagnosing PID include the following conditions:

- Endometrial biopsy with histopathologic evidence of endometritis
- Transvaginal sonography or magnetic resonance imaging techniques showing thickened, fluid-filled tubes with or without free pelvic fluid or tubo-ovarian complex, or Doppler studies suggesting pelvic infection (e.g., tubal hyperemia)
- Laparoscopic abnormalities consistent with PID

Abbreviations: PID, pelvic inflammatory disease; STIs, sexually transmitted infections.
Modified from Centers for Disease Control and Prevention (CDC). (2015d). Sexually transmitted diseases treatment guidelines, 2015. *Morbidity and Mortality Weekly Report, 64*(3), 1–137.

clinical response to oral antimicrobial therapy; inability to follow or tolerate an outpatient oral regimen; severe illness, nausea and vomiting, or high fever; and tubo-ovarian abscess. At present, no data exist to suggest that adolescents would benefit from hospitalization for treatment due to their age alone.

Although treatment regimens vary with the infecting organism, broad-spectrum antibiotics are generally administered. Several antimicrobial regimens have proved to be effective, and no single therapeutic regimen appears to be superior to the others (**Table 20-6**). Substantial clinical improvement should occur within 72 hours of beginning treatment. Women who do not respond within this time frame should be reevaluated to confirm the diagnosis of PID; they may also need hospitalization (if being treated on an outpatient basis), additional testing, and surgical intervention. Women who do not respond to oral therapy and have a confirmed diagnosis of PID should be treated with an inpatient or outpatient parenteral regimen. Women on parenteral regimens can usually be transitioned to oral therapy 24 to 48 hours after they begin to show clinical improvement.

Minimal pelvic examinations should be done during the acute phase of PID, and analgesics can be given for pain. During the recovery phase, the woman should restrict her activity and make every

TABLE 20-6	Treatment of Pelvic Inflammatory Disease

Parenteral Regimens	Oral/Intramuscular Regimens
Cefotetan 2 gm IV every 12 hours **plus** Doxycycline 100 mg orally or IV every 12 hours **or** Cefoxitin 2 gm IV every 6 hours **plus** Doxycycline 100 mg orally or IV every 12 hours **or** Clindamycin 900 mg IV every 8 hours **plus** Gentamicin loading dose IV or IM (2 mg/kg of body weight), followed by a maintenance dose (1.5 mg/kg) every 8 hours. Single-day dosing (3–5 mg/kg) may be substituted. ***Alternative parenteral regimen:*** Ampicillin/sulbactam 3 gm IV every 6 hours **plus** Doxycycline 100 mg orally or IV every 12 hours	Ceftriaxone 250 mg IM in a single dose **plus** Doxycycline 100 mg orally 2 times a day for 14 days **with[a] or without** Metronidazole 500 mg orally 2 times a day for 14 days **or** Cefoxitin 2 gm IM in a single dose and probenecid 1 gm orally administered concurrently in a single dose **plus** Doxycycline 100 mg orally 2 times a day for 14 days **with or without** Metronidazole 500 mg orally 2 times a day for 14 days **or** Other parenteral third-generation cephalosporin (e.g., ceftizoxime or cefotaxime) **plus** Doxycycline 100 mg orally twice a day for 14 days **with[a] or without** Metronidazole 500 mg orally twice a day for 14 days

Abbreviation: IM, intramuscularly; IV, intravenously.
[a] Recommended third-generation cephalosporins provide limited anaerobe coverage. If it is not known whether extended anaerobe coverage is necessary, the addition of metronidazole to the treatment regimens that include third-generation cephalosporins should be considered.
Modified from Centers for Disease Control and Prevention (CDC). (2015d). Sexually transmitted diseases treatment guidelines, 2015. *Morbidity and Mortality Weekly Report, 64*(3), 1–137.

effort to obtain adequate rest and consume a nutritionally sound diet. Women with PID who had a positive test for gonorrhea or chlamydia should have repeat testing for these pathogens 3 to 6 months after treatment (CDC, 2015d).

Patient Education

Health education is central to effective management of PID. Women should abstain from sexual activity until treatment has been completed, symptoms have resolved, and sexual partners have been adequately treated. Male sexual partners within the past 60 days preceding the onset of symptoms should be evaluated, tested, and treated presumptively for gonorrhea and chlamydia (CDC, 2015d). Clinicians should explain to women the nature of their infection and encourage them to adhere to all therapy and prevention recommendations, emphasizing the necessity of taking all medication, even if their symptoms resolve before the course of therapy is completed.

Any potential problems that would prevent a woman from completing a course of treatment, such as lack of money for prescriptions or lack of transportation to return to a clinic for follow-up appointments, should be identified and the importance of follow-up visits emphasized.

The woman diagnosed with PID will need supportive care, because PID is so closely tied to sexuality, body image, and self-concept. Her feelings need to be discussed, and her partners included in the counseling when appropriate (Hawkins et al., 2016).

Special Considerations

Pregnancy

Pregnant women who have PID are at significant risk for maternal morbidity and preterm birth. They should be hospitalized and treated as inpatients with parenteral antibiotics. Doxycycline is known to discolor teeth and should be avoided in the second and third trimesters. Consultation with an infectious disease specialist is warranted when a woman has multiple antibiotic allergies (CDC, 2015d).

Women Using an Intrauterine Device

Many women use either copper-containing or levonorgestrel-releasing IUDs for contraception (see Chapter 11). An increased risk of PID is seen in the first 21 days after IUD insertion. If a woman who is using either type of IUD is also diagnosed with PID, the device does not need to be removed immediately; indeed, it often does not need to be removed at all. Treatment should be initiated with a recommended antibiotic regimen. If no improvement is seen with 48 to 72 hours after beginning treatment, the IUD should be removed (CDC, 2015d).

SYPHILIS

Syphilis is a systemic disease caused by *Treponema pallidum*, a motile spirochete. In 2013, more than 55,000 cases of syphilis were reported in the United States, including more than 17,000 cases of primary and secondary syphilis (CDC, 2014b). Syphilis rates are higher among black women than they are among white and Hispanic women. In 2013, the male-to-female ratio for primary and secondary syphilis was 11.3:1, a rate that doubled during the previous 10 years. This difference is largely due to the number of men who have sex with men who are unaware they have syphilis. In contrast to other bacterial STIs that affect mostly adolescents and adults younger than 25 years, syphilis rates are highest among men between the ages of 20 and 29 (CDC, 2014b).

Syphilis is a complex infection that can lead to serious systemic disease and even death when untreated. The infection can affect any tissue or organ in the body. Transmission is thought to occur by entry into the subcutaneous tissue through microscopic abrasions that can be created during sexual intercourse. The infection can also be transmitted through kissing, biting, or oral–genital sex.

Syphilis is characterized by periods of active symptoms and periods of asymptomatic latency. It is divided into stages based on clinical findings, which helps guide treatment decisions (**Table 20-7**).

Primary syphilis is characterized by a primary lesion, or a chancre, which often begins as a painless papule at the site of inoculation and then erodes to form a nontender, shallow, indurated, clean ulcer that is several millimeters to a few centimeters in size (see **Color Plate 26A**). The chancre contains spirochetes and is most commonly found on the genitalia, although it may also occur on the cervix, perianal area, or mouth (Hawkins et al., 2016).

Secondary syphilis is characterized by a widespread, symmetrical maculopapular rash on the palms of the hands and soles of the feet (see **Color Plate 26B**) and generalized lymphadenopathy. The woman may also experience fever, headache, and malaise. Condylomata lata (wart-like lesions) may develop on the vulva, perineum, or anus. (Hawkins et al., 2016; Marrazzo & Cates, 2011).

If a woman with syphilis is untreated, she enters a latent phase, which is asymptomatic for the majority of individuals. At this point, if the infection is still not treated, approximately one-third of patients will develop tertiary syphilis. Cardiovascular (chest pain, cough), dermatologic (multiple nodules or ulcers; see **Color Plate 26C**), skeletal (arthritis, myalgia, myositis), and neurologic (headache, irritability, impaired balance, memory loss, tremor) symptoms can all develop in this stage. Neurologic complications are not limited to tertiary syphilis; rather, a variety of syndromes (e.g., meningitis, meningovascular syphilis, general paresis, and tabes dorsalis) may span all stages of the disease (Hawkins et al., 2016; Youngkin et al., 2013).

TABLE 20-7	Stages of Syphilis

	Primary	**Secondary**	**Early Latent**	**Late Latent**	**Tertiary**
Time After Exposure	3–90 days (average 21)	4–10 weeks	≤ 1 year	> 1 year	Years (usually 15–30)
Infectious Routes	Sexual Vertical Chancre	Sexual Vertical	Sexual Vertical	Vertical	None
Clinical Symptoms[a]	Chancre Regional lympha- denopathy	Chancre may still be present Skin lesions (papular rash of soles and palms, patchy alopecia, condylomata lata) Symptoms of systemic illness (fever, malaise, anorexia, weight loss, headache, myalgias) Lymphadenopathy	None	None	Cardiovascular syphilis (aortitis) Skin lesions (gumma)

[a]In addition, neurosyphilis (central nervous system infection) can occur at any stage.
Data from Centers for Disease Control and Prevention (CDC). (2015d). Sexually transmitted diseases treatment guidelines, 2015. *Morbidity and Mortality Weekly Report, 64*(3), 1–137; Markle, W., Conti, T., & Kad, M. (2013). Sexually transmitted diseases. *Primary Care: Clinics in Office Practice, 40*(3), 557–587. doi:10.1016/j.pop.2013.05.001.

Assessment

Women with primary syphilis may be asymptomatic, or they may report an anogenital lesion that is typically raised, painless, and indurated. Most women (70%) with secondary syphilis will give a history of flu-like symptoms, including sore throat, malaise, headache, fever, myalgias, arthralgias, hoarseness, and anorexia. These women may also report skin rashes on the trunk, extremities, palms, and soles that may be pruritic (Markle, Conti, & Kad, 2013), Approximately 25% of women report a persistent primary chancre. Some women experience alopecia and have a "moth-eaten" look or lose the lateral one-third of an eyebrow. Occasionally women will have a history of low-grade fever. When syphilis is suspected, a comprehensive sexual risk history should be obtained (Hawkins et al., 2016).

The physical assessment includes a general examination of the skin for alopecia, rash on the feet and palms, and condylomata lata. Additionally, the clinician should conduct a pharyngeal examination and inspect for enlarged inguinal nodes. Inspect the external genitalia for vulvar lesions and chancre at the point of inoculation. A speculum examination is performed to assess for lesions on the vaginal walls and cervix and for vaginal and cervical discharge. A bimanual examination is conducted to assess uterine size, shape, consistency, mobility, and tenderness, and to palpate for adnexal masses and tenderness. When history and clinical findings suggest the need, a neurologic examination may be performed as well (Hawkins et al., 2016).

Dark-field examination and direct fluorescent antibody for *T. pallidum* (DFA-TP) of lesion exudates or tissue will provide a definitive diagnosis of early syphilis, although these tests are not commercially available (CDC, 2015b). The ability to confirm the diagnosis of syphilis depends on serology results obtained during the disease's latency and late infection phases. Any test for antibodies may not be reactive in the presence of active infection, as it takes time for the body's immune system to develop antibodies to any antigens. A presumptive diagnosis is possible with the use of two serologic tests: nontreponemal and treponemal.

Nontreponemal antibody tests such as the VDRL and RPR are used as screening tests and are relatively inexpensive, sensitive, moderately nonspecific, and fast. False-positive results are not unusual with these tests and can occur in the setting of increased age, autoimmune disorders, malignancy, pregnancy, injection drug use, and recent vaccination (CDC, 2015d). Sequential serologic tests should be obtained by using the same method (VDRL or RPR), preferably by the same laboratory. A high titer (more than 1:16) usually indicates active infection. A fourfold change in the titer (e.g., from 1:16 to 1:4 or from 1:8 to 1:32) is considered clinically significant. Treatment of syphilis usually causes a progressive decline in the pathogen's presence that may result in a negative VDRL or RPR, but low titers may persist. Rising titer (fourfold) or failure of titer to decrease fourfold within 6 to 12 months suggests reinfection or treatment failure (CDC, 2015d).

The treponemal tests—the fluorescent treponemal antibody absorbed (FTA-ABS) test and the *T. pallidum* passive particle agglutination (TP-PA) assay—are used to confirm positive nontreponemal test results. Some clinical laboratories now also use a reverse screening protocol and are beginning to test samples with treponemal tests—a practice that may decrease the risk of false-positive results and identify individuals who have been previously treated for syphilis. Individuals with early primary or incubating syphilis may have negative test results.

Seroconversion usually takes place 6 to 8 weeks after exposure, so testing should be repeated in 1 to 2 months when a suspicious genital lesion exists. Treponemal antibody tests frequently stay positive for the remainder of the patient's life regardless of treatment or disease activity; therefore, treatment is monitored by VDRL or RPR titers. Tests for concomitant STIs, including HIV, should be offered as well (CDC, 2015d; Youngkin et al., 2013).

No single test can confirm the diagnosis of neurosyphilis. Confirmation of this infection depends on a combination of tests, including cerebrospinal fluid (CSF) and reactive serologic tests in the presence of neurologic symptoms. Both a CSF-VDRL and CSF FTA-ABS can be performed, although routine CSF analysis in patients with primary or secondary syphilis is not recommended. Instead, testing of the

CSF should be performed in specific situations—for example, in individuals with symptoms or signs of neurologic or ophthalmic disease, in individuals with persistent or recurring signs or symptoms, when titers increase fourfold, with high initial titers (1:32 or greater) that fail to decrease fourfold, in individuals with symptomatic late syphilis, and when evidence of active tertiary syphilis is found (CDC, 2015d).

Differential Diagnoses

Differential diagnoses include HSV, chancroid, scabies, HIV, genital warts, and drug eruptions or reactions (Hawkins et al., 2016; Youngkin et al., 2013).

Prevention

There is no vaccine for syphilis. General STI prevention strategies are detailed in **Box 20-4** and **Table 20-2**.

Management

Parenteral penicillin G is the preferred drug for treating women and men with all stages of syphilis (**Table 20-8**). It is the only proven therapy that has been widely used for individuals with neurosyphilis, congenital syphilis, and syphilis during pregnancy. Single-dose therapy is used to treat primary, secondary, and early latent syphilis. Women who have late latent, tertiary, or unknown-duration syphilis require weekly treatment for 3 weeks. Women with primary or secondary syphilis should have repeat clinical evaluation and serologic testing at 6 and 12 months after treatment. Women with latent or unknown-duration syphilis should have repeat clinical evaluation and serologic testing at 6, 12, and 24 months after treatment. Information on follow-up of individuals with tertiary syphilis is limited. Partner treatment is imperative, and management depends on the stage of the woman's infection and the timing of partner's exposure. Detailed recommendations can be found in the CDC treatment guidelines (CDC, 2015d).

Patient Education

Significant education is necessary to improve adherence to treatment and monitoring, and to reduce the risk of transmission to sexual partners. The primary treatment for syphilis involves parenteral

| TABLE 20-8 | Treatment of Syphilis for Women Who Are HIV-Negative and Not Pregnant |

Recommended	Alternatives if Penicillin Allergic[a]
Primary, secondary, and early latent syphilis: Benzathine penicillin G 2.4 million units IM in a single dose	*Primary, secondary, and early latent syphilis:* Doxycycline 100 mg orally 2 times a day for 14 days **or** Tetracycline 500 mg orally 4 times a day for 14 days
Late latent syphilis, latent syphilis of unknown duration, and tertiary syphilis: Benzathine penicillin G 7.2 million units total, administered as three doses of 2.4 million units IM each at 1-week intervals	*Late latent syphilis or latent syphilis of unknown duration:* Doxycycline 100 mg orally 2 times a day for 28 days **or** Tetracycline 500 mg orally 4 times a day for 28 days *Tertiary syphilis:* Consult an infectious diseases specialist

Abbreviation: IM, intramuscularly.
[a] There are limited data to support these regimens, so close follow-up is essential. Penicillin desensitization and treatment should be considered for persons with a penicillin allergy whose adherence to therapy or follow-up cannot be ensured.
Data from Centers for Disease Control and Prevention. (2015d). Sexually transmitted diseases treatment guidelines, 2015. *Morbidity and Mortality Weekly Report, 64*(3), 1–137.

administration of penicillin; therefore, women need to return to the office or clinic for the IM injection. This return visit, in addition to the other visits necessary for serologic monitoring, may present a hardship for some women. Any potential barriers to care and follow-up should be identified early and discussed.

Allergy history should be reviewed carefully. Even without a documented history of a penicillin allergy, such reactions are still possible. Women need to be aware that although rare, a Jarisch-Herxheimer reaction may occur. This sudden febrile episode typically happens within 24 hours of beginning treatment for syphilis. The fever is accompanied by other systemic symptoms including myalgia and headache. Jarisch-Herxheimer reaction can be misinterpreted as a medication allergy. Treatment is supportive and includes antipyretics (CDC, 2015d).

Partner notification when the woman has syphilis is essential. Transmission is most common during the first year of infection, especially when syphilitic lesions are present. State departments of public health can often assist with confidential partner notification. All sexual partners within 90 days

preceding diagnosis of early, secondary, or early latent syphilis should be treated presumptively, even if serologic testing is negative. Partners outside of the 90-day window should be tested and treated if positive. If serologic testing is not possible or partners are unable to complete follow-up, they should be treated presumptively.

Sexual contact should be avoided until the chancre has completely healed. Consistent condom use is important until follow-up serologic testing has demonstrated a response to treatment. The importance of HIV testing for women and their partners should be stressed (CDC, 2015d).

Special Considerations

Pregnancy

All women should be screened for syphilis during their initial prenatal visit. Additional screening for women who live in geographic areas with high baseline rates of syphilis and for women who are at high risk for contracting the infection should be considered at 28 weeks' gestation and again at birth. Women who have experienced an intrauterine fetal demise (IUFD) after 20 weeks' gestation should be tested for syphilis (CDC, 2015d).

Pregnant women who have been diagnosed with syphilis and are allergic to penicillin should be desensitized and treated with penicillin. Although women should be treated with the penicillin regimen that corresponds to their disease stage, women with primary, secondary, or early latent infections can receive a second dose of benzathine penicillin 2.4 million units intramuscular injection 1 week after the initial dose. Doxycycline and tetracycline are contraindicated in pregnancy and do not prevent maternal transmission of syphilis. All pregnant women with syphilis should receive care that is coordinated with infectious disease and obstetric specialists (CDC, 2015d).

HEPATITIS B

HBV is a blood-borne pathogen that is transmitted by percutaneous or mucosal exposure to infectious blood or body fluids (e.g., semen, saliva). In 2013, approximately 3,000 cases of acute hepatitis B were reported in the United States. After accounting for asymptomatic infections and underreporting, the CDC estimated that there were nearly 20,000 new infections in this country in 2013. The overall incidence (1.0/100,000) currently reported is the lowest ever recorded and has declined significantly from the rate found in 1990 (8.5/100,000). The widespread use of HBV vaccination has contributed to this decline (CDC, 2015d).

Hepatitis B infection is caused by a large DNA virus, and is associated with three antigens and their antibodies. Screening for active or chronic disease or disease immunity is based on testing for these antigens and their antibodies (**Table 20-9**). HBV is more infectious than HIV and hepatitis C virus, with HBV being able to survive outside the body for at least 7 days (CDC, 2015d). HBV infection may be transmitted both parenterally and through intimate contact. In particular, hepatitis B surface antigen (HBsAg) has been found in blood, saliva, sweat, tears, wound exudate, vaginal secretions, and semen. Perinatal transmission does occur, but the fetus is not at risk of contracting the infection until making contact with contaminated blood at birth. HBV has also been transmitted by artificial insemination (CDC, 2015d; Hawkins et al., 2016).

Factors considered to place a woman at increased risk for HBV are those associated with STI risk in general (e.g., history of multiple sexual partners, multiple STIs, unprotected sex with a partner who has HBV), injection drug use, living in a household with one or more persons who have chronic HBV infection, and being born in or traveling to a country with a high incidence of HBV infection. With routine vaccination, occupational exposure to blood and body fluids (e.g., public safety workers exposed to blood in the workplace, healthcare workers) occurs less commonly. Although HBV can be transmitted via blood transfusion, the incidence of such infections has decreased significantly since testing of blood for the presence of HBsAg became possible (CDC, 2015a, 2015d).

TABLE 20-9	Hepatitis B Serologic Tests

Name	Abbreviation	Purpose
Hepatitis B surface antigen	HBsAg	Indicates the patient has acute or chronic hepatitis B virus infection and can transmit it to others
Hepatitis B surface antibody	Anti-HBs	Indicates the patient has immunity resulting from vaccination or previous infection
Total hepatitis B core antibody	Anti-HBc	Indicates the patient has previous or ongoing infection in an undefined time frame
Immunoglobulin M antibody to hepatitis B core antigen	IgM anti-HBc	Indicates the patient has had an acute infection within the past 6 months

Modified from Centers for Disease Control and Prevention (CDC). (2015a). Hepatitis B FAQs for health professionals. Retrieved from http://www.cdc.gov/hepatitis/hbv/hbvfaq.htm.

HBV infection primarily affects the liver. It remains asymptomatic in as many as half of all individuals with the infection. When symptoms occur, they begin an average of 90 days after HBV exposure and usually last for several weeks. Symptoms of HBV infection include arthralgias, fatigue, anorexia, nausea, vomiting, fever, abdominal pain, clay-colored stools, dark urine, and jaundice. Approximately 5% of adults with HBV infection become chronically infected, and 15% to 25% of individuals with chronic HBV infection will die prematurely from liver cancer or cirrhosis (CDC, 2015a).

Assessment

Components of the history to be obtained when hepatitis B is suspected include symptoms of the infection and risk factors. Physical examination includes inspection of the skin for rashes, inspection of the skin and conjunctiva for jaundice, and palpation of the liver for enlargement and tenderness. Weight loss, fever, and general debilitation should be noted as well (Hawkins et al., 2016).

Interpretation of test results for hepatitis B is complex (**Table 20-9**). Women who have negative HBsAg, anti-HBc, and anti-HBs tests are susceptible to infection, and vaccination should be considered. A woman with a positive anti-HBs test with negative HBsAg and anti-HBc tests has immunity from vaccination. A woman with a negative HBsAg test and positive anti-HBc and anti-HBs tests has immunity from previous infection that is now resolved. A woman with acute hepatitis B infection will have positive HBsAg, anti-HBc, and IgM anti-HBc tests and a negative anti-HBs test. A woman with chronic hepatitis B infection will have positive HBsAg and anti-HBc tests and negative IgM anti-HBc and anti-HBs tests. A woman with a positive anti-HBc test and negative HBsAg and anti-HBs tests should be referred for further evaluation, as this result has multiple interpretations, including resolved infection, false-positive anti-HBc, low-level chronic infection, and resolving acute infection (CDC, 2015a).

Women who have hepatitis B should be prepared to undergo repeat testing, as HBV serologic markers may also be used to monitor the progression of the disease. Testing for other STIs, including HIV, should be performed as well.

Differential Diagnoses

Differential diagnoses include other forms of hepatitis (including hepatitis A and C as well as those caused by viruses, medications, and alcohol), biliary disease, and hemochromatosis (Hawkins et al., 2016; Youngkin et al., 2013).

Prevention

Hepatitis B is a vaccine-preventable infection. All nonimmune women at risk of hepatitis B should be informed of the existence of a hepatitis B vaccine. Vaccination is recommended for all individuals who have had more than one sex partner within the past 6 months as well as for anyone being evaluated or treated for an STI. In addition, all children younger than 19 years; individuals who use injection drugs; residents and staff of facilities for developmentally disabled persons; individuals who have a sexual partner or household contact who is HBsAg positive; individuals with end-stage renal disease, chronic liver disease, or HIV; persons whose occupation exposes them to blood or body fluids; travelers to areas with high rates of HBV infection; and anyone who wants protection from HBV infection should be vaccinated (CDC, 2015a, 2015d). Multiple vaccinations are available, including one that protects against both the hepatitis B and hepatitis A viruses. Clinicians should consult current immunization schedules (http://www.cdc.gov/vaccines/schedules/hcp/imz/adult.html) and product information to determine the appropriate vaccine, dose, and frequency based on the patient's age; individual factors, such as immunocompromised status; and need to complete the vaccine series. The vaccine should be injected into the deltoid muscle.

Management

Women with a definite exposure to hepatitis B should be given hepatitis B immunoglobulin intramuscularly in a single dose as soon as possible, and preferably within 24 hours after exposure. There is no specific treatment for acute hepatitis B; recovery is usually spontaneous. For persons with chronic infections, several antiviral drugs are available; women can discuss treatment options for viral suppression with their healthcare providers (CDC, 2015a).

Education

Education about preventing transmission of HBV to others is paramount. Women with chronic HBV should be referred to a specialist for management. Condom use with unvaccinated partners is important to prevent transmission. Other mechanisms to prevent transmission include covering cuts, not donating body fluids or organs, and not sharing household items that could be infected with blood. To avoid any further liver injury, women with HBV should avoid or limit alcohol consumption, refrain from taking any medications they have not discussed with their healthcare providers, and receive vaccinations for hepatitis A (CDC, 2015a).

Women who are beginning the HBV vaccine should be aware that completion of the series involves three injections, which are typically administered over a 6-month period. Schedules and doses can vary slightly based on manufacturer guidelines. Most adults (90%) aged 40 and younger achieve a protective antibody response after the third dose. Booster vaccination is not currently recommended. Women should be informed that reported side effects of vaccination are infrequent, with most involving pain at injection site and mild fever. The HBV vaccine can be administered with other vaccines.

Special Considerations

Pregnancy

All pregnant women should be tested for HBsAg at their initial prenatal visit, regardless of their previous vaccination status. Pregnant women who have not been vaccinated and are at risk for acquiring the virus can be vaccinated during pregnancy. Pregnant women with HBV should be managed by infectious disease and obstetric specialists, and newborns whose mothers have HBV need to receive immunoprophylaxis after birth (CDC, 2015a, 2015d).

HEPATITIS C

HCV infection is the most common chronic blood-borne infection in the United States. In 2013, slightly more than 2,000 acute cases were reported, although the CDC (2015b) estimates that the actual number is closer to 30,000 when underreporting and undiagnosed infections are considered. An estimated 3 million persons in the United States have chronic HCV, which is most prevalent in the 1945 to 1965 birth cohort. Although most transmission occurs via infected blood, sexual transmission can occur, especially in certain subgroups, including men who have sex with men (MSM), cocaine and intravenous drug users, and those who engage in group sex or traumatic sexual practices (CDC, 2015d).

Hepatitis C is caused by a single-stranded RNA virus. Parenteral transmission is most common. Those individuals at greatest risk for contracting the virus include current or former injection drug users, recipients of blood or solid-organ transplants prior to 1992, those who received clotting factor concentrate prior to 1987, and persons who have HIV (CDC, 2015b). Approximately 15% to 25% of all individuals with an acute infection will clear the virus spontaneously and not develop chronic HCV, but the infection will become chronic in more than 75% of patients. HCV infection is the leading cause of liver transplantation in the United States.

Assessment

Symptoms of acute HCV infection are often vague and nonspecific. Women may report fatigue, fever, abdominal pain, nausea, vomiting, anorexia, jaundice, dark urine, or clay-colored stool. The average time from exposure to emergence of symptoms is 4 to 12 weeks, but symptoms can occur as late as 24 weeks post exposure. Women should be asked about specific risk factors (described in previous section) and sexual contact with a partner known to have HCV.

Decisions regarding testing for HCV are based on the history and physical examination findings. Interpretation of HCV laboratory values can be found at http://www.cdc.gov/hepatitis/hcv/pdfs/hcv_graph.pdf.

Differential Diagnoses

Differential diagnoses include other forms of hepatitis (including hepatitis A and B as well as those caused by viruses, medications, and alcohol), biliary disease, and hemochromatosis (Hawkins et al., 2016; Youngkin et al., 2013).

Prevention

Unlike for hepatitis B, there is no vaccine for HCV. Prophylaxis with immune globulin is not effective in preventing infection after exposure (CDC, 2015d). Prevention relies on avoiding contact with infected blood. Although the risk of this virus's transmission is smaller than that for HBV, HCV can be transmitted via sexual activity with a partner who has HCV, especially among individuals with HIV infection (CDC, 2015d). In heterosexual, monogamous partners without HIV infection, sexual transmission to a discordant partner is rare (Webster, Klenerman, & Dusheiko, 2015).

Management

The goal of treatment is to reduce all-cause mortality and prevent or halt liver injury. Multiple medications exist that can be used to treat HCV infection. The mainstay of treatment has been a combination of interferon and ribavirin with or without protease inhibitors, although newer medications with an improved side-effect profile now exist. Members of this class of medications, called direct-acting antiviral (DAA) agents, target viral enzymes and proteins throughout the viral life cycle and have a less complicated dosing regimen and higher tolerability. They include sofosbuvir and simeprevir as well as fixed-dose combination drugs. A full discussion of all treatment options is beyond the scope of this chapter but is available from the American Association for the Study of Liver Diseases (2014).

Virologic cure is defined as the absence of HCV RNA 12 weeks after the completion of treatment. The optimal treatment regimen and timing of treatment are unclear, although the success rate for viral clearance appears to be higher when treatment begins in the acute phase of the infection. Treatment is recommended for all persons except those with a short life expectancy due to comorbid conditions. Coordination with a specialist in hepatitis management is advisable. Evaluation of chronic liver disease is imperative. Individuals who have HCV can receive vaccination for hepatitis A and B if not already vaccinated.

Education

Education about preventing transmission of HCV to others is important. Women with HCV should be referred to a specialist for management. To reduce the risk of transmitting this virus to others, women should be advised not to share personal household items (e.g., toothbrushes, razors) that may have blood on them. Any cuts or sores should be covered, and women with HCV should not donate blood, organs, or tissue. Sexual transmission is possible, although the risk is lower than with direct contact with infected blood. To protect partners, sexual activity in the presence of vaginal bleeding should be avoided. Condoms can be used with multiple partners or in the presence of coinfection with HIV. The benefit of condom use with low-risk, steady partners is uncertain. To avoid any further liver injury, women with HCV should avoid or limit alcohol consumption and refrain from taking any medications they have not discussed with their healthcare providers (CDC, 2015b).

Rates of HCV infection are high among injection drug users. Counseling about the risks of continuing drug use is important, as well as providing resources for substance abuse treatment. For those individuals who are not ready or not willing to discontinue drug use, the importance of using clean drug injection equipment and not sharing drug equipment with others should be stressed (CDC, 2015b).

Special Considerations

Pregnancy

Routine screening for HCV among all pregnant women is currently not recommended. Testing for HCV should be offered to pregnant women with known risk factors. The risk of maternal transmission of the virus to neonates varies, with the highest rates of transmission being reported among women who have both HIV and HCV. Newborns whose mothers have HCV infection should be tested for this infection as well. HCV is not transmitted through breastmilk, but women with cracked and bleeding nipples should avoid this method of feeding until complete healing has taken place (CDC, 2015b).

Women with HIV

All women who are diagnosed with HIV should also be tested for HCV during their initial evaluation. If negative, women with HIV should be screened annually if at high risk for infection (e.g., high-risk sexual behavior, injection drug use, high prevalence of HCV in the community) (CDC, 2015b).

HUMAN IMMUNODEFICIENCY VIRUS

In the early summer of 1981, the occurrence of several rare illnesses such as *Pneumocystis carinii* (now called *P. jiroveci*) pneumonia, *Mycobacterium* and *M. intracellulare* infections, cryptosporidiosis, Kaposi's sarcoma, and non-Hodgkin's lymphoma in a cluster of gay and bisexual men presented a medical mystery, which was subsequently solved by the identification of a single infectious agent that was destroying the immune system of persons who acquired it—the human immunodeficiency virus (CDC, 1981). Although the earliest identified victims of the HIV/AIDS epidemic were typically homosexual men, symptoms of the syndrome were identified in a woman within 2 months of the earliest reports of the infection in men. Within the first year of the epidemic, female partners of hemophiliacs with HIV, women using injection drugs, and female partners in heterosexual relationships in poor countries, notably Haiti, were diagnosed with HIV/AIDS.

Deeply ingrained social and cultural forces that tend to devalue women, and particularly poor women of color, perpetuated the tendency for HIV and AIDS to be considered a "men's disease," and more specifically, a disease of men who have sex with men (MSM); as a consequence, HIV/AIDS has typically been underdiagnosed in women. Twenty percent of the estimated 47,500 new cases of HIV in the United States in 2010 occurred in women (CDC, 2015c). Black women are disproportionately affected by HIV. Of the total estimated new infections among women, 64% occurred in black women, while 18% occurred among white women (CDC, 2015c).

As of 2011, 23% of all persons living with HIV in the United States were women (CDC, 2015c). Most (84%) of the new HIV infections diagnosed in women are acquired through heterosexual contact. The remaining infections are attributed to injection drug use or other factors, such as hemophilia, blood transfusion, or unreported or unknown transmission (CDC, 2015c).

HIV's Effects on the Immune System

The human immune system protects the body from invasion by a variety of microbes and tumor cells. The immune system is composed of two arms: humoral immunity, involved with antibody production, and cellular immunity, effected largely through T-helper lymphocytes (also known as CD4 cells). Central components of the cellular arm of the immune system are macrophages and CD4 cells.

HIV specifically targets CD4 cells, binding to the cell surface protein known as the CD4 receptor. The virus affects the cells in two ways: The absolute numbers of these cells are depleted and the function of the remaining cells is impaired, resulting in a gradual loss of immune function. Progressive depletion of CD4 cells in peripheral blood occurs with advancing HIV infection, such that CD4 cell counts are used to estimate the cumulative immunologic damage caused by HIV. If its course is unimpeded, HIV can destroy as many as one billion CD4 cells per day. In addition to its aggressive destruction of the immune system, HIV is genetically highly variable, mutating with apparent ease (CDC, 2014d).

HIV Transmission Issues Specific to Women

As noted earlier in this chapter, several factors increase women's risk for acquiring STIs, including HIV. In addition to the anatomically driven susceptibility of the female genitalia, the integrity of the tissues of the lower genital tract influences HIV transmission risk. Trauma during intercourse (including both vaginal and anal-receptive intercourse), STI-related inflammation or cervicitis, and an STI lesion (e.g., HSV ulcer or syphilitic chancre) may all increase susceptibility to HIV infection, as does any activity or condition that disrupts the tissues of the vagina. HIV can also be transmitted through receptive oral sex with ejaculation. Any condition that interrupts the integrity of oral tissues, including periodontal disease, increases the risk of HIV transmission in this manner (Hawkins et al., 2016; Youngkin et al., 2013).

Assessment

The CDC (2015b) now recommends HIV screening be a routine part of clinical care for patients aged 13 to 64 years in all healthcare settings. Patients presenting for STI treatment should be screened for HIV at each visit where they have new symptoms. Individuals at high risk for HIV should be tested for the presence of the virus at least once a year. Patients must be informed orally or in writing that HIV testing will be performed unless they decline (opt-out screening). Consent for HIV testing should be incorporated into the general consent for care. A separate consent form specific for HIV screening is neither required nor recommended (CDC, 2015c).

All 50 states collect HIV surveillance data using confidential name-based reporting standards. Some states offer only confidential testing, whereas others also offer anonymous testing. State laws regarding HIV testing vary, and clinicians must be fully informed of regulations where they practice. Information about state HIV testing and reporting laws can be found on the CDC website (http://www.cdc.gov/hiv/policies/law/states/index.html).

HIV infection can be diagnosed by serologic tests that detect antibodies to HIV-1 and HIV-2 and by virologic tests that detect antigens to HIV or RNA. HIV screening is conducted with standard enzyme-linked immunosorbent assay (ELISA) or enzyme immunoassay (EIA) tests that are sent to a laboratory, or with newer rapid HIV tests that can be performed at the point of care and yield results within minutes. If the screening test is reactive, then a more specific confirmatory test such as the Western blot (WB) or an indirect immunofluorescence assay (IFA) is conducted. Although a negative antibody test usually indicates that a person does not have HIV, these tests cannot always detect an acute infection. A patient with a negative test who has known or suspected exposure to HIV should be retested at a time determined by history and possible exposure (CDC, 2015d).

The CDC recommendations no longer require prevention counseling as part of a screening program. Nevertheless, such counseling is strongly encouraged for patients who are seronegative for HIV but at increased risk for infection. Patients who are at high risk for HIV or who have known or suspected exposure to the virus should also be counseled about the need for repeat testing (CDC, 2015d).

If a screening test is positive for HIV, the clinician must explain the need for confirmatory testing. If confirmatory testing is positive for HIV, the woman must be given time to react emotionally. She must assimilate a lot of information at the time of this visit. Allowing her to express her feelings prior to discussing issues related to partner notification, treatments, and other issues may allow her to take in some of the important information that must be conveyed at this time. Women with HIV must understand that although they may exhibit no signs or symptoms of HIV disease, they are still infectious, and will remain so for life. Basic information regarding minimizing transmission risk must be relayed to the patient at the time of diagnosis.

A plan for treatment must be established, which includes prompt referral to a clinician with HIV expertise. Unless the woman is clearly immunocompromised and in need of immediate treatment for opportunistic infection, there is likely to be an interval between diagnosis and treatment decisions. The woman can use this period to begin to adapt emotionally and psychologically to her diagnosis. She can make decisions about who must be told about her infection, and implement behaviors that are required of her to minimize the risk of transmitting the virus to others. Sensitive and nonjudgmental care at this time can assist the woman to make healthy accommodations in the face of her HIV diagnosis.

Differential Diagnoses

HIV infection is difficult to diagnose based on symptoms alone because signs of acute infection are often nonspecific, including fever, malaise, rash, myalgias, lymphadenopathy, sore throat, and headache (Fogel & Black, 2008). Other conditions that must be considered are upper respiratory infections, including influenza and tuberculosis, and viral infections, including mononucleosis. Immune disorders that place women at risk for opportunistic infections should also be considered (Hawkins et al., 2016; Youngkin et al., 2013).

Prevention

Prevention of HIV can occur through different mechanisms, including behavioral change to reduce exposure to HIV and pharmacologic intervention through the use of pre-exposure prophylaxis (PrEP) (CDC, 2014d). General guidelines to reduce the risk of all STIs, including HIV, can be found in **Box 20-4** and **Table 20-2**.

A complete discussion of PrEP is beyond the scope of this chapter, but full guidelines for eligibility, medication use, and monitoring are available from the CDC (2014d). Briefly, PrEP is recommended as one preventive option for women who are HIV negative and use injection drugs, women whose sexual partners are known to have HIV, and all other women who are at substantial risk for contracting HIV (e.g., commercial sex workers, partner with HIV, inconsistent or absent condom use, high number of sexual partners) (CDC, 2014d). PrEP, which is taken every day, is composed of an oral fixed-dose combination of tenofovir disoproxil fumarate (TDF) 300 mg and emtricitabine (FTC) 200 mg. Prophylactic medication should be used in conjunction with risk-reduction services and behavior changes, including safer-sex practices, to most effectively reduce HIV risk.

Management

Effective management and treatment of the patient with HIV involves the use of antiretroviral therapy (ART) to improve health, decrease morbidity, prolong life, and reduce the risk of transmission to others (CDC, 2014e). More than 25 different antiretroviral medications are available, which belong to six classes: nucleoside reverse transcriptase inhibitors (NRTIs), nonnucleoside reverse transcriptase inhibitors (NNRTIs), protease inhibitors (PIs), fusion inhibitors (FIs), CCR5 antagonists, and integrase strand transfer inhibitors (INSTIs).

Combination therapy with multiple ARTs is recommended (Panel on Antiretroviral Guidelines for Adults and Adolescents, 2015). Detailed treatment of HIV is beyond the scope of this chapter and is best provided by clinicians experienced in HIV management and infectious disease. Research activities directed toward development of new therapies and testing of different combinations of therapies can quickly change the state of the science. The AIDSinfo website (http://www.aidsinfo .nih.gov) contains the most current recommendations for HIV/AIDS management. Clinicians with questions about HIV/AIDS management can also contact the National HIV Telephone Consultation Service free of charge at 800-933-3413.

Although ART is the primary treatment for persons living with HIV, multiple complementary and alternative therapies exist that may assist women in reducing their level of stress, increasing their overall sense of wellness, and better managing the potential side effects of medications. All adjunct therapies should be discussed with healthcare providers. Some supplements, such as St. John's wort and garlic, can interfere with the effectiveness of ART. A comprehensive list of complementary and alternative therapies is available from the U.S. Department of Health and Human Services (2015).

Patient Education

Clinicians providing gynecologic care to women with HIV must be aware of the fact that the infection may necessitate adjustments to the usual standards of care, including STI screening, Pap test screening, and contraceptive choice (American College of Obstetricians and Gynecologists, 2010a, reaffirmed 2012; CDC, 2013b, 2015d; Saslow et al., 2012). Women need to be educated on the rationale for increased visits, screening, and disease surveillance, as such ongoing care may be burdensome for women, especially in addition to the self-management needed during HIV care.

Very few diseases in history have been associated with the high levels of stigmatization that may accompany an HIV diagnosis. Many persons with HIV choose to keep their diagnosis a secret from family, friends, and coworkers. Although this decision means they must hide clinic visits, medications, and HIV-related illnesses, women may feel this course of action is preferable to experiencing the stigma that accompanies this diagnosis. Persons with HIV may face the dissolution of important relationships when and if the diagnosis becomes known. Clinicians can assist patients in identifying supportive persons who can be helpful as the patient adapts to the diagnosis and treatment (Youngkin et al., 2013).

Clinicians can help women reframe their understanding of HIV, particularly in terms of perceiving it as a chronic condition that can be managed, rather than as a terminal illness. Taking care of her physical and emotional health, staying connected with others in supportive relationships, and nurturing her spiritual well-being can assist the woman with HIV to regain a sense of control and hope (Fogel & Black, 2008). Clinicians are in a unique position to understand the multiplicity of factors and issues that confront persons with HIV. Awareness of these factors can enhance health care by improving both the physical and mental health of patients, as well as the long-term health outcomes for women with HIV.

In addition to assisting with education on social issues surrounding HIV, educating woman about the importance of medication adherence, laboratory assessment, and follow-up is extremely important. Multiple healthcare visits with different providers can place a burden on women and impact childcare coordination.

Special Considerations

Pregnancy

All pregnant women should be tested for HIV at their initial prenatal visit, regardless of whether they were tested previously. Repeat testing at 36 weeks' gestation can be considered for women at high risk for HIV or for women who live in geographic areas where there is a high incidence of HIV among women. All pregnant women with a new diagnosis of HIV during pregnancy should be educated about the benefits of ART and offered treatment. Without treatment, rates of maternal transmission of HIV to infants are approximately 30%, but can decrease to 2% or less with specific interventions, including antiretroviral medication, planned cesarean birth, and avoidance of breastfeeding. All pregnant women with HIV should be comanaged with obstetric specialists and HIV/infectious disease specialists. Updated guidelines on management of HIV in pregnancy can be found at http://aidsinfo.nih.gov/guidelines (CDC, 2015c).

Additional STI Testing

All women who receive an initial diagnosis of HIV should be tested for other STIs and screened annually as part of comprehensive HIV care. Notably, trichomoniasis is common among women who have HIV. Pap testing may be required at more frequent intervals, and clinicians should review current guidelines (CDC, 2015d; Massad et al., 2013; Panel on Opportunistic Infections in HIV-Infected Adults and Adolescents, 2015). Treatment of STIs in a woman diagnosed with HIV may require prolonged or different medications—an issue addressed in the most current STI treatment guidelines (CDC, 2015d).

CONCLUSION

STIs are among the most common health problems experienced by women in the United States and around the world. Women experience a disproportionate amount of the burden associated with these illnesses, including complications of infertility, perinatal infections, poor pregnancy outcomes, chronic pelvic pain, genital tract neoplasms, and potentially death. Additionally, these infections may interfere with a woman's lifestyle and cause considerable distress, both emotional and physical. Clinicians can help to ameliorate the misery, morbidity, and mortality associated with STIs and other common infections by providing accurate, safe, sensitive, and supportive care.

Knowledge of STIs is constantly increasing and changing, with new and improved prevention, diagnostic, and treatment modalities being developed and reported on an ongoing basis. All clinicians have a responsibility to stay up-to-date on these developments by reviewing journals, attending conferences, and being knowledgeable about recommendations and bulletins from the CDC. Furthermore, it is important that clinicians be aware of policies, recommendations, and guidelines of the state in which they practice, which also may change frequently.

References

Alan Guttmacher Institute. (2011). Facts on American teens' sexual and reproductive health. Retrieved from http://www.guttmacher.org/pubs/FB-ATSRH.html

Alcaide, M. L., Feaster, D. J., Duan, R., Cohen, S., Diaz, C., Castro, J. G., . . . Metsch, L. R. (2015). The incidence of *Trichomonas vaginalis* infection in women attending nine sexually transmitted diseases clinics in the USA. *Sexually Transmitted Infections, 92*(1), 58–62. doi:10.1136/sextrans-2015-052010

American Association for the Study of Liver Diseases. (2014). Recommendations for testing, managing, and treating hepatitis C. Retrieved from http://www.hcvguidelines.org/fullreport

American College of Obstetricians and Gynecologists. (2010a, reaffirmed 2012). Gynecologic care for women with human immunodeficiency virus. ACOG Practice Bulletin No. 117. *Obstetrics & Gynecology, 116*, 1492–1509.

American College of Obstetricians and Gynecologists. (2010b). Human papillomavirus vaccination. Committee Opinion No. 467. *Obstetrics & Gynecology, 116*, 800–803.

Archer, D. F. (2015). Vaginal atrophy and disease susceptibility: The role of leukocytes. *Menopause, 22*(8), 804–805. doi:10.1097/GME.0000000000000513

Blankenship, K. M., Reinhard, E., Sherman, S. G., & El-Bassel, N. (2015). Structural interventions for HIV prevention among women who use drugs: A global perspective. *Journal of Acquired Immune Deficiency Syndromes, 69*, S140–S145. doi:10.1097/QAI.0000000000000638

Brunham, R. C., Gottlieb, S. L., & Paavonen, J. (2015). Pelvic inflammatory disease. *New England Journal of Medicine, 372*(21), 2039–2048. doi:10.1056/NEJMra1411426

Carcio, H. A., & Secor, M. C. (2015). *Advanced health assessment of women* (3rd ed.). New York, NY: Springer.

Centers for Disease Control and Prevention (CDC). (1981). *Pneumocystis* pneumonia—Los Angeles. *Mortality and Morbidity Weekly Review, 30*, 250–252.

Centers for Disease Control and Prevention (CDC). (2013a). CDC fact sheet: Incidence, prevalence, and cost of sexually transmitted infections in the United States. Retrieved from http://www.cdc.gov/std/stats/sti-estimates-fact-sheet-feb-2013.pdf

Centers for Disease Control and Prevention. (2013b). U.S. selected practice recommendations for contraceptive use, 2013. *Morbidity and Mortality Weekly Report, 62*(5), 1–60.

Centers for Disease Control and Prevention (CDC). (2014a). CDC fact sheet: Reported STDs in the United States: 2013 National Data for chlamydia, gonorrhea, and syphilis. Retrieved from http://www.cdc.gov/std/stats13/std-trends-508.pdf

Centers for Disease Control and Prevention (CDC). (2014b). Sexually transmitted disease surveillance 2013. Retrieved from http://www.cdc.gov/std/stats13/surv2013-print.pdf

Centers for Disease Control and Prevention (CDC). (2014c). Genital HPV infection: CDC fact sheet. Retrieved from http://www.cdc.gov/std/HPV/HPV-factsheet-March-2014.pdf

Centers for Disease Control and Prevention (CDC). (2014d). Preexposure prophylaxis for the prevention of HIV infection in the United States—2014. Retrieved from http://www.cdc.gov/hiv/pdf/prepguidelines2014.pdf

Centers for Disease Control and Prevention (CDC). (2014e). Recommendations for HIV prevention with adults and adolescents with HIV in the United States, 2014. Retrieved from http://stacks.cdc.gov/view/cdc/26062

Centers for Disease Control and Prevention (CDC). (2015a). Hepatitis B FAQs for health professionals. Retrieved from http://www.cdc.gov/hepatitis/hbv/hbvfaq.htm

Centers for Disease Control and Prevention (CDC). (2015b). Hepatitis C FAQs for health professionals. Retrieved from http://www.cdc.gov/hepatitis/HCV/HCVfaq.htm

Centers for Disease Control and Prevention (CDC). (2015c). HIV among women. Retrieved from http://www.cdc.gov/hiv/risk/gender/women/facts/index.html?s_cid=fb-dhap-nwghad-002

Centers for Disease Control and Prevention (CDC). (2015d). Sexually transmitted diseases treatment guidelines, 2015. *Morbidity and Mortality Weekly Report, 64*(3), 1–137.

Cunningham, F. G., Leveno, K. J., Bloom, S. L., Hauth, J. C., Rouse, D. J., & Spong, C. Y. (2010). *Williams obstetrics* (23rd ed.). New York, NY: McGraw-Hill.

Dholakia, S., Buckler, J., Jeans, J. P., Pillai, A., Eagles, N., & Dholakia, S. (2014). Pubic lice: An endangered species? *Sexually Transmitted Diseases, 41*(6), 388–391. doi:10.1097/OLQ.0000000000000142

Edwards, A. E., & Collins, C. B. (2014). Exploring the influence of social determinants on HIV risk behaviors and the potential application of structural interventions to prevent HIV in women. *Journal of Health Disparities Research and Practice, 7*(7), 141–155.

Fantasia, H. C. (2012). Sinecatechins ointment 15% for the treatment of external genital warts. *Nursing for Women's Health, 16*(5), 418–422. doi:10.1111/j.1751-486X.2012.01765.x

Fantasia, H. C., Fontenot, H. B., Sutherland, M. A., & Harris, A. L. (2011). Sexually transmitted infections in women. *Nursing for Women's Health, 15*, 48–58. doi:10.1111/j.1751-486X.2011.01610.x.

Fantasia, H. C., Sutherland, M., Fontenot, H. B., & Lee-St. John, T. (2012). Chronicity of partner violence, contraceptive patterns, and pregnancy risk. *Contraception, 86*(5), 530–535. doi:10.1016/j.contracpetion.2012.03.005.

Fogel, C. I. (2008). Sexually transmitted infections. In C. I. Fogel & N. F. Woods (Eds.), *Women's health care in advanced practice nursing* (pp. 475–526). New York, NY: Springer.

Fogel, C. I., & Black, B. P. (2008). Women and HIV/AIDS. In C. I. Fogel & N. F. Woods (Eds.), *Women's health care in advanced practice nursing* (pp. 527–552). New York, NY: Springer.

Fontenot, H. B., Fantasia, H. C., Sutherland, M. A., & Lee-St. John, T. (2014). The effects of intimate partner violence duration on individual and partner-related sexual risk factors among women. *Journal of Midwifery and Women's Health, 59*, 67–73. doi:10.1111/jmwh.12145

Gaby, A. R. (2006). Natural remedies for herpes simplex. *Alternative Medicine Review, 11*(2), 93–101.

Giuliano, A. R., Nyitray, A. G., Kreimer, A. R., Campbell, C. M. P., Goodman, M. T., Sudenga, S. L., . . . Franceschi, S. (2015). EUROGIN 2014 roadmap: Differences in human papillomavirus infection natural history, transmission and human papillomavirus–related cancer incidence by gender and anatomical site of infection. *International Journal of Cancer, 136*(12), 2752–2760. doi:10.1002/ijc.29082

GlaxoSmithKline. (2015). Highlights of prescribing information. Retrieved from https://www.gsksource.com/pharma/content/dam/GlaxoSmithKline/US/en/Prescribing_Information/Cervarix/pdf/CERVARIX-PI-PIL.PDF

Goyal, M., Hersh, A., Luan, X., Localio, R., Trent, M., & Zaoutis, T. (2013). National trends in pelvic inflammatory disease among adolescents in the emergency department. *Journal of Adolescent Health, 53*(2), 249–252. doi:10.1016/j.jadohealth.2013.03.016

Hamilton, D. T., & Morris, M. (2015). The racial disparities in STI in the US: Concurrency, STI prevalence, and heterogeneity in partner selection. *Epidemics, 11*, 56–61. doi:10.1016/j.epidem.2015.02.003

Hassan, S. T. S., Masarcikova, R., & Berchova, K. (2015). Bioactive natural products with anti-herpes simplex virus properties. *Journal of Pharmacy and Pharmacology.* doi:10.1111/jphp.12436

Hawkins, J. W., Roberto-Nichols, D. M., & Stanley-Haney, J. L. (2016). *Guidelines for nurse practitioners in gynecologic settings* (11th ed.). New York, NY: Springer.

Henneke, B., Marijn, V., Ferdinand, W., Evgeni, T., Ndayisabe, G. F., Rita, V., . . . van de Wijgert, J. (2015). The impact of hormonal contraception and pregnancy on sexually transmitted infections and on cervicovaginal microbiota in African sex workers. *Sexually Transmitted Diseases, 42*(3), 143–152. doi:10.1097/OLQ.0000000000000245

Heslop, R., Jordan, V., Trivella, M., Papastamopoulos, V., & Roberts, H. (2013). Interventions for men and women with their first episode of genital herpes. *Cochrane Database of Systematic Reviews, 7*(CD010684), 1–15. doi:10.1002/14651858.CD010684

Jackson, J. A., McNair, T. S., & Coleman, J. S. (2015). Over-screening for chlamydia and gonorrhea among urban women age ≥ 25 years. *American Journal of Obstetrics and Gynecology, 212*(1), 40.e1–40.e6. doi:10.1016/j.ajog.2014.06.051

Jackson, J. M., Seth, P., DiClemente, R. J., & Lin, A. (2015). Association of depressive symptoms and substance use with risky sexual behavior and sexually transmitted infections among African American female adolescents seeking sexual health care. *American Journal of Public Health, 105*(10):2137–2142. doi:10.2105/AJPH.2014.302493

Kogan, S. M., Cho, J., Barnum, S. C., & Brown, G. L. (2015). Correlates of concurrent sexual partnerships among young, rural African American men. *Public Health Reports, 130*(4), 392–399.

Lebrun-Vignes, B., Bouzamondo, A., Dupuy, A., Guillaume, J. C., Lechat, P., & Chosidow, O. (2007). A meta-analysis to assess the efficacy of oral antiviral treatment to prevent genital herpes outbreaks. *Journal of the American Academy of Dermatology, 57*(2), 238–246. doi:10.1016/j.jaad.2007.02.008

Le Cleach, L., Trinquart, L., Do, G., Maruani, A., Lebrun-Vignes, B., Ravaud, P., & Chosidow, O. (2014). Oral antiviral therapy for prevention of genital herpes outbreaks in immunocompetent and nonpregnant patients. *Cochrane Database of Systematic Reviews, 8*, CD009036. doi:10.1002/14651858.CD009036.pub2

Lilleston, P. S., Hebert, L. E., Jennings, J. M., Holtgrave, D. R., Ellen, J. M., & Sherman, S. G. (2015). Attitudes towards power in relationships and sexual concurrency within heterosexual youth partnerships in Baltimore, MD. *AIDS and Behavior*, 1–11. doi:10.1007/s10461-015-1105-z

Markle, W., Conti, T., & Kad, M. (2013). Sexually transmitted diseases. *Primary Care: Clinics in Office Practice, 40*(3), 557–587. doi:10.1016/j.pop.2013.05.001

Marrazzo, J. M., & Cates, W. (2011). Reproductive tract infections, including HIV and other sexually transmitted infections. In R. A. Hatcher, J. Trussell, A. L. Nelson, W. Cates, D. Kowal, & M. S. Policar (Eds.), *Contraceptive technology* (20th ed., pp. 571–620). New York, NY: Ardent Media.

Marrazzo, J. M., & Gorgos, L. M. (2012). Emerging sexual health issues among women who have sex with women. *Current Infectious Disease Reports, 14*(2), 204–211. doi:10.1007/s11908-012-0244-x

Massad, L. S., Einstein, M. H., Huh, W. K., Katki, H. A., Kinney, W. K., Schiffman, M., . . . Lawson, H. W. (2013). 2012 updated consensus for the management of abnormal cervical cancer screening tests and cancer precursors. *Journal of Lower Genital Tract Disease, 17*(5), S1–S17.

Masson, L., Passmore, J., Leibenberg, L. J., Werner, L., Baxter, C., Arnold, K. B., . . . Karim, S. S. A. (2015). Genital inflammation and the risk of HIV acquisition in women. *Clinical Infectious Diseases, 61*(2), 260–269. doi:10.1093/cid/civ298

Minnis, A. M., Doherty, I. A., Kline, T. L., Zule, W. A., Myers, B., Carney, T., & Wechsberg, W. M. (2015). Relationship power, communication, and violence among couples: Results of a cluster-randomized HIV prevention study in a South African township. *International Journal of Women's Health, 7*, 517–525. doi:10.2147/IJWH.S77398

Nelson, A. L., & Cwiak, C. (2011). Combined oral contraceptives (COCs). In R. A. Hatcher, J. Trussell, A. L. Nelson, W. Cates, D. Kowal, & M. S. Policar (Eds.), *Contraceptive technology* (20th ed., pp. 249–341). New York, NY: Ardent Media.

Panel on Antiretroviral Guidelines for Adults and Adolescents. (2015). Guidelines for the use of antiretroviral agents in HIV-1–infected adults and adolescents. Retrieved from https://aidsinfo.nih.gov/contentfiles/lvguidelines/adultandadolescentgl.pdf

Panel on Opportunistic Infections in HIV-Infected Adults and Adolescents. (2015). Guidelines for the prevention and treatment of opportunistic infections in HIV-infected adults and adolescents: Recommendations from the Centers for Disease Control and Prevention, the National Institutes of Health, and the HIV Medicine Association of the Infectious Diseases Society of America. Retrieved from https://aidsinfo.nih.gov/contentfiles/lvguidelines/adult_oi.pdf

Perfect, M. M., Bourne, N., Ebel, C., & Rosenthal, S. L. (2005). Use of complementary and alternative medicine for treatment of genital herpes. *Herpes, 12*, 38–41.

Prah, P., Copas, A. J., Mercer, C. H., Nardone, A., & Johnson, A. M. (2015). Patterns of sexual mixing with respect to social, health and sexual characteristics among heterosexual couples in England: analyses of probability sample survey data. *Epidemiology and Infection, 143*(7), 1500–1510. doi:10.1017/S0950268814002155

Rogers, S. M., Turner, C. F., Hobbs, M., Miller, W. C., Tan, S., Roman, A. M., . . . Erbelding, E. (2014). Epidemiology of undiagnosed trichomoniasis in a probability sample of urban young adults. *PloS One, 9*(3), e90548. doi:10.1371/journal.pone.0090548

Saslow, D., Solomon, D., Lawson, H. W., Killackey, M., Kulasingam, S. L., Cain, J., . . . Myers, E. R. (2012). American Cancer Society, American Society for Colposcopy and Cervical Pathology, and American Society for Clinical Pathology screening guidelines for the prevention and early detection of cervical cancer. *CA: A Cancer Journal for Clinicians, 62*(3), 147–172. doi:10.3322/caac.21139

Sastre, F., De La Rosa, M., Ibanez, G. E., Whitt, E., Martin, S. S., & O'Connell, D. J. (2015). Condom use preferences among Latinos in Miami–Dade: Emerging themes concerning men's and women's culturally-ascribed attitudes and behaviours. *Culture, Health & Sexuality, 17*(6), 667–681. doi:10.1080/13691058.2014.989266

Savaris, R. F., Ross, J., Fuhrich, D. G., Rodriguez-Malagon, N., & Duarte, R. V. (2013). Antibiotic therapy for pelvic inflammatory disease (PID) (Protocol). *Cochrane Database of Systematic Reviews, 1*, CD010285. doi:10.1002/14651858.CD010285

Senie, R.T. (2014). *Epidemiology of women's health*. Burlington, MA: Jones & Bartlett Learning.

Silver, B. J., Guy, R. J., Kaldor, J. M., Jamil, M. S., & Rumbold, A. R. (2014). *Trichomonas vaginalis* as a cause of perinatal morbidity: A systematic review and meta-analysis. *Sexually Transmitted Diseases, 41*(6), 369–376. doi:10.1097/OLQ.0000000000000134

Soper, D. E. (2010). Pelvic inflammatory disease. *Obstetrics & Gynecology, 116*, 419–428.

Sutherland, M., Fantasia, H. C., Fontenot, H. B., & Harris, A. (2012). Safer sex and partner violence in a sample of women. *Journal for Nurse Practitioners, 8*(9), 717–724.

Sutherland, M., Fantasia, H. C., & McClain, N. (2013). Abuse experiences, substance use, and sexual health in women seeking care at an emergency department. *Journal of Emergency Nursing, 39*(4), 326–333. doi:10.1016/j.jen.2011.09.011

Tat, S. A., Marrazzo, J. M., & Graham, S. M. (2015). Women who have sex with women living in low- and middle-income countries: A systematic review of sexual health and risk behaviors. *LGBT Health, 2*(2), 91–104. doi:10.1089/lgbt.2014.0124

Teitelman, A. M., Calhoun, J., Duncan, R., Washio, Y., & McDougall, R. (2015). Young women's views on testing for sexually transmitted infections and HIV as a risk reduction strategy in mutual and choice-restricted relationships. *Applied Nursing Research, 28*(3), 215–221. doi:10.1016/j.apnr.2015.04.016

Ulibarri, M. D., Roesch, S., Rangel, M. G., Staines, H., Amaro, H., & Strathdee, S. A. (2014). "Amar te Duele" ("love hurts"): Sexual relationship power, intimate partner violence, depression symptoms and HIV risk among female sex workers who use drugs and their non-commercial, steady partners in Mexico. *AIDS and Behavior, 19*(1), 9–18.

U.S. Department of Health and Human Services. (2015). Living with HIV/AIDS: Complementary and alternative therapy. Retrieved from http://aids.nlm.nih.gov/topic/1141/living-with-hiv-aids/1142/complementary-and-alternative-therapy

Van Der Pol, B., Kwok, C., Pierre-Louis, B., Rinaldi, A., Salata, R. A., Chen, P. L., . . . Morrison, C. S. (2008). *Trichomonas vaginalis* infection and human immunodeficiency virus acquisition in African women. *Journal of Infectious Diseases, 197*(4), 548–554. doi:10.1086/526496

Vasilenko, S. A., Kugler, K. C., Butera, N. M., & Lanza, S. T. (2015). Patterns of adolescent sexual behavior predicting young adult sexually transmitted infections: A latent class analysis approach. *Archives of Sexual Behavior, 44*, 705–714. doi:10.1007/s10508-014-0258-6

Webster, D. P., Klenerman, P., & Dusheiko, J. M. (2015). Hepatitis C. *Lancet, 385*, 1124–1135. doi:10.1016/S0140-6736(14)62401-6

Wechsberg, W. M., Deren, S., Myers, B., Kirtadze, I., Zule, W. A., Howard, B., & El-Bassel, N. (2015). Gender-specific HIV prevention interventions for women who use alcohol and other drugs: the evolution of the science and future directions. *Journal of Acquired Immune Deficiency Syndromes, 69*, S128–S139. doi:10.1097/QAI.0000000000000627

Woolf-King, S. E., & Maisto, S. A. (2015). The effects of alcohol, relationship power, and partner type on perceived difficulty implementing condom use among African American adults: An experimental study. *Archives of Sexual Behavior, 44*(3), 571–581. doi:10.1007/s10508-014-0362-7

Youngkin, E. Q., Davis, M. S., Schadewald, D. M., & Juve, C. (2013). *Women's health: A primary care guide* (4th ed.). Boston, MA: Pearson.

CHAPTER 21

Urinary Tract Infections

Mickey Gillmor-Kahn

Urinary tract infection (UTI) continues to be a major health problem for women worldwide. In this type of infection, bacteria ascend from the colonized urethra into the bladder, and they can continue to ascend into the kidneys. Many UTIs will resolve spontaneously without sequelae if left untreated (Knottnerus, Geerlings, Moll van Charante, & ter Reit, 2013); however, untreated UTIs can cause lasting damage to the kidneys, severe morbidity, and even mortality. Few UTIs arrive through the bloodstream. Women experience UTIs much more often than men, owing to women's pelvic anatomy and shorter urethras.

SCOPE OF THE PROBLEM

Clinicians who provide women's gynecologic health care will frequently diagnose and treat UTIs regardless of the type of healthcare setting. Half of all women have experienced a UTI by age 32 (Foxman & Brown, 2003). The burden of this disease on women and on society is great. In 2007 (most recent data available), there were 8.6 million ambulatory care visits (84% by women) with a primary diagnosis of UTI in the United States, and 23% of these occurred in hospital emergency departments (Schappert & Rechtsteiner, 2011). Litwin et al. (2005) estimate that expenditures related to UTI totaled $2.5 billion in 2000, which is equivalent to $3.4 billion in 2015.

Whatever clinicians can do to treat UTI rapidly and inexpensively will reduce these burdens. Of course, prevention would be even better, but unfortunately knowledge of effective strategies for prevention remains in its infancy.

ETIOLOGY

Urinary tract infection requires a susceptible host and an active pathogen. At least 50% of UTIs in non-hospitalized women can be ascribed to *Escherichia coli* (Foxman & Brown, 2003). In fact, some strains of *E. coli* are specifically adapted to growth in the bladder and, therefore, are designated as uro-pathogenic *E. coli*. In addition to *E. coli*, many other pathogens grow well in the bladder and can cause a symptomatic infection. These organisms include *Staphylococcus saprophyticus*, which may account for as many as 15% of UTIs (Foster, 2008); *Enterobacter* species; *Pseudomonas* species; and *Proteus mirabilis*. In addition to the presence of a uropathogen, the bladder epithelium must provide a hospitable environment for growth of the pathogen. Part of that hospitable environment may, in fact, include a genetic predisposition toward developing UTI (Hooton, 2012).

Women's increased susceptibility to UTI derives from their anatomy. The female urethra is short; there is a short distance between the urethra and the anus; and the perineal environment is moist, encouraging migration of bacteria from the rectum to the urethra (Foxman & Brown, 2003). Women whose mothers have had frequent UTIs also seem to be more susceptible to these infections. **Box 21-1** lists risk factors for UTI.

TYPES OF URINARY TRACT INFECTIONS

Urinary tract infections can be divided into two general classifications: cystitis, a relatively simple infection involving only the urinary bladder, and

---

BOX 21-1 Risk Factors for Urinary Tract Infection

- Previous UTI, including UTI as a child
- Maternal history of UTI in first-degree relative
- Women in professions in which frequent urination may be impeded (e.g., military, nurses, teachers)
- Incomplete bladder emptying
- Urinary incontinence
- Rectocele, cystocele, urethrocele, or utero-vaginal prolapse
- Urinary tract calculi
- Neurologic disorders or medical conditions requiring indwelling or repetitive bladder catheterization
- Anatomic congenital abnormalities of the urinary tract
- Frequent or recent sexual activity
- Diaphragm contraceptive use
- Use of vaginal spermicidal agents
- Vaginal atrophy
- Obesity
- Diabetes mellitus
- Sickle cell trait or disease
- ABO blood group non-secretor status

Abbreviation: UTI, urinary tract infection.
Data from American College of Obstetricians and Gynecologists. (2008, reaffirmed 2014). ACOG Practice Bulletin No. 91: Treatment of urinary tract infections in nonpregnant women. *Obstetrics & Gynecology, 111*, 785–794; Hooton, T. M. (2012). Uncomplicated urinary tract infection. *New England Journal of Medicine, 366*(11), 1028–1037; Wagenlehner, F. M. E., Weidner, W., & Naber, K. G. (2009). An update on uncomplicated urinary tract infections in women. *Current Opinion in Urology, 19*, 368–374. doi:10.1097/MOU.0b013e32832ae18c

---

upper tract infection or pyelonephritis, an infection involving one or both kidneys (**Table 21-1**). Many women also experience transient asymptomatic bacteriuria that either may eventually lead to infection or may resolve on its own. Even symptomatic UTIs may spontaneously resolve without treatment (Knottnerus et al., 2013).

Asymptomatic Bacteriuria

Asymptomatic bacteriuria, by definition, does not cause the patient to experience any symptoms, but is identified when a coincidental urinalysis shows bacteria in the urine. Treatment is not needed unless the woman is pregnant or major urinary tract surgery is planned (Wagenlehner & Naber, 2012). Additionally, treatment of asymptomatic bacteriuria in the nonpregnant woman may cause harm by damaging her microbiota, which may be protective, and selecting for antibiotic-resistant organisms (Cai et al., 2012; Cai et al., 2015; Foxman, 2010). For these reasons, screening of asymptomatic women who are not pregnant or planning major urinary tract surgery should be avoided (Gross & Patel, 2007; Nicolle, 2014; Wagenlehner & Naber, 2012).

Cystitis

Acute bacterial cystitis is the most common type of UTI affecting women. Its symptoms typically include dysuria with urinary frequency and urgency. Hematuria may also be present. Usually there is no fever, no costovertebral angle tenderness, and no flank pain. Uncomplicated cystitis occurs in a woman who is not pregnant, has not had any recent treatment with antibiotics, has not had another UTI in the last 6 months (or two UTIs in the last 12 months), has no decreased immunity due to other conditions, and has no signs of upper tract infection. Uncomplicated acute bacterial cystitis can be treated without a culture; in fact, it can be treated without a urinalysis in women who have had UTIs frequently in the past and have classic symptoms (American College of Obstetricians and Gynecologists, 2008, reaffirmed 2014).

Complicated bacterial cystitis occurs in women who are pregnant, have had recent antibiotics, have had another UTI within the last 6 months (or two other UTIs in the past 12 months), or have decreased immunity from another condition. These women require culture and sensitivity tests for diagnosis and to determine the appropriate treatment.

Pyelonephritis

When infection in the bladder ascends to the kidneys, the patient has pyelonephritis. Some authors

TABLE **21-1**	Types of Urinary Tract Infections

Infection	Definition	Uncomplicated	Complicated
Asymptomatic bacteriuria	Bacteria present in the urine with no symptoms	NA	NA
Cystitis	Involves only the urinary bladder and urethra	No fever, costovertebral angle tenderness, or flank pain None of the conditions listed under "Complicated"	Pregnant Recent antibiotics Previous UTI in last 6 months or two UTIs in last 12 months Decreased immunity No fever, costovertebral angle tenderness, or flank pain
Pyelonephritis	Involves one or both kidneys	Fever, costovertebral angle tenderness, and/or flank pain Not pregnant No vomiting No significant underlying disease that could affect treatment	Pregnant Vomiting Immunodeficient

Abbreviations: NA, not applicable; UTI, urinary tract infection.

distinguish between pyelitis (an infection in the renal pelvis that does not extend into the parenchyma) and pyelonephritis (an infection extending into the renal parenchyma). This chapter uses the term *pyelonephritis* for both conditions because they are impossible to differentiate clinically. Rarely, upper tract infection will arrive by descending through the bloodstream rather than ascending from the bladder. Like lower tract infection, upper UTI is most commonly the result of colonization with *E. coli*, although other organisms can also be involved (Colgan, Williams, & Johnson, 2011).

Like the other forms of UTI, pyelonephritis may be divided into uncomplicated and complicated infections. Uncomplicated pyelonephritis occurs in a woman who has symptoms of upper tract infection, but is not pregnant and is not nauseated or vomiting. Most of these infections can be treated on an outpatient basis. Patients who are pregnant, vomiting, hypotensive, or immunodeficient should usually be hospitalized for treatment.

Good studies of the incidence of pyelonephritis, the organisms responsible for this type of UTI, the relative efficacy of inpatient and outpatient treatment, and the epidemiology of pyelonephritis are lacking (Foxman, Ki, & Brown, 2007). One epidemiologic study suggests that many cases of pyelonephritis are actually treated without culture, although this practice is not recommended (Czaja, Scholes, Hooton, & Stamm, 2007).

Symptoms of pyelonephritis typically include fever, chills, back pain, costovertebral angle tenderness, and flank pain. Some women will have dysuria, urinary frequency and urgency, and hematuria as well. Occasionally, pyelonephritis will be silent until the patient presents with hypotension and even septic shock. Some patients experience nausea, vomiting, and diarrhea. Silent pyelonephritis should be considered in any woman who presents with illness and has a history of repeated UTI, especially if the UTI ascended to the kidneys. Untreated pyelonephritis may lead to kidney damage, including secondary hypertension and renal failure, sepsis, and death (Piccoli et al., 2008).

ASSESSMENT

History

Uncomplicated, nonrecurrent bacterial cystitis can be treated based on the patient's history alone; no laboratory testing is required. A report of nonrecurrent dysuria, frequency, and urgency is adequate to diagnose lower UTI (American College of Obstetricians and Gynecologists, 2008, reaffirmed 2014; Hooton, 2012) To rule out upper tract infection or a complicated UTI, other history must be elicited, however (**Box 21-2**).

Physical Examination

Physical examination of the woman with urinary symptoms is useful primarily to rule out more complicated disease. Some women with uncomplicated UTI have suprapubic tenderness. Flank pain may be present, but usually is not with uncomplicated UTI. Its presence would raise the index of

---

suspicion for pyelonephritis. Typically, the woman with pyelonephritis feels acutely ill. She may have fever, chills, nausea, vomiting, and costovertebral angle tenderness, as well as the symptoms of cystitis—namely, dysuria, frequency, urgency, and suprapubic pain (Colgan et al., 2011).

Laboratory Testing

If the clinician cannot rule out a complicated UTI or an upper tract infection by history alone, laboratory testing is necessary. Tools available for this purpose include the urine dipstick, microscopic urinalysis, and urine culture with sensitivities, each of which has its own place in the diagnostic process.

The urine dipstick is an inexpensive screening tool that may be used to confirm the UTI diagnosis if the history is ambiguous. A concentrated first-voided specimen is most reliable, but not always available. A dipstick that is positive for leukocyte esterase or nitrite is 75% sensitive and 82% specific for UTI (American College of Obstetricians and Gynecologists, 2008, reaffirmed 2014). Symptomatic women with a negative dipstick should have a microscopic urinalysis and/or a urine culture and sensitivity test because the dipstick may be falsely negative for a number of reasons—often because the sample is too dilute or because the leukocytes have lysed due to the passage of time (Kupelian et al., 2013).

Leukocyte esterase found on dipstick indicates that leukocytes are present in the urine, but cannot determine whether the leukocytes came from the bladder or from the vagina. While clinicians have long requested a clean midstream-voided sample, some studies have found little difference in contamination from vaginal and perineal secretions between women who washed prior to voiding and those who did not (Blake & Doherty, 2006). Extensive teaching about perineal cleansing prior to collecting a midstream sample is not necessary. With this change in practice, it is possible to collect the first part of the urine stream to use in nucleic acid amplification testing (NAAT) or polymerase chain reaction (PCR) testing for gonorrhea and chlamydia; the second midstream part can then be used for urine culture.

Nitrites are produced in the urine when bacteria present in the urine convert the normally present

---

> ## BOX 21-2 Questions to Identify Complicated Cystitis and Pyelonephritis
>
> - Are you or could you be pregnant?
> - Have you had any fever or chills?
> - Do you have any flank pain or back pain?
> - Are you nauseated or have you vomited?
> - Have you ever had a urinary tract (bladder or kidney) infection before? If so, when? How was it treated?
> - Have you taken any medicines recently? Antibiotics? Pain relievers? Over-the-counter products?
> - Do you have any other medical problems?
> - Do you take any medications on a regular basis?
> - Are you having any vaginal discharge or other vaginal problems?

nitrates to nitrites. Although *E. coli* (the most common uropathogen) does convert nitrates to nitrites, not all uropathogens do so. Therefore, failure to identify nitrites on dipstick or urinalysis does not rule out a UTI.

Urine microscopy for the woman with pyelonephritis will usually reveal red blood cells, white blood cells, and white blood cell casts (**Color Plate 27**). Samples from patients with cystitis alone usually do not show casts.

Urine culture is the reference standard for diagnosis of a UTI. Sensitivities to antibiotics ascertained at the time of the culture will guide appropriate treatment. Culture and sensitivity tests are expensive and time-consuming, however, and empiric treatment should not be delayed to wait for these results. A 2011 retrospective cohort study of nondiabetic, nonpregnant adult women aged 18 to 65 years with UTI symptoms found no increase in follow-up visits between those who did and did not have urine cultures performed (Johnson, O'Mara, Durtschi, & Kobjar, 2011). According to the researchers, these findings support the current recommendation to avoid urine culture in such patients.

Urine culture is not needed for symptomatic women who meet the criteria for uncomplicated bacterial cystitis (American College of Obstetricians and Gynecologists, 2008, reaffirmed 2014); these patients can be treated based on history alone. **Box 21-3** lists indications for urine culture. Increasing concern about empiric treatment with antibiotics and the development of resistant uropathogens may mean that in the future urine culture will again be recommended prior to treatment (Wagenlehner, Weidner, & Naber, 2009), but the recommendations do not support routine urine culture for UTI symptoms at this time.

In contrast, a urine culture and sensitivity test are indicated in any woman with a complicated cystitis or symptoms of upper tract disease. Empiric treatment must be initiated prior to obtaining the culture and sensitivity results; it should be modified later if the results indicate resistance or the patient is not improving. Blood cultures have not been shown to be useful unless the diagnosis is uncertain, the patient is immunocompromised, or assessment of the patient suggests the presence of descending infection from the blood to the kidney (American College of Obstetricians and Gynecologists, 2008, reaffirmed 2014).

DIFFERENTIAL DIAGNOSES

The differential diagnosis of dysuria/urgency/frequency in women includes bacterial cystitis, pyelonephritis, interstitial cystitis/painful bladder syndrome (see Chapter 28), and urethritis related to a sexually transmitted infection—usually gonorrhea or chlamydia (see Chapter 20). The differential diagnosis for a woman with pyelonephritis symptoms should also include nephrolithiasis. Usually fever associated with pyelonephritis will resolve within 72 hours of treatment with appropriate antibiotics. Failure to resolve may indicate abscess, obstruction, or a resistant organism.

MANAGEMENT

Cystitis

Antibiotic Treatment
Treatment of an uncomplicated lower UTI will depend largely on resistance patterns in the community, if known, and on the patient's history and allergies. **Table 21-2** shows the treatment regimens recommended by the American College of Obstetricians and Gynecologists for an uncomplicated acute bacterial cystitis.

Indiscriminate prescribing of antibiotics has led to resistance patterns in many communities. Given this fact, clinicians should consult infectious

---

BOX **21-3** **Indications for a Urine Culture in a Woman with Urinary Tract Infection Symptoms**

- Pregnancy
- Signs of upper tract infection (fever, costovertebral angle tenderness, and/or flank pain)
- Recent urinary tract infection
- Recent antibiotic treatment
- Chronic disease affecting the immune system

TABLE 21-2	Treatment Regimens for Uncomplicated Acute Bacterial Cystitis

Antimicrobial Agent	Dose	Adverse Events
Trimethoprim–sulfamethoxazole	One tablet (160 mg trimethoprim + 800 mg sulfamethoxazole), twice daily for 3 days	Fever, rash, photosensitivity, neutropenia, thrombocytopenia, anorexia, nausea and vomiting, pruritus, headache, urticaria, Stevens-Johnson syndrome, toxic epidermal necrosis, and hemolysis in individuals with glucose-6-dehydrogenase deficiency
Trimethoprim	100 mg, twice daily for 3 days	Rash, pruritus, photosensitivity, exfoliative dermatitis, Stevens-Johnson syndrome, toxic epidermal necrosis, and aseptic meningitis
Ciprofloxacin	250 mg, twice daily for 3 days	Rash, confusion, seizures, restlessness, headache, severe hypersensitivity, hypoglycemia, hyperglycemia, and Achilles tendon rupture (in patients older than 60 years)
Levofloxacin	250 mg, once daily for 3 days	Same as for ciprofloxacin
Norfloxacin	400 mg, twice daily for 3 days	Same as for ciprofloxacin
Gatifloxacin	200 mg, once daily for 3 days	Same as for ciprofloxacin
Nitrofurantoin macrocrystals	50–100 mg, 4 times daily for 7 days	Anorexia, nausea, vomiting, hypersensitivity, peripheral neuropathy, hepatitis, hemolytic anemia, and pulmonary reactions
Nitrofurantoin mono-hydrate macrocrystals	100 mg, twice daily for 7 days	Same as for nitrofurantoin macrocrystals
Fosfomycin tromethamine	3 g dose (powder), single dose	Diarrhea, nausea, vomiting, rash, and hypersensitivity

Reproduced from American College of Obstetricians and Gynecologists. (2008, reaffirmed 2014). ACOG Practice Bulletin No. 91: Treatment of urinary tract infections in nonpregnant women. *Obstetrics & Gynecology, 111,* 785–794. Reprinted with permission.

disease experts in their communities, if available, to become aware of the prevalence of resistance and alter their prescribing practices as needed. Frequent review of these patterns is appropriate, because resistance changes over time. Whenever possible, however, clinicians should prescribe the least expensive and narrowest-spectrum drug to avoid increasing the problem of microbial resistance and to decrease costs for both patients and the health system (American College of Obstetricians and Gynecologists, 2008, reaffirmed 2014; Fihn, 2003; Gross & Patel, 2007).

Although 7-day treatment has been the norm in the past, research has shown that 3-day regimens of many of these drugs have equal effectiveness in women; thus the shorter-duration regimens are now recommended (see **Table 21-2**). Overprescribing leads to unnecessary costs to both the patient and the health system (American College of Obstetricians and Gynecologists, 2008, reaffirmed 2014; Hooton, 2012; Kahan, Chinitz, & Kahan, 2004).

Treatment of Pain

An acute UTI can be extremely painful and cause significant disruption of a woman's life. Symptoms should resolve within 72 hours of the initiation of antibiotic treatment. If they do not, the clinician must consider a change in therapy or another diagnosis. Some women will desire treatment of the dysuria for 1 or 2 days with phenazopyridine, which is now available in the United States on an over-the-counter (OTC) basis. This drug will color the urine orange and is associated with numerous adverse effects, including gastrointestinal upset, headaches, rash, hemolysis in those women with glucose-6-dehydrogenase deficiency, and nephrotoxicity (Fihn, 2003; Scheurer, 2006; Youngster et al., 2010). Patients should be cautioned against chronic use of phenazopyridine. Those choosing to use this agent should also be made aware of the danger associated with its accidental ingestion by children (Gold & Bithoney, 2003).

Pyelonephritis

Uncomplicated pyelonephritis is diagnosed in the woman who has clinical evidence of upper tract disease but is not pregnant, is able to tolerate oral treatment, and has no concurrent conditions leading to immunocompromise. Most authorities agree that uncomplicated pyelonephritis may be treated on an outpatient basis if the woman is likely to be able to complete the treatment regimen and is able to return for follow-up. Treatment for 10 to 14 days is recommended, usually with a fluoroquinolone if the level of resistance to this antibiotic does not exceed 10% in the community (American College of Obstetricians and Gynecologists, 2008, reaffirmed 2014; Colgan et al., 2011; Wagenlehner et al., 2009). Knowledge of local patterns of resistance should guide initial treatment, followed by evaluation of treatment results and the culture and sensitivity test. Severely ill women with pyelonephritis may need hospitalization to receive parenteral antibiotics.

> **BOX 21-4** Indications for Hospitalizing a Woman with Pyelonephritis
>
> - Severe illness
> - Pregnancy
> - Immunocompromise
> - Inability to tolerate oral treatment due to vomiting
> - Inability to adhere to oral treatment or return for follow-up due to age, living situation, or lack of social support

Piccoli et al. (2006), in an extensive review of randomized controlled trials of pyelonephritis treatment, found little solid evidence for determining what the ideal length of treatment is, which drugs are better, or even whether renal scarring post pyelonephritis results in negative long-term effects.

Hospitalization is appropriate when parenteral treatment is needed, other conditions warrant increased surveillance, or the woman is unable to manage an outpatient regimen (Wagenlehner et al., 2009); **Box 21-4** summarizes these criteria. Decisions about hospitalization for pregnant women will depend on the woman's social support network, age, and degree of illness. Most clinicians prefer at least a brief period of hospitalized observation while initial doses or parenteral antibiotics are given to the pregnant woman, along with monitoring for preterm labor and respiratory sufficiency.

Patient Education

Clinicians treating women with UTIs can share with them what is known and unknown about prevention of UTIs. While forcing fluids is not recommended, drinking to alleviate thirst can be helpful as well as not delaying voiding. The importance of completing the treatment regimen even if symptoms resolve before all medications are taken should be emphasized to avoid the development of resistant organisms. Most importantly, a woman who has been diagnosed with a UTI should be advised to contact the clinician if her symptoms persist after 48 hours of antibiotic treatment.

Prevention

Many women develop frequent UTIs. In fact, as many as 20% to 30% of women with a UTI will have at least one additional infection within 12 months; recurrent UTI is defined as three or more UTIs in a 12-month period (Albert et al., 2004). Risk factors for UTI should be investigated and altered where possible to prevent such infections.

Clinicians and the lay public have promoted many recommendations regarding how to avoid UTIs, but there is little evidence that most of these strategies are effective. Increasing fluids, wiping front to back, and avoidance of delayed urination have not been adequately studied. These simple measures will, no doubt, still be recommended by many clinicians, because they make empiric sense and are inexpensive. Aggressive hydration could, however, be harmful if large volumes of urine encourage retrograde flow into the ureters. Similarly, no studies have demonstrated the efficacy of postcoital voiding in women whose UTIs appear to be associated with sexual activity (Fiore & Fox, 2014).

Antibiotic prophylaxis has been studied in the form of several different regimens (Albert et al., 2004; Geerlings, Beerepoot, & Prins, 2014). Single-dose postcoital antibiotics may be helpful for women who find an association between sexual activity and UTIs. Trimethoprim–sulfamethoxazole (TMP/SMX), trimethoprim alone, nitrofurantoin, and fluoroquinolones have all been shown to be effective for this purpose. Alternatively, continuous daily or every-other-day prophylaxis with nitrofurantoin, TMP/SMX, or a fluoroquinolone can decrease recurrence rates. Some women will prefer to self-initiate a 3-day course of treatment only if symptoms develop. Concerns regarding resistance patterns and the promotion of increased resistance as previously described for acute treatment apply equally to prophylactic uses of these drugs. Additionally, concerns have been raised about the use of sulfonamides in early pregnancy.

Most UTIs derive from intestinal and/or vaginal bacteria. On the theory that ingestion of lactobacilli could potentially change the flora of the intestine or the vagina, various forms of lactobacilli have been suggested as a preventive measure. The use of lactobacilli vaginal suppositories or oral capsules has been studied, albeit with inconsistent results being found depending on the strain used (Geerlings et al., 2014; Grin, Kowalewska, Alhazzan, & Fox-Robichaud, 2013). The most promising formulations are *L. crispatus* vaginal suppositories and *L. rhamnosus* GR-1 and *L. reuteri* RC-14 oral capsules (Geerlings et al., 2014).

Cranberry products contain several substances that may help to prevent UTIs. Early theories focused on the conversion of quinic acid in the cranberries to hippuric acid, which would then inhibit growth of bacteria. Measurement of the levels of hippuric acid in the bladder after ingestion of cranberry does not support this theory, however. Current theories suggest that the fructose in cranberries may keep *E. coli* from adhering to the bladder cell walls or that substances called proanthocyanidins do the same by a different process. In vitro studies have demonstrated inhibition of *E. coli* attachment for both fructose and proanthocyanidins (Jepson & Craig, 2008). Multiple trials have shown an association between ingestion of cranberry products and decreased rates of UTIs (Dugoua, Seely, Perri, Mills, & Koren, 2008; Jepson & Craig, 2008; Kontiokari et al., 2001). Disappointingly, however, the most recent Cochrane review of cranberry as prophylaxis for UTI concluded that there is no evidence of its efficacy (Jepson, Williams, & Craig, 2012). The authors of the review raised questions about the doses of cranberry used, the active ingredients in cranberry delivered by capsules or tablets, and the difficulty with long-term compliance. In the more controlled setting of a long-term care facility, Caljouw et al. (2014) found administration of cranberry capsules twice a day decreased UTI incidence in older women at high risk for UTI (e.g., diabetes, catheterization for more than 1 month, UTI within the previous year) but had no effect on UTI incidence in low-risk women. At this time, the evidence does not support use of cranberry products as a UTI-preventive measure in the general population (Jepson, Williams, & Craig, 2012).

Chinese herbal medicine has also been used for prevention of recurrent UTI. A recent Cochrane review suggests Chinese herbal medicine, used independently or in conjunction with antibiotics, may be beneficial for treating recurrent UTIs and reducing recurrence (Flower, Wang, Lewith, Liu, & Li, 2015). Tong, Jia, and Han (2013), on the one hand, report a case of chronic use of Chinese herbal therapy leading to development of a resistant strain of *E. coli*.

Tong, Sun, and Wang (2014), on the other hand, report a case of pyelonephritis associated with multidrug-resistant *Pseudomonas aeruginosa* that was successfully treated with Chinese herbal medicine.

SPECIAL CONSIDERATIONS

Adolescents

Because of the association between sexual activity and UTI, a UTI in a teenager may indicate the initiation of sexual activity. A discussion of pregnancy risk and sexually transmitted infection prevention is appropriate for adolescents. Whether an adolescent with pyelonephritis needs to be hospitalized will depend on the clinician's judgment of whether she will be able to adhere to outpatient treatment.

Postmenopausal Women

The strongest predictor of UTI in a study of postmenopausal women was premenopausal lifetime history of more than six UTIs (Jackson et al., 2004). Studies suggest topical—but not oral—estrogen therapy decreases the risk of recurrent UTIs in postmenopausal women (Mody & Juthani-Mehta, 2014; Rahn et al., 2014). A review of studies of asymptomatic and symptomatic UTI in older women found no support for treating asymptomatic bacteriuria in older community-dwelling women (Mody & Juthani-Mehta, 2014).

Pregnant Women

Anatomic and physiologic changes related to pregnancy place the pregnant woman at increased risk of UTI, including pyelonephritis. A urine culture is recommended for all women at the first prenatal visit, regardless of symptoms, and bacteriuria should be treated whether symptomatic or not (Nicolle, 2014). Pyelonephritis during pregnancy is associated with preterm labor, sepsis, acute respiratory failure, and even death (Jolley, Kim, & Wing, 2012). Many clinicians will choose to hospitalize the pregnant woman with pyelonephritis to monitor for complications and ensure adequate treatment.

Influences of Culture

Women in professions where frequent urination is impeded have higher rates of UTIs. For example, women in the military, nurses, teachers, and factory workers, who often work in settings where voiding on demand is restricted or difficult, are all susceptible to UTIs. Education about the need for voiding when the urge is present can decrease the incidence of UTIs in these women. They should also be cautioned against limiting fluids to decrease the need to urinate. Some who have worked under these conditions for a long time will no longer feel a need to urinate until the bladder is already overdistended. For them, timed voiding may be helpful in reestablishing normal bladder responsivity and avoiding UTI (Steele & Yoder, 2013; Su, Wang, Lu, & Guo, 2006).

References

Albert, X., Huertas, I., Pereiró, I. I., Sanfélix, J., Gosalbes, V., & Perrota, C. (2004). Antibiotics for preventing recurrent urinary tract infection in non-pregnant women. *Database of Systematic Reviews, 3*, CD001209. doi:10.1002/14651858.CD001209.pub2

American College of Obstetricians and Gynecologists. (2008, reaffirmed 2014). ACOG Practice Bulletin No. 91: Treatment of urinary tract infections in nonpregnant women. *Obstetrics & Gynecology, 111*, 785–794.

Blake, D. R., & Doherty, L. F. (2006). Effect of perineal cleansing on contamination rate of mid-stream urine culture. *Journal of Pediatric & Adolescent Gynecology, 19*(1), 31–34. doi:10.1016/j.jpag.2005.11.003

Cai, T., Mazzoli, S., Mondaini, N., Meacci, F., Nesi, G., D'Elia, C., . . . Bartoletti, R. (2012). The role of asymptomatic bacteriuria in young women with recurrent urinary tract infections: To treat or not to treat? *Clinical Infectious Diseases, 55*(6), 771–777. doi:10.1093/cid/cis534

Cai, T., Nesi, G., Mazzoli, S., Meacci, F., Lanzafame, P., Caciagli, P., . . . Bartoletti, R. (2015). Asymptomatic bacteriuria treatment is associated with a higher prevalence of antibiotic resistant strains in women with urinary tract infections. *Clinical Infectious Diseases, 61*(11), 1655–1661. doi:10.1093/cid/civ696

Caljouw, M. A. A., van den Hout, W. B., Putter, H., Achterberg, W. P., Cools, H. J. M., & Gussekloo, J. (2014). Effectiveness of cranberry capsules to prevent urinary tract infections in vulnerable older persons: A double-blind randomized placebo-controlled trial in long-term care facilities. *Journal of the American Geriatrics Society, 62*(1), 103–110. doi:10.1111/jgs.12593

Colgan, R., Williams, M., & Johnson, J. (2011). Diagnosis and treatment of acute pyelonephritis in women. *American Family Physician, 84*(5), 519–526.

Czaja, C. A., Scholes, D., Hooton, T. M., & Stamm, W. E. (2007). Population-based epidemiologic analysis of acute pyelonephritis. *Clinical Infectious Diseases, 45*(3), 273–280. doi:10.1086/519268

Dugoua, J., Seely, D., Perri, D., Mills, E., & Koren, G. (2008). Safety and efficacy of cranberry (*Vaccinium macrocarpon*) during pregnancy and lactation. *Canadian Journal of Clinical Pharmacology, 15*(1), e80–e86.

Fihn, S. D. (2003). Clinical practice: Acute uncomplicated urinary tract infection in women. *New England Journal of Medicine, 349*, 259–266. doi:10.1056/NEJMcp030027

Fiore, D. C., & Fox, C. L. (2014). Urology and nephrology update: Recurrent urinary tract infection. *FP Essentials, 416*, 30–37.

Flower, A., Wang, L. Q., Lewith, G., Liu, J. P., & Li, Q. (2015). Chinese herbal medicine for treating recurrent urinary tract infections in women. *Cochrane Database of Systematic Reviews, 6*, CD010446. doi:10.1002/14651858.CD010446.pub2

Foster, R. T. (2008). Uncomplicated urinary tract infections in women. *Obstetrics and Gynecology Clinics of North America, 38*, 235–248. doi:10.1016/j.ogc.2008.03.003

Foxman, B. (2010). The epidemiology of urinary tract infection. *Nature Reviews: Urology, 7*, 653–660. doi:10.1038/nrurol.2010.190

Foxman, B., & Brown, P. (2003). Epidemiology of urinary tract infections: Transmission and risk factors, incidence, and costs. *Infectious Disease Clinics of North America, 17*(2), 227–241. doi:10.1016/S0891-5520(03)00005-9

Foxman, B., Ki, M., & Brown, P. (2007). Antibiotic resistance and pyelonephritis. *Clinical Infectious Diseases, 45*(3), 281–283. doi:10.1086/519267

Geerlings, S. E., Beerepoot, M. A. J., & Prins, J. M. (2014). Prevention of recurrent urinary tract infections in women: Antimicrobial and nonantimicrobial strategies. *Infectious Disease Clinics of North America, 28*(1), 135–147.

Gold, N. A., & Bithoney, W. G. (2003). Methemoglobinemia due to ingestion of at most three pills of pyridium in a 2-year-old: Case report and review. *Journal of Emergency Medicine, 25*(2), 143–148. doi:10.1016/S0736-4679(03)00162-8

Grin, P. M., Kowalewska, P. M., Alhazzan, W., & Fox-Robichaud, A. E. (2013). *Lactobacillus* for prevention recurrent urinary tract infections in women: Meta-analysis. *Canadian Journal of Urology, 20*(1), 6607–6614.

Gross, P. A., & Patel, B. (2007). Reducing antibiotic overuse: A call for a national performance measure for not treating asymptomatic bacteriuria. *Clinical Infectious Diseases, 45*(10), 1335–1337. doi:10.1086/522183; PMid:17968830

Hooton, T. M. (2012). Uncomplicated urinary tract infection. *New England Journal of Medicine, 366*(11), 1028–1037.

Jackson, S. L., Boyko, E. J., Scholes, D., Abraham, L., Gupta, K., & Fihn, S. D. (2004). Predictors of urinary tract infection after menopause: A prospective study. *American Journal of Medicine, 117*, 903–911.

Jepson, R. G., & Craig, J. C. (2008). Cranberries for preventing urinary tract infections. *Cochrane Database of Systematic Reviews, 1*, CD001321. doi:10.1002/14651858.CD001321.pub4

Jepson, R. G, Williams, G., & Craig, J. C. (2012). Cranberries for preventing urinary tract infections. *Cochrane Database of Systematic Reviews, 10*, CD001321. doi:10.1002/14651858.CD001321.pub5

Johnson, J. D., O'Mara, H. M., Durtschi, H. F., & Kobjar, B. (2011) Do urine cultures for urinary tract infections decrease follow-up visits? *Journal of the American Board of Family Medicine, 24*(6), 647–655. doi:10.3122/jabfm.2011.06.100299

Jolley, J. A., Kim, S., & Wing, D. A. (2012). Acute pyelonephritis and associated complications during pregnancy in 2006 in US hospitals. *Journal of Maternal–Fetal & Neonatal Medicine, 25*(12), 2494–2498.

Kahan, N. R., Chinitz, D. P., & Kahan, E. (2004). Longer than recommended empiric antibiotic treatment of urinary tract infection in women: An avoidable waste of money. *Journal of Clinical Pharmacology & Therapeutics, 29*(1), 59–63. doi:10.1111/j.1365-2710.2003.00537.x

Knottnerus, B. J., Geerlings, S. E., Moll van Charante, E. P., & ter Reit, G. (2013). Women with symptoms of uncomplicated urinary tract infection are often willing to delay antibiotic treatment: A prospective cohort study. *BMC Family Practice, 14*, 71. Retrieved from http://www.biomedcentral.com/1471-2296/14/71

Kontiokari, T., Sundqvist, K., Nuutinen, M., Pokka, T., Koskela, M., & Uhari, M. (2001). Randomised trial of cranberry–lingonberry juice and *Lactobacillus* GG drink for the prevention of urinary tract infections in women. *British Medical Journal, 322*(7302), 1571. doi:10.1136/bmj.322.7302.1571

Kupelian, A. S., Horsley, H., Khasriya, R., Amussah, R. T., Badiani, R., Courtney, A. M., . . . Malone-Lee, J. (2013). Discrediting microscopic pyuria and leucocyte esterase as diagnostic surrogates for infection in patients with lower urinary tract symptoms: Results from a clinical and laboratory evaluation. *British Journal of Urology International, 112*(2), 231–238. doi:10.1111/j.1464-410X.2012.11694.x

Litwin, M. S., Saigal, C. S., Yano, E. M., Avila, C., Geschwind, S. A., Hanley, J. M., . . . Wang, M. (2005). Urologic Diseases in America Project: Analytical methods and principal findings. *Journal of Urology, 173*, 933–937. doi:10.1097/01.ju.0000152365.43125.3b

Mody, L., & Juthani-Mehta, M. (2014). Urinary tract infections in older women: A clinical review. *Journal of the American Medical Association, 311*(8), 844–854. doi:10.1001/jama.2014.303

Nicolle, L. E. (2014). Asymptomatic bacteriuria. *Current Opinion in Infectious Diseases, 27*(1), 90–96.

Piccoli, B. G., Cresto, E., Ragni, F., Veglio, V., Scarpa, R. M., & Frascisco, M. (2008). The clinical spectrum of acute "uncomplicated" pyelonephritis from an emergency medicine perspective. *International Journal of Antimicrobial Agents, 31*(suppl 1), S46–S53. doi:10.1016/j.ijantimicag.2007.09.017

Piccoli, G. B., Consiglio, V., Colla, L., Mesiano, P., Magnano, A., Burdese, M., . . . Piccoli, G. (2006). Antibiotic treatment for acute "uncomplicated" or "primary" pyelonephritis: A systematic, "semantic revision." *International Journal of Antimicrobial Agents, 28S*, S49–S63. doi:10.1016/j.ijantimicag.2006.05.017

Rahn, D. D., Carberry, C., Sanses, T. V., Mamik, M. M., Ward, R. M., Meriwether, K. V. . . . Murphy, M. (2014). Vaginal estrogen for genitourinary syndrome of menopause: A systematic review. *Obstetrics & Gynecology, 124*(6), 1147–1156.

Schappert, S. M., & Rechtsteiner, E. A. (2011). Ambulatory medical care utilization estimates for 2007. *Vital Health Statistics, 13*(169), 1–38.

Scheurer, D. B. (2006). An over-the-counter omission. *Southern Medical Journal, 99*, 1005–1006. doi:10.1097/01.smj.0000215641.58901.4c

Steele, N., & Yoder, L. H. (2013). Military women's urinary patterns, practices, and complications in deployment settings. *Urologic Nursing, 33*(2), 61–71, 78.

Su, S., Wang, J., Lu, C., & Guo, H. (2006). Reducing urinary tract infections among female clean room workers. *Journal of Women's Health, 15*, 870–876. doi:10.1089/jwh.2006.15.870

Tong, Y., Jia, S., & Han, B. (2013). Chinese herb–resistant clinical isolates of Escherichia coli. *Journal of Alternative and Complementary Medicine, 19*(4), 387–388. doi:10.1089/acm.2011.0955

Tong, Y., Sun, M, & Wang, C. (2014). Multidrug-resistant *Pseudomonas aeruginosa*: A case of pyelonephritis and herbal therapy. *Journal of Alternative and Complementary Medicine, 20*(2), 142–144. doi:10.1089/acm.2012.0864

Wagenlehner, F. M. E., & Naber, K. G. (2012). Asymptomatic bacteriuria: Shift of paradigm. *Clinical Infectious Diseases, 55,* 778–780. doi:10.1093/cid/cis541

Wagenlehner, F. M. E., Weidner, W., & Naber, K. G. (2009). An update on uncomplicated urinary tract infections in women. *Current Opinion in Urology, 19,* 368–374. doi:10.1097/MOU.0b013e32832ae18c

Youngster, I., Arcavi, L., Schechmaster, R., Akayzen, Y., Popliski, H., Shimonov Beig, S., & Berkovitch, M. (2010). Medications and glucose-6-phosphatase dehydrogenase deficiency: An evidence-based review. *Drug Safety, 33*(9), 713–726.

CHAPTER 22

Urinary Incontinence

Ying Sheng
Janis M. Miller
The editors acknowledge Sandra H. Hines, who was a coauthor of the previous edition of this chapter.

INTRODUCTION

Many women experience urinary incontinence (UI) at some point in their life. Urinary incontinence is one of the lower urinary tract symptoms (LUTS) and is among the more general classification of pelvic floor disorder—a category that also includes pelvic organ prolapse and pelvic pain. Midwives and adult nurse practitioners specializing in incontinence are the nurses most prepared to care for women experiencing pelvic floor disorders. In medicine, urogynecologists are physicians who have completed a residency in obstetrics and gynecology or urology, and have become specialists through additional years of fellowship training and certification in female pelvic medicine and reconstructive surgery, a subspecialty newly accredited by the American Urogynecologic Society in 2015.

Although most forms of UI are not directly related to birthing, women's unique ability to give birth means there are anatomic differences between women and men. These differences include greater pliability of the pelvic structures and a much shorter urethra located within (rather than outside) the pelvis. In addition, social constructs around female genitalia and toileting behaviors drive UI as an issue that disproportionately affects women's quality of life. A woman with UI can experience issues ranging in severity from a minor annoyance or inconvenience to a changed perception of herself as a social and sexual partner. Urinary incontinence can undermine a woman's body image and sense of control. It can also consume considerable amounts of her resources, through both purchases of expensive self-care products and healthcare expenses incurred. In many resource-scarce areas of the world, a woman may not be able to afford or even find appropriate care, and she can risk serious social isolation from her community as a result of UI-related issues.

Thus, caring for a woman with UI requires a holistic approach, including assessment of commonly associated LUTS and other pelvic floor disorders. Such care requires paying close attention to whether UI is imposing difficult social, psychologic, community, emotional, and financial consequences as uniquely experienced by each woman. Specialty care referral should be expedited, rather than delayed unnecessarily.

The current definition of UI is "the complaint of any involuntary leakage of urine." This definition evolved through consensus-based work from the International Continence Society and the International Urogynecological Association (Abrams et al., 2010; Abrams et al., 2002; Haylen et al., 2010). Urinary incontinence also is defined a social or hygienic problem when searching for the prevalence of bothersome UI (Abrams et al., 2010). The 2002 definition of "involuntary loss of urine *that is a social or hygienic problem*" is also still recognized (Abrams et al., 2010; Haylen et al., 2010). The simple one-sentence UI definition belies the complexity of this syndrome, and its interrelationships with many other health issues.

SCOPE OF THE PROBLEM

Epidemiology

Urinary incontinence occurs in women of all ages, although prevalence estimates vary widely, ranging from 5% to 69% for women experiencing some degree of UI, and from 5% to 15% for "daily" leakage (Buckley & Lapitan, 2010). A systematic review claimed different urgency UI prevalence by geography, with ranges of 1.8% to 30.5% in Europe, 1.7% to 36.4% in the United States, and 1.5% to 15.2% in Asia (Milsom et al., 2014). Estimates of incidence rates also vary widely. As Legendre, Ringa, Panjo, Zins, and Fritel (2015) have observed, the incidence of UI increases with age among middle-aged women.

Problematically, the prevalence of UI depends on survey estimates that utilize different UI definitions and study designs, and precise, up-to-date prevalence rates as measured by validated standardized surveys are generally lacking (Bedretdinova, Fritel, Panjo, & Ringa, 2016). Suffice it to say that UI is common and may be transient, but is experienced by a majority of women at some point in life.

Etiology and Pathophysiology

The etiology of UI may be described as any occurrence or condition (excepting a voluntary micturition) that elicits a moment of bladder pressure exceeding urethral pressure and hence results in unwanted urine loss. Thus, a simple continence equation is at work: Continence is maintained as long as bladder pressure is less than urethral pressure. However, many factors influence this equation. To understand the full etiology of UI, it is first necessary to understand the anatomic relationships that maintain urethral pressure higher than bladder pressure.

The muscle of the bladder is called the detrusor. When the smooth muscle of the detrusor contracts, the otherwise low-pressure zone within the bladder is converted to a high-pressure zone, which is needed when a woman wishes to expel urine. Whenever a woman wishes to not expel urine, the bladder serves as a low-pressure holding tank.

Relative to the bladder, the urethra is a high-pressure zone that is maintained largely by striated muscle contraction. The urethral length spans the distance from the bladder to the outside world, which for women is a mere 3 to 3.6 cm (Krantz,

1950). It is a misperception that there is a circular ring of tight muscle at the neck of the woman's bladder; likewise, there is no prostate gland encircling the upper portion of the urethra as there would be in men. Rather, the smooth muscle of the bladder transitions into smooth musculature extending longitudinally along the bladder to the most proximal 20% of its length. Circumferential muscle that is striated (hence under volitional control) is thickest at the midpoint of the urethra and though it extends proximally toward the bladder, it does not extend all the way up to the bladder neck and it is preferentially lost on aging closest to the bladder neck and atrophying down toward midurethra (Perucchini, DeLancey, Ashton-Miller, Peschers, & Kataria, 2002). Because of the striated nature of the circumferential urethral muscle, it is under voluntary control, and volitional pelvic muscle contraction elicits increased urethral closure pressure (Miller, Umek, DeLancey, & Ashton-Miller, 2004). The most distal 20% of the urethra, ending at the urinary meatus, has minimal impact on continence (Perucchini et al., 2002).

The urethra rests on the anterior vaginal wall, which is supported by the levator ani muscle (commonly referred to as the pelvic floor or Kegel muscle) and its fibrous attachments. The anterior portion of the levator ani connects to the superior aspect of the pubic bone. Lifting, upwardly oriented forces of the levator ani form a resistive plate onto which the urethra is compressed when driven downward by increasing intra-abdominal pressure, such as occurs with, for instance, coughing, sneezing, and lifting. The dynamic interrelationships among these factors are shown by the arrows in **Figure 22-1**. When a woman consciously contracts the pelvic floor muscles (i.e., striated urethral sphincteric muscle, levator ani muscle, and external anal sphincter), the urethra is closed, the bladder is lifted, and the anus is closed. DeLancey and Ashton-Miller (2004) provide a summative overview article of this anatomy.

In this dynamic system, several things can go wrong and alter the continence equation to the extent that unwanted urine leakage occurs. The concept of "detrusor instability" causing a woman's urge and within-bladder pressure increase is commonly discussed, but it has not been clearly demonstrated in all of its hypothesized applications.

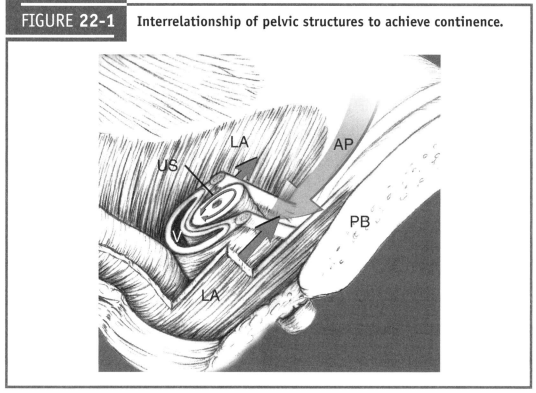

FIGURE 22-1 Interrelationship of pelvic structures to achieve continence.

Abbreviations: AP, abdominal pressure; LA, levator ani; PB, pubic bone; US, urethral sphincter; V, vagina.

Indeed, the underlying pathophysiology of detrusor overactivity largely remains unexplained. Myogenic causes are attributed to abnormal electrical activity affecting the bladder's smooth muscle and interstitial cells. Neurogenic detrusor instability is associated with neurologic lesions of either central mechanisms or peripheral afferent/efferent bladder innervation (Osman et al., 2014). The woman experiences this "overactivity" as symptoms of urgency and responds with frequency of micturition but typically low-volume voids. Likewise, detrusor "underactivity" is felt by women as very strong urgency, albeit without prior warnings in the form of smaller urge signaling that a woman would normally experience with gradual bladder filling. This detrusor "underactivity" is largely unrecognized in the literature but is commonly referred to by clinicians as "teacher's bladder" or "nurse's bladder"—labels referring to the situation in which a woman must adapt to a nonoptimal toileting pattern of long duration between voids due to job or environment restrictions.

Alternatively, some women may experience a nonoptimal bladder adaptation of detrusor activity (hyperactivity or hypoactivity) due to a "kinked urethra." Similar to the reduced flow of water that occurs with kinking of a garden hose, bladder descent (cystocele) mechanically reduces emptying; over time, this reduction affects the rate and degree of urge experienced before micturition. Most commonly, sensations of strong urgency with or without frequency are associated with the aging detrusor and the aging muscle at the bladder/urethral junction. The latter allows urine to funnel into the upper urethra, a condition felt as urgency.

A strong aging effect is observed with the striated circumferential urethral muscle. Aging-related striated urethral muscle loss begins with muscle volume decrease where the urethra merges with the bladder—that is, the urethrovesical junction (Perucchini et al., 2002). The reduced muscle volume at the urethrovesical junction translates into a loss of overall urethral pressure or a more open urethra. This functional loss is termed urethral sphincter deficiency (also referred to as bladder neck funneling, shortened urethra, or loss of urethral sphincteric mechanism). The resultant low urethral pressure increases a woman's risk of UI when the urine passively funnels into the upper portion of the urethra. This event reduces the distance between the bladder "holding zone" for urine and allows the urine to escape to the outside world at the slightest provocation. Such pronounced extrinsic sphincter deficiency is a highly distressing situation for a woman and can be debilitating. Her perceived sense of control and actual control over urine loss are greatly diminished, such that leakage can occur simply when walking across the room.

The levator ani muscle is a secondary control mechanism, which operates through (1) its functional capacity to support the bladder and urethra from below and (2) its felt accessibility to a woman for eliciting a volitional contraction that simultaneously prompts urethral striated muscle contraction. The levator ani muscle, however, is vulnerable to detachment from its origin at the pubic bone during childbirth (Lien, Mooney, DeLancey, & Ashton-Miller, 2004; Miller et al., 2015); such detachment can be documented by magnetic resonance imaging (MRI) or three-dimensional (3-D) ultrasound. Approximately 5% to 10% of women who give birth vaginally for the first time are observed to have some degree of levator ani laceration (DeLancey, Kearney, Chou, Speights, & Binno, 2003), and as many as 40% of women who give birth and have a demographic or obstetric high-risk factor for levator ani laceration develop this condition (Low et al., 2014; Shek & Dietz, 2010). The risk is greatest in women whose birthing experience includes use of forceps (Kearney et al., 2010). Varying degrees of levator ani lacerations are possible, and level of severity is associated with reduced ability to dynamically increase force and contract the levator ani. With complete laceration, there is complete loss of this muscle's ability to contract. As documented by MRI, levator ani lacerations, when they occur, are chronic in duration (Miller et al., 2015).

A woman who experiences compromises to both of the striated muscles in her urinary system—that is, both the urethral and levator ani muscles—is increased risk for UI during the stressor conditions of increased intra-abdominal pressure (DeLancey, Miller et al., 2007).

Genetic Factors

Several genes have been identified as contributing to a woman's risk for UI. For example, a case-control study conducted by Cornu et al. (2011) showed that androgen receptor polymorphism is a predisposing factor to UI. Studies have also confirmed the influence of genetic factors on alterations of the extracellular matrix, which impacts structural support of the urethra and bladder neck resulting in UI (McKenzie, Rohozinski, & Badlani, 2010). Familial UI has been underestimated in the past, but researchers have now realized that there is an association between UI in parents and their children (von Gontard, Heron, & Joinson, 2011). Racial variance is known (as discussed later in this chapter), although more definitive work is required to determine the underlying reasons for these differences.

Pregnancy

In pregnancy, increasing pressure of the enlarged uterus and fetal weight on the bladder, along with pregnancy-related hormonal changes including increased progesterone, decreased relaxin, and decreased collagen levels, may contribute to altering the continence equation during the period of gestation (Sangsawang & Sangsawang, 2013).

Lifestyle Factors

In societies that consume large amounts of beverages, as is the case in the United States, intake habits—both amount and type of beverage—may contribute to UI. Some women inadvertently exacerbate or cause their UI by overconsumption of beverages without matching void intervals to these higher intake amounts. Data are inconclusive about whether volume or ingredients, or some interaction of the two, contributes to UI (Jura, Townsend, Cuhan, Resnick, & Grodstein, 2011; Miller, Garcia, Hortsch, Guo, & Schimpf, 2016). In most studies of UI in women, the common behavior of undervoiding in relation to high fluid intake is seldom considered, perhaps because data on beverage intake are difficult to obtain and manage, given that their collection relies almost exclusively on participants keeping a detailed diary of intake.

Field studies of normal, healthy adult voiding patterns in relation to individual beverage intake could not be found. In contrast, normative void frequency and its relationship to bladder capacity is well studied in children. Healthy children typically void three to seven times per day, with bladder capacity increasing from prenatal to postnatal to toilet-training and later stages of development (De Gennaro & Capitanucci, 2015).

There is a common assumption that the healthy bladder requires large volume intake, but no evidence is available to substantiate this assumption. If a woman struggles with repeated urinary tract infections, she may be told to increase her consumption of beverages until the infection clears, but this is commonly misconstrued to continuously push a woman to drink, drink, drink, even though data supporting this recommendation are lacking.

Urinary Incontinence Comorbidities
Urinary incontinence may sometimes be a symptom of broader system pathology. Coexisting diseases have been confirmed as precipitating risk factors that may independently or interdependently influence continence of urine (Wagg et al., 2015). Such conditions include bacterial urinary tract infection, diabetes mellitus, neurologic disorders (e.g., multiple sclerosis, Parkinson's disease, cognitive impairment such as dementia or Alzheimer's disease), traumatic injury (e.g., back injury, pelvic trauma, surgical trauma), heart disease and stroke, arthritis, back problems, hearing or visual impairments, and major depressive disorders. Women who smoke cigarettes, either currently or in the past, have a higher risk of experiencing UI. In addition, many medications are associated with UI, such as diuretics, estrogen, benzodiazepines, tranquilizers, antidepressants, hypnotics, laxatives, and antibiotics. Additionally, UI is identified as a significant independent risk factor for falls (Bresee et al., 2014; Rafiq et al., 2014). Older age is one of the risk factors most strongly associated with development of UI (Bresee et al., 2014; Coyne et al., 2011; Kepenekci et al., 2011).

High body mass index (BMI) or obesity has also been identified as a significant predictor for

development of UI (Bresee et al., 2014; Buckley & Lapitan, 2010; Whitcomb & Subak, 2011). A systematic review found that women aged 50 years and older with a BMI of 35 or greater are 1.6 times more likely to develop moderate–severe urge UI over 2 years, compared with women whose BMI is 25 or less (Coyne et al., 2013). Whitcomb and Subak (2011) found that, for each 5-unit increase in their BMI, women become 20% to 70% more likely to develop UI. Conversely, Wing, West, and their colleagues (2010) reported that a 12-month weight-loss intervention reduces the frequency of stress UI episodes. Overweight and obese women who lose between 5% and 10% of their body weight have significant improvement of their UI (Wing, Creasman et al., 2010).

Pregnancy, childbirth, and increased parity have long been associated with UI (Kocaoz, Talas, & Atabekoglu, 2010; Sangsawang & Sangsawang, 2013). The prevalence and severity of UI are higher in parous women who had an instrumental birth compared to vaginal birth without instrumentation (Elbiss, Osman, & Hammad, 2013), and comparatively higher when a woman gives birth vaginally compared to by cesarean section or not birthing at all (Brown, Donath, MacArthur, McDonald, & Krastev, 2010; Buckley & Lapitan, 2010; Kepenekci et al., 2011; Ko et al., 2011; Kocaoz et al., 2010; Thom & Rortveit, 2010).

Levator ani lacerations at birth are associated with pelvic organ prolapse later in life, and prolapse is widely viewed as an independent risk factor for UI. Prolapse is clearly associated with levator ani lacerations (DeLancey, Morgan et al., 2007; Dietz & Simpson, 2008), but there is not a clear cause-and-effect relationship between symptoms of UI and levator ani lacerations (Miller et al., 2015). Constipation is also commonly viewed as associated with UI, but data on this topic are surprisingly scant and a cause-and-effect relationship has not been clearly established (Averbeck & Madersbacher, 2011; Carter & Beer-Gabel, 2012; Elbiss et al., 2013).

Clinical Presentation

With the broad definition of UI as "the complaint of any involuntary leakage of urine," actual symptoms can vary widely from one woman to another. This variance is captured by factors such as leakage symptom duration, frequency and severity, triggers for the leakage, and identification of situations that create the most bother. It can take many years for a woman to present to the clinician for care; more than 50% of women with this condition never do report UI to their healthcare providers (Burgio, Matthews, & Engel, 1991; Elbiss et al., 2013). Reasons for this reluctance vary, including lack of belief that there are effective treatments, negative physician–patient interaction, and severity of UI (Berger, Patel, Miller, DeLancey, & Fenner, 2011).

ASSESSMENT

History

The first steps in assessing UI in a holistic manner include asking a woman about her experiences while keeping in mind the broad array of symptom presentations and what is of most bother. For instance, although a woman may experience leakage with coughing, that may not be her symptom of concern. Instead, her primary concern may be the extreme urgency she experiences on arriving home, even though she rarely or never actually leaks urine at that time. It is important to ascertain the full scope of both urgency and UI in terms of their presence, frequency, severity, bother, and impact on quality of life; past medical history such as previous treatment, coexisting diseases as precipitating factors, medications, obstetric and menstrual history, and physical impairment; social history such as environmental issues and lifestyle; any measures currently being used to contain the leakage; and the extent to which the individual is seeking or desiring treatment, varying from conservative to aggressive options (Abrams et al., 2010).

A long-standing screening questionnaire has just two questions: "How often do you experience urinary leakage?" and "How much urine do you lose each time?"; a later version further specifies severity via a four-level index (Sandvik, Seim, Vanvik, & Hunskaar, 2000). An alternative questionnaire is the International Consultation on Incontinence Questionnaire, which contains four items to assess both UI and its effect on quality of life (Avery et al., 2004). One study asked a simple question about bother: "On a scale of 0 to 10, with 0 being 'not a problem,' 1 to 4 being 'a small

nuisance,' 5 being 'somewhat bothered,' 6 to 8 being 'very bothered,' and 9 to 10 being 'extremely bothered,' how much does this leakage of urine bother you?" (García-Pérez, Harlow, Sampselle, & Denman, 2013). To quantify low-level leakage in pregnant or postpartum women or others experiencing leakage onset, the eight-item Leakage Index Questionnaire (Low et al., 2013) is particularly appropriate (**Figure 22-2**). If in the history-taking a woman reports leakage with bending or reaching, or says, "I just find myself wet," this is an important indicator of likely intrinsic sphincter deficiency, especially when combined with older age.

A 3-day voiding diary is a highly valuable assessment tool for illuminating patterns that contribute to leakage in daily life, particularly as related to urge UI, exercise-induced UI, or intake and output habits that are contributory. Many styles of bladder diaries are available; **Figure 22-3** provides one example. Regardless of the type of voiding diary used, four components are critical to record:

- Time of day and amount of voiding (provide a measurement hat for the toilet)
- Time of day when an episode of UI occurs
- A place to write a brief description of the UI episode and associated events
- Types and amount of beverage intake

Although a diary can be inconvenient for women to fill out, willingness is typically improved when the woman understands the value of the tool in portraying the true nature of her daily struggles with UI to her provider. A clinic visit devoted entirely to a review of the diary helps reinforce the message from the clinician to the patient that the diary data are important and a driving factor for choosing best treatment.

Physical Examination and Diagnostic Testing

Assessing bladder capacity is done least invasively through a 3-day voiding diary. The largest void on the diary is an estimate of bladder capacity. Alternatively, a filling cystometrogram can be performed. However, this procedure is invasive and uncomfortable, and it requires equipment that is typically not available in the nonspecialty clinical environment.

FIGURE 22-2   **Leakage index questionnaire.**

Other than the few drops right after urinating, have you involuntarily lost or leaked any amount of urine or been unable to hold your water and wet yourself?

	YES	NO
	1	0

Next is a list of things that some people say can cause them to leak urine and wet themselves. Tell me whether each one has caused you to lose urine since we last saw you [date of last visit].

	YES	NO
Coughing hard	1	0
Laughing	1	0
Sneezing	1	0
Not being able to wait at least 5 minutes until it is convenient to go to the toilet...	1	0
Arriving at your door or putting your key in the lock	1	0
Suddenly finding that you are losing or about to lose urine with very little warning	1	0

Imagine that you are standing in the check-out line at the grocery store with a full bladder that you would like to empty as soon as possible. Now imagine that you have to sneeze or cough several times very hard. What is most likely to happen about urine leakage?

Check One

0   Stay dry
1   Leak a few drops, *or*
         Wet underpants but not soak through, *or*
         Possibly drip onto the floor

         TOTAL SCORE
         (Sum All Items)

Modified from Low, L. K., Miller, J. M., Guo, Y., Ashton-Miller, J. A., DeLancey, J. O. L., & Sampselle, C. M. (2013). Spontaneous pushing to prevent postpartum urinary incontinence: A randomized, controlled trial. *International Urogynecology Journal, 24*(3), 453–460. doi:10.1007/s00192-012-1884-y. PMCID: PMC3980478. Copyright 2013 by Springer. Modified with permission.

To determine whether the urethra is able to maintain a high margin of continence under "stress conditions" of intra-abdominal pressure rise, a quantified standing stress test can be performed (Miller, Ashton-Miller, & DeLancey, 1998b). This test is commonly referred to as the "paper towel test." It is a quick, inexpensive, and noninvasive way to estimate the severity of stress-type leakage. The woman does this test while standing with a comfortably full bladder; she coughs very hard three times while holding a trifold paper towel against her perineum. Urine loss onto the paper towel can be quantified—that is, visually or measured as wetted area (**Figure 22-4**). With any stress-type leakage elicited by intra-abdominal pressure rise, the cause is some combination of low urethral pressure, poor support from the levator ani muscle, and intra-abdominal pressure

FIGURE 22-3   Voiding diary.

Instructions:
Please record each time you drink fluids, you empty your bladder, you lose urine accidentally, and you perform pelvic muscle contractions for 3 consecutive days.
- "Time" columns: Be sure to write AM or PM.
- "Type" column: Write caffeinated or decaf for beverages such as coffee, tea, and cola. Other examples of beverage types include milk, juice, water, alcohol, milkshakes, etc.
- "Amount" column: Write one of the following numbers to indicate the amount of accidental urine loss:
  - 1 – leak a few drops
  - 2 – wet underpants, but not soak through
  - 3 – soak all the way through to outer clothes
  - 4 – possibly drip onto the floor
- "Urge" column: Write 'yes' if you had a sudden urge and couldn't get to the bathroom in time.
- "Activity" column: Please describe what you were doing when you accidentally lost urine (i.e., coughing, sneezing, laughing, reaching, jumping, lifting a heavy object, rising from chair, heard running water, etc.).

DATE BEGUN _____/_____/_____

Day 1

Awakening Time: _____   Bedtime: _____

Fluids I Drank Today:			Urinated in Toilet:			
Time (AM/PM)	Type	Amount (oz/ml)	Time (AM/PM)	Time (AM/PM)	Time (AM/PM)	Time (AM/PM)

Accidental Leakage of Urine:			
Time (AM/PM)	Amount	Urge (yes/no)	Activity

(how hard she is coughing). If urine pools onto the paper towel and completely saturates it, this finding is a strong indicator of likely low urethral pressure. Although a more definitive test for urethral sphincter deficiency is a urethral pressure profile, the equipment required to obtain such a profile is expensive and typically not readily accessible outside of specialty practices, and it is an invasive procedure.

It is important for the woman to validate the finding of stress-type leakage on the paper towel test as consistent with her experience of symptoms,

FIGURE 22-4   Use of a paper towel to quantify volume of urine loss upon coughing.

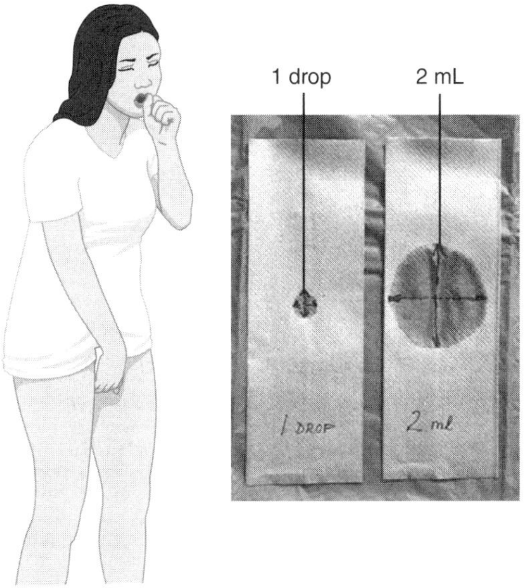

and the reason that she is seeking treatment. If she demonstrates a wetted area on the paper towel corresponding to just a couple of drops of urine, this may not be the scenario that is troublesome to her at home. The clinician should ask, "Do you routinely cough this hard outside of the clinic setting, or undertake activities that would impose an equal level of pressure?" and "Is this the type of leakage that you experience and that you find bothersome?" If not, further assessment should be undertaken to determine the scenarios and additional causative factors that might account for the leakage of bother to her.

Varying degrees of levator ani muscle laceration can be definitively ascertained only by MRI (Miller et al., 2015), although recent developments with 3-D ultrasound show promise for screening purposes. Palpation at the site of the levator ani to assess for presence and bulk (no laceration) is a commonly used clinical approach, but even when performed by experts this palpation option has shown poor reliability and poor validity as measured against MRI or 3-D ultrasound assessments for levator ani laceration (Kearney, Miller, & DeLancey, 2006; Kruger, Dietz, Budgett, & Dumoulin, 2014).

Levator ani functional capacity to lift and stabilize the continence structures can be readily observed on 2-D ultrasound. The test uses an external perineal probe and sagittal view of the bladder. This comfortable, simple assessment doubles as a quick and effective teaching aid in instructing a woman in pelvic muscle contraction technique. If ultrasound equipment is not available, the best clinical guess at functional loss (whether from levator ani muscle laceration or genetic weakness) is obtained when a woman continues to bear down or use the gluteal muscles when asked to contract her pelvic floor muscles. Specialty referral is appropriate to determine the cause in such a case.

DIFFERENTIAL DIAGNOSES

The diagnosis of UI is straightforward by definition. However, the diagnosis of UI is typically further

| TABLE 22-1 | Clarification of Urinary Incontinence |

Type of Incontinence	Definition
Stress (urinary) incontinence	Involuntary leakage with effort or physical exertion, sneezing, or coughing
Urgency (urinary) incontinence	A strong desire to urinate that is difficult to postpone (involuntary leakage associated with urgency)
Postural (urinary) incontinence	Involuntary leakage associated with change of body position
Nocturnal enuresis	Involuntary leakage during sleep
Mixed (urinary) incontinence	Involuntary urine leakage associated with symptoms of both stress and urgency urinary incontinence
Continuous (urinary) incontinence	Continuous involuntary urine leakage
Insensible (urinary) incontinence	Leakage of urine when women unaware
Coital incontinence	Involuntary urine leakage with coitus

Data from Abrams, P., Andersson, K. E., Birder, L., Brubaker, L., Cardozo, L., Chapple, C., . . . Wyndaele, J. J., & Members of the Committees. (2010). Fourth international consultation on incontinence recommendations of the international scientific committee: Evaluation and treatment of urinary incontinence, pelvic organ prolapse, and fecal incontinence. *Neurourology & Urodynamics, 29*(1), 213–240. doi:10.1002/nau.20870; Haylen, B. T., De Ridder, D., Freeman, R. M., Swift, S. E., Berghmans, B., Lee, J., . . . Schaer, G. N. (2010). An International Urogynecological Association (IUGA)/International Continence Society (ICS) joint report on the terminology for female pelvic floor dysfunction. *International Urogynecology Journal, 21*(1), 5–26. doi:10.1007/s00192-009-0976-9.

refined. The more specific definitions shown in **Table 22-1** were reconfirmed by the fourth International Consultation on Incontinence Recommendations of the International Science Committee (Abrams et al., 2010) and in a joint report by the International Urogynecological Association (IUGA) and the International Continence Society (ICS) (Haylen et al., 2010).

Careful elucidation of the numerous underlying factors that can contribute to leakage, along with the woman's indication of which leakage situation is most important to address, can provide information to establish which of these more precise subcategories of UI is present and to determine treatment priorities. Treatment follows logically in the direction of correcting the causative pathology (**Figure 22-5**). Referral for specialty care may be an important consideration.

Scope and standards of practice for nurses and other clinicians working with patients diagnosed with UI have been defined by the Society of Urologic Nurses and Associates (SUNA, 2013). In addition, competencies that are specific to urology nurse practitioners have been proposed (Quallich, Bumpus, & Lajiness, 2015). Urogynecologists have specialty training in treating women who are experiencing UI. Because of the comorbid nature of UI, full assessment and therapeutic plans for treatment may require collaboration with numerous healthcare professionals.

PREVENTION

Prevention of UI may focus on a woman addressing the following risk factors: obesity, diabetes, and excessive beverage intake. In addition, avoiding certain ingredients in beverages may be emphasized, along with gaining an understanding or awareness of optimal voiding patterns and pelvic floor health. Behavioral practices have been recommended to prevent UI, but clear evidence with replication studies supporting that advice remains lacking.

Phelan and colleagues (2012) conducted a study of association between weight loss and prevention

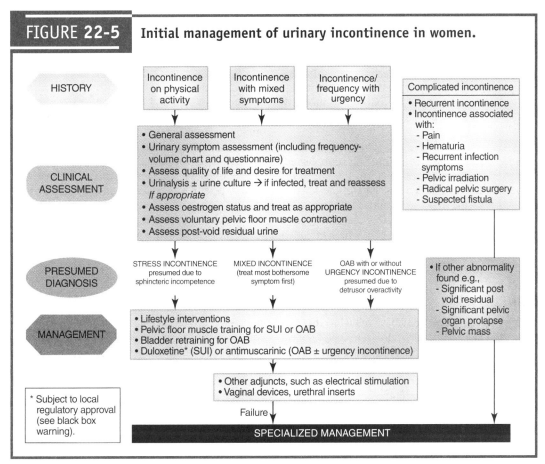

FIGURE 22-5 Initial management of urinary incontinence in women.

Abbreviations: OAB, overactive bladder; SUI, stress urinary incontinence.
Modified with permission from Abrams, P., Andersson, K. E., Birder, L., Brubaker, L., Cardozo, L., Chapple, C., . . . Wyndaele, J. J., & Members of the Committees. (2010). Fourth international consultation on incontinence recommendations of the international scientific committee: Evaluation and treatment of urinary incontinence, pelvic organ prolapse, and fecal incontinence. *Neurourology & Urodynamics, 29*(1), 213–240. doi:10.1002/nau.20870.

of UI in obese women with type 2 diabetes. In this investigation, weight loss of 1 kg was associated with a 3% reduction in the odds of incidence of UI; the incidence odds of UI were decreased by 47% when women lost 5% to 10% of their total body weight. Thus, weight loss has been recommended as a means to reduce the incidence of UI. Additionally, prevention of diabetes and effective management of diabetes may decrease the risk of developing UI, at least among women in the United States (Markland, Richter, Fwu, Eggers, & Kusek, 2011).

Considering the type of beverage intake as a factor in UI development, Jura, Townsend, Curhan, Resnick, and Grodstein (2011) conducted a study of the association between caffeine intake and risk of UI. Their data showed that women with more than 450 mg daily caffeine intake had a greater risk of UI compared with women with less than 150 mg daily caffeine intake.

Performing pelvic muscle exercises and developing the Knack skill (discussed later in this chapter) also has benefits in preventing stress UI during pregnancy and postpartum (Sangsawang & Sangsawang, 2013), UI in later pregnancy (Miller, Sampselle, Ashton-Miller, Hong, & DeLancey, 2008; Stafne, Salvesen, Romundstad, Torjusen, & Mørkved, 2012), or postpartum UI (Mørkved & Bø, 2014).

A clear understanding of what constitutes a healthy bladder has yet to be fully established, although a consensus statement of the issues involved has been published and state-of-the-science findings from the National Institutes of Health (NIH) highlight the lack of data in this area (Landefeld et al., 2008; Lukacz et al., 2011). A new initiative from the NIH is aimed at addressing this gap in basic knowledge over the next decade (NIH, 2014).

MANAGEMENT

Management of UI is aimed at reducing the factors that allow bladder pressure to exceed urethral pressure. Evaluation and treatment of a woman with UI was fully reviewed in 2010 by the fourth International Consultation on Incontinence (ICI) International Scientific Committee, representing key leaders in the field. The fifth ICI reported updates of treatment of UI from the fourth ICI report (Dumoulin et al., 2016). The ICI's step-by-step management recommendations were summarized by Abrams et al. (2010).

Nonpharmacologic Treatment

Lifestyle Interventions

Women often choose behavioral interventions as a first step for treatment of UI because these measures are less invasive and lower in risk than other treatments. Interventions related to beverage management and healthy toilet habits form the basis for initial treatment, but are dependent on evaluation of a voiding diary. The diary, although certainly an assessment tool, can be viewed equally as an intervention in and of itself. A woman may not be fully aware of her own patterns and can find the self-monitoring experience to be illuminating. "I had no idea that my bladder volumes at night were this high" represents the type of comment that might

be heard from a first-time diary keeper. The diary also serves to monitor progress over time when a repeat diary is recorded later in treatment (Arya, Heidi, Cory, Segal, & Northington, 2011).

Beverage Management

Despite scant data to determine the mechanism by which the ingredients produce UI, highly respected organizations (National Association for Continence, 2015; National Institute for Health and Care Excellence, 2013) advise women who experience UI to eliminate beverages containing caffeine, artificial sweeteners, and alcohol. In one study, instructions to reduce these ingredients did indeed result in perceived symptom improvement within the first week, and symptoms resumed with reintroduction of the beverages later in the study (Miller et al., 2016). However, volume of intake also went down and up accordingly, despite instructions to swap in water, raising the question of "Is it the ingredient or the volume change that makes the difference?" Regardless of which mechanism is at work, instructions to decrease intake of caffeinated, artificially sweetened, or alcoholic beverages can be effective for reducing symptoms in women with high overall consumption of these beverage types (Miller et al., 2016).

Bladder Training

As a rule of thumb, women should aim for approximately one cup of urine every 3 to 4 hours, with the urine having a yellow color, neither dark nor nearly colorless. Providing women with a container that fits into their toilet for urine collection to monitor color and amount of output is a valuable tool. This rule-of-thumb guideline helps monitor both intake and voiding intervals. Adjusting for healthy levels is called bladder training (also known as retraining) and is especially recommended for women experiencing urge UI (overactive bladder or detrusor instability). A voiding diary should be evaluated prior to recommending bladder training, so that baseline patterns can be established and the most appropriate adjustments identified.

On the one hand, for women who habitually empty their bladders on initial urge or whenever a toilet is available, bladder training may be as simple as holding back until approximately 8 ounces is produced on voiding. On the other hand, such training may be as complicated as voiding by the clock every hour and increasing in increments of 15 minutes weekly, until the woman can achieve normal bladder capacity through extending the time interval between voids. A woman can adopt the practice of contracting the pelvic floor muscles to suppress sensation (Knack skill) and use distraction strategies (such as counting backward) to ignore the urge. The goal is to gradually retrain the bladder to have a normative capacity of 8 to 10 ounces without fear of leakage. Steps for strict bladder retraining are described in **Box 22-1**.

BOX 22-1 **Steps in Teaching/ Learning Strict Bladder Retraining**

1. The voiding diary helps determine baseline voiding frequency. The initial bladder retraining interval should start 15 minutes earlier than the individual woman's normal voiding time to preempt urge sensation. For instance, if baseline voids occur hourly, begin strict bladder retraining at voids every 45 minutes.

2. If the urge to urinate occurs prior to the scheduled time, the woman should attempt to delay emptying until the scheduled time (or at least delay 5 minutes past the initial urge). Each week (or longer if necessary to become comfortable with the new interval), she should try to increase the interval by 15 to 30 minutes until the interval is, on average, 3 to 4 hours between voiding.

3. For most women, an average interval of 3 to 4 hours between voids means 2 to 3 hours in the morning, 4 to 5 hours in the afternoon, and 3 to 4 hours in the evening, assuming normal fluid intake.

4. The scheduled voiding is followed only during waking hours. Women who take diuretics or have a high fluid intake may have to adjust their voiding to a realistic level that accommodates an increased voiding frequency.

Reverse Bladder Retraining

Reverse bladder retaining is appropriate for selected women with urge UI experienced as late signaling or detrusor underactivity (no urge sensation until the bladder is excessively full, and only then a strong and uncontrollable urge). These women routinely report high volumes per void (greater than 350 cc) and describe themselves as having no early warning of bladder filling. Bladder training in such a case involves voiding by the clock until normalized urge sensations can be relied upon. The time interval to begin reverse bladder retraining is again established by the baseline diary. The woman should reduce her interval void time to the level that will produce no more than 300 cc per void (the first morning void may be larger).

The Knack Skill

The Knack skill is a pelvic muscle contraction (incorporating both the urethral striated muscle and the levator ani) strategically timed to a moment of expected loss of urine, whether from urge or stress-type triggers. Awareness of the triggers and learned Knack coordination skill allows a woman to volitionally increase her margin of continence (urethral pressure higher than bladder pressure) at any moment of need during her day-to-day activities (Miller, Ashton-Miller, & DeLancey, 1998a; Miller et al., 2008). Steps for Knack learning are described in **Box 22-2**.

Women who are unable to achieve a voluntary pelvic muscle contraction due to striated muscle loss or who have pelvic organ prolapse below the hymenal ring will probably be unable to effectively perform the Knack maneuver, due to mechanical misalignment for the latter problem.

Pelvic Muscle Exercise

Pelvic muscle exercises, commonly known as Kegel exercises, constitute a repetitive pelvic floor muscle contraction regimen. The goal is to increase muscle mass and strength. Kegel exercises offer rehabilitation for women whose muscles are weakened but not torn.

Assessment of a woman's ability to contract the levator ani muscle must be completed prior to recommending any pelvic muscle exercise for UI, as such exercises are likely be ineffective (and frustrating) if a woman is unable to voluntarily contract

---

BOX 22-2 Steps in Teaching/Learning the Knack

1. *Confirm voluntary control.* The clinician palpates the levator ani muscle bilaterally through the vaginal wall while the woman attempts a pelvic muscle contraction. A bulking of the muscle should be felt. If not, or if she bears down (Valsalva maneuver), instruct her in an easy flick of the muscles, the same maneuver she would use to hold back gas, to see if this elicits correct isolation. If unable to contract, Knack instruction should be discontinued.

2. *Maximize the contraction.* The woman should be taught to contract the pelvic muscles as deeply into the vagina as she is able. In some women, this is most easily accomplished by learning a stacking contraction. Start with a small flick-and-release maneuver and then build into stacking two to three small flicks. This is commonly known as the "elevator" technique (imagined as moving from one floor to the next). For other women, a smooth continuous inward pull of the muscles seems to work better. Teach the woman to maintain a steady hold of the pelvic muscle contraction while inhaling and exhaling. Remind her to avoid the tendency to incorrectly hold her breath during the pelvic muscle contraction.

3. *Begin to coordinate.* Two different coordination maneuvers are required for suppression of leakage risk scenarios. The first maneuver is to be able to reduce urge sensations. The Knack urge suppression skill uses small, gentle, pelvic muscle contractions (not strong holds). Several contractions (three to five) are usually sufficient for urge suppression. After a few seconds' rest, an additional set of three to five contractions may be needed. The second maneuver is to be able to reduce leakage during a moment of intra-abdominal pressure rise. The Knack stress suppression skill uses a single strong pelvic muscle contraction timed precisely with a secondary activity that increases intra-abdominal pressure, such as a cough or sneeze.

4. *Establish the habit.* Women can practice the Knack urge suppression skill prior to turning on the water faucet, upon arriving home to suppress latchkey urgency, or at the end of toileting to suppress postvoid dribbling. Practicing the Knack stress suppression skill can be done during planned maneuvers such as blowing the nose, voluntary coughing, lifting, rising from a chair, or momentarily stopping exercise (e.g., jogging) for a moment to "reset the pelvic floor" with a volitional pelvic muscle contraction. As skills with this technique develop, women will be ready to handle the triggers for urge UI and the surprise cough, sneeze that typifies stress UI.

Data from Miller, J. M., Ashton-Miller, J. A., & DeLancey, J. O. L. (1998a). A pelvic muscle precontraction can reduce cough-related urine loss in selected women with mild SUI. *Journal of the American Geriatrics Society, 46*(7), 870–874.

---

her levator ani muscle—for instance, if she has experienced a levator ani laceration. It is important to ascertain that the woman is not bearing down (a potential indicator of levator ani laceration) during her attempt to contract the pelvic floor muscles.

The National Association for Continence (2015) recommends a pelvic muscle exercise regimen such as the following: Sustain a contraction for 10 seconds, followed by at least 10 seconds of rest, with at least 3 sets of 10 repetitions per day. An alternative individualized protocol prescribes one of five levels of training matched to a particular woman's muscle ability, as the majority of women who need pelvic muscle exercise typically cannot sustain a contraction for a full 10 seconds (Miller, 2002). Most women will notice improvement in strength and control within 1 month, although it may require 3 months or more to see the full results. If there is no improvement within 3 months, referral to a specialist for further evaluation is important to evaluate for levator ani laceration or other problems.

Weight Management

Women who are overweight are at risk for development of UI. A longitudinal epidemiologic study clarified that weight is the major modifiable risk factor related to UI incidence in midlife-aged women (Legendre et al., 2015). Additionally, weight reduction has shown benefit in treatment of UI for overweight and obese women. A systematic review found that nonsurgical weight-loss interventions to address UI in overweight women have the potential to improve UI symptoms (Vissers et al., 2014).

Barrier Devices for UI

Incontinence pessaries are devices that are worn vaginally. They are designed to increase a woman's urethral pressure by supporting the anterior vaginal wall on which the urethra rests, especially in cases of nonfunctional levator ani muscle or extrinsic sphincter deficiency. Pessaries come in many forms, and fitting may require a number of visits to find the correct size and type. While these devices are effective for many women, some women are not satisfied by pessary support. In a study conducted by Richter and colleagues (2010), patients with UI were evaluated at 3 and 12 months for satisfaction and bothersome UI symptoms while wearing pessaries; their results were compared to women treated with behavioral therapy or a combination of pessary and behavioral therapy. At 3 months, the pessary wearers were less satisfied and reported more bother, but no significant difference was observed at 12 months. Combined behavioral and pessary therapies did not show better results than either single therapy. A state-of-the-art review reports that guidelines have not been established for determining who will achieve satisfactory results by wearing a pessary (Wood & Anger, 2014).

Pharmacologic Treatment

Pharmacologic treatment for UI varies according to the underlying etiology of this condition. For urge-type UI, anticholinergic antimuscarinic agents have been approved as therapies. They target the parasympathetic muscarinic cholinergic receptor sites of smooth muscle in the bladder. These drugs purportedly reduce the involuntary contractions of the detrusor muscle of the urinary bladder and increase the bladder capacity. The most common side effects of the antimuscarinic agents include dry mouth, blurred vision, constipation, nausea, dizziness, and headaches.

As many as 91% of women discontinue use of an anticholinergic drug for UI after one year of therapy, suggesting that these drugs have questionable long-term effectiveness (Brostrom & Hallas, 2009; Sexton et al., 2011). If a short trial is not effective, specialty referral is warranted before long-term continuation of the medication is recommended.

The drugs approved for treatment of urge UI consist of oxybutynin (Ditropan) in various forms, including extended-release oral and patch products: tolterodine (Detrol), fesoterodin (Toviaz), darifenacin (Enablex), and solifenacin (Vesicare). Immediate-release oxybutynin is considered the gold standard of treatment based on its long-time use, but the most frequently reported side effect with this agent is dry mouth—a side effect less often associated with immediate-release and extended-release tolterodine (Madhuvrata, Cody, Ellis, Herbison, & Hay-Smith, 2012). Tricyclic antidepressants, usually imipramine (Tofranil), have also been used on an off-label basis for urge-type UI, but are not considered first-line pharmacologic agents for this indication. In 2012, mirabegron came onto the market for urge UI; this drug targets detrusor muscle relaxation through activation of β_3 adrenoceptors (Wood & Anger, 2014).

There are no drugs approved specifically for stress UI in the United States. Although off-label use of some agents occurs, these medications should be prescribed only in conjunction with full evaluation by a continence specialist. Drugs used on an off-label basis to treat a woman's stress UI are selected for their purported ability to increase urethral pressure. Alpha-adrenergic agonists act on the $alpha_1$-receptor sites in the bladder neck and proximal urethra; ephedrine and pseudoephedrine (Sudafed) are the most often prescribed of these agents. Potential side effects include elevated blood pressure, headaches, dry mouth, insomnia, anxiety, nervousness, tachycardia, and palpitations (Li et al., 2013). Duloxetine is a dual serotonin and norepinephrine reuptake inhibitor that is also known to be used on an off-label basis for stress incontinence (Cardozo et al., 2010; Cipullo et al., 2014).

Vaginal estrogen may help to relieve symptoms of UI in postmenopausal women. As yet, the risks posed to the endometrium by such sustained vaginal estrogen therapy and by serum estradiol are unclear (Rahn et al., 2014; Rahn et al., 2015).

Surgical Treatment

Implantation of a sacral nerve stimulator is one approach to urge incontinence that requires a surgical procedure. Injection of botulinum toxin (Botox) into a patient's bladder—another surgical procedure to treat urge UI—was approved in 2013 (Chapple et al., 2013). Its potential side effects include bacteriuria, urinary retention, and residual urine volume (Sun, Luo, Tang, Yang, & Shen, 2015). Other forms of surgery are contraindicated for urge UI and can exacerbate urge symptoms that are related to detrusor instability.

A number of good surgical treatments for stress UI are available when this condition is related to extrinsic sphincter deficiency or urethral hypermobility or both. Injection of bulking agents is used for urethral sphincter deficiency when stress UI is primarily caused by poor urethral closure pressure and without hypermobility. Bulking agents are injected under local anesthesia by direct vision into the proximal urethra. Although the means by which bulking agents improve UI is not fully understood, they are believed to work by adding bulk to the periurethral tissue, which increases urethral closure pressure and improves resistance to urine outflow (Kavia, Rashid, & Ockrim, 2013). Bovine collagens, carbon bead particles (Durasphere), and Dextranomer/hyaluronix copolymer (Zuidex) are approved injectable agents (Kavia et al., 2013). The efficacy of bulking agents may be transient, but the procedure is repeatable.

Surgical treatments for stress UI also include a number of variations on surgical suspensions and slings (Garely & Noor, 2014). The aim of these procedures is to support and stabilize the urethra. The tension-free vaginal tape (TVT) sling procedure is the least invasive and is typically performed on an outpatient basis. The current trend is to perform a TVT, pubovaginal sling, or retropubic urethropexy.

More-traditional surgeries, including the Marshall-Marchetti-Krantz or Burch procedure and transvaginal bladder neck suspensions such as the Stamey-Raz or Gittes surgical approach, are also still performed.

Surgical repair of stress UI may also improve the frequency and urge UI components of mixed UI (Dieter, Edenfield, Weidner, Levin, & Siddiqui, 2014; Jain, Jirschele, Botros, & Latthe, 2011). This effect is likely explained by surgical correction of urine funneling into the urethra for a woman whose urge symptom etiology was striated sphincter insufficiency, not detrusor instability (which is typically worsened by surgery).

Surgery choices can differ depending on whether the patient is a very young or very old woman with stress UI (Robinson et al., 2015). Priorities for young women when considering a surgical treatment can relate to expectations of future pregnancy and childbirth. In contrast, minimally invasive procedures with low morbidity are typically the important consideration for older women, especially for frail older women with comorbidities.

Complementary and Alternative Therapies

Many women use complementary and alternative therapies for UI, including biofeedback, acupuncture, yoga, Pilates, and Tai Chi. Data on these interventions' effectiveness are scant at best.

Biofeedback uses an electronic machine to help women properly contract the right pelvic floor muscles. This adjunct therapy is used along with pelvic muscle exercise to facilitate skill development, particularly in the early stages of such treatment. Although studies demonstrate no statistically significant difference in reduction of urine leakage between groups undertaking pelvic muscle exercise with or without biofeedback, the biofeedback does improve motivation (Herderschee, Hay-Smith, Herbison, Roovers, & Heineman, 2013).

Randomized controlled trials have been conducted to explore the effect of acupuncture for UI, but have failed to find statistically significant improvement of UI with this intervention (Paik et al., 2013). Similarly, there is no strong evidence that yoga, Pilates, and Tai Chi improve stress UI (Bø & Herbert, 2013). Further research is also required to assess the efficacy of herbal medications for UI, none of which can be recommended at this time (Arunachalam & Rothschild, 2015).

When to Refer

Many women with UI will respond positively to behavioral instruction, pharmacologic treatments, or pessary use; some may be satisfied with education about UI, even if their symptoms persist. If management is ineffective, if it does not meet the woman's expectations for improvement, or if complicating factors are suspected, women should be referred to a UI specialist or specialty clinic. If possible, referral to a urogynecologist or advanced practice nurse in urogynecology should be prioritized given these professionals' specialty training and practice. A listing of urogynecologists and continence nurse practitioners can be found at http://www.voicesforpfd.org/p/cm/ld/fid=81.

Education about the various etiologies that underlie UI and the full scope of treatment modalities is important in the evaluation of UI. Some women will choose an intervention because the results are more immediate and require less personal involvement; others prefer to exhaust the full complement of behavioral approaches before considering pharmaceutical or surgical options. It is important to fully recognize UI as a nonspecific symptom of widely varying etiology and impact for each individual woman's situation. Choice of treatment modalities must be made by partnering with the woman to determine her goals and the context of her particular symptom manifestation.

Emerging Evidence That May Change Management

New instrumentation—particularly MRI and ultrasound imaging technologies—and various histologic and anatomic studies are rapidly advancing understanding about the complex continence mechanism, the pathologic factors involved, predictive variables for dysfunction, and improved prevention and treatment modalities. Given that these research findings are accumulating on a nearly daily basis, the literature should be reviewed routinely to keep abreast of the rapidly unfolding advancements.

Notably, stem cell therapy has been hypothesized as a future treatment of stress UI. The concept of cell-based therapy for stress UI is based on replenishing the sphincter muscle by injection of skeletal myoblasts into weakened urethra (Lin & Lue, 2012). A clinical trial reported improvements in 70% to 80% of 39 women in whom allogeneic cord blood stem cells were used to treat their stress UI (Lee et al., 2010).

Along with the advancing knowledge about the physiologic and mechanical factors, new understandings of women's lived experiences of UI are informing practice in this area. Further development of a language and public knowledge of UI and continence-mechanism understanding is still needed. Currently, clinicians have only limited knowledge with which to answer the postpartum woman's questions: "Why do I feel different down there? Is this degree of change normal? Must I live with it?" There is even less certainty in answering another key question: "Why does my bladder trigger unexpectedly, and will this ever completely go away?" New advances are bringing hope and a larger body of knowledge to draw from to reduce or cure UI.

PATIENT EDUCATION

During educational counseling, the following components need to be considered: how health providers diagnose UI and type of UI, available treatments, and healthy bladder behavior or lifestyle, including type and amount of fluid intake and appropriate bladder emptying time intervals to foster healthy bladder capacity. The continence mechanism is most effective when all parts function smoothly together. Overall, the etiology of UI tracks back to the situation in which any of these factors is insufficient or overcome by an adverse condition, or when ready-state redundancy in the system is compromised by stressed, injured, weakened, or aged structures, to the point where the woman is experiencing lack of urinary control that is affecting her quality of life. Current and accurate information can be difficult for women to find; hence education often involves correcting misinformation or myths. For instance, the need for all women to drink eight 8 oz glasses of water per day is a myth, with no data-based evidence to support it.

SPECIAL CONSIDERATIONS

Women living their lives within a broad biological and contextual arena find that the relevance of UI varies depending on their unique situation. Hence, it is not sufficient to explore bladder health at only one point in time. Rather, the goal is for healthcare providers to form partnerships with women so options for individually optimized bladder health, and a sense of control, can be self-determined.

Age, BMI, weight change, and parity are reported to influence the incidence and prevalence of UI (Ebbesen, Hunskaar, Rortveit, & Hannestad, 2013). In addition, differences in prevalence (Buckley & Lapitan, 2010) and incidence (Townsend, Curhan, Resnick, & Grodstein, 2010) of UI between racial groups have been reported. One review of 30 publications claimed there were associations between UI in women and race (Leroy, Lopes, & Shimo, 2012). Specifically, white and Hispanic women had higher prevalence of UI compared with black and Asian women. Moreover, stress UI was more common in white women, while urgency UI was more common in black women. Additionally, there were more risk factors of UI with white and Hispanic women than with black and Asian women. Another study conducted by Bliss and colleagues (2013) turned up different findings: When focusing on women living in nursing homes, Asian, black, and Hispanic women, as compared to white and American Indian women, had a higher prevalence of any type of UI. Despite these specific differences, the studies are in agreement that UI crosses all age, race, and ethnic groups. Indeed, all women deserve to be asked about their current satisfaction with their bladder health and control.

Variations in Management

Adolescents

Adolescents should receive information about healthy bladder practices. Learning about their own physiologic self-control mechanisms, such as developing the Knack habit and sensible beverage and eating habits, will provide them with tools to use for good bladder health over the course of their entire adult lives.

Some adolescents may have experienced UI as a child, which engendered lasting worries about bladder control. Leakage of urine is, in fact, the most common urine symptom in both children and adolescents. Urinary incontinence can lead to psychologic and psychiatric issues that are reflected in behavioral disorders among some children experiencing UI (von Gontard, Baeyens, Van Hoecke, Warzak, & Bachmann, 2011). A large epidemiologic study showed that the prevalence of UI among children aged 7.5 years was 7.8% (von Gontard, Heron, & Joinson, 2011). Moreover, this study stated that leakage of urine for those children may have genetic association, as their parents may have suffered from UI and nocturnal enuresis, defined as "intermittent incontinence while sleeping" by the International Children's Continence Society (Nevéus et al., 2006). Von Gontard, Baeyens, Van Hoeche, Warzak, and Bachmann (2011) recommend that UI management for children include a combination of psychologic intervention and UI treatment, so as to ensure optimal outcomes.

Pregnant Women

The prevalence of UI significantly increases from before pregnancy to the third trimester of pregnancy (Brown et al., 2010). Childbirth classes frequently emphasize the importance of practicing pelvic muscle exercises during pregnancy. Ko et al. (2011) and other researchers (Mørkved & Bø, 2014; Sangsawang & Sangsawang, 2013) have reported that primiparous women who practice pelvic muscle exercises during pregnancy and on a postpartum basis experience earlier recovery from symptoms of UI compared to members of a control group. Additionally, pelvic muscle exercises and the Knack skill have been shown to reduce the severity of stress UI in pregnant women (Miller et al., 2008; Sangsawang & Serisathien, 2012).

Older Women

Age is a proven etiologic risk factor for developing UI in women. Pelvic muscle exercise with or without combined bladder training and noninvasive transcutaneous electrical posterior tibial nerve stimulation may help improve UI in older women (Pereira, Escobar, & Driusso, 2012). Well-constructed incontinence pads (not menstrual pads, which are made of a different material) can be effective management aids for UI in older women. Healthcare providers also need to consider hydration, skin care, and maintenance of mobility in older women who experience UI (Roe, Flanagan, & Maden, 2015). In addition, some medications may help older women by improving their UI symptoms. However, many considerations must be paid addressed when prescribing medications in older women, as noted in the following section "Women with Disabilities."

Women with Disabilities

Urinary incontinence and disabilities are often logically associated—that is, UI is a significant cause of disabilities, and disabilities make UI more serious. For example, UI is correlated with lower back disabilities and balance impairment (Kim, Kim, Oh, & Choi, 2010). Women with urge UI are more likely than continent women to have poorer lower extremity physical functioning (Kafri, Shames, Golomb, & Melzer, 2012). Moreover, many comorbid conditions (e.g., diabetes mellitus, chronic pulmonary disease, stroke, and Parkinson's disease) may cause UI in frail elder women. Women with disabilities such as spine problems may not be able to perform a pelvic muscle contraction, or have the ability to control their bladder or urine system.

Although some medications may improve symptoms of UI for older and disabled women, a number of considerations must be taken into account before prescribing these agents. According to the fifth ICI conclusions (Wagg et al., 2015), for older women who have renal/hepatic impairment, there are many prohibitions to using these medications. For older women who take multiple medications, drug interactions are difficult to avoid. Older women also have a higher risk of experiencing retention, so post-void residual evaluation prior to and potentially after prescription needs to be careful considered. In frail older women, antimuscarinic agents can exacerbate cognitive impairment. For older women with dementia or with decreasing sensation, prompted voiding aimed at increasing toileting has shown more usefulness for control and management of UI, considering the low effectiveness and problematic side-effect profiles of medications.

Influences of Culture

Cultures may influence women's perception of UI. Non-white women (i.e., black, Arab, Asian, and Hispanic) often believe UI is a negative outcome from childbirth or prior sexual experience and blame themselves for its development (Siddiqui, Levin, Phadtare, Pietrobon, & Ammarell, 2014). Among certain religious groups, it is required that women perform ritual cleansing before prayer. An episode of UI renders unclean a woman who has cleansed herself; thus, she must cleanse herself again before she can resume prayer rituals (Hamid, Pakgohar, Ibrahim, & Dastjerdi, 2015). Women in this situation may hesitate to discuss UI, out of a concern that they may be perceived as unclean.

In addition, cultural divides may exist regarding who is willing to seek medical help for UI. In one study, women who were Jewish were relatively more likely to seek medical advice about their UI, whereas women who were Christian, Muslim, Buddhist, and Hindu did not seek medical help because they felt embarrassed and believed UI was a normal part of aging (Chaliha & Stanton, 1999). Furthermore, women with UI in Taiwan have been shown to be less likely to seek help for their UI compared with women in Western cultures (Beji, Ozbas, Aslan, Bilgic, & Erkan, 2010).

For most women who experience UI, this condition is distressing and affects their health-related quality of life (Kwon, Kim, Son, Roh, & You, 2010). Nevertheless, some women do not find UI to be of enough bother to warrant medical intervention. Instead, they may select simple self-care management strategies, such as placing a pad or tissue in their underwear to catch urine loss.

The appropriate degree of diagnostic testing and management strategies should always be determined in conjunction with the individual woman, based on her unique experience with UI. This perception can vary dramatically both within the woman over time and compared to other women. In the care of the woman with UI, she is the expert in understanding the degree of bother from her symptoms. Identifying the most bothersome aspect offers a starting point from which to prioritize efforts to sort out the complex etiology that will inform step-by-step management.

INTERNET RESOURCES

American Urogynecologic Society (Information for Women):

http://www.augs.org or

http://www.voicesforpfd.org

Diagnosis and Treatment of Overactive Bladder (Non-neurogenic) in Adults: AUA/SUFU Guideline: http://www.auanet.org/common/pdf/education/clinical-guidance/Overactive-Bladder.pdf

Guidelines on Urinary Incontinence: http://uroweb.org/wp-content/uploads/20-Urinary-Incontinence_LR.pdf

National Association for Continence: http://www.nafc.org

National Institute of Diabetes & Digestive & Kidney Diseases: http://kidney.niddk.nih.gov/kudiseases/pubs/uiwomen

Simon Foundation for Continence: http://www.simonfoundation.org

Women's Health Foundation: http://www.womenshealthfoundation.org

References

Abrams, P., Andersson, K. E., Birder, L., Brubaker, L., Cardozo, L., Chapple, C., . . . Wyndaele, J. J., & Members of the Committees. (2010). Fourth international consultation on incontinence recommendations of the international scientific committee: Evaluation and treatment of urinary incontinence, pelvic organ prolapse, and fecal incontinence. *Neurourology & Urodynamics, 29*(1), 213–240. doi:10.1002/nau.20870

Abrams, P., Cardozo, L., Fall, M., Griffiths, D., Rosier, P., Ulmsten, U., . . . Wein, A. (2002). The standardisation of terminology of lower urinary tract function: Report from the standardisation subcommittee of the International Continence Society. *Neurourology & Urodynamics, 21*(2), 167–178. doi:10.1002/nau.10052

Arunachalam, D., & Rothschild, J. (2015). Complementary alternative medicine and therapies for overactive bladder symptoms: Is there evidence for benefit? *Current Bladder Dysfunction Reports, 10*, 20–24. doi:10.1007/s11884-014-0280-5

Arya, L. A., Heidi, H., Cory, L., Segal, S., & Northington, G. M. (2011). Construct validity of a questionnaire to measure the type of fluid intake and type of urinary incontinence. *Neurourology & Urodynamics, 30*(8), 1597–1602. doi:10.1002/nau.21091

Averbeck, M. A., & Madersbacher, H. (2011). Constipation and LUTS: How do they affect each other? *International Brazilian Journal Urology, 37*(1), 16–28. doi:10.1590/S1677-55382011000100003

Avery, K., Donovan, J., Peters, T. J., Shaw, C., Gotoh, M., & Abrams, P. (2004). ICIQ: A brief and robust measure for evaluating the symptoms and impact of urinary incontinence. *Neurourology & Urodynamics, 23*(4), 322–330. doi:10.1002/nau.20041

Bedretdinova, D., Fritel, X., Panjo, H., & Ringa, V. (2016). Prevalence of female urinary incontinence in the general population according to different definitions and study designs. *European Urology, 69*(2), 256–264. doi:10.1016/j.eururo.2015.07.043

Beji, N. K., Ozbas, A., Aslan, E., Bilgic, D., & Erkan, H. A. (2010). Overview of the social impact of urinary incontinence with a focus on Turkish women. *Urologic Nursing, 30*(6), 327–334.

Berger, M. B., Patel, D. A., Miller, J. M., DeLancey J. O., & Fenner, D. E. (2011). Racial differences in self-reported healthcare seeking and treatment for urinary incontinence in comminity-dwelling women from the EPI study. *Neurourology & Urodynamics, 30*(8), 1442–1447. doi:10.1002/nau.21145

Bliss, D. Z., Harms, S., Garrard, J. M., Cunanan, K., Savik, K., Gurvich, O., . . . Virnig, B. (2013). Prevalence of incontinence by race and ethnicity of older people admitted to nursing homes. *Journal of the American Medical Directors Association, 14*(6), 451. e451–e457. doi:10.1016/j.jamda.2013.03.007

Bø, K., & Herbert, R. D. (2013). There is not yet strong evidence that exercise regimens other than pelvic floor muscle training can reduce stress urinary incontinence in women: A systematic review. *Journal of Physiotherapy, 59*(3), 159–168. doi:10.1016/S1836-9553(13)70180-2

Bresee, C., Dubina, E. D., Khan, A. A., Sevilla, C., Grant, D., Eilber, K. S., & Anger, J. T. (2014). Prevalence and correlates of urinary incontinence among older community-dwelling women. *Female Pelvic Medicine & Reconstructive Surgery, 20*(6), 328–333. doi:10.1097/spv.0000000000000093

Brostrom, S., & Hallas, J. (2009). Persistence of antimuscarinis drug use. *European Journal of Clinical Pharmacology, 65*(3), 309–314. doi:10.1007/s00228-008-0600-9

Brown, S. J., Donath, S., MacArthur, C., McDonald, E. A., & Krastev, A. H. (2010). Urinary incontinence in nulliparous women before and during pregnancy: Prevalence, incidence, and associated risk factors. *International Urogynecology Journal, 21*(2), 193–202. doi:10.1007/s00192-009-1011-x

Buckley, B. S., & Lapitan, M. C. M. (2010). Prevalence of urinary incontinence in men, women, and children—current evidence: Findings of the Fourth International Consultation on Incontinence. *Urology, 76*(2), 265–270. doi:10.1016/j.urology.2009.11.078

Burgio, K. L., Matthews, K. A., & Engel, B. T. (1991). Prevalence, incidence and correlates of urinary incontinence in healthy, middle-aged women. *Journal of Urology, 146*(5), 1255–1259.

Cardozo, L., Lange, R., Voss, S., Beardsworth, A., Manning, M., Viktrup, L., & Zhao, Y. D. (2010). Short- and long-term efficacy and safety of duloxetine in women with predominant stress urinary incontinence. *Current Medical Research Opinion, 26*(2), 253–261. doi:10.1185/03007990903438295

Carter, D., & Beer-Gabel, M. (2012). Lower urinary tract symptoms in chronically constipated women. *International Urogynecology Journal, 23*(12), 1785–1789. doi:10.1007/s00192-012-1812-1

Chaliha, C., & Stanton, S. L. (1999). The ethnic cultural and social aspects of incontinence: A pilot study. *International Urogynecology Journal, 10*(3), 166–170.

Chapple, C., Sievert, K-D., MacDiarmid, S. Khullar, V., Radziszewski, P., Nardo, C., . . . Haag-Molkenteller, C. (2013). Onabotulinumtoxin A 100 U significantly improves all idiopathic overactive bladder symptoms and quality of life in patients with overactive bladder and urinary incontinence: A randomised, double-blind, placebo-controlled trial. *European Urology, 64*(2), 249–256. doi:10.1016/j.eururo.2013.04.001

Cipullo, L. M., Zullo, F., Cosimato, C., Di Spiezio Sardo, A., Troisi, J., & Guida, M. (2014). Pharmacological treatment of urinary incontinence. *Female Pelvic Medicine & Reconstructive Surgery, 20*(4), 185–202. doi:10.1097/spv.0000000000000076

Cornu, J. N., Merlet, B., Cussenot, O., Cancel-Tassin, G., Ciofu, C., Amarenco, G., & Haab, F. (2011). Genetic susceptibility to urinary incontinence: Implication of polymorphisms of androgen and oestrogen pathways. *World Journal of Urology, 29*(2), 239–242. doi:10.1007/s00345-010-0585-8

Coyne, K. S., Sexton, C. C., Vats, V., Thompson, C., Kopp, Z. S., & Milsom, I. (2011). National community prevalence of overactive bladder in the United States stratified by sex and age. *Urology, 77*(5), 1081–1087. doi:10.1016/j.urology.2010.08.039

Coyne, K. S., Wein, A., Nicholson, S., Kvasz, M., Chen, C. I., & Milsom, I. (2013). Comorbidities and personal burden of urgency urinary incontinence: A systematic review. *International Journal of Clinical Practice, 67*(10), 1015–1033. doi:10.1111/ijcp.12164

De Gennaro, M., & Capitanucci, M. L. (2015). Lower urinary tract dysfunction. In M. Lima & G. Manzoni (Eds.), *Pediatric urology: Contemporary strategies from fetal life to adolescence* (pp. 197–206). Milan, Italy: Springer.

DeLancey, J. O. L., & Ashton-Miller, J. A. (2004). Pathophysiology of adult urinary incontinence. *Gastroenterology, 126*(1, Suppl. 1), S23–S32. doi:10.1053/j.gastro.2003.10.080

DeLancey, J. O., Kearney, R., Chou, Q., Speights, S., & Binno, S. (2003). The appearance of levator ani muscle abnormalities in magnetic resonance images after vaginal delivery. *Obstetrics & Gynecology, 101*(1), 46–53.

DeLancey, J. O., Miller, J., Kearney, R., Howard, D., Reddy, P., Umek, W., . . . Ashton-Miller, J. A. (2007). Vaginal birth and de novo stress incontinence: Relative contributions of urethral dysfunction and support loss. *Obstetrics & Gynecology, 110*(2, Pt. 1), 354–362. doi:10.1097/01.AOG.0000270120.60522.55

DeLancey, J. O., Morgan, D. M., Fenner, D. E., Kearney, R., Guire, K., Miller, J. M., . . . Ashton-Miller, J. A. (2007). Comparison of levator ani muscle defects and function in women with and without pelvic organ prolapse. *Obstetrics & Gynecology, 109*(2, Pt. 1), 295–302. doi:10.1097/01.AOG.0000250901.57095.ba

Dieter, A. A., Edenfield, A. L., Weidner, A. C., Levin, P. J., & Siddiqui, N. Y. (2014). Does concomitant anterior/apical repair during midurethral sling improve the overactive bladder component of mixed incontinence? *International Urogynecological Journal, 25*(9), 1269–1275. doi:10.1007/s00192-014-2400-3

Dietz, H. P., & Simpson, J. M. (2008). Levator trauma is associated with pelvic organ prolapse. *International Journal of Obstetrics & Gynaecology, 115*(8). doi:10.1111/j.1471-0528.2008.01751.x

Dumoulin, C., Hunter, K. F., Moore, K., Bradley, C. S., Burgio, K. L., Hagen, S., . . . Chambers, T. (2016). Conservative management for female urinary incontinence and pelvic organ prolapse review 2013: Summary of the 5th International Consultation on Incontinence. *Neurourology & Urodynamics, 35*(1), 15–20. doi:10.1002/nau.22677

Ebbesen, M., Hunskaar, S., Rortveit, G., & Hannestad, Y. (2013). Prevalence, incidence and remission of urinary incontinence in women: Longitudinal data from the Norwegian HUNT study (EPINCONT). *BMC Urology, 13*(1), 27. doi:10.1186/1471-2490-13-27

Elbiss, H. M., Osman, N., & Hammad, F. T. (2013). Social impact and healthcare-seeking behavior among women with urinary incontinence in the United Arab Emirates. *International Journal of Gynecology & Obstetrics, 122*(2), 136–139. doi:10.1016/j.ijgo.2013.03.023

García-Pérez, H., Harlow, S. D., Sampselle, C. M., & Denman, C. (2013). Measuring urinary incontinence in a population of women in northern Mexico: Prevalence and severity. *International Urogynecology Journal, 24*(5), 847–854. doi:10.1007/s00192-012-1949-y

Garely, A. D., & Noor, N. (2014). Diagnosis and surgical treatment of stress urinary incontinence. *Obstetrics & Gynecology, 124*(5), 1011–1027. doi:10.1097/aog.0000000000000514

Hamid, T. A., Pakgohar, M., Ibrahim, R., & Dastjerdi, M. V. (2015). "Stain in life": The meaning of urinary incontinence in the context of Muslim postmenopausal women through hermeneutic phenomenology. *Archives of Gerontology and Geriatrics, 60*(3), 514–521. doi:10.1016/j.archger.2015.01.003

Haylen, B. T., De Ridder, D., Freeman, R. M., Swift, S. E., Berghmans, B., Lee, J., . . . Schaer, G. N. (2010). An International Urogynecological Association (IUGA)/International Continence Society (ICS) joint report on the terminology for female pelvic floor dysfunction. *International Urogynecology Journal, 21*(1), 5–26. doi:10.1007/s00192-009-0976-9

Herderschee, R., Hay-Smith, E. C. J., Herbison, G. P., Roovers, J. P., & Heineman, M. J. (2013). Feedback or biofeedback to augment pelvic floor muscle training for urinary incontinence in women: Shortened version of a Cochrane systematic review. *Neurourology & Urodynamics, 32*(4), 325–329. doi:10.1002/nau.22329

Jain, P., Jirschele, K., Botros, S. M., & Latthe, P. M. (2011). Effectiveness of midurethral slings in mixed urinary incontinence: A systematic review and meta-analysis. *International Urogynecology Journal, 22*(8), 923–932. doi:10.1007/s00192-011-1406-3

Jura, Y. H., Townsend, M. K., Curhan, G. C., Resnick, N. M., & Grodstein, F. (2011). Caffeine intake, and the risk of stress, urgency and mixed urinary incontinence. *Journal of Urology, 185*(5), 1775–1780. doi:10.1016/j.juro.2011.01.003

Kafri, R., Shames, J., Golomb, J., & Melzer, I. (2012). Self-report function and disability: A comparison between women with and without urgency urinary incontinence. *Disability and Rehabilitation, 34*(20), 1699–1705. doi:10.3109/09638288.2012.660597

Kavia, R., Rashid, T. G., & Ockrim, J. L. (2013). Stress urinary incontinence. *Journal of Clinical Urology, 6*(6), 377–390. doi:10.1177/2051415813510115

Kearney, R., Fitzpatrick, M., Brennan, S., Behan, M., Miller, J., Keane, D., . . . DeLancey, J. O. (2010). Levator ani injury in primiparous women with forceps delivery for fetal distress, forceps for second stage arrest, and spontaneous delivery. *International Journal of Gynecology & Obstetrics, 111*(1), 19–22. doi:10.1016/j.ijgo.2010.05.019

Kearney, R., Miller, J. M., & DeLancey, J. O. (2006). Interrater reliability and physical examination of the pubovisceral portion of the levator ani muscle, validity comparisons using MR imaging. *Neurourrology & Urodynamics, 25*(1), 50–54. doi:10.1002/nau.20181

Kepenekci, I., Keskinkilic, B., Akinsu, F., Cakir, P., Elhan, A. H., Erkek, A. B., & Kuzu, M. A. (2011). Prevalence of pelvic floor disorders in the female population and the impact of age, mode of delivery, and parity. *Disease of the Colon & Rectum, 54*(1), 85–94. doi:10.1007/DCR.0b013e3181fd2356

Kim, J. S., Kim, S. Y., Oh, D. W., & Choi, J. D. (2010). Correlation between the severity of female urinary incontinence and concomitant morbidities: A multi-center cross-sectional clinical study. *International Neurourology Journal, 14*(4), 220–226. doi:10.5213/inj.2010.14.4.220

Ko, P. C., Liang, C. C., Chang, S. D., Lee, J. T., Chao, A. S., & Cheng, P. J. (2011). A randomized controlled trial of antenatal pelvic floor exercises to prevent and treat urinary incontinence. *International Urogynecology Journal, 22*(1), 17–22. doi:10.1007/s00192-010-1248-4

Kocaoz, S., Talas, M. S., & Atabekoglu, C. S. (2010). Urinary incontinence in pregnant women and their quality of life. *Journal of Clinical Nursing, 19*(23-24), 3314–3323. doi:10.1111/j.1365-2702.2010.03421.x

Krantz, K. E. (1950). The anatomy of the urethra and anterior vaginal wall. *American Journal of Obstetrics & Gynecology, 62*(2), 374–386.

Kruger, J. A., Dietz, H. P., Budgett, S. C., & Dumoulin, C. L. (2014). Comparison between transperineal ultrasound and digital detection of levator ani trauma: Can we improve the odds? *Neurourology & Urodynamics, 33*(3), 307–311. doi:10.1002/nau.22386

Kwon, B. E., Kim, G. Y., Son, Y. J., Roh, Y. S., & You, M. A. (2010). Quality of life of women with urinary incontinence: A systematic literature review. *International Neurourology Journal, 14*(3), 133–138. doi:10.5213/inj.2010.14.3.133

Landefeld, C. S., Bowers, B. J., Feld, A. D., Hartmann, K. E., Hoffman, E., Ingber, M. J., . . . Trock, B. J. (2008). National Institutes of Health state-of-the-science conference statement: Prevention of fecal and urinary incontinence in adults. *Annals of Internal Medicine, 148*(6), 449–458. doi:10.7326/0003-4819-148-6-200803180-00210

Lee, C. N., Jang, J. B., Kim, J. Y., Koh, C., Baek, J. Y., & Lee, K. J. (2010). Human cord blood stem cell therapy for treatment of stress urinary incontinence. *Journal of Korean Medical Science, 25*(6), 813–816. doi:10.3346/jkms.2010.25.6.813

Legendre, G., Ringa, V., Panjo, H., Zins, M., & Fritel, X. (2015). Incidence and remission of urinary incontinence at midlife: A cohort study. *International Journal of Obstetrics & Gynaecology, 122*(6), 816–823. doi:10.1111/1471-0528.12990

Leroy, L. d. S., Lopes, M. H. B. d. M., & Shimo, A. K. K. (2012). Urinary incontinence in women and racial aspects: A literature review. *Texto & Contexto: Enfermagem, 21*, 692–701. doi:10.1590/S0104-07072012000300026

Li, J., Yang, L., Pu, C., Tang, Y., Yun, H., & Han, P. (2013). The role of duloxetine in stress urinary incontinence: A systematic review and meta-analysis. *International Urology & Nephrology, 45*(3), 679–686. doi:10.1007/s11255-013-0410-6

Lien, K. C., Mooney, B., DeLancey, J. O., & Ashton-Miller, J. A. (2004). Levator ani muscle stretch induced by simulated vaginal birth. *Obstetrics & Gynecology, 103*(1), 31–40. doi:10.1097/01.AOG.0000109207.22354.65

Lin, C. S., & Lue, T. F. (2012). Stem cell therapy for stress urinary incontinence: A critical review. *Stem Cells & Development, 21*(6), 834–843. doi:10.1089/scd.2011.0621

Low, L. K., Miller, J. M., Guo, Y., Ashton-Miller, J. A., DeLancey, J. O. L., & Sampselle, C. M. (2013). Spontaneous pushing to prevent postpartum urinary incontinence: A randomized, controlled trial. *International Urogynecology Journal, 24*(3), 453–460. doi:10.1007/s00192-012-1884-y. PMCID: PMC3980478

Low, L. K., Zielinski, R., Tao, Y., Galecki, A., Brandon, C. J., & Miller, J. M. (2014). Predicting birth-related levator ani tear severity in primiparous women: Evaluating maternal recovery from labor and delivery (EMRLD Study). *Open Journal of Obstetrics & Gynecology, 4*(6), 266–278. doi:10.4236/ojog.2014.46043

Lukacz, E. S., Sampselle, C., Gray, M., MacDiarmid, S., Rosenberg, M., Ellsworth, P., & Palmer, M. H. (2011). A healthy bladder: A consensus statement. *International Journal of Clinical Practice, 65*(10), 1026–1036. doi:10.1111/j.1742-1241.2011.02763.x

Madhuvrata, P., Cody, J. D., Ellis, G., Herbison, G. P., & Hay-Smith, E. J. (2012). Which anticholinergic drug for overactive bladder symptoms in adults. *Cochrane Database Systematic Reviews, 1*, CD005429. doi:10.1002/14651858.CD005429.pub2

Markland, A. D., Richter, H. E., Fwu, C-H., Eggers, P., & Kusek, J. W. (2011). Prevalence and trends of urinary incontinence in adults in the United states, 2001 to 2008. *Adult Urology, 186*(2), 589–593. doi:10.1016/j.juro.2011.03.114

McKenzie, P., Rohozinski, J., & Badlani, G. (2010). Genetic influences on stress urinary incontinence. *Current Opinion Urology, 20*(4), 291–295. doi:10.1097/MOU.0b013e32833a4436

Miller, J. M. (2002). Criteria for therapeutic use of pelvic floor muscle training in women. *Journal of Wound Ostomy & Continence Nursing, 29*(6), 301–311.

Miller, J. M., Ashton-Miller, J. A., & DeLancey, J. O. L. (1998a). A pelvic muscle precontraction can reduce cough-related urine loss in selected women with mild SUI. *Journal of the American Geriatrics Society, 46*(7), 870–874.

Miller, J. M., Ashton-Miller, J. A., & DeLancey, J. O. L. (1998b). Quantification of cough-related urine loss using the paper towel test. *Obstetrics & Gynecology, 91*, 705–709.

Miller, J. M., Garcia, C. E., Hortsch, S. B., Guo, Y., & Schimpf, M. O. (2016). Does instruction to eliminate coffee, tea, alcohol, carbonated, and artificially sweetened beverages improve lower urinary tract symptoms: A prospective trial. *Journal of Wound Ostomy Continence Nurses, 43*(1), 69–79.

Miller, J. M., Low, L. K., Zielinski, R., Smith, A. R., DeLancey, J. O. L., & Brandon, C. (2015). Evaluating maternal recovery from labor and delivery: Bone and levator ani injuries. *American Journal of Obstetrics & Gynecology, 213*(2), 188.e1–188.e11. doi:10.1016/j.ajog.2015.05.001

Miller, J. M., Sampselle, C. M., Ashton-Miller, J. A., Hong, G-R. S., & DeLancey, J. O. L. (2008). Clarification and confirmation of the effect of volitional pelvic floor muscle contraction to preempt urine loss (the Knack maneuver) in stress incontinent women. *International Urogynecology Journal and Pelvic Floor Dysfunction, 19*(6), 773–782. doi:10.1007/s00192-007-0525-3

Miller, J. M., Umek, W. H., DeLancey, J. O., & Ashton-Miller, J. A. (2004). Can women increase urethral closure pressures without their pubococcygeus muscles? *American Journal of Obstetrics & Gynecology, 191*(1), 171–175.

Milsom, I., Coyne, K. S., Nicholson, S., Kvasz, M., Chen, C-I., & Wein, A. J. (2014). Global prevalence and economic burden of urgency urinary incontinence: A systematic review. *European Urology, 65*(1), 79–95. doi:10.1016/j.eururo.2013.08.031

Mørkved, S., & Bø, K. (2014). Effect of pelvic floor muscle training during pregnancy and after childbirth on prevention and treatment of urinary incontinence: A systematic review. *British Journal of Sports Medicine, 48*(4), 299–310. doi:10.1136/bjsports-2012-091758

National Association for Continence. (2015). Can your diet affect your bladder or bowel control. Retrieved from http://www.nafc.org/bladderirritants

National Institutes of Health (NIH). (2014). RFA-DK-14-004: Prevention of lower urinary tract symptoms in women: Bladder Health Clinical Centers. Retrieved from http://grants.nih.gov/grants/guide/rfa-files/RFA-DK-14-004.html

National Institute for Health and Care Excellence. (2013, September). Urinary incontinence: The management of urinary incontinence in women. Retrieved from http://www.nice.org.uk/guidance/cg171/chapter/1-recommendations

Nevéus, T., von Gontard, A., Hoebeke, P., Hjälmås, K., Bauer, S., Bower, W., . . . Djurhuus, J. C. (2006). The standardization of terminology of lower urinary tract function in children and adolescents: Report from the Standardisation Committee of the International Children's Continence Society. *Journal of Urology, 176*(1), 314–324. doi:10.1016/S0022-5347(06)00305-3

Osman, N. I., Chapple, C. R., Abrans, P., Dmochowski, R., Haab, F., Nitti, V., . . . Wein, A. J. (2014). Detrusor underactivity and the underactive bladder: A new clinical entity? A review of current terminology, definitions, epidemiology, aetiology, and diagnosis. *European Urology, 65*(2), 389–398. doi:10.1016/j.eururo.2013.10.015

Paik, S., Han, S., Kwon, O., Ahn, Y., Lee, B., & Ahn, S. (2013). Acupuncture for the treatment of urinary incontinence: A review of randomized controlled trials. *Experimental and Therapeutic Medicine, 6*(3), 773–780. doi:10.3892/etm.2013.1210

Pereira, V. S., Escobar, A. C., & Driusso, P. (2012). Effects of physical therapy in older women with urinary incontinence: A systematic review. *Brazilian Journal of Physical Therapy, 16*(6), 463–468. doi:10.1590/S1413-35552012005000050

Perucchini, D., DeLancey, J. O. L., Ashton-Miller, J. A., Peschers, U., & Kataria, T. (2002). Age effects on urethral striated muscle. *American Journal of Obstetrics & Gynecology, 186*(3), 351–355. doi:10.1067/mob.2002.121090

Phelan, S., Kanaya, A. M., Subak, L. L., Hogan, P. E., Espeland, M. A., Wing, R. R., . . . Brown, J. S. (2012). Weight loss prevents urinary incontinence in women with type 2 diabetes: results from the Look AHEAD trial. *Journal of Urology, 187*(3), 939–944. doi:10.1016/j.juro.2011.10.139

Quallich, S. A., Bumpus, S. M., & Lajiness, S. (2015). Competencies for the nursing practitioner working with adult urology patients. *Urologic Nursing, 35*(5), 221–230.

Rafiq, M., McGovern, A., Jones, S., Harris, K., Tomson, C., Gallagher, H., & de Lusignan, S. (2014). Falls in the elderly were predicted opportunistically using a decision tree and systematically using a database-driven screening tool. *Journal of Clinical Epidemiology, 67*(8), 877–886. http://dx.doi.org/10.1016/j.jclinepi.2014.03.008

Rahn, D. D., Carberry, C. Sanses, T. V., Mamik, M. M., Ward, R. M., Meriwether, K. V., . . . Society of Gynecologic Surgeons Systematic Review Group. (2014). Vaginal estrogen for genitourinary syndrome of menopause: A systematic review. *Obstetrics & Gynecology, 124*(6), 1147–1156. doi:10.1097/AOG.0000000000000526

Rahn, D. D., Ward, R. M., Sanses, T. V., Carberry, C., Mamik, M. M., Olivera, C. K., . . . Murphy, M. (2015). Vaginal estrogen use in postmenopausal women with pelvic floor disorders: Systematic review and practice guidelines. *International Urogynecology Journal, 26*(1), 3–13. doi:10.1007/s00192-014-2554-z

Richter, H. E., Burgio, K. L., Brubaker, L., Nyaard, I. E., Ye, W., Weidber, A., . . . Spino, C. (2010). A trial of continence pessary vs. behavioral therapy vs. combined therapy for stress incontinence. *Obstetrics & Gynecology, 115*(3), 609–617. doi:10.1097/AOG.0b03e81d055d4

Robinson, D., Castro-Diaz, D., Giarenis, I., Toozs-Hobson, P., Anding, R., Burton, C., & Cardozo, L. (2015). What is the best surgical intervention for stress urinary incontinence in the very young and very old? An International Consultation on Incontinence Research Society updated. *International Urogynecology Journal, 26*(11), 1599–1604. doi:10.1007/s00192-015-2783-9

Roe, B., Flanagan, L., & Maden, M. (2015). Systematic review of systematic reviews for the management of urinary incontinence and promotion of continence using conservative behavioural approaches in older people in care homes. *Journal of Advanced Nursing, 71*(1), 1464–1483. doi:10.1111/jan.12613

Sandvik, H., Seim, A., Vanvik, A., & Hunskaar, S. (2000). A severity index for epidemiological surveys of female urinary incontinence: Comparison with 48-hour pad-weighing tests. *Neurourology & Urodynamics, 19*(2), 137–145. doi:10.1002/(SICI)1520-6777(2000)19:2<137::AID-NAU4>3.0.CO;2-G

Sangsawang, B., & Sangsawang, N. (2013). Stress urinary incontinence in pregnant women: A review of prevalence, pathophysiology, and treatment. *International Urogynecology Journal, 24*(6), 901–912. doi:10.1007/s00192-013-2061-7

Sangsawang, B., & Serisathien, Y. (2012). Effect of pelvic floor muscle exercise programme on stress urinary incontinence among pregnant women. *Journal of Advanced Nursing, 68*(9), 1997–2007. doi:10.1111/j.1365-2648.2011.05890.x

Sexton, C. C., Notte, S. M., Maroulis, C., Dmochowski, R. R., Cardozo, L., Subramanian, D., & Coyne, K. S. (2011). Persistence and adherence in the treatment of overactive bladder syndrome with anticholinergic therapy: A systematic review of the literature. *International Journal of Clinical Practice, 65*(5), 567–585. doi:10.1111/j.1742-1241.2010.02626.x

Shek, K. L., & Dietz, H. P. (2010). Intrapartum risk factors for levator trauma. *BJOG: An International Journal of Obstetrics & Gynaecology, 117*(12), 1485–1492. doi:10.1111/j.1471-0528.2010.02704.x

Siddiqui, N. Y., Levin, P. J., Phadtare, A., Pietrobon, R., & Ammarell, N. (2014). Perceptions about female urinary incontinence: A systematic review. *International Urogynecology Journal, 25*(7), 863–871. doi:10.1007/s00192-013-2276-7

Society of Urologic Nurses and Assoicates (SUNA). (2013). *Scope and standards of urologic nursing practice.* Pitman, NJ: Author.

Stafne, S. N., Salvesen, K., Romundstad, P. R., Torjusen, I. H., & Mørkved, S. (2012). Does regular exercise including pelvic floor muscle training prevent urinary and anal incontinence during pregnancy? A randomised controlled trial. *BJOG: An International Journal of Obstetrics & Gynaecology, 119*(10), 1270–1280. doi:10.1111/j.1471-0528.2012.03426.x

Sun, Y. Luo, D., Tang, C., Yang, L., & Shen, H. (2015). The safety and efficiency of onabotulinumtoxinA for the treatment of overactive bladder: A systematic review and meta-analysis. *International Urology and Nephrology, 47*(11), 1779–1788. doi:10.1007/sl1255-015-1125-7

Thom, D. H., & Rortveit, G. (2010). Prevalence of postpartum urinary incontinence: A systematic review. *Acta Obstetricia et Gynecologica Scandinavica, 89*(12), 1511–1522. doi:10.3109/00016349.2010.526188

Townsend, M. K., Curhan, G. C., Resnick, N. M., & Grodstein, F. (2010). The incidence of urinary incontinence across Asian, black, and white women in the United States. *American Journal of Obstetrics & Gynecology, 202*(4), 378. e371–378. e377. doi:10.1016/j.ajog.2009.11.021

Vissers, D., Neels, H., Vermandel, A., Wachter, S. D., Tjalma, W. A. A., Wyndaele, J-J., & Taeymans, J. (2014). The effect of nonsurgical weight loss interventions on urinary incontinence in overweight women: A systematic review and meta-analysis. *Obesity Reviews, 15*(7), 610–617. doi:10.1111/obr.12170

von Gontard, A., Baeyens, D., Van Hoecke, E., Warzak, W. J., & Bachmann, C. (2011). Psychological and psychiatric issues in urinary and fecal incontinence. *Journal of Urology, 185*(4), 1432–1437. doi:10.1016/j.juro.2010.11.051

von Gontard, A., Heron, J., & Joinson, C. (2011). Family history of nocturnal enuresis and urinary incontinence: Results from a large epidemiological study. *Journal of Urology, 185*(6), 2303–2307. doi:10.1016/j.juro.2011.02.040

Wagg, A., Gibson, W., Ostaszkiewicz, J., Johnson, T. III, Markland, A., Palmer, M. H., . . . Kirschner-Hermanns, R. (2015). Urinary incontinence in frail elderly persons: Report from the 5th International Consultation on Incontinence. *Neurourology & Urodynamics, 34*(5), 398–406. doi:10.1002/nau.22602

Whitcomb, E. L., & Subak, L. L. (2011). Effect of weight loss on urinary incontinence in women. *Open Access Journal of Urology, 3,* 123–132. doi:10.2147/OAJU.S21091

Wing, R. R., Creasman, J. M., West, D. S., Richter, H. E., Myers, D., Burgio, K. L., . . . Subak, L. L. (2010). Improving urinary incontinence in overweight and obese women through modest weight loss. *Obstetrics & Gynecology, 116*(2, Pt. 1), 284–292. doi:10.1097/AOG.0b013e3181e8fb60

Wing, R. R., West, D. S., Grady, D., Creasman, J. M., Richter, H. E., Myers, D., . . . Subak, L. L. (2010). Effect of weight loss on urinary incontinence in overweight and obese women: Results at 12 and 18 months. *Journal of Urology, 184*(3), 1005–1010. doi:10.1016/j.juro.2010.05.031

Wood, L. N., & Anger, J. T. (2014). Urinary incontinence in women. *British Medical Journal, 394,* g4531. doi:10.1136/bmj.g4531

CHAPTER 23

Menstrual-Cycle Pain and Premenstrual Conditions

Ruth Zielinski

Sandra Lynne

The editors acknowledge Diana Taylor, Kerri Durnell Schuiling, and Beth A. Collins Sharp, who were the authors of the previous edition of this chapter.

OVERVIEW

Since the time of Hippocrates, physicians, philosophers, and scientists have written about the links between menstruation, the brain, and behavior (Epperson, 2012). Once thought to "purge bad humors," menstruation has always been surrounded by mystery, myth, and taboos. Tortula of Salerno, an 11th-century female gynecologist, wrote that "there are young women who are relieved when the menses are called forth" (Mason-Hohl, 1940). In ancient Greece, the prevailing belief was that the uterus moved through a woman's body and that the perimenstrual discomforts reflected where the uterus had traveled (Rowlandson, 1998). Using this concept as a context for understanding and treating illness, it was believed that a headache, for example, was caused by the uterus floating near or actually residing in the head (Rowlandson, 1998). The treatment to cure the headache, then, was to hold a woman over a fire with the hot flame near her genitals so the uterus would descend to where it belonged (Rowlandson, 1998). While many advances have been made since that time, there is still a long way to go in understanding the menstrual cycle, the pain it can cause, and perimenstrual conditions. This chapter focuses on menstrual-cycle pain and accompanying discomforts within a women-centered, normalizing context.

Most women will experience some sort of functional cyclic pain and other related symptoms during the premenstrual and menstrual phases of their menstrual cycles (Shulman, 2010; Witt, Strickland, Cheng, Curtis, & Calkins, 2013). While the cyclic changes (and often the accompanying discomforts) are a normative process, they can disrupt a woman's sense of well-being.

The menstrual cycle has three phases and is typically described in the context of a 28-day cycle, although the range of normal and other aspects often vary (see Chapter 5 for a comprehensive review of the menstrual cycle). Premenstrual symptoms may include psychological, physical, and behavioral changes—collectively termed premenstrual syndrome (PMS). While many recognize that these symptoms are often normal and are experienced by a number of women during their menstrual cycles, others, particularly those operating from within a biomedical context, tend to pathologize the symptoms. Interestingly, for the medical community to acknowledge women's pain and discomforts, menstrual variations tend to be identified as a disorder, thereby validating their existence and providing justification for research and formulation of treatment modalities.

PMS is a term often used derisively in Western culture, with its use implying that women are incapable of rational thought during the premenstrual phase of their cycle. In that context, PMS is described as including a variety of symptoms such as food cravings, irritability, mood swings, irrational behavior, and sometimes violence. Unfortunately, other conditions are often misdiagnosed as PMS and may actually be part of a serious mental health condition. However, the growing body of research and the visibility of PMS in our culture has educated women about this phenomenon, offering some solutions and validation of the symptoms, distress, and the discomfort they feel.

SCOPE AND PREVALENCE OF THE PROBLEM

Menstrual pain is the most common gynecologic problem in women of all ages and ethnicities (Osayande & Mehulic, 2014). Significant menstrual pain—often debilitating—that disrupts a woman's lifestyle is termed dysmenorrhea. Dysmenorrhea is a common occurrence among women; indeed, primary dysmenorrhea affects almost half of all women during their menses (Burbeck & Willig, 2014; Lasco, Catalano, & Benvenga, 2012; Shulman, 2010; Westling, Tu, Griffith, & Hellman, 2013). Yet, while much can be found in the medical literature about dysmenorrhea, very few studies have focused on understanding dysmenorrhea from a woman's perspective. Historically, paternalistic views of menstrual-related experiences prevailed and biomedical language predominated, with little attention being paid to alternative perspectives from other disciplines or, more important, from a woman's perspective (Burbeck & Willig, 2014). Shifting the focus of dysmenorrhea and other relevant menstrual-cycle changes to a woman's point of view provides the clinician with a woman-centered context for understanding the changes.

Menstruation and its accompanying symptoms have been "taboo" subjects, often not discussed in the transfer of wisdom from grandmother to mother and then to daughter (Schooler, Ward, Merriwether, & Caruthers, 2005). Even within the context of health education, menstruation is presented as a medical problem to be treated (Burbeck & Willig, 2014). Often women have felt ruled by their biology and believed that menstrual discomforts were a rite of passage, something that must be endured but not talked about (Dennerstein, Lehert, & Heinemann, 2011). Means of coping with these symptoms were considered "women's knowledge," rather than medically or scientifically valid practices.

During the women's movement of the 1960s and the homebirth movement of the 1970s, advocates for women's health began to bring menstruation and other women's health issues to the forefront of the cultural consciousness. More women entered the medical field and advocated more vigorously for women's health; their voices were, to some extent, heard. The Women's Health Equity Act of 1993 required that research include women, and funding was provided for research that focused on women's health. Large studies of women's health were conducted, including studies that focused on menstrual irregularities and menstrual dysphoria.

Studies about menstrual pain and the psychological and behavioral changes that occurred during menstruation documented prevalence rates ranging from 16% to 90% (Burbeck & Willig, 2014; Shulman, 2010). With such findings, it became clear that a number of women experienced cyclical pelvic pain and the sequelae of symptoms that often accompany it. It was also recognized that, even though the pain and accompanying symptoms that occur with menstruation may cause significant discomfort and affect a woman's quality of life for a time, these symptoms are more often a normal variation of the menstrual cycle rather than indicative of pathology (Burbeck & Willig, 2014). Identifying that the symptoms experienced during menstruation are often nonpathologic, however, does not mean that women should be discounted when they seek care and treatment for these symptoms. On the contrary, lifestyle modifications and therapies can, at least in part, alleviate the discomforts associated with normal menstrual-cycle changes.

DYSMENORRHEA

Dysmenorrhea—defined as painful cramps that occur with menstruation—is the most commonly reported menstrual disorder, affecting as many as 81% of women (Latthe et al., 2006). Approximately 11% to 57% of women with dysmenorrhea report moderate to severe pain that interferes with the quality of their lives and requires the use of pharmacologic methods of pain relief (Burbeck & Willig, 2014). While dysmenorrhea may accompany premenstrual syndrome and dysphoric disorders, it is often the primary and most troubling symptom that women experience.

The pain of dysmenorrhea originates from intense uterine contractions during the menstrual phase of the cycle, triggering endometrial prostaglandin production and release. The excessive amount of prostaglandins causes the uterus to contract further, reducing uterine blood flow and causing ischemia and pain. While the etiology of dysmenorrhea is not completely understood, studies support the hypothesis that uterine inflammation with menstrual cycles may also promote cross-organ pain sensitization, a mechanism by which dysfunction in one organ elicits neurogenic inflammation in another organ (Westling et al., 2013). The uterus lies in close proximity to the bladder, the bowel, and the peritoneum, and its contraction may elicit pain in those structures during the menstrual cycle. This theory, along with the current knowledge about prostaglandins' major role in dysmenorrhea, may help explain the chronicity of pain that may occur throughout the pelvic area during the menstrual cycle.

The incidence of dysmenorrhea is as high as 80% among women in their teens and early 20s, with half of these women experiencing loss of time from school or work as a result of this condition (Dawood & Yusof, 2006; Smith, 2015). Dysmenorrhea may, or may not, be accompanied by heavy bleeding. While dysmenorrhea can be experienced by any woman during the menstrual cycle, certain factors and conditions may increase the likelihood of its development (**Box 23-1**).

Dysmenorrhea is classified into two broad categories: primary (absence of pelvic pathology) and secondary (occurring from identifiable organic pathology).

Primary Dysmenorrhea

Primary dysmenorrhea, which is more common than secondary dysmenorrhea, often begins 6 to 12 months after menarche. Typically symptoms are experienced with the onset of bleeding and continue for 8 to 72 hours into the menstrual cycle. Increased endometrial prostaglandin production is believed to be the cause of the associated pain (Lentz, 2007). It is associated with multiple symptoms, including abdominal cramps, headache,

---

BOX 23-1 **Risk Factors for Dysmenorrhea**

- Age < 30 years
- Body mass index < 20
- Smoking
- Early menarche
- History of sexual abuse
- Premenstrual emotional symptoms (dysphoria)
- History of pelvic surgery
- Pelvic pain history
- Depression

Reproduced from Burbeck, R., & Willig, C. (2014). The personal experience of dysmenorrhea: An interpretive phenomenological analysis. *Journal of Health Psychology, 19*(10), 1334–1344.

---

backache, general body aches, continuous abdominal pain, and other somatic discomforts. The difference between primary dysmenorrhea and normal somatic and psychological changes prior to menses is that primary dysmenorrhea is perceived as more severe, with chronic, sometimes debilitating symptoms. There is no evidence of organic pathology in the uterus, fallopian tubes, or ovaries with primary dysmenorrhea. Women usually report repeated symptomology with each cycle. When charting their cycles, it is evident that that pain, bleeding, and disruption of lifestyle occur at regular times in the cycle.

There is a higher prevalence of depression and anxiety in women who experience pelvic pain or dysmenorrhea (Kiesner, 2011). Depression, stress, and anxiety increase circulating cortisol levels in women who experience this menstrual-related condition. Cyclic hormonal changes cause alterations in endorphins and serotonin levels. Heightened somatic sensitivity in some women is thought to play a part of primary dysmenorrhea as well as being a significant risk factor for long-term chronic pelvic pain (Westling et al., 2013). Abnormal levels of cortisol correlate with pain sensitivity in women diagnosed with dysmenorrhea (Vincent et al., 2011).

BOX 23-2 Open-Ended Question About Symptomology

Question for discussion with the woman:
Do underlying anxiety and depression contribute to dysmenorrhea, or do the pain and dread of menses cause anxiety and depression?

Pain is subjective, and the relationships among premenstrual symptoms, perimenstrual pain, and psychological symptoms such as depression and anxiety have led to the somatization or labeling of dysmenorrhea as psychosomatic. Studies have identified relationships among chronic pelvic pain, depression, and anxiety in women with somatic sensitivity (Westling et al., 2013), leading to a variety of treatments for pelvic pain such as psychologic therapy and psychotropic medications. While the relationship between dysmenorrhea and psychologic symptoms such as depression and anxiety does exist, it does not minimize the significance of the pain and discomfort of women experiencing dysmenorrhea. Understanding that these symptoms can coexist while also taking care to differentiate menstrual-cycle changes from depression and anxiety is the responsibility of a sensitive clinician (**Box 23-2**).

It is also important that the clinician distinguish primary dysmenorrhea from secondary dysmenorrhea by eliciting a thorough history and conducting a physical examination (**Box 23-3**).

Secondary Dysmenorrhea

Dysmenorrhea that is caused by pelvic pathology is referred to as secondary dysmenorrhea. Diagnosis of secondary dysmenorrhea includes pelvic pathology such as adenomyosis, leiomyomata, irritable bowel syndrome, interstitial cystitis, and endometriosis (Hoffman, 2008). Almost any process that can affect the pelvic viscera and cause acute or intermittent recurring pain might be a source of cyclic premenstrual pain, including urinary tract infection, pelvic inflammatory disease, hernia, and pelvic relaxation or prolapse (Dawood & Yusof,

---

BOX 23-3 Dysmenorrhea and Menstrual History to Collect During the Office Visit

Dysmenorrhea history:
- Pain
- Treatments used, past and present
- Duration of dysmenorrhea both cyclically and historically (i.e., when the woman first began having dysmenorrhea symptoms; during her present cycles, how often and when does it occur)

Menstrual history:
- Age at menarche
- Family history of menstrual cycles and endometriosis
- Menstrual frequency
- Contraceptive history
- Length of menses
- Estimated menstrual flow (moderate to heavy, number of pads/tampons needed)
- Presence of intermenstrual bleeding

Pain:
- Onset and duration (before or just after menses begins)
- Associated symptoms
- Location of pain: lower abdominal pain, radiating to the back or thighs
- Factors that exacerbate the pain
- Pain control measures taken
- Influence of pain on physical, sexual, and social activity

Sexual and obstetric history:
- Age at coitarche (first intercourse)
- Obstetric history of complications
- History of contraception
- History of sexual partners
- History of sexually transmitted infections
- History of sexual abuse or interpersonal trauma

2006). Clinical findings may differ from primary dysmenorrhea in that they may include reports of dyspareunia (pain with intercourse), postcoital bleeding, and abnormal uterine bleeding. The pelvic pain associated with secondary dysmenorrhea may occur before, during, or after menses.

Assessing for secondary dysmenorrhea would include the same information elicited for assessment of primary dysmenorrhea along with the history and physical examination (**Box 23-4**).

The most common cause of secondary dysmenorrhea is endometriosis—a chronic condition in which the endometrial lining is implanted outside the uterus. Tissue from the lining of the uterus (the endometrium) may attach to the ovaries, adnexa, peritoneum, and other organs such as the bowel and bladder. Just as the lining of the uterus responds to hormonal influence, so endometrial tissue breaks down and bleeds, causing pain. Scar tissue (adhesions) forms inside the pelvic cavity where the endometrial lining exists and bleeding occurs. Adhesions can attach to each other and result in chronic pelvic pain. Other symptoms often include dysuria, dyspareunia, infertility, and gastrointestinal (GI) disturbance such as constipation, diarrhea, and bloating.

Another cause of secondary dysmenorrhea is uterine fibroids (leiomyomas, myomas). Symptoms that occur with uterine fibroids are similar to those experienced with endometriosis and may also include heavy menstrual bleeding. Endometriosis and uterine fibroids are discussed in greater detail in Chapter 26.

The pain associated with either primary or secondary dysmenorrhea may be similar, although pain that has increased over time is more often associated with secondary dysmenorrhea.

Management Options for Dysmenorrhea

For centuries, women have tried alternative treatments, home remedies, and pharmaceutical agents to minimize the pain associated with their menstrual cycles. Just as menstruation was a taboo subject, so too were effective treatment and understanding of why the pain occurred and which methods of treatment actually relieved the discomforts. At menarche, many adolescent girls were given some type of pads or "protection" and a hot water bottle, while others were left to figure it out for themselves. Many women consider even severe menstrual pain as inevitable and do not seek medical care or advice. Of those who do, many do not continue with prescribed medications (Society of Obstetricians & Gynecologists of Canada [SGOC], 2005).

An emerging research base is focusing on herbal medicine and alternative treatments for dysmenorrhea. Many resources suggest the benefits of homeopathy or herbal medicine in relieving menstrual pain, but only a few research studies have actually sought to determine their efficacy. While resources such as websites often include testimonials, these anecdotes do not provide strong evidence of treatment efficacy. Ideally, clinicians should be able to provide evidence-based information that will guide women in choosing treatments to provide the best relief of their symptoms. However, while there may not be strong evidence to support herbal and alternative treatments, it is important for clinicians to support women's choices within the realm of safety.

Nonpharmacologic Treatments for Dysmenorrhea

Treatments that do not require the use of medications (either hormonal or analgesic) can help reduce the symptoms of dysmenorrhea. These treatments are referred to as alternative therapies when used alone or as complementary therapies if used in addition to pharmacologic or other therapies. Further information about complementary and alternative medicine is available from the National Center for Complementary and Alternative Medicine (http://nccam.nih.gov).

Heat Heating pads, hot water bottles, and other forms of heat therapy have long been used to reduce pelvic pain (SGOC, 2005). Use of heat either as a solo treatment modality or as a complementary therapy to nonsteroidal anti-inflammatory drugs (NSAIDs) often results in a significant amount of pain relief (Kannan & Claydon, 2014). Advise women that a temperature of approximately 104°F (40°C) is recommended. The heat can be applied as often as needed.

Lifestyle Changes Research focusing on regular exercise to decrease dysmenorrhea symptoms found that women who engaged in vigorous exercise (more than 3 times per week) reported approximately 30% less pain and noticed a decrease in other physical symptoms during menses compared to sedentary women who did not exercise (SGOC, 2005). A statistically significant finding of a cross-sectional descriptive study of 300 nursing students at an Egyptian university was that women who ate breakfast every day had more regular menstrual cycles, less pelvic pain, and less dysmenorrhea (Eittah, 2014).

Vitamin and Herbal Treatments There is a paucity of well-designed, published studies of the efficacy of complementary and herbal therapies, although the number of studies is on the rise. The effectiveness of vitamin E in reducing pelvic pain from primary dysmenorrhea was evaluated in a double-blind, randomized trial involving 120 women who were diagnosed with dysmenorrhea. The women were randomly assigned to two groups: a control group, in which women received a placebo, and the study group, in which women took vitamin E, 400 IU/day. Pain severity was analyzed using a visual analog scale (VAS) at 1 month prior to the beginning of the study and during the 2-month span of the study. The findings revealed that both groups had lower pain levels during the 2 months of the study than during the first month when no intervention was used.

However, the group using vitamin E had the lowest pain scores during the course of the study, leading to the suggestion that while placebo may work, vitamin E seems to cause a greater reduction in pain (Kashanian, Lakeh, Ghasemi, & Noori, 2013).

The impact of the herbal product Shirzai Thymus Vulgaris versus ibuprofen (an NSAID) on primary dysmenorrhea was studied in a group of 18- to 25-year-old female students at Illam University of Medical Sciences in Iran (Direkvand-Moghadam & Khosravi, 2012). The 120 participants were divided into two groups, with one group taking ibuprofen three times a day and the study group taking 5 mL of Shirazi Thymus Vulgaris five times daily. Pain severity was measured using a VAS. As in the previously mentioned study, the pain level of both groups decreased from the initial intervention-free period, with no significant differences between the groups being observed. These findings suggest that the herbal medicine Shirzai Thymus Vulgaris is just as effective as ibuprofen as a treatment for dysmenorrhea. Unfortunately, the dosage of ibuprofen was not identified in the article.

Acupuncture A systematic review of all randomized controlled trials (RCTs) that evaluated the effect of acupuncture was undertaken by Cho and Hwang in 2010. Of the 27 RCTs reviewed, only 9 could be used for the meta-analysis; the others did not describe the methodology used. The main finding was that acupuncture, when compared with either herbal treatments or pharmacologic treatments, significantly lowered pain from dysmenorrhea.

A pilot study focused on acupuncture-point injection of vitamin K_1 as a treatment for dysmenorrhea. The findings suggest that acupuncture-point injection with vitamin K_1 may provide greater pain relief when compared with placebo (Chao, Callens, Wade, Abercrombie, & Gomolak, 2014). Only 14 women completed all three visits in this study, however, so generalizations cannot be made from the findings.

In an RCT ($n = 94$) evaluating the effectiveness of ibuprofen (400–600 mg) with the efficacy of vibratory stimulation through direct stimulation of direct intravaginal tampon application (VIPON), researchers found that while both treatments reduced the pain of dysmenorrhea, the VIPON group achieved statistically greater pain relief (Witt et al.,

2013). An additional finding was that the group treated with VIPON experienced pain relief more rapidly than the group who took ibuprofen.

Pharmacologic Treatment Options

Nonsteroidal Anti-inflammatory Drugs Currently, pharmacotherapy is the most common and effective (as evidenced by clinical trials) treatment for dysmenorrhea. Of the pharmacologic choices for dysmenorrhea, NSAIDs are considered the front-line analgesics (Marjoribanks, Ayeleke, Farquhar, & Proctor, 2015). NSAIDs inhibit cyclooxygenase (COX) enzymes, thereby inhibiting the production of prostaglandins. Clinical trials have demonstrated that NSAIDs are effective in treating menstrual-cycle pain, including reducing restriction of activities of daily life and reducing days of work and school missed (SOGC, 2005). Side effects of NSAIDs may include gastrointestinal upset, headaches, and drowsiness.

NSAIDs specifically approved by the Food and Drug Administration (FDA) for treatment of dysmenorrhea include the following agents:

- Diclofenac
- Ibuprofen
- Ketoprofen
- Meclofenamate
- Mefenamic acid
- Naproxen

Clinical guidelines suggest trying one or more NSAIDs when a woman reports dysmenorrhea and then assessing her pain and cycle control after the trial (SGOC, 2005). Counsel women to begin taking NSAIDs 2 to 3 days before menses is expected, as this regimen will decrease prostaglandin production. NSAIDs are more likely to be effective for primary dysmenorrhea than for secondary dysmenorrhea because of the associated underlying pathology that often accompanies the latter (Braverman, 2007).

Oral Contraceptives Contraceptives are often used in the treatment of dysmenorrhea, particularly for women who also desire both cycle control and contraception. Combined oral contraceptives (COCs) include both estrogen and progestin and act to suppress ovulation, which in turn reduces prostaglandin production and relieves dysmenorrhea in as many as 70% to 80% of women (American College of Obstetricians and Gynecologists, 2010b, reaffirmed 2014). As early as 1937, researchers demonstrated that dysmenorrhea is reduced when ovulation is inhibited. Studies since then have yielded similar results, with a reduction in dysmenorrhea symptoms stemming from COC use (Biggs & DeMuth, 2011; SGOC, 2005). For example, one RCT demonstrated that COCs containing 30 mcg of ethinyl estradiol and 3 mg drospirenone reduced the incidence of dysmenorrhea from 19% to 6.4% (American College of Obstetricians and Gynecologists, 2010b, reaffirmed 2014).

Oral contraceptives suppress ovulation and endometrial tissue growth, thereby decreasing the amount of menstrual volume and prostaglandin secretion. The decrease in menstrual volume in turn decreases the amount of uterine pressure, which then decreases the amount of cramping felt. Reducing prostaglandin secretion during the menstrual cycle inhibits the entire cascade of symptoms described earlier. A continuous COC regimen (i.e., 84 days of continuous COC use, followed by 7 hormone-free days) may increase the benefits for women with dysmenorrhea by eliminating menses for a longer period of time. Both the risks and benefits of COCs need to be assessed prior to recommending their use for dysmenorrhea.

Progestin Implants Currently, progestin implants consist of a single rod placed intradermally in the arm. Early studies indicate that this form of contraception decreases dysmenorrhea incidence from 59% at baseline to 21% after treatment (American College of Obstetricians and Gynecologists, 2010b, reaffirmed 2014). Of those women with dysmenorrhea, 81% show a decrease in symptoms with the progestin implant. Like COCs, progestin implants suppress ovulation and often suppress ovulation and menses, thus reducing dysmenorrhea.

Levonorgestrel Intrauterine Device The levonorgestrel (progestin) intrauterine device (IUD) is a highly effective contraceptive method that offers additional noncontraceptive benefits in women with menstrual disorders such as heavy menstrual bleeding, dysmenorrhea, adenomyosis, leiomyomas, and pain due to endometriosis

(Zieman & Hatcher, 2012). Menstrual bleeding is decreased by 74% to 97% with the levonorgestrel IUD. The beneficial effects of decreasing menses and suppressing prostaglandin production result in a reduction of dysmenorrhea in many women. The volume of blood loss per cycle also becomes reduced over time (Fritz & Speroff, 2011). The progestogenic side effects are greater with the IUD than with COCs (American College of Obstetricians and Gynecologists, 2010b, reaffirmed 2014) but less than with high-dose progestin (Fritz & Speroff, 2011). Women should be counseled that side effects of the levonorgestrel IUD include irregular bleeding or spotting for up to 6 months, with approximately 20% of women becoming amenorrheic by one year of use (Dean & Schwarz, 2011).

Depot Medroxyprogesterone Acetate This contraceptive method, which consists of depot medroxyprogesterone acetate (DMPA) injections every 12 weeks, suppresses ovulation—an outcome that can be effective in treating dysmenorrhea and heavy menstrual bleeding. DMPA also induces endometrial atrophy, decreased menstrual flow, and secretion of prostaglandins. Amenorrhea with DMPA injections occurs in 55% to 60% of women by 12 months of use and as many as 68% of women by 24 months of use (SGOC, 2005). Because DMPA does not offer immediate relief of dysmenorrhea and other menstrual symptoms, it is rarely chosen as an option specifically for this indication by women. In addition, DMPA injections may result in an increased risk for side effects such as irregular bleeding and weight gain when compared to other hormonal contraceptive methods (Zieman & Hatcher, 2012).

Surgical Intervention While at least two surgical procedures have been developed to treat dysmenorrhea, these should be considered to be extreme measures that are generally not recommended (SOGC, 2005). Both of these surgeries involve dissecting or destroying the uterine nerves, which prevents the transmission of pain signals. The surgery itself can be associated with adhesions and chronic pelvic pain, and has not been found to provide long-term benefits for dysmenorrhea (SOGC, 2005).

Focusing on dysmenorrhea as a symptom or source of discomfort rather than as a disease-oriented syndrome provides a model for understanding complex gender-specific conditions that include biologic, psychosocial, and sociocultural factors. This holistic model can also be applied to other women's health problems, such as stress-related conditions (e.g., heart disease, arthritis, and immune system disorders), psychiatric disorders, and normative menstrual-cycle transitions (e.g., menarche, postpartum, and menopause).

PREMENSTRUAL-CYCLE SYNDROME AND DYSPHORIC DISORDER: AN OVERVIEW

Symptoms such as mood, weight, and appetite changes have long been associated with the menstrual cycle. However, to provide validity to the symptoms women experience, premenstrual syndrome and premenstrual dysphoric disorder had to be identified, classified, and supported with evidence gathered through scientific studies. While the lack of understanding of menstrual disorders needed to be addressed in the clinical arena, these classifications led to the pathologizing of what many women have been experiencing for hundreds of years. Recognized in the 1992 edition of the *International Classification of Diseases* manual developed by the World Health Organization, premenstrual syndrome (PMS) describes the cyclical recurrence of symptoms that impair a woman's health, relationships, and occupational functioning. Premenstrual dysphoric disorder (PMDD) is a diagnostic label that applies to a much smaller number of menstruating women experiencing severe PMS with predominantly negative affective symptoms.

The advantage of the current and emerging evidence about menstrual disorders is that it has led to better treatments and options for women. Nevertheless, there remains a lack of evidence to support many alternative and nonpharmacologic remedies, resulting in them often being discounted by the medical community. Groups of international health experts are now weighing in with consensus statements and guidelines that have provided a more integrative, woman-centered approach to treatment modalities by combining alternative treatments such as acupuncture with traditional treatments such as analgesics (Epperson et al., 2012; O'Brien et al., 2011).

In the mid-1980s, professional organizations in the United States and the United Kingdom met to define PMS, and the published proceedings established the medical basis for the presentation and clinical existence of PMS as a disease classification (Dawood, McGuire, & Demers, 1985; Halbreich, 1997). The research into PMS and PMDD has lagged behind the study of other brain disorders for more than 40 years. In an appendix to its *Diagnostic and Statistical Manual, Fourth Edition* (*DSM-IV*), the American Psychiatric Association (APA) noted that this area "required further study" (Epperson et al., 2012). Although its decision met with much controversy, the APA recognized the diagnostic term *premenstrual dysphoric disorder* in the third, fourth, and fifth editions of *Diagnostic and Statistical Manual* (APA, 1987, 1994, 2000, 2013). Previously referring to this condition as late luteal phase dysphoric disorder (LLPDD), the APA conducted an extensive literature review in 1994 and an LLPDD subcommittee concluded that very little research supported the existence of premenstrual mental illness (in contrast to PMS). Nevertheless, the term LLPDD was revised to PMDD and was included in the *DSM-IV-TR* in the research appendix and in the main text under the heading "Depressive Disorders" (APA, 2000).

In 2008, the first meeting of the International Society for Premenstrual Disorders (ISPMD) was held, with the membership of ISPMD including experts in women's health. Their goal was to reach a consensus on the diagnostic criteria to be used in research studies and guidelines for clinical trials (O'Brien et al., 2011). The APA appointed a Mood Disorders Work Group for *DSM-5* that included an international panel of experts in women's mental health to evaluate previous criteria and organize standard methods of diagnosing women with this disorder. Both of these groups recommended that PMS and PMDD have distinct diagnosis criteria in the WHO's *International Classification of Diseases* (ICD-11).

Since 2009, many studies have been conducted that have identified similar symptoms of cyclical dysphoria and provided evidence of PMS and PMDD. Once the diagnoses were "matured sufficiently," they were granted their own category in *DSM-5* as a mood disorder (APA, 2013). There is now a growing body of research regarding

---

> **BOX 23-5** **Discussion Question**
>
> Has the diagnosis of PMS and PMDD pathologized the normal premenstrual physical, emotional, and behavioral changes that possibly the majority of women experience? Or does the diagnosis give it a "voice"?

---

menstrual-cycle phases and related hormonal changes.

Inclusion of the PMS/PMDD diagnoses in *DSM-5* has validated what many women have known for years: Fluctuating hormonal changes have physiologic and behavioral impacts. Differentiating between PMS and PMDD is challenging for many women because the criteria are rather subjective. PMS includes psychological factors that vary in severity and affect women and their ability to cope differently. While now recognized by the scientific community, PMS and PMDD may still be taboo subjects or derisively regarded (**Box 23-5**).

Incidence

As many as 80% of all women report one or more physical, psychological, or behavioral symptoms during the luteal phase of their cycles, although these women may not report a severe disruption of their lifestyle (Biggs & DeMuth, 2011). PMS has mild to moderate symptoms (**Table 23-1**) and occurs in 20% to 32% of women (Biggs & DeMuth, 2011). Early studies of PMDD prevalence used different definitions to diagnose and assess the severity of symptoms, with reported rates of this condition ranging widely—from 1% (Gehlert & Hartlage, 1997) to 45% (Hurt et al., 1992). Using the *DSM-5* workgroup on PMDD's recommendation for standardized rating tools to determine the prevalence of this disorder, it is estimated that PMDD affects 3% to 8% of women (Biggs & DeMuth, 2011).

Women who have severe symptoms of PMS or PMDD suffer significant emotional and behavioral changes that can be debilitating. Epidemiological and clinical research have consistently demonstrated that many women experience various

TABLE 23-1	Symptoms of Premenstrual Syndrome and Premenstrual Dysphoric Disorder	

Symptoms	PMS	PMDD
Physical symptoms	Abdominal bloating and pain Mild weight gain from water retention Constipation followed by diarrhea at the onset of the menses Headache Pelvic pain and cramping Fatigue Extremity edema Nausea/food cravings	Physical: same as PMS but may be more severe Symptoms can begin immediately after ovulation Abdominal bloating and pain Headache Pelvic pain and cramping Fatigue Extremity edema Nausea/food cravings
Psychologic symptoms	Depression Anxiety Anger/irritability Insomnia Changes in libido Confusion, decrease in mental sharpness Social withdrawal Feelings of low self-esteem/poor self-image	Marked affective lability Marked irritability or anger or increased interpersonal conflicts Markedly depressed mood, feelings of hopelessness, or self-deprecating thoughts Marked anxiety, tension, feelings of being "keyed up" or "on edge" Decreased interest in usual activities Subjective sense of difficulty concentrating Lethargy Insomnia or hypersomnia A subjective sense of being overwhelmed or out of control
Diagnostic criteria	Symptoms begin up to 7 days prior to menses Remission of symptoms occurs from cycle days 4–13 Symptoms are significant enough to impair activities of daily living Symptoms are charted in at least 2 cycles Symptoms are not due to another disorder	Symptoms are associated with clinically significant distress or interference with work, school, social activities, or relationships with others The disturbance is not an exacerbation of the symptoms of another disorder (e.g., major depressive disorder) Criteria should be confirmed by prospective daily ratings during at least 2 symptomatic cycles (the diagnosis may be made provisionally prior to this confirmation) Symptoms are not due to the direct physiological effects of a substance (e.g., drug abuse, medications other than treatment) or a general medical condition

Abbreviations: PMDD, premenstrual dysphoric disorder; PMS, premenstrual syndrome.

symtoms in the beginning of the luteal phase of the menstrual cycle. This pattern ends with the onset of menses, usually by day 2 or 3 (Biggs & DeMuth, 2011). The key characteristic of PMS is the timing of symptoms: They should follow a predictable, identifiable pattern that is associated with the menstrual cycle.

Differentiating PMS and PMDD

PMS can be defined as a cluster of mild to moderate physical and psychological symptoms that occur during the late luteal phase of menses and resolve with menstruation (Baller et al., 2013; Biggs & DeMuth, 2011). PMDD encompasses cognitive, behavioral, emotional, and negative symptomatic changes that severely impair daily functioning, relationships, parenting, and ability to work in the late luteal menstrual phase (Baller et al., 2013; Biggs & DeMuth, 2011; Kelderhouse & Taylor, 2013). An accurate diagnosis of PMS or PMDD is the most important step in treatment. The severity of the symptoms is what differentiates PMS from PMDD (see **Table 23-1**).

Etiology

The etiology of PMS and PMDD is not well delineated, although theories abound. Many researchers and clinicians suspect that development of PMS probably involves a variety of factors that create synergies among themselves. Diet, hormones, and behavioral factors probably all play strong roles in its development. Some evidence suggests that psychosocial factors such as early exposure to physical, emotional, and sexual abuse probably contribute to the development of PMS (Bertone-Johnson et al., 2014; Biggs & DeMuth, 2011).

Physiologic Factors

Although the etiology is not completely understood, women with PMS or PMDD appear to be more physiologically sensitive to normal cycling of estrogen and progesterone (Biggs & DeMuth, 2011). Increases in aldosterone and plasma renin activity are the hypothetical mechanisms for fluid retention, weight gain, and bloating. Neurotransmitters, particularly serotonin and gamma-amino-butyric acid, also may be involved (Biggs & DeMuth, 2011). Studies of PMDD have identified serotonin as a potential causative factor (Shulman, 2010), and this theory has found further confirmation in that serotonin reuptake inhibitors (SSRIs) can be beneficial in treating PMDD (Marjoribanks, Brown, O'Brien, & Wyatt, 2013).

There may also be a genetic predisposition to PMS or PMDD, although the exact etiology of this predisposition is not known (Magnay & Ismail, 2007). Other biological theories include dysregulation of the serotonergic system. The brain disturbance that triggers PMS or PMDD may not be due to the hormonal levels but rather due to the shift, or fluctuations, in the hormonal level. Potentially, changes in the levels of gonadal steroids that are released by the pituitary gland might trigger changes in some women's moods, or otherwise predispose them to mood instability.

Based on this limited understanding of PMDD, treatments that minimize hormonal fluctuations, such as those that suppress ovulation, have been explored (American College of Obstetricians and Gynecologists, 2010b, reaffirmed 2014). Readjusting the neurotransmitter dysregulation with antidepressant or anxiolytic medications has also been effective in treating PMDD (Kelderhouse &Taylor, 2013).

Psychosocial Stressors and Sociocultural Factors

A number of studies have suggested that the manifestations of PMS, particularly premenstrual mood discomforts, may result from a combination of multiple stressors, a heightened stress response, lack of support, and a vulnerable period of biologic reactivity. A higher prevalence of depression, anxiety, and somatic complaints is noted in women with chronic pelvic pain. Many labels have been given to this set of stressors, including "brain-gut" neuroendocrine and decreased serotonin production syndromes (Latthe et al., 2006; Mykletun et al., 2010). Stress perception and stressful experiences appear to influence the reporting of premenstrual symptoms, and biopsychosocial factors (e.g., altered stress hormones, low self-esteem, negative life changes, increased sensitivity to stress) may increase the severity of PMS. Premenstrual syndrome has also been shown to be associated with psychological conditions such as overall reduced psychological well-being and mood disorders including anxiety and depression. Women with more than one condition are at greater risk of not only physical stress, but also psychological stress (Forrest-Knauss, Stuz, Weiss, & Tschudin, 2011).

Bertone-Johnson et al. (2014) assessed the relationship between early-life abuse and the incidence of moderate to severe PMS in later life by using data from the Nurses' Health Study 2 (NHS2). All women who self-reported PMS prior to 1991 were excluded from the study. Women who had a new PMS diagnosis (n = 4,108) sometime between 1991 and 2005 were then compared with a group of women (n = 3,248) randomly selected from the same study who had no PMS diagnosis during the same time frame. The researchers found that a history of sexual abuse, particularly in childhood, was more common among women seeking treatment for severe PMS (Bertone-Johnson et al., 2014. These findings provide strong support for the belief that early-life abuse is strongly related to development of PMS.

Numerous studies in other countries suggest that premenstrual discomfort and mood changes are experienced by women across different cultures (Nooh, Abdul-Hady, & El-Attar, 2015; Takeda, Imoto, Nagasawa, Muroya, & Shiina, 2015). However sociocultural factors such as geographic location, marital status, education, and occupation appear to influence the prevalence, which symptoms women experience, and which symptoms women consider to be problematic (Vigod, Frey, Soares, & Steiner, 2010).

It is unlikely that any single theory can adequately explain the complex and myriad premenstrual symptoms that many women experience. Although PMS and PMDD have been predominantly regarded as biologically based illnesses, the evidence published to date suggests that variables such as life stress, individual response to stress, history of sexual abuse, and cultural socialization are important determinants of premenstrual symptoms. The prevailing medical view, however, is that women with PMS may be more sensitive to what are essentially normal hormonal shifts, and as a result develop symptoms that do not affect other menstruating women.

Translating Research into Practice

Cyclic premenstrual pain and discomfort represent a cluster of symptoms that require the clinician and the woman to balance several seemingly dichotomous views: normative versus pathologic, one-dimensional versus multidimensional, acute versus chronic, and protocol versus individualized care. The goal for providing care related to the menstrual cycle and premenstrual experience is to explore what is normal and acceptable for each woman. Listening to women and helping them understand PMS and PMDD in the context of their life transitions, personal characteristics, and environmental stressors provides the support they need to make informed decisions for treatment.

Assumptions that underpin the assessment and therapeutic strategies for women experiencing premenstrual pain and discomforts include the following:

- Personal and social circumstances (e.g., a supportive partner) have health effects that are as important as—if not more important than—the biologic changes of the menstrual cycle.
- Biologic changes should not be ignored, but rather viewed in the context of biobehavioral relationships (e.g., shifting levels of hormones).
- Many factors (e.g., financial resources) may both promote or prevent women from being proactive in their own healthcare decisions.

Clinicians can have a significant influence on the health and well-being of women with cyclic premenstrual pain, mood and behavioral changes, the moderate symptoms known as PMS, and the more severe PMDD. Care of women with these issues must be individualized and woman centered, while also utilizing an evidence-based approach to assessing, diagnosing, and managing cyclic premenstrual pain and discomfort (Collins Sharp, Taylor, Kelly-Thomas, Killeen, & Dawood, 2002; Tschudin, Bertea, & Zemp, 2010). While these conditions are separate diagnoses, assessment approaches and therapeutic options can be similar for PMS and PMDD.

Assessment

The conventional medical approach to assessment and diagnosis focuses on ruling out pathology. Data for assessment and diagnosis are collected during the medical history, physical examination, laboratory assessments, and differential diagnoses. The evolution of diagnostic criteria for PMS and PMDD, however, has been confusing and controversial. The 10th revision of the *International Classification of Diseases* (ICD-10) places PMS under diseases of the genitourinary system, "Pain and other conditions associated with female genital organs and menstrual cycle," and labels it as "premenstrual tension syndrome (N94.3)" (Lustyk & Gerrish, 2010). PMDD is identified by the ICD-10 in the category "Other {affective} disorders (F38)." The ICD does not require a minimum number or description of symptoms or functional impairment for a diagnosis of PMS or PMDD.

The challenge for women's health clinicians is to integrate the strengths of a feminist approach to clinical practice with biomedical knowledge and skills. A feminist model of intervention focuses on women-centered care, advocacy, health promotion, and self-care. PMS and PMDD are individualized experiences requiring a dynamic and personalized assessment and diagnosis, which includes self-monitoring of symptoms, rating of symptom severity, and identification of symptom clusters and patterns specific to the particular woman. Screening should assess for pelvic pain at or around the time of menstruation, other related discomforts, and the effectiveness of currently used therapies.

Much of the information currently used in PMS/PMDD assessment is based on older research. The Association of Women's Health, Obstetric and Neonatal Nurses (AWHONN, 2003) suggests completing a focused assessment that includes screening questions, a health history, and a focused physical examination. Many PMS and PMDD questionnaires are available online—some of them well researched, while many others are actually advertisements for various products. Consequently, many women will come into the clinic setting with lists of already "diagnosed" conditions that they have found while searching the Internet.

The Patient Health Questionnaire 9 (PHQ-9) offers an opportunity for opening a dialog and creating a trusting environment to discuss the woman's symptoms of PMS or PMDD from a psychological perspective. The PHQ-9 can provide a baseline of symptoms and can be used for follow-up testing and assessment of treatment progress. Any woman with depressive symptoms should be screened for suicidal thoughts or ideations.

Symptom Assessment and Monitoring

The goal for assessment is to understand each woman's premenstrual experience and to help her define and manage her distressing symptoms and their concomitant problems. Prospective assessment of individual symptoms or symptom clusters—the recommended method—can be accomplished by the use of a calendar or symptom checklist kept for one or two consecutive cycles (Biggs & DeMuth, 2011).

A woman-centered approach relies on the woman as the expert knower of what her symptoms and condition mean to her as an individual. Her description of her symptoms, their severity, and their effect on her life assists in the diagnosis and management of those symptoms. Using an integrated approach to assess, diagnose, and treat premenstrual symptoms encourages the use of both pharmacologic and nonpharmacologic treatment modalities. In addition, an integrated approach encourages women to participate in the decision-making process and to take responsibility for those aspects of the treatment regimen within their control, such as nutrition and exercise.

A better understanding by both the clinician and the woman of the type, timing, and effects of individual symptoms can be obtained by record keeping. American College of Obstetricians and Gynecologists and other professional organizations that focus on women's health care suggest using a calendar of symptoms or a checklist for this purpose. Women can do this record keeping themselves, which allows them to describe their unique symptoms and to consider and reflect on the severity of the symptoms. The American College of Obstetricians and Gynecologists' symptom record is especially helpful (**Figure 23-1**), although many other tools can be used to log symptoms.

Prospective record keeping provides the practitioner and the woman seeking care with documentation to rule out other possible diagnoses and to observe the symptoms that occur cyclically. Women who complete such a record are able to understand their symptoms better, and identifying the patterns that develop validates their experiences. This record gives them a strong voice

FIGURE 23-1	PMS symptom record.

Keeping a Symptom Record

A symptom record can help your healthcare provider decide what treatment is best for you. Keeping a record is easy. Write your symptoms on a calendar, or use a chart like the one shown below. Keep a record for 2–3 months.

Instructions:

- Record up to five symptoms that are bothersome.
- At the end of each day, rate each symptom as mild (1), moderate (2), or severe (3).
- If you have no symptoms, leave the space for that day blank.
- For the row labeled "Menses," put an "M" in the box of each day you have menstrual bleeding.

The following are common PMS symptoms that you can use in your record:

Emotional Symptoms

Depression
Angry outbursts
Irritability
Crying spells
Anxiety
Confusion
Social withdrawal
Poor concentration
Insomnia
Increased nap taking
Changes in sexual desire

Physical Symptoms

Thirst and appetite changes (food cravings)
Breast tenderness
Bloating and weight gain
Headache
Swelling of the hands or feet
Aches and pains
Fatigue
Skin problems
Gastrointestinal symptoms
Abdominal pain

Example of a completed record:

MONTH <u>November</u>

Day of month	1	2	3	4	5	6	7	8	9	10	11	12	13	14	15	16	17	18	19	20	21	22	23	24	25	26	27	28	29	30	31
Menses																M	M	M	M	M											
Insomnia								1	1	2	2	3	3	3	1																
Irritability								2	2	2	3	3	3	3	3	2	1														
Depression								2	2	2	3	3	3	3	3																
Fatigue								1	1	1	2	2	3	3	3	2	1														
Breast tenderness								1	1	1	1	1	1	1	1	1															

Blank record:

MONTH _____

Day of month																															

when discussing the findings with their clinician and can guide treatment options. Continuing the record keeping during treatment is also key to understanding their individual responses to pharmacologic as well as nonpharmacologic remedies.

Symptom monitoring essentially consists of educating women in self-diagnosis. Getting in touch with their symptoms includes simply listing and rating feelings, symptoms, and behavioral changes, as well as focusing on social and physical environmental factors. Women can see their own patterns of symptoms and identify the relationship between these symptoms and the circumstances of their lives as well as the menstrual cycle. Not only will daily monitoring of these factors help women determine the severity and pattern of their symptoms, but it will also provide them with a basis for making healthy changes all month long.

Although prospective assessment is the recommended method of assessing symptom severity, distress, and pattern, retrospective assessment can be an initial first step in determining symptom distress. Retrospective symptom severity reports are likely to overestimate severity and do not provide data about symptom patterns, but they can assist with diagnosis and ruling out other chronic illnesses. Retrospective assessment can include the following questions:

- In your own words, describe the pain and discomforts that are the most severe and distressing to you.
- What is the pattern of pain and discomforts during a typical menstrual cycle? How many days before, during, or after your period do you notice symptoms? Do the symptoms occur around ovulation?
- Does anything in particular—such as work stress, dietary influences, or exercise—worsen or alleviate symptoms?

Determining Symptom Severity and Distress Patterns

It is important to clearly delineate symptoms, their patterns, and the ways that they may be related to the menstrual cycle, because PMS and premenstrual symptoms have no clearly defined cause. A number of investigators have found that many women who believed they had PMS were later found to

have another problem, such as endometriosis, that worsened around the time of menstruation. In other instances, a woman's mood or behavior changes—which may have been heightened during the premenstrual phase—were attributed to PMS when, in fact, they were a result of external problems such as work-related stress, relationship difficulties, problems with children, on-the-job harassment, violence, and other legitimate sources of anxiety, fear, and frustration. Alternatively, when examining a completed symptom record, women may discover that certain symptom clusters—pain and fatigue, for example—continue all month long but just worsen prior to menstruation. Recording symptoms helps a woman to gain a sense of self-awareness and become more attuned to how her perimenstrual experiences manifest themselves as symptoms, feelings, or behaviors, as well as the degree to which they affect her life.

The diagnostic criteria for PMS are as follows:

- Symptoms consistent with PMS (see **Table 23-1**)
  - Affective symptoms
    - ‣ Depression
    - ‣ Angry outbursts
    - ‣ Irritability
    - ‣ Anxiety
    - ‣ Confusion
    - ‣ Social withdrawal
  - Somatic symptoms
- Breast tenderness or swelling, abdominal bloating, headache, joint or muscle pain, weight gain, swelling of extremities
- Consistent occurrence of the symptoms only during the luteal phase of the menstrual cycle
- Negative impact of the symptoms on some facet of the woman's life
- Exclusion of other diagnoses that may better explain the symptoms (American College of Obstetricians and Gynecologists, 2014; Association of Reproductive Health Professionals, 2008)

If the woman reports at least one of these symptoms during the premenstrual phase and has had the same symptoms occur for at least three prior cycles, a diagnosis of PMS can be made (American College of Obstetricians and Gynecologists, 2014).

The diagnostic criteria for PMDD are as follows:

I. In the majority of cycles, five or more symptoms, including affective and physical symptoms, are present during the week before menses and are absent in the follicular phase.

II. One (or more) of the following symptoms is present: irritability, depressed mood, marked anxiety, tension, or affective lability.

III. One or more of the following symptoms must additionally be present (the combination of symptoms in I and II must total five): decreased interest in usual activities, difficulty concentrating, fatigue, appetite change (decreased or increased), changes in sleep patterns (hypersomnia or insomnia), sense of feeling overwhelmed, physical symptoms such as breast tenderness, joint or muscle pain, bloating, or weight gain.

IV. The symptoms markedly interfere with occupational or social functioning.

V. The symptoms are not due to an exacerbation of another disorder.

VI. The preceding criteria have been confirmed by prospective daily ratings over at least two menstrual cycles (American College of Obstetricians and Gynecologists, 2014; Association of Reproductive Health Professionals, 2008).

Laboratory Assessments
There are no specific tests for CPP, PMS, or PMDD, although some laboratory tests can be helpful in ruling out underlying problems. Simple blood tests can identify conditions such as anemia, thyroid disorders, diabetes, or hypoglycemia. Ovarian hormone testing is unnecessary unless premature menopause (before the age of 40 years) is suspected.

Differential Diagnoses

The patterns and severity of symptoms are the best guide for sorting out whether a woman has PMS or PMDD and whether there is an underlying etiology. Symptom-tracking charts and calendars along with menstrual and health history data will provide essential clues for making a diagnosis. PMS and PMDD need to be distinguished from endocrine, psychiatric, and other disorders. Furthermore, the transition to menopause may be a vulnerable period when women experience the onset or a worsening of CPP or PMS, especially mood disturbances and fatigue.

Many medical and psychiatric conditions may be exacerbated in the premenstrual or menstrual phase of the cycle, leading a woman to believe that she must be experiencing PMS. For example, hypothyroidism, anemia, endometriosis, and physiologic ovarian cysts can mimic the signs and symptoms of PMS (Biggs & DeMuth, 2011). Other psychiatric disorders, such as substance abuse and eating disorders such as bulimia, can be exacerbated during the luteal phase of the menstrual cycle. Many women with epilepsy experience changes in seizure frequency and severity with changes in reproductive cycles, including at puberty, over the menstrual cycle, with pregnancy, and at menopause.

Musculoskeletal pain syndromes, such as arthralgias, arthritis, and fibromyalgia, can cause symptoms that mimic those of PMS (e.g., generalized pain, fatigue, sleep disturbances, or cognitive impairment) and may be misdiagnosed or undiagnosed in women with moderate to severe PMS. Cyclic premenstrual pain that is severe and begins at midcycle or worsens premenstrually may indicate an underlying gynecologic condition such as pelvic inflammatory disease, endometriosis, or chronic pelvic pain. In addition, migraine-type headaches appear to increase during the premenstrual and menstrual phases. Menstrual migraines tend to occur 1 to 3 days before menstruation begins or during the first day or two of menstruation, when hormone levels drop significantly.

Women who are menstruating report that gastrointestinal (GI) symptoms, such as stomach pain, nausea, and loose stools, are highest during menses, and almost 50% of women with irritable bowel syndrome (IBS) report a premenstrual increase in their symptoms (Pinkerton, Guico-Pabia, & Taylor, 2010). Women with Crohn's disease report more premenstrual and menstrual GI symptoms, such as diarrhea, abdominal pain, and constipation, than women with other types of bowel disease. Women with functional bowel disease (FBD)—that is, bowel disease not yet classified as a GI disorder—report more stomach pain, nausea, and diarrhea at menses than women without FBD (Pinkerton et al., 2010).

Beginning the Therapeutic Process: Setting Goals

Sometimes the process of assessment is therapeutic in itself—raising self-awareness and validating women's symptom experience. Setting goals and outcome criteria formalizes the plan of care and encourages the woman's participation in her self-care. Goals should include both health-related outcomes and other outcomes, such as functional status and economic impact. In terms of functional status, the detrimental effects of inadequately treated PMS and PMDD range from missed life opportunities, such as work, school, or other activities, to economic costs, including missed work opportunities and urgent healthcare visits (Dawood & Yusof, 2006).

Women, in collaboration with their clinicians, can facilitate the therapeutic process, which is dependent on the following elements:

- Desired outcome
- Characteristics of the diagnosis
- Evidence-based efficacy of the intervention
- Feasibility of successfully implementing the intervention
- Acceptability and motivation of the woman
- Education and experience of the clinician (Bulechek & McCloskey, 1999)

Therapeutic Options

For many years, the focus on singular (usually pharmacologic) therapy has dominated treatments for premenstrual symptoms including PMS (Baller et al., 2013; Freeman, Sammel, Hui, Rickles, & Sondheimer, 2011). However, clinical research suggests that combination therapy may be more beneficial than single therapies (Burbeck & Willig, 2014). Moreover, outcomes from symptom-management programs suggest that when symptoms are comprehensively managed, women are more likely to remain in treatment and demonstrate improved outcomes. Models of symptom management that combine self-care, social support, medical therapies, and psychosocial strategies applied to specific conditions have shown promising results. In a clinical trial of multimodal symptom-management strategies for women experiencing severe PMS, Taylor (1999) found that women prefer to select multiple strategies for symptom management, that

premenstrual symptom severity declined markedly within the first few months with this approach, and that this effect could be maintained over the long term.

Health-Promoting Strategies

Strategies that are generally health promoting, such as eating a balanced diet, getting sufficient exercise, and reducing stress may also result in premenstrual symptom relief. Ideally, establishing healthy dietary and exercise habits and managing personal and environmental stress during early adulthood will lead to lifelong healthy behaviors that result in chronic disease prevention in later adult life. However, women at any age can make lifestyle changes that may be beneficial for symptom management. Symptom-management interventions can also be considered as complementary to pharmacologic therapy in women with a dual diagnosis or a depressive disorder that regularly worsens during a specific menstrual-cycle phase.

No particular diet has been shown to consistently offer women relief from PMS. Often, clinicians or self-help books recommend decreasing refined sugar, salt, or caffeine intake despite little evidence to support these recommendations (Rapkin & Lewis, 2013; Sadler et al., 2010). Anecdotally, women may report an improvement with certain dietary changes, in which case they should be encouraged to continue those modifications. Rather than focusing on specific restrictive dietary changes, recommending a balanced diet with evidence to support overall health would be of greater benefit.

Many clinicians and professional organizations recommend regular aerobic exercise as a way to relieve PMS/PMDD symptoms. Preliminary evidence supports these recommendations, although there are not enough to studies to say that this treatment is truly "evidence-based" (Biggs & DeMuth, 2011; Witt et al., 2013). The lack of a strong evidence base should not preclude clinicians from encouraging women with PMS/PMDD to exercise regularly because of the overall health benefits.

Cognitive-behavioral therapy (CBT) is a type of psychotherapy that is typically short term in duration and focused on identifying and modifying dysfunctional thoughts and behaviors. While some evidence indicates that CBT may be beneficial in reducing PMS/PMDD symptoms, it has been gleaned from studies that show CBT is effective in reducing other affective disorders such as anxiety and pain. Thus its suggested effectiveness for treating either PMS or PMDD is theoretical (Biggs & DeMuth, 2011).

Nonpharmacologic Therapies

Acupuncture Studies of acupuncture as an intervention for alleviating PMS symptoms vary in the type of treatment administered (some including moxibustion) as well as the number of sessions and the treatment period within the menstrual cycle (Jang, Kim, & Choi, 2014). Symptom improvement has been reported to be greater in the area of physical symptoms (e.g., headache, cramps, breast pain, hot flashes) than in psychological symptoms (Jang et al., 2014). The variation in methods used in the studies of acupuncture creates challenges in recommending the most effective method for treating PMS/PMDD symptoms, although this intervention does appear to have the potential to effect symptom reduction.

Dietary Supplements Research suggests that supplemental calcium may be beneficial in the treatment of PMS (American College of Obstetricians and Gynecologists, 2010b, 2014; Bertone-Johnson, Hankinson, Johnson, & Manson, 2007; Canning, Waterman, & Dye, 2006). Canning et al.'s (2006) systematic review of dietary and herbal treatments used by women with PMS revealed that use of calcium and continuous vitamin B_6 may be helpful in treating the symptoms of PMS. Specifically, vitamin B_6 doses in the range of 50 to 150 mg/day may be beneficial, whereas intermittent usage does not appear to improve symptoms (Wyatt, Dimmock, & O'Brien, 1999).

Preliminary data indicate that curcumin (found in turmeric) dietary supplements may be beneficial in treatment of PMS (Khayat et al., 2015). In a double-blind RCT, women with PMS who took curcumin 100 mg twice daily for 7 days before until 3 days after their menstrual cycle reported a significant improvement in both physical and mood symptoms (Khayat et al., 2015).

Herbs, Botanicals, and Traditional Therapies Several herbs may have beneficial effects on both PMS and menstrual cramps, including Vitex (chaste tree berry), cramp bark, and evening primrose oil.

These herbs are available without a prescription at pharmacies and health food stores, but not all of them have clinical or research evidence to document their safety or efficacy. Herbs that have been recommended by the German Commission E (which was established more than 20 years ago and has reviewed all the available literature on more than 300 herbs) or by the late Varro Tyler, a professor of pharmacognosy at Purdue University and author of Tyler's Honest Herbal (Foster & Tyler, 2000), are included here. Additional information can be obtained from the following resources:

- *The American Pharmaceutical Association Practical Guide to Natural Medicines* (Pierce, 1999)
- The American Botanical Council's *The ABC Guide to Herbal Medicine* (http://abc.herbalgram.org/site/PageServer?pagename=The_Guide)
- The National Center for Complementary and Alternative Medicine (http://nccam.nih.gov)

Native to the Mediterranean and central Asia, the chaste tree (also called Vitex) is a shrub that produces dark brown to black fruit the size of a peppercorn. Preparations of the fruit as an extract or in powdered form have been approved by German health authorities for the treatment of menstrual irregularities, such as PMS and breast pain associated with a woman's menstrual period. This herb appears to have a dopamine-like activity and effect on the pituitary gland, helping to reinstate the normal balance between estrogen and progesterone during the luteal phase of the menstrual cycle. Clinical trials suggest that chaste tree berry reduces breast pain and other somatic and emotional symptoms associated with the menstrual cycle by 50% or more (Jang et al., 2014). Preliminary research suggests that for some women chaste tree berry extracts may be as beneficial as pharmacologic (fluoxetine) therapy with fewer sexual side effects (Atmaca, Kumru, & Tezcan, 2003; Kloss, Marcom, Odom, Tuggle, & Weatherspoon, 2012), although additional research is needed to confirm this finding. Reports of side effects during these studies were rare and included acne, skin rash, and intermenstrual bleeding. Although chaste tree berry extracts do not contain hormones, they should not be used with combined contraceptives or other hormone therapies. It is important to obtain a complete history of all medications used and understand interactions of this herb to ensure optimal care.

In traditional Chinese medicine (TCM), both herbs and acupuncture are used separately or in combination to treat health conditions that result from disruptions to the flow of the body's vital energy (qi or chi), which represent an imbalance between the eternal opposites of yin and yang. An important requirement of TCM is that the treatment is tailored to the patterns or signs and symptoms the woman experiences (Woo & McEneaney, 2010). Most TCM practitioners use a combination of acupuncture and herbs in the treatment of severe PMS. There is little evidence of the efficacy of TCM in alleviating PMS symptoms (Jing, Yang, Ismail, Chen, & Wu, 2009; Woo & McEneaney, 2010).

The seed oil of the evening primrose, a weed that is native to North America, contains high concentrations of the essential fatty acid gamma-linolenic acid, which is a precursor to prostaglandin. Two well-controlled studies failed to show any beneficial effects from evening primrose oil in PMS/PMDD symptom relief, although because the trials were relatively small, modest effects cannot be excluded. Current research does not show any benefit from evening primrose oil in the treatment of PMS or PMDD (Biggs & DeMuth, 2011; National Center for Complementary and Integrative Health, 2013).

SAM-e *S*-Adenosylmethionine, or SAM-e, is neither a drug nor an herb. Rather, SAM-e is a molecule manufactured in the body from the amino acid methionine during metabolism (Deligiannidis & Freeman, 2010, 2014). A double-blind, placebo-controlled trial found no difference between the antidepressive efficacy of 1,600 mg of SAM-e and 400 mg of imipramine, except that SAM-e was more easily tolerated (Delle Chiaie, Pancheri, & Scapicchio, 2002). SAM-e, in doses of 200 to 1,600 mg, can be effective in treating symptoms associated with PMS and PMDD (Deligiannidis & Freeman, 2010, 2014). Nevertheless, it has been reported to cause mild and transient insomnia, nervousness, lack of appetite, constipation, headaches, heart palpitations, nausea, dry mouth, sweating, and dizziness. Because SAM-e is converted into homocysteine (a protein associated with heart disease) in the body, it is unclear whether rising levels of homocysteine secondary to SAM-e metabolism will increase the risk of heart disease.

SAM-e must be taken with a daily multivitamin, along with a diet high in fruits and vegetables. Three of the B vitamins (folic acid [B_3], B_6, and B_{12}) can lower the homocysteine levels that SAM-e elevates (Bottiglieri, 2002). Because raw SAM-e degrades quickly unless stored at proper temperatures, there is no guarantee that the pills available for sale will include the recommended dosage. SAM-e is also very expensive, with daily doses ranging in price from $2.50 to $18.00.

SAM-e may potentiate or augment the effect of SSRIs, and may be used as adjuvant therapy with those medications (Papakostas, Mischoulon, Shyu, Alpert, & Fava, 2010).

Homeopathy Homeopathy is a holistic treatment system based on the principle that taking the right dose of a natural substance that might disturb the body if administered in the wrong amount can actually trigger healing. Studies of homeopathy in treating PMS/PMDD to date have been small and are of only fair quality; recent studies are not available in the literature. In a meta-analysis of 105 clinical trials of homeopathic treatments, researchers found that 75% of interpretable trials showed some improvement of symptoms with homeopathy (Chapman, Angelica, Spitalny, & Strauss, 1994). In a randomized, controlled, double-blind clinical trial in Israel, 90% of the women participating in the study experienced an improvement of more than 30% in their premenstrual symptoms after an oral dose of a homeopathic medication (Yakir et al., 2001). Although homeopathic remedies have no side effects and are available without a prescription, it is wise to consult a professional homeopath who can help choose the most appropriate treatments.

Pharmacologic Therapies

Selective Serotonin Reuptake Inhibitors Selective serotonin reuptake inhibitors are a highly effective treatment for the symptoms of PMS and PMDD. While only three SSRIs— fluoxetine, sertraline, and paroxetine—have FDA indications for use with PMS/PMDD, essentially all SSRIs have been shown in randomized controlled trials to be efficacious in reducing PMS/PMDD symptoms (Rapkin & Lewis, 2013). Across 31 randomized controlled trials, SSRIs reduced the symptoms of PMDD significantly compared with placebo, with 60% to 75% of women reporting such symptom improvement

(Marjoribanks et al., 2013). This symptom improvement included not only psychological symptoms but also physical and functional symptoms.

Premenstrual cyclic disorders can be treated with either continuous SSRIs or intermittent therapy (i.e., taking the SSRI only during the second half of the menstrual cycle). A newer method of treatment may be to take the SSRI at the onset of symptoms or 2 to 3 days prior to the expected onset of symptoms and then discontinue it when menstruation begins (Rapkin & Lewis, 2013). This type of dosing may decrease medication-related side effects and minimize exposure to pharmacotherapy. Paroxetine is the only medication that should not be taken cyclically, because it produces the most pronounced discontinuation effects.

SSRIs should be taken for at least two menstrual cycles to adequately assess their benefit or lack of benefit. Approximately 15% of women do not experience relief with these drugs after two cycles, in which case an alternative treatment should be recommended.

While improvement of symptoms has been seen with use of low doses, some women experience greater improvement with moderate doses (20 mg versus 10 mg of escitalopram), particularly if intermittent or symptom-onset dosing is used (Rapkin & Lewis, 2013). As when treating other conditions, the recommendation is to initially prescribe lower doses of SSRIs and increase them after 1 to 2 months if indicated.

Side effects associated with SSRIs may include headaches, sleep disturbances, dizziness, weight gain, dry mouth, and decreased libido. Some women have sexual side effects with SSRIs, the most common of which is difficulty achieving orgasm. If this occurs, using a lower dose, intermittent therapy, or a trial of an alternative agent in the same drug class is recommended. Less frequently reported side effects include decreased appetite, weight loss, drowsiness, impaired concentration, altered taste, nausea, diarrhea, and nervousness. If these problems occur, they can usually be lessened by prescribing lower dosages of the medication.

Anxiolytic Drugs The most commonly prescribed antianxiety medication for noncyclic anxiety or panic disorders is alprazolam (Xanax). Other agents in this class include diazepam (Valium), lorazepam (Ativan), buspirone (BuSpar), and clonazepam (Klonipin). Research on the use of antianxiety medications to relieve PMS symptoms has shown mixed results. In the only two randomized, crossover, placebo-controlled clinical trials of alprazolam for use during the premenstrual phase, women taking this drug experienced less anxiety, depression, and headaches (Freeman, Rickels, Sondheimer, & Polansky, 1995). However, alprazolam has also been shown to stimulate increased appetite premenstrually, which could make it difficult to control food cravings or binges. Furthermore, alprazolam has the potential to produce addiction, tolerance, and bothersome sedation; for this reason, it is not recommended as a first-line treatment.

Anxiolytic medications are intended for short-term use only, and continued use should not exceed 8 weeks without medical or psychiatric evaluation, because physical and psychological dependencies can occur quickly with these drugs. Indeed, relying on pills may impede the development of nonpharmacologic stress-management strategies. Side effects of anxiolytic agents may include visual problems, mood swings, and joint stiffness. Other, less frequently reported side effects include drowsiness, headaches, dizziness, blurred vision, dry mouth, weakness, confusion, nausea, constipation, agitation, and depression. Oral contraceptives can increase the potency of antianxiety drugs, which in turn may increase the risk of side effects. By contrast, alcohol, if consumed while taking an antianxiety drug, increases depression of the central nervous system.

Oral Contraceptive Pills Combined oral contraceptives (COCs) contain both estrogen and progesterone. They have been widely used to treat symptoms of PMS/PMDD, although they are more apt to relieve physical symptoms, such as pain, than psychological symptoms, such as mood or anxiety disruptions. A number of investigators have found that temporarily suppressing ovulation can reduce dysmenorrhea pain as well as cyclic premenstrual physical and mood discomforts in some women (Björn et al., 2002; Björn, Bixo, Nöjd, Nyberg, & Bäckström, 2000; Freeman et al., 2001; Sanders, Graham, Bass, & Bancroft, 2001). Level III evidence indicates that COCs can reduce premenstrual negative mood symptom severity and variability (Oinonen & Mazmanian, 2002).

While the benefit from oral contraceptives is mainly in the form of relief of physical symptoms, a meta-analysis of randomized controlled trials of COCs containing drospirenone as the progestational agent indicates that these therapies may provide additional benefit for PMS/PMDD psychosocial symptoms such as loss of productivity (Lopez, Kaptein, & Helmerhorst, 2012). Symptoms may be improved by taking COCs continuously rather than the traditional 21/7 method. To do this, the woman takes all of the active pills in a pack and then opens a new pack; the placebo pills are discarded. Similarly, COCs that contain 24 active pills and 4 placebos may be more efficacious than the 21/7 versions (Rapkin & Lewis, 2013).

Progesterone deficiency has not been shown to be a causal mechanism for PMS, and results of research using progesterone-only formulations as a treatment for PMS are inconsistent. A systematic review of 14 trials with progestogens administered orally, vaginally, or rectally did not support the use of progestogen therapy for this indication (Wyatt, Dimmock, Jones, Obhrai, & O'Brien, 2001).

Other methods of ovarian suppression have also been studied to determine their utility in treating PMDD. High doses of estrogen (100–200 mg per day through transdermal patches) demonstrated improvement in symptoms—but due to the risk of unopposed estrogen, progesterone must be added to the regimen, which then can cause PMS-like symptoms (Rapkin & Lewis, 2013). Danazol is an androgen agonist/antagonist that inhibits ovulation, albeit one that is associated with high rates of side effects (acne, weight gain, and hirsutism). Only limited and inconsistent evidence supports the utility of hormonal ovulation suppression with gonadotropin-releasing hormone (GnRH) agonists in treating PMS and related disorders. Although some women have benefited from these therapies, these pharmacologic agents are associated with significant side effects as well as potential for increased risk. Surgical oophorectomy is an irreversible therapeutic option that should be considered only as a last resort.

Diuretics Diuretics have been widely prescribed for severe premenstrual bloating and fluid retention. However, no evidence exists to show that thiazide diuretics are of benefit in this indication, and they can actually make symptoms worse via potassium depletion, which results in stimulation of the autonomic nervous system. An aldosterone antagonist with antiandrogenic properties, spironolactone, is the only diuretic that has demonstrated evidence in reducing severe premenstrual bloating and headaches (American College of Obstetricians and Gynecologists, 2010b).

CONCLUSION

Menstrual-cycle disorders, including dysmenorrhea, PMS, and PMDD, are better understood now than they were in the past. **Table 23-2** summarizes the effectiveness of the various therapeutic options for these disorders. Further study, particularly

---

| TABLE 23-2 | Effectiveness of Various Therapies for Menstrual-Cycle Pain, Premenstrual Syndrome, and Premenstrual Dysphoric Disorder |

General Category	Specific Intervention	Dysmenorrhea	PMS	PMDD
Lifestyle modification	Aerobic exercise	Effective	Effective	May be effective
	Yoga	May be effective	May be effective	No studies
	Decreased caffeine, sugar, or alcohol intake		May be effective	No studies

(continues)

TABLE 23-2 Effectiveness of Various Therapies for Menstrual-Cycle Pain, Premenstrual Syndrome, and Premenstrual Dysphoric Disorder (*continued*)

General Category	Specific Intervention	Dysmenorrhea	PMS	PMDD
Dietary supplements	Calcium		May be effective	No studies
	B-complex vitamins		May be effective	No studies
	Magnesium	May be effective		
	Fish oil	May be effective		
Herbal supplements	*Agnus castus* (chaste berry)		May be effective	May be effective
	Hypericum perforatum (St. John's wort)		May be effective	May be effective
Nonpharmaco-logic therapies	Cognitive-behavioral therapy		May be effective	May be effective
	Bright light therapy		May be effective	May be effective
	Heat	Effective		
	TENS	May be effective		
	Acupuncture/ massage	May be effective	May be effective	May be effective
Analgesics	Acetaminophen	May be effective		
	NSAIDs	Effective	May be effective	May be effective
Hormonal therapies	Combined estrogen/ progesterone oral contraceptives	Effective	May be effective if drospirenone is the progesterone	May be effective if drospire-none is the progesterone
	Progesterone-only therapies	Effective	Not effective	Not effective
Other phar-macologic therapies	SSRIs, either contin-uous or cyclical		Effective	Effective
	Anxiolytics (short-term use only)			May be effective if anxiety is primary symptom

Abbreviations: NSAIDs, nonsteroidal anti-inflammatory drugs; PMDD, premenstrual dysphoric disorder; PMS, premenstrual syndrome; SSRIs, selective serotonin reuptake inhibitors; TENS, transcutaneous electrical nerve stimulation.

related to lifestyle and nonpharmacologic options for their treatment, is needed. Women working collaboratively with their clinicians will ensure that their voice and opinions are heard and validated in this quest. Integration of pharmacologic and complementary therapies is essential to treat these conditions holistically and within the context of women's experiential knowledge.

References

American College of Obstetricians and Gynecologists. (2010a). *ACOG education pamphlet AP057: Premenstrual syndrome.* Washington, DC: Author. Retrieved from http://www.acog.org

American College of Obstetricians and Gynecologists. (2010b, reaffirmed 2014). *ACOG Practice Bulletin: Nonhormonal uses of hormonal contraceptives.* Washington, DC. Author.

American College of Obstetricians and Gynecologists. (2014). *Guidelines for women's health.* (4th ed.). Washington, DC. Author.

American Psychiatric Association (APA). (1987). *Diagnostic and statistical manual of mental disorders* (3rd ed., revision) (*DSM-III-R*). Washington, DC: Author.

American Psychiatric Association (APA). (1994). *Diagnostic and statistical manual of mental disorders* (4th ed., revision) (*DSM-IV-R*). Washington, DC: Author.

American Psychiatric Association (APA). (2000). *Diagnostic and statistical manual of mental disorders* (4th ed., text revision) (*DSM-IV-TR*). Washington, DC: Author.

American Psychiatric Association (APA). (2013). *Diagnostic and statistical manual of mental disorders* (5th ed.) (*DSM-5*). Arlington, VA: Author.

Association of Reproductive Health Professionals. (2008). Managing premenstrual symptoms. Retrieved from http://www.arhp.org/Publications-and-Resources/Quick-Reference-Guide-for-Clinicians/PMS

Association of Women's Health, Nurses and Neonatal Nursing (AWHONN). (2003). *Evidence-based clinical practice guideline: Nursing management for cyclic perimenstrual pain and discomfort.* Washington, DC: Author.

Atmaca, M., Kumru, S., & Tezcan, E. (2003). Fluoxetine versus *Vitex agnus castus* extract in the treatment of premenstrual dysphoric disorder. *Human Psychopharmacology, 18*(3), 191–195.

Baller, E. B., Wei, S. M., Kohn, P. D., Rubinow D. R., Alarcon, G., Schmidt, P. J., & Berman, K. F. (2013). Abnormalities of dorsolateral prefrontal function in women with premenstrual dysphoric disorder: A multimodal neuroimaging study. *American Journal of Psychiatry, 170,* 305–314.

Bertone-Johnson, E., Hankinson, S., Johnson, S., & Manson, J. (2007). Assessing premenstrual syndrome in large prospective studies. *Journal of Reproductive Medicinc, 52*(9), 779–786.

Bertone-Johnson, E., Whitcomb B. W., Missmer, S. A., Manson, J. E., Hankinson, S. E., & Rich-Edwards J. W. (2014). Early life emotional, physical, and sexual abuse and the development of premenstrual syndrome: A longitudinal study. *Journal of Women's Health, 23*(9), 729–739.

Biggs, W. S., & DeMuth, R. H. (2011). Premenstrual syndrome and premenstrual dysphoric disorder. *American Family Physician, 84*(8), 918–924.

Björn, I., Bixo, M., Nöjd, K., Collberg, P., Nyberg, S., Sundstrom-Poromaa, I., & Bäckström, T. (2002). The impact of different doses of medroxyprogesterone acetate on mood symptoms in sequential hormonal therapy. *Gynecology and Endocrinology, 16*(1), 1–8.

Björn, I., Bixo, M., Nöjd, K., Nyberg, S., & Bäckström, T. (2000). Negative mood changes during hormone replacement therapy: A comparison between two progestogens. *American Journal of Obstetrics & Gynecology, 183*(6), 1419–1426.

Bottiglieri, T. (2002). S-Adenosyl-L-methionine (SAMe): From the bench to the bedside: Molecular basis of a pleiotrophic molecule. *American Journal of Clinical Nutrition, 76*(5), 1151S–1157S.

Braverman, P. K. (2007). Premenstrual syndrome and premenstrual dysphoric disorder. *Journal of Pediatric & Adolescent Gynecology, 20*(1), 3–12. doi:10.1016/j.jpag.2006.10.007

Bulechek, G. M., & McCloskey, J. C. (1999). *Nursing interventions: Effective nursing treatments* (3rd ed.). Philadelphia, PA: Saunders.

Burbeck, R., & Willig, C. (2014). The personal experience of dysmenorrhea: An interpretive phenomenological analysis. *Journal of Health Psychology, 19*(10), 1334–1344.

Canning, S., Waterman, M., & Dye, L. (2006). Dietary supplements and herbal remedies for premenstrual syndrome (PMS): A systematic research review of the evidence for their efficacy. *Journal of Reproductive and Infant Psychology, 24*(4), 363–378.

Chao, M. T., Callens, M. L., Wade, C. M., Abercrombie, P. D., & Gomolak, D. (2014). An innovative acupuncture treatment for primary dysmenorrhea: A randomized crossover pilot study. *Alternative Therapies in Health & Medicine, 20*(1), 49–56.

Chapman, E., Angelica, J., Spitalny, G., & Strauss, M. (1994). Results of a study of the homeopathic treatment of PMS. *Journal of the American Institute of Homeopathy, 87,* 14–21.

Cho, S. H., & Hwang, E. W. (2010). Acupuncture for primary dysmenorrhea: A systematic review. *British Journal of Obstetrics & Gynaecology, 117,* 509–521.

Collins Sharp, B., Taylor, D., Kelly-Thomas, K., Killeen, M. B., & Dawood, M.Y. (2002). Cyclic perimenstrual pain and discomfort: The scientific basis for practice. *Journal of Obstetric, Gynecological, and Neonatal Nursing, 31,* 637–649.

Dawood, M. Y., McGuire, J. L., & Demers, L. M. (1985). *Premenstrual syndrome and dysmenorrhea.* Baltimore, MD/Munich, Germany: Urban & Schwarzenberg.

Dawood, M., & Yusof, M. D. (2006). Primary dysmenorrhea: Advances in pathogenesis and management. *Obstetrics & Gynecology, 108*(2), 428–441.

Dean, G., & Schwarz, E. B. (2011). Intrauterine contraceptives (IUCs). In R. A. Hatcher, J. Trussell, A. L. Nelson, W. Cates, D. Kowal, M. S. Policar (Eds.), *Contraceptive technology* (20th ed., pp. 147–191). New York, NY: Ardent Media.

Deligiannidis, K. M., & Freeman, M. P. (2010). Complementary and alternative medicine for the treatment of depressive disorders in women. *Psychiatric Clinics of North America, 33*(2), 441–463.

Deligiannidis, K. M., & Freeman, M. P. (2014). Complementary and alternative medicine therapies for perinatal depression. *Clinical Obstetrics & Gynecology, 28*(1), 85–95.

Delle Chiaie, R., Pancheri, P., & Scapicchio, P. (2002). Efficacy and tolerability of oral and intramuscular -S-adenosyl-L-methionine

1,4-butanedisulfonate (SAMe) in the treatment of major depression: Comparison with imipramine in 2 multicenter studies. *American Journal of Clinical Nutrition, 76*(5), 1172S–1176S.

Dennerstein, L., Lehert, P., & Heinemann, K. (2011). Global study of women's experiences of PMS symptoms and their effects on daily life. *Post Reproductive Health, 17*(3), 88–95.

Direkvand-Moghadam, A., & Khosravi, A. (2012). The impact of a novel herbal Shirazi Thymus Vulgaris on primary dysmenorrhea in comparison to the classical Ibuprofen. *Journal of Research in Medical Societies, 17*(7), 668–670.

Eittah, H. F. A. (2014). Effect of breakfast skipping on young females' menstruation. *Health Science Journal, 8*(4), 469–484.

Epperson, C. N. (2012). Premenstrual dysphoric disorder and the brain. *American Journal of Pediatrics.* doi:10.1176/appi.ajp.2012.12121555

Epperson, C. N., Steiner, M., Hartlage, S. A., Eriksson, R., Schmidt, P. J., Jones, I., & Yonkers, K. A. (2012). Premenstrual dysphoric disorder: Evidence for a new category for *DSM-5*. *American Journal of Psychiatry, 169*(5), 465–475.

Forrester-Knauss, C., Stutz, E. Z., Weiss, C., & Tschudin, S. (2011). The interrelation between premenstrual syndrome and major depression: Results from a population based sample. *BMC Public Health, 11,* 795–806.

Foster, S., & Tyler, V. (2000). *Tyler's honest herbal: A sensible guide to the use of herbs and related remedies.* Binghamton, NY: Haworth Press.

Freeman, E., Kroll, R., Rapkin, A., Pearlstein, T., Brown, C., Parsey, K., . . . Foegh, M. (2001). Evaluation of a unique oral contraceptive in the treatment of premenstrual dysphoric disorder. *Journal of Women's Health & Gender Based Medicine, 10*(6), 561–569.

Freeman, E., Rickels, K., Sondheimer, S., & Polansky, M. (1995). A double-blind trial of oral progesterone, alprazolam, and placebo in treatment of severe premenstrual syndrome. *Journal of the American Medical Association, 274*(1), 51–57.

Freeman, E. W., Sammel, M. D., Hui, L., Rickles, K., & Sondheimer, S. J. (2011). Clinical subtypes of premenstrual syndrome and responses to sertraline treatment. *Obstetrics & Gynecology, 118*(6), 1293–1300.

Fritz, M. A., & Speroff, L. (2011). *Endometriosis in clinical gynecologic endocrinology and infertility* (8th ed., pp. 1221–1248). Philadelphia, PA: Lippincott, Williams and Wilkins.

Gehlert, S., & Hartlage, S. (1997) A design for studying the *DSM-IV* research criteria of premenstrual dysphoric disorder. *Journal of Psychosomatic Obstetrics & Gynecology, 18*(1), 36–44.

Halbreich, U. (1997). Menstrually related disorders: Towards interdisciplinary international diagnostic criteria. *Cephalalgia, 17,* 1–4.

Hoffman, B. (2008). Pelvic pain. In B. L. Hoffman, J. O. Schorge, J. I. Schaffer, L. M. Halvorson, K. D. Bradshaw, F. G. Cunningham, & L. E. Calver (Eds.), *Williams gynecology* (pp. 244–268). New York, NY: McGraw-Hill.

Hurt, S. W., Schnurr, P. P., Severino, S. K., Freeman, E. W., Gise, L. H., Rivera-Tovar, A., & Steege, J. F. (1992). Late luteal phase dysphoric disorder in 670 women evaluated for premenstrual complaints. *American Journal of Psychiatry, 149*(4), 525–530.

Jang, S. H., Kim, D. I., & Choi, M.-S. (2014). Effects and treatment methods of acupuncture and herbal medicine for premenstrual syndrome/premenstrual dysphoric disorder: systematic review. *BMC Complementary and Alternative Medicine, 14,* 11. doi:10.1186/1472-6882-14-11

Jing, Z., Yang, X., Ismail, K. M., Chen, X., & Wu, T. (2009). Chinese herbal medicine for premenstrual syndrome. *Cochrane Database of Systematic Reviews, 1,* CD006414. doi:10.1002/14651858.CD006414.pub2

Kannan, P., & Claydon, L. S. (2014). Some physiotherapy treatments may relieve menstrual pain in women with primary dysmenorrhea: A systematic review. *Journal of Physiotherapy, 60*(1), 13–21.

Kashanian, M., Lakeh, M. M., Ghasemi, A., & Noori, S. (2013). Evaluation of the effect of vitamin E on pelvic pain reduction in women suffering from dysmenorrhea. *Journal of Reproductive Medicine, 58*(1–2), 35–38.

Kelderhouse, K., & Taylor, J. S. (2013). A review of treatment and management modalities for premenstrual dysphoric disorder. *Nursing for Women's Health, 17*(4), 294–305.

Kiesner, J. (2011). One woman's low is another woman's high: Paradoxical effects of the menstrual cycle. *Psychoneuroendocrinology, 36,* 68–76.

Khayat, S., Fanaei, F., Kheirkhah, M., Moghadam, Z. B., Kasaeian, A., & Javadimehr, M. (2015). Curcumin attenuates severity of premenstrual syndrome symptoms: A randomized, double-blind, placebo-controlled trial. *Complementary Therapies in Medicine, 23,* 318–324.

Kloss, B. A., Marcom, L. A., Odom, A. M., Tuggle, C. L., & Weatherspoon, D. (2012). PMS treatment through the use of CAM. *International Journal of Childbirth Education, 27*(3), 60–63.

Lasco, A., Catalano, A., & Benvenga, S. (2012). Improvement of primary dysmenorrhea caused by a single oral dose of vitamin D: Results of a randomized, double-blind, placebo-controlled study. *Archives of Internal Medicine, 172*(4), 366–367.

Latthe, P., Latthe, M., Say, L., Gülmezoglu, M, & Khan, K. S. (2006). WHO systematic review of prevalence of chronic pelvic pain: A neglected reproductive health morbidity. *BMC Public Health, 6,* 177.

Lentz, G. (2007). Primary and secondary dysmenorrheal, premenstrual syndrome, and premenstrual dysphoric disorder. In V. Katz, G. Lentz, R. Lobo, & D. Gershenson (Eds.), *Comprehensive gynecology* (pp. 901–914). Maryland Heights, MO: Mosby Elsevier.

Lopez, L. M, Kaptein, A., & Helmerhorst, F. M. (2012). Oral contraceptives containing drospirenone for premenstrual syndrome. *Cochrane Database of Systematic Reviews, 2,* CD006586. doi:10.1002/14651858.CD006586.pub4

Lustyk, M. K., & Gerrish, W. G. (2010). Premenstrual syndrome and premenstrual dysphoric disorder: Issues of quality of life, stress and exercise. In V. R. Preedy & R. R. Watson (Eds.), *Handbook of disease burdens and quality of life measures* (pp. 1951–1971). New York, NY: Springer.

Magnay, J. L. & Ismail, K. M. (2007). Genetics of premenstrual dysphoric disorder. In S. O'Brien, A. J. Rapkin, & P. J. Schmidt (Eds.), *The premenstrual syndromes PMS and PMDD* (pp. 161–170). Boca Raton, FL: CRC Press.

Marjoribanks, J., Ayeleke, R. O., Farquhar, M., & Proctor, M. (2015). Nonsteroidal anti-inflammatory drugs for dysmenorrhea. *Cochrane Database Systematic Reviews, 7,* CD001751. doi:10.1002/14651858.CD001751.pub3

Marjoribanks, J., Brown, J., O'Brien, P. M. S., & Wyatt, K. (2013). Selective serotonin reuptake inhibitors for premenstrual syndrome. *Cochrane Database of Systematic Reviews, 6,* CD001396. doi:10.1002/14651858.CD001396.pub3

Mason-Hohl, E. (1940). *The diseases of women: : A translation of* Passionibus Mulierum Curandorum. Los Angeles, CA: Ward Ritchie Press.

Mykletun, A., Jacka, F., Williams, L., Pasco, J., Henry, M., Nicholson, G.C., . . . Berk, M. (2010). Prevalence of mood and anxiety disorder in self reported irritable bowel syndrome (IBS): An epidemiological population based study of women. *Biomedcentral Gastroenterology, 10*(88). Retrieved from: http://www.ncbi.nlm.nih.gov/pmc/articles/PMC2928181/pdf/1471-230X-10-88.pdf

National Center for Complementary and Integrative Health. (2013, May). Evening primrose oil. Retrieved from https://nccih.nih .gov/health/eveningprimrose

Nooh, A. M., Abdul-Hady, A., & El-Attar, N. (2015). Nature and prevalence of menstrual disorders among teenage female students at Zagazig University, Zagazig, Egypt. *Journal of Pediatric & Adolescent Gynecology, 29*(2), 137–142.

O'Brien, P. M., Bäckström, T., Brown, C., Dennerstein L., Endicott, J., Epperson C. N., . . . Yonkers, K. (2011). Towards a consensus on diagnostic criteria, measurement and trial design of the premenstrual disorders: The ISPMD Montreal consensus. *Archives of Women's Mental Health, 14*(1), 13–21.

Oinonen, K. A., & Mazmanian, D. (2002). To what extent do oral contraceptives influence mood and affect? *Journal of Affective Disorders, 70,* 229–240.

Osayande, A. S., & Mehulic, S. (2014). Diagnosis and initial management of dysmenorrhea. *American Family Physician, 89*(5), 341–346.

Papakostas, G. I., Mischoulon, D., Shyu, I., Alpert, J., & Fava, M. (2010). *S*-Adenosyl methionine (SAMe) augmentation of serotonin reuptake inhibitors for antidepressant nonresponders with major depressive disorder: A double-blind, randomized clinical trial. *American Journal of Psychiatry, 167,* 942–948.

Pierce, A. (1999). *The American Pharmaceutical Association practical guide to natural medicines.* New York, NY: William Morrow.

Pinkerton, J. V., Guico-Pabia, C. J., & Taylor, H. S. (2010). Menstrual cycle–related exacerbation of disease. *American Journal of Obstetrics & Gynecology, 202*(3), 221–231. doi:10.1016/j.ajog.2009.07.061

Rapkin, A. J., & Lewis, E. I. (2013). Treatment of premenstrual dysphoric disorder. *Women's Health, 9*(6), 537–556.

Rowlandson, J. (1998). *Women and society in Greek and Roman Egypt.* Cambridge, UK: Cambridge University Press.

Sadler, C., Smith, H., Hammond, J., Bayly, R., Borland, S., Panay, N., . . . Inskip, H. (2010). Lifestyle factors, hormonal contraception, and premenstrual symptoms: The United Kingdom Southhampton Women's Survey. *Journal of Women's Health, 19*(3), 391–396.

Sanders, S., Graham, C., Bass, J., &, Bancroft, J. (2001). A prospective study of the effects of oral contraceptives on sexuality and well-being and their relationship to discontinuation. *Contraception, 64*(1), 51–58.

Schooler, D., Ward, L. M., Merriwether, A., & Caruthers, A. S. (2005). Cycles of shame: Menstrual shame, body shame, and sexual decision-making. *Journal of Sex Research, 42*(4), 324–334.

Shulman, L. P. (2010). Gynecological management of premenstrual symptoms. *Current Pain and Headache Reports, 14,* 367–375.

Smith, R. P. (2015). Managing dysmenorrhea. Retrieved from http://contemporaryobgyn.modernmedicine.com/contemporary -obgyn/news/managing-dysmenorrhea

Society of Obstetricians & Gynecologists of Canada (SOGC). (2005). Clinical practice guideline: Primary dysmenorrhea consensus guidelines. *Journal of Obstetrics and Gynaecology Canada, 169,* 1117–1130.

Takeda, T., Imoto, Y., Nagasawa, H., Muroya, M., & Shiina, M. (2015). Premenstrual syndrome and premenstrual dysphoric disorder in Japanese collegiate athletes. *Journal of Pediatric & Adolescent Gynecology, 28*(4), 215–218.

Taylor, D. (1999). Effectiveness of professional-peer group treatment: Symptom management for women with PMS. *Research in Nursing & Health, 22*(6), 496–511.

Tschudin, S., Bertea, P. C., & Zemp, E. (2010). Prevalence and predictors of premenstrual syndrome and premenstrual dysphoric disorder in a population based sample. *Archives of Women's Mental Health, 13*(6), 485–494.

Vigod, S. N., Frey, B. N., Soares, C. N., & Steiner, M. (2010). Approach to premenstrual dysphoria for the mental health practitioner. *Psychiatric Clinics of North America, 33*(2), 257–272.

Vincent, K., Warnaby, C., Stagg, C. J., Moore, F., Kennedy, S., & Tracey, I.. (2011). Dysmenorrhoea is associated with central changes in otherwise healthy women. *Pain, 152*(9), 1966–1975.

Westling, A. M., Tu, F. F., Griffith, J. W., & Hellman, K. M. (2013). The association of dysmenorrhea with noncyclic pelvic pain accounting for psychological factors. *American Journal of Obstetrics & Gynecology, 209*(11), 422–431.

Witt, J., Strickland, J., Cheng, A., Curtis, C., & Calkins, J. (2013). A randomized trial comparing the VIPON tampon and ibuprofen for dysmenorrhea pain relief. *Journal of Women's Health, 22*(8), 702–705.

Woo, P., & McEneaney, M.J. (2010). New strategies to treat primary dysmenorrhea. *Clinical Advisor, 11:* 43–49.

World Health Organization. (1992). International classification of diseases. Geneva, Switzerland: Author. Retrieved from www. who.int/classifications

Wyatt, K., Dimmock, P., Jones, P., Obhrai, M., & O'Brien, S. (2001). Efficacy of progesterone and progestogens in management of premenstrual syndrome: Systematic review. *British Medical Journal, 323*(7316), 776–780.

Wyatt, K., Dimmock, P., & O'Brien, P. (1999). Efficacy of vitamin B-6 in the treatment of premenstrual syndrome: Systematic review. *British Medical Journal, 318,* 1375–1381.

Yakir, M., Kreitler, S., Brzezinski, A., Vithoulkas, G., Oberbaum, M., & Bentwich, Z. (2001). Effects of homeopathic treatment in women with premenstrual syndrome: A pilot study. *British Homeopathic Journal, 90,* 148–153.

Zieman, M., & Hatcher, R. A. (2012). *Managing contraception.* Tiger, GA: Bridging the Gap Foundation.

CHAPTER 24

Normal and Abnormal Uterine Bleeding

Ruth Zielinski

Tanya Vaughn

The editors acknowledge Mary Ann Faucher and Kerri Durnell Schuiling, who were the authors of the previous edition of this chapter.

INTRODUCTION

A feminist perspective of health care views women holistically and avoids reducing a woman to her "parts" or medicalizing symptoms that are, in fact, representations of normal. A medical model inscripts the disorder on the body, necessitating symptom interpretation from the single perspective of the clinician's expertise (Bordo, 1993). For example, the term *abnormal uterine bleeding* suggests pathology and the need to fix a "problem." Nevertheless, for continuity of terminology, abnormal uterine bleeding (AUB) will be the term used throughout this chapter to describe bleeding that is considered out of the ordinary by either the woman or the clinician. That said, it is important to appreciate that some of the knowledge about women's cyclicity has been medicalized, socially constructed, or both. In some cases, "abnormal" bleeding actually represents a variation of normal, signifying the physiologic passage of a woman's body into the next stage of development—for example, menarche or menopause. For this reason, it is important to look beyond the biomedical model when caring for women with concerns regarding their menstrual-cycle bleeding.

Medical intervention—particularly surgical intervention—should be the last resort in many cases of abnormal uterine bleeding. It is important to consider the woman's goals for treatment when collaborating with her to develop a plan of care.

When the uterine bleeding diagnosed as irregular or abnormal is actually a variation of normal, treatment with education, reassurance, and nonpharmacologic intervention such as dietary changes or relaxation techniques is most often appropriate. As more clinicians embrace the normalcy of menstrual variations, there will be less temptation to "cure" normal female processes (Tavris, 1992). The expert clinician is one who actively listens, values input provided by the woman, and then carefully evaluates all available information before determining whether the bleeding is truly abnormal or just a variation of normal. A feminist approach to women's health care using a health-oriented, normalizing model allows normalcy to be validated. This paradigm enables assessment, diagnosis, and treatment that is woman centered and that values the woman's standpoint, background, ethnicity, and culture.

PHYSIOLOGY AND PATTERNS OF NORMAL MENSES

The physiology of normal menstrual processes and the anatomic and functional structure of the genital tract provide a foundation for understanding AUB (see Chapter 5). Normal menses results from a functional hypothalamic–pituitary–ovarian axis (HPOA) and a precise sequence of hormonal events that lead to ovulation. If conception does not occur

TABLE 24-1	Ranges of Normal Menstrual Cycles

Parameter	Terminology	Normal Limits
Cycle interval/frequency	Frequent Normal Infrequent	< 24 days 24–38 days > 38 days
Cycle variation over 12 months	Absent Regular Irregular	No bleeding Variation ± 2–20 days Variation > 20 days
Duration of flow	Prolonged Normal Shortened	> 8 days 4.5–8.0 days < 4.5 days
Amount of flow	Heavy Normal Light	> 80 mL 5–80 mL < 5 mL

Modified from Munro, M. G., Critchley, H. O. D., & Fraser, I. S. (2012). The FIGO systems for nomenclature and classification of causes of abnormal uterine bleeding in the reproductive years: Who needs them? *American Journal of Obstetrics & Gynecology, 207*(4), 259–265. Copyright 2012, with permission from Elsevier.

and if the outflow tract is patent, menses ensues. Normal menses may vary in length, duration, and amount of flow from woman to woman; reflecting this fact, normal parameters are provided as ranges (**Table 24-1**). It is wise to ask women who present with a concern about abnormal bleeding, "What is a normal pattern for you?"; the woman is always the best authority in describing her cycles.

Menses resulting from ovulatory cycles tend to demonstrate the same interval, amount, and duration from cycle to cycle unless significant health changes occur that negatively affect the HPOA. Menses in individual women tend to have consistent patterns once ovulation is established. Women who have regular, ovulatory menstrual cycles often experience premenstrual symptoms such as bloating, fatigue, constipation, and mood changes. These symptoms (collectively called *molimina*) are a result of higher levels of progesterone in the body. The progesterone surge in the luteal phase sustains the corpus luteum for a finite period of time. When conception does not occur, the corpus luteum atrophies, with resultant progesterone withdrawal bleeding. The withdrawal of progesterone also causes the production of arachidonic acid, which in turn stimulates the production of PGF_2 alpha. Although

the pathology of dysmenorrhea is not entirely understood, it is believed that dysmenorrhea associated with ovulatory bleeding results from the effects of PGF_2 alpha that cause vasoconstriction and contraction of smooth muscle (Smith, 2015). Chapter 23 of this text describes menstrual-cycle pain and premenstrual syndrome in greater detail.

ABNORMAL UTERINE BLEEDING

Abnormal uterine bleeding is one of the more common reasons women seek health care. It accounts for as many as one-third of all annual gynecologic visits (American College of Obstetricians and Gynecologists, 2012, reaffirmed 2014). AUB has a significant impact on the quality of life for the women it affects. Bleeding patterns range from amenorrhea (no menses) to heavy menstrual bleeding (HMB).

Current costs of HMB to employers and use of resources in the U.S. healthcare system were updated in a study of women ($n = 29,842$) who had a diagnosis of HMB matched with control participants who were not diagnosed with HMB. The findings revealed that women diagnosed with HMB had significantly higher annual all-cause healthcare resource use compared to the controls, and that average annual healthcare costs were significantly higher for the women with HMB than for women in the control group; in fact, almost 80% of women diagnosed with HMB had higher average annual costs for health care (Jensen et al., 2012). These findings do not include intangible costs or productivity losses, such as time lost from work. Clearly, even by conservative estimates, AUB imposes a heavy economic burden.

ABNORMAL UTERINE BLEEDING CLASSIFICATION AND TERMINOLOGY

Abnormal uterine bleeding is an all-encompassing term referring to any uterine bleeding that is irregular in amount, frequency, duration, or timing (i.e., cycle irregularity). It may or may not be related to a woman's menstrual cycle. AUB can occur as a normal physiologic event, such as the irregular bleeding that often accompanies menarche or perimenopause due to irregular ovulation. However, it can also signal pathologic, life-threatening conditions such as an ectopic pregnancy or endometrial cancer. Historically, it has been difficult to investigate the etiologies of AUB due to inconsistencies in definitions. The nomenclature surrounding AUB has evolved over the years but remains confusing, making this condition difficult to adequately study, diagnose, and treat.

In 2009, the International Federation of Gynecology and Obstetrics (FIGO) set out to standardize classifications of AUB via a system called PALM-COEIN (**Figure 24-1**). **PALM** is the acronym for the basic system made up of four categories that are defined by visually objective structural criteria: **P**olyp, **A**denomyosis, **L**eiomyoma (which is divided further into women who have at least one submucosal myoma and those whose myomas do not impact the endometrial cavity), and **M**alignancy and hyperplasia. **COEIN** (pronounced as *coin*) consists of five categories unrelated to structural abnormalities: **C**oagulopathy, **O**vulatory dysfunction, **E**ndometrial, **I**atrogenic, and **N**ot yet classified (FIGO, 2011).

The new nomenclature no longer includes the term *dysfunctional uterine bleeding*, instead replacing it with an evidence-based set of categories to define nonstructural causes of AUB—that is, causes not related to structural abnormalities of the uterus (Munro, Critchley, Broder, & Fraser, 2011; Munro, Critchley, & Frasier, 2012). Many other poorly defined and confusing terminologies have also been abandoned and replaced with a set of terms that are clearer in definition and can be more easily translated into other languages (Munro et al., 2011) (**Box 24-1**).

ETIOLOGY AND PATHOPHYSIOLOGY OF ABNORMAL UTERINE BLEEDING

The causes of abnormal bleeding can be physiologic, pathologic, or pharmacologic. Disruption of endocrine function at any level of the HPOA can disrupt normal menstrual physiology and disturb menstrual-cycle regularity, frequency, duration, or volume. In women of reproductive age, the most common cause of a bleeding pattern that suddenly

---

FIGURE 24-1 The PALM-COEIN classification for abnormal uterine bleeding.

PALM – Structural Abnormalities
Polyps AUB-P
Adenomyosis AUB-A
Leiomyoma-submucosal/other AUB-L
Malignancy and hyperplasia AUB-M

COEIN – Nonstructural Abnormalities
Coagulopathy AUB-C
Ovulatory Dysfunction AUB-O
Endometrial AUB-E
Iatrogenic AUB-I
Not yet classified AUB-N

Hand: © Tatiana Popova/Shutterstock
Coin: © marekuliasz/Shutterstock

Data from International Federation of Gynecology and Obstetrics (FIGO). (2011). FIGO classification system (PALM-COEIN) for causes of abnormal uterine bleeding in nongravid women of reproductive age. *International Journal of Gynecology and Obstetrics, 113*, 3–13. http://dx.doi.org/10.1016/j.ijgo.2010.11.011

BOX 24-1 Terms No Longer Used to Describe or Define Abnormal Uterine Bleeding

- Dysfunctional uterine bleeding
- Epimenorrhagia
- Epimenorrhea
- Functional uterine bleeding
- Hypermenorrhea
- Hypomenorrhea
- Menometrorrhagia
- Menorrhagia (all uses of this term)
- Metrorrhagia
- Metropathica hemorrhagica
- Oligomenorrhea
- Polymenorrhagia
- Polymenorrhea
- Uterine hemorrhage

Data from Munro, M. G., Critchley, H. O. D., Broder, M. S., & Fraser, I. S. (2011). FIGO classification system (PALM-COEIN) for cause of abnormal uterine bleeding in nongravid women of reproductive age. *International Journal of Gynecology & Obstetrics, 113,* 3–13; Munro, M. G., Critchley, H. O. D., & Fraser, I. S. (2012). The FIGO systems for nomenclature and classification of causes of abnormal uterine bleeding in the reproductive years: Who needs them? *American Journal of Obstetrics & Gynecology, 207*(4), 259–265.

---

differs from a woman's established menstrual pattern is a complication of pregnancy, including threatened or incomplete abortion, ectopic pregnancy, retained products of conception, or gestational trophoblastic disease (Fritz & Speroff, 2011). As a consequence, clinicians treating women of childbearing age who present with AUB—especially adolescents who may not be forthcoming about their sexual activity—should always first exclude pregnancy or a complication of pregnancy as a cause of the bleeding.

Once complications of pregnancy have been ruled out, a multitude of etiologies must be considered that can cause AUB. The PALM-COEIN classification system can help guide evaluation, diagnosis, and treatment of AUB by organizing specific categories of AUB systematically. The various etiologies are discussed here in the PALM-COEIN format.

PALM: Structural Abnormalities

AUB-P (Polyps)

Endocervical polyps are commonly occurring benign growths on the cervix. They are easily visualized with a speculum, appearing as smooth, deep to bright red growths that are fragile and bleed with little encouragement during examination. Women with cervical polyps may present with a concern about vaginal bleeding. With further investigation, the bleeding associated with polyps often occurs after sexual intercourse.

Endometrial polyps are usually benign growths of the endometrium consisting of connective, glandular, or muscular tissue; they are usually asymptomatic, but are generally thought to contribute to AUB in some women. Rarely, polyps can resemble atypical or cancerous cells (FIGO, 2011). Within the FIGO classification system, polyps are classified as either present or not. The FIGO system does not indicate how many polyps must be present or how large they must be, although this information can be added as a subcategory and should be documented by the provider. (See Chapter 26 for further information regarding polyps.)

AUB-A (Adenomyosis)

Adenomyosis is a common condition that typically affects women who are multiparous and older than age 40 (Levy et al., 2013). Adenomyosis is characterized by small areas of endometrial tissue within the myometrium. The predominant predisposing factor for this condition is more than one pregnancy as well as history of miscarriage, curettage, endometrial resection, cesarean section, or tamoxifen use (Levy et al., 2013). The connection between adenomyosis and AUB is not well understood.

Ultrasonography and occasionally magnetic resonance imaging (MRI) have been used to detect the severity of the adenomyosis, which may include uterine enlargement. It is proposed that ultrasound evaluation meets the minimum requirements for diagnosis, as MRI diagnosis is not readily available worldwide (FIGO, 2011). Imaging guidelines and histopathologic detection have yet to be standardized. (See Chapter 26 for further discussion about AUB-A.)

AUB-L (Leiomyoma)

Leiomyomas, commonly known as "fibroids," are fibromuscular benign tumors in the myometrium. Leiomyoma is a more accurate term than either fibroid or myoma for these benign tumors of the myometrium (FIGO, 2011). Leiomyomas are the most common benign pelvic tumors in women and the leading indication for hysterectomy (American College of Obstetricians and Gynecologists, 2008, reaffirmed 2014). Women who have leiomyomas generally have no symptoms and do not require treatment, although depending on their locations within the uterus the fibroids may have the potential to contribute to AUB. The primary classification system accounts for only the presence or absence of leiomyomas.

Leiomyomas are further classified by a secondary category that labels their location within the uterus. It is important to determine if the leiomyoma interferes with the endometrium (submucosal), because this type is most likely to cause AUB. The "other" category includes subserosal and intramural leiomyomas. The sizes of leiomyomas are not included in the current classification system, but could be considered with a tertiary classification system. This would further standardize the classifications of leiomyomas, thereby providing a reliable, accurate system for research studies and patient documentation. (See Chapter 26 for further discussion about AUB-L.)

AUB-M (Malignancy and Hyperplasia)

Malignancy and atypical hyperplasia are rare in women of reproductive age and in women who have a normal body mass index (BMI) and who do not have polycystic ovarian syndrome (PCOS). However, these conditions must still be considered as a potential cause of AUB, particularly if a women is obese or has PCOS. It is well established that women who are obese and those who have PCOS have an increased risk of endometrial cancer (American College of Obstetricians and Gynecologists, 2015; Cass, 2015; Farrell-Turner, 2011). In fact, women who are either overweight or obese have estimated odds ratios of 1.43 and 3.3, respectively, of developing endometrial cancer when compared with women of normal weight (Cass, 2015). Furthermore, while African American women have a 30% decreased incidence of being diagnosed with endometrial cancer (when compared to Caucasian women),

they have a 2½ times higher risk of death if they are diagnosed with endometrial cancer (Cass, 2015). This finding is probably a result of healthcare disparities and the reality that African American women are more likely to be diagnosed with a more advanced stage of the disease (American College of Obstetricians and Gynecologists, 2015).

The most common symptoms of endometrial cancer are AUB and postmenopausal bleeding (American College of Obstetricians and Gynecologists, 2015). Therefore, a malignancy must be ruled out in all women who are experiencing postmenopausal vaginal bleeding. Any woman diagnosed with AUB-M will also have a subclassification of her condition using the World Health Organization (WHO) or FIGO oncology staging systems. The PALM-COEIN AUB classification system is not meant to replace the oncology staging system.

COEIN: Nonstructural Abnormalities

AUB-C (Coagulopathy)

The coagulopathy category encompasses a wide range of blood clotting disorders that can potentially cause AUB. Approximately 13% of women who present with AUB will have a blood clotting disorder, with von Willebrand's disease (VWD) being one of the more commonly inherited bleeding disorders. Among young women with heavy bleeding, approximately 20% to 30% will have a diagnosis of VWD (American College of Obstetricians and Gynecologists, 2013a; Khamees, Klima, & O'Brien, 2015). Women presenting with complaint of heavy menstrual bleeding who have history of easy bruising and prolonged bleeding following dental work or surgery warrant further follow-up for VWD.

Conversely, some women with coagulopathy disorders take anticoagulant medications that could contribute to AUB. Although this type of bleeding could be considered iatrogenic in nature, it is still termed AUB-C because of the rationale (coagulopathy disorder) for the drug therapy (American College of Obstetricians and Gynecologists, 2013a).

The diagnosis of AUB-C is usually made by thoroughly reviewing the woman's history and confirmed by hematologic testing. Treatment includes consultation with a hematologist or other provider experienced in caring for coagulopathy disorders.

AUB-O (Ovulatory Dysfunction)

Ovulatory dysfunction AUB is the new name for the category that was once termed dysfunctional uterine bleeding (FIGO, 2011). This category encompasses many different presentations of AUB, including amenorrhea as well as light or heavy menses that can be more frequent, less frequent, or occurring in regular menstrual patterns. Depending on the severity of the bleeding, the woman may need pharmacologic or surgical intervention. Many cases of AUB-O stem from endocrinopathies including thyroid disorders, polycystic ovarian syndrome, excessive exercise, or extreme mental distress. Subcategories of AUB-O are defined as anovulatory uterine bleeding, amenorrhea (absence of bleeding), and ovulatory uterine bleeding.

Anovulatory Uterine Bleeding Anovulatory bleeding, in contrast to the typically regular, predictable bleeding experienced with ovulatory cycles, frequently leads to abnormal cycle intervals, excessively heavy bleeding, or lighter than normal amounts of bleeding. This type of bleeding tends to be heavy secondary to the high and sustained levels of unopposed estrogen that can result in endometrial hyperplasia. Endometrial hyperplasia, in turn, can result in episodes of amenorrhea, heavy menstrual bleeding, and intermenstrual bleeding (IMB). Anovulatory cycles characterized by a lack of progesterone in the luteal phase lead to an unstable, excessively vascular endometrium. Fritz and Speroff

(2011) provide a clear description of anovulation and its effect on a woman's cycle:

> By definition, the anovulatory woman is always in the follicular phase of the ovarian cycle and in the proliferative phase of the endometrial cycle. There is no luteal or secretory phase because there is no ovulation or cycle. The only ovarian steroid signal the endometrium receives is estrogen, levels of which constantly fluctuate, rising and falling as each new cohort of follicles begins to grow but ultimately loses its developmental momentum and, sooner or later, lapses into atresia. Although the amplitude of the signal may vary, the message, growth, stays the same. (p. 599)

Table 24-2 identifies recognized physiologic and pathologic causes of anovulation (American College of Obstetricians and Gynecologists, 2013b).

Evidence from histologic and molecular studies suggests that anovulatory bleeding is the result of an increased density of abnormal vessels that have a fragile structure prone to focal rupture, which is then followed by the release of lysosomes (proteolytic enzymes) from surrounding epithelial and stromal cells and migratory leukocytes and macrophages (Fritz & Speroff, 2011). This condition is generally caused by one of three hormonal imbalances: estrogen withdrawal, estrogen breakthrough, or progesterone breakthrough (American College of Obstetricians and Gynecologists, 2012, reaffirmed 2014).

TABLE 24-2   Physiologic and Pathologic Causes of Anovulation

Physiologic Causes	Pathologic Causes
Pregnancy	Hyperandrogenic disorders (e.g., polycystic ovarian syndrome)
Lactation	Hypothalamic dysfunction (secondary to anorexia nervosa)
Perimenarche	Hyperprolactinemia
Perimenopause	Iatrogenic (secondary to radiation therapy, chemotherapy or
Obesity	medications)
BMI < 18	Thyroid disorders
Excessive exercise	Primary pituitary disorders

Data from American College of Obstetricians and Gynecologists. (2013b). ACOG Practice Bulletin No. 136: Management of abnormal uterine bleeding associated with ovulatory dysfunction. *Obstetrics & Gynecology, 122*(1), 176–185.

Estrogen levels increase the thickness of the endometrium; thus women with high sustained levels of estrogen tend to experience the heaviest menstrual bleeding. Estrogen breakthrough bleeding occurs as a result of the endometrium being stimulated by long-term, chronic unopposed estrogen, such as that observed in women experiencing chronic anovulation. These women often include those who have PCOS, are obese, or are perimenopausal (Fritz & Speroff, 2011). Women with PCOS often experience estrogen breakthrough bleeding because of chronic anovulation (Fritz & Speroff, 2011). Diseases or syndromes causing insulin resistance, such as PCOS, increase circulating levels of insulin, which in turn leads to an elevation in androgen production and concomitant anovulation (American College of Obstetricians and Gynecologists, 2009a, reaffirmed 2013). The relationship between insulin and androgens is believed to be an underlying cause of PCOS. (See Chapter 25 for additional information about PCOS.)

Endocrine disorders may cause bleeding abnormalities; consequently, they should always be considered when evaluating a woman for AUB. Thyroid disorders (both hypothyroidism and hypothyroidism) can cause AUB (Sweet, Schmidt-Dalton, Weiss, & Madsen, 2012). Hyperthyroidism can result in a range of bleeding patterns, including vaginal spotting, heavy menstrual bleeding, or amenorrhea. Pituitary disease and some pituitary tumors may result in elevated levels of prolactin. Amenorrhea associated with elevated prolactin levels is due to prolactin inhibition of the pulsatile secretion of gonadotropin-releasing hormone (GnRH) (Fritz & Speroff, 2011). Prolactin-secreting pituitary adenomas are the most common type of pituitary tumor (Fritz & Speroff, 2011). Approximately one-third of women with elevated prolactin levels will also have galactorrhea. Nevertheless, many individuals (10%) have silent pituitary masses that are not endocrinologically active and have no adverse impact on health and well-being. If there is no evidence of hormonal disturbance, no immediate intervention is probably necessary, although long-term surveillance is appropriate (Fritz & Speroff, 2011).

Progesterone breakthrough bleeding occurs when the progesterone–estrogen ratio becomes elevated (American College of Obstetricians and Gynecologists, 2012, reaffirmed 2014). This type of AUB is sometimes seen in women using progestin-only pills or other forms of progestin-only contraception (Fritz & Speroff, 2011). Heavy and/or irregular bleeding results from an imbalance in both the vasoconstricting and vasodilating properties of prostaglandins and platelet aggregation and inhibition (American College of Obstetricians and Gynecologists, 2012, reaffirmed 2014). The abnormal microvasculature is probably the cause of the abnormal bleeding that results from this phenomenon (Fritz & Speroff, 2011).

The most common times for a woman to experience irregular menstrual cycles are at the beginning and the end of her reproductive life cycle: postmenarche and perimenopause. The HPOA is most affected by the normal life-cycle transitions that occur during the first 2 years after menarche and 3 years prior to menopause (Fritz & Speroff, 2011); thus irregular bleeding during this time may be a reflection of normal functioning.

The least amount of variation in menses occurs during the childbearing years, which generally encompass ages 20 to 40, although most women will experience some variation from their established normal pattern from time to time. Even though bleeding patterns may fall within the range of normal, it is important to listen to the woman's description prior to making a diagnosis, because for her, the bleeding may be abnormal and require some amount of reassurance, education, or follow-up.

Amenorrhea Amenorrhea simply means absence of menses and is part of the spectrum of ovulatory disorders classified as AUB-O. The most common causes of amenorrhea are pregnancy, hypothalamic amenorrhea, and PCOS (American College of Obstetricians and Gynecologists, 2014). According to Fritz and Speroff (2011, p. 436), women meeting any of the following criteria should be evaluated for amenorrhea:

- No menses by age 14 in the absence of growth or development of secondary sexual characteristics
- No menses by age 16 regardless of the presence of normal growth and development of secondary sexual characteristics
- In women who have menstruated previously, no menses for an interval of time equivalent to a total of at least three previous cycles, or 6 months

Amenorrhea typically is categorized as either primary or secondary. Primary amenorrhea is the failure to begin menses by the age of 16. A number of disorders can be treated as soon as they are diagnosed, however, so any girl who has not reached menarche by age 15 years or who has not had a menses within 3 years of thelarche should be evaluated (American College of Obstetricians and Gynecologists, 2014). Secondary amenorrhea is defined as 3 months without a menses once menses has been established. The American Society for Reproductive Medicine recommends that any woman experiencing 3 months of amenorrhea once the menses is established should be evaluated (American College of Obstetricians and Gynecologists, 2014). Because primary and secondary amenorrhea can have the same causes, the initial investigation for both is similar.

Physiologic causes of amenorrhea include anatomic defects, ovarian failure, chronic anovulation, anterior pituitary disorders, and central nervous system disorders. Age is an important criterion in making the differential diagnosis of primary versus secondary amenorrhea, and is relevant in determining the types of questions to ask when taking the medical history. Primary amenorrhea in a young woman may be indicative of HPOA disorder or anatomic factors, such as outflow tract obstruction. With primary amenorrhea, the physical examination should focus on identifying the maturation of secondary sex characteristics (e.g., Tanner staging for breast development and pubic hair pattern; see Chapter 2) and establishing outflow tract patency. The question "Have you had any bleeding from the vagina?" can assist in determining primary, secondary, and potential causes. Other important interview questions to consider relate to lifestyle patterns (e.g., exercise, medication, and drug use) and eating habits (e.g., possible eating disorders). A family history of anatomic or genetic abnormalities should be explored as well.

Normal menstrual function requires that four anatomic and structural components are in working order: uterus, ovary, pituitary, and hypothalamus (Fritz & Speroff, 2011). The clinician can then categorize the amenorrhea according to the site or level of disturbance (Fritz & Speroff, p. 438):

- Disorders of the genital outflow tract

- Disorders of the ovary
- Disorders of the anterior pituitary
- Disorders of the hypothalamus or central nervous system

The differential diagnosis for women who are not pregnant and who present with amenorrhea is either primary amenorrhea or secondary amenorrhea, although Fritz and Speroff (2011) warn that premature categorization of amenorrhea can lead to diagnostic omissions and, in many cases, unnecessary and expensive diagnostic testing.

Athletic women, particularly long-distance runners, gymnasts, and professional ballet dancers, are at risk for amenorrhea, as are women who have anorexia and other eating disorders (Fritz & Speroff, 2011; Polotsky, 2010). Typically, amenorrhea occurs as the menstrual cycle stops after the start of an intensive training regimen, although some reports indicate that when intensive training begins prior to menarche, menarche can be delayed by as much as 3 years (Fritz & Speroff, 2011). It is important to understand that it is not exercise in general that causes the amenorrhea, but rather the specific type of exercise (Fritz & Speroff, 2011). For example, swimming is less likely to cause amenorrhea than long-distance running. Women with a low BMI and low percentage of body fat combined with a high level of intensive physical activity have the highest risk for amenorrhea (Fritz & Speroff, 2011).

The pathophysiology of exercise-induced amenorrhea is complex and most likely due to the combination of low body fat and diminished secretion of GnRH. Lower GnRH levels result in fewer luteinizing hormone (LH) and follicle-stimulating hormone (FSH) pulses, which in turn decreases the amount of estrogen produced by the ovaries. The critical weight theory hypothesizes that some critical weight and amount of body fat exist that must be maintained for women to experience regular menstrual cycles (Fritz & Speroff, 2011).

Ovulatory Abnormal Uterine Bleeding Ovulatory dysfunction (AUB-O) includes a spectrum of disorders from amenorrhea to irregular heavy menstrual periods that are usually caused by an endocrinopathy such as PCOS (American College of Obstetricians and Gynecologists, 2012, reaffirmed 2014). Ovulatory AUB, one of the disorders of AUB-O, occurs significantly less often than abnormal bleeding due to anovulation; it is typically observed in the post-adolescent years and during the premenopausal years. Ovulatory abnormal bleeding tends to be cyclic and regular, although the bleeding patterns are often abnormal. The HPOA is intact and the steroid hormone profile is normal in ovulatory AUB (American College of Obstetricians and Gynecologists, 2012, reaffirmed 2014).

Prolonged, heavy menstrual bleeding is the pattern most frequently observed with ovulatory abnormal bleeding that is commonly associated with pelvic pathology such as uterine fibroids (leiomyomas), adenomyosis, or endometrial polyps (American College of Obstetricians and Gynecologists, 2008, reaffirmed 2014). Therefore, in women with ovulatory abnormal bleeding, an evaluation to rule out endometrial lesions and other pathology is indicated. HMB is also frequently associated with bleeding dyscrasias, and as many as 20% of adolescents who present with HMB have a bleeding disorder (Fritz & Speroff, 2011).

AUB-E (Endometrial)

Endometrial AUB usually occurs in a predictive and cyclical manner and includes heavy menstrual bleeding (FIGO, 2011). AUB-E can also present with intermenstrual or prolonged bleeding patterns.

All women of childbearing age who present with AUB should be considered pregnant until proven otherwise. A thorough history and physical examination (including pelvic examination and cultures) will assist in ruling out pregnancy or infection as a cause of the abnormal bleeding. Although the role of infection is not discussed extensively in the current literature (FIGO, 2011), *Chlamydia trachomatis* has been found to be associated with endometritis, which can produce intermenstrual bleeding as observed with this type of AUB. Thus the clinician should discuss testing with the woman as a means of possibly ruling this out as the causative factor (Munro et al., 2011). Other infections, such as gonorrhea, and endometritis may cause irregular spotting due to irritation and inflammation of the tissues of the cervix or endometrium.

The endometrium is a unique tissue that releases blood as a part of normal physiology. The etiology of AUB-E can involve a premature release of blood from the endometrium or disorders of local endometrial hemostasis. Platelets are involved in endometrial hemostasis very marginally at the time of menstruation. There can be a decrease of local endometrial vasoconstrictors (endothelin-1 and prostaglandin F_2), thereby causing vasodilation and HMB. Excessive amounts of plasminogen activator or decreased amounts of plasminogen activator inhibitor can also lead to HMB. The exact processes that happen during AUB-E are not well defined in the current literature. Consequently, there are no diagnostic tests that clinicians can use to confirm the presence of AUB-E; rather, it is a diagnosis of exclusion.

AUB-I (Iatrogenic)

Medications or devices that act on the endometrium can cause iatrogenic AUB. The Mirena, Skyla, Liletta, and Paragard intrauterine systems can also cause irregular spotting and bleeding after placement, although this phenomenon usually resolves within 3 to 6 months after the device's placement. Any medication that acts on the endometrium itself or interferes with the ovulation cycle can cause AUB-I. A large portion of women in this category will have breakthrough bleeding (BTB) related to the use of gonadal steroidal medications (hormonal contraception) (FIGO, 2011). Other hormonal methods of contraception may also result in irregular or breakthrough bleeding. For more information regarding contraceptives please refer to Chapter 11.

Antidepressant therapies including the tricyclics and phenothiazines can cause AUB-I related to a disturbance in the HPOA (FIGO, 2011). Any medications that alter the serotonin reuptake process can potentially cause AUB-I as well.

Any woman taking anticoagulants for a blood clotting disorder is placed in the AUB-C category rather than AUB-I because the disorder is the rationale for needing anticoagulant therapy, which can then cause dysfunctional bleeding (FIGO, 2011).

AUB-N (Not Yet Classified)

The AUB-N category may be used when possible causes of AUB, other than those previously mentioned, are being explored. For example, some women may experience AUB related to conditions such as arterial–venous malformations that do not fit into any of the other AUB categories (FIGO, 2011). This category also leaves room for yet unidentified causes of AUB.

Special Considerations for Evaluating Abnormal Uterine Bleeding

Trauma to the genital tract can also cause AUB. Tampons can irritate the cervix and cause spotting. In addition, hymeneal tearing with tampon use or consensual intercourse can cause bleeding. Women who have been sexually assaulted, particularly those who have not had sexual intercourse prior to the assault, may experience abnormal bleeding from lacerations and other injuries affecting the internal organs and genitals (American College of Obstetricians and Gynecologists, 2014).

Outflow Tract Causes of AUB

A properly functioning outflow tract (i.e., a patent uterus, cervix, and vagina) is a necessary component for normal menstrual flow. Anatomic abnormalities at any level of the outflow tract can interfere with normal menstrual flow and often result in amenorrhea. For example, uterine or cervical congenital structural abnormalities can cause obstruction and make menstrual flow impossible or abnormal. Rarely, segments of the Müllerian tube may fail to develop, resulting in abnormalities such as imperforate hymen, lack of a vaginal orifice, lapses in the continuity of the vaginal canal, or an absent uterus, cervix, uterine cavity, or endometrium. Obstruction of menses may lead to painful distention due to a menstrual blood collection such as hematometra (blood in the uterus), hematocolpos (vagina), or hemoperitoneum (peritoneum). Affected women are genotypically and phenotypically normal females with functioning ovaries. Such abnormalities are uncommon, except in women whose mothers were given diethylstilbestrol (DES) during pregnancy typically between the years of 1938 and 1971 (Fritz & Speroff, 2011). Women with a history of multiple cervical procedures such as dilation and curettage (D & C) or significant endometrial infections are at risk for scarring that may cause outflow tract AUB.

If a woman presents with amenorrhea with no history of infection or trauma and her pelvic examination and bimanual examination are normal, then an abnormality of the outflow tract is not likely.

ASSESSMENT OF NORMAL AND ABNORMAL BLEEDING

History

Interview questions should be guided by the PALM-COEIN classification system. Evaluation begins with the clinician obtaining a medical history and then proceeding with a careful physical examination (see Chapter 6). During the history, the clinician explores the woman's general overall health, her lifestyle, and any chronic diseases, history of trauma, or stress factors in her life. Factors such as age (adolescence), family history of eating disorders, and participation in competitive athletics or extreme exercise are risks for lifestyle stress that can interrupt the function of the HPOA and lead to amenorrhea (American College of Obstetricians and Gynecologists, 2014). Contraceptive history may reveal long-term use of hormonal contraceptives and, therefore, suggest the likelihood of amenorrhea due to endometrial atrophy (Fritz & Speroff, 2011). Changes in body weight or body distribution (e.g., large waist circumference) suggest PCOS and chronic anovulation, whereas weight gain and temperature intolerance suggest thyroid disorders. A history of headaches and galactorrhea may be related to a prolactin-secreting tumor or hypothyroidism. A woman's report of hot flushes, cessation of menses, or vaginal dryness suggests menopause as a possible etiology for amenorrhea. History of multiple D & C procedures, significant endometrial infections, or cervical treatments (e.g., cryotherapy) may indicate cervical stenosis related to Asherman syndrome and subsequent amenorrhea.

A detailed menstrual history provides the most useful information to differentiate between types of abnormal uterine bleeding and may be enough to confidently make a diagnosis and proceed with treatment without further testing. For example, the diagnosis of AUB can be confidently made in women with a history of irregular, unpredictable bleeding for 6 months or longer in the absence of premenstrual symptoms (FIGO, 2011). However, in women with regular, heavy bleeding that is prolonged, menstrual history alone is likely to be inadequate for making an accurate diagnosis (Fritz & Speroff, 2011). It is critical to remember that women of reproductive age presenting with abnormal uterine bleeding must first have pregnancy ruled out before proceeding to other testing.

Begin the history interview by asking the woman to describe in detail what brought her in for the visit and then obtain a detailed menstrual history. Questions should include her current age as well as her age at menarche and menopause (if appropriate); cycle length, duration, and estimated amount of flow; and when the menstrual pattern changed.

When questioning women about cycle length, duration, and flow, it is important to understand how the woman calculates each of these factors. Some women do not include the first day of spotting or may not include the days when the flow is light when determining cycle length. Reviewing the parameters of what is considered normal may also provide the woman with a useful guide for describing her cycles. Her observation about how the current bleeding deviates from her established pattern is a valuable tool to use in the assessment. Many studies have demonstrated that estimating the amount of blood loss during the menses can be highly imprecise (Chimbira, Anderson, & Turnball, 1980; Halberg, Hogdahl, Nillson, & Rybo, 1966). The current biomedical standard for measuring the amount of blood lost during menstruation is the alkaline hematin method, which is quite expensive and can be inconvenient for women (Schumacher et al., 2012). It requires a woman to collect all menstrual products (pads, tampons) used during a menses and bring them to a lab, where these materials are then tested to determine how much blood they contain, enabling a calculation of the amount of blood lost during the menses. The products are treated with sodium hydroxide for 48 hours to convert the menstrual blood hemoglobin to alkaline hematin and then the optical density of the alkaline hematin is measured spectrophotometrically (Hasson, 2012). Next, venous blood is drawn from the woman and the optical density of the alkaline hematin in that peripheral blood is measured. The ratio of the hemoglobin concentration in the total menstrual discharge to the peripheral blood is considered the volume of menstrual blood loss (Davies, Anderson, & Turnball, 1981).

It is particularly helpful to determine whether the bleeding occurs at regular or irregular intervals, as the pattern of bleeding provides clues to its etiology. For example, if a woman is postmenopausal and reports that she experienced spontaneous, painless, and irregular bleeding, the clinician must include endometrial hyperplasia in the differential diagnosis and undertake prompt endometrial evaluation. A woman who reports having regular cycles that have now become heavy, accompanied by the passage of clots, and who says she has noticed a sensation of pelvic fullness, may be experiencing AUB secondary to uterine fibroids. Listening to the woman is important for making an accurate diagnosis and allows the clinician to find ways to provide her with needed support during the assessment.

Ask the woman about the dates of her last six menstrual periods and the date of her last *normal* menses. Often, providing her with a calendar will assist her in answering these questions accurately. Inquire about the color and character of her flow and related signs and symptoms such as pain, odor, and postcoital spotting for the majority of the last 6 months. Inquire whether hot flushes or the sensation of a racing heartbeat are present—these signs accompanied by abnormal bleeding may indicate menopause is approaching, particularly if the woman is in the perimenopausal years. Inquiring about other associated symptoms is important. For example, the presence of premenstrual symptoms may indicate ovulation, whereas reports of dyspareunia or IMB lead to a different set of differential diagnoses. The gynecologic history may reveal other episodes of abnormal bleeding as well as previous treatment modalities. Inquire about cervical cancer screening history (human papillomavirus [HPV] DNA and Papanicolaou test), gynecologic surgeries, sexually transmitted infections, and other infections of the genital tract or organs.

If the woman is currently using or has used contraception in the past, obtain information about the type, the length of use, and any side effects encountered. Contraceptive history may reveal that her abnormal bleeding is mechanically caused by an intrauterine device (IUD) or is related to the use of hormonal contraception, such as oral contraceptives or injectable depot medroxyprogesterone acetate (Depo-Provera). In addition, inquire about hormone therapy in postmenopausal women to rule out a history of taking unopposed estrogen—a therapy that can lead to endometrial hyperplasia.

A medical history or general health history, including family history, provides information that may reveal underlying medical conditions that might be the cause of the abnormal bleeding. Ask about symptoms of thyroid disorders (e.g., cold intolerance, fatigue, hyperactivity, weight gain or loss) and hormone-secreting tumors (e.g., hair loss, changes in breast size, hirsutism, headache, breast discharge). Findings in the health history may suggest the presence of a systemic disease; therefore, pay particular attention to signs and symptoms such as easy bruising, presence of petechiae, weight or appetite changes, and changes in elimination patterns. Given that bleeding and endocrine disorders can be inherited, it is important to look for familial patterns.

Including questions about lifestyle is also important to obtain information about drug use or abuse, exercise patterns, and nutrition. Obtain a complete medication history. Glucocorticoids, tamoxifen, and anticoagulants may predispose women to abnormal uterine bleeding. Ask about use of over-the-counter and herbal medications. Notably, the herb bromelain may increase the risk of bleeding.

Physical Examination

The physical examination should include an overall body assessment, noting general habitus, weight, body fat distribution, and hair patterns. Data obtained during the physical examination may be suggestive of systemic disease, particularly organic pathology. Height, weight, body BMI, vital signs, hair, and body fat distribution are important parameters to include. Note signs of possible androgen excess, including hirsutism, acne, and alopecia (see Chapter 25). Tanner staging (see Chapter 2) is helpful when examining adolescents because it can validate information from the history and may help to determine ovulatory status. A breast examination can rule out the presence of galactorrhea, which may indicate an elevated prolactin level. The amount of breast development is an indicator of estrogen production or exposure to exogenous estrogen (Fritz & Speroff, 2011). Assessing for the presence of galactorrhea and performing a visual field evaluation are particularly important when women present with headaches or galactorrhea, both of which are suggestive of pituitary disease.

Observe the woman for signs of anemia, such as pale skin tone and delayed capillary refill.

Palpating the thyroid may identify enlargement, nodules, or tumors related to either hypothyroidism or hyperthyroidism. Vital signs, particularly the pulse rate and skin changes, may be helpful in diagnosing thyroid disease.

A pelvic examination is essential for a woman of any age who is (or has been) sexually active or has abdominal pain, anemia, irregular bleeding, or bleeding that is so heavy her hemodynamic stability is compromised. In contrast, if the patient is an adolescent who is not sexually active, has only recently began menstruating, and has a normal hematocrit, a pelvic examination is most likely unnecessary. Prior to the pelvic examination, visually assess the external genitalia and the presence of pubic hair, which indicates androgen production or exposure (Fritz & Speroff, 2011). Absence of pubic hair is not always indicative of abnormality, as pubic hair removal is relatively common (Smolak & Murnen, 2011). Observe for bruising, lacerations, lesions, or evidence of infection. Visual inspection of the external genitalia may reveal clitoral hypertrophy and other signs of androgen excess (Kathiresan, Carr, & Attia, 2011). The pelvic examination is helpful in identifying whether the genital anatomy is normal, the outflow tract is patent, and estrogen depletion is present.

A speculum examination enables observation of the vagina and cervix for evidence of infection, trauma, or foreign objects. Cervical cultures to rule out infection and cervical cancer screening (if indicated) should be obtained at this time. Clinicians caring for young or developmentally disabled clients who are not sexually active but who require a pelvic examination to rule out the cause of the abnormal bleeding should use a pediatric speculum, inserting it with great care and gentleness. Rarely, a pelvic examination in these instances may need to be done under anesthesia if the woman is too uncomfortable, either physically or emotionally. A bimanual examination provides the opportunity to assess for the presence of tumors, cervical polyps, ovarian cysts, uterine tenderness or enlargement, and adnexal pain or masses. If the bimanual examination is performed on a young adolescent, the clinician should use only one digit and, again, proceed with great care and gentleness.

Laboratory and Diagnostic Testing

Laboratory tests used to diagnose AUB can be invasive and expensive. Decisions regarding which tests to perform should be based on the differential diagnosis and directed by the information collected during the history and physical examination, including the woman's age and her reproductive status (**Table 24-3**).

General tests to consider for all types of AUB include the following:

1. A pregnancy test (if the woman is of child-bearing age):
   - Qualitative urine human chorionic gonadotropin (hCG).

- Serial serum quantitative β-hCG to diagnose specific pregnancy disorders.
2. Complete blood count (CBC):
   - Order if indicated or anemia is suspected.
3. Thyroid-stimulating hormone (TSH):
   - Order especially if hypothyroidism or hyperthyroidism or other thyroid abnormality is suspected.
4. Prolactin level:
   - Order if the woman reports headaches and has galactorrhea and/or peripheral vision changes.

| TABLE 24-3 | Laboratory Testing for Abnormal Uterine Bleeding |

Test	Differential Diagnosis	Abnormal Results
Qualitative urine: hCG	Pregnancy; threatened, missed, or incomplete spontaneous abortion	May be positive or negative
Quantitative serum hCG	Ectopic pregnancy or impending spontaneous abortion	Level lower than expected for gestational age, lack of significant increase in 48 hours and/or plateauing
CBC with platelets	Anemia	Hemoglobin < 10 mg/dL
	Clotting abnormalities	Platelets < 150,000 cells/mm^3
PT, aPTT, bleeding time	Von Willebrand's disease, leukemia, prothrombin deficiency	Increased bleeding time
Serum iron/ferritin	Iron-deficiency anemia secondary to bleeding	Decreased levels
FSH	Amenorrhea due to menopause; premature ovarian failure	Levels > 30 mIU/mL, some texts cite 40 mIU/mL
Progesterone	Anovulatory	Levels < 10 ng/mL
TSH	Hypothyroidism or hyperthyroidism	Levels < 0.8 or > 4.0
Papanicolaou (Pap) test	Dysplasia; carcinoma	Atypical cells suggestive of dysplasia and/or carcinoma
Prolactin	Pituitary adenoma	Levels > 100 ng/mL
Cultures and/or microscopic examination of vaginal secretions	Vaginal infection (e.g., gonorrhea, chlamydia, trichomoniasis, vulvovaginal candidiasis)	Positive test or microscopy (see Chapters 20 and 21)

Abbreviations: aPTT, activated partial thromboplastin time; CBC, complete blood count; FSH, follicle-stimulating hormone; hCG, human chorionic gonadotropin; PT, prothrombin time; TSH, thyroid-stimulating hormone.

5. Papanicolaou test (unless the woman is younger than age 21 per current cervical screening guidelines).
6. Nucleic acid amplification test (NAAT) for gonorrhea and chlamydia if the woman is sexually active.
7. Microscopic examination of vaginal secretions with normal saline and potassium hydroxide.
8. Coagulation studies if there is suspicious history of bleeding or easy bruising; unexplained menorrhagia.
   - Include both a prothrombin time (PT) and an activated partial thromboplastin time (aPTT).
9. A serum progesterone if the menstrual history does not indicate whether the woman is ovulating. Obtain between cycle days 22 and 24.

Additional tests should be ordered only for specific indications (**Table 24-4**). For example, if the woman says she is experiencing heavy bleeding, is passing clots greater than 1 inch in diameter, and has to change her pads or tampons frequently, particularly during the night, a serum ferritin test should be considered.

Although menstrual history alone is often sufficient to make the diagnosis of AUB, after organic, systemic, and iatrogenic causes are ruled out, other diagnostic tests may be required for definitive diagnosis of endometrial pathology. If a woman is experiencing AUB-O and is older than 45 years of age, then endometrial biopsy and pelvic sonography are recommended (American College of Obstetricians and Gynecologists, 2013b). If she is younger than 45 years and has a history of unopposed estrogen exposure, failed medical management, and persistent AUB, then an endometrial biopsy should also be performed (American College of Obstetricians and Gynecologists, 2013b).

TABLE 24-4 Differential Diagnosis and Laboratory Assessment of Abnormal Uterine Bleeding

To Rule Out . . .	Laboratory Tests to Order
Endocrine causes of AUB	General labs + prolactin, FSH and LH levels (if premature ovarian failure is suspected)
Adrenal causes (see Chapter 25)	General labs + adrenal studies, testosterone levels Adjunct: CT scan of abdomen, cortisol levels
Hormone-producing tumor	General labs + MRI, CT scan, cortisol levels
Structural abnormalities	General labs + ultrasound
Infection	General labs + gonorrhea and chlamydia tests + wet mount; consider need for WBC
Cervical or uterine pathology	General labs + colposcopy with biopsy; endometrial biopsy; hysteroscopy
Amenorrhea	General labs + FSH, LH, prolactin levels, TSH, T_3, and T_4
VWD	Ristocetin cofactor assay
Liver disease	Liver function tests
Renal disease	Renal function tests
Coagulation disorders other than VWD	PTT, PT, assessment of platelet function

Abbreviations: AUB, abnormal uterine bleeding; CT, computed tomography; FSH, follicle-stimulating hormone; LH, luteinizing hormone; MRI, magnetic resonance imaging; PT, prothrombin time; PTT, partial thromboplastin time; T_3, triiodothyronine; T_4, thyroxine; TSH, thyroid-stimulating hormone; VWD, von Willebrand's disease; WBC, white blood cell count.
Data from Fritz, M., & Speroff, L. (2011). *Clinical gynecologic endocrinology and infertility.* Philadelphia, PA: Wolters Kluwer Lippincott Williams & Wilkins.

Transvaginal ultrasonography (abbreviated TVS for transvaginal scan) of the pelvis is one of the first-line diagnostic tools used because it is convenient and reliable for detecting polyps and submucosal fibroids, measuring endometrial thickness, evaluating pregnancy complications, and assessing ovarian masses (Abou-Salem, Elmazny, & El-Sherbiny, 2010). In women who are premenopausal, TVS should be performed between days 4 and 6 of the menstrual cycle. In women who are postmenopausal, this method can reliably measure endometrial thickness and rule out endometrial carcinoma in women with a thin endometrium, defined as 5 mm or less. Endometrial thickness of greater than 5 mm on TVS in a postmenopausal woman warrants follow-up.

An endometrial evaluation in the form of a biopsy should be performed (preferably in the clinician's office) for women ages 30 to 45 with a negative β-hCG who have not responded to medical treatment and should be considered for those ages 19 to 29 (American College of Obstetricians and Gynecologists, 2013b). Women age 45 and older who present with suspected AUB-O should have a β-hCG to rule out pregnancy; if this test is negative, the clinician should follow up with an endometrial biopsy prior to initiating medical management (American College of Obstetricians and Gynecologists, 2013b).

An endometrial biopsy is easily accomplished in the office setting and can be performed by clinicians who have had the education and training required to carry out this test accurately and safely. Endometrial biopsy can be useful in the diagnosis of both ovulatory and anovulatory AUB. It has a high overall accuracy in diagnosing endometrial cancer if an adequate specimen is obtained; however, this procedure can also miss the cancer if less than 50% of the surface area of the endometrium is occupied by the cancer (American College of Obstetricians and Gynecologists, 2012, reaffirmed 2014). Essentially, a positive endometrial biopsy is more reliable than a negative one. Endometrial biopsy can also sometimes miss fibroids and polyps; thus, if these growths are suspected or need to be ruled out, imaging should be done. Use of additional evaluative methods such as transvaginal ultrasonography, sonohysterography, or office hysteroscopy is suggested when the endometrial biopsy returns an insufficient tissue sample, is nondiagnostic, or cannot be performed (American College of Obstetricians and Gynecologists, 2012, reaffirmed 2014).

Hysteroscopy is highly accurate in diagnosing endometrial cancer because it allows for direct visualization of the endometrial cavity and permits the clinician to take directed biopsies (American College of Obstetricians and Gynecologists, 2012, reaffirmed 2014). Saline infusion sonohysterography (SIS) may offer an even more complete evaluation of the endometrium, but cannot be undertaken if the woman has an IUD in place. A study comparing the diagnostic accuracy of TVS and SIS in the evaluation of the endometrial cavity in women who were premenopausal ($n = 100$) and women who were postmenopausal ($n = 33$) found that the sensitivity and specificity of TVS in diagnosing endometrial pathologies were 83% and 70.6%, respectively, whereas the sensitivity and specificity of SIS in the diagnosis were 97.7% and 82.4%, respectively (Erdem, Bilgin, Bozkurt, & Erdem, 2007). The sensitivity and specificity of SIS in the diagnosis of endometrial polyps were 100% and 91.8%, respectively (Erdem et al., 2007). These findings suggest that SIS is more accurate than TVS alone when used to evaluate the endometrial cavity of women with AUB. Women should be instructed to take an anti-inflammatory such as ibuprofen prior to undergoing SIS to reduce the cramping associated with this procedure.

Magnetic resonance imaging (MRI) and computed tomography (CT) scan may be used to diagnose adnexal masses, adenomyosis, uterine fibroids, and pituitary adenomas. The costs of these technologies may be considered excessive, however, if other types of evaluation methods would provide the same information (American College of Obstetricians and Gynecologists, 2012, reaffirmed 2014; Fritz & Speroff, 2011). MRI should be ordered if ovarian or endometrial cancer is suspected.

As mentioned earlier, none of these diagnostic tests is generally necessary for evaluation of a woman with anovulatory AUB, because often the menstrual history is sufficient for making a diagnosis. Nevertheless, an endometrial biopsy or hysteroscopy should always be included in the assessment of abnormal bleeding in women who are perimenopausal, those who are postmenopausal, obese adolescents with long-term (3 or more years) unexplained abnormal bleeding, or any woman whose endometrium has been exposed to unopposed estrogen.

MANAGEMENT

Management goals for treating AUB are to (1) normalize the bleeding, (2) correct any anemia, (3) prevent cancer, and (4) restore quality of life. The clinician should always consider the woman's choice of treatment when developing a plan of care. Concomitant therapy may be necessary to achieve these goals, particularly if the bleeding is severe and threatens hemodynamic stability. For example, a woman who presents with severe bleeding from a raw and denuded endometrium may require high-dose estrogen to stop the bleeding. Estrogen therapy will provide rapid growth of a denuded endometrium. Once the acute bleeding is under control, additional treatment options such as oral contraceptives, use of the levonorgestrel intrauterine system, and progestin therapy (among others) are available for long-term treatment (American College of Obstetricians and Gynecologists, 2012, reaffirmed 2014). If testing reveals that the woman is anemic because of the bleeding, she will need iron therapy.

Age, desire for future fertility, and the woman's preferences all need to be considered when determining treatment options for women with AUB. Treatment falls into two categories: treatment of acute bleeding and treatment of chronic bleeding. Women who present with excessive HMB and who have a dangerously low hematocrit require physician consultation. All episodes of acute hemorrhagic bleeding should be managed by a physician in a hospital setting. Usually intravenous estrogen therapy is instituted in such cases. Following intravenous administration of estrogen, high-dose estrogen therapy should be continued orally, tapering to once daily when bleeding is under control and adding a progestogen such as medroxyprogesterone acetate (Fritz & Speroff, 2011). This same treatment is effective for the woman whose bleeding is acute but not yet considered an emergency.

Pharmacologic Management of Acute Non-Life-Threatening Heavy Menstrual Bleeding

A variety of pharmacologic choices are available for women with HMB, including combined oral contraceptives (COCs), progestogen-only therapy, and levonorgestrel-releasing intrauterine devices

(Schuiling & Brucker, 2011). **Table 24-5** describes medical therapies for HMB.

Estrogen Therapy

If a significantly denuded endometrium is suspected as the cause of the heavy bleeding, then administration of high-dose estrogen usually will stop the bleeding and allow for further evaluation. Estrogen therapy stimulates rapid endometrial proliferation and resolves the bleeding from a denuded endometrium (Fritz & Speroff, 2011). Concomitant use of antiemetics is indicated when high-dose estrogen is administered because of the nausea that often accompanies its use. The clinician needs to be mindful that estrogens—particularly high-dose estrogens—may precipitate thromboembolism and, therefore, are contraindicated in women with a history of thrombosis, other coagulopathies, or family history of idiopathic venous thromboembolism. Conjugated equine estrogens (Premarin) 2.5 mg every 6 hours can be given until the bleeding decreases or subsides, although therapy should not continue past 25 days. After estrogen therapy has been completed, a progesterone such as medroxyprogesterone acetate 10 mg should be given for 10 days.

Combined Oral Contraceptives

For a woman who is hemodynamically stable, a monophasic COC administered twice daily should also result in the reduction of bleeding within 24 hours. If the flow does not stop with 48 hours, further evaluation is indicated. The COC is typically tapered to once daily after 5 to 7 days and continued with 21 days of active pills, followed by 7 days of placebo pills or no pills. An alternative to the 21/7-day cycle is an extended regimen of 84 days of monophasic COCs followed by a 7-day pill-free interval (Schuiling & Brucker, 2011). When the bleeding stops, 2.5 mg of conjugated equine estrogen (CEE; Premarin) can be administered daily, followed by the addition of 10 mg of medroxyprogesterone acetate (MPA; Provera), taken during the last 10 days of therapy to initiate withdrawal bleeding.

Progestogen Therapy

Progestogens can be used to treat chronic heavy bleeding that is due to anovulation (**Box 24-2**). An endometrial biopsy should be repeated within 3 to 6 months once treatment has been initiated to be certain there is no longer endometrial hyperplasia

TABLE 24-5	Medical Therapies for Heavy Menstrual Bleeding
Acute Bleeding: Estrogen Therapy[a]	• Replenish intravascular volume • CEE 25 mg IV q 4–6 h as needed, then CEE 2.5 mg–5 mg PO 4×/day for 2–3 days, then add MPA 10 mg for 10–14 days (continue CEE) • COCs 2×–3×/day, then taper
Acute Bleeding: Progestin Therapy	• (Use only if endometrium is normal or increased in thickness. Treatment should continue for 3 weeks, decreasing to once-daily treatment after 7–10 days.) • Medroxyprogesterone acetate 10–20 mg 2×/day or • Megestrol 20–40 mg 2×/day or • Norethindrone 5 mg 2×/day
Acute Prolonged Bleeding: Estrogen–Progestin Therapy	• Any monophasic COC beginning with 1 pill 2×/day, decreasing to 1 pill daily. Continue treatment for a minimum of 2 weeks.
Long-term/Chronic Management	• Cyclic MPA 10 mg/day for 10–14 days, every 30–40 days • Combined contraceptives (oral, patch, ring) • Oral micronized progesterone 300 mg for 10–14 days, every 30–40 days • Depo medroxyprogesterone acetate (Depo-Provera) 150 mg IM every 3 months • LNG-IUS (Mirena) • NSAIDs • Tranexamic acid

Note: High doses of estrogen may precipitate a thrombotic event and, therefore, are contraindicated in women with a history of thrombosis or a family history of idiopathic venous thromboembolism. Also, warn the woman using progestin therapy that withdrawal of progestin will result in heavy menses. In women who desire contraception, treatment with an estrogen–progestin contraceptive is a better choice (Fritz & Speroff, 2011).
Abbreviations: CEE, conjugated equine estrogen; COC, combined oral contraceptive; LNG-IUS, levonorgestrel intrauterine system; MPA, medroxyprogesterone acetate; NSAIDs, nonsteroidal anti-inflammatory drugs; OCP, oral contraceptive pill .
[a] High-dose estrogen often causes nausea; therefore, concurrent treatment with an antiemetic is recommended.

BOX 24-2 Progestogen Therapy for Chronic Anovulation

• Medroxyprogesterone acetate (Provera) 10 mg × 10 days
• Norethindrone 5 mg 2×/day × 10 days
• Oral micronized progesterone (Prometrium) 200 mg/day × 10 days
• Depo medroxyprogesterone acetate (Depo-Provera) 150 mg IM every 12 weeks
• Levonorgestrel-releasing intrauterine system (LNG-IUS; Mirena, Skyla)

(Sweet et al., 2012). Women with chronic menorrhagia can be offered cyclic MPA at doses of 10 mg/day for 10 to 14 days, with the therapy being repeated every 30 to 40 days. Oral micronized progesterone (Prometrium) 200 mg should be taken at night due to its potential to induce fatigue. Use Prometrium with caution in women with peanut allergies, as peanut oil is used in the manufacturing process.

Progestogens are not as effective as estrogen in stopping acute bleeding, but are effective for long-term treatment once the acute bleeding episode has been resolved. Additionally, progestogens may be the management regimen of choice if the woman has contraindications to taking estrogen.

To induce normal bleeding, a progestogen is given for 7 to 12 days each month. Withdrawal bleeding should occur within 2 to 7 days of discontinuing the progestogen. If bleeding fails to occur or if irregular bleeding persists, diagnostic reevaluation is necessary and physician consultation is recommended. Do not use progestogen therapy if the woman thinks she might be pregnant, even if her pregnancy test is negative.

If the woman has no contraindications to their use, intrauterine devices containing levonorgestrel are a particularly effective therapy for HMB caused by fibroids (see Chapter 11 for more information on intrauterine devices). Women with fibroids are candidates for the LNG-IUS if the fibroid does not distort the uterine cavity and the uterus is less than 12 weeks' gestation in size.

Gonadotropin-Releasing Hormone Agonists

Gonadotropin-releasing hormone agonists (GnRHas) such as leuprolide acetate (Lupron), nafarelin acetate (Synarel), and goserelin acetate (Zoladex) may be used for a short period of time while a woman is awaiting surgical treatment for her heavy bleeding. Because GnRHas have many side effects related to estrogen deficiency, they are not considered for long-term treatment (Willemsen, Elleri, Williams, Ong, & Dunger, 2014). GnRHa use in women who are anemic needs to be carefully considered. GnRHa therapy is also quite expensive—another reason for using it on only a short-term basis. Nevertheless, these agents are very effective in stemming the bleeding with resultant amenorrhea. In the interim, the woman's hemoglobin has time to rise, thereby optimizing surgical outcomes.

Nonhormonal Pharmacologic Management for Acute Heavy Menstrual Bleeding

Nonsteroidal anti-inflammatory drugs are useful for ovulatory–idiopathic HMB. The heavier the bleeding, the better the effectiveness of NSAIDs, although their mechanism of action in curtailing HMB remains poorly understood. It is suspected that the NSAIDs interfere with the transformation of arachidonic acid to cyclic endoperoxidases, thereby blocking the production of prostaglandins. Because they can also be an effective treatment for dysmenorrhea, NSAIDs may be a good option for women who have both HMB and painful menstrual bleeding. Optimally, an NSAID should be initiated 3 days

---

> **BOX 24-3** **NSAID Therapy for Heavy Menstrual Bleeding**
>
> - Mefanamic acid 500 mg 3×/day[a]
> - Ibuprofen 600 mg 3×/day
> - Naproxen sodium 550 mg loading dose, then 275 mg every 6 hours
>
> [a] FDA approved.

---

prior to the start of menses, although some experts suggest waiting until the onset of menses to start treatment (Schuiling & Brucker, 2011). All NSAIDs are contraindicated in women with ulcers or bronchospastic lung disease. **Box 24-3** identifies NSAIDs that are commonly used to manage HMB.

In 2009, tranexamic acid (Lysteda), an antifibrinolytic agent that reduces menstrual bleeding by 45% to 60%, was approved in the United States for the treatment of heavy bleeding (Fritz & Speroff, 2011). This drug is particularly useful as a second-line option for women who cannot or do not wish to use hormonal options ("New Option," 2010; "Pharmacological Treatment," 2008). It is also effective in managing the severe bleeding that accompanies von Willebrand's disease. Tranexamic acid treatment results in a significant reduction in blood loss when compared to placebo (Lukes et al., 2010). A concern with use of this therapy is venous thromboembolism (VTE). Cases of venous and arterial thrombosis have been reported while using tranexamic acid, as have arterial and venous retinal occlusions (Tengborn, Blomback, & Berntorp, 2015). Use of tranexamic acid is contraindicated in women with a history or who are at risk of thrombosis. The prescribed dose is 1,300 mg taken 3 times daily for a maximum of 5 days per menstrual cycle. Side effects are rare but include nausea and leg cramps.

Surgical Management of Heavy Menstrual Bleeding

When medical therapy fails, surgical management options for HMB include D & C, endometrial ablation, uterine artery embolization, and hysterectomy. In the presence of a thin endometrium, medical therapy for excessive uterine bleeding is reasonable.

Although D & C is the quickest way to stop acute bleeding, the choice of surgical modality is based on a number of factors, including the woman's initial response to medical management and her desire for future fertility (American College of Obstetricians and Gynecologists, 2013b). D & C is a temporary measure and not considered a long-term treatment for HMB (Duckitt & Collins, 2012).

Endometrial Ablation
Endometrial ablation was introduced in the 1990s as an alternative to hysterectomy. A less invasive operative procedure, it results in destruction of the endometrium using heated fluid (either contained within a balloon or circulating freely within the uterine cavity), tissue freezing, microwave, or radiofrequency electricity (American College of Obstetricians and Gynecologists, 2007a, reaffirmed 2015). Endometrial ablation should not be performed on a woman who desires to maintain her fertility. A potential issue with this therapeutic approach is that methods of screening for endometrial cancer post ablation, such as endometrial biopsy, may be challenging (American College of Obstetricians and Gynecologists, 2007a, reaffirmed 2015). Women at risk for endometrial cancer should be counseled prior to endometrial ablation about this potential risk.

Several devices can be used to perform uterine ablation. The most commonly employed is a modified urological resectoscope that uses radiofrequency current (American College of Obstetricians and Gynecologists, 2007a, reaffirmed 2015). The types of electrodes used range from loop electrodes to grooved or spiked electrodes, all of which serve to destroy the endometrium and cause coagulation of adjacent tissues (American College of Obstetricians and Gynecologists, 2007a, reaffirmed 2015).

Nonresectoscopic systems destroy the endometrium using various devices and techniques. Cryotherapy essentially freezes the endometrial tissues. The application of heated free fluid (as is used in the Hydro ThermAblator) achieves endometrial ablation with heated normal saline (American College of Obstetricians and Gynecologists, 2007a, reaffirmed 2015) and results in tissue necrosis. Hysteroscopic monitoring enables the clinician to visualize the progress during the procedure.

Two approved ablation devices employ microwaves; one is disposable, while the other is reusable. The probe used in this technique transmits information about the temperature of the surrounding tissues back to the control module.

The NovaSure system (**Figure 24-2**) uses radiofrequency electricity; its probe also provides a feedback system to monitor the endometrial cavity. A NovaSure ablation can be performed in the hospital or office setting and is usually performed with conscious sedation. This procedure is fairly simple to perform:

1. The microarray expands to the shape of the uterus (Hologic, n.d.).
2. The NovaSure system performs a safety test to assess the integrity of the endometrial cavity (Hologic, n.d.).
3. The NovaSure system results in electrosurgical vaporization and desiccation of endometrial tissues in approximately 90 seconds (American College of Obstetricians and Gynecologists, 2007b, reaffirmed 2009).

FIGURE 24-2 **NovaSure endometrial ablation.**

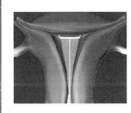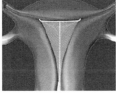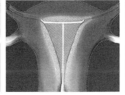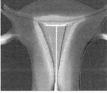

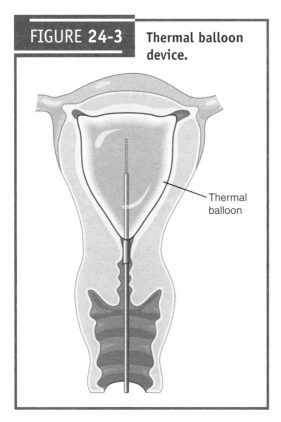

FIGURE 24-3 **Thermal balloon device.**

Thermal balloon

4. The electrode array is then retracted and removed.

The woman is then observed for a short time and is usually sent home the same day.

The thermal balloon (**Figure 24-3**) is a probe with a balloon tip; this tip is extended with heated fluid, which then results in destruction of the endometrium.

Complications, although rare, have been associated with resectoscopic ablation devices, including distention media fluid overload, with the excess fluid being absorbed into the systemic circulation and causing hyponatremia, hyposmolality, brain edema, permanent neurologic damage, and death (American College of Obstetricians and Gynecologists, 2007a, reaffirmed 2015). Other potential complications include uterine trauma due to cervical injury or perforation of the uterus during the procedure, burns to the vagina and vulva, post-ablation tubal ligation syndrome, and pregnancy

complications. Although pregnancy after ablation is rare, it does occur; thus endometrial ablation should not be considered a sterilization procedure. Women who become pregnant post endometrial ablation and elect to continue the pregnancy have a high rate of malpresentation, prematurity, placenta accreta, and perinatal mortality (American College of Obstetricians and Gynecologists, 2007a, reaffirmed 2015). Complications associated with use of nonresectoscopic devices are rarer than those with use of resectoscopic devices.

Some authorities do not recommend ablation in women 50 years or older because of the increased risk of endometrial cancer in this age group. This guideline is a subject of debate, however, and no consensus of opinion on this topic has been achieved as yet. Women with abnormal bleeding who are considering ablation should undergo hysteroscopy before ablation to rule out the presence of endometrial disease. Use of endometrial ablation for AUB is limited to women who meet very specific candidate criteria (**Table 24-6**).

Uterine Artery Embolization
Because 20% to 50% of all women have fibroids, uterine artery embolization was introduced as a surgical intervention that addresses fibroids and may provide relief from HMB. Typically uterine artery embolization is performed as an overnight hospital procedure by a radiologist. The objective is to occlude blood flow to the fibroids, shrinking the fibroids and decreasing their associated symptoms (Goodwin & Spies, 2009). Uterine artery embolization may be an option for women who desire to retain their fertility (American College of Obstetricians and Gynecologists, 2007a, reaffirmed 2015). Women considering a pregnancy after this procedure, however, should be counseled that there may be a higher rate of miscarriage and pregnancy complications (Goodwin & Spies, 2009). If the indication for this intervention is fibroids, myomectomy may result in improved fertility (Gupta, Sinha, Lumsden, & Hickey, 2014). Women should be counseled that they will have moderate to intense cramping and light vaginal bleeding for about a week after treatment. They should expect to see an improvement in menstrual bleeding approximately two to three months after the uterine artery embolization.

TABLE 24-6	Candidates and Contraindications for Endometrial Ablation

Candidates	Contraindications
Cancer has been ruled out	Known or suspected uterine cancer
No previous myomectomy	Uterine hyperplasia
Nondistorted uterine cavity	Thin myometrium
Completed childbearing	Intrauterine device
Refractory to medical therapy	Pregnancy
	Previous classical cesarean birth
	Pelvic, uterine, cervical, or vaginal infection
	Uterus sounds to < 4 cm or uterus sounds outside of the device parameter
	Disorders of Müllerian fusion or absorption

Data from American College of Obstetricians and Gynecologists. (2007a, reaffirmed 2015). ACOG Practice Bulletin No. 81: Endometrial ablation. *Obstetrics & Gynecology, 109*, 1233–1248.

Hysterectomy

Each year, more than 600,000 women in the United States have a hysterectomy (Wright et al., 2013). This procedure should be reserved as the last resort for women who experience ongoing HMB that has not resolved with other treatments and who do not wish to preserve their fertility (Sweet et al., 2012). Advantages of hysterectomy have been reported, including improved quality of life, but postoperative morbidity, including postsurgical fatigue, weight change, and changes in sexual satisfaction, are widespread.

Women facing the decision to undergo hysterectomy, as with all surgeries, want their clinician to provide them with full information about the physical and emotional effects of the procedure and potential body image issues that may arise, including those related to perceptions of sexuality and femininity.

Alternative Treatments for Heavy Menstrual Bleeding

A systematic review of Chinese herbal medicine (CHM) as compared to conventional Western medicine was performed to determine the efficacy and safety of using CHM for AUB. Four randomized clinical trials (RCTs) involving 452 women were reviewed. The conclusion was that all but one of the RCTs had methodological problems that rendered their findings unsuitable for use as evidence for practice (Tu, Huang, & Tan, 2009). No adverse effects with the use of CHM were identified, however, and findings in one of the trials that used an appropriate methodology suggest that CHM may be effective. More research is needed in this area.

It is common for women in Iran to use purslane to treat symptoms of AUB. Purslane seeds are obtained from the purslane plant. These seeds are washed, dried, and ground into a powder, which is then distributed in 5-gm bags. The powder is mixed in hot water (sugar is often added) and taken orally every 4 hours, beginning 48 hours after the start of the menses and continuing for 3 days. To date, one small study of this therapy has been conducted (*n* = 10), in which 8 of 10 participants reported an improvement in symptoms (Shobeiri, Sharei, Heidari, & Kianbakht, 2009). There were no adverse effects, and there are no known risks associated with purslane. Until further studies confirm this therapy's efficacy, women should be counseled that it may be beneficial but that studies are lacking.

EVIDENCE FOR PRACTICE

Level I evidence consistently demonstrates that the treatment of choice for abnormal uterine bleeding is pharmacologic treatment with combined contraceptives. Cyclic progestogens also work well

(American College of Obstetricians and Gynecologists, 2013b). Recommendations that are based primarily on consensus and expert opinion (Level III) are as follows: Underlying coagulopathies should be considered in all women (particularly adolescents) with abnormal bleeding if the bleeding does not respond to treatment and is not able to be explained. The efficacy of using CEE therapy in anovulatory bleeding is based on limited evidence, but this strategy is effective in controlling the abnormal bleeding (American College of Obstetricians and Gynecologists, 2013b).

DIAGNOSIS AND MANAGEMENT OF AMENORRHEA

While outflow tract abnormalities due to abnormal development of the Müllerian duct are uncommon, they should be considered in primary amenorrhea if the cervix is not visible or if the vagina is not patent. Obstruction of the vagina in the presence of a bulging, bluish-colored membrane indicates imperforate hymen. An obstructed bimanual examination warrants referral and follow-up for the possibility of either a vaginal septum or blind pouch.

Ovarian function abnormalities are the most common cause of amenorrhea, and estrogen production is the most reliable measure of ovarian function (Fritz & Speroff, 2011). Laboratory tests to assess estrogen production include serum estradiol levels, progestogen challenge test, measurement of endometrial thickness, and serum FSH concentration. A random serum estradiol level that is greater than 40 pg/mL indicates functioning ovaries. If the level is low, the woman may be amenorrheic because of ovarian failure or have hypothalamic amenorrhea.

A progesterone challenge test that produces withdrawal bleeding is indicative of functioning ovaries, because bleeding will occur only if a sufficient amount of circulating estrogen is present. A progesterone challenge can be accomplished by administering micronized progesterone (Prometrium) 400 mg daily for 7 to 10 days or medroxyprogesterone acetate (Provera) 10 mg daily for 7 to 10 days. Withdrawal bleeding should occur within 7 to 10 days after the progesterone is discontinued if the level of endogenous estrogen is appropriate to produce a withdrawal bleed and the outflow tract is patent. If the

woman chooses to use micronized progesterone, it is suggested that she take this medication at bedtime, because it can cause drowsiness in some women. If the response to the progesterone challenge is positive (withdrawal bleeding occurs), the woman does not have galactorrhea, and her prolactin level is normal, the possibility of a pituitary tumor is effectively ruled out (Fritz & Speroff, 2011). In this case, the diagnosis is anovulation, and the treatment is a progestogen for the first 10 days of each month or a combined contraceptive (pill, patch, or vaginal ring). The woman should also be evaluated for PCOS. If the woman does not have a positive progestogen challenge, then a physician consult is warranted for further evaluation and management options.

Serum FSH indirectly measures ovarian function, with lower levels of FSH indicating normally functioning ovaries. In contrast, an elevated result may indicate ovarian function disorder or disease and warrants further investigation. If the aforementioned tests reveal that the ovaries are producing estrogen and the FSH level is normal, the diagnosis is chronic anovulation (Fritz & Speroff, 2011).

Thyroid disease and hyperprolactinemia are also common causes of anovulation. A TSH level can detect either hypothyroidism (TSH is elevated) or hyperthyroidism (TSH is low), both of which can cause amenorrhea. Menstrual cycles almost always return to normal once the thyroid level is normalized.

Hyperprolactinemia is not always accompanied by galactorrhea (discharge from the nipples), but can be diagnosed by obtaining a serum prolactin level in women with amenorrhea. Some medications, including antidepressants, opiates, calcium-channel blockers, and estrogens, can cause an elevated prolactin level; therefore, it is important to ask about medications when obtaining the health history. Hyperprolactinemia has many causes (see Chapter 16), but if it and the accompanying amenorrhea cannot be attributed to medication or another condition, then further evaluation to rule out pituitary tumors and hypothalamic mass lesions is necessary (Fritz & Speroff, 2011). A dopamine agonist is the treatment of choice for hyperprolactinemia (Fritz & Speroff, 2011).

Table 24-7 lists the causes of primary and secondary amenorrhea.

TABLE 24-7	Causes of Primary and Secondary Amenorrhea

Primary Amenorrhea	Secondary Amenorrhea
Pregnancy	Pregnancy
Upper genital tract causes	Asherman syndrome
Müllerian agenesis (absence of uterus and vagina, normal secondary sex characteristics)	Cervical stenosis
	Hormonal contraception
Testicular feminization (absence of uterus, blind ending vaginal pouch, normal breast development, scant pubic and axillary hair)	Hyperthyroidism/hypothyroidism
	Polycystic ovary syndrome (PCOS)
	Pituitary tumor
Lower genital tract causes	Premature ovarian failure
Labial agglutination	Menopause
Imperforate hymen	Hypothalamic/central nervous system (CNS)
Transverse vaginal septae	disorders (e.g., lifestyle stress, eating
Hypergonadotropic-hypogonadism	disorder, extreme athleticism)
Follicle-stimulating hormone (FSH) > 40 mIU/L	
Gonadal dysgenesis	
Ovarian enzyme disorder	
Resistant ovarian syndrome	

All women with anovulation require management of this condition: If left untreated, endometrial cancer can occur, regardless of the woman's age. Typically treatment consists of inducing menses using a progestogen such as medroxyprogesterone acetate 5 to 10 mg daily for the first 12 to 14 days of the cycle. It is important for the woman to know she is not protected against pregnancy during this treatment. If she does not have her menses, she should have a pregnancy test if she has engaged in intercourse during the treatment period. Oral contraceptive pills can also be used to induce a menstrual cycle.

Ovarian failure is diagnosed when low estrogen production is identified while the serum FSH is high. Premature ovarian failure can be due to many causes, including genetic conditions. For this reason, Fritz and Speroff (2011) recommend a karyotype test for all women younger than the age of 30 years who have a diagnosis of ovarian failure. Ovarian failure may also be due to autoimmune diseases, particularly Addison's disease. Consequently, it is reasonable to test for anti-adrenal antibodies in women who have premature ovarian failure (Fritz & Speroff, 2011).

MRI assessment is suggested in those instances where there is no clear explanation for either hypogonadism or hyperprolactinemia (Fritz & Speroff, 2011). If no lesions are found, there is no need to perform further pituitary testing, and the diagnosis is functional hypothalamic amenorrhea (Fritz & Speroff, 2011).

Functional hypothalamic amenorrhea is characterized by "the absence of menses due to the suppression of HPOA in which no anatomic organic disease is identified" (Gordon, 2010, p. 365). The typical picture of a woman diagnosed with functional amenorrhea is the adolescent who is underweight, overexercises, and is experiencing a great deal of stress. In this setting, an energy deficit occurs, with a resultant negative impact on the HPOA (Gordon, 2010). Treatment generally focuses on weight gain and exercise reduction, although psychological counseling may also be helpful. A goal of treatment is to offset the bone loss that occurs during the estrogen-deficient periods of time (Gordon, 2010). The underlying pathophysiology of functional hypothalamic amenorrhea is not well understood, however, and more research about this condition is needed.

SPECIAL CONSIDERATIONS

Adolescents

The American College of Obstetricians and Gynecologists Committee on Adolescent Health and the American Academy of Pediatrics encourage using the menstrual cycle as a vital sign because of the important information it provides about overall health (American College of Obstetricians and Gynecologists, 2006, reaffirmed 2009).

Nutrition has a considerable impact on the gynecologic health of adolescents. Adolescent females with eating disorders such as anorexia, bulimia nervosa, or obesity frequently have menstrual abnormalities (Rosenfield, 2013) and, therefore, history and physical assessment are important diagnostic tools in these young women. It is also important for clinicians to make no assumptions about an adolescent's sexual activity. It is essential to question teens about their sexual and gynecologic histories. Confidentiality is an important part of therapeutic interactions with all teens.

Once a thorough history is obtained, decide if a pelvic examination is necessary. The new cervical cytology guidelines do not recommend a Papanicolaou test for any woman younger than age 21 (see Chapter 7). Therefore, a pelvic examination should be done only if there is a specific indication for it, such as infection.

Most adolescents with anovulatory bleeding can be treated with medical therapy (American College of Obstetricians and Gynecologists, 2013b) and nutritional counseling. Teaching women with significant anemia about consumption of a diet rich in iron and folic acid is important, and often a short course of iron supplementation is appropriate (Benjamin, 2009).

Women with Disabilities

Women with physical or mental disabilities and their caregivers may be particularly challenged by menstruation. It is important for the clinician to assess the level of knowledge the adolescent or adult has about her body and about menstruation. Communication should be directed to the adolescent or adult, not to the caregiver (American College of Obstetricians and Gynecologists, 2009b, reaffirmed 2012). It is important to ascertain if

specific concerns need to be addressed. It is also important to use developmentally appropriate education to teach the woman about hygiene, contraception, sexually transmitted infections, and abuse prevention (American College of Obstetricians and Gynecologists, 2009b, reaffirmed 2012).

When the evaluation is complete, communicating with the woman and her parents or caregiver is important. There may be a need to treat dysmenorrhea, or contraception may be desired. If contraception is desired, the level of cognitive disability will help to determine which method might work best. Some contraceptives may not be suggested if the woman is immobile (e.g., those contraceptives that have venous thromboembolism risks associated with their use); therefore, the clinician should assess the risk–benefit profile prior to prescribing any option (American College of Obstetricians and Gynecologists, 2009b, reaffirmed 2012).

If the family or caregiver is requesting a hysterectomy or sterilization procedure for the adolescent, it is important to find out the specific reason for the request. States have different laws about surgical procedures resulting in sterilization of minors (American College of Obstetricians and Gynecologists, 2007b, reaffirmed 2009; 2009b, reaffirmed 2012).

Perimenopause

The incidence of AUB increases as women approach menopause. The onset of anovulatory cycles actually represents a continuation of declining ovarian function. Women should be educated early about health-promoting activities that can offset the risks associated with menopause, such as osteoporosis. They should be encouraged to exercise regularly and modify their diets to include foods rich in iron and calcium; in addition, if they smoke, they should be counseled about quitting (American College of Obstetricians and Gynecologists, 2013b).

Older Women

One of the most important goals in the assessment of AUB is to rule out endometrial cancer, particularly in older women. The risk of developing endometrial cancer increases with age. The overall incidence is 10.2 cases per 100,000 in women aged

---

BOX 24-4 **Risk Factors for Endometrial Cancer**

- Age 40 years or older
- Anovulation
- Polycystic ovary syndrome (PCOS)
- Family history of endometrial cancer
- New onset of heavy irregular bleeding, particularly after menopause
- Nulliparity
- Overweight
- Unopposed estrogen stimulation of endometrium
- Tamoxifen therapy
- Infertility
- Type 2 diabetes

---

19 to 39 years, increasing to 36.5 cases per 100,000 in women aged 40 to 49 years (Albers, Hull, & Wesley, 2004). The American College of Obstetricians and Gynecologists (2013b) recommends endometrial evaluation in women aged 35 years and older who present with abnormal bleeding.

Box 24-4 lists the risk factors for endometrial cancer. Notably, estrogen stimulation resulting in endometrial hyperplasia increases a woman's risk for developing endometrial cancer. Symptoms of endometrial cancer include postmenopausal bleeding; thus all uterine bleeding in a woman who is postmenopausal should be considered cancer until proven otherwise.

Cultural Factors

Culturally, regular menses seems to be an essential part of their health for many women, such that deviations from established regular patterns are often perceived as pathologic (Livingstone & Fraser, 2002). Previous studies have demonstrated that some women will reject modes of contraception that do not produce a regular bleeding cycle (Thomas & Ellerton, 2000), although other studies indicate women are interested in avoiding bleeding (Andrist et al., 2004; Hardy, Hebling, deSousa, Kneuper, & Snow, 2009). It is important for the clinician to listen to the woman who presents with a concern about abnormal bleeding and to ascertain her perception of the bleeding, to learn how her individual culture defines abnormal bleeding, and to learn which modes of management and treatment might be acceptable to her.

CONCLUSION

The clinical management of AUB is complex and requires the clinician to consider not only the physical etiology, but also the individual, emotional, and economic aspects of management. Age, history, and physical examination are reliable tools that suggest etiologic factors. For the clinician, it is essential to always rule out pregnancy first, and to never assume the cause of the bleeding. Be thorough and consider all aspects of the PALM-COEIN classification system. If bleeding persists even in the face of negative or reassuring tests, re-instigate the investigation and consider consultation and referral. Order laboratory tests selectively, and always involve the woman actively in the decision-making process and management plan.

References

Abou-Salem, N., Elmazny, A., & El-Sherbiny, W. (2010). Value of 3-dimensional sonohysterography for detection of intrauterine lesions in women with abnormal uterine bleeding. *Journal of Minimally Invasive Gynecology, 17,* 200–204. doi:10:1016/j .jmig.2009.12.010

Albers, J., Hull, S., & Wesley, R. (2004). Abnormal uterine bleeding. *American Family Physician, 69,* 1915–1926.

American College of Obstetricians and Gynecologists. (2006, reaffirmed 2009). Menstruation in girls and adolescents: Using the menstrual cycle as a vital sign. (ACOG Committee Opinion No. 349). *Obstetrics & Gynecology, 108,* 1323–1328.

American College of Obstetricians and Gynecologists. (2007a, reaffirmed 2015). ACOG Practice Bulletin No. 81: Endometrial ablation. *Obstetrics & Gynecology, 109,* 1233–1248.

American College of Obstetricians and Gynecologists. (2007b, reaffirmed 2009). Sterilization of women, including those with mental disabilities (ACOG Committee Opinion No. 371). *Obstetrics & Gynecology, 110,* 217–220.

American College of Obstetricians and Gynecologists. (2008; reaffirmed 2014). Alternatives to hysterectomy in the management of leiomyomas: ACOG Practice Bulletin No. 96. *Obstetrics & Gynecology, 112,* 387–400.

American College of Obstetricians and Gynecologists. (2009a, reaffirmed 2013). ACOG Practice Bulletin No. 108: Polycystic ovary syndrome. *Obstetrics & Gynecology, 114,* 936–949.

American College of Obstetricians and Gynecologists. (2009b, reaffirmed 2012). Menstrual manipulation for adolescents with disabilities (ACOG Committee Opinion No. 448). *Obstetrics & Gynecology, 114,* 1428–1431.

American College of Obstetricians and Gynecologists. (2012, reaffirmed 2014). Diagnosis of abnormal uterine bleeding in reproductive-aged women: Practice Bulletin No. 128. *Obstetrics & Gynecology, 120,* 197–206.

American College of Obstetricians and Gynecologists. (2013a). Von Willebrand disease in women (ACOG Committee Opinion No. 580). *Obstetrics & Gynecology, 122*(6), 1368–1373.

American College of Obstetricians and Gynecologists. (2013b). ACOG Practice Bulletin No. 136: Management of abnormal uterine bleeding associated with ovulatory dysfunction. *Obstetrics & Gynecology, 122*(1), 176–185.

American College of Obstetricians and Gynecologists. (2014). *Guidelines for women's health care: A resource manual* (4th ed.). Washington, DC: American College of Obstetricians and Gynecologists.

American College of Obstetricians and Gynecologists. (2015). Endometrial cancer: Practice Bulletin No. 149. *Obstetrics & Gynecology, 125,* 1006–1026.

Andrist, L. C., Arias, R. D., Nucatola, D., Kaunitz, A. M., Musselman, B. L., Reiter, S., . . . Emmert, S. (2004). Women's and providers' attitudes toward menstrual suppression with extended use of oral contraceptives. *Contraception, 70,* 359–363.

Benjamin, L. J. (2009). Practice guideline: Evaluation and management of abnormal uterine bleeding in adolescents. *Journal of Pediatric Health, 23,* 189–193.

Bordo, S. (1993). *Unbearable weight: Feminism, Western culture, and the body.* Berkeley, CA: University of California Press.

Cass, I. (2015). Endometrial cancer 2005–2015. Commentary. *ContemporaryOBGYN.net.* Retrieved from http://contemporary obgyn.modernmedicine.com/contemporary-obgyn/news/acog-guidelines-glance-endometrial-cancer

Chimbira, T., Anderson, A., & Turnball, A. (1980). Relation between measured menstrual blood and patient's subjective assessment of loss during bleeding, number of sanitary towels used, uterine weight, and endometrial surface area. *British Journal of Obstetrics & Gynaecology, 87,* 603–609.

Davies, A. J., Anderson, A. B., & Turnball, A. C. (1981). Reduction by naproxen of excessive menstrual bleeding in women using intrauterine devices. *Obstetrics & Gynecology, 57,* 74–78.

Duckitt, K., & Collins, S. (2012). Menorrhagia. *British Medical Journal of Clinical Evidence.* Retrieved from http://www.ncbi.nlm.nih.gov/pmc/articles/PMC3285230

Erdem, M., Bilgin, U., Bozkurt, N., & Erdem, A. (2007). Comparison of transvaginal ultrasonography and saline infusion sonohysterography in evaluating the endometrial cavity in pre- and postmenopausal women with abnormal uterine bleeding. *Menopause, 14,* 846–852.

Ethicon. (2015). Gynecare Thermachoice III uterine balloon therapy system. Retrieved from http://www.ethicon.com/healthcare-professionals/products/uterine-pelvic/endometrial-ablation/gynecare-thermachoice#!science-and-technology

Farrell-Turner, K. A. (2011). Polycystic ovarian syndrome: Update on treatment options and treatment considerations for the future. *Clinical Medicine Insights: Women's Health, 4,* 67–80.

Fritz, M., & Speroff, L. (2011). *Clinical gynecologic endocrinology and infertility.* Philadelphia, PA: Wolters Kluwer Lippincott Williams & Wilkins.

Goodwin, S. C., & Spies, J. B. (2009). Uterine fibroid embolization. *New England Journal of Medicine, 361,* 690–697.

Gordon, C. (2010). Functional hypothalamic amenorrhea. *New England Journal of Medicine, 363,* 365–371.

Gupta, J. K., Sinha, A., Lumsden, M. A., & Hickey, M. (2014). Uterine artery embolization for symptomatic uterine fibroids. *Cochrane Library, 12,* CD005073. doi:10.1002/14651858.CD005073.pub3

Halberg, L., Hogdahl, A., Nillson, L., & Rybo, G. (1966). Menstrual blood loss: A population study. *Acta Obstetrics Gynecology Scandinavia, 44,* 347–351.

Hardy, E., Hebling, E. M., deSousa, M. H., Kneuper, E., & Snow, R. (2009). Association between characteristics of current menses and preference for induced amenorrhea. *Contraception, 80,* 266–269.

Hasson, K. A. (2012). From bodies to lives, complainers to consumers: Measuring menstrual excess. *Social Science & Medicine, 75,* 1729–1738.

Hologic. (n.d.). NovaSure endometrial ablation. Retrieved from http://www.hologic.com/products/intervention-and-treatment/gynecologic-surgery/novasure-endometrial-ablation

International Federation of Gynecology and Obstetrics (FIGO). (2011). FIGO classification system (PALM-COEIN) for causes of abnormal uterine bleeding in nongravid women of reproductive age. *International Journal of Gynecology and Obstetrics, 113,* 3–13. http://dx.doi.org/10.1016/j.ijgo.2010.11.011

Jensen, J. T., Lefebvre, P., Laliberte, F., Sarda, S. P., Law, A., Pocoski, J., & Duh, M. S. (2012). Cost burden and treatment patterns associated with management of heavy menstrual bleeding. *Journal of Women's Health, 21*(5), 539–547.

Kathiresan, A. S. Q., Carr, B. R., & Attia, G. R. (2011). Virilization from partner's use of topical androgen in a reproductive-aged woman. *American Journal of Obstetrics & Gynecology, 205*(3), e3–e4.

Khamees, D., Klima, J., & O'Brien, S. H. (2015). Population screening for von Willebrand's disease in adolescents with heavy menstrual bleeding. *Journal of Pediatrics, 166*(1), 195–197.

Levy, G., Dehaene, A., Laurent, N., Lernout, M., Collient, P., Lucot, J., . . . Poncelet, E. (2013, January). An update on adenomyosis. *Diagnostic and Interventional Imaging, 94*(1), 3–25. doi:10.1016/j.diii.2012.10.012

Livingstone, M., & Fraser, I. (2002). Mechanisms of abnormal uterine bleeding. *Human Reproduction Update, 8*(1), 60–67.

Lukes, A. S., Moore, K. A., Muse, K. N., Gersten, J. K., Hecht, B. R., Edlund, M., . . . Shangold, G. A.. (2010). Tranexamic acid treatment for heavy menstrual bleeding. *Obstetrics & Gynecology, 116,* 865–875.

Munro, M. G., Critchley, H. O. D., Broder, M. S., & Fraser, I. S. (2011). FIGO classification system (PALM-COEIN) for cause of abnormal uterine bleeding in nongravid women of reproductive age. *International Journal of Gynecology & Obstetrics, 113,* 3–13.

Munro, M. G., Critchley, H. O. D., & Fraser, I. S. (2012). The FIGO systems for nomenclature and classification of causes of abnormal uterine bleeding in the reproductive years: Who needs them? *American Journal of Obstetrics & Gynecology, 207*(4), 259–265.

New option available for heavy menstrual bleeding. (2010, March). *Contraceptive Technology,* 30.

Pharmacological treatment of heavy menstrual bleeding varies according to the need for contraception and the presence of haemostatic impairment. (2008). *Drugs & Therapy Perspectives, 24*, 13–16.

Polotsky, A. (2010). Amenorrhea caused by extremes of body mass: Pathophysiology and sequelae. *ContemporaryOBGYN.net*. Retrieved from http://www.modernmedicine.com/modernmedicine/Modern+Medicine+Now/Amenorrhea-caused-by-extremes-of-body-mass-pathoph/ArticleStandard/Article/detail/682086

Rosenfield, R. (2013). Adolescent anovulation: Maturational mechanisms and implications. *Journal of Clinical Endocrinology Metabolism, 98*(9), 3572–3583.

Schuiling, K., & Brucker, M. (2011). Pelvic and menstrual disorders. In T. King & M. Brucker (Eds.), *Pharmacology for women's health* (pp. 916–949). Sudbury, MA: Jones and Bartlett.

Schumacher, U., Schumacher, J., Mellinger, U., Gerlinger, C., Wienke, A., & Endrikat, J. (2012). Estimation of menstrual blood loss volume based on menstrual diary and laboratory data. *BMC Women's Health, 12*, 24. doi:10.1186/1472-6874-12-24

Shobeiri, S. F., Sharei, S., Heidari, A., & Kianbakht, S. (2009). *Portulaca oleracea L.* in the treatment of patients with abnormal uterine bleeding: A clinical trial. *Phytotherapy Research, 23*, 1411–1414.

Smith, R. P. (2015). Managing dysmenorrhea: therapy for pain relief. *Contemporary OBGYN, 60*(4). 18–24.

Smolak, L., & Murnen, S. (2011). Gender, self-objectification and pubic hair removal. *Sex Roles, 65*, 506–517.

Sweet, M. G., Schmidt-Dalton, G. A., Weiss, P. M., & Madsen, K. P. (2012). Evaluation and management of abnormal uterine bleeding in premenopausal women. *American Family Physician, 85*(1), 35–43.

Tavris, C. (1992). *The mismeasure of woman*. New York, NY: Simon & Schuster.

Tengborn, L., Blomback, M., & Berntorp, E. (2015). Tranexamic acid: An old drug still going strong and making a revival. *Thrombosis Research, 135*, 231–242.

Thomas, S., & Ellerton, C. (2000). Nuisance or natural and healthy: Should monthly menstruation be optional for women? *Lancet, 355*, 922–924.

Tu, X., Huang, G., & Tan, S. (2009). Chinese herbal medicine for dysfunctional uterine bleeding: A meta-analysis. *eCAM, 6*, 99–105. doi:10.1093/ecam/nem063

Willemsen, R. H., Elleri, D., Williams, R. M., Ong, K. K., & Dunger, D. G. (2014). Pros and cons of GnRHa treatment for early puberty in girls. *Nature Reviews Endocrinology, 10*(6), 352–363.

Wright, J. D., Herzog, T. J., Tsui, J., Ananth, C. V., Lewin, S. N., Lu, Y., . . . Hereshman, D.L. (2013). Nationwide trends in the performance of inpatient hysterectomy in the United States. *Obstetrics & Gynecology, 122*(201), 233–241.

CHAPTER 25

Hyperandrogenic Disorders

Leslye Stewart Kemp

The editors acknowledge Christine L. Anderson, who was the author of the previous edition of this chapter.

In the past, clinicians often regarded women with hirsutism, acne, alopecia, irregular menses, and other symptoms of hyperandrogenemia as suffering from a cosmetic or reproductive disorder requiring only symptomatic treatment. Fortunately, it is now well understood that the hyperandrogenic state is also associated with cardiometabolic dysfunction and psychological distress. As a result, hyperandrogenism is a driver for dyslipidemias, hypertension, diabetes mellitus, and mood disorders, in addition to infertility/subfertility and clinical signs of hyperandrogenemia. Due to advances in the understanding and management of hyperandrogenic disorders, clinicians now have the opportunity to positively affect the quality and duration of life for women with these conditions by providing screening, treatment, and education.

Hyperandrogenism is both a complex endocrine disorder and a cosmetic problem. The woman with hyperandrogenemia may have multifaceted concerns regarding her general health, sexuality, fertility, appearance, and social acceptance. Given these broad implications, it is important for clinicians to approach a woman who has symptoms of hyperandrogenism with empathy and concern. This chapter reviews the pathophysiology, clinical presentation, diagnostic evaluation, and therapy for hyperandrogenism, with a focus on the most common hyperandrogenic disorder—polycystic ovary syndrome—and its sequelae.

DESCRIPTION OF HYPERANDROGENIC DISORDERS

Scope of the Condition

Hyperandrogenism in reproductive-aged women is most frequently associated with polycystic ovary syndrome (PCOS), the most common endocrinopathy in women in this age cohort. A condition with variable phenotypic expression, PCOS occurs in 6% to 15% of all women, with the prevalence depending on the diagnostic criteria used, and in approximately 70% of women presenting with clinical signs of hyperandrogenism (Azziz et al., 2009; Fauser et al., 2012). Women with PCOS may experience a variety of symptoms, including clinical hyperandrogenism (e.g., hirsutism, acne, and androgenic alopecia), menstrual irregularity, or subfertility/infertility. Women with PCOS also have an increased risk for adverse health outcomes such as endometrial cancer, type 2 diabetes, and cardiovascular disease (Goodarzi, Dumesic, Chazenbalk, & Azziz, 2011; Teede, Deeks, & Moran, 2010). Women with PCOS need to have regular, comprehensive, preventive health care and education to decrease the long-term sequelae associated with this syndrome.

Other causes of hyperandrogenism, such as nonclassical adrenal hyperplasia and androgen-producing tumors, are rarely seen. Nevertheless, they must be included in the diagnostic evaluation of women with hyperandrogenism.

Etiology

Androgen production occurs in the ovaries and adrenal glands, as well as by peripheral conversion in adipose tissue, skin, and the liver. The major circulating androgens in women are dehydroepiandrosterone sulfate (DHEA-S), dehydroepiandrosterone (DHEA), androstenedione, testosterone, and dihydrotestosterone (DHT), which is the active metabolite of testosterone. Testosterone is the most potent androgen. DHEA-S, DHEA, and androstenedione must be converted to testosterone to cause androgenic effects. Women normally produce amounts of testosterone in the range of 0.2 to 0.3 mg per day, 50% of which is derived from the peripheral conversion of androstenedione. The ovaries are the most common source of increased testosterone and androstenedione. By comparison, adrenal causes of excess production of these particular hormones are relatively rare (Fritz & Speroff, 2011).

The bioactivity and androgenicity of testosterone are determined by sex hormone–binding globulin (SHBG). Circulating testosterone is bound to SHBG, which is produced in the liver. It is normal for approximately 80% of circulating testosterone to be bound to SHBG, 19% to be loosely bound to albumin, and the remaining 1% to be left unbound. The unbound, free testosterone is mainly responsible for androgenicity, although the fraction associated with albumin makes some contribution to this condition.

SHBG levels are increased by estrogens and thyroid hormone, and suppressed by androgens and insulin. Therefore, in the presence of high levels of thyroid hormone or estrogen, more testosterone is bound, making less biologically available. If SHBG is suppressed or androgen production increases, the amount of free (unbound) testosterone will increase without necessarily increasing the total testosterone level, and the woman may develop symptoms of hyperandrogenism. Thus, because of the interplay among SHBG, insulin, thyroid hormone, estrogen, and androgen production, the total testosterone concentration may remain in the normal range, with symptoms reflecting only the decreased binding capacity of the SHBG and the increased percentage of unbound testosterone (Fritz & Speroff, 2011).

Although testosterone is the major circulating androgen, DHT is the hormone responsible for the clinical expression of androgen stimulation in many androgen-sensitive tissues, such as the skin, the pilosebaceous unit, and the hair follicles (see **Color Plate 28**). Conversion of testosterone to DHT is accomplished by 5α-reductase, an enzyme that is present in these target tissues. Racial and ethnic differences have been noted both in the number of hair follicles present on the body and in the degree of 5α-reductase activity present in the hair follicles. The sensitivity of the hair follicle to the effect of androgens depends on the degree of 5α-reductase activity and is genetically predetermined. In women who are genetically predisposed to excessive 5α-reductase activity, even normal levels of androgen can stimulate hair growth, leading to idiopathic hirsutism (Fritz & Speroff, 2011).

The symptoms of hyperandrogenism—that is, hirsutism, acne, alopecia, and frequently, anovulation—can all be traced to an increase in androgen levels, a decrease in production of SHBG, or an increase in 5α-reductase activity in the skin and hair follicles that has caused an initial stimulus to androgen-sensitive areas and subsequently acts to sustain continued sensitivity (Fritz & Speroff, 2011). The source of the increased androgen production is the key to determining the cause of hyperandrogenism.

Biochemical Features of Polycystic Ovary Syndrome

The pathogenesis of PCOS is complex and not completely understood, although many hormonal pathways have been identified as contributors to the syndrome. Women with PCOS are predominantly anovulatory, and they typically maintain relatively steady levels of gonadotropins and sex steroids instead of experiencing the fluctuations in these levels characteristic of the normal menstrual cycle. Serum concentrations of luteinizing hormone (LH) are higher than those found in women who ovulate normally. The elevated LH levels are a result of increased pulse frequency and amplitude. Women with PCOS have a relatively constant LH pulse frequency of approximately one pulse per hour, whereas women who are ovulatory experience cyclic variations in LH frequency. The increased LH pulse frequency is caused by increased gonadotropin-releasing hormone (GnRH) pulse frequency, which also causes follicle-stimulating hormone (FSH) levels to be at the low end of the normal range. FSH levels are also decreased because of the increased estrone levels resulting from peripheral conversion of increased androstenedione. Women with PCOS generally exhibit an increased LH:FSH ratio (Fritz & Speroff, 2011).

Most of the increased androgen production seen with PCOS occurs in the ovaries as a result of increased LH stimulation, as increased LH pulse frequency stimulates ovarian theca cell production of androgens (Burt et al., 2012). Many women with PCOS also have some increased androgen production in the adrenal glands. Insulin resistance, which results in compensatory hyperinsulinemia, is common in women with PCOS and can further contribute to hyperandrogenism. Increased insulin levels stimulate androgen production in the ovaries, both in isolation and by potentiating LH, and suppress SHBG production in the liver. A vicious cycle is created in which the elevated androgens and insulin suppress SHBG synthesis, resulting in an increase in free testosterone, which in turn exacerbates the insulin resistance (Fritz & Speroff, 2011). In addition, the lower FSH levels found in women with PCOS impair follicle maturation and ovulation (Burt et al., 2012).

CLINICAL PRESENTATION

Hirsutism

Hirsutism is defined as excessive terminal hair growth in women occurring in anatomic areas where the hair follicles are most androgen sensitive. Androgens cause transformation of fine, soft, unpigmented, vellus hair to coarse, dark, terminal hair in androgen-dependent areas of hair growth (Escobar-Morreale et al., 2012; Goodman et al., 2015a). Hirsutism is present in approximately 70% of women with PCOS (Fauser et al., 2012). Common sites of involvement include the face and chin, upper lip, areolae, lower abdomen, inner thighs, and perineum. The presence of significant amounts of terminal hair in these areas is considered abnormal.

The degree and extent of hirsutism are commonly evaluated using a modified version of the Ferriman–Gallwey scale (Ferriman & Gallwey, 1961; Hatch, Rosenfield, Kim, & Tredway, 1981). See **Color Plate 29** for the scale. Hirsutism is typically defined as a score of 8 or greater on this scale, although the interpretation of scores varies by ethnicity, with scores of 9 or greater for women of Mediterranean descent and 2 or greater for women of Asian descent being used to define hirsutism in these populations (Escobar-Morreale et al., 2012).

Not all women with PCOS have hirsutism. Hirsutism is a product of the interaction between circulating androgens, local androgen concentrations, hormonal variables including insulin resistance, and the sensitivity of hair follicles to androgens. The severity of hirsutism does not correlate with the severity of androgen excess, and women with significant biochemical hyperandrogenemia may present with only mild or no hirsutism (Escobar-Morreale et al., 2012). In addition, use of the Ferriman–Gallwey scale can be limited by the fact that many women who present with hirsutism are already removing excess hair. Assessment of the types and frequency of hair removal methods can be more useful for assessment and follow-up of the response to therapy (Fritz & Speroff, 2011).

Alopecia

In contrast to hirsutism, prolonged exposure to circulating androgens may paradoxically cause hair loss due to miniaturization of androgen-sensitive scalp hair (decreased density) and reduced scalp coverage (decreased volume). This process typically results in diffuse alopecia that includes hair loss at the vertex and crown with preservation of the frontal hairline, although bitemporal and frontal hair loss can be seen with more severe hyperandrogenemia (Goodman et al., 2015a). The majority of women who present with hirsutism will be found to have PCOS, whereas only 10% of women who present with alopecia alone will be found to have PCOS. Thus, isolated alopecia is not a clear marker of hyperandrogenemia (Azziz et al., 2009; Fauser et al., 2012).

Acne

Androgen stimulation of the pilosebaceous unit can cause enlargement of the sebaceous glands and increased secretion of sebum, leading to acne. Acne is a common finding in adolescents and usually regresses by the time affected individuals reach their mid-20s. In contrast, acne that persists beyond this time or that presents when a woman is in her mid-20s or 30s may be considered a sign of hyperandrogenemia, particularly if acne presents with hirsutism or menstrual dysfunction or is treatment resistant (Goodman et al., 2015a).

Virilization

Virilization is characterized by clitoral hypertrophy, severe hirsutism, deepening of the voice, increased muscle mass, breast atrophy, and male pattern baldness. This condition may indicate the presence of one of the less common causes of hyperandrogenism, such as adrenal or ovarian tumor, congenital adrenal hyperplasia, or hyperthecosis. It may also be associated with severe hyperinsulinemia. If the onset of virilization is sudden or the progression is rapid, this condition is particularly concerning for neoplasm (Rosenfield, Barnes, & Ehrmann, 2015).

Menstrual Dysfunction and Infertility

Women with hyperandrogenism may have various degrees of ovulatory dysfunction. Indeed, menstrual irregularity is a hallmark feature of PCOS. Oligomenorrhea (cycle length is 35–199 days) is the most common presentation of overt menstrual dysfunction. Women with PCOS may also present with amenorrhea (cycle length greater than 199 days), and these women have been noted to have more significant endocrinopathies, including more severe hyperandrogenemia, increased serum LH and cortisol levels, and increased incidence of hyperinsulinemia (Burt et al., 2012; Strowitzki, Capp, & von Eye, 2010). More rarely, women with PCOS may present with polymenorrhea, which may induce iron-deficiency anemia (Goodman et al., 2015a). Bleeding is generally irregular and unpredictable, and can be heavy as a result of continuous estrogenic stimulation of the endometrium and resultant endometrial hyperplasia. Typically, menstrual irregularity begins at menarche, but it can occur after regular cycles (Fritz & Speroff, 2011).

Regular menses do not rule out the possibility of oligo-anovulation. Subclinical menstrual dysfunction, in which women have regularly occurring menses but chronic anovulation, is common in individuals with PCOS (Azziz et al., 2009). With either type of menstrual function, women may be unaware of the impending arrival of menses before bleeding begins due to a lack of premenstrual symptoms, which is a clinical indicator of anovulation.

Many women with hyperandrogenism experience infertility as a result of anovulation, although women with PCOS can ovulate intermittently. More than half of women with PCOS are fertile (i.e., they will become pregnant within 12 months of trying), although it may take them longer to conceive (Teede at al., 2010).

Polycystic Ovaries

Since Stein and Leventhal originally described the thickened, glistening, white, enlarged multicystic ovary in 1935, it has been clear that PCOS is associated with a classic ovarian morphology. In women with PCOS, polycystic ovaries are a result of chronic anovulation (Fritz & Speroff, 2011). In 2003, a consensus definition of PCOS was developed at a joint European Society for Human Reproduction and Embryology (ESHRE) and American Society for Reproductive Medicine (ASRM) meeting; this new definition represented a revision of the consensus statement on PCOS sponsored by the National Institutes of Health (NIH) in 1990. At the 2003 meeting, the following description of the morphology of the polycystic ovary was agreed upon: one or both ovaries with 12 or more follicles measuring 2 to 9 mm in diameter and/or increased ovarian volume of more than 10 mL (Balen, Laven, Tan, & Dewailly, 2003). These criteria were based on dated ultrasound technology, but more recent Androgen Excess and PCOS Society guidelines, based on new ultrasound technology, have increased the threshold from 12 follicles to 25 ovarian follicles measuring 2 to 9 mm in the whole ovary (Dewailly et al., 2014; Goodman et al., 2015a).

While the majority of women with PCOS have polycystic ovaries, the presence of this morphology is not required if other diagnostic criteria for the syndrome are met (Azziz et al., 2009). The definition of polycystic ovaries does not apply to women who take combined oral contraceptives (COCs), because COCs modify ovarian morphology. In addition, women who do not meet the diagnostic criteria for PCOS can have polycystic-appearing ovaries on ultrasound (Sirmans & Pate, 2014).

Obesity

Approximately half of women with PCOS are obese, and obesity increases the risk for developing PCOS. Typically the obesity occurs in the abdominal region (android obesity or "apple shape"), with an increase in the waist–hip ratio (WHR), as opposed to the lower body (gynoid obesity or "pear shape"). Obesity is associated with three alterations that interfere with normal ovulation:

- Increased peripheral aromatization of androgens, resulting in chronically elevated estrogen concentrations
- Decreased levels of hepatic SHBG, resulting in increased circulating concentrations of free estradiol and testosterone
- Insulin resistance, leading to a compensatory increase in insulin levels that stimulates androgen production in the ovarian stroma, resulting in high local androgen concentrations that impair follicular development (Fritz & Speroff, 2011, p. 500)

As a result, obesity increases the likelihood of menstrual dysfunction and infertility (Fritz & Speroff, 2011). Women with PCOS who are also obese have been found to have worsened metabolic and reproductive outcomes, including increased testosterone and free androgen index, decreased SHBG, increased fasting glucose and fasting insulin, and a worsened lipid profile (Lim, Norman, Davies, & Moran, 2013). Women with PCOS who are obese are more likely to develop impaired glucose tolerance, type 2 diabetes, hypertension, dyslipidemias, and estrogen-dependent tumors than women with PCOS who are of normal or low weight (Baldani, Skrgatic, & Ougouag, 2015; Goodman et al., 2001).

Insulin Resistance

Approximately 50% to 70% of women with PCOS are insulin resistant—a condition that often results in compensatory hyperinsulinemia (Azziz et al., 2009). Hyperinsulinemia plays a pathogenic role in the etiology of PCOS by stimulating ovarian androgen production and decreasing serum SHBG concentrations. Obesity further complicates the condition by increasing insulin resistance due to excess adiposity (Goodarzi & Korenman, 2003). Insulin resistance occurs in both normal-weight and overweight women with PCOS, but its frequency and magnitude are increased in obese women with PCOS (Moran, Arriaga, Rodriguez, & Moran, 2012). Insulin resistance occurs in 95% of obese women

with PCOS and 30% of lean women with PCOS (Randeva et al., 2012; Wild et al., 2010).

Insulin resistance increases the risk for both impaired glucose tolerance and type 2 diabetes. A systematic review and meta-analysis found that women with PCOS have more than twice the odds of impaired glucose tolerance (odds ratio, 2.48; 95% confidence interval, 1.63–3.77) and more than four times the odds of type 2 diabetes mellitus (odds ratio, 4.43; 95% confidence interval, 4.06–4.82) compared to women without PCOS (Moran et al., 2010). In recognition of this relationship, the American Diabetes Association (2014) has designated PCOS as a nonmodifiable risk factor for type 2 diabetes.

Dyslipidemia

Most women with PCOS (70%) have at least one lipid level that is borderline or high (Azziz et al., 2009). Dyslipidemias commonly found in women with PCOS include decreased high-density lipoprotein (HDL) cholesterol and increased triglycerides, low-density lipoprotein (LDL) cholesterol, and non-HDL lipoproteins, reflecting more arthrogenic apolipoprotein ratios (Burt et al., 2012). While dyslipidemias are typically more severe in women with PCOS who have a higher body mass index (BMI), the prevalence of dyslipidemias is higher in women with PCOS regardless of BMI than in women without PCOS (Wild, Rizzo, Clifton, & Carmina, 2011).

Metabolic Syndrome

Obesity, insulin resistance, and dyslipidemia are part of metabolic syndrome, which is a cluster of risk factors for cardiovascular disease and diabetes (Alberti et al., 2009). Criteria for diagnosing this condition are found in **Box 25-1**. One-third to one-half of women with PCOS have metabolic syndrome (Essah, Wickham, & Nestler, 2007). A systematic review and meta-analysis found that women with PCOS have nearly three times the odds of developing metabolic syndrome (odds ratio, 2.88; 95% confidence interval, 2.40–3.45) compared to women without PCOS (Moran et al., 2010).

Cardiovascular Disease Markers

In addition to an increased risk for insulin resistance, dyslipidemias, obesity, and hypertension, women with PCOS have been found to have an excess of numerous biochemical inflammatory and

BOX 25-1 Diagnostic Criteria for Metabolic Syndrome in Women

Three or more of the following:

- Waist circumference ≥ 88 cm (35 in.)
- Triglycerides ≥ 150 mg/dL or drug treatment for elevated triglycerides
- HDL-C < 50 mg/dL or drug treatment for reduced HDL-C
- Systolic BP ≥ 130 mm Hg and/or diastolic BP of ≥ 85 mm Hg or drug treatment for hypertension
- Fasting glucose ≥ 100 mg/dL or drug treatment for elevated glucose

Abbreviations: BP, blood pressure; HDL-C, high-density lipoprotein cholesterol.
Data from Alberti, K. G. M. M., Eckel, R. H., Grundy, S. M., Zimmet, P. Z., Cleeman, J. I., Donato, K., . . . Smith, S. C. (2009). Harmonizing the metabolic syndrome: A joint statement of the International Diabetes Federation Task Force on Epidemiology and Prevention; National Heart, Lung, and Blood Institute; American Heart Association; World Heart Federation; International Atherosclerosis Society; and International Association for the Study of Obesity. *Circulation, 120,* 1640–1645.

thrombotic markers of cardiovascular disease, including circulating cytokines and pro-arthrogenic factors, such as C-reactive protein, homocysteine, vascular endothelial growth factor, and plasminogen activator inhibitor-1. Women with PCOS have a higher incidence of systemic inflammation associated with endothelial vascular dysfunction, as well as a higher incidence of coronary artery calcification (Burt et al., 2012; Deligeoroglou et al., 2012; Toulis et al., 2011).

Psychological Impact

The expression of hyperandrogenism (hirsutism, alopecia, and acne), the annoyance and unpredictability of irregular menstrual bleeding, and the pain of infertility can have significant negative impacts on a woman's psychological health and well-being. Additionally, the frequent occurrence of obesity with

hyperandrogenism can have a negative effect on self-esteem and self-image. Rates of depressive disorders, anxiety disorders, and binge eating are higher among women with PCOS than among those without the condition (Barry, Kuczmiercyk, & Hardiman, 2011; Veltman-Verhulst, Boivin, Eijkemans, & Fauser, 2012). Moreover, it appears that PCOS is associated with decreased sexual satisfaction and lowered health-related quality of life (Fauser et al., 2012; Mansson et al., 2011).

Cancer Risks

Women with PCOS are at a threefold increased risk of developing endometrial cancer because of chronic, unopposed estrogen stimulation of the endometrium (Haoula, Salman, & Atiomo, 2012). Women who are obese are thought to be at the greatest risk of developing endometrial cancer because the peripheral conversion of androgens to estrogen occurs in adipose tissue (Rotterdam ESHRE/ASRM-Sponsored PCOS Consensus Workshop Group [Rotterdam PCOS Consensus Group], 2004). Although some data collected in earlier studies suggested the possibility of a link between PCOS and ovarian cancer, a recent meta-analysis reveals no increased risk for ovarian or breast cancer in women with PCOS (Barry, Azizia, & Hardiman, 2014).

ASSESSMENT

Women with hyperandrogenism can have a range of clinical manifestations and associated problems. Therefore, appropriate diagnosis, therapeutic management, and follow-up are essential. A thorough history and physical examination will give clues to the etiology of hyperandrogenism.

History

During the history taking, the clinician should ask about the woman's age at thelarche (onset of breast development), adrenarche (onset of pubic hair), and menarche, and the menstrual pattern since menarche. Obtain a complete pregnancy history, including time to conceive and history of miscarriages. Note the age of onset and progression of obesity, hirsutism, seborrhea, acne, and alopecia, along with any treatments for these conditions and their success or failure. If alopecia is present, assess for other causes of hair loss, such as nutritional deficiencies, iron-deficiency anemia, thyroid dysfunction, recent surgery, rapid weight loss, or major illness (Gordon & Tosti, 2011).

A complete medication history is important to seek a pharmacologic cause of the symptoms. Medications that have been associated with hyperandrogenism include testosterone, anabolic steroids, danazol, certain progestins, glucocorticoids, and valproic acid (Brodell & Mercurio, 2010; Rosenfeld et al., 2015).

An especially important component of the history is determining whether the woman has experienced rapid development of symptoms of hirsutism and any rapid progression to virilization over the course of several months. Ask the woman if she has experienced increased libido, increased muscle bulk, voice deepening, breast atrophy, or clitoromegaly. Although rare, these symptoms should raise the suspicion for an androgen-producing tumor (Escobar-Morreale et al., 2012; Fritz & Speroff, 2011).

In addition, assess the woman for polydipsia or polyuria, which suggest glucose intolerance; galactorrhea, visual disturbance, or headache, which are associated with hyperprolactinemia and pituitary tumor; hot or cold intolerance and weight loss or gain, which suggest thyroid dysfunction; and striae, mood changes, easy bruisability, or weight gain, which suggest Cushing syndrome (Schmidt & Shinkai, 2015). Identify cardiovascular and metabolic risk factors, including cigarette smoking, history of hypertension, dyslipidemia, or diabetes mellitus (Wild et al., 2010). Ask about family history of hirsutism, acne, infertility, diabetes mellitus, cardiovascular disease (especially first-degree relatives with premature cardiovascular disease, occurring before age 55 in men and before age 65 in women), dyslipidemia, or obesity (American College of Obstetricians and Gynecologists, 2009, reaffirmed 2015; Wild et al., 2010).

Physical Examination

The physical examination should be geared toward establishing the degree of severity of hyperandrogenism and its related symptoms. In addition to assessing height and weight, measurement of the waist circumference and BMI (see Chapter 6) are important in assessing the degree of obesity in women with hyperandrogenism. It is also important to measure blood pressure, as abnormalities may indicate an increased risk for morbidity and mortality related to the metabolic syndrome (Wilson, 2011).

Conduct a thorough skin examination, paying particular attention to the presence of hirsutism, acne, and alopecia. The pattern of body hair distribution and degree of hirsutism may be evaluated using a grading tool such as the modified Ferriman–Gallwey scale (see **Color Plate 29**). Racial, familial, genetic, and hormonal influences that affect body hair distribution and amount should be considered, however. Northern Europeans, natives of North and South America, and African Americans generally have less hair than persons of Mediterranean descent. East Asians tend to have less hair than Euro-Americans, albeit with no difference in testosterone levels (Escobar-Morreale et al., 2012). In some women, acanthosis nigricans (skin that is velvety, warty, and hyperpigmented), which is associated with insulin resistance, may be present in the neck area or axillae or under the breasts.

Perform a thyroid examination and breast examination to evaluate for thyroid conditions or evidence of galactorrhea. Observe for signs of Cushing syndrome such as moon facies, dorsocervical fat pad (buffalo hump), and abdominal striae. Perform a complete pelvic examination, including evaluation of the clitoris for hypertrophy and bimanual examination to determine the size of the uterus and ovaries as well as the presence of masses (American College of Obstetricians and Gynecologists, 2009, reaffirmed 2015).

Diagnostic Testing

Laboratory tests for women with evidence of hyperandrogenism should be selected based on the individual's history and physical examination. There is some disagreement in the literature regarding which tests are essential and which are superfluous. The following recommendations for laboratory studies to be completed during the initial assessment of hyperandrogenism are based on guidance from the American Association of Clinical Endocrinologists (Goodman et al., 2015a, 2015b), the American College of Endocrinology (Goodman et al., 2015a, 2015b), the American College of Obstetricians and Gynecologists (2009, reaffirmed 2015), the Androgen

Excess and PCOS Society (Azziz et al., 2009; Dewailly et al., 2014; Goodman et al., 2015a, 2015b), the Endocrine Society (Legro et al., 2013), and Fritz and Speroff (2011).

All women who have hyperandrogenism with ovulatory dysfunction should have a serum prolactin, serum thyroid-stimulating hormone (TSH), fasting lipid profile, and 2-hour oral glucose tolerance test (American College of Obstetricians and Gynecologists, 2009, reaffirmed 2015; Fritz & Speroff, 2011; Goodman et al., 2015b; Legro et al., 2013). The prolactin and TSH levels are used to exclude hyperprolactinemia and thyroid disorders, both of which can cause ovulatory dysfunction. The prevalence of dyslipidemias in women with PCOS warrants baseline assessment of a fasting lipid profile. The 2-hour oral glucose tolerance test is used to identify impaired glucose tolerance (i.e., result in the range of 140–200 mg/dL) and diabetes mellitus (i.e., result of 200 mg/dL or greater). Routine screening for insulin resistance is not recommended due to the lack of a uniformly accepted test (Fritz & Speroff, 2011).

Women who have clinical signs of hyperandrogenism with regular menstrual cycles should be evaluated for ovulatory dysfunction by obtaining a serum progesterone level between days 20 and 24 of the menstrual cycle (Azziz et al., 2009; Goodman et al., 2015b; Legro et al., 2013). If this luteal-phase progesterone level is less than 3 ng/mL, the cycle is considered oligo-anovulatory. Repeating the progesterone level during a second cycle can confirm the diagnosis of chronic oligo-anovulation and PCOS.

Routine measurement of androgen levels in women with clinical signs of hyperandrogenism is controversial due to the limitations in accuracy and sensitivity of testosterone assay methods. Given that no standardized assay exists, clinicians must be aware of the type and quality of assay being used as well as the particular laboratory's reference ranges (Goodman et al., 2015a; Legro et al., 2013; Rosner, Auchus, Azziz, Sluss, & Raff, 2007). The American Association of Clinical Endocrinologists, American College of Endocrinology, and Androgen Excess and PCOS Society endorse the assessment of free testosterone levels, which are more sensitive than the measurement of total testosterone when establishing a diagnosis of hyperandrogenemia; however, these organizations recommend that the calculated free testosterone be used if the clinician is uncertain about the quality of free testosterone assay being used, as direct analogue radioimmunoassays for free testosterone are inaccurate, and equilibrium dialysis techniques are the standard for assessing free testosterone (Goodman et al., 2015a). The American College of Obstetricians and Gynecologists (2009, reaffirmed 2015) recommends routine free testosterone measurement either directly by equilibrium dialysis or calculated from high-quality measurements of total testosterone and SHBG. According to Fritz and Speroff (2011), routine testosterone measurement is unnecessary when clinical signs of hyperandrogenism are present. These authors recommend reserving testosterone testing for women who have moderate or severe hirsutism, sudden onset or rapid progression of hirsutism, or signs of virilization, as these findings suggest the presence of an androgen-producing tumor. Women in whom a tumor is suspected should have a serum total testosterone, ideally performed after extraction and chromatography by mass spectrometry or immunoassay rather than on whole serum (Fritz & Speroff, 2011; Rosner et al., 2007). Women with a serum total testosterone level of 150 ng/dL or greater (100 ng/dL or greater in postmenopausal women) need evaluation for an androgen-producing tumor (discussed in detail in the next section on imaging studies). Routine DHEA-S testing is not recommended (American College of Obstetricians and Gynecologists, 2009, reaffirmed 2015; Fritz & Speroff, 2011; Goodman et al., 2015a; Legro et al., 2013).

Measurement of serum 17-hydroxyprogesterone (17-OHP) is performed to assess for nonclassical or "late-onset" congenital adrenal hyperplasia, which is characterized by excessive adrenal androgen production and can present very similarly to PCOS. The American College of Obstetricians and Gynecologists (2009, reaffirmed 2015), the Androgen Excess and PCOS Society (Dewailley et al., 2014), and the Endocrine Society recommend routine 17-OHP testing. According to Fritz and Speroff (2011), routine testing is reasonable, but it is also safe to reserve 17-OHP testing for women who have pre- or peri-menarcheal onset of hirsutism, have a family history of nonclassical congenital adrenal hyperplasia, or are members of a high-risk ethnic group (Hispanic, Mediterranean, Slavic,

Ashkenazi Jew, or Yupik Eskimo). 17-OHP testing is performed in the morning during the follicular phase. Values less than 200 ng/dL exclude the diagnosis of PCOS, whereas values greater than 800 ng/dL establish the diagnosis. Values from 200 to 800 ng/dL warrant referral to an endocrinologist for an adrenocorticotropic hormone (ACTH) stimulation test (Fritz & Speroff, 2011).

The American Association of Clinical Endocrinologists, the American College of Endocrinology, and the Androgen Excess and PCOS Society best practice guidelines endorse the usefulness of anti-Müllerian hormone (AMH) assessment in the diagnosis of PCOS, particularly when no accurate ultrasound is available (Goodman et al., 2015a). AMH levels greater than 4.5 ng/mL are associated with PCOS (Dewailly et al., 2011; Goodman et al., 2015a).

Testing for Cushing syndrome, which results from excess adrenal cortisol secretion, should be reserved for women with symptoms of this condition (American College of Obstetricians and Gynecologists, 2009, reaffirmed 2015; Fritz & Speroff, 2011; Legro et al., 2015). Screening for Cushing syndrome consists of the overnight dexamethasone suppression test, which is performed by giving the woman 1 mg of dexamethasone orally between 11 p.m. and 12 a.m., and then drawing a serum cortisol at 8 a.m. the next morning. Values less than 1.8 mcg/dL are considered normal (Fritz & Speroff, 2011).

Imaging Studies and Endometrial Biopsy

Pelvic ultrasonography can be used to assess for polycystic ovary morphology and identify endometrial hyperplasia in women who are oligomenorrheic or amenorrheic (American College of Obstetricians and Gynecologists, 2009, reaffirmed 2015; Fritz & Speroff, 2011; Goodman et al., 2015b; Legro et al., 2013). Recent guidelines from the Androgen Excess and PCOS Society recommend the use of transvaginal ultrasound with machines using new software for automatic follicle numbering and probes with a frequency of at least 8 mHz for optimal views of ovarian morphology (Dewailly et al., 2014). When this kind of ultrasound technology is used, a threshold of 25 or more follicles of 2 to 9 mm is recommended for a diagnosis of PCO morphology (Dewailly et al., 2014; Goodman et al., 2015a).

An endometrial biopsy is recommended for any woman who has longstanding anovulation because of the risk for endometrial carcinoma. The decision to perform an endometrial biopsy should not be based on a woman's age, as endometrial cancer can be encountered in young anovulatory women. It is the duration of exposure to unopposed estrogen that is critical, rather than the woman's age (Fritz & Speroff, 2011).

If a virilizing tumor is suspected but an adnexal mass is not palpable, transvaginal ultrasound of the ovaries is indicated. If no ovarian tumor is identified on ultrasound, adrenal computed tomography (CT) imaging should be performed. Routine adrenal imaging should be avoided because it can lead to unnecessary evaluation of nonfunctioning adrenal masses (incidentalomas) (Fritz & Speroff, 2011).

MAKING THE DIAGNOSIS OF POLYCYSTIC OVARY SYNDROME

The diagnosis of PCOS is one of exclusion (Sirmans & Pate, 2014). If history, physical examination, and laboratory testing rule out all other possible causes of hyperandrogenism, the most likely diagnosis is PCOS. It is important to remember that PCOS is a syndrome; thus, no single diagnostic criterion is sufficient for clinical diagnosis. Three sets of diagnostic criteria have been developed for PCOS (**Table 25-1**). Of these, the Rotterdam criteria and the Androgen Excess and PCOS Society criteria are the most widely used.

In addition to the diagnostic criteria, four specific phenotypes of PCOS have been identified (**Box 25-2**), and some evidence suggests that these subgroups differ biologically (Baldani et al., 2015). At a 2012 evidence-based methodology workshop on PCOS, the NIH endorsed the broad Rotterdam diagnostic criteria, which encompass the NICHD and Androgen Excess and PCOS Society criteria, and recommended specifically identifying these phenotypes of PCOS in future research and data collection (NIH, 2012). Clinicians should be aware which diagnostic criteria were used when reviewing research studies and should further clarify subgroups by phenotype in future studies (Fritz & Speroff, 2011; NIH, 2012).

TABLE 25-1	Diagnostic Criteria for Polycystic Ovary Syndrome

Source	Diagnostic Criteria
National Institute of Child Health and Human Development (Zawadzki & Dunaif, 1992)	• Clinical and/or biochemical hyperandrogenism • Menstrual dysfunction
Rotterdam PCOS Consensus Group (2004)	Exclusion of other etiologies and two out of three of the following: • Oligo- or anovulation • Clinical and/or biochemical signs of hyperandrogenism • Polycystic ovaries
Androgen Excess and Polycystic Ovary Syndrome Society (Azziz et al., 2009)	• Hyperandrogenism: hirsutism and/or hyperandrogenemia • Ovarian dysfunction: oligo-anovulation and/or polycystic ovaries • Exclusion of other androgen excess or related disorders

---

BOX 25-2 Polycystic Ovary Syndrome Phenotypes

- Androgen excess + ovulatory dysfunction
- Androgen excess + polycystic ovarian morphology
- Ovulatory dysfunction + polycystic ovarian morphology
- Androgen excess + ovulatory dysfunction + polycystic ovarian morphology

Reproduced from National Institutes of Health (NIH). (2012). Evidence-based methodology workshop on polycystic ovary syndrome December 3–5, final report. Retrieved from https://prevention.nih.gov/docs/programs/pcos/FinalReport.pdf.

DIFFERENTIAL DIAGNOSES

Differential diagnoses for hyperandrogenism include PCOS; congenital adrenal hyperplasia; hyperandrogenism, insulin resistance, and acanthosis nigrans (HAIR-AN) syndrome; androgen-producing ovarian or adrenal tumors; idiopathic hirsutism; Cushing syndrome; thyroid disorders; androgenic medications; conditions associated with pregnancy; and hyperprolactinemia. The most likely of these is PCOS. Key points for differential diagnoses can be found in **Table 25-2**.

PREVENTION

PCOS cannot be prevented. Early detection and management are critical to appropriately manage metabolic and cardiovascular disease risk factors, as well as cosmetic and psychologic issues (Goodman et al., 2015a).

MANAGEMENT

Management goals in women with PCOS are to treat current clinical manifestations and ameliorate long-term sequelae. Management should address any cosmetic manifestations of hyperandrogenism that the woman finds distressing as well as the psychological stress associated with PCOS.

Nonpharmacologic Management

Lifestyle Modification

All women with PCOS, regardless of their weight, must be aware of the importance of a healthy diet,

TABLE 25-2	Differential Diagnoses for Hyperandrogenism
Polycystic ovary syndrome (PCOS)	• Most common cause of hyperandrogenism, occurs in approximately 80% of women with androgen excess • Clinical and/or biochemical evidence of hyperandrogenism • Oligo-anovulation • Polycystic ovaries • Exclusion of other etiologies
Nonclassical congenital adrenal hyperplasia	• Occurs in approximately 2% of women with androgen excess • Clinically indistinguishable from PCOS • Elevated 17-hydroxyprogesterone (17-OHP), greater than 800 ng/dL
Hyperandrogenism, insulin resistance, and acanthosis nigrans (HAIR-AN) syndrome	• Occurs in approximately 4% of women with androgen excess • Severe hyperandrogenism, possible virilization • Acanthosis nigricans • Severe hyperinsulinemia/insulin resistance
Androgen-producing tumors (ovarian or adrenal)	• Rare • Acute, rapid course of virilizing symptoms • Testosterone usually elevated to more than 150 ng/dL in premenopausal women or more than 100 ng/dL in postmenopausal women • Palpable adnexal mass or mass on imaging of ovaries or adrenal glands
Idiopathic hirsutism	• Occurs in approximately 5% of women with androgen excess • Normal serum androgen levels • Normal ovulation by basal body temperature charting or luteal-phase progesterone measurements
Cushing syndrome	• Frequent referral diagnosis, one of the least common final diagnoses • Evidence of striae over abdomen, central weight distribution, muscle weakness, altered mood, easy bruisability • Failure of cortisol suppression after overnight dexamethasone suppression test
Thyroid disorders	• Palpable thyroid enlargement or mass • Suspect with presence of alopecia • Elevated thyroid-stimulating hormone
Androgenic medication use	• May be systemic or topical • Hirsutism is common
Pregnancy	• Rapid virilization occurs during pregnancy • Common causes: pregnancy luteoma or theca-lutein cysts (hyperreactio luteinalis)
Hyperprolactinemia	• Galactorrhea • Elevated prolactin level

Data from Fritz, M. A., & Speroff, L. (2011). *Clinical gynecologic endocrinology and infertility* (8th ed.). Baltimore, MD: Lippincott Williams & Wilkins; Goodman, N. F., Bledsoe, M. B., Futterweit, W., Goldzieher, J. W., Petak, S. M., Smith, K. D., . . . Steinberger, E. (2001). American Association of Clinical Endocrinologists medical guidelines for clinical practice for the diagnosis and treatment of hyperandrogenic disorders. *Endocrine Practice, 7*(2), 120–134; Kanova, N., & Bicikova, M. (2011). Hyperandrogenic states in pregnancy. *Physiological Research, 60*, 243–252; Legro, R. S., Arslanian, S. A., Ehrmann, D. A., Hoeger, K. M., Murad, M. H., Pasquali, R., . . . Welt, C. K. (2013). Diagnosis and treatment of polycystic ovary syndrome: An Endocrine Society clinical practice guideline. *Journal of Clinical Endocrinology Metabolism, 98*, 4565–4592; Rotterdam ESHRE/ASRM-Sponsored PCOS Consensus Workshop Group. (2004). Revised 2003 consensus on diagnostic criteria and long term health risks related to polycystic ovary syndrome (PCOS). *Human Reproduction, 19*(1), 41–47; Schmidt, T. H., & Shinkai, K. (2015). Evidence-based approach to cutaneous hyperandrogenism in women. *Journal of the American Academy of Dermatology, 73*, 672–690.

regular exercise, and weight management in controlling symptoms of PCOS and preventing sequelae. Weight loss is the first-line treatment for women who are obese. Weight loss—even in relatively small amounts (2–5%)—decreases androgen levels and increases SHBG. Additional benefits include decreased hirsutism, resumption of ovulation, improved menstrual function, increased pregnancy rates, and reduced risk of miscarriage. Weight loss also improves fasting insulin, glucose, glucose tolerance, and lipid levels, which are important for preventing and treating diabetes and cardiovascular disease (Fritz & Speroff, 2011; Goodman et al., 2015b; Moran, Pasquali, Teede, Hoeger, & Norman, 2009).

The most important dietary strategy for weight loss is decreased caloric consumption, entailing a reduction of 500 to 1,000 kcal/day. Fat intake that constitutes fewer than 30% of total calories, with fewer than 10% of calories coming from saturated fat, and an increase in consumption of fiber, whole grains, fruits, and vegetables are recommended. Specific macronutrient composition of the diet, such as high protein, low glycemic index, or very low carbohydrate consumption, has been studied, but there is not yet clear evidence to recommend any specific approach as being superior to the others (American College of Obstetricians and Gynecologists, 2009, reaffirmed 2015; Fritz & Speroff, 2011; Legro et al., 2013; Moran et al., 2009).

The weight management program should include at least 30 minutes of structured exercise per day. It appears that exercise offers benefits even if significant weight loss does not occur (Farrell & Antoni, 2010). Evidence supporting the use of anti-obesity medications (e.g., phentermine, sibutramine, and orlistat) and bariatric surgery in women with PCOS is limited, and further research is needed to assess their use when other weight management options prove unsuccessful (Moran et al., 2009; Wild et al., 2010). Structure and support for any weight management program are important, and the clinician must provide close follow-up and monitoring (Moran et al., 2009).

Mechanical Hair Removal

Contrary to popular belief, mechanically removing hair by shaving, plucking, waxing, or applying depilatory creams does not stimulate further hair growth. These methods may be used in conjunction with pharmacologic therapy to remove hair as needed. Electrolysis and photoepilation with laser or intense pulsed light (IPL) can be used for permanent hair reduction. Both strategies require several sessions of treatment and can cause pigment changes and scarring. The Endocrine Society recommends laser therapy over electrolysis because laser treatment is faster and less painful than electrolysis; however, electrolysis is less expensive than laser therapy (Martin et al., 2008).

Pharmacologic Management

This section focuses on pharmacologic treatment for women who are not trying to conceive. When selecting a medication, it is important to consider the specific treatment goals for the woman, such as improving clinical signs of hyperandrogenism (e.g., hirsutism, acne, and/or alopecia), regulating menstrual cycles, protecting the endometrium, and preventing long-term sequelae of PCOS. Most women have multiple treatment goals, and some individual medications (e.g., combined oral contraceptives and insulin sensitizing agents) address more than one treatment goal.

Combined Oral Contraceptives

Combined oral contraceptives (COCs) are recommended as a first-line pharmacologic treatment for women with PCOS (American College of Obstetricians and Gynecologists, 2009, reaffirmed 2015; Fritz & Speroff, 2011; Legro et al., 2013; Martin et al., 2008). COCs treat hyperandrogenism by inhibiting LH secretion and subsequently LH-dependent ovarian androgen production, and by raising the concentration of SHBG, which binds free testosterone. As a result, COCs provide cosmetic relief of acne and hirsutism. These medications also regulate menstrual cycles and provide protection against endometrial cancer by interrupting the steady state of estrogen stimulation of the uterus and inducing a monthly withdrawal bleed. Some concerns have been raised about the safety of COC in women with PCOS, given that COCs may increase insulin resistance. There is no evidence that these risks are substantially higher in women with PCOS, however (Fritz & Speroff, 2011).

A COC with a 20 to 35 mcg dose of ethinyl estradiol and a nonandrogenic progestin component is recommended. Formulations containing desogestrel, norgestimate, or drospirenone are commonly used because of their low androgenic effects

(Escobar-Morreale et al., 2012). Drospirenone functions as an androgen receptor agonist. Its dose in COCs (3 mg) is equivalent to approximately 25 mg of spironolactone, which may not be enough for hirsutism treatment, but should be considered if additional spironolactone is given due to the potential for hyperkalemia with such therapy (Martin et al., 2008).

The maximal effect of COCs on acne is usually observed within 2 months. In contrast, the maximal effect on hair growth may take as long as 9 to 12 months for its realization because of the length of the hair growth cycle. COCs as monotherapy may be insufficient to treat hirsutism (Goodman et al., 2015b; van Zuuren, Fedorowicz, Carter, & Pandis, 2015). Nonoral combined contraceptives—the transdermal patch and the vaginal ring—are also likely to be beneficial for women with PCOS, but evidence on their use in this population is limited.

One study found that the risk of venous thromboembolism was increased 2-fold in women who had PCOS and were using COCs and 1.5-fold in women who had PCOS and were not using COCs compared to women without PCOS (Bird, Hartzema, Brophy, Etminan, & Delaney, 2013; Goodman et al., 2015b). Given this potential increased risk, women with PCOS should be questioned about additional risk factors for venous thromboembolism. More detailed information about combined contraceptives can be found in Chapter 11.

Progestogens

Women who have contraindications to or do not wish to take COCs can use progestogens to prevent endometrial hyperplasia and cancer. Women who need contraception can use the levonorgestrel-releasing intrauterine system (LNG-IUS), progestin-only pills (POPs), the depot medroxyprogesterone acetate injection, or the subdermal implant. Women who do not need contraception can take a dose of 5 to 10 mg medroxyprogesterone acetate or 200 mg micronized progesterone daily for the first 14 days of each month. Progestational therapy alone will not treat hirsutism, however (American College of Obstetricians and Gynecologists, 2009, reaffirmed 2015; Fritz & Speroff, 2011).

Antiandrogens

Antiandrogens are effective in the treatment of hirsutism, but they should always be used in combination with effective contraception in a woman who is sexually active because of their potential for teratogenicity. Although COCs are generally used as a first-line treatment for hirsutism, in women whose hirsutism remains refractory after 6 months of COC use, the addition of an antiandrogen medication may be more effective than administration of either agent alone (Escobar-Morreale et al., 2012; Martin et al., 2008; Wilson, 2011). Conversely, antiandrogens can be used as first-line therapy in women who do not want or need to take COCs. These medications include spironolactone, finasteride, and flutamide.

Spironolactone is effective in the treatment of hirsutism and androgenic alopecia. It works by inhibiting testosterone from binding to its receptors, thereby inhibiting its action. The usual dose is 50 to 100 mg twice daily, with the effects being dose dependent. It can take 6 months or longer to see the full clinical effect from this therapy. Side effects may include lightheadedness, dizziness, fatigue, diuresis, and increased risk of hyperkalemia. Spironolactone may also cause menstrual irregularity when used as monotherapy. Combination therapy with COCs reduces this side effect, and improves clinical response (American College of Obstetricians and Gynecologists, 2009, reaffirmed 2015; Fritz & Speroff, 2011; Goodman et al., 2015a; Martin et al., 2008).

Finasteride inhibits 5α-reductase activity, which blocks the conversion of testosterone to DHT in the skin. A dose of 5 mg per day is effective in decreasing hirsutism without engendering any adverse effects. This medication should be considered when COCs and spirolactone are ineffective for hirsutism (Goodman et al., 2015a). Women who are treated with finasteride should be aware that this medication can adversely affect the development of the genital tract in male fetuses, and must be counseled to use a highly effective contraceptive method. Pregnant women should not touch crushed or broken finasteride tablets due to their teratogenicity (American College of Obstetricians and Gynecologists, 2009, reaffirmed 2015; Fritz & Speroff, 2011; Martin et al., 2008).

Flutamide is a pure antiandrogen without progestogenic effects that has shown some benefit in treating hirsutism (Badawy & Einashar, 2011). Unfortunately, this medication is associated with hepatotoxicity that can cause liver failure and rarely death. Neither the Androgen Excess and PCOS Society nor the Endocrine Society recommends flutamide for hirsutism treatment (Escobar-Morreale et al., 2012; Martin et al., 2008).

Insulin-Sensitizing Agents

Metformin is an oral antihyperglycemic agent whose primary mechanisms of action are inhibition of hepatic glucose production and increased peripheral insulin sensitivity. Metformin has been shown to increase ovulatory frequency and decrease androgen levels in women with PCOS, but it has minimal effects on weight loss. In women with PCOS and hyperinsulinemia, metformin decreases fasting insulin levels, blood pressure, and LDL cholesterol levels (American College of Obstetricians and Gynecologists, 2009, reaffirmed 2015; Nathan & Sullivan, 2014).

While metformin can treat some clinical manifestations of PCOS and has the potential to prevent or delay the onset of diabetes mellitus, routine therapy with this medication in all women with PCOS is not recommended. Metformin should be considered for women with impaired glucose tolerance whose weight does not respond to diet and exercise or whose weight is normal such that weight loss is not appropriate (Goodman et al., 2015a; Legro et al., 2013; Wild et al., 2010). Metformin has also been used in infertility treatment for women with PCOS, but is now recommended mainly as an adjuvant therapy to prevent ovarian hyperstimulation in women undergoing in vitro fertilization (Legro et al., 2013). This medication should not be given solely to treat hirsutism or promote weight loss (Escobar-Morreale et al., 2012; Legro et al., 2013).

The usual dose of metformin is 1,500 to 2,550 mg per day, with the dose being started low (500 mg per day) and then gradually increased over 4 to 6 weeks. It is taken with meals to reduce this medication's abdominal side effects. It is contraindicated in cases of impaired renal function, congestive heart failure, hepatic dysfunction, sepsis, or history of alcohol abuse. The most serious side effect of metformin is the development of lactic acidosis, although this is rare. Vitamin B_{12} deficiency can also occur. Gastrointestinal side effects, which are more common, include nausea, abdominal discomfort, diarrhea, and anorexia (Nathan & Sullivan, 2014).

The thiazolidinediones (TZDs), which are also known as glitazones, lower glucose levels by increasing the utilization of glucose by the skeletal muscles and decreasing hepatic glucose synthesis.

Most studies of this class of drugs have investigated troglitazone, which was withdrawn from the market because of its propensity to cause significant hepatocellular toxicity. Two related drugs, rosiglitazone and pioglitazone, have been investigated for use in PCOS. Both can cause or worsen congestive heart failure, and rosiglitazone has been associated with increased risk of myocardial infarction (Katsiki & Hatzitolios, 2010). Use of TZDs for PCOS is not recommended (Legro et al., 2013).

Topical Preparations

Eflornithine HCl 13.9% (Vaniqa) is a topical cream approved for the treatment of facial hirsutism. It is applied to affected areas twice daily, with noticeable improvements occurring in 6 to 8 weeks. This medication's primary mechanism of action is inhibition of the enzyme ornithine decarboxylase in human skin, which slows the rate of hair growth. It is not a depilatory, and hair growth returns after discontinuation of the cream. The main side effects associated with eflornithine HCl are itching and dry skin (Brodell & Mercurio, 2010; Martin et al., 2008).

Additional Medications

Gonadotropin-releasing hormone (GnRH) analogs, such as leuprolide, have been used in the treatment of hirsutism. These medications work by inhibiting gonadotropin secretion and subsequent ovarian hormone secretion, which results in not only a slowing of hair growth, but also severe estrogen deficiency. GnRH treatment is expensive, requires injections and estrogen therapy, and may not be more effective than COCs and antiandrogens. For these reasons, the Endocrine Society recommends reserving use of GnRH analogs for women with severe hyperandrogenemia, such as ovarian hyperthecosis, that has not responded to COCs and antiandrogens (Escobar-Morreale et al., 2012; Martin et al., 2008).

Follow-Up

Patient education and comprehensive woman-centered care are crucial to the successful management of PCOS and the reduction of negative long-term sequelae. Long-term follow-up with routine visits is appropriate to monitor response to treatment and development of complications. Screening for evidence of development of metabolic consequences must be undertaken at regular intervals. The clinician should assess the woman's BMI, waist circumference, and blood pressure at every visit (Wild et al., 2010). Weight loss should be encouraged in women who are overweight or obese. If the baseline fasting lipid profile is normal, repeat this test every 2 years or sooner if the woman gains weight. If the baseline 2-hour oral glucose tolerance test is normal, repeat this test every 2 years or sooner if the woman develops additional risk factors. Women with impaired glucose tolerance should undergo annual screening for diabetes mellitus (Wild et al., 2010). Diabetes mellitus, hypertension, and dyslipidemia require prompt treatment (or referral for treatment) after diagnosis. Advise women that cigarette smoking further increases their risk for cardiovascular disease, and provide smoking cessation interventions for women who smoke.

Complementary and Alternative Therapies

Complementary therapies such as acupuncture, reflexology, homeopathy, and herbal medicine are increasingly available in the United States. However, few studies have been conducted to assess the efficacy of these modalities for PCOS (Badawy & Einashar, 2011). A randomized controlled trial investigated the effect of electro-acupuncture and physical exercise on hyperandrogenism and oligo-anovulation in women with PCOS and found that both low-frequency electro-acupuncture and physical exercise improved hyperandrogenism and oligo-anovulation in women with PCOS better than no intervention, and low-frequency electro-acupuncture was superior to physical exercise (Jedel et al., 2011).

When to Refer Patients

Endocrinopathies

If diagnostic testing reveals that a woman has congenital adrenal hyperplasia, HAIR-AN syndrome, Cushing syndrome, hyperprolactinemia, or androgen-producing tumors, she should be referred to an endocrinologist. An endocrinology consultation should also be considered for women who are refractory to treatment for PCOS. Clinicians who are not experienced in the management of metabolic syndrome should seek appropriate consultation for treating women with PCOS who meet the criteria for metabolic syndrome.

Treatment of Infertility

Treatment of infertility in women with PCOS can be challenging and is beyond the scope of this chapter. Information about infertility treatment can be found in Chapter 18. Women with PCOS and infertility require care from a clinician experienced in treating these conditions concomitantly.

SPECIAL CONSIDERATIONS

Adolescents

Unfortunately, the symptoms of hyperandrogenism are not usually brought to the attention of the clinician until the woman is in her late teens, early 20s, or even older. The most common causes of hyperandrogenism, however, usually become active in early adolescence. Premature adrenarche may be a consequence of hyperinsulinemia. These adolescents go on to develop clinical signs of hyperandrogenism and/or irregular menses, for which they often are treated symptomatically without undergoing a thorough assessment of the causes of symptoms. Menstrual irregularity is common soon after menarche but warrants investigation if it persists for more than 2 years. Every attempt should be made to diagnose and treat hyperandrogenic conditions as early as possible, as early treatment may help ameliorate symptoms and prevent the development of adverse sequelae and psychological dysfunction (Fritz & Speroff, 2011).

Pregnant Women

Virilization presenting in pregnancy should raise the suspicion for a luteoma—a condition that is an exaggerated reaction of the ovarian stroma to normal levels of chorionic gonadotropin and not a true tumor. The solid luteoma is associated with a normal pregnancy and is usually unilateral. Maternal virilization occurs in 25% to 35% of pregnancies affected by a luteoma. If the mother is virilized as a result of the luteoma, there is a 60% to 70% chance that her female fetus will show some signs of masculinization. The luteoma does not cause other maternal effects and regresses postpartum. Virilization may be recurrent in subsequent pregnancies (Kanova & Bicikova, 2011).

In contrast, a theca-lutein cyst or hyperreactio luteinalis is usually bilateral and is seen with

trophoblastic disease or with the high human chorionic gonadotropin levels associated with a multiple gestation. Maternal virilization occurs in 30% of
pregnancies affected with a theca-lutein cyst, but
does not carry any risk of fetal masculinization.

If a woman is experiencing virilization during
pregnancy, a pelvic ultrasound can be very helpful
in making the diagnosis. If a solid unilateral ovarian
lesion is present, malignancy is likely (Fritz & Speroff,
2011; Kanova & Bicikova, 2011).

Women with PCOS are at increased risk of several pregnancy complications (preeclampsia, gestational diabetes, and preterm birth), with this risk
being exacerbated by obesity. Therefore, precon-
ceptional assessment of BMI, blood pressure, and
oral glucose tolerance are recommended (Legro
et al., 2013). Women being treated for hyperandrogenism who become pregnant should be aware
of the benefits and risks of any medications they
are taking. Although metformin may prove beneficial during pregnancy by reducing the risk of gestational diabetes mellitus, evidence is insufficient
to recommend its routine use during pregnancy
(Fauser et al., 2012). Some medications, such as
finasteride, flutamide, and spironolactone, are contraindicated in pregnancy and should be discontinued immediately upon suspicion that the woman is
pregnant. A woman who becomes pregnant while
taking antiandrogens needs counseling regarding
these medications' potential effects on her fetus.

Perimenopause and Older Women

Women with PCOS often develop improved menstrual function with age, and evidence indicates that
women with PCOS have prolonged reproductive
function and increased ovarian reserve when compared to women who do not have PCOS. Age may
improve other manifestations of PCOS, including
ovarian morphology and serum testosterone levels.
More studies need to be done regarding the general health of women with PCOS as they transition
into menopause, but it is suspected that these
women have increased rates of obesity, diabetes,
and cardiovascular disease risk factors (Fauser
et al., 2012).

Cultural Influences

PCOS is a complex, multifactorial disorder arising in
the presence of various genetic and environmental
factors. It affects the reproductive, endocrine, cardiovascular, dermatologic, and psychosocial health of
a large number of women, but is often not well understood by clinicians or the public. Experts have
proposed changing the name of the syndrome to
better incorporate the multiple interactions (e.g.,
metabolic, hypothalamic, pituitary, ovarian, adrenal)
that characterize the syndrome, as the current name
focuses only on ovarian morphology and is, in some
experts' opinion, a distraction to progress (NIH,
2012). Experts also recommend increased multidisciplinary awareness programs for clinicians and
the public, as the syndrome represents a major
public health concern (NIH, 2012; Sanchez, 2014).
Indeed, women with PCOS who are provided with
detailed education regarding the syndrome, related
health risks, and lifestyle changes and pharmacologic management strategies for symptoms report
increased knowledge and motivation, as well as
physical and psychological benefits (Colwell, Lujan,
Lawson, Pierson, & Chizen, 2010).

References

Alberti, K. G. M. M., Eckel, R. H., Grundy, S. M., Zimmet, P. Z., Cleeman, J. I., Donato, K., . . . Smith, S. C. (2009). Harmonizing the metabolic syndrome: A joint statement of the International Diabetes Federation Task Force on Epidemiology and Prevention; National Heart, Lung, and Blood Institute; American Heart Association; World Heart Federation; International Atherosclerosis Society; and International Association for the Study of Obesity. *Circulation, 120*, 1640–1645.

American College of Obstetricians and Gynecologists. (2009, reaffirmed 2015). Polycystic ovary syndrome. American College of Obstetricians and Gynecologists Practice Bulletin No. 108. *Obstetrics & Gynecology, 114*, 936–949.

American Diabetes Association. (2014). Screening for type 2 diabetes. *Diabetes Care, 27*, s11–s14.

Azziz, R., Carmina, E., Dewailly, D., Diamanti-Kandarakis, E., Escobar-Morreale, H. F., Futterweit, W., . . . Witchel, S. F. (2009). The Androgen Excess and PCOS Society criteria for the poly-cystic ovary syndrome: The complete task force report. *Fertility and Sterility, 91*(2), 456–488.

Badawy, A., & Einashar, A. (2011). Treatment options for polycystic ovary syndrome. *International Journal of Women's Health, 3*, 25–35.

Baldani, D. P., Skrgatic, L., & Ougouag, R. (2015). Polycystic ovary syndrome: Important underrecognised cardiometabolic risk factor in reproductive-age women. *International Journal of Endocrinology, 2015*, 1–17.

Balen, A. H., Laven, J. S., Tan, S., & Dewailly, D. (2003). Ultrasound assessment of the polycystic ovary: International consensus definitions. *Human Reproduction Update, 9*(6), 505–514.

Barry, J. A., Azizia, M. M., & Hardiman, P. J. (2014). Risk of endometrial, ovarian and breast cancer in women with polycystic ovary syndrome: A systematic review and meta-analysis. *Human Reproduction Update, 20*(5), 748–758.

Barry, J. A., Kuczmierczyk, A. R., & Hardiman, P. J. (2011). Anxiety and depression in polycystic ovary syndrome: A systematic review and meta-analysis. *Human Reproduction Update, 26*(9), 2442–2451.

Bird, S. T., Hartzema, A. G., Brophy, J. M., Etminan, M., & Delaney, J. A. (2013). Risk of venous thromboembolism in women with polycystic ovary syndrome: A population-based matched cohort analysis. *Canadian Medical Association Journal, 185*, e115–e120.

Brodell, L. A., & Mercurio, M. G. (2010). Hirsutism: Diagnosis and management. *Gender Medicine, 7*, 79–87.

Burt, C. M., Solorzano, J. P., Beller, M. Y., Abshire, J. S., Collins, J. C., McCartney, C. R., . . . Marshall, J. C. (2012). Neuroendocrine dysfunction in polycystic ovary syndrome. *Steroids, 77*, 332–337.

Colwell, K., Lujan, M. E., Lawson, K. L., Pierson, R. A., & Chizen, D. R. (2010). Women's perceptions of polycystic ovary syndrome following participation in a clinical research study: Implications for knowledge, feelings, and daily health practice. *Journal of Obstetrics and Gynaecology Canada, 32*(5), 453–459.

Deligeoroglou, E., Vrachnis, N., Athanasopoulos, N., Illodromiti, Z., Sifakis, S., Illodromiti, S., . . . Creatsas, G. (2012). Mediators of chronic inflammation in polycystic ovary syndrome. *Gynecological Endocrinology, 28*, 974–978.

Dewailly, D., Gronier, H., Poncelet, E., Robin, G., Leroy, M., Pigney, P., . . . Catteau-Jonard, S. (2011). Diagnosis of polycystic ovary syndrome (PCOS): Revisiting the threshold values of follicle count on ultrasound and of the serum AMH level for the definition of polycystic ovaries. *Human Reproduction, 26*(11), 3123–3129.

Dewailly, D., Lujan, M. E., Carmina, E., Cedars, M., Laven, J., Norman, R., & Escobar-Morreale, H. F. (2014). Definition and significance of polycystic ovarian morphology: A task force report from the Androgen Excess and Polycystic Ovary Syndrome Society. *Human Reproduction Update, 20*(3), 334–352.

Escobar-Morreale, H. F., Carmina, E., Dewailly, D., Gamineri, A., Kelestimur, F., Moghetti, P., . . . Norman, R. J. (2012). Epidemiology, diagnosis and management of hirsutism: A consensus statement by the Androgen Excess and Polycystic Ovary Syndrome Society. *Human Reproduction Update, 18*(2), 146–170.

Essah, P. A., Wickham, E. P., & Nestler, J. E. (2007). The metabolic syndrome in polycystic ovary syndrome. *Clinical Obstetrics and Gynecology, 50*, 205–225.

Farrell, K., & Antoni, M. H. (2010). Insulin resistance, obesity, inflammation, and depression in polycystic ovary syndrome: Biobehavioral mechanisms and interventions. *Fertility and Sterility, 94*(5), 1565–1574.

Fauser, B. C., Tarlatzis, B. C., Rebar, R. W., Legro, R. S., Balen, A. H., Lobo, R., . . . Barnhart, K. (2012). Consensus on women's health aspects of polycystic ovary syndrome (PCOS): The Amsterdam ESHRE/ASRM-sponsored 3rd PCOS consensus workshop group. *Fertility and Sterility, 97*(1), 28-38.e25.

Ferriman, D., & Gallwey, J. D. (1961). Clinical assessment of body hair growth in women. *Journal of Clinical Endocrinology and Metabolism, 21*, 1440–1447.

Fritz, M. A., & Speroff, L. (2011). *Clinical gynecologic endocrinology and infertility* (8th ed.). Baltimore, MD: Lippincott Williams & Wilkins.

Goodarzi, M. O., Dumesic, D. A., Chazenbalk, G., &Azziz, R. (2011). Polycystic ovary syndrome: Etiology, pathogenesis, and diagnosis. *Nature Reviews Endocrinology, 7i*(4), 219–231.

Goodarzi, M. O., & Korenman, S. G. (2003). The importance of insulin resistance in polycystic ovary syndrome. *Fertility and Sterility, 80*(2), 255–258.

Goodman, N. F., Bledsoe, M. B., Futterweit, W., Goldzieher, J. W., Petak, S. M., Smith, K. D., . . . Steinberger, E. (2001). American Association of Clinical Endocrinologists medical guidelines for clinical practice for the diagnosis and treatment of hyperandrogenic disorders. *Endocrine Practice, 7*(2), 120–134.

Goodman, N. F., Cobin, R. H., Futterweit, W., Glueck, J. S., Legro, R. S., & Carmina, E. (2015a). American Association of Clinical Endocrinologists, American College of Endocrinology, and Androgen Excess and PCOS Society disease state clinical review: Guide to the best practices in the evaluation and treatment of polycystic ovary syndrome—part 1. *Endocrine Practice, 21*(11), 1291–1300.

Goodman, N. F., Cobin, R. H., Futterweit, W., Glueck, J. S., Legro, R. S., & Carmina, E. (2015b). American Association of Clinical Endocrinologists, American College of Endocrinology, and Androgen Excess and PCOS Society disease state clinical review: Guide to the best practices in the evaluation and treatment of polycystic ovary syndrome—part 2. *Endocrine Practice, 21*(12), 1415–1426.

Gordon, K. A., & Tosti, A. (2011). Alopecia: Evaluation and treatment. *Clinical, Cosmetic and Investigational Dermatology, 4*, 101–106.

Haoula, Z., Salman, M., & Atiomo, W. (2012). Evaluating the association between endometrial cancer and polycystic ovary syndrome. *Human Reproduction, 27*(5), 1327–1331.

Hatch, R., Rosenfield, R. L., Kim, M. H., & Tredway, D. (1981). Hirsutism: Implications, etiology, and management. *American Journal of Obstetrics and Gynecology, 140*, 815–830.

Jedel, E., Labrie, F., Oden, A., Holm, G., Nillson, L., Janson, P. O., . . . Stener-Victorin, E. (2011). Impact of electro-acupuncture and physical exercise on hyperandrogenism and oligo/anovulation in women with polycystic ovary syndrome: A randomized controlled trial. *American Journal of Physiology—Endocrinology and Metabolism, 300*(1), E37–E45.

Kanova, N., & Bicikova, M. (2011). Hyperandrogenic states in pregnancy. *Physiological Research, 60*, 243–252.

Katsiki, N., & Hatzitolios, A. I. (2010). Insulin-sensitizing agents in the treatment of polycystic ovary syndrome: An update. *Current Opinion in Obstetrics and Gynecology, 22*, 466–476.

Legro, R. S., Arslanian, S. A., Ehrmann, D. A., Hoeger, K. M., Murad, M. H., Pasquali, R., . . . Welt, C. K. (2013). Diagnosis and treatment of polycystic ovary syndrome: An Endocrine Society clinical practice guideline. *Journal of Clinical Endocrinology Metabolism, 98*, 4565–4592.

Lim, S. S., Norman, R. J., Davies, M. J., & Moran, L. J. (2013). The effect of obesity on polycystic ovary syndrome: A systematic review and meta-analysis. *Obesity Reviews, 14*(2), 95–109.

Mansson, M., Norstrom, K., Holte, J., Landin-Wilhelmsin, K., Dahlgren, E., & Landen, M. (2011). Sexuality and psychological well-being in women with polycystic ovary syndrome compared with healthy controls. *European Journal of Obstetrics & Gynecology and Reproductive Biology, 155*, 161–165.

Martin, K. A., Chang, J., Ehrmann, D. A., Ibanez, L., Lobo, R. A., Rosenfield, R. L., . . . Swiglo, B. A. (2008). Evaluation and treatment of hirsutism in premenopausal women: An Endocrine Society clinical practice guideline. *Journal of Clinical Endocrinology & Metabolism, 93*, 1105–1120.

Moran, C., Arriaga, M., Rodriquez, G., & Moran, S. (2012). Obesity differentially affects phenotypes of polycystic ovary syndrome. *International Journal of Endocrinology, 2012*, article ID 317241, 1–7.

Moran, L. J., Misso, M. L., Wild, R. A., & Norman, R. J. (2010). Impaired glucose tolerance, type 2 diabetes and metabolic syndrome in polycystic ovary syndrome: A systematic review and meta-analysis. *Human Reproduction Update, 16*(4), 347–363.

Moran, L. J., Pasquali, R., Teede, H. J., Hoeger, K. M., & Norman, R. J. (2009). Treatment of obesity in polycystic ovary syndrome: A position statement of the Androgen Excess and Polycystic Ovary Syndrome Society. *Fertility and Sterility, 92*(6), 1966–1982.

Nathan, N., & Sullivan, S. D. (2014). The utility of metformin therapy in reproductive-aged women with polycystic ovary syndrome. *Current Pharmaceutical Biotechnology, 15*(1), 70–83.

National Institutes of Health (NIH). (2012). Evidence-based methodology workshop on polycystic ovary syndrome December 3–5, final report. Retrieved from https://prevention.nih.gov/docs/programs/pcos/FinalReport.pdf

Randeva, H. S., Tan, B. K., Weickert, M. O., Lois, K., Nestler, J. E., Sattar, N., & Lehnert, H. (2012). Cardiometabolic aspects of the polycystic ovary syndrome. *Endocrine Reviews, 33*, 812–841.

Rosenfeld, R. C., Barnes, R. B., & Ehrmann, D. A. (2015). Hyperandrogenism, hirsutism, and polycystic ovary syndrome. In J. L. Jameson & L. J. DeGroot (Eds.), *Endocrinology: Adult and pediatric* (7th ed., pp. 2275–2296). Philadelphia, PA: Saunders.

Rosner, W., Auchus, R. J., Azziz, R., Sluss, P. M., & Raff, H. (2007). Utility, limitations, and pitfalls in measuring testosterone: An Endocrine Society position statement. *Journal of Clinical Endocrinology & Metabolism, 92*, 405–413.

Rotterdam ESHRE/ASRM-Sponsored PCOS Consensus Workshop Group. (2004). Revised 2003 consensus on diagnostic criteria and long term health risks related to polycystic ovary syndrome (PCOS). *Human Reproduction, 19*(1), 41–47.

Sanchez, N. (2014). A lifecourse perspective on polycystic ovary syndrome. *International Journal of Women's Health, 6*, 115–122.

Schmidt, T. H., & Shinkai, K. (2015). Evidence-based approach to cutaneous hyperandrogenism in women. *Journal of the American Academy of Dermatology, 73*, 672–690.

Sirmans, S. M., & Pate, K. A. (2014). Epidemiology, diagnosis, and management of polycystic ovary syndrome. *Clinical Epidemiology, 6*, 1–13.

Strowitzki, T., Capp, E., & von Eye, C. H. (2010). The degree of cycle irregularity correlates with the grade of endocrine and metabolic disorders in PCOS patients. *European Journal of Obstetrics and Gynecology and Reproductive Biology, 149*(2), 178–181.

Teede, H., Deeks, A., & Moran, L. (2010). Polycystic ovary syndrome: A complex condition with psychological, reproductive and metabolic manifestations that impacts health across the lifespan. *BMC Medicine, 8*, 41.

Toulis, K. A., Goulis, D. G., Mintziori, G., Kintiraki, E., Eukarpidis, E., Mouratoglou, S. A., . . . Tarlatzis, B. C. (2011). Meta-analysis of cardiovascular disease risk markers in women with polycystic ovary syndrome. *Human Reproduction Update, 17*(6), 741–760.

van Zuuren, E. J., Fedorowicz, Z., Carter, B., & Pandis, N. (2015). Interventions for hirsutism (excluding laser and photoepilation therapy alone). *Cochrane Database of Systematic Reviews, 4*, CD010334.

Veltman-Verhulst, S. M., Boivin, J., Eijkemans, M. J., & Fauser, B. J. (2012). Emotional distress is a common risk in women with polycystic ovary syndrome: A systematic review and meta-analysis of 28 studies. *Human Reproduction Update, 18*(6), 638–651.

Wild, R. A., Carmina, E., Diamanti-Kandarakis, E., Dokras, A., Escobar-Morreale, H. F., Futterweit, W., . . . Dumesic, D. A. (2010). Assessment of cardiovascular risk and prevention of cardiovascular disease in women with the polycystic ovary syndrome: A consensus statement by the Androgen Excess and Polycystic Ovary Syndrome (AE-PCOS) Society. *Journal of Clinical Endocrinology & Metabolism, 95*, 2038–2049.

Wild, R. A., Rizzo, M., Clifton, S., & Carmina, E. (2011). Lipid levels in polycystic ovary syndrome: Systematic review and meta-analysis. *Fertility and Sterility, 95*(3), 1073–1079.

Wilson, J. F. (2011). In the clinic: The polycystic ovary syndrome. *Annals of Internal Medicine, 154*, ITC2-2–ITC2-15.

Zawadzki, J. K., & Dunaif, A. (1992). *Diagnostic criteria for polycystic ovary syndrome: Towards a rational approach*. Boston, MA: Blackwell Scientific.

CHAPTER 26

Benign Gynecologic Conditions

Katharine K. O'Dell

The editors acknowledge Carol A. Verga, who was the author of the previous edition of this chapter.

While they are not life threatening, many benign gynecologic conditions severely diminish quality of life for affected women. This chapter addresses several benign, bothersome conditions that bring women to clinicians' offices seeking relief. The following are topics included in this chapter:

- Conditions of the vulva
  - Skin cysts
    - Folliculitis, furuncles, carbuncles
    - Epidermoid and sebaceous cysts
    - Hidradenitis suppurativa
  - Dermatoses
    - Contact dermatitis
    - Lichen sclerosus
    - Lichen planus
    - Lichen simplex chronicus
    - Psoriasis
- Conditions of the uterus and cervix
  - Cervical and endometrial polyps
  - Uterine fibroids
  - Endometriosis and adenomyosis
- Conditions of the adnexa
  - Ovarian cysts

For reasons that are still unclear, several of these diagnoses are associated (e.g., endometrial and cervical polyps, uterine fibroids, and endometriosis) and often appear in tandem in individual women (American Association of Gynecologic Laparoscopists [AAGL], 2012). Some are easily curable, such as polyps and ovarian cysts, while others can be chronic or recurring, such as endometriosis and certain vulvar dermatoses. Clinicians will better serve women if they have a solid understanding of these common gynecologic conditions.

Those conditions that are chronic and/or unpredictable place a special burden on women, their families, and their healthcare providers. The etiologies of these disorders are often poorly understood. In some cases, the symptoms may be more debilitating to the woman than her physical findings would otherwise suggest. In addition, symptoms of any of these conditions can vary markedly in affected women over time and between women with the same diagnoses, and can improve spontaneously with no intervention. These factors make it very difficult to build an evidence base for optimal management using standardized clinical trials. For all of these reasons, chronic gynecologic conditions can frustrate everyone involved and challenge relationships between affected women, their families, and their clinicians.

At all healthcare visits, clinicians should listen to women, complete a thorough assessment, and provide up-to-date, condition-specific information and management. In addition, women affected by aggravating chronic or recurring gynecologic symptoms will need special assistance to help them develop realistic expectations and goals for treatment, and monitor symptom changes over time to guide ongoing management (Hooten et al., 2013).

CONDITIONS OF THE VULVA

Vulvar skin includes both keratinized and mucocutaneous surfaces. To help women with aggravating skin changes, clinicians need a thorough understanding of this complex anatomy (see Chapter 5) and basic history and physical examination skills (see Chapter 6). This section reviews two vulvar findings often seen in primary care: skin cysts and dermatoses. Infection of the mucous-secreting glands of the vulva and vulvar pain syndromes are discussed elsewhere in this text. See Chapters 19 and 20 for infections and Chapter 16 for vulvar pain.

At least 20% of women experience seriously bothersome vulvar discomfort, including itching, burning, pain, rashes, and lesions (British Association for Sexual Health and HIV, 2014). Some of these symptoms and signs are limited to the genital area, whereas others are manifestations of diffuse chronic diseases of the skin or mucous membranes. Differentiating between normal variations, benign disease, and malignancy is paramount. Optimal management planning is complicated because many vulvar skin conditions have similar appearances and symptoms, and a woman may have multiple conditions simultaneously. Examples of the numerous differential diagnoses for vulvar skin conditions are presented in **Table 26-1**. A systematic approach

TABLE 26-1   Differential Diagnoses of Vulvar Skin Conditions

Erosions and Ulcers	Erythematous Papules and Plaques	Depigmentation
Aphthosis (oral–genital)	Basal cell carcinoma	Severe atrophy
Atrophic vaginitis	Candidiasis	Congenital hypopigmentation
Basal cell carcinoma	Condyloma acuminata (genital warts)	Halo nevus
Bechet's disease	Contact dermatitis	Lichen sclerosus
Chancroid	Crohn's disease	Lichen simplex chronicus
Chemotherapy-induced reaction	Eczema	Tinea versicolor
Contact dermatitis	Erythema multiforme	Vitiligo
Herpes simplex	Folliculitis/epidermoid cysts	
Herpes zoster	Hemangiomas	
Impetigo	Hidradenitis suppurativa	
Melanoma	Intertrigo	
Stevens-Johnson syndrome	Lichen planus	
Syphilis	Lichen sclerosus	
Tuberculosis (genital)	Lichen simplex chronicus	
	Melanoma	
	Molluscum contagiosum	
	Nevi (moles)	
	Paget's disease	
	Pemphigus/pemphigoid	
	Pityriasis versicolor	
	Psoriasis/inverse psoriasis	
	Scabies	
	Seborrheic dermatitis	
	Squamous cell carcinoma	
	Syphilis	
	Vulvar intraepithelial neoplasia	
	Vulvodynia/vestibulitis	

Data from British Association for Sexual Health and HIV. (2014). 2014 UK national guideline on the management of vulval conditions. Retrieved from http://www.bashh.org; Schlosser, B. J., & Mirowski, G. W. (2015). Lichen sclerosus and lichen planus in women and girls. *Clinical Obstetrics & Gynecology, 58,* 125–142.

to assessment should be used to avoid delay in identifying malignant changes and improve symptoms expediently. This section provides an overview of key points for evaluation and treatment needed to help women manage these benign conditions. Premalignant and malignant vulvar lesions are addressed in Chapter 27.

Assessment of Vulvar Skin Disorders

History

Women should be asked essential elements of their related health history, including onset and progression of symptoms; aggravating or alleviating factors, including any relationship to sexual activity; prior self- or prescribed treatments and their outcomes; and concomitant systemic changes, such as lymphadenopathy or skin, perianal, or oral mucosal disease. Increased risk of malignancy should be considered when women report a prior history of high-risk human papillomavirus (HPV) or genital warts, or personal or close family history of skin malignancies, such as malignant melanoma. Personal or family history of systemic skin conditions, such as lupus, eczema, or psoriasis, may also guide diagnosis. Associated skin symptoms in sexual partner(s) or close family members suggest a potential infectious process. See Chapter 20 for information about sexually transmitted infections.

Physical Examination

Assessment of the woman's skin should go beyond the vulvar and perianal skin surfaces. Include palpation for systemic lymphadenopathy; careful inspection of the scalp, eyes, nasal mucosa, and oral mucosa; and examination of the abdominal, inguinal, and gluteal skin folds (British Association for Sexual Health and HIV, 2014). All surface inspection requires excellent lighting, augmented by magnifying glass or colposcope, if necessary. A speculum examination should be included to identify vaginal involvement.

Diagnostic Testing

Selective testing may aid diagnosis. For example, testing for concomitant infections may be helpful (e.g., cultures for yeasts or sexually transmitted infections, microscopy for scabies or vaginal pathogens). Vulvar biopsy should be performed if women have any atypical, nonresponding, or otherwise

concerning findings (American College of Obstetricians and Gynecologists [ACOG], 2008b, reaffirmed 2013). A technique for vulvar punch biopsy suggested by Mayeaux and Cooper (2013) is summarized in **Box 26-1**. If the woman is at increased risk for autoimmune disorders based on her personal or family history, appropriate blood tests include thyroid evaluation, serum ferritin, and fasting blood sugar (British Association for Sexual Health and HIV, 2014). Referral for allergy or patch testing may also be warranted.

Differential Diagnoses

A list of differential diagnoses for common vulvar lesions is provided in **Table 26-1**. Additionally, there are a wide variety of rare conditions affecting the vulva that are beyond the scope of this chapter. Unusual findings or inadequate response to standard treatment suggest need for expedient referral to a dermatology specialist. It is also important to remember that concomitant skin conditions are common, and more than one therapy may be necessary. For example, lichen sclerosus can be present with incontinence-associated dermatitis and/or vulvovaginal candidiasis.

Prevention

There is scant to no evidence to support common genital skin care recommendations. For this reason, expert opinion continues to guide recommendations. **Box 26-2** summarizes the general advice for genital skin care that should be provided to women with vulvar irritation (International Society for the Study of Vulval Diseases, 2013a, 2013b). As sensitivities to products vary, women may need to experiment to find their optimal self-care regimen.

Vulvar Skin Cysts

Cysts are closed cavities lined by epithelium and filled with fluid or semisolid material. They are common on the vulva (Lynch, Moyal-Barracco, Scurry, & Stockdale, 2012). Many women also have normal vulvar findings that can be confused with cystic pathology, so clinicians should be aware of these variations. Examples include vulvar papillomatosis (asymmetrical finger-like projections around the vestibule or minora), Fordyce spots (prominent sebaceous glands), and angiokeratomas (benign blood vessel growths often seen on the labia majora)

BOX 26-1 Technique for Vulvar Punch Biopsy

A successful biopsy provides a nondistorted specimen for optimal pathologic interpretation. Cutting or shaving with a scalpel blade or scissors may be used to obtain samples of raised or pedunculated lesions. For flat to slightly raised lesions, a 3- to 6-mm Keyes punch biopsy is often used as follows:

1. Identify the area(s) to be biopsied; typically this includes either the entirety of a small lesion or the most suspicious area(s) of all larger lesions (e.g., atypically pigmented, raised, or irregularly contoured margins).
2. Cleanse the area with povidone–iodine or chlorhexidine.
3. To decrease the woman's discomfort from the local anesthetic injected into this sensitive area, consider initial superficial desensitization with ice or a topical anesthetic (e.g., 2.5% lidocaine with 2.5% prilocaine in a cream base, left in place up to 60 minutes on keratinized skin or 20 minutes on mucous membranes; application on mucous membranes is an off-label use).
4. Lidocaine solution (1–2%) with epinephrine is commonly used as the injected local anesthetic, although epinephrine should be avoided near the clitoris. A tuberculin or 30-gauge needle is held bevel up, with the solution injected slowly to form a bleb under and just beyond the margins of the chosen biopsy site(s).
5. The punch biopsy is held directly perpendicular to the skin surface to avoid distortion and rotated back and forth 180 degrees to just reach the subcutaneous adipose (full thickness); the sample should then be lifted with a tissue forceps, released with a small surgical scissors, and placed in preserving medium, such as formalin.
6. Specimen sites smaller than 4 mm typically do not require closure; any bleeding can be stopped with pressure or application of aluminum chloride or silver nitrate. If a suture is used, removable silk may be more pliable and comfortable on sensitive surfaces than dissolvable suture (e.g., 4-0 chromic). Removable suture is typically removed in 5 to 14 days depending on the amount of stress on the site.

Data from Mayeaux, E. J., & Cooper, D. (2013). Vulvar procedures. *Obstetrics and Gynecology Clinics of North America, 40*, 759–772.

(Schlosser & Mirowski, 2015). Other common, benign changes are reviewed in this section.

Folliculitis, Furuncles, and Carbuncles

Infected hair follicles on the vulvar skin are a common source of vulvar skin cysts. Small, scattered lesions, such as shaving folliculitis, are easily identified and will resolve with elimination of the precipitating factors, in conjunction with warm compresses and/or application of topical antibacterial or antifungal agents if indicated by surrounding erythema. Larger infected cysts, such as vulvar furuncles and carbuncles, may require incision and drainage, culture, and/or systemic antibiotic treatment in women with additional risks, such as

immunosuppression, systemic signs of infection, or inadequate response to other treatments.

Epidermoid and Sebaceous Cysts

Epidermoid (keratin-filled) or similar sebaceous gland cysts can form on vulvar hair-bearing surfaces, with their prevalence increasing with aging. Women often report concerns about these nodules and need reassurance of their benign nature. Both types of cysts are typically slow growing, rarely drain, often resolve spontaneously over weeks or months, and usually require no intervention. Women should be advised to avoid any squeezing and manipulation of these cysts. If a woman reports serious discomfort due to size or site, surgical

---

BOX 26-2 General Skin Care Advice for Women Affected by Vulvar Irritation

- Avoid contact with irritants, which can include chronic irritative moisture (perspiration, incontinence, semen, antiseptics); feminine hygiene products; topical medications (anesthetics such as benzocaine, antifungals); soaps, shampoos, and bubble bath; and hair removal products.
- Simple emollient soap-substitutes are often better tolerated and can be used to both clean and moisturize. If they do seem irritating, use water with a small amount of non-perfumed cream or ointment to avoiding excessive dryness.
- Shower no more than once a day, rather than bathing; avoid over-cleaning or over-drying. Use just a hand (rather than a sponge or washcloth) for cleaning, avoid scrubbing, and pat gently dry.
- Remoisturize throughout the day with any non-perfumed, well-tolerated emollient; cold (refrigerated) moisturizers may help stop itching. Each woman may need to do her own skin test to find an emollient she can tolerate. Skin with a high moisture content will feel less irritated and is better able to avoid infection.
- Avoid use of spermicides.
- Avoid tight-fitting clothing that can cause friction and perspiration buildup.
- Sleep without underwear.

Data from British Association for Sexual Health and HIV. (2014). 2014 UK national guideline on the management of vulval conditions. Retrieved from http://www.bashh.org; International Society for the Study of Vulval Diseases. (2013a). Genital itch in women. Retrieved from http://issvd.org/wordpress/wp-content/uploads/2014/09/GenitalCare-2013-final.pdf; International Society for the Study of Vulval Diseases. (2013b). Genital skin care. Retrieved from http://issvd.org/wordpress/wp-content/uploads/2014/09/GenitalCare-2013-final.pdf.

---

excision can be performed, remembering that new cysts are common.

Hidradenitis Suppurativa

Hidradenitis suppurativa is a chronic, relapsing inflammatory disorder of the hair follicles that can have a similar appearance to sebaceous cysts in its early stages (see **Color Plate 30**). In women, hidradenitis suppurativa is more likely to occur under the breasts and in the axillae, as well as in the genital hair-bearing areas (Margesson & Danby, 2014). Unlike epidermoid cysts, hidradenitis suppurativa can be very painful, disfiguring, and odiferous, and it can have a profound negative effect on quality of life. As many as 4% of women are affected, with an average age of onset of 23 years. Optimal outcomes from treatment require early diagnosis and intervention, with appropriate referral as needed.

Lesions of hidradenitis suppurativa arise due to genetically and hormonally mediated defects in the support structure within the base of the folliculopilosebaceous unit (Margesson & Danby, 2014).

Plugged follicular units become distended with keratin and sebum and can rupture, resulting in inflammation, scarring, and formation of permanent draining sinus tracts. The inflammation is locally mediated, and removal of the contents will resolve individual lesions. Because the lesions are sterile, associated cellulitis and septicemia are rare.

In women, androgen sensitivity plays a role in the expression of hidradenitis suppurativa. Symptoms are often limited to the reproductive years, may be premenstrually cyclic, and may be exacerbated by use of androgenic progestins. Symptoms are also exacerbated by obesity, smoking, lithium use, and dietary sensitivities (e.g., high-glycemic carbohydrates and the androgen precursors in dairy products). In contrast, this condition often improves temporarily during pregnancy and lactation, presumably due to estrogen dominance.

Early symptoms of hidradenitis suppurativa include deep-seated, painful nodules. They can become abscessed or draining sinuses, with bridging and scarring occurring over time (Margesson &

Danby, 2014). Symptoms can be either chronic or recurring. Unlike furuncles, these lesions typically do not respond to antibiotic treatment and do tend to rupture and track subcutaneously, rather than coming to a head and discharging to the surface. For this reason, symptoms are exacerbated by squeezing, pinching, friction, and pressure, which promote rupture and inflammation of the underlying cyst.

In early disease, the differential diagnosis includes epidermoid cysts, folliculitis, and furuncles. Bartholin's duct abscess and anogenital fistulae associated with Crohn's disease are included in the differential diagnosis for advanced disease.

Due to a dearth of evidence, treatment strategies are based on expert opinion. Typically, they are multimodal, including behavioral, metabolic, medical, and surgical strategies (Margesson & Danby, 2014). Behavioral strategies center on avoidance of injury to the skin, and limiting other exacerbating factors. Recommendations include gentle, friction-free local hygiene with a mild, non-soap cleansing bar; antiseptic cleansing, which may be helpful if the odor is bothersome; avoidance of pinching or squeezing; weight control; use of tampons rather than pads; avoidance of nicotine-related products, overheating, tight clothing, and excessive perspiration; zinc supplementation (e.g., zinc gluconate 90 mg/day); and comprehensive avoidance of dietary triggers, especially dairy (due to androgenic properties) and high-glycemic load products (Margesson & Danby, 2014).

Pharmacologic treatments include metformin to aid weight loss; antibiotics for their anti-inflammatory effect and odor control, administered either topically (e.g., clindamycin 1% solution) or systemically (e.g., minocycline); antiandrogens such as drospirenone-containing oral contraceptives or finasteride 5–10 mg/day (the latter is used on an off-label basis with precautions due to teratogenicity); and adjunct immunosuppressives (e.g., high-dose, rapidly tapered prednisone for acute flares). These and other potential agents, including retinoids and phototherapy, may be more comprehensively available through a dermatologic referral. Androgenic progestins should be avoided.

Surgical management options include unroofing of fluctuant lesions, both for early active nodules and branching severe lesions of advanced disease.

Unroofing enhances drainage, resolution, and pain control, and can be done by trained clinicians in primary care settings, using only local anesthesia. It is typically accomplished by snipping with sturdy surgical scissors, held parallel to the skin surface, or, for small lesions, punch biopsy (see **Box 26-1**). The need for more invasive surgical options may be reduced by early intervention. In women with advanced disease, bariatric surgery to aid weight loss and wide excision of severely affected areas can be performed (Margesson & Danby, 2014).

Vulvar Dermatoses

Most dermatoses that affect either skin or mucous membranes can appear on the vulva. This section reviews general management of several vulvar dermatoses. Benign skin changes are differentiated from malignancy either clinically (by response to treatment) or by biopsy. Dermatoses by definition are noninfectious, and they generally involve an inflammatory reaction. They are often treated with high-potency topical corticosteroid preparations; **Boxes 26-3** and **26-4** provide general use instructions for women and clinicians.

While treatments may be similar, expectations for response to treatment can be very different, making it especially important that clinicians are able to achieve an accurate diagnosis. This section addresses specific considerations for management of contact dermatitis, lichenoid disorders (sclerosus, planus, and simplex chronicus), and psoriasis. *Lichen* and *lichenoid* are dermatologic terms applied to inflammatory skin disorders that include flat, scaly patches with an appearance similar to plant lichen.

Clinicians should remember that vulvar dermatoses can result in both physical symptoms and psychological consequences. Women often suffer for years with symptoms and may present for care already feeling frustrated or hopeless. Body image and sexual function can be deeply affected and should be assessed. It is important to spend time reviewing realistic expectations for often long-term care, and to explain that multiple dermatoses may be superimposed and require multiple treatments. At the same time, the clinician should express a commitment to helping each woman obtain relief of symptoms and improve her quality of life. Women with chronic dermatoses may benefit from joining local or online support groups.

BOX 26-3 Instructions for Women Using High-Potency Corticosteroid Products

- Surface application of a strong corticosteroid ointment can be a very safe, effective way to treat inflammation that causes genital skin irritation, but these preparations can cause serious side effects if misused.
- Apply a very small amount of your prescribed product to clean skin, just enough to put a very thin layer onto the area(s) of skin pointed out to you by your clinician. Usually a dab the size of a small pea is enough for one treatment; a small, 30-gram tube of ointment is likely to last several months. Gently massage the product into your skin until it disappears.
- Some women will be allergic to these products. If your rash, irritation, itching, or burning get worse instead of better over the first week, stop using the product and call your clinician. Ointments usually are better tolerated and stay on better than creams; creams generally have more additives.
- Do not use this product on your face, near your eyes or mouth, or on acne or rosacea. Check with your clinician before you use the ointment on any open sores.
- If you are to use the product once a day, try to use it at night, and do not cover the treated skin with tight dressings or clothing.
- Wash your hands after application.
- Keep this product away from children and ask your clinician about continuing use if you become pregnant or are breastfeeding.
- While use as directed is generally safe, overuse can result in too much steroid being absorbed into your body, which can cause several problems, including thinning, weakening, stretch marks, and changes in color of treated skin. In addition, symptoms such as rapid weight gain, skin thinning, and new depression can result from high steroid levels (Cushing's syndrome), and your adrenal glands may stop making normal hormones when the medicine is absorbed in high levels. If you have a tendency toward diabetes or high blood sugar, this can become worse.

Data from British Association for Sexual Health and HIV. (2014). 2014 UK national guideline on the management of vulval conditions. Retrieved from http://www.bashh.org; Schlosser, B. J., & Mirowski, G. W. (2015). Lichen sclerosus and lichen planus in women and girls. *Clinical Obstetrics & Gynecology, 58*, 125–142.

Contact Dermatitis

Irritant contact dermatitis (ICD) and allergic contact dermatitis (ACD) are often referred to collectively as contact dermatitis (ACOG, 2008b, reaffirmed 2013) (see **Color Plate 31)**. These two forms have some distinguishing characteristics, which are summarized in **Table 26-2**. A detailed assessment will help differentiate the various types and develop a plan for prevention. Women with either form of contact dermatitis should avoid provoking agents, and use prescribed topical corticosteroids appropriately until symptoms resolve. Based on the severity of symptoms, a low- to very high-potency steroid

ointment can be selected (**Table 26-3**), typically starting with use once or twice daily until the irritation has resolved.

Lichen Sclerosus

Table 26-4 compares benign, lichenoid disorders. Lichen sclerosus (LS), one of the most common of these conditions, is a chronic mucocutaneous disorder that is characterized by inflammation, epithelial thinning and depigmentation, and dermal changes, which often include agglutination of the labia minora. It can be progressive or relapsing and remitting. While most often genital, LS is

---

BOX 26-4 Guidelines for Prescribing Topical Corticosteroid Therapy

- Treat concomitant candidiasis (e.g., topical nystatin), as steroids can worsen candidal infection.
- Safety in pregnancy and breastfeeding has not been established; the smallest effective dose should be used if indicated.
- Ointments are typically preferred over creams, which are less adherent and more likely to have potentially irritating additives.
- Potent or superpotent steroid therapy is often required for vulvar conditions because the modified mucous membranes of the vulva can be steroid resistant. Caution should be used when corticosteroids are applied to surrounding areas that are not steroid resistant (e.g., hair-bearing areas, perianal skin, and medial thighs) because atrophy can occur more easily in those areas.
- Taper protocols are typically used: corticosteroid (e.g., clobetasol propionate 0.05% ointment or similar agent) applied sparingly once at night for one month, then tapered to every other day for one month, and then twice weekly for one month.
- Carefully instruct the woman in use; a 30-gram tube should last 3 months.
- If symptoms recur with reduced frequency of application during tapering, use can be increased again to control symptoms.
- The woman should be reevaluated 3 months after initiating therapy: persistent or increased symptoms imply need for biopsy and/or referral. If the desired response is achieved, a low to medium potency may be sufficient for maintenance (typically one to three applications per week), or the woman may choose to stop treatment and restart when symptoms recur.
- Ongoing assessment for vulvar status should occur at least annually. Referral should be considered when symptoms are severe, involve the vagina, or are unresponsive to therapy, or if management requires medications with which the clinician is unfamiliar.

Data from American College of Obstetricians and Gynecologists. (2008b, reaffirmed 2013). Diagnosis and management of vulvar skin disorders. Practice Bulletin No. 93. *Obstetrics & Gynecology, 111*, 1243–1253; British Association for Sexual Health and HIV. (2014). 2014 UK national guideline on the management of vulval conditions. Retrieved from http://www.bashh.org; Schlosser, B. J., & Mirowski, G. W. (2015). Lichen sclerosus and lichen planus in women and girls. *Clinical Obstetrics & Gynecology, 58*, 125–142.

---

occasionally identified in other body areas, including the trunk, neck, forearms, axillae, and under the breasts, often occurring on tissue that has undergone trauma (Schlosser & Mirowski, 2015). LS was once thought to be primarily hormonally mediated, as it is most often evident in young girls and in women after menopause. While affected women have been found to have variant hormone receptors, LS is now known to occur in both men and women at any age; it is likely predominantly an autoimmune disorder that manifests in genetically susceptible individuals (Fistarol & Itin, 2013; Schlosser & Mirowski, 2015). Young girls who develop LS prior to puberty are no longer thought to outgrow it, and they should be followed through adolescence and adulthood for surveillance and maintenance therapy as needed. Some affected women may also have other autoimmune disorders, such as thyroid disease, vitiligo, or alopecia areata. While events such as hormonal changes of menopause, infections, trauma, or persistent moisture from occlusive garments may act as precipitating factors, they are not causative. A small increased risk (less than 5%) of vulvar cancer has been noted in women with LS (Schlosser & Mirowski, 2015).

Women with LS can have a range of symptoms, from none to severely debilitating. Early symptoms

TABLE 26-2	Differentiation of Contact Dermatitis

Factor	Irritant Contact Dermatitis	Allergic Contact Dermatitis
Etiology	Non-immunologic	Hypersensitivity reaction to a preexisting allergen; other known systemic or skin allergies common
Common irritants	Perfumed soaps, feminine hygiene sprays and deodorants, bath bubbles and oils, colored or scented toilet paper, laundry detergents, sanitary napkins, tampons, condoms, spermicides, tight clothing, adult wipes, topical medications, and body fluids	Medications (e.g., anesthetics, antibiotics, antifungals, antiseptics, corticosteroids), douches, emollients, fragrances, nail polish, nickel, preservatives, rubber, sanitary napkins, spermicides
Symptom onset	Within 12 hours of exposure	Delayed (48–72 hours post exposure)
Symptoms	Burning, pruritus, pain	Similar to ICD
Signs	Acute: Erythema, edema, vesicles, ulcerations Chronic or subacute: Scale, excoriation	Similar to ICD
Management	Avoidance of provoking agent Cool packs or sitz baths, wet dressings with Burrow's solution to decrease itching and burning Avoidance of scratching Topical corticosteroids until resolution of symptoms	Similar to ICD Severe cases: Oral corticosteroids and antihistamines may be warranted
Resolution	More rapid after elimination of irritant(s)	Slower resolution after elimination of irritant(s)

Abbreviation: ICD, irritant contact dermatitis.
Data from American College of Obstetricians and Gynecologists. (2008b, reaffirmed 2013). Diagnosis and management of vulvar skin disorders. Practice Bulletin No. 93. *Obstetrics & Gynecology, 111*, 1243–1253.

may include dull, nonspecific vulvar irritation, whereas progressive disease often manifests with severe pruritus, burning, and associated dyspareunia. Perianal symptoms, including pruritus ani, painful defecation, and anal fissures, may also occur. Introital stenosis and loss of the structural architecture of the vulva occur with progressive disease. Phimosis of the labia minora over the clitoris can diminish sexual sensation and may result in a pseudocyst due to collection of keratin debris (Schlosser & Mirowski, 2015). Introital stenosis may preclude sexual activity. Dribbling and dysuria may occur from fusion of the minora over the urethra, which may become completely obstructed.

On physical examination, women with LS may have a range of genital skin findings, from maculopapular lesions to coalescing plaques to a classic, pale atrophic figure-eight depigmented formation surrounding the vulva and perianal area (see **Color Plate 32**). The depigmented tissue has a "cigarette paper" appearance and is susceptible to fissuring, ecchymosis, and erosion with minimal trauma. The labia minora may agglutinate and fuse with the labia majora, and eventual phimosis may

TABLE 26-3	Topical Corticosteroid Ointments Used for Vulvar Dermatoses	
Potency	**Medication**	**Strength**
Low	Alclometasone dipropionate (Aclovate)	0.05%
	Desonide (DesOwen)	0.05%
	Hydrocortisone (Hytone)	2.5%
Medium	Betamethasone valerate (Beta-Val, Valisone)	0.1%
	Fluticasone propionate (Cutivate)	0.005%
	Mometasone furoate (Elocon)	0.1%
	Triamcinolone (Aristocort, Kenalog)	0.1%
High	Betamethasone dipropionate (Diprosone, Maxivate)	0.05%
	Desoximetasone (Topicort)	0.05%, 0.25%
	Fluocinonide (Lidex)	0.05%
	Halcinonide (Halog)	0.1%
Very high Superpotent	Betamethasone dipropionate (Diprolene)	0.05%
	Clobetasol propionate (Temovate)	0.05%
	Diflorasone diacetate (Psorcon)	0.05%
	Halobetasol propionate (Ultravate)	0.05%

obscure the clitoris, urethra, and/or introitus. Irregular, patchy post-inflammatory hyperpigmentation is often present, and biopsy may be needed to rule out malignant change (Schlosser & Mirowski, 2015). Nongenital lesions on the neck, upper back, breasts, axillae, scalp, abdomen, or thighs are typically asymptomatic, but may appear as pale, wrinkled papules or plaques (Schlosser & Mirowski, 2015).

In the absence of atypical genital findings, biopsy is generally deferred pending a 12-week treatment trial (Fistarol & Itin, 2013). Biopsy is often inconclusive in early-stage disease, but is generally indicated for persistent areas of unusual pigmentation, hyperkeratosis, erosion, erythema, friability, or focal atypical papules. Additional evaluation could include thyroid testing due to the association of LS with other autoimmune diseases.

A condensed differential diagnosis for vulvar lesions is presented in **Table 26-1**. LS is most often confused with lichen planus, lichen simplex chronicus, vitiligo, immunobullous disorders such as pemphigoid, and vulvar intraepithelial neoplasia.

Goals of treatment of LS include relief of symptoms, potential reversal of agglutination, prevention of further architectural distortion with loss of

function, and prevention of potential malignant changes (Fistarol & Itin, 2013; Schlosser & Mirowski, 2015). First-line treatment consists of high- or very high-potency topical steroid ointment (e.g., clobetasol propionate 0.05%). The optimal regimen has not been determined, but a 3-month tapered dosing schedule is a common recommendation (British Association for Sexual Health and HIV, 2014). Sample guidelines for tapering are presented in **Box 26-4**.

Women with LS should be informed that this skin condition is chronic, that recurrence of symptoms is expected even after successful treatment, and that reuse of treatment has not been found to result in adverse effects. Recommendations for follow-up therapy vary: Some clinicians recommend maintenance corticosteroid application once or twice weekly, whereas others recommend discontinuation of such therapy pending symptom recurrence (ACOG, 2008b, reaffirmed 2013; Fistarol & Itin, 2013).

Although evidence supporting this practice is limited, women with LS may benefit from a yearly vulvar examination to provide for early detection of potential malignant skin changes (Schlosser & Mirowski, 2015). In addition, women should be

TABLE 26-4 **Differentiation of Lichenoid Disorders of the Vulva**

Factor	Lichen Sclerosus	Lichen Planus	Lichen Simplex Chronicus	Psoriasis
Etiology	Autoimmune, hereditary; hormone-receptor variant present	Autoimmune, hereditary, inflammatory condition	Local variant of atopic dermatitis; spontaneous onset or response to chronic friction/scratch	Autoimmune, hereditary
Incidence	Approximately 2%	Rare (less than 1% of women)	Varies; typically reported to be less than 10%	Approximately 3%; most common autoimmune disorder
Age at onset	Bimodal age peak (prepuberty and early postmenopause); 20% of onset is in young adults	Most commonly midlife (ages 40–60)	Any age	Any age; peak onset is adolescence to young adulthood
Distribution	Primarily affects genitalia; anal and perineal involvement common; extragenital and vaginal involvement are rare	Diverse; variant: oral and vaginal involvement	Vulva and periclitoris are commonly affected, but can occur on any chronically irritated skin	Generally scattered (knees, elbows, scalp), but may be only vulvar
Symptoms	Asymptomatic to severe itching, burning, dysuria, dyspareunia; chronic or remitting	Asymptomatic to severe pain; vulvar itching, dysuria, dyspareunia; chronic or remitting	Severe itching; temporary relief by scratching or rubbing; excoriations are common as scratching feels so good	Asymptomatic or mild itch, burning, soreness; intermittent flares; common triggers: cold, dry climate, dry skin, stress; joint pain with related arthritis

(continues)

TABLE 26-4 Differentiation of Lichenoid Disorders of the Vulva (continued)

Factor	Lichen Sclerosus	Lichen Planus	Lichen Simplex Chronicus	Psoriasis
Signs	Onset: Maculopapular coalescing plaques. Advanced: Ivory, "cigarette paper" skin; pale figure-of-eight around vulva and anus; fissures, ecchymosis, erosion, phimosis, and atrophy; agglutination may obscure clitoris, introitus, and/or urethra; lichenification if scratching; post-inflammatory hyperpigmentation common	Type 1 (classic): Pruritic papular lesions of vulva, perineum, perianus; may have white reticulation/striae Type 2 (hypertrophic): Rare; white hypertrophic, rough vulvar plaques, which may have ulcers Type 3 (erosive): Pain; erythematous erosions; serosanguinous discharge; white striae; friable, eroded vagina; adhesions, stenosis, with vaginal and/or clitoral obliteration possible; may have oral involvement	Onset: Mild erythema Advanced: Thickened patch(es), fissures, pallor, excoriations, hyperpigmentation; area may be denuded of pubic hair due to scratching	On vulva: Thin plaques, typically highly erythematous with scant scaling due to maceration; satellite lesions common Inverse psoriasis: predominantly in skin folds
Malignant potential	Less than 5%	Isolated case reports	Not identified	Not identified
Differentiating factors	Symmetrical depigmentation in a figure-of-eight of pale, tissue-paper thin tissue around vulva and perianal area Loss of vulvar architecture with agglutination is common and supports the diagnosis	Vaginal and/or oral involvement; can also affect scalp, skin, and nails Other diagnostic criteria: Well-demarcated erosions; white, hyperkeratotic borders; pain, burning, scarring, loss of genital architecture	Temporary relief with scratching; thickened keratinized skin; excoriations	Family or personal history; thick, pale red to white scaly plaques outside the genital area; typically thin, bright red, well-demarcated plaques without scaling on genitals; milder itch typical, excoriations uncommon

Management	Rule out other auto-immune disorders (thyroid, ferritin, diabetes) Defer biopsy of symmetrical classic signs pending 3-month treatment trial First-line: High- or very high-potency steroid ointment tapered (e.g., daily for 1 month, every other day the next month, then twice weekly) Nonresponse warrants biopsy and/or referral Maintenance therapy after successful treatment is often needed (continuous or intermittent)	Type 1: May resolve spontaneously or may use emollient and medium-potency topical steroid Type 2: Superpotent topical steroid over 3 months or intralesional injection (triamcinolone) repeated in 6–8 weeks as needed Type 3: Superpotent topical steroid for 3 months; taper as symptoms improve, then maintenance (once or twice weekly); second-line: tacrolimus, pimecrolimus, intralesional corticosteroid injection, oral prednisolone, antibiotics, or immunosuppressive (e.g., azathioprine, cyclosporine)	Eliminate identifiable irritants Rule out secondary infection (e.g., yeast culture) Topical xylocaine and oral antihistamine/anxiolytic (e.g., hydroxyzine) to break nighttime itch–scratch–itch cycle Superpotent topical steroid ointment, tapered over 3–4 months until lichenification is totally resolved Cognitive-behavioral therapy for concomitant mental illness	Biopsy seldom required for diagnosis Keep skin moist with emollients; careful exposure to sunlight may be helpful; topical steroids
Other considerations	Ongoing yearly vulvar examination warranted to identify early skin changes due to the small increased risk of vulvar cancer	Specialist referral for erosive or vaginal disease, as condition is highly debilitating Early use of progressive vaginal dilators may improve and preserve vaginal integrity	Consider psychological component if resolution is atypical (e.g., obsessive–compulsive disorder)	Referral and online support groups may be helpful for women with extensive disease

Data from British Association for Sexual Health and HIV. (2014). 2014 UK national guideline on the management of vulval conditions. Retrieved from http://www.bashh.org; Schlosser, B. J., & Mirowski, G. W. (2015). Lichen sclerosus and lichen planus in women and girls. *Clinical Obstetrics & Gynecology, 58*, 125–142.

asked to contact the clinician if they notice interim changes in vulvar symptoms or appearance.

For women with atypical findings, equivocal biopsy, or poorly controlled symptoms with appropriate topical corticosteroid treatment, referral to a specialist is warranted. Surgery is typically reserved for release of phimosis, introital stenosis, or excision of malignancy. Other experimental treatments include phototherapy, topical or systemic retinoids, and the topical calcineurin inhibitors pimecrolimus and tacrolimus (Fistarol & Itin, 2013). Use of such experimental treatments, especially immunosuppressive agents, is done on an off-label basis and remains controversial, because of the already small elevation in malignant potential attributed to LS.

Lichen Planus

Fewer than 1% of all women are affected by lichen planus (LP), but it has the potential to be the most debilitating type of autoimmune-mediated, lichenoid inflammatory condition (Schlosser & Mirowski, 2015). While LP can affect men, it is more common in women, where it is typically identified on the vulva, scalp, skin, nails, and/or epithelial linings of the mouth and vagina (Fistarol & Itin, 2013). LS and LP can be very similar clinically and histologically, and some women may not receive a differentiated diagnosis (Schlosser & Mirowski, 2015).

Clinical findings are used to differentiate three types of LP: type 1 (classical), type 2 (hypertrophic), and type 3 (erosive) (British Association for Sexual Health and HIV, 2014; Schlosser & Mirowski, 2015) (see also **Table 26-4**). Type 3 (erosive) LP is the most likely to cause severe vulvovaginal symptoms (see **Color Plate 33**). Its presentation can include severe genital pain with vaginal involvement, brightly erythematous erosions, white striae on erosion borders (Wickham's striae), and serosanguinous discharge. Eroded vaginal epithelium can bleed easily with any penetration. Purulent-appearing discharge is common, and adhesion, stenosis, and obliteration of the vagina can occur.

Some women have a variant of erosive LP called vulvovaginal–gingival syndrome, which involves similar highly erythematous, erosive, striated lesions on the gingivae, buccal mucosa, and tongue, as well as small papules or rough plaques. A second variant, inverse LP, results in erythematous papules

and/or diffuse erythema without scale within moist skin folds (e.g., inguinal, axillary, gluteal, intramammary) (Schlosser & Mirowski, 2015).

LP is typically treated with corticosteroids topically, intralesionally, and/or systemically, and women can expect to experience a treatment response based on their type of LP (**Table 26-4**). Erosive LP is most often managed by multidisciplinary specialists, as it is the most painful, debilitating, and difficult-to-treat type. One treatment specific to erosive vaginal involvement is the use of vaginal dilators to help manage agglutination and stenosis, and improve the woman's ability to resume or continue sexual penetration. For this treatment, the woman is taught to use progressively sized vaginal dilators, often in conjunction with intravaginal topical steroid ointment, holding the dilator in her vagina overnight with snug-fitting underwear. Once the appropriate-size dilator is reached, she may need to continue its use at least weekly for maintenance of her vaginal patency. If labial or vaginal agglutination is bothersome, surgical intervention may be helpful once active inflammation is controlled (ACOG, 2008b, reaffirmed 2013).

Lichen Simplex Chronicus

Lichen simplex chronicus (LSC; formerly called squamous hyperplasia, hyperplastic dystrophy, and leukoplakia) is a localized variant of atopic dermatitis (British Association for Sexual Health and HIV, 2014). LSC can arise spontaneously, often in women with other atopic conditions such as allergies or asthma, or it can be triggered by a vulvar disorder that causes pruritus. As the woman scratches, epidermal thickening and hyperproliferation of the cells (lichenification) occur. As the tissue thickens, blood flow is further compromised, and itching becomes increasingly intense as the itch–scratch–itch cycle progresses.

Presenting symptoms and signs of LSC typically facilitate the differentiation of this condition from LS and LP (**Table 26-4**). Affected women often report prior ineffective treatments for vague diagnoses, such as chronic yeast infections. Symptoms of itching can be continuous or recurrent, often for years, and typically are unique in that scratching or rubbing offer an intensely pleasurable temporary relief of the itch, especially at night.

Initial signs may include localized edema and erythema, and mild exaggeration of the skin architecture. As the disease progresses, fissures, excoriation, epidermal thickening, and lichenified plaques will become visible (see **Color Plate 34**). Hyperpigmentation or unusual whiteness of the tissue (from scale) may also be evident. Pubic hair may be broken or eliminated by chronic scratching (British Association for Sexual Health and HIV, 2014).

Affected women should be screened for secondary infections, if suspected; if such an infection is identified, oral therapy should be considered to minimize potential vulvar irritation. For the LSC itself, superpotent topical corticosteroid ointment (e.g., clobetasol propionate 0.05%) is again the first-line treatment (**Table 26-3** and **Boxes 26-3** and **26-4**). Corticosteroids are typically not effective immediately, however, so 2% lidocaine jelly may be used initially to relieve itching until the steroids take effect (British Association for Sexual Health and HIV, 2014). Second-line treatments, such as tacrolimus or pimecrolimus, are typically reserved for specialist referral.

Itching and scratching are often worse at night, and medications that provide sedation may be helpful in managing these nocturnal symptoms. Low-dose tricyclic antidepressants, such as amitriptyline or doxepin, may provide better and longer sedation than antihistamines (e.g., hydroxyzine, diphenhydramine), while also improving anxiety and depression, which are common associated symptoms in many women with LSC. Wearing gloves at night may also be helpful to interrupt the itch–scratch–itch cycle (British Association for Sexual Health and HIV, 2014).

Psoriasis

Psoriasis is a chronic, immune-mediated, genetic disease that manifests in the skin and/or joints. While the peak incidence of this disease is adolescence through the 20s, it can develop at any age.

The most common form of psoriasis is characterized by well-demarcated, pale, erythematous papules or plaques covered with silvery-white, often thick scale. These lesions are frequently found on the knees, elbows, and scalp. Vulvar psoriasis (see **Color Plate 35**) can occur as an isolated manifestation, or coexist with psoriasis on other body areas. On genital skin, which is typically moister,

psoriasis-related plaques tend to be thinner and more intensely erythematous, with minimal scaling due to maceration (British Association for Sexual Health and HIV, 2014). Inverse psoriasis is a variant that involves the development of red, well-demarcated plaques only in skin folds (e.g., natal, inguinal, gluteal). Satellite lesions are often present, and women with inverse psoriasis are often misdiagnosed and ineffectively treated for candidal intertrigo or incontinence-associated dermatitis.

While vulvar psoriasis may be asymptomatic, symptoms may also include itching, burning, soreness, and fissuring of skin folds. Symptoms are typically less intense than with other lichenoid conditions. Many women report triggers of disease recurrence, including emotional stress; cold, dry weather, with limited sunlight; and skin dryness. Affected skin may benefit from regular use of emollients and/or moisture barriers to improve skin moisture content. When flares occur, topical corticosteroids are again the mainstay of therapy, but weak- to moderate-potency agents may be sufficient to control symptoms in many women (**Table 26-3** and **Boxes 26-3** and **26-4**). Referral is indicated if vulvar psoriasis is unresponsive to corticosteroids.

Special Considerations

Specific Populations

Women Who Are Pregnant or Breastfeeding Most management strategies for genital skin care do not vary by age. However, recommendations related to treatment in pregnancy and lactation may vary by country. In the United States, clobetasol and other topical steroids remain Category C drugs, to be used with caution, whereas in the United Kingdom these agents are recommended as safe for use as directed in pregnancy and lactation (British Association for Sexual Health and HIV, 2014). Other second-line potential treatment agents, such as calcineurin inhibitors and retinoids, are contraindicated in pregnancy and lactation. When topical steroids are not sufficiently effective in treating vulvar conditions, a woman who is pregnant should be referred to a specialist.

Postmenopausal Women In women who are post menopause, treatment of concomitant genital atrophy with a topical estrogen product may play and important role in symptom relief. See Chapters 12 and 19 for more information about vulvovaginal atrophy and hormone therapy).

Influences of Culture

Ideas of genital health and beauty vary markedly between cultures. Women presenting with bothersome genital skin symptoms may have strongly held and divergent beliefs about the importance of activities such as genital shaving, hygiene products, piercing, tattooing, cosmetic surgeries or genital cutting, and self-touch. Couples may have difficulty understanding which skin conditions are infectious and which are not. Environmental factors, such as cold, dry weather, or heat and humidity, can aggravate many genital skin conditions. Continence care and basic hygiene can be very problematic in resource-scarce cultures, and highly effective steroid ointments may be unavailable or prohibitively expensive. Clinicians need to be sensitive and respectful of cultural norms, while helping women find safe and nonirritating care routines to attain and maintain healthy genital skin.

CONDITIONS OF THE UTERUS AND CERVIX

Women with non-pregnancy-related concerns about their uterus and uterine cervix often have pain or bleeding, or worry about the potential for malignancy. This section addresses evaluation and management options for women experiencing several common conditions that may raise those concerns: polyps of the cervix and uterus, uterine fibroids, and the ectopic endometrial conditions of endometriosis and adenomyosis. Further information about normal variations on physical examination, such as cervical changes such as ectropion and Nabothian cysts, are described in Chapter 6. Infections and malignancy of the cervix and endometrium are addressed Chapters 20 and 27, while management of abnormal uterine bleeding is addressed in Chapter 24.

Polyps

Polyps formed within the endocervical canal or endometrium are focal hyperplastic protrusions of epithelial tissue with a vascular core, not true neoplasia (Buyukbayrak et al., 2011). Their etiology is unknown, but both hormonal and chronic inflammatory stimuli

may play a role in their formation. Although typically benign, they do have malignant potential, and women with such polyps need careful education as they consider their treatment options.

Cervical Polyps

Cervical polyps occur in as many as 10% of women, but fewer than 1% of those polyps are malignant. They can be single or multiple in number, and typically are less than 3 cm in diameter, but can be larger. Usually lobular or pear shaped, their stalk arises from the cervical canal and may be either short or long. Cervical polyps range in color from flesh colored to reddish-purple if vascular congestion is present (see **Color Plate 36**).

Cervical polyps are often asymptomatic and incidentally diagnosed on routine speculum examination. If symptoms occur, they typically include postcoital or intermenstrual bleeding. Differential diagnosis includes endometrial polyps, cervical carcinoma, and cervical leiomyomata, all of which also may protrude through the cervical os. Approximately 10% of women with cervical polyps will have concomitant endometrial pathology (e.g., atypia, cancer, or polyps) (Buyukbayrak et al., 2011), and evaluation of the endometrium should be considered whenever women present with irregular bleeding.

When cervical polyps are identified, women will need to choose between observation and removal for histology (Nelson, Papa, & Ritchie, 2015). Up-to-date cytology, HPV testing, and colposcopy are important aids to rule out high risk for dysplasia or malignancy. If the polyp is asymptomatic and the woman prefers the option of observation, she should be asked to report irregular or postcoital bleeding. If a woman with cervical polyps experiences symptoms (e.g., irregular or postcoital bleeding, increased discharge) or has an atypical polyp (e.g., larger than 3 cm, necrotic, friable, irregular color), removal for histology is indicated (Nelson et al., 2015). The woman should also be informed that if the polyp is removed, recurrence is not uncommon.

If the stalk insertion is clearly visible, removal of a simple cervical polyp may be accomplished in the office setting by an experienced clinician. Typically, the polyp is grasped gently at the stalk with a ring forceps, clamped pressure is applied for 3 to 5 minutes to achieve homeostasis, and then the forceps is twisted with gentle traction to remove the polyp. The vascular core of the polyp may sometimes bleed heavily with this procedure, so an option for cautery must be available. Cautery may also decrease the risk of recurrence. If the woman opts for removal or it is otherwise indicated but the polyp base is not clearly identifiable, transvaginal ultrasound may facilitate the differential diagnosis and/or referral for operative hysteroscopy may be required for safe removal.

Endometrial Polyps

Endometrial polyps are similar to cervical polyps in that they are a hyperplastic overgrowth of the endometrial glandular and stromal cells with a vascular core. They are also most often asymptomatic, can be single or multiple in number, and are a common cause of abnormal vaginal bleeding (Matthews, 2015). Endometrial polyps are typically smaller than 10 mm in size, and approximately 25% of the smaller polyps resolve spontaneously within one year (AAGL, 2012).

Endometrial polyps are most common in women 30 to 50 years of age, but their prevalence does not appear to change after menopause. Because they are often asymptomatic, their incidence is unknown; estimates range from 7% to 35% of women. One-third of women of any age who are evaluated for infertility have endometrial polyps, but causation is not established and age may be a factor (AAGL, 2012). Women who have symptoms most typically report abnormal (e.g., intermenstrual or postmenopausal) bleeding. Malignant transformation appears to be uncommon, but such polyps share similar risk factors with endometrial cancer, including increasing age, obesity, hypertension, and use of selective estrogen receptor modulators that stimulate the endometrium (e.g., tamoxifen). For this reason, unexpected bleeding in women with these risk factors should raise the level of concern (AAGL, 2012; Ricciardi et al., 2014).

Endometrial polyps are most commonly identified and evaluated using transvaginal ultrasound. In menstruating women, this imaging is optimally done when the endometrium is thinnest (in the early follicular phase, cycle days 4–6) to improve detection of polyps smaller than 10 mm (AAGL, 2012; Matthews, 2015). Both color or power Doppler and contrast with or without 3-D imaging may improve visualization. If the findings are ambiguous, repeat

imaging at a more optimal cycle time may be appropriate, or referral may be warranted. Saline infusion sonohysterogram is often used to facilitate visualization during ultrasound, and hysteroscopy (i.e., placement of a thin telescopic tube through the cervix and into the uterine canal) can be used for identification and biopsy.

For asymptomatic endometrial polyps identified incidentally on ultrasound imaging, conservative management, such as repeat imaging to establish stability, is an appropriate option (AAGL, 2012). Medications have a limited role in treating symptomatic polyps. Gonadotropin-releasing hormone (GnRH) agonists are sometimes used to shrink large polyps prior to hysteroscopic resection, but the cost-effectiveness of this therapy is not clear. The levonorgestrel intrauterine system (LNG-IUS) does not have a role in treatment but may prevent endometrial polyp formation in high-risk women, such as those using tamoxifen (AAGL, 2012). For women who report abnormal bleeding, blind biopsy is inadequate; hysteroscopic polypectomy is the removal method of choice (AAGL, 2012).

Specific Populations

Pregnant Women Pregnancy is a contraindication to removal of either cervical or endometrial polyps. Unless there is an urgent indication, removal should be deferred or performed only by a specialist.

Postmenopausal Women Malignancy risk increases with aging; postmenopausal women with atypical polyps and/or vaginal bleeding warrant a thorough endometrial evaluation (e.g., imaging and guided biopsy or polypectomy).

Uterine Fibroids

Uterine fibroids, also known as myomas or leiomyomatas, are benign growths that arise from the smooth muscle of the uterus. They are classified based on the uterine layer most involved in their location: *Subserosal* fibroids arise on the external surface of the uterus, *intramural* or *myometrial* fibroids lie completely within the myometrium, and *submucosal* fibroids make contact with the endometrium (see **Color Plate 37**). When fibroids are pedunculated, they are vulnerable to torsion, necrosis, or prolapse through the cervical canal, where they can be confused with cervical polyps. Fibroids range in size from microscopic to large tumors weighing several pounds. Multiple fibroids are common, but they can also occur singularly.

Incidence

The majority of women have fibroids present in their uterus by menopause, but only approximately 25% become symptomatic (Aissani, Zhang, & Weiner, 2015; Segars et al., 2014). Even so, fibroids are the most common indication for hysterectomy in the United States.

Heredity and cumulative exposure to estrogen both play roles in fibroid growth. Symptomatic fibroids are more common in the decade prior to menopause, in obese and primiparous women, and in women with African ancestry; they are uncommon after menopause. While most women with fibroids do not have infertility or related pregnancy loss, fibroids can impede fertility in some women, depending on their size and location (e.g., via blockage of sperm migration or of implantation due to the decreased blood supply and hypoestrogenic environment of the fibroids themselves) (Patel, Malik, Britten, Cox, & Catherino, 2014).

Etiology and Pathophysiology

The etiology of fibroids remains poorly understood (Segars et al., 2014). The extent of their expression in an individual woman's uterus appears to depend on a convergence of genetic, environmental, and lifestyle factors. They are known to arise from uterine smooth muscle (myometrium). The myometrial cells in fibroids are more similar to gravid rather than nongravid cells, suggesting they may be a manifestation of the type of myometrial stem cell stimulation and hyperproliferation normally seen in a pregnant uterus. The cells of fibroids also display disorganization of collagen fibrils very similar to that seen in keloids, suggesting a potential common etiology, which is supported by the more common occurrence of both keloids and fibroids in women of African ancestry. It is surprisingly unclear why fibroids, which result from highly hormone-sensitive cellular hyperproliferation, so rarely involve malignancy (less than 1%) (Segars et al., 2014).

Clinical Presentation

The majority of fibroids are asymptomatic and identified incidentally at ultrasound or pathology.

Women who have symptoms typically report heavy or irregular menses, dysmenorrhea, pelvic pressure or pain, dyspareunia, or change in urine or bowel control (Segars et al., 2014). Some women with fibroids may also have associated pregnancy-related problems, including infertility and pregnancy loss. When women report pain, it is often dull, crampy, and mild to moderate, but pain may become acute if torsion or necrosis occurs. Women with very enlarged fibroids may report an increase in abdominal girth, and occasionally incorrectly assume they are pregnant. Fibroids (subserosal, intramural, or submucosal), can occasionally involve the cervix or protrude through the cervical canal, being visible or palpable as a mass on pelvic examination.

Assessment

Key factors in the health history of women presenting with symptoms suggestive of uterine fibroids (e.g., abnormal uterine bleeding, pelvic pain or pressure) include a detailed menstrual and bleeding history, and clear descriptors of related pain or pressure, helping to define any cyclic relationship. Women should be asked about any difficulty achieving or maintaining pregnancy and any personal or family history of uterine fibroids or keloid formation.

Typically, fibroids are firm to palpation and nontender. Whether or not they are palpable will depend on their location and size. The uterus may be palpable abdominally if the fibroids are very large. On bimanual examination, the uterus may feel normal, smoothly enlarged, or irregular. Rectal examination may facilitate the identification of posterior fibroids. A pedunculated subserosal fibroid may be confused with a firm adnexal mass. Guarding or rebound tenderness can indicate irritation of the peritoneum related to torsion.

Definitive diagnosis of fibroids is usually made by ultrasound. In perimenopausal and postmenopausal women, endometrial cancer should be ruled out even if fibroids are identified, as they may be a concomitant condition. Any woman who reports frequent, heavy bleeding should have a hematocrit to evaluate the extent of blood loss.

Differential Diagnoses

Uterine fibroids are part of the differential diagnosis for abnormal uterine bleeding (see Chapter 24).

Women can experience similar symptoms of pelvic pain and pressure with endometriosis and adenomyosis as well as non-uterine conditions, such as ascites; disorders of the gastrointestinal tract (e.g., constipation, irritable bowel syndrome) or urinary tract (e.g., bladder diverticula, benign tumors); other gynecologic abnormalities (e.g., benign adnexal tumors); and neoplasia at any abdominal or pelvic location.

Management

No effective strategies for prevention or early intervention for fibroids have been identified, and conversion to malignancy is rare (Segars et al., 2014). For these reasons, asymptomatic uterine fibroids are managed expectantly. When fibroids become symptomatic, treatment options include medical therapies, surgery (minimally invasive procedures or hysterectomy), uterine artery embolization, and magnetic resonance imaging (MRI)-guided focused ultrasound. There are very limited comparative outcomes data for these modalities (Marret et al., 2012), and even fewer studies have been conducted that included a representative number of women of African ancestry (Segars et al., 2014). Generally, decisions about the timing and type of treatment are based on the number, size, and location of fibroids; the type and severity of symptoms; the woman's age and proximity to menopause; future childbearing plans; and preference regarding uterine preservation (Matthews, 2015).

No available medical treatments make fibroids disappear. To be the optimal treatment for women with symptomatic fibroids, an agent would need to reduce fibroid size and symptoms over the long term, with minimal side effects and fertility preservation, if desired. Current options, summarized in **Table 26-5**, do not meet these criteria, but rather are expected to modify symptoms and/or shrink fibroids temporarily (Marret et al., 2012; Segars et al., 2014; Song, Lu, Navaratnam, & Shi, 2013).

If a woman chiefly desires control of fibroid-related heavy bleeding, oral progestogens, an LNG-IUS, or a short-term GnRH agonist may be sufficient (Marret et al., 2012). The LNG-IUS may improve dysmenorrhea as well. The LNG-IUS is contraindicated for women who have fibroids that are submucosal, distort the uterine cavity, or are large (total uterine size greater than 12 cm). Chapter 11 contains additional information about the LNG-IUS.

Leuprolide, a GnRH agonist, is approved by the U.S. Food and Drug Administration (FDA) as a medical treatment to shrink fibroids temporarily (e.g., preoperatively or prior to attempting to become pregnant), and may temporarily control bleeding (see **Tables 26-5** and **26-6**). Preoperative GnRH agonist treatment not only reduces fibroid volume (35% to 65% within 3 months of initiating treatment), but also increases systemic blood volume, thereby lowering the risks associated with surgery (Matthews, 2015). Major concerns for women using GnRH agonists include vasomotor symptoms and decreases in bone density, so only short-term treatment is approved. The effect of a GnRH agonist is temporary: Fibroids will begin to regrow within months of discontinuation, and surgery or pregnancy attempts should ensue as soon as therapy is completed to maximize the benefits.

Although surgery is rarely indicated for women with asymptomatic fibroids, women may choose surgical treatment if they have pedunculated fibroids, due to the higher risk for torsion; related symptoms poorly controlled by medical treatments; or fibroids that obstruct other treatments (e.g., fertility or cancer interventions). Surgical options for the treatment of fibroids include myomectomy and hysterectomy (ACOG, 2008a, reaffirmed 2014; Marret et al., 2012; Matthews, 2015). Hysterectomy is a definitive option for women who have severe symptoms, are distant from menopause, and feel they have completed childbearing. Laparoscopically assisted and transvaginal hysterectomies have been shown to reduce postoperative recovery time and infection risk. Nevertheless, open abdominal procedures continue to be performed for women with large fibroids, especially since the FDA issued warnings about power morcellation (debulking of large fibroids in situ to aid removal) carrying a risk of disseminating rare uterine sarcomas (Liu, Galvan-Turner, Pfaenler, Longoria, & Bristow, 2015).

Myomectomy, in contrast, preserves the uterus, and can be performed laparoscopically, abdominally, or hysteroscopically depending on fibroid quantity, size, and location (Matthews, 2015). This procedure can be performed in conjunction with a cesarean birth if indicated. Myomectomy does not prevent the growth of new lesions, however, and women

TABLE 26-5	Medical Treatment Options for Uterine Fibroids

Class	Target Symptom(s)	Considerations
Progestogens	Heavy bleeding	Reduce fibroid-associated endometrial hyperplasia Intrauterine system may improve dysmenorrhea also but is contraindicated with submucosal fibroids or an irregularly shaped endometrial cavity
Gonadotropin-releasing hormone agonist	Used to shrink fibroid prior to fertility treatment or surgery May control heavy bleeding	Only approved for short term (3 months) due to adverse-effect profile Fibroids can regrow quickly after treatment
Selective estrogen reuptake modulators	Shrink fibroid volume	Off-label use May increase cancer risk in other cells
Selective progesterone receptor modulators	Shrink fibroid volume	Off-label use May increase cancer risk in other cells
Aromatase inhibitors	Shrink fibroid volume	Off-label use, limited data, and high adverse-effect profile
Combined oral contraceptives	May improve periodic bleeding control and/or dysmenorrhea	No evidence they enhance fibroid growth; not contraindicated for women with fibroids
Nonsteroidal anti-inflammatory drugs	May improve periodic bleeding control and/or dysmenorrhea	Rare but serious risks include gastrointestinal bleeding, acute renal failure, and congestive heart failure

Data from American College of Obstetricians and Gynecologists. (2008b, reaffirmed 2013). Diagnosis and management of vulvar skin disorders. Practice Bulletin No. 93. *Obstetrics & Gynecology, 111,* 1243–1253; Matthews, M. L. (2015). Abnormal uterine bleeding in reproductive-aged women. *Obstetrics and Gynecology Clinics of North America, 42,* 103–115; Segars, J. H., Parrott, E. C., Nagel, J. D., Guo, X. C., Gao, X., Birnbaum, L. S., & Pinn, V. W. (2014). Proceedings from the Third National Institutes of Health International Congress on Advances in Uterine Leiomyoma Research: Comprehensive summary and future recommendations. *Human Reproduction Update, 20,* 309–333.

choosing this option should be aware that they may require future procedures if symptomatic fibroids recur.

Additional nonmedical, minimally invasive treatments are currently available or in development to resolve or decrease the size of fibroids through necrosis. These options include the FDA-approved procedures of uterine artery embolization (UAE) and MRI-guided focal ultrasonography ablation, as well as cryomyolysis and temporary transvaginal occlusion of the uterine arteries, which are not yet approved (Matthews, 2015; Patel et al., 2014). UAE is performed by interventional radiology and involves a guided injection of embolic particles to obstruct vascular supply of the fibroid(s). The limited evidence comparing UAE to surgery suggests that women who undergo UAE may be equally satisfied with their outcome but are more likely to have additional surgical treatment for fibroids within 5 years (32% versus 7% respectively) (Gupta, Sinha,

TABLE 26-6	Gonadotropin-Releasing Hormone Agonists		

Product Names	Approved Indication(s)	Route of Administration	Dosage
Leuprolide (Lupron)	Endometriosis and uterine fibroids	Intramuscular injection	3.75 mg monthly or 11.25 mg every 3 months
Nafarelin (Synarel)	Endometriosis	Nasal spray, 200 mcg per spray	400–800 mcg per day 400 mcg: One spray in one nostril in the morning and one spray in the other nostril in the evening 800 mcg: One spray in each nostril twice a day
Goserelin (Zoladex)	Endometriosis	Subcutaneous injection in the upper abdomen	3.6 mg monthly

Note: These medications are contraindicated in pregnancy and must be used in conjunction with contraception. See the specific prescribing reference for full information on doses, side effects, contraindications, and cautions.
Data from American College of Obstetricians and Gynecologists. (2008b, reaffirmed 2013). Diagnosis and management of vulvar skin disorders. Practice Bulletin No. 93. *Obstetrics & Gynecology, 111,* 1243–1253; Matthews, M. L. (2015). Abnormal uterine bleeding in reproductive-aged women. *Obstetrics and Gynecology Clinics of North America, 42,* 103–115; Segars, J. H., Parrott, E. C., Nagel, J. D., Guo, X. C., Gao, X., Birnbaum, L. S., & Pinn, V. W. (2014). Proceedings from the Third National Institutes of Health International Congress on Advances in Uterine Leiomyoma Research: Comprehensive summary and future recommendations. *Human Reproduction Update, 20,* 309–333.

Lumsden, & Hickey, 2014). MRI-guided, focused high-frequency ultrasound therapy is a thermoablative option for inducing fibroid necrosis and was FDA approved for treatment of fibroids in 2004 (Patel et al., 2014). Cryomyolysis involves the use of a probe to apply a cooling agent to necrose the fibroid. Temporary transvaginal occlusion of uterine arteries is an outpatient technique to achieve ischemia of the fibroid(s). No comparisons of important outcomes, such as cost-effectiveness and future pregnancy risks, are available for these procedures (Marret et al., 2012). Fertility outcomes after these uterus-sparing procedures have not been well studied.

While most uterine fibroids present as a chronic subacute condition, emergencies can occur. Torsion, which can cause acute, severe abdominal pain and necrosis, is a surgical emergency requiring immediate referral. Acute hemorrhage may also occur. Women with symptomatic fibroids who do not improve with medical management or are attempting pregnancy and meet the criteria for infertility

should be referred for general gynecologic or specialist intervention.

Specific Populations

Pregnant Women Many women with fibroids have normal pregnancy outcomes. Even so, close observation is indicated in pregnancy, as women with fibroids have a higher risk of poor pregnancy outcomes, including infertility, failed implantation, spontaneous abortion, preterm labor, placental abruption, malpresentation, cesarean birth, peripartum hysterectomy, and postpartum hemorrhage (Segars et al., 2014). Some of these associations may be explained by advanced maternal age (Marret et al., 2012).

Pre-pregnancy, fibroidectomy may be considered in women with fibroids that appear to be impairing fertility and for submucosal fibroids (Marret et al., 2012). Approximately 70% of fibroids grow during pregnancy (De Vivo et al., 2011), suggesting a role for serial reevaluation of enlarging fibroids when women become pregnant. Any other intervention during pregnancy typically involves a response to specific symptoms, such as acute pain. Women who have undergone a prior myomectomy have a small increased risk of uterine rupture in labor, and should be carefully counseled and monitored related to their individual history (Marret et al., 2012).

Perimenopausal and Postmenopausal Women
After menopause, the spontaneous decrease in hormone production typically results in reduction in fibroid size and resolution of symptoms. Exogenous hormone therapy after menopause is not contraindicated for women with fibroids if that treatment is otherwise warranted (ACOG, 2008a, reaffirmed 2014; Marret et al., 2012). For women who are perimenopausal or postmenopausal and present with enlarging fibroids, hysterectomy is indicated. Myomectomy, especially via power morcellation, is contraindicated in such women because the risk of occult cancers of the uterine corpus increases with aging.

Influences of Culture
Abnormal, irregular bleeding can cause significant social and sexual difficulties for women from cultures that have activity taboos related to menstrual bleeding. In addition, the lack of proven alternative therapies for treatment of uterine fibroids and the potential need for surgery may be problematic for women who prefer to avoid allopathic medicine. Fertility preservation may be of primary importance for women from some cultures and may warrant special consideration in treatment planning. All of these concerns may also play a role in assessment and treatment planning for women with the benign conditions discussed in the remainder of this chapter, including endometriosis, adenomyosis, and ovarian cysts.

Endometriosis and Adenomyosis

Endometriosis is the presence of endometrial glands and stroma outside of the uterus. Adenomyosis includes the presence of similarly atypical diffuse or localized endometrial cells within the myometrium and is a variant of endometriosis. Outside of the uterus, endometrial implants have been identified in diverse sites, including the ovaries, anterior and posterior cul-de-sac, posterior broad ligaments, uterosacral ligaments, fallopian tubes, sigmoid colon, appendix, and round ligaments. Less commonly, histology has confirmed cases in other genital organs (e.g., vagina, vulva, cervix, perineum), the urinary tract, inguinal canals, elsewhere in the gastrointestinal tract, the respiratory system and diaphragm, the pericardium, surgical scars, and the umbilicus (Machairiotis et al., 2013). Women affected by endometriosis at any site may have cyclic or noncyclic pain that severely impairs their quality of life and are also at increased risk for infertility and poor pregnancy outcomes.

Incidence
The true incidence of endometriosis is unknown, but it is thought to affect at least 10% of women (Kodaman, 2015). This condition, which can be very burdensome, is present in more than 80% of women with chronic pelvic pain, 50% of women with infertility, and 50% of adolescents with dysmenorrhea (ACOG, 2010, reaffirmed 2014). Adenomyosis has been identified in 20% to 30% of pathology specimens at hysterectomy (Cockerham, 2012).

Risk factors for endometriosis include genetic factors (sevenfold risk increase in women with symptomatic first-degree relatives), Caucasian race, early menarche, short menstrual cycles, and active ovarian function (symptoms are uncommon in premenarche and after menopause) (Kodaman, 2015). In addition, women with a diagnosis of endometriosis are more likely to have other pain syndromes (e.g., interstitial cystitis, fibromyalgia) and other autoimmune conditions (e.g., thyroid dysfunction, asthma), suggesting this condition may involve both underlying alterations in immune surveillance and central sensitization (Smorgick, Marsh, As-Sanie, Smith, & Quint, 2013).

Etiology
Understanding of the etiology of endometriosis continues to evolve. Multiple mechanisms—hereditary, environmental, immunologic, mechanical, and hormonal—have been proposed to account for the ectopic distribution and activation of endometrial cells (Machairiotis et al., 2013; Signorile & Baldi, 2015); they are summarized in **Box 26-5**. These mechanisms may be responsible for the varied phenotypes of endometriosis, which include adenomyosis; the often asymptomatic superficial

BOX 26-5 Proposed Mechanisms for the Development of Endometriosis

- Implantation of otherwise normal retrograde menstruation (observed as early as neo-natally), which becomes activated in girls and women with genetic or environmentally mediated susceptibility
- Spontaneous metaplasia of coelomic epithe-lium (the lining cells of body cavities) or mesenchymal stem cells
- Atypical differentiation of epithelial cells; triggers may include endogenous or exog-enous biochemical or immunologic factors
- Mechanical spread, as during surgery (e.g., adenomyosis or the implants identified in abdominal surgical or episiotomy scars)
- Distant seeding of endometrial or stem cells via the lymphatic or circulatory system
- Dysregulation of organogenesis (especially of the uterine wall) in embryonic females (hereditary or environmentally mediated endocrine disruptors)

Data from Machairiotis, N., Stylianaki, A., Dryllis, G., Zarogoulidis, P., Kouroutou, P., Tsimais, N., . . . Machairiotis, C. (2013). Extrapelvic endometriosis: A rare entity or an under-diagnosed condition? *Diagnostic Pathology, 8*, 194; Signorile, P. G., & Baldi, A. (2015). New evidence in endometriosis. *International Journal of Biochemistry & Cell Biology, 60,* 19–22.

implants seen incidentally on the peritoneum at surgery; severely pain-evoking, deep infiltrating en-dometriosis; and endometriomas (cyst-like structures, usually in the ovaries, and containing endometrial tissue and blood) (Kodaman, 2015).

Recent molecular studies have suggested addi-tional insights. Women with endometriosis have been shown to have biochemically atypical endome-trial cells, whether they are intrauterine or ectopic. Ectopic endometrial implants appear to function independently from the ovaries, producing their own endogenous estrogen de novo from cholesterol con-version, but lacking progesterone receptors to bal-ance this estrogen activity (Signorile & Baldi, 2015).

This progesterone resistance may play a more im-portant role in disease progression and related infertility than estrogen dependence does (Brosens, Puttemans, & Benagiano, 2013). In addition, the increased density and variation in typology of nerve cells in the endometrium and myometrium of women with endometriosis suggest potential mech-anisms for related pain intensity. Some women with endometriosis also display abnormalities in central pain sensitivity processing, suggested by the increased incidence of coexisting syndromes such as anxiety and depression, migraine headaches, fi-bromyalgia, bladder pain syndrome, and irritable bowel syndrome (Hooten et al., 2013; Smorgick et al., 2013).

Clinical Presentation

Endometriosis can result in a wide range of often unpredictable symptoms, which may not correlate with the extent of visible implants and may ob-scure and delay diagnosis. On the one hand, endo-metrial implants may be seen incidentally during surgery performed on asymptomatic women. On the other hand, women may present with severe to debilitating dysmenorrhea, dyspareunia, dys-chezia, dysuria, or chronic or intermittent dull, throbbing, or sharp pelvic, abdominal or back pain, and can experience associated infertility (ACOG, 2010, reaffirmed 2014). Women with ade-nomyosis may have menorrhagia as well as dys-menorrhea, dyspareunia, and pelvic pain (Cockerham, 2012). Endometriomas may result in acute pain episodes (see the section on ovarian masses later in this chapter). Because of the di-verse locations in which endometrial implants have been identified, extrapelvic endometriosis should be included in the differential diagnosis whenever women report cyclic symptoms in any organ (Machairiotis et al., 2013).

Assessment

A detailed history should be obtained from any woman reporting chronic pelvic pain (see Chapters 6 and 28), including full descriptors and a pain scale (Hooten et al., 2013). The location and character of any dyspareunia should be assessed, along with menstrual cycle patterns, associated symptoms (e.g., dysmenorrhea, nausea and vomiting, diarrhea), fertility history, and family history of endometriosis.

Discovery of the effects of this condition on quality of life and response to treatments may help with the differential diagnosis and facilitate a better understanding of the woman's attitude toward her symptoms.

Findings on physical examination may be limited or absent, but abdominal and pelvic examination, including a rectal examination, are indicated. When pelvic pain is present, it may be less traumatic to the woman to begin with a gentle single-digit vaginal examination to map foci of pain, rather than with a speculum examination. Women with adenomyosis may have a diffusely enlarged, boggy, and/or tender uterus, which may be asymmetrical, but lacking the firm nodularity of fibroids. Women with endometriosis may exhibit condition-specific signs such as pain or nodules at palpation of the posterior fornix or rectovaginal septum, tenderness or induration of the uterosacral ligaments, a tender nonmobile uterus, and a tender enlarged adnexal mass (consistent with endometrioma). Palpation of the vaginal side walls and ancillary pelvic floor muscles may aid in differentiation of endometriosis from pelvic-floor myalgias. Occasionally, endometrial implants are seen on the cervix or vaginal walls during speculum examination, appearing as nonblanching red or brownish/blackish areas or firm nodules. Asymptomatic lesions do not require treatment, although biopsy for histology is appropriate if the diagnosis is unclear.

There are no specific laboratory tests for endometriosis (Signorile & Baldi, 2015). Biomarkers have been proposed, but reliable ones have not yet been identified. Women with irregular, heavy, or irregular bleeding may warrant endometrial biopsy and testing for anemia.

Transvaginal ultrasound is a relatively low-cost technology that can play a role in ruling out other diagnoses and that may identify endometriomas, adenomyosis, and, occasionally, deeply infiltrating endometriosis in the bladder, uterosacral ligaments, rectum, or rectovaginal septum. Transrectal ultrasound may identify bowel involvement and aid in surgical planning (Kodaman, 2015). MRI appears to add little to high-resolution ultrasound findings (ACOG, 2010, reaffirmed 2014; Signorile & Baldi, 2015), but it may be useful if other uterine abnormalities are suspected (Cockerham, 2012).

Endometriosis and adenomyosis are really diagnoses of histology and require surgical biopsy for confirmation. Diagnostic laparoscopy for staging is no longer recommended, however, because the extent of visible disease does not correlate well with either a woman's symptoms or her prognosis for future fertility (ACOG, 2010, reaffirmed 2014).

Differential Diagnoses

Other gynecologic and nongynecologic causes of chronic pelvic pain include bladder pain syndromes, irritable bowel syndrome, pelvic-floor muscle myalgias, and other gynecologic anatomic abnormalities (e.g., uterine fibroids, ovarian cysts, hydrosalpinx). See Chapter 29 for a detailed discussion of pelvic pain.

Management

Women experiencing symptoms of endometriosis variants generally can choose among expectant management, medical therapies, and surgery. In planning treatment, the woman and her provider(s) must consider both symptom management and any desire to preserve future fertility (ACOG, 2010, reaffirmed 2014). Considerations relating to fertility are discussed in the "Special Populations" subsection.

Goals of medical management include both symptom management and maintenance of desired fertility. Ovulation suppression is a primary target of medical therapy, with the goal being to eliminate or reduce ectopic endometrial activity. **Table 26-7** identifies several agents that have been shown to decrease women's reported pain in randomized controlled trials, including combined estrogen and progestin contraceptives; progestins; GnRH agonists (e.g., goserelin, leuprorelin); and the synthetic, androgenic hormone ethisterone (Danazol) (Brown & Farquhar, 2014; Kodaman, 2015). There is insufficient evidence to compare the pain relief effectiveness of specific agents or specific regimens, either as initial treatment or for postsurgical maintenance. There is also insufficient evidence to support the use of acupuncture and other alternative or herbal treatments (American Society for Reproductive Medicine [ASRM], 2014; Brown & Farquhar, 2014). Of equal importance to many women, there is insufficient evidence to affirm that any medical treatments will improve their chances of successful pregnancy outcomes (ACOG, 2010, reaffirmed 2014; ASRM, 2014; Brown & Farquhar, 2014). In addition, pain symptoms that do improve with such

TABLE 26-7 Medical Treatments for Endometriosis

Category	Agents	Regimens	Adverse Effects	Considerations
Combined oral contraceptives	Pill, vaginal ring, transdermal patch	Cyclic or continuous (continuous may be more effective for pain management); no data to define optimal oral dosage	Minimal, compared to other agents (mood swings, low increased clot risk)	Long-term safety is well documented Inexpensive Limited data on pain management but appear comparable to other methods No data to support fertility preservation
Progestins	Oral (norethindrone, megestrol, or medroxyprogesterone acetate) Intramuscular injection (DMPA) Implant (etonogestrel rod) LNG-IUS	Continuous (implant or LNG-IUS), long-acting (injection every 3 months), or short-acting (daily oral) agents Medroxyprogesterone acetate and norethindrone acetate are FDA approved for endometriosis treatment	Irregular menstrual bleeding, breast tenderness, fluid retention, weight gain, and depression or mood instability	Pain reduction of typically 70–100% Decreased bone mineral density with long-term DMPA use LNG-IUS may be optimal for adenomyosis or postsurgical suppression due to low adverse effects
GnRHa	Depot injectable with quicker onset (leuprolide, goserelin) Nasal spray (nafarelin) Norethindrone acetate is FDA approved only as add-back therapy	Combine with add-back estrogen and/or progestogen, tibolone, bisphosphonates, or selective estrogen receptor modulators to limit bone loss and hot flashes	Hypoestrogenic symptoms (bone loss, vaginal atrophy, vasomotor symptoms,	Pain reduction as high as 100%, with 50% recurrence post discontinuation Decreases size of endometriomas Significantly more expensive than other treatments, with no evidence of superior outcomes Backup nonhormonal contraception is recommended Approval of an oral agent is pending; may decrease bone loss

(continues)

TABLE 26-7 Medical Treatments for Endometriosis (*continued*)

Category	Agents	Regimens	Adverse Effects	Considerations
Synthetic androgenic hormones	Ethisterone (Danazol)	Oral daily	Hyperandrogenic and hypoestrogenic: Weight gain, muscle cramps, decreased breast size, acne, hirsutism, hot flashes, mood changes, depression, permanently lower voice	Pain relief similar to GnRHa but less well tolerated Concomitant use of effective contraception is imperative due to risks of virilization of female fetus

Abbreviations: DMPA, depot medroxyprogesterone acetate; FDA, U.S. Food and Drug Administration; GnRHa, gonadotropin-releasing hormone agonists; LNG-IUS, levonorgestrel intrauterine system.

Data from Brown, J., & Farquhar, C. (2014). Endometriosis: An overview of Cochrane Reviews. *Cochrane Database of Systematic Reviews, 3*, CD009590; Kodaman, P. H. (2015). Current strategies for endometriosis management. *Obstetrics and Gynecology Clinics of North America, 42*(1), 87–101.

treatments may recur when the medical therapy is discontinued. Additional medications directed at pain control, including neurotransmitter modulators and opioids, are used for chronic pelvic pain associated with endometriosis. They may improve a woman's quality of life if used judiciously, but play no role in control of the disease or fertility preservation.

While surgery is required for definitive diagnosis of endometriosis, this modality is now reserved for treatment for women with debilitating symptoms and poor response or intolerance to medical therapy. Surgical options include laparoscopic conservative management (e.g., removal of endometrial implants, focal areas of adenomyosis, endometriomas, and distorting adhesions), and definitive surgery (e.g., complete hysterectomy with bilateral salpingo-oophorectomy).

Laparoscopic removal of implants and adhesions is effective for pain management and resolution of symptomatic endometriomas, although removal may decrease ovarian reserve (Brown & Farquhar, 2014). Excision is recommended over ablation to allow for histologic diagnosis. In addition, moderate-quality evidence supports a role for laparoscopic interventional surgery in increasing pregnancy and live birth rates for women with endometriosis and infertility. Following conservative surgery, medical suppression is often restarted, as pelvic pain symptoms may recur in as many as 40% of women (Kodaman, 2015). Repeat procedures increase risks of postoperative adhesions and damage to ovarian reserve. Endometriomas larger than 4 cm are typically removed, even if asymptomatic, as they have been associated with ovarian cancers (Kodaman, 2015).

Women who have severe pain, but wish to preserve their fertility and have not responded to other treatments, may consider a presacral neurectomy (excision of the portion of the superior hypogastric plexus that provides sympathetic innervation to the uterus) (Kodaman, 2015). This complex procedure is done infrequently, but provides better long-term pain control when compared to laparoscopic procedures alone.

The definitive surgery for endometriosis is hysterectomy with salpingo-oophorectomy. Women may be most likely to choose hysterectomy if they do not desire a future pregnancy and have resistant symptoms that are severely impacting their quality of life. They should know that pain persists after definitive surgery in as many as 15% of women, and may increase again over time in as many as 5% more (Kodaman, 2015). Women who elect ovarian preservation have the benefit of bone preservation and positive cardiovascular effects, but increase their risk of persistent or recurrent symptoms six-fold (Kodaman, 2015). In contrast, use of add-back estrogen post oophorectomy appears to have minimal effects on the risk of persistent or recurrent symptoms.

For isolated adenomyosis, women may choose to undergo complete hysterectomy with ovarian preservation. This procedure is typically curative. Endometrial ablation for superficial disease, UAE, and excision of localized disease may also be effective in selected situations (Cockerham, 2012; Popovic, Puchner, Berzaczy, Lammer, & Bucek, 2011).

Aromatase inhibitors (AIs) are being investigated as a potential therapy for all types of endometriosis (Brosens et al., 2013; Usluogullari, Duvan, & Usluogullari, 2015). AIs may be able to suppress the endogenous estrogen production of ectopic endometrial implants (Kodaman, 2015; Signorile & Baldi, 2015). Unfortunately, evidence of their effectiveness remains limited, the cost–benefit ratio is unclear, and the adverse effects of AIs can be severe, including loss of bone density, joint and muscle pain, hot flashes, mood swings, depression, cardiovascular disease, and genital atrophy. Consequently, AIs should be reserved for severely affected women (Dunselman et al., 2014). In premenopausal women, AIs may induce ovulation and should be used with ovarian suppression (Kodaman, 2015).

Other potential agents under investigation for endometriosis management include statins, given that blocking cholesterol biosynthesis may inhibit bioconversion activity in implants; immunomodulators, to modify immune surveillance for ectopic cells; angiogenesis inhibitors, to limit implant proliferation; synthetic steroids, which are used in other countries to treat endometriosis, but are currently banned in the United States due to their risk of abuse as performance-enhancing drugs; and valproic acid, which appears to reverse silencing of apoptotic genes that effect endometriosis (Quass, Weedin, & Hansen, 2015). Nonpharmaceutical agents under investigation include the antioxidant hormone melatonin; certain isoflavones (e.g., pycnogenols), which may compete for and block estrogen receptors; and herbal agents with anticytokine, antioxidant properties. Results for these modalities remain preliminary, however, and the preparations are nonstandardized, so they may contain varying amounts of active ingredients (Quass et al., 2015).

Special Populations

Adolescents Endometriosis should be considered in the differential diagnosis of even premenarcheal girls with chronic pelvic pain, as cases of biopsy-confirmed symptomatic implants have been reported (Brosens et al., 2013). Also, endometriosis is more common in girls with imperforate hymen or other obstructive Müllerian anomalies.

When combined oral contraceptives are recommended to young adolescents as the first-line treatment, some families may object, assuming this use may be a license to sexual activity. However, an open discussion with the adolescent and her family to review concerns, treatment safety profiles, and the expected potential benefits of endometriosis treatment (e.g., improved quality of life, prevention of central sensitization by good pain management, but no clear role in preventing infertility) may facilitate achievement of an optimal plan. Diagrams to demonstrate anatomy and physiology, along with handouts that can be reviewed at home, may be particularly helpful when caring for adolescents. Unsuccessful symptom management using medications alone indicates a need for referral for potential surgery at any age (Brosens et al., 2013).

Women with Infertility Despite the clear association between endometriosis and infertility, the mechanisms of this relationship remain unclear (Pfeifer et al., 2012). Distortion of anatomy, inflammation, abnormal tubal transit, progesterone resistance, and implantation defects may all be involved (Brosens et al., 2013; Kodaman, 2015). There is not universal agreement on the indications for surgical evaluation and therapy during infertility treatment. Age, duration of infertility, family history, pelvic pain, and stage of endometriosis should be taken into account when developing the management plan. For women with infertility and endometriosis, treatment may include expectant

management after laparoscopy, superovulation (with gonadotropins) and intrauterine insemination, or in vitro fertilization (see Chapter 18). The use of GnRH agonists to suppress endometriotic activity for 3 to 6 months prior to in vitro fertilization may improve outcomes, but not always (Pfeifer et al., 2012).

Pregnant Women Although the etiology is unclear, women with either endometriosis or adenomyosis have increased risks when they do achieve pregnancy, including late miscarriage, preterm birth, fetal growth restriction, and antepartum hemorrhage (Brosens et al., 2013). These outcomes may be related to progesterone resistance and/or the increased risk of subclinical atherosclerosis, a condition that is also associated with endometriosis.

Older Women In postmenopausal women, emerging evidence suggests that while symptom resolution is typical, endometriosis-related problems may sometimes persist (Brosens et al., 2013). For example, women with endometriosis-associated infertility may have early-onset menopause; as many as 4% of women, especially obese women, continue to have active symptoms after menopause, even in the absence of hormone therapy; use of hormone therapy or tamoxifen has been implicated in symptom recurrence after menopause for some women; and there is a low (less than 1%) but increased risk of malignant transformation of endometrial implants, especially on the ovaries (Brosens et al., 2013). For symptomatic women with a history of endometriosis who request hormone therapy, use of combined estrogen and progestin or AIs have been suggested (Kodaman, 2015).

CONDITIONS OF THE ADNEXA

Adnexal Masses

While benign adnexal masses can arise in the fallopian tubes (e.g., hydrosalpinx, related to tubal occlusion from surgery or infection), the majority are ovarian. Ovarian masses can occur in any of the differentiated tissues of the ovary. Most adnexal masses are benign, but vigilance is always essential to allow for early identification of life-threatening conditions, such as malignancy and ectopic pregnancy (see Chapters 27 and 31). Even benign ovarian tumors can cause women severe distress, including physical symptoms (e.g., pain, dyspareunia), and significant anxiety. Appropriate education about the etiology; likely outcomes, including course with and without treatment, any expected effect on future fertility, and risk of recurrence; and reassurance about the benign nature of the condition can often allay unspoken anxiety and smooth the course of follow-up for women and their families.

Incidence

The incidence of ovarian masses is unknown, as it is likely that many are asymptomatic. They frequently appear as incidental findings on pelvic imaging. In one large U.S. study, 39,000 women were followed via serial transvaginal ultrasounds over 25 years, and 17% had at least one abnormal adnexal finding (Pavlik et al., 2013). As expected, cystic masses were approximately twice as common in actively menstruating women, and most abnormal findings resolved spontaneously.

Etiology and Pathophysiology

Common benign ovarian masses include functional (physiologic) ovarian cysts, mature cystic teratomas, serous or mucinous cystadenomas, and endometriomas (ACOG, 2007, reaffirmed 2013; Liu & Zanotti, 2011). Functional ovarian cysts are typically asymptomatic and resolve without intervention. Occasionally, they may rupture and produce the transient, acute pain of peritoneal irritation. In addition, the involved ovary, when enlarged by any type of cyst, is more susceptible to the surgical emergency of torsion.

Functional cysts include follicular, corpus luteal, and hemorrhagic cysts. Follicular cysts develop early in the menstrual cycle from unruptured follicles, are common, and are often asymptomatic. The pain that accompanies spontaneous follicular cyst rupture with ovulation is termed *mittelschmerz*. If ovulation does not occur, the follicular cyst may continue to enlarge, with the already noted risks of symptomatic rupture or torsion.

A corpus luteal cyst develops within the corpus luteum that forms in the ovary normally after ovulation. These cysts may persist into pregnancy and are also typically not symptomatic. Again, rupture-related pain is likely to be self-limiting, but severe pain may signal torsion.

A hemorrhagic cyst can occur when a small vessel within any cyst lining erodes. The bleeding may be contained within the cyst or extrude into the peritoneal cavity and cause transient pain if rupture occurs. Although symptoms are typically self-limiting, heavy or continued bleeding may require emergent surgery (Liu & Zanotti, 2011).

Mature cystic teratomas, also called dermoid cysts, arise from the ovarian germ cell and are the most common ovarian tumors. They are filled with sebaceous material and often contain hair, bone, teeth, or other tissues from the germ layers. They can grow to be many centimeters in diameter, and ovarian torsion occurs with as many as 10% (Liu & Zanotti, 2011).

Serous or mucinous cystadenomas arise from glandular tissue within the ovarian epithelium. One-fourth of benign ovarian tumors are serous cystadenomas. They often persist, but can be managed expectantly if they are small and have no concerning features. Mucinous cystadenomas can become very large, again increasing the risk of torsion (Liu & Zanotti, 2011).

Endometriomas, also known as chocolate cysts, are a form of endometriosis (see the previous section).

Clinical Presentation

The presentation of ovarian masses varies. They may be asymptomatic and identified as an incidental finding on imaging. When identified, the mass can range in size from less than a centimeter to basketball size and several pounds. Any size of ovarian mass may produce symptoms, which typically include pressure, unilateral or bilateral pelvic pain, dyspareunia, irregular vaginal bleeding, and changes in bladder or bowel habits. Women may report diverse quality of discomfort— dull, cramping pressure; sharp and intermittent stabbing; cyclic, bilateral, or abrupt and persistent pain; or any combination of these forms. Pain with abrupt onset often represents spilling of cystic fluid (serous and/or sanguineous) into the peritoneal cavity. Abrupt onset of severe pain may represent ovarian torsion, which occurs more commonly if the ovary is enlarged by a mass. When masses become large, abdominal girth can increase from the tumor and may be mistaken for pregnancy.

Assessment

Women with pelvic pain symptoms that suggest adnexal mass should be asked sufficient history questions to allow the clinician to rule out the most morbid or life-threatening conditions quickly, including ectopic pregnancy, appendicitis, ovarian torsion or infection, and malignancy. Key topics from the general health and gynecologic history include the specific characteristics of the symptoms the woman is experiencing; her menstrual, sexual, and contraceptive history; any changes in vaginal bleeding or discharge; a pain scale; and a family history of risk factors such as malignancy or endometriosis.

Taking the woman's vital signs will aid in ruling out infection, fever, and severe pain or shock. Systemic or atypical lymphadenopathy may suggest malignancy or infection. Unexplained weight gain or a disproportionate change in abdominal girth without weight gain may indicate large tumor growth.

Inspect, auscultate, and palpate the abdomen. Large masses may cause visible changes in the abdomen or may be palpable abdominally or on bimanual vaginal and rectal examination. Guarding or rebound tenderness can indicate peritoneal irritation.

Perform a complete pelvic examination, documenting the location, size, shape, texture, mobility, and tenderness of any palpable mass. While pelvic and/or rectal examination are indicated, be aware that their sensitivity is limited, especially in women with higher body mass index (ACOG, 2007, reaffirmed 2013).

Pregnancy testing is essential in women of reproductive age. Gonorrhea and chlamydia testing and complete blood count are warranted if a tuboovarian abscess is suspected. While imaging is the first-line assessment for adnexal pathology, blood testing plays a role in multivariate index assays that have been developed in an attempt to predict malignant potential reliably and limit unnecessary intervention (Dodge et al., 2012; Elder et al., 2014). Tests appropriately ordered in primary care while specialist consultation is pending include cancer antigen 125 (CA-125), alpha fetoprotein (AFP), lactate dehydrogenase (LDH), and human chorionic gonadotropin (hCG) (ACOG, 2007, reaffirmed 2013). The CA-125 test is not reliable as a stand-alone modality for distinguishing benign and malignant masses, especially in premenopausal women, as the level of this protein is also elevated by endometriosis, fibroids, pelvic inflammatory disease, and other benign findings (ACOG, 2007, reaffirmed 2013). In addition, no biomarkers have been demonstrated to be accurate for screening purposes, as they can lead to unacceptably high rates of unnecessary intervention, without significant reduction in mortality.

Transvaginal ultrasound remains the first-line imaging modality for evaluation of ovarian masses (ACOG, 2007, reaffirmed 2013). Ultrasound will classify a mass as cystic, solid, or complex. Three-dimensional ultrasound may improve acuity, while color Doppler ultrasound as an adjunct can assess measurement of blood flow in and around a mass (Dodge et al., 2012). MRI and computed tomography (CT) imaging are typically reserved for specific indications such as determination of the origin of an associated non-ovarian pelvic mass (MRI) or evaluation for potential metastases (CT) (ACOG, 2007, reaffirmed 2013).

Differential Diagnoses

Table 26-8 offers an overview of the differential diagnoses for adnexal masses and some typical characteristics that may aid in achieving accurate diagnosis.

Management

Asymptomatic simple ovarian cysts less than 10 cm in diameter, including functional cysts and benign neoplasms, have a low probability of malignancy and can be followed with serial imaging. There is little evidence-based guidance for timing of repeat ultrasounds, but they are generally obtained at 3- or 6-month intervals to establish stability (Ackerman, Irshad, Lewis, & Munazza, 2013). Many functional cysts will resolve within 3 months. In one study, benign-appearing cysts (e.g., unilocular or cysts with septations but no solid component) resolved within 1 year of follow-up in approximately 40% of participating women (Pavlik et al., 2013). Women who are receiving serial follow-up should be educated to report any increase in pain or other symptoms (e.g., bowel or bladder status). While unlikely to promote resolution of an existing cyst, hormonal contraceptives can be used to control repeated episodes of symptomatic functional cysts.

TABLE 26-8	Differential Diagnoses for Adnexal Masses	

Diagnosis	Distinguishing Typical Characteristics	Diagnostic Aids
Appendicitis, diverticular abscess	Gradual onset; fever, vomiting, unilateral pain	Complete blood count
Benign ovarian cysts (functional, cystadenoma)	Dull cramping pressure; sharp sudden pain with activity or on rupture—typically transient	Vaginal ultrasound
Bladder diverticulum	Palpable mass, urinary symptoms	Imaging
Ectopic pregnancy	Symptoms vary and may include pelvic pain, vaginal bleeding, or missed menses	Pregnancy testing Vaginal ultrasound
Endometrioma, endometritis	Dyspareunia, cyclic menstrual pain	Vaginal ultrasound
Hydrosalpinx/fallopian tube tumor	Pain, watery discharge	Vaginal ultrasound
Malignancy	Symptoms may be vague, such as bloating, pelvic or abdominal pain, difficulty eating, early satiety, change in urine/bowels; women who have an adnexal mass prior to puberty or post menopause are at higher risk	Vaginal ultrasound Blood assay/tumor markers (CA-125)
Mittelschmerz	Midcycle pain; temporary, predictable, may alternate sides	Typically none, possible vaginal ultrasound
Ovarian torsion	Sudden onset pain, severe, often unilateral; associated nausea or vomiting	Complete blood count Vaginal ultrasound
Pelvic inflammatory disease, tubo-ovarian abscess	Gradual onset; fever, vomiting, purulent discharge	Complete blood count Chlamydia and gonorrhea testing
Ruptured cyst (follicular or corpus luteum)	Sudden onset, post activity or intercourse	Hematocrit Vaginal ultrasound if needed
Teratoma	Dull, cramping, persistent, noncyclic	Vaginal ultrasound
Uterine fibroid	Predominantly menstrual symptoms: Cyclic pain, dysmenorrhea; menorrhagia	Vaginal ultrasound

Data from American College of Obstetricians and Gynecologists. (2007, reaffirmed 2013). Management of adnexal masses. Practice Bulletin No. 83. *Obstetrics & Gynecology, 110*, 201–214; Dodge, J. E., Covenx, A. L., Lacchetti, C., Elit, L. M., Le, T., Devries-Aboud, M., & Fung-Kee-Fung, M.; Gynecology Cancer Disease Site Group. (2012). Management of a suspicious adnexal mass: A clinical practice guideline. *Current Oncology, 19*, e244–e257.

Women can be informed that complex and solid ovarian masses have been shown to resolve spontaneously in as many as 80% of women (Pavlik et al., 2013). This type of mass does have a higher risk for malignancy, however, and the woman should be referred from primary care to general gynecologic or gynecologic oncology for in-depth assessment (Ackerman et al., 2013; ACOG 2007, reaffirmed 2013).

Specific Populations

Adolescents When girls who are premenarche have an adnexal mass, they should be referred to a specialist; adnexal masses in this age group have a higher risk of malignancy. Adolescent girls often have functional cysts, both follicular and luteal, simply because of their higher prevalence of anovulatory cycles. These cysts typically resolve spontaneously. If they are recurrently symptomatic, the adolescent may benefit from medical prevention, typically with combined hormonal contraceptives.

In adolescents who also have irregular menses, hirsutism, or severe acne, polycystic ovary syndrome should be considered (see Chapter 25).

Pregnant Women As ultrasound in pregnancy has become routine, more ovarian masses are being identified during early pregnancy. Corpus luteal cysts and mature cystic teratomas are the most commonly reported adnexal masses during pregnancy. The risk of malignancy and acute complications from an ovarian mass during pregnancy is low, and expectant management is appropriate in the absence of rapid or atypical growth (ACOG, 2007, reaffirmed 2013).

Postmenopausal Women Postmenopausal women are at increased risk for ovarian cancer, and benign functional cysts are rare in this age group. Any adnexal mass in a postmenopausal woman should be considered highly suspicious for malignancy and thoroughly evaluated.

References

Ackerman, S. Irshad, A., Lewis, M., & Munazza, A. (2013). Ovarian cystic lesions: A current approach to diagnosis and management. *Radiologic Clinics of North America, 51,* 1067–1085.

Aissani, B., Zhang, K., & Wiener, H. (2015). Follow-up to genome-wide linkage and admixture mapping studies implicates components of the extracellular matrix in susceptibility to and size of uterine fibroids. *Fertility and Sterility, 103,* 528–534.

American Association of Gynecologic Laparoscopists (AAGL). (2012). AAGL practice report: Practice guidelines for the diagnosis and management of endometrial polyps. *Journal of Minimally Invasive Gynecology, 19,* 3–10.

American College of Obstetricians and Gynecologists. (2007, reaffirmed 2013). Management of adnexal masses. Practice Bulletin No. 83. *Obstetrics & Gynecology, 110,* 201–214.

American College of Obstetricians and Gynecologists. (2008a, reaffirmed 2014). Alternatives to hysterectomy in the management of leiomyomas. Practice Bulletin No. 96. *Obstetrics & Gynecology, 112,* 387–400.

American College of Obstetricians and Gynecologists. (2008b, reaffirmed 2013). Diagnosis and management of vulvar skin disorders. Practice Bulletin No. 93. *Obstetrics & Gynecology, 111,* 1243–1253.

American College of Obstetricians and Gynecologists. (2010, reaffirmed 2014). Management of endometriosis. Practice Bulletin No. 114. *Obstetrics & Gynecology, 116,* 223–236.

American Society for Reproductive Medicine (ASRM). (2014). Treatment of pelvic pain associated with endometriosis: A committee opinion. *Fertility and Sterility, 101,* 927–935.

British Association for Sexual Health and HIV. (2014). 2014 UK national guideline on the management of vulval conditions. Retrieved from http://www.bashh.org

Brosens, I., Puttemans, P., & Benagiano, G. (2013). Endometriosis: A life cycle approach? *American Journal of Obstetrics & Gynecology, 209,* 307–316.

Brown, J., & Farquhar, C. (2014). Endometriosis: An overview of Cochrane Reviews. *Cochrane Database of Systematic Reviews, 3,* CD009590.

Buyukbayrak, E., Karageyim Karsidag, A. Y., Kars, B., Sakin, O., Ozyapi Alper, A. G. Pirimaglu, M., . . . Turan, C. (2011). Cervical polyps: Evaluation of routine removal and need for accompanying D&C. *Archives of Gynecology & Obstetrics, 283,* 581–584.

Cockerham, A. Z. (2012). Adenomyosis: A challenge in clinical gynecology. *Journal of Midwifery & Women's Health, 57,* 212–220.

DeVivo, A., Macuso, A., Giacobbe, A., Savasta, L. M., De Dominici, R., Dugo, N., . . . Vaiarelli, A. (2011). Uterine myomas during pregnancy: A longitudinal sonographic study. *Ultrasound in Obstetrics & Gynecology, 37,* 361–365.

Dodge, J. E., Covenx, A. L., Lacchetti, C., Elit, L. M., Le, T., Devries-Aboud, M., & Fung-Kee-Fung, M.; Gynecology Cancer Disease Site Group. (2012). Management of a suspicious adnexal mass: A clinical practice guideline. *Current Oncology, 19,* e244–e257.

Dunselman, G. A., Vermeulen, N., Becker, C., Calhaz-Jorge, C., D'Hooghe, T., DeBie, B., . . . Nelen, W.; European Society of Human Reproduction and Embryology. (2014). ESHRE guideline:

Management of women with endometriosis. *Human Reproduction, 29,* 400–412.

Elder, J. W., Pavlik, E. J., Long, A., Miller, R. W., DeSimone, C. P., Hoff, J. T., . . . Ueland, F. R. (2014). Serial ultrasonographic evaluation of ovarian abnormalities with a morphology index. *Gynecologic Oncology, 135,* 8–12.

Fistarol, S. K., & Itin, P. H. (2013). Diagnosis and treatment of lichen sclerosus: An update. *American Journal of Clinical Dermatology, 14,* 27–47.

Gupta, J. K., Sinha, A., Lumsden, M. A., & Hickey, M. (2014). Uterine artery embolization for symptomatic uterine fibroids. *Cochrane Database of Systematic Reviews, 12,* CD005073.

Hooten, W. M., Timming, R., Belgrade, M., Gaul, J., Goertz, M., Haake, B., . . . Walker, N.; Institute for Clinical Systems Improvement. (2013). Assessment and management of chronic pain. Retrieved from https://www.icsi.org/_asset/bw798b /ChronicPain.pdf

International Society for the Study of Vulval Diseases. (2013a). Genital itch in women. Retrieved from http://issvd.org /wordpress/wp-content/uploads/2014/09/GenitalCare -2013-final.pdf

International Society for the Study of Vulval Diseases. (2013b). Genital skin care. Retrieved from http://issvd.org/wordpress /wp-content/uploads/2014/09/GenitalCare-2013-final.pdf

Kodaman, P. H. (2015). Current strategies for endometriosis management. *Obstetrics and Gynecology Clinics of North America, 42*(1), 87–101.

Liu, F. W., Galvan-Turner, V. B., Pfaendler, K .S., Longoria, T. C., & Bristow, R. E. (2015). A critical assessment of morcellation and its impact on gynecologic surgery and the limitations of the existing literature. *American Journal of Obstetrics & Gynecology, 212,* 717–724.

Liu, J. H., & Zanotti, K. M. (2011). Management of the adnexal mass. *Obstetrics & Gynecology, 117,* 1413–1428.

Lynch, P. J., Moyal-Barracco, M., Scurry, J., & Stockdale, C. (2012) 2011 ISSVD terminology and classification of vulvar dermatological disorders: An approach to clinical diagnosis. *Journal of Lower Genital Tract Disease, 16,* 339–344.

Machairiotis, N., Stylianaki, A., Dryllis, G., Zarogoulidis, P., Kouroutou, P., Tsimais, N., . . . Machairiotis, C. (2013). Extrapelvic endometriosis: A rare entity or an underdiagnosed condition? *Diagnostic Pathology, 8,* 194.

Margesson, L. J., & Danby, W. F. (2014). Hidradenitis suppurativa. *Best Practice & Research Clinical Obstetrics & Gynaecology, 28,* 1013–1027.

Marret, H., Frital, X., Ouldamer, L., Bendifallah, S., Brun, J. L., DeJesus, I., . . . Farnandez, H.; CNGOF (French College of Gynecology & Obstetrics). (2012). Therapeutic management of uterine fibroid tumors: Updated French guidelines. *European Journal of Obstetrics, Gynecology, & Reproductive Biology, 165,* 156–164.

Matthews, M. L. (2015). Abnormal uterine bleeding in reproductive-aged women. *Obstetrics and Gynecology Clinics of North America, 42,* 103–115.

Mayeaux, E. J., & Cooper, D. (2013). Vulvar procedures. *Obstetrics and Gynecology Clinics of North America, 40,* 759–772.

Nelson, A. L., Papa, R. R., & Ritchie, J. J. (2015). Asymptomatic cervical polyps: Can we just let them be? *Women's Health, 11,* 121–126.

Patel, A., Malik, M., Britten, J., Cox, J., & Catherino, W. H. (2014). Alternative therapies in management of leiomyomas. *Fertility and Sterility, 102,* 649–655.

Pavlik, E. J., Ueland, F. R., Miller, R. W., Ubellacker, J. M., Desimone, C. P., Elder, J., . . . van Nagell, J. Jr. (2013). Frequency and disposition of ovarian abnormalities followed with serial transvaginal ultrasonography. *Obstetrics& Gynecology, 122,* 210–217.

Pfeifer, S., Fritz, M., Goldberg, J., McClure, R., Lobo, R., Thomas, M., . . . Barbera, A. L.; Practice Committee of the American Society of Reproductive Medicine. (2012). Endometriosis and infertility: A committee opinion. *Fertility and Sterility, 98,* 591–598.

Popovic, M., Puchner, S., Berzaczy, D., Lammer, J., & Bucek, R. A. (2011). Uterine artery embolization for the treatment of adenomyosis: A review. *Journal of Vascular and Interventional Radiology, 22,* 901–909.

Quass, A. M., Weedin, E. A., & Hansen, K. R. (2015). On-label and off-label drug use in the treatment of endometriosis. *Fertility and Sterility, 103,* 612–625.

Ricciardi, E., Vecchione, A., Marci, R., Schimberni, M., Frega, A., Maniglio, P., . . . Moscarini, M. (2014). Clinical factors and malignancy in endometrial polyps. *European Journal of Obstetrics, Gynecology, and Reproductive Biology, 183,* 121–124.

Schlosser, B. J., & Mirowski, G. W. (2015). Lichen sclerosus and lichen planus in women and girls. *Clinical Obstetrics & Gynecology, 58,* 125–142.

Segars, J. H., Parrott, E. C., Nagel, J. D., Guo, X. C., Gao, X., Birnbaum, L. S., & Pinn, V. W. (2014). Proceedings from the Third National Institutes of Health International Congress on Advances in Uterine Leiomyoma Research: Comprehensive summary and future recommendations. *Human Reproduction Update, 20,* 309–333.

Signorile, P. G., & Baldi, A. (2015). New evidence in endometriosis. *International Journal of Biochemistry & Cell Biology, 60,* 19–22.

Smorgick, N., Marsh, C. A., As-Sanie, S., Smith, Y. R., & Quint, E. H. (2013). Prevalence of pain syndromes, mood conditions, and asthma in adolescents and young women with endometriosis. (2013). *Journal of Pediatric & Adolescent Gynecology, 26,* 171–175.

Song, H., Lu, D., Navaratnam, K., & Shi, G. (2013). Aromatase inhibitors for uterine fibroids. *Cochrane Database of Systematic Reviews, 10,* CD009505.

Usluogullari, B., Duvan, C., & Usluogullari, C. (2015). Use of aromatase inhibitors in practice of gynecology. *Journal of Ovarian Research, 8*(1), 4.

CHAPTER 27

Gynecologic Cancers

Nancy Maas

Kristi Adair Robinia

The editors acknowledge Mary Wallace and Alison Boehm Barlow, who were the authors of the previous edition of this chapter.

Gynecologic cancers are serious, life-threatening diseases. Many symptoms of these diseases are vague and subtle, making early diagnosis, treatment, and successful recovery difficult. A humanistic approach that integrates patient-centered care with medical and sociopsychological perspectives serves to equalize the power imbalance between a woman and her clinician. Clinicians using this approach actively listen to their patients and assess them in the context of their lived experiences, ethnicity, culture, and socioeconomic class. Such clinicians are less likely to miss hearing a woman as she describes vague symptoms that may be warnings of underlying disease, and instead encourage her to provide more information that may be helpful in making an accurate diagnosis. Clinicians using a humanistic approach are cautious and thoughtful, and think critically, using the most recent evidence in assessing and formulating treatment for the disease. They arm their patients with information that is critical to informed consent and decision making. Sensitive clinicians who use good listening skills are the practitioners who have helped decrease the number of cancer deaths in women who were misdiagnosed when their voices were ignored.

In the United States, gynecologic cancers account for approximately 98,280 new cases of cancer each year and are responsible for 30,440 deaths of women annually (American Cancer Society [ACS], 2015e). Prevention of health problems such as gynecologic cancers is the primary goal of clinicians who provide health care for women. For each woman, genetic, behavioral, and environmental factors will influence her risk of developing a gynecologic malignancy.

VULVAR CANCERS

Description of the Problem

Vulvar cancer accounted for approximately 4% of all reproductive-organ cancers and 0.6% of all cancers in women in 2015 (ACS, 2015d; Hacker, Eifel, & van der Velden, 2015). The age-adjusted rate of new cases of vulvar cancer in 2014 was 2.4 per 100,000 women (National Cancer Institute [NCI], n.d.). The overall 5-year survival rate for a woman with vulvar cancer is 87% if it is confined to the primary site (NCI, n.d.). Lymph node involvement is an important prognostic factor (Deppe, Mert, & Winer, 2014). The overall 5-year survival rate for women with regional lymph node involvement ranges from 50% to 60%, but this rate decreases to 15.9% when the cancer has metastasized to distant sites (NCI, n.d.).

Carcinoma of the vulva is primarily a disease of women who are postmenopausal (Hacker et al., 2015). The average age of women diagnosed with vulvar cancer is 68 to 70 years (ACS, 2015d; NCI, n.d.), with more than two-thirds of cases all occurring in women older than 60 years (Reyes & Cooper, 2014). Fewer than 20% of vulvar cancers occur in women younger than age 50 (ACS, 2015d). Women who are older (60 years or older) and who are diagnosed with vulvar cancer have a greater mortality risk compared to women who are younger. After controlling for race, tumor grade, and surgical treatment, older age is associated with almost a fourfold risk for death from vulvar cancer (Brown, 2013; Rauh-Hain et al., 2014).

Etiology and Pathophysiology

Both genetic and epigenetic changes are associated with the pathogenesis of vulvar cancer, and mutations are detected more often with increasing tumor stage (Trietsch, Nooij, Gaarenstroom, & van Poelgeest, 2015). DNA mutations resulting in vulvar cancer are acquired over the course of an individual's life; consequently, the risk for vulvar cancer is not inheritable.

The majority of vulvar malignancies are squamous cell carcinomas. Less common forms include malignant melanomas, adenocarcinomas, and basal cell carcinomas (Porth, 2015). Research suggests that squamous cell vulvar cancer evolves from two separate types of vulvar intraepithelial neoplasia (VIN) that differ in terms of their etiology, pathogenesis, and clinical significance (Reyes & Cooper, 2014):

- Usual-type VIN (warty, basaloid, and mixed) is related to human papillomavirus (HPV) infection in most cases, and tends to occur in younger women. It may be associated with similar lesions of the cervix and vagina (Hacker et al., 2015).
- Differentiated-type VIN is usually diagnosed in women 65 to 75 years of age and is associated with vulvar dermatologic conditions such as lichen sclerosus, squamous cell hyperplasia, and Paget's disease of the vulva (American College of Obstetricians and Gynecologists 2011a, reaffirmed 2014; Brown, 2013; Hacker, Eifel, & van der Velden, 2012, 2015; Trietsch et al., 2015).

Infection with HPV types 16, 18, 31, and others confers a high risk of developing vulvar cancer and appears to play a role in 30% to 60% of diagnosed cases of usual-type VIN (ACS, 2015d; Deppe et al., 2014; Reyes & Cooper, 2014). Women who have HPV as a risk factor tend to be younger and frequently have multiple elevated lesions on examination (Preti, Scurry, Marchitelli, & Micheletti, 2014). Risk factors are similar to those for cervical neoplasia related to acquisition of the HPV virus, including multiple sex partners and impaired immunologic status. Early sexual contact and infection with HPV provides more time for malignant transformation of usual-type VIN to vulvar cancer. Women who smoke cigarettes and have HPV infection are at an even higher risk of developing vulvar cancer (American College of Obstetricians and Gynecologists 2011a, reaffirmed 2014; Deppe et al., 2014; Reyes & Cooper, 2014). Vulvar cancer associated with high-risk HPV types initially presents as a premalignant, usual-type VIN that is either basaloid or warty in tissue histology (Reyes & Cooper, 2014; Trietsch et al., 2015). The presence of usual-type VIN confers an increased risk of vulvar cancer, even though most cases do not progress to squamous cell cancer. An estimated 9% to 16% of women with untreated usual-type VIN develop invasive disease (Trietsch et al., 2015).

Differentiated-type VIN is considered a high-grade precursor lesion for vulvar squamous cell carcinoma and occurs primarily in older women (older than age 60). It has a higher risk of progression to squamous cell vulvar cancer than usual-type VIN, and is associated with chronic inflammatory conditions such as lichen sclerosus (Reyes & Cooper, 2014). Approximately 4.5% of women with lichen sclerosus will develop vulvar cancer (Stiles, Redmer, Paddock, & Schrager, 2012). Reyes and Cooper (2014) note that pruritus has been observed in as many as 60% of women with lichen sclerosus (see Chapter 26). The pruritus leads to a severe itch–scratch cycle, which is thought to cause squamous cell hyperplasia, which then progresses to cellular atypia and finally to invasive squamous cell carcinoma. Vulvar cancer, on average, develops 10 years after the onset of lichen sclerosus in affected women (Stiles et al., 2012). Aggressive evaluation and treatment have the potential to decrease the incidence of vulvar cancer in this subgroup of women (Wedel & Johnson, 2014).

Genetic research indicates that women with differentiated-type VIN often have a genetic mutation involving the *p53* tumor suppressor gene, which plays a key role in the carcinogenesis of vulvar cancer (Deppe et al., 2014; Trietsch et al., 2015). The p53 protein stops cell growth and division in DNA-damaged cells. When the damage cannot be repaired, the p53 protein triggers cell apoptosis, thereby preventing unregulated cell growth by damaged cells (ACS, 2015d). Mutation of the *p53* gene appears to be an early event in the development of differentiated-type VIN, and research indicates that the same mutation may be present in cases of lichen sclerosus (Reyes & Cooper, 2014). Differentiated-type VIN has a higher risk of progression to squamous cell vulvar cancer, with an estimated 33% of women diagnosed with this type of VIN eventually developing invasive disease (Reyes & Cooper, 2014).

Additional risk factors for vulvar cancer include infection with human immunodeficiency virus (HIV) and previous gynecologic malignancy (ACS, 2015d; Centers for Disease Control and Prevention [CDC], 2010). HIV infection causes immunosuppression, thereby making tissues susceptible to persistent HPV infections, which in turn increases the risk of vulvar cancer (ACS, 2015d).

Clinical Presentation

Vulvar cancer is often asymptomatic. If signs and symptoms do become apparent, however, the most common presentation is a woman's report of a vulvar lump or mass that may or may not be painful. There is often a prolonged history of vulvar pruritus, and vulvar bleeding, discharge, and dysuria may be present (ACS, 2015d; Hacker et al., 2012). On physical examination, the lesion is usually raised, and may be ulcerated, warty, or fleshy in appearance; alternatively, it may appear to be an area of squamous cell hyperplasia (see Chapter 26). Lesions may be single or multiple in number, and color can vary from white to gray, red to brown, or black. Most squamous cell carcinomas occur on the labia majora, although the labia minora, clitoris, and perineum are other possible primary sites. Women with advanced disease may present with a lump in the groin related to lymph node metastasis (American College of Obstetricians and Gynecologists, 2011a, reaffirmed 2014; Hacker et al., 2012; Porth, 2015).

Malignant melanoma of the vulva, which accounts for 10% of all vulvar cancers, appears as unusual macules or papules on the labia majora, and less commonly on the labia minora or clitoris (Murzaku, Penn, Hale, Pomeranz, & Polsky, 2014). Extra-mammary Paget's disease is an adenocarcinoma of the vulva characterized by asymmetrical white and red scaly plaques on the vulva

(Edey, Murdoch, Cooper, & Bryant, 2013). Although rare, adenocarcinoma can develop in the Bartholin's glands and can easily be mistaken for a cyst; therefore a delay in accurate diagnosis is common (Hacker et al., 2012).

Assessment

History and Physical Examination

Early identification of women at risk for developing vulvar cancer is important. Because HPV infection is a known risk factor for vulvar cancer, the clinician should ask about sexual activity and relationships, use of barrier protection, previous history or exposure to sexually transmitted infections (STIs), and HPV immunization status. Additionally, clinicians need to ask about a history of lichen sclerosis, previous VIN, Paget's disease, malignant melanoma, or Bartholin's cyst, as each of these conditions increases a woman's risk of developing vulvar cancer (Hacker et al., 2012, Reyes & Cooper, 2014).

Thorough patient education about when and how to perform a vulvar self-examination and visual inspection of the external genitalia during the clinical pelvic examination are essential to early identification. Although annual Papanicolaou tests (Pap tests) are no longer recommended for all women (see Chapter 7), the American College of Obstetricians and Gynecologists (2012) recommends an annual pelvic examination for all women starting at age 21 regardless of the age of onset of sexual activity. In addition, pelvic examination is an appropriate component of a comprehensive physical examination for any woman with known risk factors for vulvar cancer or one who reports symptoms suggestive of gynecologic malignancy (American College of Obstetricians and Gynecologists, 2012, reaffirmed 2014).

Genital neoplasia in women is often multifocal. Thus careful examination of the entire vulva, vagina, cervix, perineum, and perianal area, including the anus, should be performed as part of the routine pelvic examination. In addition, the femoral and inguinal lymph nodes should be palpated routinely during pelvic examination.

Diagnostic Testing

Currently, there is no identified screening test for vulvar cancer. Women with a past history of cervical or vaginal cancer or those with lichen sclerosis should be examined regularly, and all women reporting or found to have a vulvar lesion must be thoroughly evaluated to rule out malignancy (American College of Obstetricians and Gynecologists, 2011a; Deppe et al., 2014; Hacker et al., 2012). Diagnosis of vulvar cancer is made by identifying a lesion through visual inspection and then obtaining confirmation with a biopsy.

Colposcopy may assist in defining the extent of disease (American College of Obstetricians and Gynecologists, 2011a, reaffirmed 2014; Preti et al., 2014). Additional diagnostic testing may include colposcopy of the cervix and vagina because of the association of vulvar cancer with other gynecologic neoplasia. A CT scan, magnetic resonance imaging (MRI), or positron emission tomography (PET) scan of the pelvis and groins may be helpful in detecting any enlarged lymph nodes or erosion of underlying bony structures, and may assist in staging the cancer (if detected) (ACS, 2015d; Deppe et al., 2014; Hacker et al., 2012).

Both women and clinicians may contribute to the delay in diagnosis of vulvar cancers. Common causes of late-stage diagnosis of vulvar cancer include women not seeking treatment when initial symptoms occur, and clinicians providing symptomatic treatment for months prior to obtaining a biopsy (Rauh-Hain et al., 2014). Experts recommend that a biopsy be performed in women who are postmenopausal who present with an apparent condyloma, particularly if it has not responded to therapy (American College of Obstetricians and Gynecologists, 2011a).

Differential Diagnoses

When establishing differential diagnoses for vulvar disorders, the clinician should consider basic vulvar changes and move up in complexity to inflammatory conditions and neoplasia (Hoffstetter, 2014). The following are potential differential diagnoses to consider prior to making a diagnosis of vulvar cancer:

- Papillomatosis
- Lichen simplex chronicus
- Vulvar psoriasis
- Lichen planus
- Lichen sclerosus
- Vulvar nevi, melanosis, or melanoma
- HPV infection
- Paget's disease
- Vulvar neoplasia

Prevention

The quadrivalent HPV vaccine, which protects against HPV genotypes 6, 11, 16, and 18, is indicated to prevent intraepithelial cancers of the vulva, cervix, anus, and vagina. With increasing use of HPV vaccination, it is expected that there will be a significant reduction in the incidence of VIN, usual type, as well as incidence of invasive vulvar cancer in women who are premenopausal (Hacker et al., 2015). The CDC (2015a) recommends that the HPV vaccine routinely be given to females and males ages 11 to 12 years. The vaccine may be given to individuals as young as 9 years, and catch-up vaccination is recommended until an individual is 26 years old. Although sexually active women can receive the vaccine, it may be less effective in those who have already been exposed to HPV. It is important for clinicians to provide education to their patients (or to their patients' parents or guardian if patients are younger than the age of consent) about the target age range for HPV-related cancers. It is important for them to know that vaccination is an important preventive measure against vulvar cancer (American College of Obstetricians and Gynecologists, 2015b).

Prevention of vulvar cancer should also focus on its other risk factors. Sexually active women should receive education on limiting the number of sexual partners and using barrier protection to limit their risk of exposure to HPV and HIV infection. Cigarette smoking is strongly associated with the development of usual-type VIN, and smoking cessation should be encouraged. Identification and treatment of vulvar dermatologic disorders such as lichen sclerosis may also reduce the risk of differentiated-type VIN and subsequent cancer (American College of Obstetricians and Gynecologists, 2011a, reaffirmed 2014). Clinicians should emphasize the importance of vulvar self-examination and routine gynecologic visits to ensure prompt evaluation and treatment of all precancerous and cancerous lesions (ACS, 2015d; Rauh-Hain et al., 2014; Tergas, Tseng, & Bristow, 2013).

Management

Staging, using the tumor–node–metastasis (TNM) classification system, classifies vulvar cancer growth by direct tumor extension first, local lymph node involvement second, and finally presence or absence of distant metastasis. The TNM classification is a widely used carcinoma classification system that provides a concise way of describing the clinical and anatomic spread of a tumor (American Joint Committee on Cancer [AJCC], 2016):

- The "T" describes the primary tumor according to its size and location.
- The "N" refers to the extent of cancer in the regional lymph nodes that drain fluid from the area of the tumor.

- The "M" identifies whether the cancer has spread to distant areas in the body (e.g., from the vulva to the lungs) by vascular or lymphatic channels.

The AJCC's TNM categories correspond to the stages accepted by the International Federation of Gynecology and Obstetrics (FIGO). Vulvar cancer staging according to the FIGO guidelines (2014) is outlined in **Table 27-1**.

Vulvar cancer lesions that are well differentiated tend to be minimally invasive, whereas poorly differentiated, anaplastic lesions are more likely to

TABLE 27-1	FIGO Staging for Carcinoma of the Vulva, Cervix, and Corpus Uteri

FIGO Stage	Description
I	Tumor confined to the vulva
IA	Lesions ≤ 2 cm in size, confined to the vulva or perineum and with stromal invasion ≤ 1.0 mm,[a] no nodal metastasis
IB	Lesions > 2 cm in size with stromal invasion > 1.0 mm,[a] confined to the vulva or perineum, with negative nodes ′
II	Tumor of any size with extension to adjacent perineal structures (lower third of urethra, lower third of vagina, anus) with negative nodes
III	Tumor of any size with or without extension to adjacent perineal structures (lower third of urethra, lower third of vagina, anus) with positive inguinofemoral nodes
IIIA	(i) With 1 lymph node metastasis (≥ 5 mm), or (ii) With 1–2 lymph node metastasis(es) (< 5 mm)
IIIB	(i) With 2 or more lymph node metastases (≥ 5 mm), or (ii) With 3 or more lymph node metastases (< 5 mm)
IIIC	With positive nodes with extracapsular spread
IV	Tumor invades other regional (upper two-thirds of urethra, upper two-thirds of vagina), or distant sites
IVA	Tumor invades any of the following: (i) Upper urethral and/or vaginal mucosa, bladder mucosa, rectal mucosa, or fixed pelvic bone, or (ii) Fixed or ulcerated inguinofemoral lymph nodes
IVB	Any distant metastasis including pelvic lymph nodes

Abbreviation: FIGO, International Federation of Gynecology and Obstetrics.
[a] The depth of invasion is defined as the measurement of the tumor from the epithelial–stromal junction of the adjacent most superficial dermal papilla to the deepest point of invasion.

be deeply invasive (NCI, 2015b). Local spread may extend to the urethra, vagina, perineum, and anus. Lymphatic spread usually occurs first in the inguinal lymph nodes, then involves the femoral lymph nodes, and finally spreads to the external iliac chain of the pelvic lymph nodes (AJCC, 2010). The incidence of lymph node involvement is approximately 30% (Deppe et al., 2014). Hematogenous spread to distant sites appears to be uncommon (NCI, 2015b).

Referral

Patients presenting with symptoms or questionable lesions need to be referred to a gynecologist or gynecologic oncologist who has expertise in cancer surgery. Treatment is recommended for all women with vulvar cancer and for those with either type of precancerous VIN. When invasion is not a concern, VIN can be treated with surgical therapy, laser ablation, or medical therapy (American College of Obstetricians and Gynecologists, 2011a). Management of invasive cancer is highly individualized and emphasis is on selecting the most conservative and appropriate treatment consistent with cure of the disease (Hacker et al., 2012).

Pharmacologic Treatment

Topical therapy with imiquimod, which is an immune modulator, or chemotherapeutic agents such as 5-fluorouracil (5-FU) may be used for women who have VIN that has not progressed to invasive disease. Topical therapy may have adverse skin effects and may be less effective than other treatment modalities (ACS, 2015d).

Laser Treatment

Laser excision is also an acceptable option for the treatment of precancerous VIN. It can be used for single or multifocal lesions, although the risk of recurrence may be higher than with surgical wide excision. Regular follow-up is important because women treated for VIN are considered to remain at risk for recurrent VIN and vulvar cancer throughout their lifetime (American College of Obstetricians and Gynecologists, 2011a, reaffirmed 2014; NCI, 2015b; Preti et al., 2014).

Surgical Treatment

Surgical resection is the standard treatment for patients with vulvar cancer regardless the stage of the disease (Deppe et al., 2014; Preti et al., 2014). Localized wide excision involves removing the tumor and at least a 1-cm margin of normal tissue surrounding the tumor to limit recurrence. Such surgery is the preferred intervention for women with early-stage vulvar cancer (American College of Obstetricians and Gynecologists, 2011a; Hacker et al., 2012; Preti et al., 2014; Woelber et al., 2013). Lymph node exploration is recommended when higher-grade vulvar tumors are present or when diagnostic testing indicates cancer spread (Preti et al., 2014). Because groin invasion of vulvar cancer carries a much higher mortality risk, appropriate lymph node management is the single most important factor in reducing mortality from early-stage vulvar cancer (Hacker et al., 2012). Sentinel node biopsy and dissection is the preferred method of lymph node evaluation and treatment. It carries less risk of wound breakdown and the lower-extremity lymphedema that is seen following more invasive inguinofemoral node dissection (Deppe et al., 2014; Hacker et al., 2012; NCI, 2015b; Woelber et al., 2013).

Radical vulvar excision with removal of inguinal and femoral nodes may be required in women who are diagnosed with stage III–IV vulvar cancer (Woelber et al., 2013). Chemotherapy and radiation treatment options for vulvar cancer have been limited to adjuvant use for locally advanced or metastatic disease, but both are being increasingly used in patients with earlier stages of the disease (Deppe et al., 2014; Woelber et al., 2013).

Emerging Evidence That May Change Management

Research into the genetic and epigenetic changes that play a role in the carcinogenesis of vulvar cancer may lead to greater insight into the etiology of vulvar cancer, assist in predicting prognosis, and guide development of new targeted therapies (Trietsch et al., 2015). Identified characteristics and capabilities of cancer cells have been used to develop new cancer-fighting drugs that disrupt cellular signaling pathways or utilize cells of the immune system to modify cell functions affecting cancer growth and spread (Porth, 2015). Targeted therapy approaches are at the forefront of improving treatment and outcomes for all women who have gynecologic cancers.

Patient Education

Treatment side effects and their impact on a woman's quality of life vary with the type of vulvar cancer treatment. Women diagnosed with vulvar cancer require anticipatory education prior to treatment about the potential complications of any therapeutic option. Evaluation and discussion should then continue with each follow-up visit. Side effects from surgical treatment may include significant changes to the physical appearance of the vulva and vagina and numbness at the site, both of which are proportional to the size and location of tumor excision (ACS, 2015d; Barlow, Hacker, Hussain, & Parmenter, 2014).

Chronic lymphedema of the lower extremities may occur in patients who have undergone radical lymph node dissection, and may develop either early or late after treatment (Deppe et al., 2014; Woelber et al., 2013). Lymphedema and surgically induced anatomic changes to the urinary meatus may cause the urinary stream to change direction, causing urine to "spray" rather than "stream." If this occurs, a cone-shaped urinal (sometimes used by women when camping outdoors) may be helpful. In addition, intrinsic sphincter deficiency (ISD), resulting from surgical damage to the innervation or anatomic structure of the urethra, may lead to urinary stress incontinence (Hillary, Osman, & Chapple, 2015). Vaginal introital stenosis related to scar formation, alterations in body image, depression, and sexual dysfunction are other late complications associated with surgery for vulvar cancer (ACS, 2015d; Barlow et al., 2014).

Regular (three times a week) use of vaginal dilators or regular sexual intercourse can help to stretch vaginal tissues and should be initiated before the vaginal introitus becomes stenotic. If introital stenosis occurs, the clinician may need to use a pediatric speculum for vaginal visualization, and insert only a single digit when palpating the vagina.

Some degree of sexual dysfunction is almost always present with definitive treatment of vulvar cancer. In particular, problems with arousal, orgasm, vaginal dryness, and sexual relationship issues are commonplace. Vaginal dryness may be helped by the use of vaginal lubricants such as Astroglide or vaginal moisturizers such as Replens. Changing positions for sexual intercourse may reduce discomfort.

Counseling that explores relationship issues, changes in body image, and possible alternatives to vaginal intercourse will allow for the woman's expression of grief over the loss of normal sexual function. It is also important to address the ever-present fear of recurrence of the disease or metastasis. If needed, the choice of a personal caregiver should be carefully considered—it is important to understand that the woman's sexual partner may not always be the best choice. Indeed, some women have attributed significant negative changes in their sexual relationship to the participation of a sexual partner in postoperative wound care.

When diagnosed and treated early, vulvar cancer has a good prognosis, but unfortunately more than one-third of patients suffer from recurrent disease (American College of Obstetricians and Gynecologists, 2011a, reaffirmed 2014; Trietsch et al., 2015). Consequently, lifelong follow-up on a regular schedule is important. Many patients can return to their primary care clinicians for follow-up after surgical recovery and resolution of any postoperative wound healing complications. Vulvar cancer is thought to have a relatively slow rate of progression, so women who have a good response to therapy and develop no new lesions at 6 and 12 months after treatment may be followed annually (American College of Obstetricians and Gynecologists, 2011a, reaffirmed 2014).

A comprehensive history and physical examination are standard components of follow-up care. New or persistent symptoms need to be reported promptly and evaluated carefully. Every follow-up visit should focus on the history of any new vulvar lesion, bladder function, bowel function, bone pain, and lower-extremity lymphedema. Post treatment, all women should be taught how to perform a monthly self-examination of the vulva. Recurrent disease is always a possibility, and its early identification offers the best chance for effective treatment and survival (ACS, 2015d; Rauh-Hain et al., 2014; Tergas et al., 2013).

Special Considerations

Women who are immunocompromised and those who are HIV positive are at increased risk for the development of neoplasia in the lower genital tract (Preti et al., 2014). HPV infection with usual-type VIN tends to be more aggressive, recur more often after treatment, and progress to squamous cell carcinoma more often in this population. Strict follow-up and rapid detection of suspicious lesions is important to minimize the need for repeated invasive treatments, which can have significant long-term physical and emotional effects (Preti et al., 2014).

CERVICAL CANCER

Description of the Problem

Globally, cervical cancer ranks as the fourth most common female malignancy in terms of both incidence and mortality (Bermudez, Bhatla, & Leung, 2015). Worldwide, cervical cancer is the second most commonly diagnosed cancer and the third most common cause of death among women who live in low-resource countries (Bermudez et al., 2015). Clearly, living in a low-resource country and being economically disadvantaged significantly increase a woman's risks of both developing cervical cancer and dying from it.

Cervical cancer death rates in the United States have decreased by more than 50% over the past 30 years, mainly due to implementation of screening protocols (ACS, 2014). Today, in the United States, it is much more likely for a woman to be diagnosed with cervical precancer than with invasive cervical cancer (ACS, 2014). Cervical cancer is responsible for approximately 0.7% of all new cancers in the United States (NCI, 2015a) and ranks 14th among all cancers affecting U.S. women (Howlader et al., 2014; National Institutes of Health [NIH], 2013). Approximately 12,900 new cases of cervical cancer and 4,100 deaths from cervical cancer were estimated to occur in the United States in 2015. Early detection is key to minimizing mortality, because women treated for precursor lesions have a 5-year survival rate of nearly 100% (ACS, 2014). When a diagnosis of cervical cancer is made, an estimated 46.9% of women will have localized cervical cancer (5-year survival rate = 90.9%), another 36% will have regional-stage cervical cancer with spread to lymph nodes (5-year survival rate = 57.4%), and 12% will have metastasized cervical cancer (5-year survival rate = 16.1%) (NCI, 2015a).

Unfortunately, cervical cancer remains a disease of socioeconomic disparity in the United States. Women who are Hispanic or African American are more likely to be diagnosed with the disease and are more likely to die of it compared to white women (ACS, 2015a, 2015b). A review of the incidence of cervical cancer rates in the United States per 100,000 women from 1999 to 2011 identified the risk percentiles for women of different race and ethnicity as follows: Asian/Pacific, 5.9%; American Indian/Alaska Native, 6.3%; white, 7.3%; black, 9.0%; and Hispanic. 9.8% (U.S. Cancer Statistics Working Group, 2014). The risk for women who identify with Asian/Pacific, American Indian/Alaska Native, or Hispanic ethnicity may well be underestimated due to a lack of a unified approach to understanding and accurately reporting race (U.S. Cancer Statistics Working Group, 2014). Higher incidence and mortality rates are indicative of barriers to health care especially for women who are members of minority groups and those who have a lower socioeconomic status, because they may not have access to adequate screening or treatments for early precancerous cervical lesions (ACS, 2014; U.S. Cancer Statistics Working Group, 2014). This disparity in access to care and subsequent treatment is experienced on a global scale, with statistics indicating that 500,000 women in low- and middle-income countries are diagnosed annually with late-stage cervical cancer, making it the second largest cancer killer among women who are poor and belong to a minority group (Bermudez et al., 2015; Saslow, 2013).

Etiology and Pathophysiology

HPV is now recognized as the most important causative agent in cervical carcinogenesis. This virus is detected in 99.7% of cervical cancers, and it is generally accepted that women must be infected by HPV before they develop cervical cancer (McCormack, 2014). HPV is the most common STI worldwide (World Health Organization [WHO], 2015) and nearly all women who are sexually active will be infected at some point with this virus, with many experiencing repeated infections (ACS, 2014, 2015b; CDC, 2015a; McCormack, 2014; WHO, 2015). Although HPV is considered an STI, it can be spread by skin-to-skin genital contact without intercourse. Most women are infected shortly after beginning their first sexual relationship, with the highest prevalence seen in women younger than 25 years. Thereafter, prevalence decreases rapidly, probably because of use of protection such as condoms, although condoms reduce but do not eliminate the risk of transmission (ACS, 2014).

Despite the significant correlation between HPV infection and cervical cancer, 80% to 90% of infections are transient, sometimes causing only mild cytologic abnormalities, and they usually become undetectable within 1 to 2 years. A successful immune response results in viral control or clearance. Nevertheless, of the 10% to 20% of women who are at risk for HPV persistence, approximately 2% will develop cervical carcinoma. A persistent infection with high-risk HPV is the most significant risk factor for the development of invasive cervical cancer (ACS, 2014).

At least 150 genotypically distinct variants of HPV have been identified, approximately 40 of which will infect the epithelium of the skin or mucous membranes of the genital area. Genital HPV types can be divided into two broad categories based on their risk of oncogenesis. The low-risk HPV types include 6, 11, 42, 43, 44, 54, 61, 70, 72, and 81. Types 6 and 11 are responsible for 90% to 100% of genital warts (condylomata acuminata) and low-grade cervical changes such as mild dysplasia. Lesions due to low-risk HPV infections have a higher likelihood of regression and rarely progress to cancer (ACS, 2014; CDC, 2015a; McCormack,

2014). Nevertheless, approximately 20% to 50% of people infected with low-risk viruses have coinfection with high-risk HPV types (McCormack, 2014). The high-risk HPV types include 16, 18, 31, 33, 35, 39, 45, 51, 52, 56, 58, 59, 68, 73, and 82. High-risk HPV types are known to cause persistent infection that leads to high-grade cervical changes such as moderate or severe dysplasia and neoplasia. At the same time, these strains are frequently found to be the etiologic factor in minor lesions and mild dysplasia. Types 16 and 18 are found in 70% of cervical cancer cases and are also found in other types of anogenital cancers (ACS, 2014) (**Table 27-2**).

Human papillomaviruses are small, nonenveloped viruses containing 72 capsomeres coating a genome of double-stranded circular DNA (CDC, 2015a; Gearhart, Higgins, Randall, & Buckley, 2015). The HPV genome has three regions:

- An early (E) region that codes for cellular transformation
- A late (L) region that codes for the structural proteins L1 and L2, which are responsible for creating the capsid
- A long control region that determines replication and gene function (Gearhart et al., 2015)

HPV types are differentiated by molecular methods according to genetic sequencing found on the outer capsid protein, L1. HPV infections begin developing when there is a break in the basal epithelium, and the virus remains latent in this region.

TABLE 27-2	Common HPV Types Associated with Benign and Malignant Disease

Risk	HPV Types	Manifestations
High risk	Types 16 and 18	Low-grade cervical changes High-grade cervical changes Cervical cancer Cancers of the vagina, vulva, anus, and penis
Low risk	Types 6 and 11	Benign low-grade cervical changes Genital warts

Abbreviation: HPV, human papillomavirus.
Data from American Cancer Society (ACS). (2014). Cervical cancer prevention and early detection. Retrieved from http://www.cancer.org/cancer/cervicalcancer/moreinformation/cervicalcancerpreventionandearlydetection/cervical-cancer-prevention-and-early-detection-pdf.

Although HPV viruses are specific to humans and have not been grown in vitro, communicability through skin-to-skin contact is assumed to be high secondary to the large numbers of new infections annually (CDC, 2015a; Gearhart et al., 2015). Cell-mediated immunity (CMI) plays an important role in containing the infection, with viral genes being activated when infected well-differentiated keratinocytes leave the basal layer (CDC, 2015a; Gearhart et al., 2015).

The major difference between low- and high-risk HPV types is that after infection is established, the low-risk HPV types are maintained as extra-chromosomal DNA episomes, while the high-risk HPV genomes become integrated into the host cells' DNA in malignant lesions. Integration of the viral genome into the host cell genome is considered a hallmark of malignant transformation. High-risk HPV produces viral protein products (E6, E7) that bind and inactivate the host's tumor suppressor genes *p53* and *pRb*. The inactivation of these genes blocks apoptosis (programmed cell death) and induces chromosomal abnormalities (Gearhart et al., 2015).

Cervical cancer is characterized by a well-defined premalignant phase that can be identified through cytologic examination of exfoliated cells (Pap test) and confirmed on histologic examination. Premalignant changes can represent a spectrum of cervical abnormalities, which are referred to as squamous intraepithelial lesions (SIL) or cervical intraepithelial neoplasia (CIN). These early lesions, which form a continuum that is divided into low-grade or high-grade SIL or CIN 1, 2, and 3, reflect the increasingly abnormal changes that occur in the cervical epithelium. Over time, the premalignant lesions can persist, regress, or progress to invasive malignancy. CIN 1 often regresses spontaneously, whereas CIN 2 and 3 are more likely to persist or progress. The premalignant changes almost always occur in the metaplastic epithelium at the squamo-columnar junction. Unfortunately, cytologic and histologic examinations cannot reliably distinguish the few women with abnormal cytology who will progress to invasive cancer from the vast majority of women whose abnormalities will spontaneously regress (ACS, 2015b; Boardman & Matthews, 2014).

The latency period between HPV exposure and the development of cervical cancer is usually measured in years or decades. Longitudinal studies have shown that in untreated patients with carcinoma in situ (CIS) lesions, 30% to 70% will develop invasive carcinoma over a period of 10 to 12 years. In approximately 10% of patients, however, lesions progress from in situ to invasive in a period of less than 1 year (NCI, 2015a, 2015c). The long natural history of this disease provides an opportunity to screen women for premalignant lesions, thereby preventing the lesions from evolving into cervical cancer.

Two main types of cervical cancer are distinguished. The most common type of cervical cancer is squamous cell carcinoma (SCC), which accounts for 80% to 90% of all cervical cancers. SCC arises from the squamous cells that cover the ectocervix, and HPV 16 has been implicated as the type most commonly associated with SCC (Woodman, Collins, & Young, 2007). Adenocarcinoma, the second most common cervical cancer type, accounts for 10% to 12% of cervical cancer cases. It most often arises from the columnar epithelium—a group of mucus-producing glandular cells—located in the endocervix and has been associated most commonly with HPV 18, followed by HPV 16 (Woodman et al., 2007). An increase in the incidence of adenocarcinomas has been observed during the past 20 to 30 years: Among women younger than 35 years, the incidence more than doubled between 1970 and the mid-1980s. On rare occasions, cervical cancers have features of both SCC and adenocarcinoma; these cases are called adenosquamous carcinomas or mixed carcinomas (ACS, 2014).

Risk Factors Associated with Acquiring HPV

Age

Early age at first intercourse (age 18 years or younger) is a risk factor for HPV: It is believed the younger-developing cervix is at a greater risk of being infected because of the normal physiologic process called squamous metaplasia. The process of squamous metaplasia occurs at the squamo-columnar junction, or transformation zone, where the more fragile columnar epithelial cells are replaced with hardier squamous epithelial cells. Squamous metaplasia is initiated by the eversion of the columnar epithelium onto the ectocervix, which occurs under the influence of estrogen and its ensuing exposure to the acidic vaginal pH. Although metaplasia may arise throughout the reproductive years, it is most active during adolescence and first pregnancy. Indeed, first-time pregnancies that occur in women younger than 17 years are associated with twice the risk of cervical cancer compared to women who develop cervical cancer later in life (ACS, 2014; American Society for Colposcopy and Cervical Pathology [ASCCP], 2014). Cells undergoing metaplasia are more vulnerable to carcinogenic agents such as HPV.

The age of greatest risk, however, is midlife, when the majority of cervical cancer diagnoses are made. An estimated 15% cases are diagnosed after 65 years of age, with most occurring in women who have not participated in regular screening (ACS, 2014).

Sexual Behavior

Having multiple sexual partners or having a partner with multiple sex partners increases the risk of multiple exposures to HPV (ACS, 2015b). Nevertheless, only a small proportion of women who become infected with HPV go on to develop cervical cancer (CDC, 2012). Cofactors, such as smoking, are thought to play a contributing role in this evolution.

Smoking

Among women infected with HPV, current and former smokers have approximately two to three times the incidence of high-grade cervical intraepithelial lesions or invasive cancer. Passive smoking is also associated with increased risk, albeit to a lesser extent (ACS, 2015b; NCI, 2015a; NIH, 2013). Women who smoke cigarettes are twice as likely as nonsmokers to develop cervical cancer. Smoking exposes the body to many carcinogens that affect more than just the lungs, as carcinogens are absorbed by the lungs and carried in the bloodstream, thereby traveling throughout the body. Tobacco by-products have been found in the cervical mucus of women who smoke, and it is believed that these by-products damage the DNA in cervical cells. Smoking may also impair the immune response, thereby interfering with the body's ability to clear the HPV infection (ACS, 2014; NCI, 2015b; NIH, 2013).

Immunosuppression

Patients who are immunocompromised from HIV, AIDS, or other causes (e.g., medications) have an increased prevalence and persistence of HPV infection. A precancerous lesion may develop more quickly into an invasive cancer if a woman is immunocompromised (ACS, 2014). The immune system plays an important role in destroying cancer cells and slowing their growth and spread (ACS, 2014).

Oral Contraceptives

The risk of cervical cancer doubles after 5 years of combined oral contraceptive (COC) use, but returns to normal about 10 years following discontinuation of oral contraceptives (ACS, 2014). Interestingly, women who have used an intrauterine device (even if for less than a year) appear to have a lower risk of developing cervical cancer (ACS, 2014).

While the connection between COCs and cervical cancer is not yet fully understood, it appears that the estrogenic effect of COCs may prevent the ectopy of the cervix from receding into the cervical canal, leaving the vulnerable area exposed. Moreover, COC users are less likely to use barrier protection, thereby increasing their risk of contracting HPV. Findings to date do not warrant discontinuing COC use in the case of an abnormal Pap test (ACS, 2015b; Bertram, 2004). Experts recommend that clinicians discuss the risks and benefits of COC use with women based on their individual history and risk factors (ACS, 2014, 2015b; Boardman & Mathews, 2014).

High Parity

Having had three or more full-term pregnancies has been associated with an increased risk for cervical cancer (ACS, 2015b; CDC, 2012). Speculation for the causes of this relationship ranges to having had more unprotected sex and therefore more opportunities for HPV exposure to the lower immunity state experienced during pregnancy coupled with hormonal changes that may facilitate cancer cell growth (ACS, 2015b).

Genetic Predisposition

Studies suggest that women whose mother or sisters have had cervical cancer are more likely to develop the disease. Twin studies also suggest a familial susceptibility to cervical cancer is possible. Some researchers suspect a familial tendency is caused by an inherited condition that makes some women more susceptible to HPV infection than others (ACS, 2015b; Boardman & Matthews,

2014). Several genetic changes have been associated with cervical cancer. Indeed, changes in genes involved in apoptosis and gene repair have been suggested as explaining why some women are not able to spontaneously clear HPV infection. Genetics, however, is estimated to affect less than 1% of cervical cancers (Boardman & Matthews, 2014).

Nutritional Status

Diets low in fruits and vegetables have been identified as potential contributing factors in the development of cervical cancer. Low levels of vitamins C and E, folate, and carotenoids have been linked to cervical cancer (ACS, 2015b; García-Closas, Castellsagué, Bosch, & González, 2005). Further research is needed to clarify these relationships.

Poverty

Many women with a lower socioeconomic status or living in developing countries continue to lack ready access to adequate screening and treatment (ACS, 2015b).

Diethylstilbestrol

Daughters of women who took diethylstilbestrol (DES) are 40 times more likely to develop clear cell adenocarcinoma (CCA) of the vagina and cervix than women who were not exposed to DES in utero. Clear cell adenocarcinoma is a rare form of vaginal and cervical cancer. The average age of women diagnosed with DES-related cervical cancer is 19 years. DES was removed from the market in 1971, so women who were exposed at age 19 years (or younger) are less likely to receive a diagnosis of cervical carcinoma. Nevertheless, it is not known how long they will remain at higher risk for contracting the disease (ACS, 2014).

Infectious Agents

The specific role of herpes simplex virus 2 (HSV-2) and other infectious agents in the pathogenesis of cervical cancer remains unclear. Nevertheless, HSV-2 and *Chlamydia trachomatis* infections are known to be associated with a chronic inflammatory response and micro-ulceration of the cervical epithelium. Such an inflammatory response is associated with the generation of free radicals, which are thought to play important roles in the initiation and progression of cancers. Free radicals directly damage DNA and DNA repair proteins and inhibit apoptosis, allowing the development of genetic instability (ACS, 2014).

Clinical Presentation

Early cervical cancer is usually asymptomatic. As many as 20% of patients who have invasive cervical cancer are asymptomatic when the disease is diagnosed. If symptoms do occur, the most commonly noted are abnormal vaginal bleeding, such as postmenopausal bleeding, irregular menses, heavy menstrual flow, painless heavy menstrual bleeding, or postcoital bleeding. An abnormal vaginal discharge that is odiferous, watery, purulent, or mucoid may also be present. Late symptoms that suggest metastatic spread include bladder outlet obstruction, constipation, back pain, pelvic pain, pain during intercourse, and leg swelling (ACS, 2015b; Boardman & Matthews, 2014; NIH, 2013).

Assessment

History

Key areas to cover in the history that can assist clinicians in identifying women at high risk for cervical cancer include the following:

- Abnormal vaginal bleeding (intermenstrual or postcoital bleeding), unusual vaginal discharge, or dyspareunia
- Sexual history—age at first intercourse, number of sexual partners in the past 6 months, number of lifetime partners, and presence of lesions in sexual partners
- Contraceptive history, including use of barrier methods
- HPV and other STIs in the woman and her partners
- Immunosuppression, including HIV infection
- Prior history of cancer or cancer therapy (e.g., radiation, chemotherapy, surgery)
- In utero DES exposure
- Date and result of the most recent Pap test
- Prior abnormal cervical cytology
- Menstrual history, including the date of the last menstrual period
- Pregnancy history
- History of tobacco, drug, or alcohol use
- Family history of cervical cancer
- HPV immunization status

Physical Examination

The physical examination should include a thorough pelvic, abdominal, inguinal lymph node, and rectal examination. Cervical cancer usually begins around the cervical os. In its earliest stages, a cancerous cervix cannot be distinguished from a normal cervix. As the disease progresses, the cervix may appear abnormal, with gross erosion, ulcers, or a mass that bleeds easily on contact. In the late stages, an extensive, irregular, cauliflower-like growth may develop. The cervix may be hard and indurated, and its mobility may be restricted or lost. As the tumor enlarges, it grows by extending upward into the endometrial cavity, downward into the vagina, and laterally to the pelvic wall. It can invade the bladder and rectum directly. A bimanual examination can detect a mass or bleeding from tumor erosion.

Common sites for distant metastasis include the pelvic lymph nodes, liver, lungs, and bones (Boardman & Matthews, 2014). Metastasis to the liver may lead to findings of hepatomegaly. Leg edema is suggestive of tumor obstruction of the lymph or vascular systems. The triad findings of leg edema, pain, and hydronephrosis are indicative of spread to the pelvic wall (Boardman & Matthews, 2014).

Diagnostic Testing

Recommendations for cervical cancer screening have changed dramatically since 2012. The belief that routine Pap testing for precancerous lesions that has led to a dramatic decline in mortality rate from cervical cancer is now being balanced against data showing that 9 of 10 abnormal Pap tests will revert to normal even without treatment. It is also theorized that women's immune system responses will resolve approximately 90% of HPV infections (ACS, 2014; NCI, 2015a; NIH, 2013). The cost of treating precancerous cells or high-risk HPV infections that may spontaneously resolve without any intervention includes the anxiety of enduring more invasive and possibly painful testing procedures that have their own potential complications.

In recognition of these considerations, in 2012 the ACS, the ASCCP, and the American Society for Clinical Pathology (ASCP) issued new screening guidelines that are in alignment with the guidelines published by the U.S. Preventive Services Task Force (see Chapter 7) and American College of Obstetricians and Gynecologists. These guidelines recommend that screening for cervical cancer start at age 21 years. The evidence suggests that women younger than 21 years have a high likelihood of spontaneous clearance of abnormal cells and, therefore, are at low risk for developing cervical cancer (National Comprehensive Cancer Network [NCCN], 2015b; NCI, 2014). Screening should start at age 21 years with a routine Pap test and continue at 3-year intervals until the age of 29 years. Between the ages of 30 years and 65 years, cotesting (Pap test with HPV DNA testing) should be performed every 5 years. Cotesting is important because it has a lower false-negative rate and therefore there is less possibility of missing an abnormality (NCI, 2016). An acceptable alternative for this age group is to complete a Pap test every 3 years. Women older than 65 years who have never had precancerous changes, who have never been diagnosed with cervical cancer, or who have had removal of the cervix and uterus with no evidence of precancerous or cancerous changes do not require further screening for cervical cancer. Women who are 65 years and older and who are at high risk for cervical cancer, such as those who were exposed to diethylstilbestrol in utero, have an immunosuppressed status, are positive for HIV, or have a history of organ transplant, should discuss alternative interval testing with their clinicians. It is important for clinicians to appreciate that while guidelines can be helpful, they are not meant to replace sound clinical judgment that is based on an individualized assessment of a woman's risk profile, her subjective concerns, and assessment findings.

The debate over the efficacy of using a conventional versus liquid-based Pap test might be largely resolved in the United States, as automated liquid-based pap cytology has largely replaced conventional Pap smears. Although both tests appear to have similar efficacy in regard to detecting cell abnormalities, the liquid-based testing enables the use of the same cell sample to test for high-risk types of HPV (NCI, 2014).

Most laboratories in the United States use the Bethesda System for reporting the results of cervical cytology. Satisfactory specimens require at least 5,000 squamous cells for a liquid-based preparation, with a minimum of 10 endocervical or squamous metaplastic cells. Unsatisfactory specimens include those in which more than 75% of the epithelial cells are obscured, which may occur due to inflammation or blood. The Bethesda System includes the general categories of "negative for intraepithelial lesion or malignancy," "epithelial cell abnormality," or "other," which may describe an unusual finding such as endometrial cells that might require further investigation. If there is an unusual or abnormal finding, the goal is to either document or rule out high-grade disease (CIN 3 or HSIL).

The Bethesda System (TBS) provides a uniform set of terminology as well as guidance for clinical management. In this system, abnormalities of squamous cells and glandular cells are considered separately (see **Table 27-3**). This distinction is important because atypical glandular cells have an increased association with high-grade disease. Glandular cells are also specified according to cell type because treatment options may vary based on the type (Solomon et al., 2002).

Table 27-3 provides a description of the Bethesda System for reporting cervical cytology results (Nayar & Wilbur, 2015). Changes from the 2001 TBS are identified.

Over the past 10 years several changes in cervical cancer prevention, screening, and management have occurred such as the increased use of liquid-based preparations for testing and cotesting (Pap test combined with high risk HPV testing). Today there is better understanding about the biology of HPV along with the approval and use of HPV vaccines. The terminology for histopathology has also changed during the last decade (Nayar & Wilbur, 2015). These changes and others led to a review and update of TBS 2001 (Nyar & Wilbur, 2015). TBS 2014 (**Table 27-4**) has only minimal

---

TABLE 27-3	2001 Bethesda Categories of Epithelial Cell Abnormalities

Category	Description
ASC-US	Atypical squamous cells of undetermined significance. This term is used when the squamous cells do not appear completely normal but it is not possible to determine the cause of the abnormal cells. An estimated 10–20% of women with ASC-UC may have CIN 2 or 3. An estimated 1 in 1,000 women with ASC-UC may have invasive cancer.
ASC-H	Atypical squamous cells—cannot exclude HSIL.
LSIL	Low-grade squamous intraepithelial neoplasia. Encompasses: • HPV transient infection • CIN 1 (mild dysplasia): Lesion involves the initial one-third of the epithelial layer
HSIL	High-grade squamous intraepithelial neoplasia. Encompasses: • HPV persistent infection • CIN 2 (moderate dysplasia): Lesion involves one-third to less than two-thirds of the epithelial layer • CIN 3 (severe dysplasia, carcinoma in situ): Lesion involves two-thirds of the epithelial layer to full thickness
Squamous carcinoma	Malignant cells penetrate the basement membrane of the cervical epithelium and infiltrate the stromal tissue (supporting tissue). In advanced cases, cancer may spread to adjacent organs such as the bladder or rectum, or to distant sites in the body via the bloodstream and lymphatic channels.

Abbreviation: HPV, human papillomavirus.
Data from Centers for Disease Control and Prevention (CDC). (2011). Cervical cancer screening for women who attend STD clinics or have a history of STDs. Retrieved from: http://www.cdc.gov/std/treatment/2010/cc-screening.htm; Solomon, D., Davey, D., Kurman, R., Moriarty, A., O'Connor, D., Prey, M., . . . Young, N. (2002). The 2001 Bethesda System: Terminology for reporting results of cervical cytology. *Journal of the American Medical Association, 287*(16), 2114–2119; Verma, I., Jain, V., & Kaur, T. (2014). Application of Bethesda system for cervical cytology in unhealthy cervix. *Journal of Clinical and Diagnostic Research, 8*(9), 26–30.

TABLE 27-4	2014 Bethesda System for Interpreting the Results of Cervical Cytologic Diagnoses (Abridged)
Speciman Type[a]	Conventional Pap test, liquid-based preparation or other
Adequacy of Specimen	Satisfactory for evaluation (note presence or absence of endocervical or transformation zone components and any other qualifiers such as inflammation, or blood on os present) Unsatisfactory for evaluation (specify reason)
General Categorization (Optional)	Negative for intraepithelial lesion or malignancy Epithelial cell abnormality: specify whether squamous or glandular cells[b] Other (e.g., endometrial cells in a woman age 45 or older)
Interpretation/Result[a]	**Non-neoplastic cellular findings (optional to report)** Non-neoplastic variations • Squamous metaplasia • Keratotic changes • Tubal metaplasia • Atrophy • Pregnancy associated changes Reactive cellular changes associated with: • Inflammation • Lymphocytic (follicular cervicitis) • Radiation • IUD Glandular status post hysterectomy **Organisms** • *Trichommonas vaginalis* • Fungal organisms with a form or structure that looks like *Candida* spp. • Change in flora (e.g. consistent with bacterial vaginosis) • Bacteria that have a form consistent with *Actinomyces* spp. • Cellular changes consistent with herpes simplex virus • Cellular changes consistent with cytomegalovirus **Other** • Such as endometrial cells in a woman age 45 or older (note that the age is changed from 40 years in 2001 to 45 years in TBS 2014). • Other findings

Epithelial Cell Abnormalities	Squamous cell
	 • ASC are divided into two categories:
	   • ASC-US: Atypical squamous cells of undetermined significance
	   • ASC-H: Cannot exclude high-grade squamous intraepithelial lesion

(continues)

TABLE 27-4	2014 Bethesda System for Interpreting the Results of Cervical Cytologic Diagnoses (Abridged) (*continued*)

	• LSIL
	   • Refers to cervical cancer precursors encompassing human papillomavirus, mild dysplasia, and CIN 1
	• HSIL
	   • Refers to cervical cancer precursors encompassing moderate and severe dysplasia, carcinoma in situ, and CIN 2 and CIN 3
	   • Includes identification of features consistent with invasion
	• Squamous cell carcinoma
	
	Glandular cell
	• Atypical
	   • Specify endocervical, endometrial, glandular cells, or NOS
	• Atypical
	   • Specify if specimen is either endocervical cells or glandular cells favoring neoplastic disease
	• Endocervical AIS
	• Adenocarcinoma
	   • Identify if endocervical, endometrial, extrauterine, or NOS

Other Malignant Neoplasms (List Is Not Comprehensive)	Endometrial cells in a woman 45 years or older

Abbreviations: AIS, adenocarcinoma in situ; ASC, atypical squamous cells; CIN cervical intraepithelial neoplasia; HSIL, high-grade squamous intraepithelial lesion; IUD, intrauterine device; LSIL, low-grade squamous intraepithelial lesion; NOS, not otherwise specified.
[a] This section is new or revised from TBS 2001.
[b] Indicate whether there is cellular evidence of neoplasia.
Modified from Nayar, R., & Wilbur, D. C. (2015). The Pap test and Bethesda 2014. *Acta Cytologica, 59*(2), 121–132. doi:10.1159/000381842.
Copyright © 2015 Karger Publishers, Basel, Switzerland.

terminology changes (therefore categories identified in **Table 27-3** remain accurate). Changes in the 2014 Bethesda System include the following:

- Reporting of benign appearing endometrial cells is now recommended for women age 45 years or older whereas in 2001 the recommended age was 40 or older
- No new category was created for squamous lesions with LSIL and few cells suggestive of concurrent HSIL
- The new system requires the clinician to identify whether the specimen type is the traditional Pap smear, liquid-based preparation or some other type.

Further Testing

Additional laboratory testing that might be indicated to rule out other causes of vaginal discharge or bleeding includes the following:

- *STI testing.* Chlamydia and gonorrhea are commonly encountered STIs that may produce symptoms similar to those of cervical cancer—namely, dysuria, urinary frequency, vaginal discharge, and postcoital bleeding. Many other women who have chlamydia or gonorrhea are asymptomatic, however, so it is wise to test for HPV, chlamydia, and gonorrhea when a woman presents with a vaginal discharge that has not resolved. Testing can be done using a single vaginal or cervical swab (Hollier & Hensley, 2011). See Chapter 6, Appendix 6-A.
- *Wet mount preparation.* Women who have vulvovaginal candidiasis, bacterial vaginosis, or trichomoniasis can present with a variety of symptoms, including vaginal discharge, malodor, irritation, burning or itching, dysuria, and dyspareunia. Accurate

identification of the pathogen requires microscopic examination of vaginal secretions. The microscopic examinations include a saline wet mount and a potassium hydroxide (KOH) preparation. See Chapter 6, Appendix 6-A.

- *Referral.* Women with suspicious lesions on physical examination require referral regardless of the cytology results (Boardman & Mathews, 2014). An abnormal Pap test may require a referral for colposcopic examination with a biopsy of the abnormal area (ACS, 2015b).
- *Endocervical curettage.* A curette is inserted into the endocervical canal to remove tissue when the transformation zone is not visible. This procedure is aided by colposcopy (ACS, 2015b).
- *Cone biopsy.* In this procedure, a cone-shaped tissue extending from the exocervix to the endocervical canal (including the transformation zone) is removed. The loop electrosurgical technique (LEEP) uses a wire hook heated by an electrical current to remove the tissue. A cold-knife biopsy uses either a surgical scalpel or laser to remove tissue under anesthesia (ACS, 2015b).

The ASCCP (2013) provides algorithms for the management of women with cervical cytologic abnormalities. The new evidence-based guidelines were influenced by the analysis of a large clinical database of 1.4 million women who received care after abnormal cytologic tests from the Kaiser Permanente Northern California Medical care plan. The guidelines assist clinicians in referral or management decisions for women who have abnormal cervical intraepithelial neoplasia or adenocarcinoma in situ results. Clinicians with an iPhone, iPad, or Android smartphone can download a mobile app of the 19 algorithms at http://www.asccp.org/store-detail2/asccp-mobile-app. Algorithms are also provided in the **Appendix 27-A**.

Differential Diagnoses

Differential diagnoses for cervical cancer include the following conditions, which must be ruled out prior to diagnosing cancer (Boardman & Matthews, 2014):

- Cervicitis: noninfectious related to trauma or chemical irritation; infectious related to STIs such as chlamydia, *Neisseria gonorrhoeae*, HSV, and *Trichomonas*
- Vaginitis
- Granulomatous (rare) or cervical polyps
- Pelvic inflammatory disease

Symptoms highly suggestive of cervical cancer may rarely be due to Paget's disease, vaginal cancer, endometrial carcinoma, or primary myeloma.

Management

Prevention

Three human papillomavirus vaccines are now available that provide effective protection against cervical cancer (**Table 27-5**). All three recombinant vaccines (bivalent [2vHPV], quadrivalent [4vHPV], and 9-valent [9vHPV]) use noninfectious virus-like particles prepared from the L1 capsid protein from the HPV types for which the vaccines provide coverage. Each of these vaccines provides coverage for HPV 16 and 18, which together are responsible for an estimated 66% of cervical cancer cases; the 9vHPV vaccine offers coverage for five additional oncogenic HPV types that are collectively responsible for an additional 15% of cervical cancer cases (Joura et al., 2015; Markowitz & Shimabukuro, 2015; McCormack, 2014).

Studies of the bivalent and 4vHPV vaccines indicate that these vaccines also produce antibodies that neutralize non-vaccine-covered high-risk HPV types, with the bivalent vaccine demonstrating greater efficacy against HPV types 31 and 45 (McCormack, 2014). Despite this, research has yet to reveal the relationship between the degree of antibody levels and the protective effect, with no difference in efficacy being seen in terms of the protective effects against oncogenic HPV types (McCormack, 2014). The 9vHPV vaccine was approved for use in December 2014 based on randomized clinical trials following more than 14,000 women who received either the 9vHPV or 4vHPV vaccine. High efficacy against HPV types 31, 33, 45, 52, and 58 was demonstrated by the 9vHPV vaccine, as well as noninferior immunogenicity to

| TABLE 27-5 | Human Papillomavirus Vaccines |

Manufacturer/Vaccine Type (Name)	Components of Vaccine	Summary of Use
GlaxoSmithKline/bivalent HPV recombinant vaccine (Cervarix)	HPV types 16, 18 Adjuvant: Aluminum hydroxide	Protects against precancer and cancer of the cervix
Merck/quadrivalent HPV recombinant vaccine (Gardasil in the United States; Silgard in some other countries)	HPV types 6, 11, 16, 18 Adjuvant: Amorphous aluminum hydroxyphosphate sulfate	Protects against precancer and cancer of the cervix, vulva, and vagina Protects against anal precancer and cancer Protects against genital warts
Merck/9-valent HPV (Gardasil 9)	HPV types 6, 11, 16, 18, 31, 33, 45, 52, 58 Adjuvant: Amorphous aluminum hydroxyphosphate sulfate	Protects against precancer and cancer of the cervix, vulva, and vagina Protects against anal precancer and cancer Protects against genital warts

Abbreviation: HPV, human papillomavirus.

the 4vHPV vaccine. Researchers reported that the 9-valent vaccine has 96.7% (95% confidence interval) efficacy against high-grade cervical, vulvar, and vaginal lesions (Joura et al., 2015). These results suggest that the 9vHPV vaccine has the potential of increasing the rate of prevention of cervical cancer from approximately 70% to 90% (Joura et al., 2015; Markowitz & Shimabukuro, 2015).

The safety of the 4vHPV and 2vHPV vaccines has been reviewed by several international agencies including WHO's Global Advisory Committee on Vaccine Safety in 2013, the European Medicines Agency's Pharmacovigilance Risk Assessment Committee in 2014, and several U.S. federal agencies and vaccine manufacturers with ongoing postlicensure surveillance studies (McCormack, 2014; Stokley et al., 2014). Placebo-controlled clinical trials indicate that HPV vaccines are generally well tolerated. The side effects most commonly reported have been pain, swelling and redness at the injection site, and systemic symptoms of headache

and fever (McCormack, 2014; Stokley et al., 2014). Rare adverse reactions found to be causally related to HPV vaccines include syncope (which can happen with any injected vaccine) and anaphylaxis (Institute of Medicine, 2011).

Extensive postmarketing surveillance data for HPV vaccines have been published (Markowitz & Shimabukuro, 2015). The CDC maintains the Vaccine Adverse Event Reporting System (VAERS)—a national vaccine safety surveillance program run by the CDC and the Food and Drug Administration (FDA). VAERS is intended to serve as an early warning system to detect possible safety issues with U.S. vaccines by collecting information about adverse events (possible side effects or health problems) that occur after vaccination (CDC, 2015b). It was created in 1990 in response to the National Childhood Vaccine Injury Act (http://www.cdc.gov /vaccinesafety/ensuringsafety/history/index.html). If any health problem occurs following a vaccination, anyone—doctors, nurses, vaccine manufacturers, and any member of the general public—can submit a report to VAERS (CDC, 2015b).

Initial reviews of the vaccine adverse event reports in 2009 indicated higher-than-expected rates of venous thrombosis (VTE), and some concern was raised when a 2011 vaccine safety datalink study reported nonsignificant elevated risk (risk ratio [RR], 1.98) for venous thromboembolism in women between 9 and 17 years of age. Subsequent national register-based cohort studies in Denmark and Sweden failed to find any relationship between 4vHPV vaccination and VTE (Markowitz & Shimabukuro, 2015). A safety review of Gardasil (which accounts for 99% of all HPV vaccinations administered in the United States) was conducted by examining VAERS reports from June 2006 to March 2014. Following administration of 67 million doses of Gardasil, 25,176 adverse event reports were recorded, with 92.4% classified as nonserious (Stokley et al., 2014). There were 96 reports of death and 21 reports of ovarian failure, but none of these outcomes appeared to be causally related to Gardasil (Stokley et al., 2014). Nationally and internationally, reports have failed to show any causal association between vaccination and anaphylaxis, autoimmune and neurologic disease, and incidence of complex regional pain syndrome (Markowitz & Shimabukuro, 2015; McCormack, 2014).

A post-surveillance general safety assessment of approximately 190,000 females from two large U.S. health plans reported an association between the 4vHPV vaccine and syncope on the same day as injection as well as skin infections reported 2 weeks post injection, some of which were determined to be localized (Markowitz & Shimabukuro, 2015). The CDC (2015a) guidelines emphasize having women sit or lie down during vaccine administration and remain supine for 15 minutes post injection so that they can be observed to minimize injury from potential syncope.

The newest HPV vaccine, 9vHPV, was licensed in December 2014 based on data from seven prelicensure studies with approximately 15,000 participants. Results indicated that the vaccine is well tolerated, with an adverse-effect profile similar to that of 4vHPV (Markowitz & Shimabukuro, 2015). Differences noted were more injection-site swelling and erythema and a higher spontaneous abortion rate than reported with the 4vHPV vaccine

(although the spontaneous abortion rate was still within expectations for rates of early loss of pregnancy and, therefore, there may not be a causal relationship). Ongoing studies of all three HPV vaccines are exploring the safety of their use during pregnancy and case reports of rare adverse events (Joura et al., 2015; Markowitz & Shimabukuro, 2015; Petrosky et al., 2015; Stokley et al., 2014).

Current recommendations from the Advisory Committee on Immunization Practices (ACIP) are to begin HPV immunization for women at 11 or 12 years (or 9 years, if deemed necessary) and to follow a 3-dose schedule at 0, 1 to 2 months, and 6 months (Markowitz & Shimabukuro, 2015; Petrosky et al., 2015). The period for women to be immunized spans from age 13 to 26 years. Early immunization is important, as 46% of women who report having only one sex partner still test positive for HPV within 3 years of first having sexual intercourse (McCormack, 2014). In addition, all women diagnosed with high-grade cervical cancer during the clinical trials of the HPV vaccines were infected with HPV at baseline (Joura et al, 2015). Clearly, it is essential to vaccinate individuals before they are potentially exposed to HPV.

Women who already have abnormal cervical cytology results are still candidates for the vaccine, as it does not treat current disease, but will provide protection from infections from other HPV types. The ACIP urges practitioners to use any available HPV vaccine to protect women against HPV 16 and 18, and advises completion of the series even if one formulation needs to be substituted for another due to availability issues. If the vaccination series schedule is interrupted, the woman does not need to restart it from the first dose (Markowitz & Shimabukuro, 2015; Petrosky et al., 2015).

One important caveat is that women who have a history of immediate hypersensitivity to yeast should not receive the 4-valent or 9-valent HPV series. Likewise, prefilled syringes of 2-valent vaccine are contraindicated for women who have a history of anaphylactic response to latex (FDA, 2014, 2015a, 2015b).

The HPV vaccine is currently contraindicated during pregnancy, but may be given to women who are breastfeeding (FDA, 2014, 2015a, 2015b). Woman who have inadvertently received a first dose during pregnancy may be reassured that there is no evidence from clinical trials or through interim analysis of 5 years of pregnancy registry data that suggests the immunization increases the risk of adverse outcomes (McCormack, 2014). However, practitioners are requested to contact the appropriate manufacturers' registry to add to the knowledge base regarding safety during pregnancy.

Following immunization, the identification and treatment of early precancerous lesions are critical to the prevention of cervical cancer. Screening is essential for both vaccinated and unvaccinated women (CDC, 2015a). Scheduling and keeping appointments for regular gynecologic examinations and Pap tests decreases the incidence and mortality of cervical cancer (NCI, 2015a). Abnormal changes in the cervix are readily detected by the Pap test and are easily cured before cancer develops. Preventive measures should include educating women that the risk of infection can be decreased by delaying the onset of sexual activity, decreasing the number of sexual partners, using condoms consistently, and eliminating tobacco use.

Definitive Treatment

The choice of treatment depends primarily on the stage of disease at the time of diagnosis, but other factors, such as a woman's general health and preferences, should also be considered (ACS, 2015f). The quest to identify the cellular events that stimulate carcinogenesis continues because this understanding ultimately will enable better tumor classification and prognostication (Binder, Prat, & Mutch, 2015). Current technology allows for analysis of DNA, RNA, and proteins; thus genetic and molecular studies can be performed on blood and tissue samples obtained during operative evaluation and treatment of the cancer (Binder et al., 2015). Findings from these studies will provide a path for the development of a classification system that is based on genomic and proteomic foundations.

Surgical Treatment

Cervical cancer is staged using the FIGO and AJCC-TNM systems. Treatment of precancerous lesions and CIS (stage 0; Tis, N0, M0) includes cryosurgery or laser ablation to kill abnormal cells. Loop electrosurgical excision or cold-knife conization can be used for definitive treatment

in women with early-stage IA1 (T1a1, N0, M0) who want to preserve fertility (ACS, 2015b; NCI, 2015a). After treatment, patients require lifelong surveillance at regular intervals. The clinician determines the timing and frequency of follow-up based on Pap test results and colposcopy examinations (NCI, 2015a).

Hysterectomy is a choice for stage IA1 cancers and some stage 0 disease if cone biopsy reveals positive margins. For cervical cancer stages IA2 (T1a2, N0, M), IB (T1b, N0M), and sometimes IIA (T2a, N0, M), a radical hysterectomy removing the uterus, parametria and uterosacral ligaments, upper part of the vagina, and sometimes lymph nodes is indicated. Postoperative complications associated with any pelvic surgery can include new-onset urinary incontinence, pelvic pain, and dyspareunia. Many times the ovaries and fallopian tubes are preserved. Women might need emotional support for issues such as loss of fertility; possible need for a catheter, as voiding can be difficult with the disruption of nerves; and concerns regarding sexuality. Clinicians can reassure women that the clitoral area is not disturbed and that their ability to have sexual relations and achieve orgasm will remain intact (ACS, 2015b; NCCN, 2015b). Women and their partners may need counseling for feelings of loss or difficulty with intimacy (NCI, 2015a). A good resource for women can be found at the American Cancer Society's website, which includes a pamphlet entitled "Sexuality for the Woman with Cancer" (ACS, 2015h).

A surgical option is available to women with IA2, IB, or IIA cervical cancer who want to preserve fertility and have lesions smaller than 2 cm. A trachelectomy removes the cervix and upper part of the vagina while preserving the body of the uterus. (ACS, 2015b; NCCN, 2015b). Women who are not eligible for this procedure should be encouraged to consult with a reproductive specialist regarding embryo or oocyte cryopreservation prior to surgery.

Other options for women with stage IA2, IB, or IIA cancer include bypassing surgery and choosing external-beam pelvic radiation plus internal brachytherapy. When biopsies have positive margins, chemotherapy is added to the radiation therapy. Definitive radiation therapy has growing support in the literature (ACS, 2015b; Carlson et al., 2014).

Advanced-stage cervical cancers—that is, IIB (T2b, N0 M0), III (T3, N0, M0), or IVA (T4, N0, M0)—are usually not treated with surgery. Instead, external pelvic radiation with internal brachytherapy is combined with chemotherapy. Special attention is given to imaging studies (MRI, PET scan) to ascertain possible metastasis. The treatment of stage IVB (any T, any N, M1) cervical cancer is primarily palliative, because cure is not possible. Palliative radiation may be used to control bleeding, pelvic pain, or urinary or bowel obstruction from pelvic disease. Current clinical trials are examining the efficacy of new chemotherapy regimens (ACS, 2015b; NCCN, 2015b).

Women with recurrent cervical cancer are candidates for total pelvic exenteration, which extends the removal of organs and tissues from the radical hysterectomy to include pelvic lymph node dissection and, depending on spread, removal of the bladder, vagina, rectum, and part of the colon. Emotional and physical recovery needs are extensive when such surgery is performed, as the woman must learn to manage urostomy and colostomy sites and may have difficulty with edema in the legs from removal of lymph nodes. A new vagina may be surgically constructed and if desired, a woman can resume a satisfactory sex life (ACS, 2015b; NCCN, 2015b).

Pharmacologic Treatment

A gynecologic oncologist will review several options, including participation in clinical trials, for women with locally advanced and advanced stages of cervical cancer (ACS, 2015b; NCCN, 2015b). Adding chemotherapy as an adjunct has been shown to boost positive response to radiation. The use of platinum compounds is standard treatment, followed by plant alkaloids and topoisomerase inhibitors. Adding bevacizumab—a monoclonal antibody that inhibits angiogenesis and slows the growth of new blood vessels supplying cancer cells—appears to increase survival rate by 3.7 months without adversely affecting quality of life (Cella, 2015). First-line single agents include cisplatin, carboplatin, and paclitaxel. First-line combination therapies include cisplatin/paclitaxel/bevacizumab; cisplatin/paclitaxel; topotecan/paclitaxel/bevacizumab; carboplatin/paclitaxel; cisplatin/topotecan; topotecan/paclitaxel; and cisplatin/gemcitabine (NCCN, 2015b).

New and Emerging Evidence for Practice

Screening Tests

Ongoing research into more specific screening tests and monitoring for disease progression is yielding promising results. One area of investigation is testing for the E6 and E7 oncoproteins, which are linked to the cellular transformations of cervical cancer; such studies may lead in the future to more specific cotests for women who are HPV positive (Wan, 2013). Another area of investigation is changes in the levels of microRNA molecules in infected tissues, which might be exploited in monitoring for disease progression (NCI, 2015a). Ongoing work is also seeking to develop low-cost, rapid HPV screening tests for use at home to encourage more women to screen themselves (WHO, 2015).

Already on the market is a cobas HPV DNA test approved by the FDA in April 2014. This test detects 14 high-risk HPV types, including HPV 16 and 18. It has been approved for women 25 and older to use as a primary method to determine the need for any additional testing. Approval was based on the ATHENA trial, which found that among 47,000 women, HPV testing alone was more effective than Pap testing in identifying severe cervical cell carcinoma. This study found that one in seven women with normal cytology results was actually positive for HPV 16 and had CIN 2 or cells indicating the presence of moderate dysplasia (Stoler et al., 2011).

The FDA indicates that women screened with the cobas HPV DNA tests who have positive results for HPV 16 or 18 should have a colposcopy with biopsy, while women who test positive for any of the other HPV high-risk types should have a Pap test to determine the need for colposcopy. Concerns related to this test—specifically, that using cobas HPV DNA testing alone is more expensive than the established and effective Pap testing, that it might lead to unnecessary colposcopies, and that approximately 5% women diagnosed with CIN 3 on Pap tests are negative for HPV—have stalled changes in the current U.S. evidence-based guidelines; these guidelines are currently under review by the ACS (ACS, 2015b; Wan, 2013).

Avoidance of unnecessary treatment is being addressed in current research studies. The

ASCUS-LSIL Triage Study (ALTS) study is trying to identify biomarkers that might predict whether a woman's immune response will effectively clear low-grade cervical lesions. The Study to Understand Cervical Cancer Early Endpoints (SUCCEED) is seeking to elucidate the molecular distinctions that occur throughout each stage of cancer progression so as to identify biomarkers that might assist with management decisions (NCI, 2015a).

Therapeutic Vaccines
Also under ongoing investigation are vaccines for treating established high-grade cervical dysplasia by triggering the immune response. These DNA recombinant vaccines use the HPV 16 E7 antigen and the HPV 16 and HPV 18 E6 and E7 antigens to stimulate an immune response that has been shown to resect cervical tissue (NCI, 2015a).

Pharmacologic Therapy
Researchers continue to study the best doses and combinations of chemotherapeutic agents that are more effective and best tolerated. One area of interest is the use of an antiviral agent, cidofovir, that may sensitize HPV-infected cervical cancer cells to chemoradiation (Harrison, 2014). Another curiosity under study is a nutritional supplement, active hexose correlated compound (AHCC); it is derived from a Japanese mushroom and has shown promise in eradicating persistent HPV infection (Nelson, 2014). Still another area of research is carrageenan, a compound extracted from seaweed and widely used for its gelatin effects in the food industry; it shows promise for inhibiting HPV as a topical microbicide (NIH, 2013).

Patient Education
Immunization rates for HPV continue to hover around 50% despite the fact that vaccinations for this virus have reduced HPV prevalence by 56% in female adolescents since 2006 (CDC, 2015a). Women who have sex with women have even lower vaccination rates (approximately 28.5%), which are attributed in part to myths that HPV cannot be transmitted from female to female (Hunter-Keller, 2015). Sensitive clinicians need to advocate for HPV vaccination through reminder contacts and by dispelling misinformation that vaccination encourages sexual activity or is not safe. Adolescents should receive HPV vaccination

with other routine tetanus–diphtheria–acellular pertussis and meningococcal vaccines, and clinicians need to strongly recommend the vaccine to their young patients' parents for cancer prevention (CDC, 2015a; Schuchat, 2015).

Women who have received the full HPV immunization series need encouragement to continue to comply with screening. Education and reeducation regarding the screening protocols, along with phone or letter reminders, are important to integrate into practice.

When discussing an abnormal Pap test with women, clinicians need to be aware that precancerous lesions are often associated with a diagnosis of cancer. Clarifying misperceptions and education regarding the treatment protocols for early lesions can alleviate stress.

Finally, clinicians need to educate women on the association between HPV infection and cervical cancer and review STI prevention strategies and safe sex practices. Young women need to understand the importance of delaying the risk of HPV exposure through delaying the onset of sexual activity, decreasing the number of sexual partners, using condoms to decrease risk, and eliminating use of tobacco products.

Special Considerations
Disparities in Screening
Studies have found that women who are from minority groups, have less than a high school education, are of lower social economic status, and are single are at higher risk for not seeking screening (Chen, Kessler, Mori, & Chauhan, 2012; Lee, Yang, Lee, & Ghebre, 2015). Providing cervical cancer literacy education to high-risk groups is essential to eliminating these disparities.

Treatment During Pregnancy
Cervical cancer is the most common gynecologic malignancy during pregnancy. Fortunately most women are diagnosed in stage I. No treatment is warranted for preinvasive lesions of the cervix during pregnancy, although expert colposcopy is recommended to exclude the possibility of invasive cervical cancer. Treatment of invasive cervical cancer depends on the stage of the cancer and the gestational age at diagnosis. When the cancer is diagnosed before fetal maturity, the traditional

approach is to recommend immediate therapy appropriate for the stage of disease. Other reports suggest that if the cancer is in the early stages, delaying therapy may be a reasonable option to allow for improved fetal viability (NCI, 2015a; NCCN, 2015b). Most experts advocate a cesarean birth at fetal viability with concurrent radical hysterectomy and pelvic node dissection (NCCN, 2015b). Management of cervical cancer during pregnancy is a complex dilemma and requires a multidisciplinary approach.

ENDOMETRIAL CANCER

Description of the Problem

The majority of cancers affecting the uterine corpus are adenocarcinomas affecting the endometrium (NCI, 2015d). Carcinoma of the endometrium is the most prevalent gynecologic malignancy and the fourth most common malignant neoplasm in women in the United States, after breast, lung, and colon cancers (ACS, 2015a). Globally, endometrial cancer ranks as the sixth most common malignancy, with approximately 290,000 new cases diagnosed annually (Amant, Mirza, Koskas, & Creutzberg, 2015). Interestingly, the incidence of endometrial cancer is greater in high-resource countries than in low-resource countries (Amant et al., 2015), although the risk of dying from endometrial cancer is greater in the latter. It is theorized that the increased incidence observed in high-resource countries is due to the larger number of women who are obese and physically inactive in such areas. Both obesity and physical inactivity are risk factors for endometrial cancer (Amant et al., 2015).

Approximately 54,870 new cases of endometrial cancer and 10,170 deaths from endometrial cancer were estimated to occur in 2015 in the United States (Amant et al., 2015; ACS, 2015a). From 2007 to 2011, the incident rate of this disease increased by 2.4% per year and the death rate increased by 1.9% per year. The incidence of endometrial cancer is higher in white women than in black women, but the mortality rate in black women is nearly twice as high as that in white women. A major factor explaining the increased mortality rate in black women is the significant occurrence of higher-grade and more aggressive histologies in this population (NCI, 2015d). Whereas the rates of new cases in white women have been stable since 1992, the rates in black women have risen over the same period (ACS, 2015a).

When endometrial cancer is diagnosed, an estimated 68% of tumors will be diagnosed in the localized stage, 20% in the regional stage, and 8% in the metastasized stage. Survival rates are based on staging, with a 95% survival rate being associated with localized tumors, a 67% rate with regional tumor, and a 16% rate with distant spread. The overall all-stage survival rate is 82% (Siegel, Naishadham, & Jemal, 2013). The average age of diagnosis in the United States is 63 years (American College of Obstetricians and Gynecologists, 2015a). Interestingly, the most common cause of death among women diagnosed with endometrial cancer is cardiovascular disease. This outcome most likely reflects the high probability of curative treatment for endometrial cancer, as well as the prevalence of cardiac disease (NCI, 2015d; Ward et al., 2012).

Etiology and Pathophysiology

Endometrial cancer is sometimes classified into two types. Type I, or estrogen-dependent endometrial cancer, is the most common and is diagnosed in more than 75% of cases. It is caused by an excess of endogenous or exogenous estrogen, unopposed by progesterone. Long-term unopposed estrogen exposure allows for continued endometrial growth as well as the development of hyperplasia with or without atypia. The resulting tumors are usually low grade and have a favorable prognosis. Histologic types include endometrioid adenocarcinomas (most cases); adenosquamous tumors, which contain elements of both glandular and squamous epithelium; and other rare variants such as ciliated carcinoma. These types of well-differentiated tumors usually limit their spread to the surface of the endometrium (ACS, 2015g; American College of Obstetricians and Gynecologists, 2015a; NCI, 2015d).

Type II endometrial cancer accounts for approximately 10% of cases and was traditionally thought to be estrogen independent, as the endometrium is generally atrophic or has polyps with this type of disease. The current thought is that estrogen may play some role in polyps' development, although the extent of this association has not been determined (ACS, 2015g; Setiawan et al., 2013). These neoplasms consist of poorly differentiated prognostic cell types (such as papillary serous or clear cell tumors), often present as higher-grade tumors, and are more aggressive (ACS, 2015g; American College of Obstetricians and Gynecologists, 2015a; NCI, 2015d). Approximately 4% of type II cancers are uterine carcinosarcomas (CS), also known as malignant mixed mesodermal tumors or malignant mixed Müllerian tumors, which have characteristics of both sarcomas and endometrial carcinomas (ACS, 2015g).

Endometrial carcinoma has been linked to a genetic predisposition to develop this disease. As many as 10% of the cases occur in women diagnosed prior to age 50 years who have the autosomal dominant syndrome known as Lynch syndrome (also called hereditary nonpolyposis colorectal cancer). Lynch syndrome manifests as heritable mutations in a germline typically affecting mismatch repair genes—*MLH1, MAH1, PMA1,* or *MSH6* (American College of Obstetricians and Gynecologists, 2015a). This disorder is also associated with an increased risk of developing colon and ovarian cancer and carries up to a 61% risk of developing endometrial cancer by age 70 years, with most cases appearing by age 50.

Cowden disease (also known as multiple hamartoma syndrome) is another autosomal dominant disorder that involves germline mutations of the tumor suppressing the phosphatase and tensin homolog (*PTEN*) gene and is associated with increased risk for endometrial, breast, and thyroid cancer. In addition, speculation about the role of genetic mutations in the *BRCA* genes in familial endometrial cancer continues, although it is unknown whether the mutation itself or prophylactic treatment for the mutation (tamoxifen) increases risk (American College of Obstetricians and Gynecologists, 2015a).

While the exact cause of endometrial cancer is unknown, the current understanding of risk factors helps to identify women at risk for type I endometrial cancer due to estrogen excess. Risk factors associated with exogenous sources of estrogen include the following:

- *Estrogen therapy (ET).* For women with a uterus, the risk of endometrial cancer

associated with unopposed estrogen use for 5 or more years is 20-fold higher compared with the risk in women not taking ET. Adding progestogen therapy continuously or for at least 10 days per month significantly mitigates this risk (American College of Obstetricians and Gynecologists, 2015a; Karageorgi, Hankinson, Kraft, & De Vivo, 2010; NCI, 2015d). Guidelines from American College of Obstetricians and Gynecologists continue to advise clinicians to limit ET use for menopausal symptoms to the lowest effective dose and shortest duration. Treatment decisions need to be individualized according to severity of symptom complaints and an analysis of risk versus benefit regardless of age (American College of Obstetricians and Gynecologists, 2015b).

- *Tamoxifen.* Tamoxifen (Nolvadex), when used for chemoprevention of breast cancer, increases the risk of endometrial cancer nearly fourfold for women 50 years and older (American College of Obstetricians and Gynecologists, 2015a). A selective estrogen receptor modulator (SERM), tamoxifen has site-specific activity in different tissues. It suppresses growth in breast tissue, but stimulates the growth of the endometrial lining (American College of Obstetricians and Gynecologists, 2015a; NCI, 2015d). Raloxifene, another SERM, has not been associated as a risk factor for endometrial cancer. The potential risk of using ospemifene, a SERM approved for treatment of dyspareunia, needs further postmarket assessment (American College of Obstetricians and Gynecologists, 2015a).

Risk factors *associated* with endogenous sources of estrogen include the following:

- *Early menarche.* Starting menstruation before the age of 12 years increases the number of years during which the endometrium is exposed to estrogen (American College of Obstetricians and Gynecologists, 2015a; Karageorgi et al., 2010; NCI, 2015d).
- *Late menopause.* Menopause occurring after the age of 52 increases the duration of estrogen exposure (American College of Obstetricians and Gynecologists, 2015a; Karageorgi et al., 2010; NCI, 2015d).

- *History of infertility or nulliparity.* During pregnancy, the hormonal balance shifts toward more progesterone, which protects the uterine lining (endometrium). Progesterone seems to expedite removal of premalignant cells, and pregnancy creates a protective immunity-mediated effect (American College of Obstetricians and Gynecologists, 2015a). As a consequence, women who have had many pregnancies have a reduced risk of developing endometrial cancer, whereas women who are infertile or who have never been pregnant have an increased risk (American College of Obstetricians and Gynecologists, 2015a; Karageorgi et al., 2010; NCI, 2015d). Late age for a last pregnancy (40 years or older) also has a protective effect by further decreasing estrogen exposure just prior to menopause (Karageorgi et al., 2010).
- *Obesity.* The majority of women who develop endometrial cancer tend to be obese. There is a 200% to 400% linear increase in risk for women who have a body mass index (BMI) greater than 25. This risk increases even further with a BMI greater than 27. Women who are young and diagnosed with endometrial cancer are very likely to be obese, be nulliparous, and have type I well-differentiated histology (American College of Obstetricians and Gynecologists, 2015a). Women who are obese have higher levels of endogenous estrogen as a result of the conversion of androstenedione to estrone and the aromatization of androgens to estradiol—both processes that occur in peripheral adipose tissue (ACS, 2015g; American College of Obstetricians and Gynecologists, 2015a; NCI, 2015d).
- *Chronic anovulation.* Anovulation is a common cause of infertility and may be attributable to several factors. One of the leading causes of chronic anovulation is polycystic ovary syndrome (PCOS; see Chapter 25). Women with PCOS have excess androgens and elevated luteinizing hormone (LH) and normal or low follicle-stimulating hormone (FSH) levels. They may also have elevated levels of free estrogen, owing to the peripheral conversion of androgens to estrogens and the decreased production of sex hormone–binding globulin (SHBG) in the liver, which serves to increase

the unopposed effects of estrogen over time (ACS, 2015g; Marrinan, 2007).
- *Diabetes.* Type 2 diabetes mellitus and hypertension have been associated with obesity and up to a threefold increased risk for endometrial cancer. Women who are not overweight and have diabetes also have an increased risk of endometrial cancer (ACS, 2015g; American College of Obstetricians and Gynecologists, 2015a).
- *High-fat diet.* Consumption of a high-fat diet may lead to obesity, and obesity is a well-documented risk factor for endometrial cancer. Some researchers believe that fatty foods may also have a direct effect on estrogen metabolism, thereby increasing the risk for endometrial cancer (ACS, 2015g).
- *Ovarian cancer.* Certain ovarian tumors, such as granulosa theca cell tumors, produce estrogen, thereby increasing a woman's risk of developing endometrial cancer (ACS, 2015g).

Other risk factors for endometrial cancer include increased age, smoking (for type II cancers), sedentary lifestyle, history of pelvic radiation to treat another cancer, and endometrial hyperplasia.

Clinical Presentation

Endometrial cancer occurs most frequently in women who are postmenopausal. The average age at diagnosis is approximately 63 years, with 15% of woman being diagnosed before age 50 and 5% before age 40 (American College of Obstetricians and Gynecologists, 2015a). Younger women usually have specific risk factors such as morbid obesity, chronic anovulation, and heredity syndromes. The most common symptom—present in 90% of women—is abnormal uterine bleeding. In women who are menstruating, this symptom can take the form of bleeding between periods or excessive, prolonged menstrual flow. In women who are postmenopausal, any bleeding is considered abnormal and should be evaluated (ACS, 2015g; American College of Obstetricians and Gynecologists, 2015a; NCI, 2015d). Advanced symptoms include pelvic pain, abdominal distention with or without pain, bloating, change in bowel or bladder pattern, and change in appetite (American College of Obstetricians and Gynecologists, 2015a).

Assessment

History

Key pieces of information that assist the clinician in identifying women at high risk for endometrial cancer include the character of the bleeding, the pattern of the flow, and the number of pads used when bleeding occurs. Inquire about accompanying problems (e.g., dyspareunia, pain, bladder or bowel problems); ask the woman if she is experiencing any unusual vaginal discharge or if she has ever been diagnosed with an STI. Obtain a menstrual history and inquire if the woman is taking any hormones. Ask about the possibility of pregnancy and whether she has experienced any symptoms of pregnancy (e.g., missed period, breast tenderness, or nausea and vomiting). If she has previously been pregnant, obtain a pregnancy history in addition to medical and family histories (see Chapter 6). Be sure to ask the woman if she has a personal or family history of breast, ovarian, or colon cancer. Ask her if she has experienced infertility problems or if she has a history of PCOS (NCI, 2015d; Porth, 2015).

Physical Examination

The physical examination should include a thorough abdominal, inguinal lymph node, pelvic, vaginal, and rectal examination. Abnormal bleeding from the genital tract can occur from the vagina, cervix, uterus, or fallopian tubes. Inspect the external genitalia for lesions or atrophic vaginitis, which may be the cause of the bleeding. Perform a vaginal examination to determine whether the bleeding is caused by vaginal or cervical infection. Note the amount, color, consistency, and odor of the vaginal discharge; determine whether the cervix is friable or has an unusual discharge; and examine the patient for cervical polyps.

Perform a bimanual examination. Palpate the cervix, which normally feels smooth, firm, evenly rounded, and mobile. Note any cervical motion tenderness. Next, palpate the uterus, ovaries, and inguinal lymph nodes. Note uterine size and contour. Endometrial cancer seldom causes much uterine enlargement, and any increase in size usually occurs slowly. Uterine fibroids usually feel firm and may make the uterus asymmetrical. Note any enlargement of the ovaries and lymph nodes. Lastly, perform a rectal examination to identify lesions or other abnormalities.

Metastatic spread of endometrial cancer occurs in a characteristic pattern, commonly to the pelvic and para-aortic nodes. Common sites for distant metastasis include the lungs, inguinal and supraclavicular lymph nodes, liver, bones, brain, and vagina (ACS, 2015g; Dunphy, Winland-Brown, Porter, & Thomas, 2015).

Diagnostic Testing

There is no screening test currently available to detect endometrial cancer. In particular, a Pap test is not effective in detecting endometrial cancer. Nevertheless, the finding of atypical glandular cells in a postmenopausal woman is suggestive of uterine malignancy and requires further investigation as does any postmenopausal bleeding (NCI, 2015d). This follow-up can be done through an endometrial biopsy or transvaginal ultrasonography.

Transvaginal Ultrasound Transvaginal ultrasound is used as an adjunctive means of evaluation for endometrial hyperplasia as well as polyps, myomas, and structural abnormalities of the uterus. An endometrial thickness of 4 mm or less indicates that biopsy can be deferred. As rare cases of type II endometrial cancer present with endometrial thickness of 3 mm or less, ongoing symptoms of bleeding require biopsy. Persistent bleeding in the face of a negative biopsy also requires further investigation. For women who are premenopausal, the value of imaging is questionable, as the measurement of endometrial thickness is irrelevant (American College of Obstetricians and Gynecologists, 2015a). The clinician must make a decision to biopsy based on the clinical presentation and symptoms.

Endometrial Biopsy Endometrial biopsy is an office procedure that is now the primary method for histologic sampling of the endometrium (American College of Obstetricians and Gynecologists, 2015a). The biopsy is obtained through the use of an endometrial suction catheter that is inserted through the cervix into the uterine cavity. Endometrial biopsy detects 80% to 90% of endometrial cancers if an adequate tissue sample is obtained. If the biopsy result fails to provide sufficient diagnostic information or if abnormal bleeding persists, a dilation and curettage (D & C) with a hysteroscopy is recommended (American College of Obstetricians and Gynecologists, 2015a; NCI, 2015d).

Dilation and Curettage Dilation and curettage is the gold standard for assessing uterine bleeding and diagnosing endometrial cancer. If endometrial biopsy findings are inadequate or negative with ongoing symptoms of bleeding, or if the endometrial thickness as assessed by transvaginal ultrasound is greater than 4 mm, or if a high degree of suspicion exists, the patient needs a D & C under anesthesia to exclude malignancy (American College of Obstetricians and Gynecologists, 2015a; NCI, 2015d).

Hysteroscopy Hysteroscopy is used in the office setting to directly visualize the uterine cavity. With this technique, a tiny telescope is introduced through the cervix into the uterus. After filling the uterus with saline, the practitioner can visualize and biopsy suspicious areas. Hysteroscopy is not required in conjunction with the D & C, but is recommended because it provides the best opportunity to examine the endometrium and confirm premalignant endometrial lesions (American College of Obstetricians and Gynecologists, 2015a).

CA-125 Levels Elevated CA-125 levels are associated with some endometrial cancers. Extremely high levels are suggestive of metastasis beyond the uterus. Evaluation of CA-125 is another assessment option for women who are poor surgical candidates (ACS, 2015g).

Referral
Women who are diagnosed with endometrial cancer require surgical staging. Exceptions would be women who are poor surgical candidates who require assessment of potential metastasis sites with imaging (CT, MRI, PET/CT). In any case, decisions made preoperatively are complex and best suited to physicians with advanced expertise in endometrial carcinoma. A referral to a gynecologic oncologist ensures a comprehensive evaluation of the need for preoperative imaging (CT, MRI, PET/CT), extent of comprehensive staging or debulking, and best treatment options (American College of Obstetricians and Gynecologists, 2015a).

Differential Diagnoses

The differential diagnoses for genital bleeding depend on the clinical picture. Bleeding from the lower genital tract can occur from the vagina (carcinoma, lacerations, trauma, infections, or atrophic changes with age) or the cervix (cervicitis, STIs, polyps, or cervical carcinoma). It may also occur from the uterus (carcinoma, fibroids, polyps, pregnancy, or dysfunctional uterine bleeding) or the fallopian tubes (pelvic inflammatory disease [PID], ectopic pregnancy). Women who are on hormone replacement therapy may experience breakthrough bleeding (Creasman, 2014; NCI, 2015d).

Management

Prevention
Although most cases of endometrial cancer cannot be prevented, several factors are associated with a decreased incidence of endometrial cancer:

- *Combined oral contraceptives.* The risk of endometrial hyperplasia is increased by the presence of unopposed estrogen. Thus using a COC instead of an estrogen-only contraceptive prevents the proliferative effect of estrogen, thereby decreasing the risk of developing abnormal endometrial hyperplasia, which might eventually result in endometrial cancer (ACS, 2015g). The chance of developing endometrial cancer due to unopposed estrogen is both risk and duration related, and it remains increased for years after stopping use of unopposed estrogen. These effects are ameliorated by adding progestins in the correct dose and duration (ACS, 2015g; NCI, 2015d). Other measures known to minimize risk include the use of depot medroxyprogesterone acetate and use of a levonorgestrel-releasing IUD (ACS, 2015g).
- *Physical activity.* Studies investigating the relationship between physical activity and the risk of endometrial cancer have shown a weak to moderate inverse relationship between the two (ACS, 2015g; NCI, 2015d). It is believed that physical activity modifies the risk of endometrial cancer by reducing obesity, a known risk factor for endometrial cancer (NCI, 2015d).
- *Low-fat diet.* A number of observational studies have demonstrated that consumption of a diet low in saturated fats and high in fruit and vegetable intake is associated with a reduced risk of developing endometrial cancer (NCI, 2015d).

Controlling Other Risk Factors

Women with PCOS need appropriate treatment to avoid the effect of unopposed estrogen on the uterus. Women who are menopausal and have an intact uterus should avoid using unopposed estrogen to relieve menopausal symptoms. Women with a history of breast or ovarian cancer or hereditary nonpolyposis colorectal cancer (HNPCC; Lynch syndrome) need to be closely monitored for endometrial cancer. The American Cancer Society recommends that women with or at increased risk for HNPCC should be offered annual testing for endometrial cancer with endometrial biopsy beginning at the age of 35 years. These women should also be counseled about preventive measures such as the option of prophylactic hysterectomy with bilateral salpingo-oophorectomy at the completion of childbearing (ACS, 2015g).

Definitive Treatment

The choice of treatment for endometrial cancer depends primarily on the type and stage of the disease, the level of differentiation, the woman's overall health, and her personal preferences (NCCN, 2015c). Treatment options for endometrial cancer include surgery, radiation therapy, chemotherapy, hormonal therapy, and biologic therapy. Chemotherapy may be used in recurrent or advanced cases of endometrial cancer (NCI, 2015d, 2015e). Extensive clinical guidelines for the management of endometrial cancer are available at the NNCN website (2015c).

Surgery Comprehensive surgical staging is achieved through total abdominal hysterectomy with bilateral salpingo-oophorectomy and peritoneal washing for cytology. The preferred extent of pelvic and para-aortic lymphadenectomy is the subject of debate, as some surgeons choose selective lymph node sampling versus full dissection. Studies to date have not fully resolved this issue, but multiple-site sampling has been associated with improved survival rates and complete pelvic and para-aortic lymphadenectomy remains the standard (American College of Obstetricians and Gynecologists, 2015). Patients with localized disease are usually cured with surgery alone. In contrast, patients with myometrial invasion are usually treated with a combination of surgery and adjuvant radiation therapy. Careful staging guides therapy (NCI, 2015d).

Staging FIGO's surgical staging system is used for surgical staging of endometrial cancer (**Table 27-6**) (American College of Obstetricians and Gynecologists, 2015a). Additional pathological findings also guide treatment and prevent overtreatment. Less favorable prognosis findings include hormone receptor status—progesterone receptor site levels greater than 100 are associated with 93% disease-free survival rate at 3 years as opposed to a 36% rate if these levels are less than 100; myometrial invasion; vascular invasion; presence of aneuploidy; oncogene (mutated gene) expression, and the fraction of cells in S-phase—the percentage of cells in a tumor that are in the phase of the cell cycle when DNA is synthesized (NCI, 2015d).

Radiation Therapy Radiation treatments may be given externally (external-beam radiation), via an intracavitary method (brachytherapy), or both. Vaginal brachytherapy has less gastrointestinal (GI) toxicity and is better tolerated by most women (American College of Obstetricians and Gynecologists, 2015a). Diarrhea and fatigue are common side effects of radiation therapy.

Pelvic radiation may also cause vaginal stenosis (narrowing of the vagina from scar tissue), which may make vaginal intercourse painful. The use of a vaginal dilator or having vaginal intercourse several times per week can help prevent scar tissue formation. Use of vaginal lubricants may also be helpful (ACS, 2015g; American College of Obstetricians and Gynecologists, 2015a; NCI, 2015d).

Chemotherapy Chemotherapy has been shown to improve outcomes for women with advanced endometrial cancer. The most common agents used for treatment include paclitaxel, carboplatin, doxorubicin, and cisplatin (ACS, 2015g). The combination of paclitaxel, doxorubicin, and cisplatin has been shown to significantly improve response rates in women with advanced or recurrent endometrial cancer, although neurotoxicity is a significant problem for many patients; paclitaxel in conjunction with carboplatin is less toxic and is an alternative regimen (American College of Obstetricians and Gynecologists, 2015a).

TABLE 27-6	FIGO Staging for Carcinoma of the Corpus Uteri

FIGO Stage	Description
I	Tumor confined to the corpus uteri
IA	Endometrial only or less than 50% invasion through the myometrium
IB	Invasion equal to or more than 50% of the myometrium
II	Growing into the supporting connection tissue of the cervix (stroma)
III	Invasion beyond the uterus and cervix; not in the pelvis
IIIA	Spread to serosa of the corpus uteri and/or fallopian tubes or ovaries (adnexal)
IIIB	Vaginal and/or parametrial involvement
IIIC1	Metastases to pelvic and/or apra-aortic lymph nodes
IIIC2	Spread to pelvic and aorta lymph nodes
IV	Invasion into the bladder or rectum, lymph nodes in groin and/or distant organs
IVA	Invasion into the bladder and/or bowel mucosa and/or distant metastases
IVB	Spread to distant lymph nodes, the upper abdomen, the omentum or organs (bones, lungs)

Abbreviation: FIGO, International Federation of Gynecology and Obstetrics.
Reproduced from Pecorelli, S. (2009). Corrigendum to "Revised FIGO staging for carcinoma of the vulva, cervix, and endometrium."
International Journal of Gynecology and Obstetrics, 105, 103–104. Reprinted with permission from Elsevier.

Hormone Therapy Patients who are not candidates for surgery or radiation, or who have advanced disease and are poor candidates or unwilling to undergo more aggressive treatment, may opt for hormonal therapy (ACS, 2015g; American College of Obstetricians and Gynecologists, 2015a). The hormonal agents most commonly used for this purpose are progestational drugs such as medroxyprogesterone (Provera) and megestrol (Megace). Response to hormones reflects the presence and level of hormone receptors and the degree of tumor differentiation (ACS, 2015g; NCI, 2015d). Other hormone therapy options include tamoxifen and aromatase inhibitors, which block the use of estrogen in fat tissue (ACS, 2015g).

Follow-Up
An important part of the treatment plan is a specific schedule of follow-up visits after surgery, chemotherapy, or radiation therapy. Follow-up visits are scheduled every 3 to 6 months during the first 2 years, then every 6 months for 3 years, and then annually (American College of Obstetricians and Gynecologists, 2015a). Most endometrial cancer recurrences are found within the first 3 years (ACS, 2015g).

An examination of the abdomen and inguinal lymph nodes, along with speculum and rectovaginal examinations, should be done at each follow-up visit. History questions should focus on symptoms that might indicate cancer recurrence, because most recurrences are discovered during evaluation of symptomatic patients. If the patient's symptoms or physical examination results suggest recurrent cancer, imaging tests such as a CT scan, ultrasound, CA-125 blood test, or biopsies should be ordered. Conversely, if no symptoms or physical examination abnormalities are identified, routine blood tests and imaging tests are not recommended (American College of Obstetricians and Gynecologists, 2015a). Practitioners need to keep in mind that the greatest risk of death in endometrial cancer survivors is associated with noncancer causes, so it is very important to encourage women to consume a healthy diet and adopt healthy lifestyle behaviors.

Emerging Evidence That May Change Management

Women with advanced or recurrent endometrial cancer, in particular, need to consider enrollment in a clinical trial. Multiple trials, with enrollment depending on staging, are examining different chemotherapeutic regimens and use of biologic agents (e.g., bevacizumab, temsirolimus) either as solo therapies or as adjuncts to chemotherapy (ACS, 2015g). Research is ongoing to find the least toxic, most effective therapeutic regimens.

Patient Education

Women need to be educated on the early symptoms of endometrial cancer and encouraged to report any postmenopausal bleeding promptly. Young women need to understand the relationship between high BMI and the risk for endometrial cancer. Clinicians need to keep in mind that most endometrial cancer survivors die due to noncancer causes (ACS, 2015g; NCI, 2015d). Encouraging weight loss and healthy diet and lifestyle behaviors is a crucial aspect of patient management.

Special Considerations

Women of childbearing age may be devastated at the loss of fertility upon receiving a diagnosis of endometrial cancer. Although there are limited data on this issue, some woman are candidates for more conservative, fertility-sparing treatment options. Women who have grade 1, well-differentiated endometrioid endometrial carcinoma without myometrial invasion or metastasis may want to discuss these options with a specialist. After careful evaluation and consideration of the risk, these woman may choose a hormonal treatment with a progestin or a gonadotropin-releasing hormone agonist (ACS, 2015g; American College of Obstetricians and Gynecologists, 2015a). Most experts continue to recommend surgical management immediately following completion of childbearing.

Other women might be interested in ovarian preservation, which is not traditionally recommended at the time of hysterectomy. The ovaries are potential sites for occult metastatic disease—a variant estimated to occur in 19% of women who are premenopausal at time of diagnosis with endometrial cancer—and the ongoing production of estrogen is a risk factor for reoccurrence (American College of Obstetricians and Gynecologists, 2015a). Once again, women need to have a conversation with a specialist to make informed treatment decisions regarding the potential for ovarian preservation.

Finally, women who are premenopausal require evaluation for quality of life issues following surgical treatment for early-stage endometrial cancer. New evidence suggests that estrogen therapy to treat menopausal symptoms might be a viable option for these women despite the conventional wisdom that exogenous estrogen is a potential risk factor for reoccurrence (American College of Obstetricians and Gynecologists, 2015a). A trial involving 1,236 women indicated no significant difference in reoccurrence rates between women receiving estrogen and those receiving a placebo (American College of Obstetricians and Gynecologists, 2015a). Although the trial closed early, the American College of Obstetricians and Gynecologists has determined that estrogen therapy to manage menopausal symptoms is a reasonable option given appropriate counseling and monitoring.

OVARIAN CANCER

Description of the Problem

Ovarian cancer has the highest mortality rate of all gynecologic cancers and is the fifth leading cause of all cancer deaths among women (Moyer & U.S. Preventive Services Task Force [USPSTF], 2012; NCI, 2015c). According to ACS (2015e) estimates, approximately 21,290 new cases of ovarian cancer were diagnosed and 14,180 women died of ovarian cancer in the United States during 2015.

Advancing age is a significant risk factor in the development of ovarian cancer, with the risk increasing at menopause and continuing into a woman's 80s (Cramer, 2012). The average age of women in the United States who are diagnosed with ovarian cancer is 63 years (ACS, 2015c; NCI, 2015c), although primary diagnoses of ovarian cancer occur most commonly in women who are 40 to 75 years of age (Hollier & Hensley, 2011).

Worldwide, ovarian cancer is the most lethal gynecologic cancer in developed countries, with more women dying from ovarian cancer than from cervical and endometrial cancer combined (American College of Obstetricians and Gynecologists, 2011b). Ovarian cancer is observed more often in industrialized and Northern European populations (Cramer, 2012). African American women have a lower lifetime risk of ovarian cancer than Caucasian women, but the 5-year survival rates are similar in both groups (ACS, 2015a).

Ovarian cancer is commonly diagnosed in late stages primarily because of its vague early symptoms and lack of reliable screening methods. The prognosis for most women with ovarian cancer remains poor: Survival rates have improved only slightly with advances in surgery and chemotherapy in the past 50 years (American College of Obstetricians and Gynecologists, 2011b; Falconer, Yin, Grönberg, & Altman, 2015; Kurman & Shih, 2011; Marcus, Maxwell, Darcy, Hamilton, & McGuire, 2014). If the disease is confined to the ovary (stage I) at the time of diagnosis, 5-year survival rates approach 95%; however, only 15% of women have localized disease at the time of their diagnosis, and women initially diagnosed with stage IV ovarian cancer have a 5-year survival rate of just 17% (ACS, 2015c; American College of Obstetricians and Gynecologists, 2011b). Overall, the 5-year survival rate for ovarian cancer is 44% (Marcus et al., 2014). Clinical and technological advances in early detection are urgently needed to decrease the morbidity and mortality associated with this disease.

Etiology and Pathophysiology

Four broad categories of ovarian tumors have been identified. Epithelial ovarian carcinomas are the most common type of ovarian cancer, accounting for approximately 80% to 90% of diagnoses. Germ cell tumors represent 20% to 25% of ovarian tumors, but only 2% to 3% of these are malignant. Stromal cell tumors arise from the supporting tissues of the ova and ovary; they are less common, accounting for 5% to 8% of ovarian neoplasms. Lastly, metastatic neoplasms, most commonly originating in the gastrointestinal tract, may invade ovarian tissue (Cramer, 2012; Dunphy et al., 2015; Zeppernick, Mainhold-Heerlein, & Shih, 2014).

Epithelial ovarian cancer arises from the single-thickness epithelial tissue that covers the surface of the ovary. This tissue closely resembles the epithelium of the female reproductive tract and peritoneum. Epithelial ovarian cancer is now grouped into two categories: types I and II.

Type I tumors include low-grade serous, endometrioid, mucinous or clear cell carcinomas. They usually are large cystic masses confined to one ovary, and are thought to develop from benign lesions that progress to atypia and finally to low-grade invasive disease. Type I tumors rarely have *p53* mutations and are relatively stable from a genetic standpoint. Epithelial tumors of low-malignancy potential (borderline ovarian carcinoma) are usually found in younger women and are often confined to the ovary at diagnosis (Berliner, Fay, Cummings, Burnett, & Tillmanns, 2013; Dunphy et al., 2015; Kurman & Shih, 2011; Zeppernick et al., 2014).

Type II tumors include high-grade serous and endometrioid carcinomas. They are aggressive and usually present as advanced disease. Genetically, mutation of the *p53* tumor suppressor gene is common. This type of ovarian cancer is also linked with mutations of the tumor suppressor genes *BRCA1* and *BRCA2*, which are involved in the cellular response to DNA damage (Berliner et al., 2013; Dunphy et al., 2015; Kurman & Shih, 2011; Zeppernick et al., 2014).

As the ovary enlarges with tumor growth, cells from the surface of the ovary are shed into the peritoneal cavity, where they may become implanted on the peritoneal surface, omentum, bowel, or bladder. Invasive spread to the regional ileac, inguinal, para-aortic, and pelvic lymph nodes may occur, and diaphragmatic and liver surface involvement is common (AJCC, 2016; NCI, 2015c). Approximately 9% of women who appear to have stage I ovarian cancer already have lymph node metastasis. Lymph node involvement is found in the majority of women who undergo node dissection and is present in 78% of advanced cases (NCI, 2015c). A finding of ascites is also common, with this fluid buildup occurring because of increased inflammation in response to metastatic cancer deposits on the peritoneum (Lanceley et al., 2011; Prat & FIGO Committee on Gynecologic Oncology, 2014).

Risk Factors

The most important risk factor for ovarian cancer is a family history in a first-degree relative. Approximately 10% to 20% of ovarian cancers have hereditary causes. Women who have two or more first- or second-degree relatives who have been diagnosed with ovarian cancer are at the highest risk of developing ovarian cancer. Gene mutations associated with the development of cancer are also more common in families that have a history of ovarian or breast cancers before the age of 50 years, in families that have a history of male breast cancer, and in specific high-risk populations such as those of Northern European or Ashkenazi Jewish descent (Berliner et al., 2013; Moyer & USPSTF, 2012; NCI, 2015c).When a woman carries the *BRCA1* or *BRCA2* genetic mutation, her risk for hereditary ovarian cancer is increased; she is also at significantly increased risk for developing breast cancer.

Women with a *BRCA1* gene mutation have an increased risk of ovarian cancer of 39% by age 70 years. For women with a *BRCA2* mutation, the ovarian cancer risk increases to 10% to 17% by age 70 years. Ovarian cancers involving *BRCA* mutations are more likely to be type II, higher grade, and at an advanced stage at the time of diagnosis (Berliner et al., 2013; Moyer & USPSTF, 2014).

Age is also a significant risk factor in the development of ovarian cancer. The risk of ovarian cancer increases with age, and half of all ovarian cancers are diagnosed in women older than the age of 63 (ACS, 2015c; NCCN, 2015a).

The risk of ovarian cancer has been linked to the number of ovulations that a woman experiences in her lifetime. Mutations seen in ovarian cancer cells are associated with the repeated injury and repair of the ovarian epithelium that occurs with ovulation (Cramer, 2012). Furthermore, cyclic hormonal stimulation by estrogen is cited as a factor in the malignant transformation to ovarian cancer (Cramer, 2012). These theories correlate the risk of ovarian cancer with reproductive factors. Women who have never been pregnant have a slightly higher risk of developing ovarian cancer than women who have gone through at least one full-term pregnancy, especially if the pregnancy was carried to term before age 26 years (ACS, 2015c; NCCN, 2015a). Short or irregular menstrual cycles and late age at menopause are also associated with increased risk of ovarian cancer. Menopausal hormone use confers a higher risk largely related to the use of estrogen-only medications (i.e., medications that are unopposed by progestin) (Cramer, 2012). Conversely, risk decreases in women who have used oral contraceptives to suppress ovulation or who have had a greater number of pregnancies (Cramer, 2012; Dunphy et al., 2015; Zeppernick et al., 2014). Breastfeeding is also believed to decrease the risk of ovarian cancer, most likely because of the suppression of pituitary gonadotropins and ovarian production of estradiol that occurs during lactation (Feng, Chen, & Shen, 2014).

A history of hysterectomy, tubal ligation, or previous salpingectomy is associated with a decreased risk of ovarian cancer (Falconer et al., 2015; Zeppernick et al., 2014), and tubal ligation may reduce the risk of ovarian cancer by approximately 60% (ACS, 2015c). Although the mechanism for decreased risk is considered unknown, important new research indicates that neoplastic cells originating in the uterus or fallopian tubes are shed through the tubal fimbriae and incorporate themselves on the ovarian surface, where they then develop into ovarian malignancy. It has been proposed that this process is the actual origin of most epithelial ovarian cancers; if so, it explains the decreased risk of ovarian cancer associated with tubal removal (Kurman & Shih, 2011; Zeppernick et al., 2014).

Women with a history of Lynch syndrome have an increased risk of developing both endometrial and ovarian cancer (ACS, 2015c; Cramer, 2012; Lanceley et al., 2011; Moyer & USPSTF, 2012). This syndrome is associated with several inherited genetic mutations that reduce the cells' ability to repair errors in DNA during replication. For a woman with Lynch syndrome, the risk of developing ovarian cancer by age 70 is 10% to 12% (ACS, 2015c; Lanceley et al., 2011).

Other risk factors associated with ovarian cancer include obesity, use of talcum powder, and smoking. Women who have a BMI greater than 30 have a higher risk of developing ovarian cancer (ACS, 2015c; Cramer, 2012). The use of talcum powder has been suggested as a possible risk factor in the development of ovarian cancer, although research results regarding the use of talcum powder as a risk factor are mixed. Some studies have shown as much as a 40% increase in the risk of ovarian cancer with the use of talcum powder, yet a large prospective study recently found no increase in ovarian cancer risk associated with duration of talcum powder use, area of application, or ovarian cancer type (Houghton et al., 2014). Although smoking does not increase an overall risk for ovarian cancer, it is linked to an increased risk for the mucinous type of ovarian cancer (ACS, 2015c).

Women who have used fertility drugs have also been suggested to be at an increased risk for ovarian cancer. The use of the fertility drug clomiphene citrate (Clomid) may increase the risk of type I ovarian tumors. According to the ACS (2015c), the magnitude of the increased risk appears to be greater in women who did not get pregnant while taking the drug. It is unknown how this finding is related to the ovarian cancer risks of nulliparity, not carrying a pregnancy to term, and lack of oral contraceptive use (ACS, 2015c).

Clinical Presentation

The majority of cases of ovarian cancer are diagnosed when the disease has already reached an advanced stage. Often referred to as a "silent disease," ovarian cancer is associated with vague symptoms that offer only subtle signs of its presence, such as abdominal bloating and discomfort, difficulty eating, and early satiety—all of which can be caused by many factors. Clinicians should suspect ovarian cancer particularly in women older

than age 50 who present with persistent or progressive symptoms (American College of Obstetricians and Gynecologists, 2011b; Dunphy et al., 2015; Lanceley et al., 2011; NCCN, 2015a). Additional symptoms that may or may not accompany ovarian cancer include back pain, changes in bowel or bladder function (e.g., constipation or diarrhea, and a sensation of urinary frequency, pressure, or urge). Signs of advanced disease include a sense of pelvic pressure or discomfort, anorexia, nausea or vomiting, ascites, vaginal bleeding, painful intercourse, an abdominal mass, or unexplained weight loss (ACS, 2015c; Dunphy et al., 2015). **Table 27-7** identifies the early and late symptoms that may occur with ovarian cancer.

Assessment

History and Physical Examination

It is important for the clinician to remember that detection of early-stage ovarian cancer results in improved survival (American College of Obstetricians and Gynecologists, 2011b). Most women present to their clinician with at least one early symptom of ovarian cancer within the year prior to diagnosis (Lanceley et al., 2011; Moyer & USPSTF, 2012). The clinician should seek clarification of any report of persistent abdominal bloating, pelvic or abdominal pain, difficulty eating, or quickly feeling full, as a woman's description of symptoms may be

TABLE 27-7	Clinical Presentation of Ovarian Cancer

Early Symptoms	Later Symptoms
Abdominal bloating/discomfort	Ascites
Early satiety	Anorexia
Indigestion	Nausea or vomiting
Fatigue/weakness	Palpable abdominal or pelvic mass
Vague abdominal pain/painful areas in abdomen on palpation	Distinct abdominal pain
Urinary frequency, pressure, or urge	Vaginal bleeding
Diarrhea or constipation	Painful intercourse
Unexplained weight loss	Unexplained weight loss
	Jaundice
	Back pain
	Pleural effusion

disregarded or attributed to normal processes such as menopause or aging (Lanceley et al., 2011). Additional history questions may include a detailed description of the woman's family history of cancer; surgical and obstetric history; dietary, bowel, and bladder habits; and menstrual history (Dunphy et al., 2015).

Women with *BRCA1* and *BRCA2* mutations and those with a family history of breast, ovarian or hereditary nonpolyposis colon cancer (Lynch syndrome) are at increased risk for ovarian cancer and should be considered candidates for genetic counseling to further evaluate their risk (Moyer & USPSTF, 2014). The clinician should explain why genetic testing is being offered, how the results relate to cancer risk, and which medical management options may be offered based on the results (Berliner et al., 2013). Genetic cancer risk assessment may create anxiety in women, as women identified as having genetic mutations may have to make difficult decisions about managing their risks. They may have to contend with reactions of family members, decisions regarding reproduction, and fear of disclosure of information (Berliner et al., 2013). For women identified as being at high risk of ovarian cancer, screening for genetic mutations should be offered starting at age 18 years, and a family history of cancer should be reviewed every 5 to 10 years (Moyer & USPSTF, 2014).

If an ovarian malignancy is suspected, a bimanual pelvic examination to palpate for tumors is indicated (American College of Obstetricians and Gynecologists, 2011b). If palpated, malignant tumors may be large, nodular, and characterized by decreased mobility (Dunphy et al., 2015). A palpable pelvic mass in a woman who is postmenopausal is always considered abnormal and should be evaluated further. If a tumor is detected with palpation, it almost always indicates advanced disease.

Diagnostic Testing

Routine population-based screening for ovarian cancer is not recommended (Moyer & USPSTF, 2012). Neither pelvic examination, nor tumor-associated antigen CA-125, nor transvaginal ultrasound is considered sufficiently sensitive or specific enough to be recommended for screening asymptomatic women for this disease. Palpation of the ovaries during pelvic examination has

not proved useful in identifying ovarian cancer in women who are premenopausal. Routine screening with transvaginal ultrasound or serum CA-125 has not been shown to decrease the number of deaths from ovarian cancer (American College of Obstetricians and Gynecologists, 2011b; Moyer & USPSTF, 2012; NCI, 2015c), and these measures have resulted in false-positive results and major surgical interventions in women who do not have cancer (Moyer & USPSTF, 2012; NCI, 2015c). Screening recommendations from Moyer and the U.S. Preventive Services Task Force (2014) do state that women who have a strong family history of breast, ovarian, or tubal cancer should be screened for *BRCA1* and *BRCA2* gene mutations. In contrast, routine genetic screening is not recommended for women whose family history does not indicate increased risk for *BRCA1* or *BRCA2* mutations (Moyer & USPSTF, 2014).

CA-125 is a tumor-associated antigen (glycoprotein) that has been used to monitor the clinical status of patients with ovarian cancer. It is found in 69% to 88% of ovarian cancers depending on tumor type and stage. The clinician must consider the cost-effectiveness and the psychological benefits and drawbacks of using this diagnostic test for ovarian cancer because of the variations in interpretation of results and the lack of evidence on its overall effect on survival (Marcus et al., 2014). The CA-125 level is elevated in only 50% of stage I tumors; consequently, its measurement has limited use in early detection because diagnosis during stage I disease is an important determinant of survival (Marcus et al., 2014). Elevation of CA-125 level (greater than 35 units) is not specific for ovarian cancer; indeed, this level may be elevated in women with endometriosis, other nongynecologic malignancies, PID, fibroids, and menstruation, and during the first trimester of pregnancy. An extremely high CA-125 level may assist in the evaluation of premenopausal women who present with signs and symptoms of ovarian cancer, and it may suggest whether further definitive testing is needed (American College of Obstetricians and Gynecologists, 2011b; Lanceley et al., 2011). For women who are postmenopausal and who have a pelvic mass, the CA-125 measurement may be helpful in predicting a higher likelihood of malignancy, but a normal finding does not preclude lack of disease.

Approximately 50% of stage I tumors and 20% of advanced disease are associated with normal CA-125 values (American College of Obstetricians and Gynecologists, 2011b).

CA-125 measurements can be useful as part of the follow-up of treated patients if the level was obtained and found to be elevated at the time of diagnosis, then was observed to drop significantly after definitive treatment of the ovarian cancer. CA-125 levels that rise to twice the normal limits approximately 3 months before imaging studies are performed reflect recurrence (Marcus et al., 2014).

Imaging studies such as transvaginal ultrasound may be helpful in determining ovarian size and general tumor composition in women with an identified pelvic mass (ACS, 2015c; American College of Obstetricians and Gynecologists, 2011b). Transvaginal ultrasound has value in the determination of advanced ovarian cancer, but its ability to provide accurate detection in the early stage of the disease is poor and as a screening method it does not reduce the number of deaths from ovarian cancer (Moyer & USPSTF, 2012). The finding of a palpable pelvic mass combined with a positive transvaginal ultrasound and elevated CA-125 level may improve the rate of accurate detection, although research is ongoing to determine how use of imaging methods such as transvaginal ultrasound combined with CA-125 measurements affect survival rates of ovarian cancer for both average- and high-risk populations (American College of Obstetricians and Gynecologists, 2011b; Moyer & USPSTF, 2012; NCCN, 2015a).

Further imaging studies such as CT scan or MRI of the abdomen, pelvic ultrasound, intravenous pyelogram, barium enema, or colonoscopy may be considered to determine metastasis. Tumor biopsy is not recommended, as it may cause tumor cells to further disseminate into the peritoneal cavity (ACS, 2015c; Dunphy et al., 2015; NCCN, 2015a).

New developments in the screening for ovarian cancer include a search for biomarkers that can be detected by a simple blood test. For example, a qualitative serum test recently approved by the FDA appears to improve the predictability of ovarian cancer in women with identified adnexal masses. It evaluates five biomarkers: (1) transthyretin, (2) apolipoprotein, (3) ß2 microglobulin, (4) transferrin, and (5) CA-125 II. The clinical utility of this test has not yet been determined (American College of Obstetricians and Gynecologists, 2011b). At this point, the Society of Gynecologic Oncology (SGO), the FDA, the Mayo Clinic, and the NCCN (2015a) do not recommend it for screening of ovarian cancer because serum levels do not increase early enough to detect the disease in its early stages. Continued research and development of reliable screening and early diagnostic methods are urgently needed to improve the survival rates of ovarian cancer.

Differential Diagnoses

Differential diagnoses in the evaluation for ovarian cancer include GI malignancy, uterine fibroid, irritable bowel syndrome, inflammatory bowel disease, ovarian cysts or benign tumors, ectopic pregnancy, tubo-ovarian abscess, endometriosis, and pelvic adhesions (Dunphy et al., 2015; Hollier & Hensley, 2011).

Prevention

Preventive strategies for ovarian cancer are individualized according to a woman's history and reproductive choices. Factors that inhibit ovulation appear to reduce the risk of developing ovarian cancer. For example, use of COCs for 5 or more years reduces the risk of ovarian cancer by as much as 50%, and the protective effect continues for several years following discontinuation of their use (ACS, 2015c). Pregnancy resulting in at least one full-term birth and breastfeeding also reduces ovarian cancer risk (ACS, 2015c; Cramer, 2012; Houghton et al., 2014; NCCN, 2015a). The more times a woman has been pregnant, the lower her risk of ovarian cancer. Tubal ligation, salpingectomy, and hysterectomy without oophorectomy also appear to reduce the risk of ovarian cancer (ACS, 2015c; Cramer, 2012; Falconer et al., 2015; NCCN, 2015a).

Risk-reduction surgeries such as bilateral mastectomy and bilateral salpingo-oophorectomy are often recommended to women who have documented mutations in the *BRCA1* or *BRCA2* gene. These procedures, which appear to reduce the risk of both breast cancer and ovarian cancer, are associated with a 55% reduction in all-cause mortality in carriers of these mutated genes (Moyer & USPSTF, 2014; NCI, 2015c). Patients who choose a risk-reducing bilateral salpingo-oophorectomy continue to have a risk of breast cancer, melanoma, and pancreatic cancer (Berliner et al., 2012), however, and need to continue to be followed. Women considering this option need genetic counseling and testing as well as education regarding the clinical effects of premature menopause so they may make informed decisions.

Management

Referral

When the physical examination, laboratory, and imaging results indicate a pelvic mass suspicious for ovarian cancer, the clinician should refer the patient to a gynecologic oncologist. Indicators for referral include elevated CA-125 levels, presence of ascites, a nodular or fixed pelvic mass, and evidence of abdominal or distant metastasis (American College of Obstetricians and Gynecologists, 2011b).

Operative procedures for ovarian cancer should be done by gynecologic oncologists trained to appropriately stage and debulk tumors. Optimally, treatment should occur in facilities that have large volumes of ovarian cancer cases and that can also offer support services to maximize patient outcomes (American College of Obstetricians and Gynecologists, 2011b; Cliby et al., 2015). Delivery of ovarian cancer care that follows current practice guidelines in facilities that treat larger case volumes can result in improved survival for women with ovarian cancer (Cliby et al., 2015). Referral often offers the woman an opportunity to work with a multidisciplinary cancer team who will develop her cancer treatment plan while taking into account her personal preferences, age, general health, renal function, tumor type, and disease stage (Lanceley et al., 2011).

In women who are premenopausal, infertility and abrupt entry into menopause as a result of surgery and chemotherapy can be devastating. All women who are premenopausal should receive education about childbearing and treatment options prior to surgery and a referral to a fertility specialist before treatment is initiated (Lanceley et al., 2011).

Surgery

Surgical exploration is the first step in ovarian cancer treatment and is required to make a definitive diagnosis of cancer, stage the extent of the disease, and debulk (remove) all of the visible tumor in the abdomen and pelvis (ACS, 2015c; NCCN, 2015a). The initial surgery is usually a staging laparotomy.

A total abdominal hysterectomy, bilateral salpingo-oophorectomy, omentectomy, pelvic and para-aortic lymph node sampling and dissection, scraping of the undersurface of the diaphragm, multiple peritoneal biopsies, and aspiration of ascites for cytology are all part of the standard surgical procedure (ACS, 2015c; Lanceley et al., 2011; NCCN, 2015a). In stage II to IV ovarian cancers, debulking is also performed. The goal of debulking is to leave tumor bulk less than 1 cm in diameter, which is referred to as optimal debulking. Patients whose tumors have been optimally debulked have a better prognosis than those left with larger tumors after surgery (ACS, 2015c; NCCN, 2015a). For women who wish to maintain fertility and those with stage I disease, a less invasive laparoscopy and unilateral salpingo-oophorectomy may be considered (American College of Obstetricians and Gynecologists, 2011b; NCCN, 2015a).

Ovarian cancer is surgically staged, and the FIGO staging system is used to provide important prognostic information that is used to determine treatment options (**Table 27-8**). High-grade epithelial serous carcinoma is the most common type of ovarian cancer and is now thought to arise from precursor lesions in the fallopian tubes. Consequently, ovarian, fallopian, and peritoneal cancers are staged together and treated similarly (NCI, 2015c; Prat & FIGO Committee on Gynecologic Oncology, 2014).

Pharmacologic Management

With the advent of personalized cancer medicine, histopathological diagnosis of ovarian cancer is an important component of successful treatment. Ovarian tumors have distinct molecular characteristics depending on the tumor type, and they respond to chemotherapy differently based on this type (Prat & FIGO Committee on Gynecologic Oncology, 2014). All women diagnosed with ovarian cancer are potential candidates for clinical trials and should be offered participation in them if they meet the selection criteria.

Women with early stage I disease with well-differentiated or moderately well-differentiated histologies require continued observation but no further treatment after surgical staging. They have a 5-year survival rate of greater than 90%, provided they have undergone total abdominal hysterectomy and bilateral salpingo-oophorectomy with

TABLE 27-8	FIGO Staging Classification for Cancer of the Ovary, Fallopian Tube, and Peritoneum

Stage	Characteristics
Stage I	Tumor confined to the ovaries or fallopian tube(s)
Stage II	Tumor involves one or both ovaries or fallopian tubes with pelvic extension (below pelvic brim) or primary peritoneal cancer
Stage III	Tumor involves one or both ovaries or fallopian tubes, or primary peritoneal cancer, with cytologically and histologically confirmed spread to the peritoneum outside the pelvis and/or metastasis to the retroperitoneal lymph nodes. and pelvis; has extended to bowel, peritoneum, or lymph nodes
Stage IV	Distant metastasis excluding peritoneal metastasis

Abbreviation: FIGO, International Federation of Gynecology and Obstetrics.
Reproduced from Prat, J., & FIGO Committee on Gynecologic Oncology. (2014). Staging classification for cancer of the ovary, fallopian tube, and peritoneum. *International Journal of Gynecology and Obstetrics, 124,* 1–5. http://dx.doi.org/10.1016/jigo.2013.10.001. Reprinted with permission from Elsevier.

omentectomy, visualization and biopsy of the undersurface of the diaphragm, pelvic and peritoneal biopsies, and peritoneal washings (NCCN, 2015a).

Stage II to IV disease is treated with a combination of staging and debulking surgery followed by postoperative chemotherapy. Standard combination chemotherapy includes intravenous platinum-based compounds and taxanes, which are given in six cycles over a 6-month period (ACS, 2015c; NCCN, 2015a). The use of intraperitoneal chemotherapy in combination with intravenous chemotherapy has been shown to improve survival in women with advanced disease and those who have had optimal debulking (NCCN, 2015a). Intraperitoneal chemotherapy allows higher doses of chemotherapy to be applied directly to the area of greatest risk of recurrence for ovarian cancer, although women may experience increased neuropathy, abdominal pain, nausea and vomiting, and risk of sepsis with this treatment (ACS, 2015c; Lanceley et al., 2011; NCCN, 2015a). The effectiveness of chemotherapy treatment is assessed at the middle and end of treatment with a CT scan or MRI of the chest, abdomen, and pelvis. A serum CA-125 may be done in patients who had an elevated CA-125 level at the time of diagnosis (Lanceley et al., 2011; NCCN, 2015a). Patients with partial remission or evidence of progression are followed up with second-line approaches such as clinical trials and different combinations and dosing of chemotherapeutic agents (NCCN, 2015a).

Alternative treatment regimens may be given in specific cases of ovarian cancer. Women with bulky stage III or IV cancer, those with distant metastasis, and those who are too weak or ill for major surgery may be offered neoadjuvant therapy, which is typically chemotherapy given to reduce tumor burden prior to staging and debulking surgery (ACS, 2015c). Women with advanced-stage disease who undergo partial tumor debulking may receive three to six cycles of chemotherapy, which is then followed by a second tumor reduction surgery (NCCN, 2015a). The role of total abdominal and pelvic radiation therapy remains controversial as adjuvant treatment and is not included in the 2015 Guidelines for Ovarian Cancer (NCCN, 2015a), although palliative radiation therapy is an option for symptom control in women with recurrent advanced disease.

Emerging Evidence That May Change Management

Research into distinct cancer cell characteristics has led to the development of new molecularly targeted drugs that have lower toxicity than conventional chemotherapy and may positively affect clinical outcomes in ovarian cancer (Banerjee & Kaye, 2013). For example, angiogenesis is the process in which cancer cells develop blood vessels for growth and metastasis. Angiogenesis inhibitors such as the drug bevacizumab inhibit vascular endothelial growth factor (VEGF), the cell mediator that signals angiogenesis in cancer cells. Use of bevacizumab in combination with standard chemotherapy has improved the period of progression-free survival for some ovarian cancer patients (ACS, 2015c; Banerjee & Kaye, 2013). Poly ADP-ribose polymerase (PARP) works in combination with *BRCA* to repair DNA damage in cancer cells. In clinical trials, PARP drugs have been able to assist in hindering the cancer cells' ability to repair DNA and continue to replicate. They have been well tolerated and have demonstrated benefit in the treatment of cancer associated with *BRCA* mutations (Banerjee & Kaye, 2013; Lanceley et al., 2011). Lastly, folate receptors have been found to be overexpressed in some ovarian cancer cells. Research is ongoing to develop folate receptor antagonists that may curtail cancer cell survival related to a decreased nutrient supply (Banerjee & Kaye, 2013).

Recent molecular and genetic studies have led to a paradigm shift in our understanding of ovarian cancer. New evidence indicates that the pathogenesis of epithelial ovarian cancer types I and II starts with precursor tissue originating in the fallopian tube or uterus, which then implants and undergoes carcinogenesis on the ovary. In addition, some ovarian cancers have been linked with endometriosis and retrograde menstruation. This new understanding of ovarian cancer may have important clinical implications for prevention strategies. Salpingectomy without oophorectomy may reduce the incidence of disease while maintaining ovarian function and fertility for women, and it may prove to be a less radical approach to risk reduction for women who are carriers of *BRCA* mutations (Falconer et al., 2015; Kurman & Shih, 2011).

Patient Education

Women with a positive family history of ovarian and breast cancer should be educated on genetic screening and counseled on the cancer risk assessment process, the genetics of cancer, and the risks, benefits, and limitations of genetic screening. Women at such increased risk should also be encouraged to seek evaluation for typical early signs of ovarian cancer such as loss of appetite, early satiety,

abdominal bloating, pain, or urinary symptoms that are either persistent or progressive in nature. While approximately 75% of women have advanced disease when diagnosed with ovarian cancer, the majority report at least one early symptom of ovarian cancer in the year prior to diagnosis (Lanceley et al., 2011; Moyer & USPSTF, 2012). Patient education can assist in earlier detection of the disease.

Factors that positively influence the prognosis for women with a diagnosis of ovarian cancer include diagnosis at a younger age, a lower stage of disease at diagnosis, a well-differentiated tumor, no ascites present, smaller tumor residual volume following debulking surgery, and a cell type other than mucinous or clear cell (NCI, 2015c). Women may benefit from a greater understanding of their prognosis and potential treatment options for ovarian cancer, and are likely to have opinions about the importance of quality of life versus length of life related to treatment (Havrilesky et al., 2014). While many women consider the progression-free interval to be the most important factor in determining their preferred treatment, some women are willing to accept a reduction in the time spent without progression in return for improvements in quality of life, side effects, and convenience (Havrilesky et al., 2014).

Post-Treatment Patient Education and Follow-Up

Because most women have widespread disease at the time of diagnosis, the 10-year survival rate in women with ovarian cancer who are treated with first-line cytoreductive surgery and chemotherapy remains approximately 10% (Marcus et al., 2014). As more effective treatments have become available, increasing numbers of women with advanced disease at diagnosis are surviving longer, and most women are achieving complete remission with initial surgery and chemotherapy. Women with stage III disease whose tumors are optimally debulked now have a median progression-free survival time of approximately 18 months. The majority of women treated for ovarian cancer relapse within 5 years (Marcus et al., 2014).

All women with all stages of ovarian cancer require follow-up after their initial treatment (NCCN, 2015a). Recurrence of disease is identified clinically through physical examination, an evaluation of new or returning symptoms, CA-125 measurements, or imaging (Marcus et al., 2014; NCCN, 2015a). Major metastatic sites include the abdomen and pelvis, pelvic and para-aortic lymph nodes, diaphragm, lungs, liver, serosa, pleura, peritoneum overlying the kidneys, adrenal glands, bladder, and spleen.

Ascites is present in two-thirds of women during the course of their disease. Intestinal obstruction with tumor or adhesions causing extrinsic compression of the bowel can occur in women with ovarian cancer. Obstruction can be either partial or complete, and either acute or chronic. The most common presenting symptom is cramping abdominal pain (Lanceley et al., 2011; Marcus et al., 2014; NCI, 2015c). Pleural effusion and lymphedema are other possible complications of recurrent disease.

The primary goal of follow-up care is the early identification of recurrence in hopes that additional treatment will offer the possibility of disease control. A therapeutic alliance and partnership between clinician and patient improves the likelihood that early, subtle signs of recurrence will be promptly reported and evaluated. Lifelong follow-up will be required at regularly scheduled intervals. Follow-up needs to be coordinated with the primary care provider and the gynecologic oncologist, or medical and radiation oncologists. Patients are usually seen for follow-up every 2 to 4 months for 2 years, then every 4 to 6 months for 3 years, and then annually for 5 years (Marcus et al., 2014).

During each follow-up visit, history taking should include questions about changes in appetite, increase in abdominal size or mass, weight gain or loss, changes in bowel or bladder function, pelvic pain, and leg edema (Marcus et al., 2014; NCCN, 2015a). Physical examination should focus on the breasts, lungs, abdomen, pelvis, and extremities. A rising CA-125 level is highly suggestive of recurrent disease. Nevertheless, it is important to keep in mind that not all ovarian carcinomas are revealed by CA-125 levels; ovarian cancer may recur without a corresponding elevation in CA-125. Options for treatment of recurrent disease include surgical debulking of the gross tumor, additional chemotherapy, and radiation therapy to decrease tumor burden, control symptoms, and improve quality of life (NCCN, 2015a).

The fear of recurrence is always present for a woman who has been treated for ovarian cancer. Periods of remission followed by recurrence and the need for retreatment keep women in an ongoing state of uncertainty and anxiety. Even in women with a good prognosis, the fear of recurrence commonly persists for years after completion of definitive treatment and may surface at some follow-up appointments and not others. All symptoms should be taken seriously by the woman and her clinician, because the initial symptoms of ovarian cancer are subtle, vague, and ill defined. The woman who reports symptoms should be seen promptly, even though the symptoms may be a result of sometimes minor, transient problems such as indigestion or a muscle strain. Each follow-up assessment must always include the consideration of the possibility of recurrent disease as well as the delayed effects of surgery, chemotherapy, and radiation therapy.

Quality of life and the meaning of life itself are important issues for ovarian cancer survivors. When the diagnosis of ovarian cancer is first received, women often feel isolated and wish to avoid others who have the disease, particularly those women whose disease is at an advanced stage. Later, many women diagnosed with ovarian cancer will seek relationships with other women who have the disease so that they can share the lived experience and find emotional support. Many women have difficulty coping with the wish that the cancer had been diagnosed sooner (Guenther, Stiles, & Dimmitt Champion, 2012). Women with ovarian cancer often will take control of their treatment by seeking out alternative and complementary therapies that they will combine with conventional treatment. Some women worry about passing a genetic predisposition for ovarian cancer on to their daughters. Relationships may be reevaluated and personal beliefs about life and death examined, as well as the woman's spirituality.

Loss of fertility and the permanent physical changes that accompany total abdominal hysterectomy and bilateral salpingo-oophorectomy, followed by chemotherapy, add to the stress that the cancer diagnosis places on women's personal relationships. Menopausal symptoms such as hot flashes and vaginal dryness, and the side effects of chemotherapy such as peripheral neuropathy and temporary hair loss, often leave women feeling as though they have lost their femininity and sexuality (Lanceley et al., 2011).

In spite of these negative aspects of the disease and the treatment process, quality of life is moderately high for most women with ovarian cancer. When faced with a bleak prognosis, women with ovarian cancer may restructure their life goals and find new meaning to life (Guenther et al., 2012). These women derive great benefit and support from the presence of consistent, sensitive clinicians who take their symptoms and concerns seriously and provide prompt, thorough follow-up that does not offer any false sense of reassurance or undue sense of alarm.

References

Amant, F., Mizra, M. R., Koskas, M., & Creutzberg, C. (2015). FIGO cancer report 2015: Cancer of the corpus uteri. *International Journal of Gynecology and Obstetrics, 131,* S96–S104.

American Cancer Society (ACS). (2014). Cervical cancer prevention and early detection. Retrieved from http://www.cancer.org/cancer/cervicalcancer/moreinformation/cervicalcancerpreventionandearlydetection/cervical-cancer-prevention-and-early-detection-pdf

American Cancer Society (ACS). (2015a). Cancer facts & figures 2015. Retrieved from http://www.cancer.org/research/cancerfactsstatistics/cancerfactsfigures2015/index

American Cancer Society (ACS). (2015b). Cervical cancer. Retrieved from http://www.cancer.org/cancer/cervicalcancer/detailedguide/cervical-cancer-pdf

American Cancer Society (ACS). (2015c). Detailed guide: Ovarian cancer. Retrieved from http://www.cancer.org/acs/groups/cid/documents/webcontent/003130-pdf.pdf

American Cancer Society (ACS). (2015d) Detailed guide: Vulvar cancer. Retrieved from http://www.cancer.org/cancer/vulvarcancer/detailedguide/index

American Cancer Society (ACS). (2015e). Estimated number of new cancer cases and deaths by sex, US, 2015. Retrieved from http://www.cancer.org/acs/groups/content/@editorial/documents/document/acspc-044514.pdf

American Cancer Society (ACS). (2015f). Treatment options for cervical cancer, by stage. Retrieved from http://www.cancer.org/cancer/cervicalcancer/detailedguide/cervical-cancer-treating-by-stage

American Cancer Society (ACS). (2015g). Endometrial cancer. Retrieved from http://www.cancer.org/cancer/endometrialcancer/index

American Cancer Society (ACS). (2015h). Sexuality for the woman with cancer. Retrieved from http://www.cancer.org/treatment/treatmentsandsideeffects/physicalsideeffects/sexualsideeffectsinwomen/sexualityforthewoman/index

American College of Obstetricians and Gynecologists. (2011a, reaffirmed 2014). Management of vulvar intraepithelial neoplasia (Committee Opinion No. 509). Retrieved from https://www.acog.org/Resources-And-Publications/Committee-Opinions/Committee-on-Gynecologic-Practice/Management-of-Vulvar-Intraepithelial-Neoplasia

American College of Obstetricians and Gynecologists. (2011b). The role of the obstetrician-gynecologist in the early detection of epithelial ovarian cancer (Committee Opinion No. 477). Retrieved from https://www.acog.org/Resources-And-Publications/Committee-Opinions/Committee-on-Gynecologic-Practice/The-Role-of-the-Obstetrician-Gynecologist-in-the-Early-Detection-of-Epithelial-Ovarian-Cancer

American College of Obstetricians and Gynecologists. (2012, reaffirmed 2014). Well–woman visit (Committee Opinion No. 534). Retrieved from http://www.acog.org/Resources-And-Publications/Committee-Opinions/Committee-on-Gynecologic-Practice/Well-Woman-Visit

American College of Obstetricians and Gynecologists. (2015a). Endometrial cancer (Committee Opinion No. 149). Retrieved from http://www.acog.org

American College of Obstetricians and Gynecologists. (2015b). Human papillomavirus vaccination (Committee Opinion No. 641). Retrieved from https://www.acog.org/Resources-And-Publications/Committee-Opinions/Committee-on-Adolescent-Health-Care/Human-Papillomavirus-Vaccination

American Joint Committee on Cancer (AJCC) (2016). Cancer staging references: What is cancer staging? Retrieved from https://cancerstaging.org/references-tools/Pages/What-is-Cancer-Staging.aspx

American Society for Colposcopy and Cervical Pathology (ASCCP). (2013). *Algorithms.* Retrieved from http://www.asccp.org/Assets/51b17a58-7af9-4667-879a-3ff48472d6dc/635912165077730000/asccp-management-guidelines-august-2014-pdf

American Society for Colposcopy and Cervical Pathology (ASCCP). (2014). Updated consensus guidelines for managing abnormal cervical cancer screening tests and cancer precursors. Retrieved from http://www.asccp.org/Assets/405b4550-593f-40a7-ae25-0c783de95b0d/635912114192570000/asccp-updated-guidelines-3-21-13-pdf

Banerjee, S., & Kaye, S. B. (2013). New strategies in the treatment of ovarian cancer: Current clinical perspectives and future potential. *Clinical Cancer Research, 19*(5), 961–966. http://dx.doi.org/10.1158/1078-0432.CCR-12-2243

Barlow, E. L., Hacker, N. F., Hussain, R., & Parmenter, G. (2014). Sexuality and body image following treatment for early-stage vulvar cancer: A qualitative study. *Journal for Advanced Nursing, 70*(8). 1856–1866. http://dx.doi.org/10.1111/jan.12346

Berliner, J. L., Fay, A. M., Cummings, S. A., Burnett, B., & Tillmanns, T. (2013). NSGC Practice guideline: Risk assessment and genetic counseling for hereditary breast and ovarian cancer, *Journal of Genetic Counselors, 22,* 155–163. http://dx.doi.org/10.1007/s10897-012-9647-1

Bermudez, A., Bhatla, N., & Leung, E. (2015). FIGO cancer report 2015: Cancer of the cervix uteri. *International Journal of Gynecology and Obstetrics, 131,* S88–S95.

Bertram, C. (2004). Evidence for practice: Oral contraception and risk of cervical cancer. *Journal of the American Association of Nurse Practitioners, 16*(10), 455–461. Retrieved from http://onlinelibrary.wiley.com/doi/10.1111/jaan.2004.16.issue-10/issuetoc

Binder, P. S., Prat, J., & Mutch, D. G. (2015). FIGO cancer report 2015: The future role of molecular stating in gynecologic cancer. *International Journal of Gynecology and Obstetrics, 131*, S127–S131.

Boardman, C. H., & Matthews, K. J. (2014). Cervical cancer. Retrieved from http://emedicine.medscape.com/article/253513-overview#aw2aab6b2b1aa

Brown, L. (2013). Pathology of the vulva and vagina. In British Association of Gynecological Pathologists, *Essentials of diagnostic gynecological pathology*. Retrieved from http://link.springer.com/chapter/10.1007/978-0-85729-757-0_7/fulltext.html

Carlson, J. A., Rusthoven, C., DeWitt, P. E., Davidson, S. A., Schefter, T. E., & Fisher, C. M. (2014). Are we appropriately selecting therapy for patients with cervical cancer? Longitudinal patterns-of-care analysis for stage IB–IIB cervical cancer. *International Journal of Radiation Oncology biology physics, 90*(4). http://dx.doi.org/10.1016/j.ijrobp.2014.07.034

Cella, D. (2015). Bevacizumab and quality of life in advanced cervical cancer. *Lancet Oncology, 16*(3), 301–311. http://dx.doi.org.10.1016/S1470-2045(15)70052-5

Centers for Disease Control and Prevention (CDC). (2010). Vaginal and vulvar cancers. Retrieved from http://www.cdc.gov/cancer/vagvulv/pdf/vagvulv_facts.pdf

Centers for Disease Control and Prevention (CDC). (2011). Cervical cancer screening for women who attend STD clinics or have a history of STDs. Retrieved from: http://www.cdc.gov/std/treatment/2010/cc-screening.htm

Centers for Disease Control and Prevention (CDC). (2012). Cervical cancer: Fact sheet. Retrieved from http://www.cdc.gov/cancer/cervical/pdf/cervical_facts.pdf

Centers for Disease Control and Prevention (CDC). (2015a). Frequently asked questions about HPV vaccine safety. Retrieved from http://www.cdc.gov/vaccinesafety/Vaccines/HPV/hpv_faqs.html

Centers for Disease Control and Prevention (CDC). (2015b). Vaccine adverse event reporting system. Retrieved from http://www.cdc.gov/vaccinesafety/ensuringsafety/monitoring/vaers/index.html

Chen, H., Kessler, C. L., Mori, N., & Chauhan, S. P. (2012). Cervical cancer screening in the United States, 1993–2010: Characteristics of women who are never screened. *Journal of Women's Health, 21*(11), 1132–1138. http://dx.doi.org/10.1089/jwh2011.3418

Cliby, W. A., Powell, M. A., Al-Hammadi, N., Chen, L., Miller, P., Roland, P. Y., . . . Bristow, R. E. (2015). Ovarian cancer in the United States: Contemporary patterns of care associated with improved survival. *Gynecologic Oncology, 136*, 11–17. http://dx.doi.org/10.1016/j.ygno.2014.10.023

Cramer, D. W. (2012). The epidemiology of endometrial and ovarian cancer. *Hematology/Oncology Clinics of North America, 26*(1), 1–12. http://dx.doi.org/10.1016/j.hoc.2011.10.009

Creasman, W. T. (2014). Endometrial carcinoma: Differential diagnosis. Retrieved from http://www.emedicine.medscape.com/article/254083-differential

Davy, D. D. (2003). Cervical classification and the Bethesda system. *The Cancer Journal, 9*(5), 327–334.

Deppe, G., Mert, I., & Winer, I. S. (2014). Management of squamous cell vulvar cancer: A review. *Journal of Obstetrics and Gynaecology Research, 40*(5), 1217–1225. http://dx.doi.org/10.1111/jog.12352

Dunphy, L. M., Winland-Brown, J. E., Porter, B. O., & Thomas, D. J. (2015). *Primary care: The art and science of advanced practice nursing.* Philadelphia, PA: F. A. Davis.

Edey, K. A., Murdoch, A. E., Cooper, S., & Bryant, A. (2013). Interventions for the treatment of Paget's disease of the vulva (review). *Cochrane Database of Systematic Reviews, 10*, 1–26. http://dx.doi.org/10.1002/14651858.CD009245.pub2

Falconer, H., Yin, L., Grönberg, H., & Altman, D. (2015). Ovarian cancer risk after salpingectomy: A nationwide population-based study. *Journal of the National Cancer Institute, 107*(2), 1–6. http://dx.doi.org/10.1093/jnci/dju410

Feng, L.-P. Chen, H.-L., & Shen, M.-Y. (2014). Breastfeeding and the risk of ovarian cancer: A meta-analysis. *Journal of Midwifery & Women's Health, 59*(4), 428–437. http://dx.doi.org/10.1111.jmwh.12085

FIGO Committee on Gynecologic Oncology. (2014). FIGO guidelines: FIGO staging for carcinoma of the vulva, cervix, and corpus uteri. *International Journal of Gynecology and Obstetrics, 125*, 97–98. http://dx.doi.org/10.1016/j.ijgo.2014.02.003

García-Closas ,R., Castellsagué, X., Bosch, X., & González, C. A. (2005). The role of diet and nutrition in cervical carcinogenesis: A review of recent evidence. *International Journal of Cancer, 117*(4), 629–637. http://dx.doi.org/10.1002/ijc.21193

Gearhart, P. A., Higgins, R. V., Randall, T. C, & Buckley, R. M., Jr. (2015). Human papillomavirus. Retrieved from http://emedicine.medscape.com/article/219110-overview#aw2aab6b2b1aa

Guenther, J., Stiles, A., & Dimmitt Champion, J. (2012). The lived experience of ovarian cancer: A phenomenological approach. *Journal of the American Academy of Nurse Practitioners, 24*, 595–603. http://dx.doi.org/10.111/j.1745-7599.2012.00732x

Hacker, N. F., Eifel, P. J., & van der Velden, J. (2012). FIGO cancer report 2012: Cancer of the vulva. *International Journal of Gynecology and Obstetrics, 119S2*, s90–s96.

Hacker, N. F., Eifel, P. J., & van der Velden, J. (2015). FIGO cancer report 2015: Cancer of the vulva. *International Journal of Gynecology and Obstetrics, 131*, S76–S83.

Harrison, P. (2014). Antiviral sensitizes HPV cervical cancer to chemoradiation. Retrieved from http://www.medscape.com/viewarticle/836418

Havrilesky, L. J., Secord, A. A., Ehrisman J. A., Berchuck, A., Valea, F. A., Lee, P. S., . . . Reed, S. D. (2014). Patient preferences in advanced or recurrent ovarian cancer. *Cancer, 120*, 3651–3659. http://dx.doi.org/10.1002/cncr.28940

Hillary, C. J., Osman, N., & Chapple, C. (2015). Considerations in the modern management of stress incontinence resulting from intrinsic urethral deficiency. *World Journal of Urology, 33*, 1251–1256. http://dx.doi.org/10.1007/s00345-015-1599-z

Hoffstetter, S. (2014). Diagnosing diseases of the vulva. Retrieved from http://www.clinicaladvisor.com/features/diagnosing-diseases-of-the-vulva/article/327908

Hollier, A., & Hensley, R. (2011). *Clinical guidelines in primary care: A reference and review book.* Lafayette, LA: Advanced Practice Education Associates.

Houghton, S. C., Reeves, K. W., Hankinson, S. E., Crawford, L., Lane, D., Wactawski-Wende, J., . . . Sturgeon, S. R. (2014). Perineal powder use and risk of ovarian cancer. *Journal of the National Cancer Institute, 106*(9), 1–6. http://dx.doi.org/10.1093/jnci/dju208

Hunter-Keller, E. (2015). Fear, assumptions heighten lesbians' cervical-cancer risk. Retrieved from http://hsnewsbeat.uw.edu/story/fear-assumptions-heighten-lesbians%E2%80%99-cervical-cancer-risk

Howlader, N., Noone, A. M., Krapcho, M., Garshell, J., Miller, D., Altekruse, S. F., . . . Cronin, K. A. (Eds.). (2014). *SEER cancer statistics review, 1975–2011.* Retrieved from http://seer.cancer.gov/csr/1975_2011

Institute of Medicine. (2011, August). Adverse effects of vaccines: Evidence and causality. Retrieved from http://www.iom.edu/~/media/Files/Report%20Files/2011/Adverse-Effects-of-Vaccines-Evidence-and-Causality/Vaccine-report-brief-FINAL.pdf

Joura, E. A., Giuliano, A. R., Iversen, O. E., Bouchard, C., Mao, C., Mehlsen, J., . . . Luxembourg, A. (2015). A 9-valent HPV vaccine against infection and intraepithelial neoplasia in women. *New England Journal of Medicine, 372*(8), 711–723. http://dx.doi.org/10.1056/NEJMoa1405044

Karageorgi, S., Hankinson, S. E., Kraft, P., & De Vivo, I. (2010). Reproductive factors and postmenopausal hormone use in relation to endometrial cancer risk in the Nurses' Health Study cohort 1976–2004. *International Journal of Cancer, 126,* 208–2016. http://dx.doi.org/10.1002/ijc.24672/epdf

Kurman, R. J., & Shih, I. (2011). Molecular pathogenesis and extraovarian origin of epithelial ovarian cancer: Shifting the paradigm. *Human Pathology, 42,* 918–931. http://dx.doi.org/10.1016/j.humpath.2011.03.003

Lanceley, A., Fitzgerald, D., Jones, V., Miles, T., Elliott, E., Darraugh, L., & Peck, L. (2011). Ovarian cancer: Symptoms, treatment and long-term patient management. *Primary Health Care, 21*(7), 31–38. http://dx.doi.org/10.7748/phc2011.09.21.7.31.c8689

Lee, H. Y., Yang, P. N., Lee, D. K., & Ghebre, R. (2015). Cervical cancer screening behavior among Hmong-American immigrant women. *American Journal of Health Behavior, 39*(3), 301–307. http://dx.doi.org/10.5993/AJHB.39.3.2

Marcus, C. S., Maxwell, G. L., Darcy, K. M., Hamilton, C. A., & McGuire, W. P. (2014). Current approaches and challenges in managing and monitoring treatment response in ovarian cancer. *Journal of Cancer, 5*(1), 25–30. http://dx.doi.org/10.7150/jca.7810

Markowitz, L. E., & Shimabukuro, T. (2015, April 3). HPV vaccine recommendation update [Webinar from the Centers for Disease Control and Prevention]. Retrieved from https://www.youtube.com/watch?v=LDvauWcDVhE

Marrinan, G. (2007). Polycystic ovarian disease (Stein-Leventhal syndrome). Retrieved from http://www.emedicine.com/radio/topic565.htm

McCormack, P. L. (2014). Quadrivalent human papillomavirus (types 6, 11, 16, 18) recombinant vaccine (Gardasil): A review of its use in the prevention of premalignant anogenital lesions cervical and anal cancers, and genital warts. *Drugs, 74,* 1253–1283. http://dx.doi.org/10.1007/s40265-014-0255-z

Moyer, V. A., & U.S. Preventive Services Task Force (USPSTF). (2012). Screening for ovarian cancer: U.S. Preventive Services Task Force reaffirmation statement. *Annals of Internal Medicine, 157*(12), 900–904.

Moyer, V. A., & U.S. Preventive Services Task Force (USPSTF). (2014). Genetic counseling, and genetic testing for BRCA-related cancer in women: U.S. Preventive Services Task Force recommendation statement. *Annals of Internal Medicine, 160*(4), 271–282.

Murzaku, E. C., Penn, L. A., Hale, C. S., Pomeranz, M. K., & Polsky, D. (2014). Vulvar nevi, melanosis and melanoma: An epidemiologic, clinical and histopathologic review. *Journal of the American Academy of Dermatology, 71,* 1241–1249. http://dx.doi.org/10.1016/j.jaad.2014.08.019

National Cancer Institute (NCI). (n.d.). SEER cancer statistics factsheets: Vulvar cancer. Retrieved from http://seer.cancer.gov/statfacts/html/vulva.html

National Cancer Institute (NCI).(2014). *Pap and HPV testing.* Retrieved from http://www.cancer.gov/types/cervical/pap-hpv-testing-fact-sheet

National Cancer Institute (NCI). (2015a). Cervical cancer treatment (PDQ): Health professional version. Retrieved from http://www.cancer.gov/types/cervical/hp/cervical-treatment-pdq#link/_532_toc

National Cancer Institute (NCI). (2015b). General information about vulvar cancer (PDQ): Health professional version. Retrieved from http://www.cancer.gov/cancertopics/pdq/treatment/vulvar/HealthProfessional/page1

National Cancer Institute (NCI). (2015c). Ovarian, epithelial, fallopian tube and peritoneal cancer treatment (PDQ): Health professional version. Retrieved from http://www.cancer.gov/cancertopics/pdq/treatment/ovarianepithelial/HealthProfessional

National Cancer Institute (NCI). (2015d). Uterine cancer for health professionals. Retrieved from http://www.cancer.gov/types/uterine/patient/endometrial-prevention-pdq#section/_4

National Cancer Institute (NCI). (2015e). Endometrial cancer treatment (PDQ®)–Patient version. Retrieved from Uterine cancer for health professionals. Treatment option overview. Retrieved from: http://www.cancer.gov/types/uterine/patient/endometrial-treatment-pdq#section/_131

National Cancer Institute (NCI). (2016). Pap and HPV testing. Retrieved from http://www.cancer.gove/types/cervical/pap-hpv-testing-fact-sheet

National Comprehensive Cancer Network (NCCN). (2015a). NCCN clinical practice guidelines version 1.2015 ovarian cancer. Retrieved from https://www.tri-kobe.org/nccn/guideline/gynecological/english/ovarian.pdf

National Comprehensive Cancer Network (NCCN). (2015b). NCCN clinical practice guidelines in oncology version 2.2015 cervical cancer. Retrieved from http://www.nccn.org/professionals/physician_gls/pdf/cervical.pdf

National Comprehensive Cancer Network (NCCN). (2015c). NCCN clinical practice guidelines version 2.2016 endometrial carcinoma. Retrieved from https://www.tri-kobe.org/nccn/guideline/gynecological/english/uterine.pdf

National Institutes of Health (NIH). (2013). NIH fact sheet: Cervical cancer. Retrieved from http://www.report.nih.gov/nihfactsheets/viewfactsheet.aspx?csid=76

Nayar, R., & Wilbur, D. C. (2015). The Pap test and Bethesda 2014. *Acta Cytologica, 59*(2), 121–132. doi:10.1159/000381842

Nelson, R. (2014). Japanese mushroom extract could help treat HPV infections. Retrieved from http://www.medscape.com/viewarticle/834183

Pecorelli, S. (2009). Corrigendum to "Revised FIGO staging for carcinoma of the vulva, cervix, and endometrium." *International Journal of Gynecology and Obstetrics, 105,* 103–104.

Petrosky, E., Bocchini, J. A., Hairiri, S., Chesson, H., Curtis, C. R., Saraiya, M., . . . Markowitz, L. (2015, March 27). Use of 9-valent human papillomavirus (HPV) vaccine: Updated HPV vaccination recommendations of the Advisory Committee on Immunization Practices. *Morbidity and Mortality Weekly Report, 64*(11), 300–304. Retrieved from http://www.cdc.gov/mmwr/preview/mmwrhtml/mm6411a3.htm?s_cid=mm6411a3_w

Porth, C. M. (2015). *Essentials of pathophysiology* (4th ed.). Philadelphia, PA: Wolters Kluwer.

Prat, J., & FIGO Committee on Gynecologic Oncology. (2014). Staging classification for cancer of the ovary, fallopian tube, and peritoneum. *International Journal of Gynecology and Obstetrics, 124,* 1–5. http://dx.doi.org/10.1016/j.jjigo.2013.10.001

Preti, M., Scurry, J., Marchitelli, C. E., & Micheletti, L. (2014). Vulvar intraepithelial neoplasia. *Best Practice & Research*

Clinical Obstetrics and Gynaecology, 28, 1051–1062. doi:10.1016/j.bpobgyn.2014.07.010

Rauh-Hain, J. A., Clemmer, J., Clark, R. M., Bradford, L. S., Growdon, W. B., Goodman, A., . . . del Carmen, M. G. (2014). Management and outcomes for elderly women with vulvar cancer over time, *BJOG, 55,* 719–726. http://dx.doi.org/10.1111/1471-0528.12580

Reyes, M. C., & Cooper, K. (2014). An update on vulvar intraepithelial neoplasia: Terminology and a practical approach to diagnosis. *Journal of Clinical Pathology, 66,* 290–294. http://dx.doi.org/10.1136/jclinpath-2013-202117

Saslow, D. (2013, January). Cervical cancer is an international issue. Retrieved from http://blogs.cancer.org/expertvoices/2013/01/30/cervical-cancer-is-an-international-issue

Schuchat, A. (2015). HPV "coverage." *New England Journal of Medicine, 372*(8), 775. http://dx.doi.org/10.1056/NEJMe1415742

Setiawan, V. W., Yang, H. P., Pike, M. C., McCann, S. E., Yu, H., Xiang, Y., . . . Horn-Ross, P. L. (2013). Type I and II endometrial cancers: Have they different risk factors? *Journal of Clinical Oncology, 31*(20), 2607–2618. http://dx.doi.org/10.1200/JCO.2012.48.2596

Siegel, R., Naishadham, D., & Jemal, A. (2013). Cancer statistics 2013. *CA A Cancer Journal for Clinicians, 63*(1), 11–30. http://dx.doi.org/10.3322/caac.21166

Solomon, D., Davey, D., Kurman, R., Moriarty, A., O'Connor, D., Prey, M., . . . Young, N. (2002). The 2001 Bethesda System: Terminology for reporting results of cervical cytology. *Journal of the American Medical Association, 287*(16), 2114–2119.

Stiles, M., Redmer, J., Paddock, E., & Schrager, S. (2012). Gynecologic issues in geriatric women. *Journal of Women's Health, 21*(1), 4–9. http://dx.doi.org/10.1089/jwh.2011.2803

Stokley, S., Jeyarajah, J., Yankey, D., Cano, M., Gee, J., Roark, J., . . . Markowitz, L. (2014, July 25). Human papillomavirus vaccination coverage among adolescents, 2007–2013, and postlicensure vaccine safety monitoring, 2005–2014—United States. *Morbidity and Mortality Weekly Report, 63*(29), 62–624. Retrieved from http://www.cdc.gov/mmwr/preview/mmwrhtml/mm6329a3.htm

Stoler, M. H., Wright, T. C., Sharma, A., Apple, R., Gutekunst, K., & Wright, T.L. (2011). High-risk human papillomavirus testing in women with ASC-US cytology: Results from the ATHENA HPV study. *American Journal of Clinical Pathologists, 135*(3), 468–475.

Tergas, A. I., Tseng, J. H., & Bristow, R. E. (2013). Impact of race and ethnicity on treatment and survival of women with vulvar cancer in the United States. *Gynecologic Oncology, 129,* 154–158. http://dx.doi.org/10.1016/j.ygyno.2012.12.032

Trietsch, M. D., Nooij, L. S., Gaarenstroom, K. N., & van Poelgeest, M. (2015). Genetic and epigenetic changes in vulvar squamous cell carcinoma and its precursor lesions: A review of the current literature. *Gynecologic Oncology, 136,* 143–157. http://dx.doi.org/10.1016/j.ygyno.2014.11.002

U.S. Cancer Statistics Working Group. (2014). *United States cancer statistics: 1999–2011 incidence and mortality web-based report.* Atlanta: U.S. Department of Health and Human Services, Centers for Disease Control and Prevention, & National Cancer Institute.

U.S. Food and Drug Administration (FDA). (2014). FDA approves Gardasil 9 for prevention of certain cancers caused by five additional types of HPV. Retrieved from http://www.fda.gov/NewsEvents/Newsroom/PressAnnouncements/ucm426485.htm

U.S. Food and Drug Administration (FDA). (2015a). Cervarix. Retrieved from http://www.fda.gov/BiologicsBloodVaccines/Vaccines/ApprovedProducts/ucm186957.htm

U.S. Food and Drug Administration (FDA). (2015b). Gardasil. Retrieved from http://www.fda.gov/downloads/BiologicsBloodVaccines/Vaccines/ApprovedProducts/UCM111266.pdf

Verma, I., Jain, V., & Kaur, T. (2014). Application of Bethesda system for cervical cytology in unhealthy cervix. *Journal of Clinical and Diagnostic Research, 8*(9), 26–30.

Wan, W. (2013). HPV testing and cancer: Will E6/E7 change the paradigm? Retrieved from http://www.mlo-online.com/articles/201304/hpv-testing-and-cancer-will-e6-e7-change-the-paradigm.php

Ward, K.K., Shah, N.R., Saenz, C.C., McHale, M.T., Alvarez, E.A., & Plaxe, S.C. (2012). Cardiovascular disease is the leading cause of death among endometrial cancer patients. *Obstetrics & Gynecology, 126*(2), 176–179. doi:10.1016/j.ygyno.2012.04.013

Wedel, N., & Johnson, L. (2014). Vulvar lichen sclerosis: Diagnosis and management. *Journal for Nurse Practitioners, 10*(1), 42–48. http://dx.doi.org/1016/j.nurpra.2013.10.009

Wilbur, D., Wright, T., & Young, N. (2002). The 2001 Bethesda System: Terminology for reporting results of cervical cytology. *Journal of the American Medical Association, 287*(16), 2114–2119.

Woelber, L., Trillsch, F., Kock, L., Grimm, D., Peterson, C., Choschzick, M., . . . Mahner, S. (2013). Management of patients with vulvar cancer: A perspective review according to tumor stage. *Therapeutic Advances in Medical Oncology, 5*(3), 183–192. http://dx.doi.org/10.1177/1758834012471699

Woodman, C. B. J., Collins, S. I., & Young, L. S. (2007). The natural history of cervical HPV infection: Unresolved issues. *National Reviews Cancer, 7,* 11–22. http://dx.doi.org/10.1038/nrc2050

World Health Organization (WHO). (2015). Human papillomavirus (HPV) and cervical cancer. Retrieved from http://www.who.int/mediacentre/factsheets/fs380/en

Zeppernick, F., Meinhold-Heerlein, I., & Shih, I-M. (2014). Precursors of ovarian cancer in the fallopian tube: Serous tubal intraepithelial carcinoma-an update. *Journal of Obstetrics and Gynaecology Research, 41*(1), 6–11. http://dx.doi.org/10.1111/jog.12550

APPENDIX 27-A

ASCCP Algorithms

Unsatisfactory Cytology

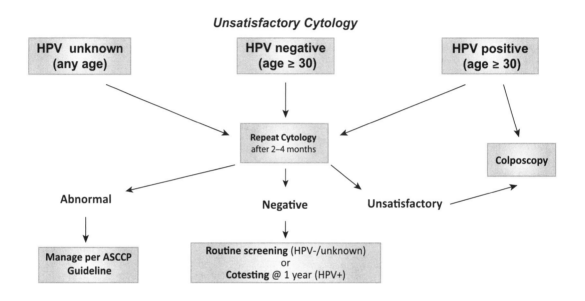

Cytology NILM* but EC/TZ Absent/Insufficient

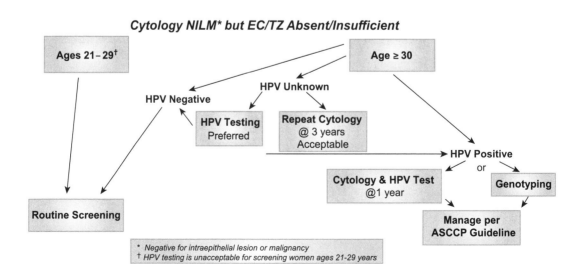

* Negative for intraepithelial lesion or malignancy
† HPV testing is unacceptable for screening women ages 21-29 years

Management of Women ≥ Age 30, who are Cytology Negative, but HPV Positive

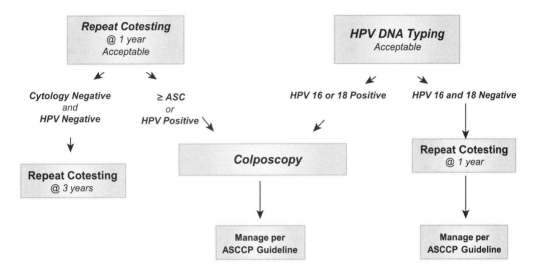

Management of Women with Atypical Squamous Cells of Undetermined Significance (ASC-US) on Cytology*

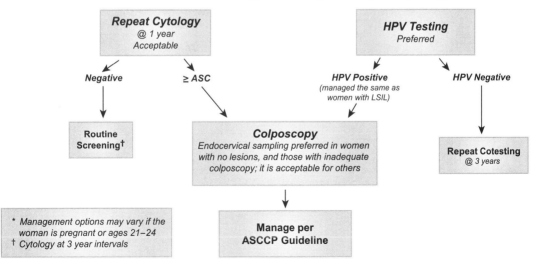

Management of Women Ages 21–24 years with either Atypical Squamous Cells of Undetermined Significance (ASC-US) or Low-grade Squamous Intraepithelial Lesion (LSIL)

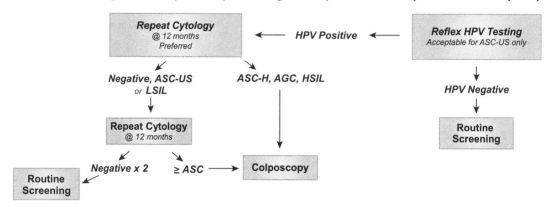

Management of Women with Low-grade Squamous Intraepithelial Lesions (LSIL)*†

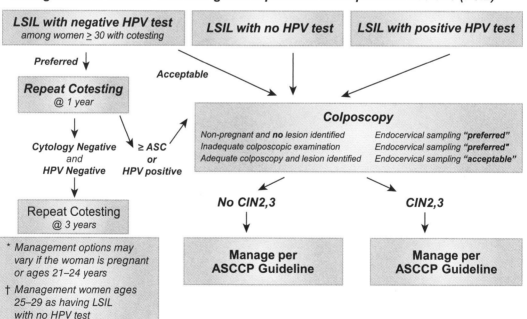

Management of Pregnant Women with Low-grade Squamous Intraepithelial Lesion (LSIL)

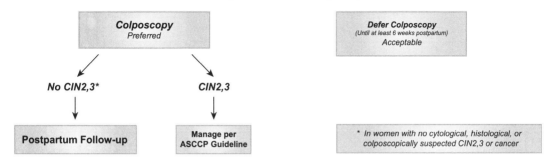

Management of Women with Atypical Squamous Cells: Cannot Exclude High-grade SIL (ASC-H)*

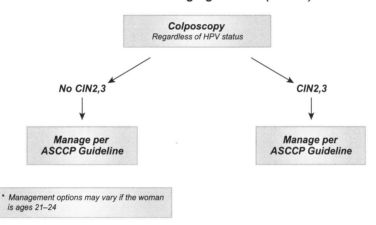

Management of Women Ages 21–24 yrs with Atypical Squamous Cells, Cannot Rule Out High Grade SIL (ASC-H) and High-grade Squamous Intraepithelial Lesion (HSIL)

Colposcopy
Immediate loop electrosurgical excision is unacceptable

No CIN2,3 → **Observation with Colposcopy & Cytology***
@ 6 month intervals for up to 2 years

CIN2,3 → **Manage per ASCCP Guideline for Young Women with CIN2,3**

Observation branches:

- **High-grade colposcopic lesion** *or* **HSIL**
  Persists for 1 year → **Biopsy** → **CIN2,3**
  (If no CIN2,3, continue observation) → **Manage per ASCCP Guideline for Young Women with CIN2,3**

- **HSIL**
  Persists for 24 months with no CIN2,3 identified → **Diagnostic Excisional Procedure†**

- **Other Results** → **Manage per ASCCP Guideline**

- **Two Consecutive Cytology Negative Results** *and* **No High-grade Colposcopic Abnormality** → **Routine Screening**

* *If colposcopy is adequate and endocervical sampling is negative. Otherwise a diagnostic excisional procedure is indicated.*

† *Not if patient is pregnant*

Management of Women with High-grade Squamous Intraepithelial Lesions (HSIL)*

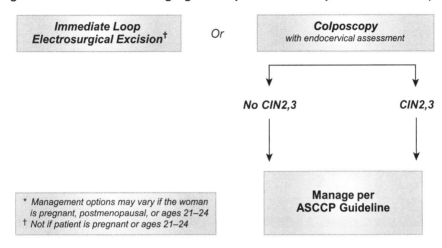

Immediate Loop Electrosurgical Excision†   Or   Colposcopy with endocervical assessment

No CIN2,3   CIN2,3

* Management options may vary if the woman is pregnant, postmenopausal, or ages 21–24
† Not if patient is pregnant or ages 21–24

Manage per ASCCP Guideline

Initial Workup of Women with Atypical Glandular Cells (AGC)

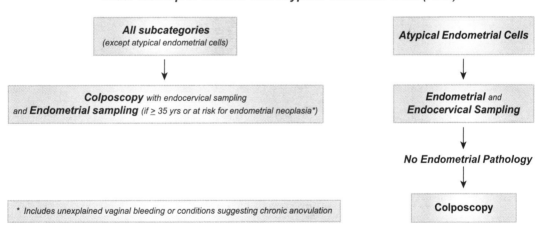

All subcategories (except atypical endometrial cells)

Atypical Endometrial Cells

Colposcopy with endocervical sampling and Endometrial sampling (if ≥ 35 yrs or at risk for endometrial neoplasia*)

Endometrial and Endocervical Sampling

No Endometrial Pathology

* Includes unexplained vaginal bleeding or conditions suggesting chronic anovulation

Colposcopy

Subsequent Management of Women with Atypical Glandular Cells (AGC)

Initial Cytology is AGC (favor neoplasia) or AIS

→ No Invasive Disease

→ **Diagnostic Excisional Procedure***

* *Should provide an intact specimen with interpretable margins. Concomitant endocervical sampling is preferred*

Initial Cytology is AGC - NOS

- *CIN2+ but no Glandular Neoplasia* → **Manage per ASCCP Guideline**

- *No CIN2+, AIS or Cancer* → **Cotest** *@ 12 & 24 months*
  - *Any Abnormality* → **Colposcopy**
  - *Both Negative* → **Cotest** *3 years later*

704

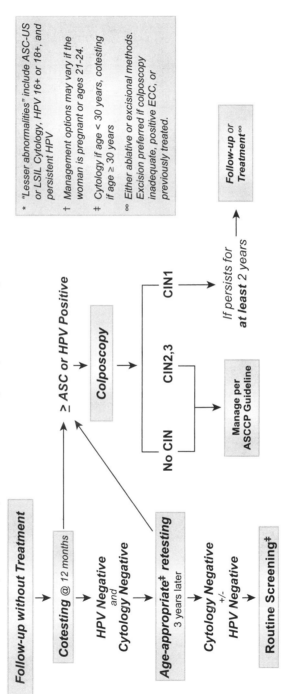

Management of Women with No Lesion or Biopsy-confirmed Cervical
Intraepithelial Neoplasia — Grade 1 (CIN1) Preceded by "Lesser Abnormalities" * †

Follow-up without Treatment

Cotesting @ 12 months

↓

HPV Negative
and
Cytology Negative

↓

Age-appropriate‡ retesting
3 years later

↓

*Cytology Negative
+/-
HPV Negative*

↓

Routine Screening‡

≥ **ASC or HPV Positive**

↓

Colposcopy

No CIN   CIN2,3   CIN1

**Manage per
ASCCP Guideline**

*If persists for
at least 2 years* →

**Follow-up or
Treatment∞**

* "Lesser abnormalities" include ASC-US
  or LSIL Cytology, HPV 16+ or 18+, and
  persistent HPV

† Management options may vary if the
  woman is pregnant or ages 21-24.

‡ Cytology if age < 30 years, cotesting
  if age ≥ 30 years

∞ Either ablative or excisional methods.
  Excision preferred if colposcopy
  inadequate, positive ECC, or
  previously treated.

705

Management of Women with No Lesion or Biopsy-confirmed Cervical Intraepithelial Neoplasia — Grade 1 (CIN1) Preceded by ASC-H or HSIL Cytology

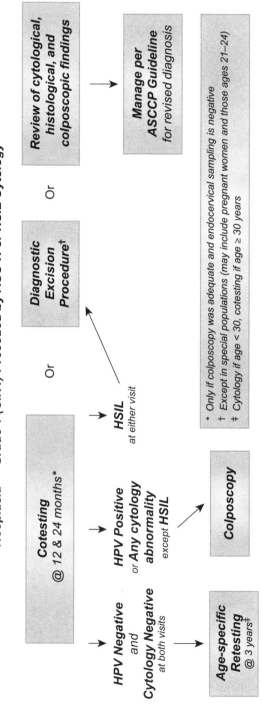

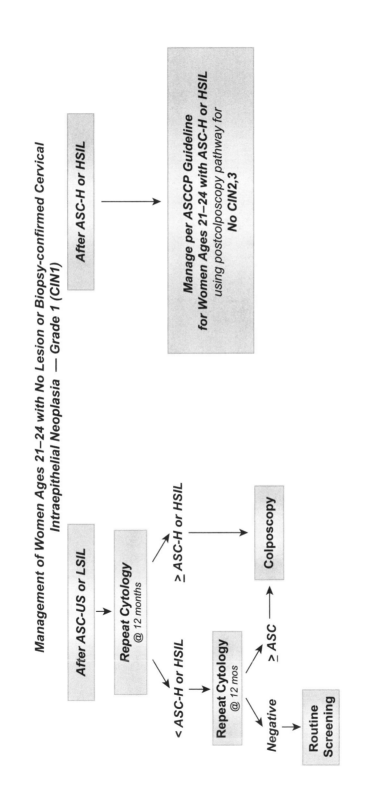

Management of Women Ages 21–24 with No Lesion or Biopsy-confirmed Cervical Intraepithelial Neoplasia — Grade 1 (CIN1)

After ASC-US or LSIL

Repeat Cytology
@ 12 months

≥ ASC-H or HSIL → **Colposcopy**

< ASC-H or HSIL →

Repeat Cytology
@ 12 mos

≥ ASC → **Colposcopy**

Negative → **Routine Screening**

After ASC-H or HSIL

Manage per ASCCP Guideline for Women Ages 21–24 with ASC-H or HSIL using postcolposcopy pathway for *No CIN2,3*

Management of Women with Biopsy-confirmed Cervical Intraepithelial Neoplasia — Grade 2 and 3 (CIN2,3)*

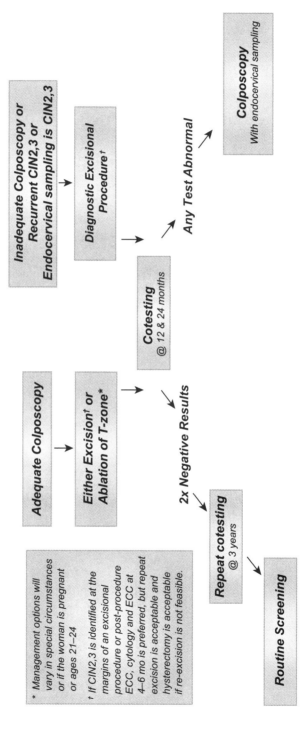

Adequate Colposcopy

Either Excision† or Ablation of T-zone*

Cotesting
@ 12 & 24 months

2x Negative Results

Repeat cotesting
@ 3 years

Routine Screening

Inadequate Colposcopy or Recurrent CIN2,3 or Endocervical sampling is CIN2,3

Diagnostic Excisional Procedure†

Any Test Abnormal

Colposcopy
With endocervical sampling

* Management options will vary in special circumstances or if the woman is pregnant or ages 21–24

† If CIN2,3 is identified at the margins of an excisional procedure or post-procedure ECC, cytology and ECC at 4–6 mo is preferred, but repeat excision is acceptable and hysterectomy is acceptable if re-excision is not feasible.

Management of Young Women with Biopsy-confirmed Cervical Intraepithelial Neoplasia — Grade 2,3 (CIN2,3) in Special Circumstances*

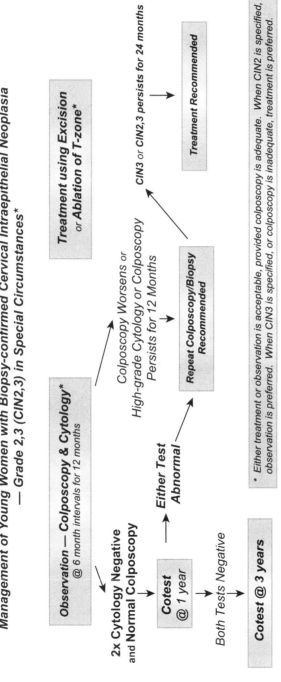

2x Cytology Negative and Normal Colposcopy

Observation — Colposcopy & Cytology* @ 6 month intervals for 12 months

Either Test Abnormal

Cotest @ 1 year

Both Tests Negative

Cotest @ 3 years

Repeat Colposcopy/Biopsy Recommended

Colposcopy Worsens or High-grade Cytology or Colposcopy Persists for 12 Months

Treatment using Excision or **Ablation of T-zone***

CIN3 or CIN2,3 persists for 24 months

Treatment Recommended

* Either treatment or observation is acceptable, provided colposcopy is adequate. When CIN2 is specified, observation is preferred. When CIN3 is specified, or colposcopy is inadequate, treatment is preferred.

Management of Women Diagnosed with Adenocarcinoma in-situ (AIS) during a Diagnostic Excisional Procedure

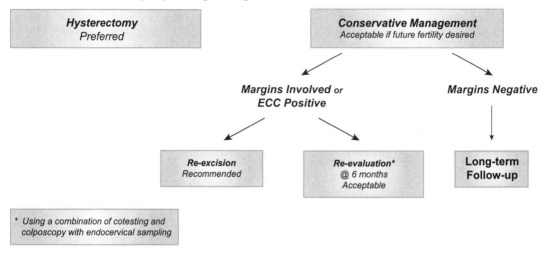

Hysterectomy
Preferred

Conservative Management
Acceptable if future fertility desired

Margins Involved or ECC Positive

Margins Negative

Re-excision
Recommended

Re-evaluation*
@ 6 months
Acceptable

Long-term Follow-up

* Using a combination of cotesting and colposcopy with endocervical sampling

Interim Guidance for Managing Reports using the Lower Anogenital Squamous Terminology (LAST) Histopathology Diagnoses

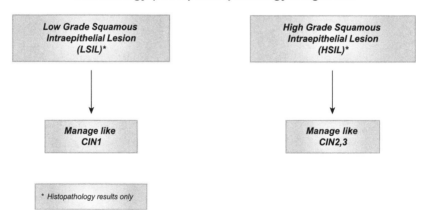

Low Grade Squamous Intraepithelial Lesion (LSIL)*

High Grade Squamous Intraepithelial Lesion (HSIL)*

Manage like CIN1

Manage like CIN2,3

* Histopathology results only

CHAPTER 28

Chronic Pelvic Pain

Nanci Gasiewicz

Melissa Romero

The editors acknowledge Kerri Durnell Schuiling, who was a coauthor of the previous edition of this chapter.

INTRODUCTION

Concern about pelvic pain is the reason for 1% to 2% of all healthcare visits made by women (Johnson, Thomas, & Porter, 2015). Historically, when a woman presented with pelvic or lower abdominal pain, the clinician automatically focused solely on the gynecologic organs, assuming they were the cause of the problem. This narrow clinical view risks categorizing normal female physiologic processes as abnormal and encourages the use of surgical interventions because it assumes pathology. A number of the causes of pelvic pain in women are unrelated to the gynecologic organs. Often pelvic pain is caused by multiple factors, requiring clinicians to take a multidisciplinary, holistic approach to its assessment and management. An appreciation for the intertwining influence of the mind and the body during assessment and in planning interventions is important. This approach places the woman at the center of her management plan, and respects her credibility as the authoritative "knower."

This chapter addresses pelvic pain that is primarily chronic and gynecologic in origin. Nongynecologic acute and chronic pelvic pain is addressed in the context of providing differential diagnoses for the clinician to consider during assessment and evaluation.

DESCRIPTION AND DEFINITION

Pelvic pain is a broad term encompassing a number of etiologies, within or across body systems. Such pain can be acute, chronic, cyclic, or noncyclic and may or may not be related to gynecologic organs. It may be symptomatic of an underlying cause, or it can be a syndrome unto itself. Pelvic pain can be so severe that it adversely affects a woman's normal functioning, keeping her from maintaining her normal lifestyle. Although seeking treatment for pelvic pain is one of the most common reasons women come to a clinician for care, diagnosing its cause and prescribing the appropriate treatment is often difficult because of the complexity of the pathophysiology and the myriad contributing factors.

Pelvic pain is divided into two types: acute and chronic. Onset of acute pelvic pain may be the result of pelvic disorders, such as pelvic inflammatory disease (PID), ruptured ovarian cyst, ectopic pregnancy, or torsion of an ovarian cyst, ovary, or fallopian tube (Johnson et al., 2015). PID accounts for approximately 20% of acute pelvic pain in women, ovarian cysts for approximately 40%, and adnexal torsion for approximately 16% (Johnson et al., 2015). Nearly 10% of women who present with concerns about acute pelvic pain are experiencing an extrapelvic condition, such as anal fissure, thrombosed external hemorrhoids, or appendicitis (Johnson et al., 2015; Stein, 2013). Acute pelvic pain typically resolves with treatment and subsequent healing. Acute pelvic pain that is gynecologically related is discussed in greater detail elsewhere in this text.

Acute pelvic pain is generally defined as pain that occurs in the pelvis or lower abdomen and is of less than 3 months' duration (Kruszka & Kruszka, 2010). Acute pain is intense and generally characterized as being sudden in onset, sharp in nature, and short in duration (Rapkin & Nathan, 2012). Almost half of all visits to the emergency department by women of reproductive age are for complaints of acute pelvic pain, pelvic inflammatory disease, and lower genital tract infections (e.g., cervicitis, candidiasis, Bartholin's abscess) (Hart & Lipsky, 2014). Given that acute pelvic pain is often associated with an identifiable cause such as PID or ectopic pregnancy, a wrong diagnosis of acute pelvic pain can lead to serious sequelae, such as impaired fertility, rupture of an ectopic pregnancy or a hemorrhagic ovarian cyst, and even death (Hart & Lipsky, 2014; Rapkin & Nathan, 2012). The incidence of heterotopic pregnancy was 1 in 30,000 in 1948 and is currently reported to be as high as 1 in 8,000 (Hart & Lipsky, 2014). Unrecognized abuse may be life threatening as well (Hart & Lipsky, 2014).

In contrast to acute pelvic pain, chronic pelvic pain (CPP) is described as pain lasting at least 6 months that can be sudden or gradual in onset and severity (Stein, 2013). Some types of chronic pelvic pain are associated with normal physiologic functions, such as menstruation and childbearing. However, a number of nongynecologic causes of pelvic pain must be considered. CPP that is primarily gynecologic in origin is the main focus of discussion in this chapter. Although CPP has traditionally been thought to encompass the peritoneal and lower abdominal viscera below the umbilicus and within the boundaries of the anatomic pelvis, various authors have also included portions of the external genitalia (vulva, vagina) and musculoskeletal system (e.g., sacroiliac joint) in close proximity to the bony pelvis (Styer, 2013). There is no universally accepted definition of chronic pelvic pain. For the purposes of this chapter, chronic pelvic pain is defined as "noncyclic pain of six or more months duration that localizes to the anatomic pelvis, anterior abdominal wall at or below the umbilicus, the lumbosacral back, or the buttocks, and is of sufficient severity to cause functional disability or lead to medical care" (American College of Obstetricians and Gynecologists, 2004, reaffirmed 2010). CPP is a malady that plagues women of all age groups, although it more commonly affects women with a mean age of approximately 30 years (Shin & Howard, 2011).

Scope and Incidence of Chronic Pelvic Pain

Chronic pelvic pain is a serious health condition that affects 15% to 20% of women aged 18 to 50 years in the United States (American College of Obstetricians and Gynecologists, 2004, reaffirmed 2010; As-Sanie et al., 2012; Beckmann et al., 2014; Stein, 2013). It often lasts longer than a year and contributes significantly to healthcare costs (Beckmann et al., 2014).

Women experiencing CPP are reported to use significantly more medications, have nongynecologic operations much more often, and are more likely to have a hysterectomy and reduced quality of life than women who do not have pelvic pain (Williams, Hartmann, Sandler, Miller, & Steege, 2004). In the United States, 10% of gynecologic visits are for treatment of chronic pelvic pain, 40% of all laparoscopies performed are attributable to this condition, and 10% to 17% of hysterectomies performed because of chronic pain have no pathologic findings (Altman & Lee, 2009; Whiteman et al., 2008).

Estimates suggest that CPP is responsible for $2.8 billion in direct care costs each year in the United States (American College of Obstetricians and Gynecologists, 2004, reaffirmed 2010; Mathias, Kuppermann, Liberman, Lipschutz, & Steege, 1996)). Many women with chronic pelvic pain are unable to work and, therefore, unable to contribute to their family's household income. The loss of daily functioning because of pelvic pain creates increased psychosocial stressors including hopelessness, marital distress, loss of interest in sexual intimacy, and despair compounded by financial stress, all of which can lead to anxiety and depression (Rapkin & Nathan, 2012). Women with CPP often have poor treatment outcomes when they are administered traditionally effective gynecologic and medical therapies and may endure multiple unsuccessful surgical procedures for pain (Rapkin & Nathan, 2012).

Etiology and Pathophysiology

Considerable debate has focused on whether acceptable symptoms for the diagnosis of CPP should include cyclic pain (e.g., dysmenorrhea associated with menses or pain during a particular phase of the menstrual cycle), sporadic pain (e.g., dyspareunia), or noncyclic pain of unpredictable onset (Styer, 2013). Unlike acute pelvic pain, CPP is often a complex affliction with coexisting gynecologic and nongynecologic origins of pain (Shin & Howard, 2011). In fact, many women with pelvic pain have more than one diagnosis as the possible cause of their pain, and women who have multiple diagnoses related to pelvic pain have been shown to suffer greater pain than their counterparts who have one diagnostic cause (American College of Obstetricians and Gynecologists, 2004, reaffirmed 2010). For example, approximately one-third of women with endometriosis also present with comorbid conditions, such as interstitial cystitis or irritable bowel syndrome (Shin & Howard, 2011). Therefore, following medical or surgical interventions for endometriosis-associated pelvic pain, women may experience only partial improvement in their symptoms if urologic and gastrointestinal components are missed in the initial assessment and diagnosis and, therefore, they are not treated correctly (Shin & Howard, 2011). Musculoskeletal dysfunction of the abdominal wall or pelvic floor can also contribute to CPP (Shin & Howard, 2011).

Pelvic pain generally arises from either a visceral source, such as the gynecologic, genitourinary, or gastrointestinal tracts, or from a somatic source, such as the pelvic bones, ligaments, muscles, and fascia (American College of Obstetricians and Gynecologists, 2004, reaffirmed 2010). For these reasons, the initial diagnostic approach to CPP should entail a comprehensive history (Shin & Howard, 2011). The physical examination is conducted in a systematic manner to connect the stated history with identified areas of pain and to distinguish between somatic and visceral types of pain (Shin & Howard, 2011).

Somatic pain may be either superficial or deep. Superficial pain occurs when the body surface is stimulated, whereas deep pain originates in muscles, joints, bones, or connective tissue. Somatic pain is often described as being either sharp or dull, and is usually localized; that is, it is found on either the right or the left within specific dermatomes that correspond to the innervations of the involved tissues (Hoffman, 2012; Stein, 2013). Chronic pelvic pain is often sensed as deep pain.

Visceral pain arises from internal organs and is often associated with strong contractions of visceral muscles (Hoffman, 2012). Stretching, distention, ischemia, or spasm of abdominal organs can stimulate visceral pain (Hoffman, 2012). Because visceral innervation of the pelvic structures share common neural pathways, isolating the source of visceral pain may prove challenging (Stein, 2013). This type of pain is transmitted through the sympathetic tracts of the autonomic nervous system, and is usually described as being dull, crampy, or poorly localized; it may be associated with autonomic phenomena such as nausea, vomiting, and sweating (Hoffman, 2012; Stein, 2013).

Nociceptive pain is "pain with a purpose" that arises from damage or injury to non-neural tissue and is a result of activation of nociceptors in a normally functioning somatosensory nervous system (Taverner, 2014). This type of pain, which is often thought of as inflammatory pain, serves as a defense mechanism that alerts the sufferer to tissue injury and/or disease (Taverner, 2014). When the noxious stimulus is removed, the activity of the sensory pain receptors (also known as nociceptors) quickly ceases (Hoffman, 2012). Nociceptive pain subsides with proper treatment and/or healing of the associated injury and/or disease.

Neuropathic pain is described as complex type of "pain without purpose" and arises as a direct consequence of a lesion or disease affecting the somatosensory system (International Association for the Study of Pain [IASP], 2014; Taverner, Closs, & Briggs, 2014). This complex pain syndrome requires a multimodal treatment approach that includes both pharmacologic and nonpharmacologic management strategies (Taverner, 2014). It occurs when noxious stimuli have sustained action, producing continuous central sensitization and loss of neuronal inhibition that becomes permanent (Hoffman, 2012). The result is a decreased pain threshold and complaints of pain that may seem disproportionate to the amount of coexisting disease. When neuropathic pain occurs in the context of chronic pelvic pain, it often presents as burning, paresthesia, or lancing pain. This phenomenon explains why it is common for a woman to experience pain that is disproportionate to the amount of coexisting disease (Hoffman, 2012; Stein, 2013).

A thorough assessment of the underlying etiology of CPP should also include evaluation of the level of functional disability (e.g., the woman's ability to work, engage in daily activities, and emotional and sexual relationships) (Stein, 2013). Psychological factors must always be considered when evaluating and treating any CPP disorder (Shin & Howard, 2011). Such factors are especially relevant in women with history of sexual abuse, physical abuse, depression, or anxiety (Meltzer-Brody & Leserman, 2011; Stein, 2013). As-Sanie, Clevenger, Geisser, Williams, and Roth (2014) found that women with CPP and a history of physical abuse as an adolescent or an adult reported substantially greater pain-related disability compared to women reporting no abuse in these categories. In addition, women with CPP who experienced childhood physical or sexual abuse reported significantly more depressive symptoms than women who reported no such history of child abuse. These findings do not diminish the need for accurate physical diagnosis, but they do point out that proper recognition and treatment of functional disabilities and psychological factors may be important components in symptom improvement (Meltzer-Brody & Leserman, 2011; Stein, 2013).

The three most frequent causal findings on laparoscopy for CPP are endometriosis (33%), adhesions (24%), and absence of pathologic condition (35%) (Nelson et al., 2011). However, the etiologies of CPP can be complex and may encompass the gastroenterologic, urologic, gynecologic, oncologic, musculoskeletal, and psychosocial systems (Stein, 2013). Unfortunately, subspecialists often lack interdisciplinary training and understanding of the multifaceted approaches necessary to properly evaluate and treat the complexities of CPP (Stein, 2013). This knowledge gap makes comprehensive evaluation, diagnosis, and treatment difficult, potentially leading to frustration among women who are sent from one specialist to another without adequate resolution of their CPP symptoms.

Given the myriad etiologic aspects of CPP, the approach to health care for the woman with pelvic pain must also be multifaceted. The process of determining the cause of pelvic pain and developing a successful treatment plan is often difficult, time consuming, and costly for the woman, and difficult and confusing, at best, for even the most experienced clinician. Many of the diseases believed to cause pelvic pain do not meet the epidemiologic criteria for causality; that is, the evidence may strongly suggest such factors as the cause, but research results do not yet provide definitive support for such a relationship. This ambiguity increases the difficulty of assessment, diagnosis, and treatment of pelvic pain (American College of Obstetricians and Gynecologists, 2004, reaffirmed 2010). Because the causes of many disorders that are associated with pelvic pain are not well established, the majority of clinicians treat the condition empirically.

Clinical Presentation

Pelvic pathology causing acute pain is common, and the presenting complaint may be diffuse or lower abdominal pain, pelvic pain, or low back pain (Hart & Lipsky, 2014). Women with CPP may also develop an acute process, either secondary to the chronic pain condition or arising from a new source (Hart & Lipsky, 2014). More than one-third of women of reproductive age will experience nonmenstrual pelvic pain. In nearly half of all women with CPP, their condition will be due to pelvic inflammatory disease and lower genital tract infections (e.g., cervicitis, candidiasis, Bartholin's abscess) (Hart & Lipsky, 2014). In the general population, ectopic pregnancy accounts for 2% of first-trimester pregnancies, but the incidence of ectopic pregnancies among those women presenting to emergency departments with vaginal bleeding and acute pelvic pain can be as high as 18% (American College of Obstetricians and Gynecologists, 2008, reaffirmed 2014).

Acute pelvic pain is generally accepted to comprise pain in the lower abdomen or pelvic region that is present for less than 7 days (Hoffman, 2012); it may or may not be recurrent or related to the menstrual cycle. The woman usually describes acute pelvic pain that has a rapid onset and a sharp intensity. The discomfort may consist of colicky pain, or it may come and go like menstrual cramps. Vital signs may be unstable because of the sharpness of the pain. The cause of acute pelvic pain must be quickly diagnosed because a delay can result in increased morbidity and death (Hart

& Lipsky, 2014; Rapkin & Nathan, 2012). If the woman is of reproductive age, the first priority is to rule out pregnancy.

Chronic pelvic pain is often classified as either gynecologic or nongynecologic. Categorizing the pain further into cyclic or noncyclic categories assists the clinician in determining whether the pain may be related to the woman's menstrual cycle. Sometimes, however, cyclic pain has no relationship to the menstrual cycle and is totally unrelated to the pelvic organs. Pelvic pain that is cyclic and gynecologic in origin is addressed in various chapters within this text, such as those dealing with dysmenorrhea and endometriosis. See Chapters 23 and 26 for further information on conditions that cause this type of pain.

Women presenting with CPP often have had the pain for some time and do not come for treatment until they are so negatively affected by the pain that they can no longer perform activities of daily living. They do not always appear to be experiencing the amount of distress that individuals with severe pain often display. This affect may reflect the fact that these women have lived with the pain for so long that they have normalized it and, therefore, do not present as the typical individual suffering from significant pain. Frequently they will describe an inability to work or function at home and a pain that is unrelenting. It is also not unusual to observe that a woman has seen a variety of clinicians over several years with a variety of concerns, all of which center on her pelvic pain.

ASSESSMENT

A detailed history and physical examination are essential to make an accurate diagnosis. This is particularly important when dealing with CPP because the signs and symptoms of many gynecologic and nongynecologic etiologies may overlap (Styer, 2013). Using a formatted, widely accepted questionnaire can be helpful in ensuring that all critical points are covered. The International Pelvic Pain Society provides the Pelvic Pain Assessment Form for this purpose; it can be downloaded at no cost from http://pelvicpain.org/docs/resources /forms/history-and-physical-form-english .aspx and is also available in **Appendix 28-A**. An

alternative pelvic pain assessment form, adapted from the Pelvic Pain Assessment Form, and designed to collect comprehensive subjective data from the woman, is available from the Institute for Women in Pain and can be downloaded at no cost from http://www.instituteforwomeninpain.com /assets/files/Initial%20Questionnaire.pdf. This Initial Female Pelvic Pain Questionnaire is available in **Appendix 28-B**.

History

History is a vital component in accurate evaluation of CPP (Stein, 2013). The approach to assessment and diagnosis of pelvic pain needs to be systematic and detailed for the cause to be identified and an appropriate treatment plan developed. Care must be taken during the first visit to validate the woman's symptoms and acknowledge her agency in the healthcare process. It is important to allow enough time during the visit so that she can tell her story in its entirety. She needs to feel that she has been listened to and heard. However, the most important endpoint to any medical history is the formulation of a comprehensive and detailed differential diagnosis prior to the physical examination (Styer, 2013). The International Pelvic Pain Society and the Institute for Women in Pain provide extensive history intake forms to facilitate this process.

Focused questioning is important for obtaining an accurate history, and active listening is essential. Valuing the woman's description of her pain and validating her feelings are paramount in developing trust and rapport. A holistic approach considers how the pain a woman describes is affecting every facet of her life. The multiple roles most women play are all altered by pain, and obtaining information about how the pain affects the individual woman physically and emotionally, how it impacts her activities of daily living, and how it changes her relationships is important.

The importance of a meticulous health history cannot be overemphasized. A pain history should be taken during the first visit, to include the nature of each pain symptom (i.e., location, radiation, severity, aggravating and alleviating factors); the effects of the menstrual cycle, stress, work, exercise, intercourse, and orgasm on the pain; the context in which pain arose; the social and occupational toll of the pain; and prior or current opioid use (Rapkin & Nathan, 2012; Styer, 2013).

Rapkin and Nathan (2012, p. 488) offer the mnemonic "OLD CAARTS" as an aid for performing a pain history:

O = Onset: When and how did the pain start?

L = Location: Specific location of the pain. Can you put a finger on it?

D = Duration: How long does it last?

C = Characteristics: What is the pain like—cramping, aching, stabbing, burning, tingling, itching, and so on?

A = Alleviating or aggravating factors: What makes the pain better (e.g., medication, position change, heat) and what makes it worse (e.g., specific activity, stress, menstrual cycle)?

A = Associated symptoms: Gynecologic (dyspareunia, dysmenorrhea, abnormal bleeding, discharge, infertility), gastrointestinal (constipation, diarrhea), genitourinary (dysuria, urgency, incontinence), and neurologic (specific nerve involvement).

R = Radiation: Does the pain move to other areas on your body?

T = Temporal: What time of day is the pain worse and better?

S = Severity (on a scale of 1 to 10).

The use of a pain-rating scale may assist the clinician to comprehend the intensity of the woman's pain. Pain-rating scales, such as the numeric-ranking scale, visual-analog scales, and verbal-descriptive scales, allow the woman to identify the severity of her pain. If there is a language barrier related to culture or mental ability, the Wong-Baker FACES pain-rating scale (smile to frown) may be helpful in conveying this information (Ignatavicius & Workman, 2002).

An accurate and nonjudgmental sexual history is very important. Clinicians should not allow heterosexism to blind their objectivity; a woman's partner may be female. Keep in mind that although a woman may believe she is monogamous with one partner, her partner may have other partners. Additionally, a woman may report a monogamous relationship, but fail to mention that it is her third monogamous relationship in the past year. Given these possibilities, it is important to ask about her number of sexual partners and the possibility of her partner having multiple partners.

A detailed obstetric history should be obtained. Pregnancy and childbirth are traumatic events for the musculoskeletal system that may cause damage to the back and pelvis (Styer, 2013). Peripartal risk factors include poor musculoskeletal conditioning, delivery of a large baby, and lumbar lordosis (Styer, 2013). Obtain a detailed obstetric history because pregnancy and vaginal birth can damage neuromuscular structures and have been linked to pelvic floor, symphyseal, and sacroiliac joint pain (Hoffman, 2012). Cesarean birth has been linked to lower abdominal wall pain and adhesions.

The surgical history provides information about the woman's risk for adhesions, peritoneal injuries, infections, and related diagnoses that may be responsible for the pain (e.g., endometriosis). In addition, certain disorders have a tendency to persist or recur; thus information about prior surgeries for endometriosis, adhesive disease, or malignancy should be sought (Hoffman, 2012).

Many studies have documented an association between acute and chronic pelvic pain and abuse (Hart & Lipsky, 2014; Karnath & Breitkopf, 2007). Unrecognized abuse may have serious or even deadly consequences (Hart & Lipsky, 2014). The reason for the association is unknown, and more research on this topic is needed. If the abuse is currently occurring, it is important that the woman be counseled appropriately (see Chapters 13 and 14). Obtaining a careful psychosocial history, then, is critically important.

The evidence also suggests that women with pelvic pain should be screened for depression (Kassab & Rollins, 2011). In Kassab and Rollins's study, women who had chronic pelvic pain were found to have depression more often than their counterparts and experienced significantly more issues with social impairment and decreased quality of life.

The risk of substance abuse among individuals with chronic pain is double that of the general population (Styer, 2013). Always inquire about the use of narcotics, alcohol, and recreational drugs when assessing clients who have chronic pelvic pain. The therapeutic goal is to administer the minimum amount of pain medication to achieve a reasonable therapeutic effect (Styer, 2013). Styer (p. 103) identifies the following key elements of care for women requiring opioid use:

1. A pain diagnosis must be established with a reasonable differential diagnosis.
2. Consider psychological factors.
3. Institute an opioid treatment agreement.
4. Assess pain level and function at each visit.
5. Avoid opioid monotherapy.
6. Monitor compliance with periodic random urine drug screens.
7. Adhere to strict documentation guidelines.
8. For new patients to the practice, obtain all previous records prior to initiating opioid therapy.

Physical Examination

Perhaps the most important aspect of the patient evaluation is the physical examination. The physical examination provides the opportunity for the clinician to connect information collected during the history to a focused examination and discovery of findings (Styer, 2013). This process may provide a good understanding of the underlying cause of CPP. A commonly overlooked facet of the physical examination is sensitivity to the acute and chronic pain that the woman may have endured for years (Styer, 2013). Always obtain baseline vital signs, including blood pressure, temperature, pulse, and respirations, prior to performing the physical examination. If the woman has not had a complete physical examination in the last year, one should be performed during the first visit (see Chapter 6). Because the examination may exacerbate anxiety, stress, and pain for many women, especially if the woman has a history of chronic pelvic pain, be sure to let her know that she has the ability to halt the examination at any time (Hoffman, 2012; Styer, 2013). This approach may allow the woman to recall aspects of the history that may have been previously omitted, and relate this information to real-time physical findings during the physical examination (Styer, 2013).

Proceed with the examination in a slow, careful, and deliberate step-by-step fashion to minimize pain and allow for the woman to relax between steps (Hoffman, 2012; Styer, 2013). Observe the woman's gait, movement, and sitting pose. Women with intraperitoneal pathology or myofascial pain syndromes may compensate for their symptoms by changing their posture or sitting off to one side (Hoffman, 2012; Stein, 2013). Also, musculoskeletal structures may be the site of referred pain from these organs; thus an orthopedic evaluation is important in women with pelvic pain.

Examine the head, neck, cardiac, and respiratory systems to rule out abnormalities. A brief, but succinct neurologic examination, including inspection, palpation, and percussion of the spinal column, can be helpful in ruling out radiculopathy. When the woman is in a supine position, inspect the abdomen, noting any scars, auscultating for bowel sounds, percussing, and palpating for organomegaly. To differentiate abdominal wall pain from visceral sources of pain perform the Carnett test: Ask the woman to raise her head off of the table while she is in the supine position and then have her straight-raise her legs (Beckmann et al., 2014; Rapkin & Nathan, 2012); the clinician then palpates the area. If the woman has tenderness to palpation, the source is most likely abdominal wall pain.

Palpating over the area the woman identifies as the origin of the pain and pain mapping may also aid diagnosis and can be accomplished during this part of the physical examination. Pain mapping enables clients who feel as if they "hurt all over" to identify the location of their pain. It is done by asking the woman to point or specify the exact location of the pain or painful areas. Sometimes it is useful to have the woman use a diagram of the body to identify the locations. It may be necessary to focus on one area at a time and move methodically to ensure that all areas that hurt are identified or mapped. Women who feel as if they hurt all over are often relieved to realize their pain is actually localized and that other areas are not painful. Conscious pain mapping is a technique performed under local anesthesia during laparoscopy. During this procedure, the woman remains awake and can be questioned about her pain (Hoffman, 2012).

One way to improve pain mapping by digital pelvic examination is through use of a tenderness-guided endovaginal ultrasound (EVUS) examination (Yong, Sutton, Suen, & Williams, 2013). This technique entails use of the EVUS probe as an extension of the clinician's digit to palpate difficult-to-reach structures while also imaging the anatomic landmarks to confirm the structure that is being palpated (Yong et al., 2013). EVUS examination is especially useful in making the differential diagnosis of endometriosis—endometriosis is found in approximately 25% of women with CPP (Morelli, Rocca, Venturella, Mocciaro, & Zullo, 2013).

The pelvic examination should begin with visual inspection, making particular note of areas of discoloration, dermatologic disorders, or signs of infection (Stein, 2013). A Q-tip examination using light touch provides evaluation of the sensory and neurologic systems of the perineum (Stein, 2013). During the pelvic examination, pay particular attention to the woman's reaction when the vagina is palpated to observe if she experiences discomfort from pressure along the pelvic floor; this finding may be indicative of myofascial pain syndrome. Tenderness of the urethra or bladder may indicate involvement of the genitourinary system. Pain with deep palpation may indicate endometriosis, whereas cervical motion tenderness is suggestive of PID, adhesions, and other conditions. A rectal examination should also be included in the pelvic examination of a woman with pelvic pain. Guidelines for the pelvic examination are provided in Chapter 6.

Diagnostic Testing

Laboratory testing for women with chronic pelvic pain should include the following elements:

- Complete blood count (CBC)
- Erythrocyte sedimentation rate (ESR)
- Serologic testing for syphilis
- Urinalysis and urine culture (where appropriate)
- Pregnancy testing (if appropriate)
- Vaginal smears or cultures to rule out infection
- Stool guaiac to evaluate gastrointestinal pathology
- Thyroid-stimulating hormone (TSH)

A TSH measurement is performed because thyroid disease affects body functions and may be found in women with bowel or bladder symptoms (Hoffman, 2012).

Historically, the evaluation of pelvic pain in women who were of reproductive and postmenopausal ages was conducted by ultrasound (US). Transvaginal ultrasound is useful for real-time assessment of the pelvis (Styer, 2013). "This modality is most effective for detection of pelvic masses (adnexal, some gastrointestinal tumors, uterine fibroids) as well as characterization of the uterus and adnexa" (Styer, 2013, p. 107). Ultrasound findings may support a diagnosis of PID if evidence of salpingitis is found, or a ruptured cyst if a characteristic ovarian appearance is combined with presence of a small amount of free fluid (Hart & Lipsky, 2014). Ultrasound may be used to examine the appendix, although it is not as reliable as computed tomography (CT) in making a diagnosis of appendicitis (Hart & Lipsky, 2014). The modality of choice for initial imaging remains US, although it is often followed by CT scan. Whereas diffuse and focal adenomyosis and pelvic varices can be identified readily with high-resolution sonography and color Doppler, endometriosis, endometriomas, adhesions, and neoplastic processes are better identified by CT because of this imaging modality's sensitivity (Olson & Schnatz, 2007; Potter & Chandrasekhar, 2008).

Additional imaging studies may be performed if the woman's symptoms indicate the need for them. For example, a barium enema study may be performed in women with bowel symptoms; in contrast, if pelvic congestion is suspected, pelvic venography is the tool of choice (Hoffman, 2012). If urinary symptoms are primarily associated with the pelvic pain, then a cystoscopy is typically advised (Hoffman, 2012). Laparoscopy is considered the gold standard for evaluation of chronic pelvic pain and is used when pelvic pathology cannot be detected by physical examination or other testing; it allows direct visualization and may enable direct treatment of intra-abdominal pathology (Hoffman, 2012).

DIFFERENTIAL DIAGNOSES

Pathology within systems (nongynecologic and gynecologic) needs to be considered when developing a list of differential diagnoses for pelvic pain. The clinician should be mindful that there may be more than one cause of pelvic pain and involvement of more than one body system. **Table 28-1** lists differential diagnoses of pelvic pain organized by system.

Evaluation of the pain must differentiate between acute and chronic etiologies as well as gynecologic and nongynecologic causes (Rapkin &

TABLE 28-1	Differential Diagnoses for Pelvic Pain

Diagnoses of Gynecologic Origin	Nongynecologic Diagnoses
Endometriosis	**Gastrointestinal**
Chronic pelvic inflammatory disease (PID)	Irritable bowel syndrome (IBS)
Dysmenorrhea, primary and secondary	Diverticulitis
Pelvic adhesions	Constipation
Pelvic congestion	Bowel obstruction
Mittelschmerz	Appendicitis
Vulvodynia	Colon cancer
Uterine prolapse	Gastroenteritis
Ovarian cyst	**Genitourinary**
Ovarian remnant syndrome	Interstitial cystitis
Adenomyosis	Urinary tract infection
Fibroids	Urinary retention
Ovarian cancer	Renal calculi
Cervical cancer	Pyelonephritis
Torsion of adnexa	Ureteral lithiasis
Tubo-ovarian abscess	Bladder neoplasm
Uterine fibroids	**Musculoskeletal**
Ectopic pregnancy	Scoliosis
Abortion, threatened or incomplete	Radiculopathy
	Arthritis
	Herniated disk
	Hernia
	Abdominal wall hematoma
	Other
	Aortic aneurysm
	Pelvic thrombophlebitis
	Acute porphyria
	Abdominal angina
	Psychiatric, depression
	Somatization disorder
	Prior or current physical or sexual abuse
	Substance abuse

Data from Berek, J. (2012). *Berek and Novak's gynecology* (15th ed.). Philadelphia, PA: Lippincott, Williams & Wilkins; Hart, D., & Lipsky, A. (2014). Acute pelvic pain in women. In J. Marks, R. Hockberger, & R. Walls (Eds.), *Rosen's emergency medicine: Concepts and practice* (8th ed., pp. 266–272). Philadelphia, PA: Elsevier Saunders; Styer, A. K. (2013). Gynecologic etiologies of chronic pelvic pain. In A. Bailey & C. Bernstein (Eds.), *Pain in women: A clinical guide* (pp. 95–141). Boston, MA: Harvard Medical School.

Nathan, 2012). **Table 28-2** lists common differential diagnoses related to acute pelvic pain of gynecologic origin, and **Table 28-3** lists common differential diagnoses of acute pelvic pain that are not related to a gynecologic problem.

After all other causes of pelvic pain are ruled out, psychogenic pain needs to be considered as a possibility. Neis and Neis (2009) identified that nearly 60% of women referred with chronic pelvic pain were found to have psychiatric problems.

TABLE 28-2	Acute Pelvic Pain of Gynecologic Origin (Noncyclic): Common Differential Diagnoses and Signs, Symptoms, and Location of Pain	
Condition	**Symptoms**	**Signs**
Abortion: threatened, inevitable, or incomplete (see also Chapter 7)	Crampy, intermittent pain that is in the midline or bilateral lower abdomen	Pregnancy test usually positive Vaginal bleeding usually present If infection: elevated WBC and ESR
Ectopic pregnancy (see also Chapter 7)	Unilateral crampy pain that is often continuous	Usually vaginal bleeding is present May have very slight elevation of temperature ESR and WBC may be slightly elevated Serum β-hCG is positive US may help with diagnosis PE may reveal an adnexal mass
Pelvic inflammatory disease (see also Chapter 21)	Lower abdominal, uterine adnexal, and cervical motion tenderness Pain is often described as dull or achy and may radiate to back or upper thighs May have nausea and vomiting due to pain	Low-grade fever Purulent discharge Elevated WBC Elevated ESR
Ovarian cysts (see also Chapter 27)	Pain is mild to moderate and self-limiting unless it is due to a hemorrhagic corpus luteum cyst, which can result in significant blood loss and hemoperitoneum Onset of pain is usually sudden and midcycle Note: corpus luteum cyst is the most prone to rupture and mimics ectopic pregnancy	Hypovolemia only if there is hemoperitoneum Most critical sign is significant abdominal tenderness, often associated with rebound tenderness due to peritoneal irritation May be able to palpate a mass during the pelvic examination if the cyst is still leaking and not entirely ruptured
Adnexal torsion	Results in ischemia and rapid onset of acute pelvic pain Pain is usually severe and constant unless torsion is intermittent, in which case the pain will come and go Pain may worsen with lifting, exercise, and intercourse	Tender abdomen with PE and localized rebound tenderness in lower abdominal quadrants Most important sign: large pelvic mass on PE Mild temperature elevation Mild elevated WBC

Condition	Symptoms	Signs
Uterine fibroids (see also Chapters 25 and 27)	Often asymptomatic, can have increased uterine bleeding, pelvic pressure or pain, and dyspareunia (pain with intercourse) Acute pain with torsion or rupture Note: may be confused with subacute salpingo-oophoritis	Palpation of abdomen reveals mass(es) arising from uterus May note tenderness with palpation May have elevated temperature and WBC
Endometriosis (see also Chapters 24 and 27)	Often asymptomatic Most common symptoms are dysmenorrhea, deep dyspareunia, and sacral backache during menses	PE findings may be absent or limited Laparoscopy with biopsy is the gold standard for diagnosis

Abbreviations: ESR, erythrocyte sedimentation rate; hCG, human chorionic gonadotropin; PE, physical examination; US, ultrasound; WBC, white blood cell.

Data from Berek, J. (2012). *Berek and Novak's gynecology* (15th ed.). Philadelphia, PA: Lippincott, Williams & Wilkins; Dunphy, L. M., Winland-Brown, J. E., Porter, B. O., & Thomas, D. J. (2015). *Primary care: The art and science of advanced practice nursing* (4th ed.). Philadelphia, PA: F.A. Davis Company; Hart, D., & Lipsky, A. (2014). Acute pelvic pain in women. In J. Marks, R. Hockberger, & R. Walls (Eds.), *Rosen's emergency medicine: Concepts and practice* (8th ed., pp. 266–272). Philadelphia, PA: Elsevier Saunders; Hoffman, B. L. (2012). Pelvic pain. In B. L. Hoffman, J. O. Schorge, J. I. Schaffer, L. M. Halvorson, K. D. Bradshaw, F. G. Cunningham, & L. E. Calver (Eds.), *Williams gynecology* (2nd ed., pp. 304–332). New York, NY: McGraw-Hill Medical; Kruszka, P. S., & Kruszka, S. J. (2010). Evaluation of acute pelvic pain in women. *American Family Physician, 82*(2), 141–147; Lentz, G., Lobo, R., Gershenson, D. M., & Katz, V. (2012). *Comprehensive gynecology* (6th ed.). Philadelphia, PA: Mosby Elsevier; Stein, S. L. (2013). Chronic pelvic pain. *Gastroenterology Clinics of North America, 42,* 785–800.

TABLE **28-3**	Acute Pelvic Pain of Nongynecologic Origin: Common Differential Diagnoses, Signs, Symptoms, and Location of Pain

Condition (System)	Symptoms	Signs	Comment
Appendicitis (GI)	Diffuse abdominal pain, generally periumbilical Anorexia, nausea, vomiting Pain usually in RLQ (McBurney's point) Chills	May have low-grade fever High fever if ruptured Chills Rebound tenderness Positive psoas sign[a] Positive obturator sign[b] Rovsing's sign[c] elicited May observe leukocyte shift to left	Most common source of acute pelvic pain in women May be confused with gastroenteritis, pelvic inflammatory disease, urinary tract infection, or ruptured ovarian cyst

(continues)

| TABLE 28-3 | Acute Pelvic Pain of Nongynecologic Origin: Common Differential Diagnoses, Signs, Symptoms, and Location of Pain (*continued*) | | |

Condition (System)	Symptoms	Signs	Comment
Diverticulitis (GI)	Often asymptomatic May experience abdominal bloating, constipation, and diarrhea Severe LLQ pain	Distended abdomen with LLQ tenderness with palpation Localized rebound tenderness May palpate a doughy, mobile mass in the LLQ Hypoactive bowel sounds May see elevated WBC	Mimics IBS Fistulas can occur Note: diverticulitis can present with perforations or abscess that produce peritonitis
Intestinal obstruction (GI)	Colicky abdominal pain Abdominal distention Vomiting Constipation and obstipation Higher and acute obstruction presents with early vomiting Colonic obstruction presents with greater degree of abdominal distention and obstipation	Significant abdominal distention Bowel sounds are abnormal: at onset they are high pitched during pain and later will decrease and may be absent due to ischemia Elevated WBC and fever are noted as the condition progresses	
Irritable bowel syndrome (GI)	Acute abdominal pain (may also cause chronic pelvic pain) Bloating Urgency of defecation Diarrhea Constipation	Abdominal pain with palpation May note blood with stool and/or rectal bleeding	IBS is the most commonly identified functional bowel disorder It is diagnosed more often in women than in men
Gastroenteritis (GI)	Vomiting Diarrhea Abdominal cramping and pain	May have systemic toxicity such as fever and tachycardia Marked abdominal tenderness with palpation	Causes generally are viral or bacterial Usually self-limited

Condition (System)	Symptoms	Signs	Comment
Ureteral lithiasis (GU)	Severe, colicky pain in suprapubic area and in pelvis Urinary frequency Dysuria Nausea, vomiting	Hematuria Flank and costovertebral angle pain	Can mimic ectopic pregnancy
Cystitis (GU)	Lower abdominal or pelvic pain usually midline Dysuria, urinary urgency and frequency	Urine dipstick positive for leukocyte esterase or nitrite	See Chapter 22
Abdominal wall hernia (MU)	Sharp pain sometimes radiates to lower back	Pain intensity is related to position Abdominal tenderness increases when abdominal wall is tensed	

Abbreviations: GI, gastrointestinal; GU, genitourinary; IBS, irritable bowel syndrome; LLQ, left lower quadrant; MU, musculoskeletal; RLQ, right lower quadrant; WBC, white blood cells.

[a] Psoas sign: Passively lift the woman's thigh against the examiner's hand above the knee. A positive sign is pain in the RLQ.
[b] Obturator sign: The woman passively flexes her right hip and knee and internally rotates her right leg at the hip. A positive sign is when the acute pain travels from the periumbilical region to the RLQ.
[c] Rovsing's sign: Pressing the LLQ produces pain in the RLQ when pressure is released.

Data from Berek, J. (2012). *Berek and Novak's gynecology* (15th ed.). Philadelphia, PA: Lippincott, Williams & Wilkins; Dunphy, L. M., Winland-Brown, J. E., Porter, B. O., & Thomas, D. J. (2015). *Primary care: The art and science of advanced practice nursing* (4th ed.). Philadelphia, PA: F. A. Davis; Hart, D., & Lipsky, A. (2014). Acute pelvic pain in women. In J. Marks, R. Hockberger, & R. Walls (Eds.), *Rosen's emergency medicine: Concepts and practice* (8th ed., pp. 266–272). Philadelphia, PA: Elsevier Saunders; Hoffman, B. L. (2012). Pelvic pain. In B. L. Hoffman, J. O. Schorge, J. I. Schaffer, L. M. Halvorson, K. D. Bradshaw, F. G. Cunningham, & L. E. Calver (Eds.), *Williams gynecology* (2nd ed., pp. 304–332). New York, NY: McGraw-Hill Medical; Kruszka, P. S., & Kruszka, S. J. (2010). Evaluation of acute pelvic pain in women. *American Family Physician, 82*(2), 141–147; Lentz, G., Lobo, R., Gershenson, D. M., & Katz, V. (2012). *Comprehensive gynecology* (6th ed.). Philadelphia, PA: Mosby Elsevier; Merlin, M. A., Shah, C. N., & Shiroff, A. M. (2010). Evidence-based appendicitis: The initial work-up. *Postgraduate Medicine, 122*(3), 189–195.

Psychiatric and psychosocial disorders may include substance abuse, depression, physical and emotional abuse, somatization, and hypochondriasis (Champaneria, Daniels, Raza, Pattison, & Khan, 2012; Demir, Ozcimen, & Oral, 2012; Styer, 2013). It is important that all other causes of the pain be ruled out first as historically women presenting with pelvic pain were too often told, "It is in your head," and no further assessment took place.

Common Noncyclic Gynecologic Causes of Chronic Pelvic Pain

The most common gynecologic-related causes of chronic pelvic pain identified by laparoscopy are endometriosis (see Chapter 26) and adhesions (Rapkin & Nathan, 2012). Other common causes include ovarian remnant, retained ovary syndrome, pelvic congestion syndrome, pelvic relaxation causing prolapse of gynecologic organs (e.g., uterine prolapse; see Chapter 25), subacute salpingo-oophoritis (see Chapter 20), cancer of gynecologic origin (see Chapter 27), and ovarian hyperstimulation syndrome (OHSS).

Pelvic adhesions are coarse bands of tissue that connect organs to other organs or to the abdominal wall in places where there should be no connection. Adhesions can be caused by previous surgeries, infection, or endometriosis (Hoffman, 2012;

Rapkin & Nathan, 2012; Styer, 2013). They may be the etiology for infertility, dyspareunia, and bowel obstruction (Styer, 2013). Currently, the causal role of adhesions in pelvic pain is unknown. The myriad of symptoms range from mild intermittent abdominopelvic pain to constant pain with gastrointestinal (constipation, bloating, dyschezia), gynecologic (dyspareunia, dysmenorrhea, focal lateral or central pelvic and adnexal pain), and musculoskeletal symptoms (abdominal wall tenderness) (Styer, 2013). If symptoms are exacerbated during specific portions of the menstrual cycle (e.g., menses, luteal phase, follicular phase), then medical therapy should be considered with use of hormonal suppression of the cycle (Styer, 2013). If symptoms are constant, then use of nonsteroidal anti-inflammatory drugs (NSAIDs) and other forms of analgesics should be considered, with possible referral to a pain specialist (Styer, 2013).

Surgical lysis of adhesions may lead to further development of adhesions and increases the risk of visceral injury (Rapkin & Nathan, 2012; Styer, 2013). Therefore, surgical lysis of adhesions is not recommended unless there is evidence of bowel obstruction or infertility (Rapkin & Nathan, 2012). If surgical lysis of adhesions is performed, barrier materials such as oxidized regenerated cellulose or hyaluronic acid with carboxymethylcellulose can be utilized to prevent renewed adhesion formation (Rapkin & Nathan, 2012). In a small study by Cheong, Reading, Bailey, Sadek, Ledger, and Li (2014), women who underwent surgical adhesiolysis did demonstrate significant improvements in pain scores, physical well-being, and emotional well-being. Unfortunately, recruitment of participants to this study was stopped before a statistically powered sample size could be reached.

Table 28-4 summarizes diagnosis and treatment recommendations related to pelvic adhesions.

Ovarian remnant syndrome and ovarian retention syndrome are two separate etiologies of chronic pelvic pain. They produce almost the same symptoms and are diagnosed and managed similarly. Ovarian remnant syndrome occurs when some of the ovarian tissue is left behind after an oophorectomy, whereas ovarian retention syndrome occurs when an ovary is purposely left behind after hysterectomy (Hoffman, 2012; Rapkin & Nathan, 2012; Styer, 2013). **Table 28-4** summarizes diagnosis and treatment recommendations related to these conditions.

Ovarian hyperstimulation syndrome (OHSS) can result from treatment for infertility. OHSS refers to a combination of ovarian enlargement caused by multiple ovarian cysts, whose rupture may create a shift of fluids from the intravascular spaces. This can potentially become a life-threatening complication of ovulation induction.

Mild OHSS is a self-limiting disease, and treatment should be conservative and aimed at symptoms. Medical therapy suffices for most women (Horwitz, Pundi, & Blankstein, 2011). Nevertheless, mild OHSS can evolve into moderate or severe disease, particularly if conception occurs (Horwitz et al., 2011). Symptoms of increasing severity include enlarging abdominal girth, acute weight gain, and abdominal discomfort. Treatment of moderate to severe disease includes careful fluid management particularly directed at maintenance of intravascular blood volume. After a few days, third-space fluid is absorbed into intravascular spaces, hemoconcentration reverses, and natural dieresis occurs (Horwitz et al., 2011). Intravenous fluids can be discontinued as oral intake of fluids becomes adequate. Complete resolution usually occurs 10 to 14 days after the initial onset of symptoms (Horwitz et al., 2011). Surgery is required in extreme cases, such as in the case of a ruptured cyst, ovarian torsion, or internal hemorrhage. Aggressive palpation of the abdomen can precipitate follicular rupture and should be avoided if OHSS is suspected.

Pelvic congestion syndrome is typically seen in women of reproductive age (Rapkin & Nathan, 2012; Stein, 2013). It occurs when uterine blood vessels remain chronically dilated, creating reflux of blood in the ovarian veins, which then causes pelvic vascular congestion (Styer, 2013). The pathophysiology involved is unclear, but the syndrome is believed to result from a malfunction or absence of functional valves within ovarian veins, resulting in retrograde blood flow and venous dilation (Styer, 2013). **Table 28-4** summarizes diagnosis and treatment recommendations related to pelvic congestion syndrome.

TABLE 28-4 Common Noncyclic Gynecologic Causes of Chronic Pelvic Pain: Signs, Symptoms, Diagnosis, and Management

Condition	Symptoms	Signs	Diagnosis	Management
Adhesions	Lower abdominal or pelvic pain that occurs or increases when the peritoneum or organ serosa is stretched Dyspareunia	May elicit abdominal pain with light palpation Decreased motility of pelvic organs Adnexal enlargement	Laparoscopy is the diagnostic tool of choice if somatic causes are ruled out and the psychosocial evaluation is negative	Surgical lysis of adhesions only after a thorough evaluation and failed medical therapy
Ovarian remnant syndrome; ovarian retention syndrome	Lateral pelvic pain described as sharp and stabbing or dull and not radiating May have dyspareunia, constipation, or flank pain May have genitourinary and/or gastrointestinal symptoms that accompany the pelvic pain	Pelvic mass identified during bimanual examination May observe that the vulva and vagina remain in a persistent estrogenized state	US Note: US may be improved by treating the woman with clomiphene citrate (Clomid) 100 mg for 5–10 days prior to the US to stimulate follicular development	Initial treatment with danazol or high-dose progestins may be helpful in some cases GnRH agonist may help but cannot be used for long-term therapy Surgical excision is often required
Pelvic congestion syndrome	Bilateral lower abdominal and back pain Dysmenorrhea Dyspareunia Abnormal uterine bleeding Chronic fatigue Irritable bowel syndrome	Bulky feeling to uterus when palpated during the bimanual examination Ovaries may be enlarged and there may be many functional cysts on the ovaries Uterus, parametria, and uterosacral ligaments are tender to touch	Transuterine venography is the primary method used for diagnosis Other methods include the following: • Ultrasound • Magnetic resonance imaging • Laparoscopy	Begin with the least invasive measures Hormonal measures include progestin or GnRH agonist administration Ovarian vein embolization or ligation Hysterectomy with bilateral salpingo-oophorectomy should be the last resort

Abbreviations: GnRH, gonadotropic-releasing hormone; US, ultrasound.
Data from Berek, J. (2012). *Berek and Novak's gynecology* (15th ed.). Philadelphia, PA: Lippincott, Williams & Wilkins; Hoffman, B. L. (2012). Pelvic pain. In B. L. Hoffman, J. O. Schorge, J. I. Schaffer, L. M. Halvorson, K. D. Bradshaw, F. G. Cunningham, & L. E. Calver (Eds.), *Williams gynecology* (2nd ed., pp. 304–332). New York, NY: McGraw-Hill Medical; Lentz, G., Lobo, R., Gershenson, D. M., & Katz, V. (2012). *Comprehensive gynecology* (6th ed.). Philadelphia, PA: Mosby Elsevier; Stein, S. L. (2013). Chronic pelvic pain. *Gastroenterology Clinics of North America, 42,* 785–800; Styer, A. K. (2013). Gynecologic etiologies of chronic pelvic pain. In A. Bailey & C. Bernstein (Eds.), *Pain in women: A clinical guide* (pp. 95–141). Boston, MA: Harvard Medical School; Tu, F. F., Hahn, D., & Steege, J. F. (2010). Pelvic congestion syndrome–associated pelvic pain: A systematic review of diagnosis and management. *Obstetrical & Gynecological Survey, 65*(5), 332–340.

Common Nongynecologic Causes of Chronic Pelvic Pain

In a number of instances, the cause of chronic pelvic pain is not gynecologic in origin. The more common nongynecologic causes are addressed here because they should be considered when the clinician is developing a list of differential diagnoses for chronic pelvic pain (see **Table 28-1**). An in-depth discussion is beyond the scope of this text; instead, the reader is referred to the appropriate references at the end of this chapter.

GASTROINTESTINAL CAUSES OF PELVIC PAIN

Irritable bowel syndrome (IBS) is the most common functional gastrointestinal disorder, accounting for as many as 60% of referrals to the gynecologist for complaints of chronic pelvic pain; women who have had a hysterectomy for chronic pelvic pain are twice as likely to have IBS (Rapkin & Nathan, 2012; Shin & Howard, 2011; Stein, 2013; Styer, 2013;). In a study conducted by Tachawiwat and Cheewadhanaraks (2012), the researchers found that approximately 20% of women with varying degrees of CPP also had IBS.

IBS is a diagnosis of exclusion (Stein, 2013). Other causes of bowel dysfunction must first be ruled out, such as Crohn's disease, diverticulitis, sprue, lactose allergy, and chronic appendicitis. IBS is characterized by a recurrent abdominal pain or discomfort at least 3 days a month for the past 3 months, and is usually accompanied by constipation or diarrhea (American College of Obstetricians and Gynecologists, 2004, reaffirmed 2010; Shin & Howard, 2011; Styer, 2013).

Clinical features of IBS include shifting abdominal pain accompanied by constipation or diarrhea, or both. Bloating, nausea, and vomiting are also common symptoms. The pain may be identified in one quadrant of the abdomen but then relocate during the next attack. Typically, defecation provides relief from the pain. Although the exact etiology of IBS is unknown, its cause is believed to involve dysregulation in interactions between the central nervous system and the enteric nervous system (Hoffman, 2012). This brain–gut dysfunction my ultimately disrupt the GI mucosal immune response, intestinal motility and permeability, and visceral sensitivity (Hoffman, 2012).

The woman's history is critical to the diagnosis of IBS because the diagnosis is based on the symptoms. The Rome criteria are used to categorize the symptoms and make the diagnosis. These criteria constitute a system developed to classify functional gastrointestinal disorders (FGIDs)—that is, disorders of the digestive system in which symptoms cannot be explained by the presence of structural or tissue abnormality—based on clinical symptoms (Rome Foundation, 2015). The Rome III Diagnostic Criteria for IBS include the following findings: recurrent abdominal pain or discomfort that has occurred for at least 3 days each month for the past 3 months and has been accompanied by at least two of the following: (1) improvement with defecation, (2) onset associated with a change in frequency of stool, and (3) onset associated with a change in form (appearance) of stool.

During physical examination of the abdomen, areas of hard feces may be felt in the transverse and descending colon, and the rectal examination may reveal the presence of a hard, lumpy stool if constipation is one of the symptoms. Women with IBS often experience bloating and general intestinal irritability. Passage of mucus rectally is common. Less frequently, women with IBS may experience blood in their stools, so guaiac testing is important. Other gastrointestinal causes of pelvic pain to keep in mind (although not as common as IBS) include chronic appendicitis, adhesions from previous bowel surgery, and abdominal wall hernia, including umbilical hernias.

Management of IBS depends on the symptoms and the presence of any comorbidities. Often psychologic support is helpful, especially education regarding stress reduction (Rapkin & Nathan, 2012; Solnik & Munro, 2014). A diet that eliminates carbohydrates—specifically, fructose, lactose, and sorbitol—is recommended (Solnik & Munro, 2014). Many clinicians recommend an increase in fiber consumed as part of the diet, although there is no evidence to support this recommendation.

In general, medications for IBS are aimed at the predominant symptoms (Hoffman, 2012). Medications to decrease anxiety have been used with some success. Low-dose tricyclic antidepressants (TCAs), selective serotonin reuptake inhibitors

(SSRIs), and serotonin/norepinephrine reuptake inhibitors (SNRIs) have all been used successfully in the treatment of IBS (Rapkin & Nathan, 2012). Other medications are prescribed to treat the symptoms of diarrhea and constipation. Antispasmodics such as dicyclomine (Bentyl) and hyoscyamine (Levsin) have been used to decrease abdominal pain due to spasm (Hoffman, 2012; Rapkin & Nathan, 2012).

Musculoskeletal disorders have not been routinely considered as causes of pelvic pain, but their importance is increasingly becoming recognized. For example, myofascial pain originating from trigger points in skeletal muscle has been identified as the cause in some cases of pelvic pain (Rapkin & Nathan, 2012; Shin & Howard, 2011). The incidence of myofascial disease is unknown. Testing for Carnett's sign assists in making the diagnosis and identifying the trigger points (Rapkin & Nathan, 2012). Once these sites have been identified, they can be injected with local anesthetic—a technique that has been shown to bring relief of the symptoms.

Urologic causes of chronic pelvic pain, such as interstitial cystitis (see Chapter 21), occur more often in women than in men. Most individuals diagnosed with this condition are between 40 and 60 years of age (Rapkin & Nathan, 2012). Cystoscopy findings of petechiae or decreased bladder capacity (less than 350 mL) are considered diagnostic for interstitial cystitis (American College of Obstetricians and Gynecologists, 2004, reaffirmed 2010). Symptoms include severe urinary frequency and pain, nocturia, and dysuria, in the absence of infection (Shin & Howard, 2011). Hematuria may also be present. Pain is frequently noted in the suprapubic area, lower back, or buttock, and 51% of women also complain of dyspareunia (Stein, 2013). Anterior pain that occurs when palpating the vaginal wall over the border of the bladder is suggestive of interstitial cystitis. Diagnosis of this disorder is made based on symptoms and findings on cystoscopy. The etiology of interstitial cystitis is unknown; thus its management is empirical. Diet changes, stress reduction, and behavior changes are often suggested, and the woman is encouraged to do pelvic floor exercises, which sometimes bring relief of urge frequency.

Urethral syndrome is associated with incomplete emptying of the bladder and burning during urination, especially after intercourse (Stein, 2013). Its etiology is uncertain but is thought to involve noninfectious, stenotic, or fibrous changes in the urethra, often associated with multiparity, delivery without episiotomy, and general pelvic relaxation (Rapkin & Nathan, 2012; Stein, 2013). Diagnosis is made by exclusion. For this reason, a clean-catch or catheterized urine specimen should be ordered to rule out urinary tract infection. Sometimes sterile pyuria is present; if it is, a course of doxycycline or erythromycin is helpful (Rapkin & Nathan, 2012). A trial of local estrogen therapy is suggested, though if there is no improvement after 2 months, urethral dilation is a consideration (Rapkin & Nathan, 2012).

MANAGEMENT

Nonpharmacologic Treatment

CPP can be a debilitating condition that is difficult to diagnose and treat (Shin & Howard, 2011). There are many possibilities for the source of the pain, which exhibit varying degrees of causality (Shin & Howard, 2011). It is very important the clinicians understand that even a distinct diagnosis does not ensure that treatment will be curative; indeed, recurrence of CPP is common. Awareness of the many causative possibilities, formulation of a differential diagnosis, and initiating appropriate treatment strategies will ensure the best possible outcomes for women with CPP.

The treatment options discussed in this section focus on gynecologic causes of chronic pelvic pain. Enlisting the woman's input in developing her treatment plan and encouraging her to take an active role in and feel ownership of the plan are encouraged and often critical to the success of the management plan. Treatment needs to be comprehensive and may include both pharmacologic and complementary approaches. The treatment plan is most often dictated by the diagnosis. If no pathology is identified, however, treatment is aimed at relieving the dominant symptoms (Hoffman, 2012).

Exercise and physical therapy have been shown to be helpful in mitigating CPP but require a specialized physiotherapist for initial evaluation to determine an appropriate plan (Bruckenthal, 2011). Physical therapy activities can restore and maintain tissue and joint flexibility, improve posture and body mechanics, restore strength and coordination, reduce nervous system irritability, and restore function (Rapkin & Nathan, 2012). Results from a study conducted by Bedaiwy, Patterson, and Mahajan (2013) indicate that pelvic floor physical therapy is an effective treatment for myofascial pelvic pain. The women in this study who completed the entire course of physical therapy had a significant improvement in pelvic pain.

Both aerobic exercises and nonaerobic exercises, such as weight lifting, have shown positive results. Determining which type of exercise a woman is likely to do and encouraging that activity may be helpful in reducing the severity of the pain, especially in cases where no known cause can be found.

Pharmacologic Treatment

Pharmacologic treatment for chronic pelvic pain frequently begins with an oral analgesic such as acetaminophen (Tylenol) or NSAIDs, and then moves to both nonselective and the cyclooxygenase 2 (COX-2) inhibitors (American College of Obstetricians and Gynecologists, 2004, reaffirmed 2010; Hoffman, 2012; Styer, 2013). If pain relief is not satisfactory with these options, the next pharmacologic agent to consider is a mild opioid such as codeine or hydrocodone, although use of opioid therapy in individuals with chronic pain is controversial (Hoffman, 2012; Rapkin & Nathan, 2012). Risk of addiction with these drugs has been shown to be low in women with chronic pain (American College of Obstetricians and Gynecologists, 2004, reaffirmed 2010). If the pain persists, stronger opioids such as morphine or fentanyl can be considered, although close and regular surveillance is important with these agents (Rapkin & Nathan, 2012).

Hormonal treatment offers another alternative, and several options are available. Combined oral contraceptives (COCs) are useful in providing relief from primary dysmenorrhea and endometriosis (American College of Obstetricians and Gynecologists, 2004, reaffirmed 2010; Hoffman, 2012). The gonadotropin-releasing hormone (GnRH) agonist goserelin may be helpful in reducing pelvic pain from endometriosis and dyspareunia (American

College of Obstetricians and Gynecologists, 2004, reaffirmed 2010; Morelli et al., 2013). Progestogen therapy can be useful in treating chronic pelvic pain that results from endometriosis and pelvic congestion syndrome (American College of Obstetricians and Gynecologists, 2004, reaffirmed 2010).

If the chronic pelvic pain is neuropathic in origin, then tricyclic antidepressants may be helpful. These agents are also useful in treating the depression that often accompanies chronic pain. Amitriptyline (Elavil) and its metabolite nortriptyline (Pamelor) have well-documented efficacy in the treatment of both neuropathic and non-neuropathic pain (Hoffman, 2012; Lindsay & Farrell, 2015; Taverner, 2014).

The clinician may also have to consider combining drugs that work via differing mechanisms of action to increase pain relief. For example, an NSAID and an opioid may be prescribed as dual therapy, particularly if inflammation is present (Hoffman, 2012). Tramadol is good alternative to opioid analgesia (Lindsay & Farrell, 2015).

Transcutaneous electrical nerve stimulation (TENS) can be useful for treatment of localized or regional chronic pelvic pain. TENS therapy involves placement of electrodes near nerve pathways; the electrodes deliver electrical impulses that may help to control or alleviate some types of pain.

Surgical Treatment

Surgical intervention may be necessary in some women with CPP and has been shown to be helpful in reducing CPP that is unrelieved by any other measure. When endometriosis is present, excision or laser ablation of the endometrial tissue may be performed, although these procedures have varying success rates (American College of Obstetricians and Gynecologists, 2004, reaffirmed 2010). Presacral neurectomy has been useful in treating CPP associated with dysmenorrhea after other treatment methods have failed.

Hysterectomy is, of course, a last resort; this option should be considered only after other methods have failed. If the woman is of reproductive age, every attempt should be made to treat her pain with nonsurgical methods before considering hysterectomy. Although 19% of hysterectomies are performed for treatment of pelvic pain, 30% of the women seen in primary care clinics have already undergone a hysterectomy without relief of pelvic pain symptoms, and 5% may experience worsening pain (Lamvu, 2011; Rapkin & Nathan, 2012). An interprofessional approach to pelvic pain treatment with a team that includes a gynecologist, physical therapist, and psychologist has been shown to reduce the frequency of hysterectomy and other surgical interventions as management for pelvic pain symptoms (Ghosh & Ojha, 2011; Lamvu, 2011; Rapkin & Nathan, 2012).

Brazilian researchers Silva et al. (2011) found that of the 147 women presenting with CPP, 97 reported the CPP was a result of abdominal surgery. In more than 40% of those cases, the abdominal surgery was a cesarean section.

A study by Gyang, Feranee, Patel, and Lamvu (2014) discovered that CPP after reconstructive pelvic surgery with transvaginal mesh occurs in as many as 30% of women. Women with a preoperative history of CPP should be carefully evaluated and counseled for vaginal mesh placement. A combination treatment regimen consisting of medication and physical therapy should be attempted.

Psychotherapy should always be considered for a woman with chronic pelvic pain. Physical and sexual abuse is a significant cause of pelvic pain, and as many as 50% of women with chronic pelvic pain have experienced either physical or sexual abuse, or both (American College of Obstetricians and Gynecologists, 2004, reaffirmed 2010). Psychotherapies found to be useful include cognitive therapy, operant conditioning, and behavioral modification (American College of Obstetricians and Gynecologists, 2004, reaffirmed 2010).

If an infection has been confirmed as the source of chronic pelvic pain, antibiotics should be prescribed. The type and length of antibiotic treatment often depend on culture and sensitivity results from the infectious source(s).

Alternative and Complementary Treatment

"Caring for women with CPP is best approached in a holistic manner that investigates all of the potential sources of pain affecting the mind, body, and spirit" (Abercrombie & Learman, 2012, p. 676). Ideally, the clinician should offer a wide range of treatment modalities that address the physical and psychosocial sources of pain, with the clinician filling the coordinating role for the various therapies (Abercrombie & Learman, 2012).

Alternative and complementary therapies are now much more widely accepted and available within developed countries. It is not unusual for even small towns to hold yoga and Tai Chi classes. Nontraditional therapies for treatment of CPP include acupuncture, biofeedback, transcutaneous nerve stimulation, and herbal and nutritional supplements (Styer, 2013). Pain causes muscular contraction; therefore, techniques that relax muscles may help to reduce some types of chronic pelvic pain. Studies indicate that both acupuncture and acupressure have promise in relieving chronic pelvic pain (Cho & Hwang, 2010; Smith, Zhu, He, & Song, 2011). Knowing what is available in the community and talking with the woman to gain an understanding of what she would favor are important parts of the multifaceted approach needed to resolve symptomatology. In turn, the woman needs to be receptive to trying these measures to obtain any degree of effectiveness.

Some clinicians have used herbal, nutritional, and other forms of complementary therapy for the treatment of pelvic pain; however, the evidence base for these treatments is lacking (American College of Obstetricians and Gynecologists, 2004, reaffirmed 2010). Although these alternatives to allopathic procedures may hold promise in the future, there are no current evidence-based recommendations for their use.

When to Refer

In many cases, CPP involves clinical overlap of gynecologic, gastrointestinal, urologic, musculoskeletal, and psychological disorders. Consequently, it is imperative that the clinician perform a comprehensive history and physical examination to determine a precise differential diagnosis and effective treatment. At times, an effective treatment plan may include referral to an appropriate specialist in a gynecologic or nongynecologic arena (**Table 28-3**).

Women with CPP have higher incidences of physical and psychological abuse, drug abuse, and alcohol abuse than women without CPP

(Champaneria et al., 2012). Consequently, psychological referrals should be considered equally as important as medical and surgical referrals.

For many women, CPP and sexuality are inextricably linked. Women must be helped to find a new level of normalcy to incorporate pleasure into their lives, despite living with CPP (Howard, 2012). Sexuality is important to relationships, self-image, and quality of life. Helping a women to adjust sexually is a way to effect change, even if the CPP is resistant to treatment. Turning the focus to sexual adjustment can provide a woman with a welcome diversion in coping with the discomfort of CPP. Offering limited information about common concerns can be accomplished through use of resources such as relevant research, books, articles, websites, and referrals to support groups; such information can provide a sense of normalcy for the woman with CPP. Clinicians do not need to become sexuality experts to make a difference—they can make referrals to trained sexuality counselors if necessary (Howard, 2012).

Current and Emergent Evidence for Practice

Recommendations based on limited or inconsistent scientific evidence (Level B) include using GnRH agonists to treat chronic pelvic pain that is not caused by endometriosis or IBS. These agents are often tried only because they have been shown to be effective in treating pelvic pain associated with endometriosis; there is no scientific evidence to support their use for relief of long-standing chronic pelvic pain. Other Level B treatments that the American College of Obstetricians and Gynecologists (2004, reaffirmed 2010, p. 11) suggests for consideration include the following:

- Surgical adhesiolysis for adhesions other than bowel adhesions
- Hysterectomy to treat chronic pelvic pain associated with gynecologic tract symptoms
- Sacral nerve stimulation
- Various physical therapies
- Nutritional supplementation with vitamin B_1 or magnesium for pain associated with dysmenorrhea
- Injection of trigger points of the abdominal wall, vagina, and sacrum with local anesthetic

- Treatment of abdominal trigger points by application of magnets to the trigger points
- Acupuncture, acupressure, and transcutaneous nerve stimulation for treatment of pain related to primary dysmenorrhea

Recommendations identified by the American College of Obstetricians and Gynecologists (2004, reaffirmed 2010, p. 11) that are based primarily on consensus and expert opinion (Level C) include the following:

- A detailed history and physical examination as the basis for differential diagnoses
- Antidepressants
- Opioid analgesics

PATIENT EDUCATION

The International Pelvic Pain Society provides a chronic pelvic pain patient education booklet (included in **Appendix 28-C**) that can be downloaded at no cost from http://pelvicpain.org/docs/patients/basic-chronic-pelvic-pain.aspx.

SPECIAL CONSIDERATIONS

Adolescents

Pelvic pain in adolescents is usually gynecologic in origin, but nongynecologic sources should also be considered (Trotman & Gomez-Lobo, 2013). Common causes of pelvic pain in adolescents, listed in order of frequency, include gynecologic, urologic, gastrointestinal, musculoskeletal, and psychological disorders (Trotman & Gomez-Lobo, 2013). Interestingly, pelvic pain is more likely to be of gynecologic origin than of gastrointestinal origin (specifically IBS) within this age group. It is important to rule out PID as a cause of pelvic pain in adolescents because this disease is so commonly diagnosed in adolescents. Clinicians should aggressively pursue the diagnosis and treatment of chronic pelvic pain in adolescents to avoid future reproductive health issues that could potentially lead to diminished quality of life (Trotman & Gomez-Lobo, 2013).

Adolescents, because of their stages of emotional and physical development, pose challenges to clinicians that are different from those associated with women in their 20s and beyond. Developing a rapport with any teenager may be the biggest challenge facing the clinician working with members of this age group. Suggestions for developing rapport include maintaining eye contact, demonstrating a nonjudgmental attitude, treating the teen with respect, and giving her undivided attention. It is important to validate her symptoms and the feelings she associates with them.

It is also important to be familiar with state and local statutes regarding health care for minors. Many states have parental consent laws. Each practice needs to have its own policy that must follow the legal parameters already in place.

Women of Reproductive Age

Modesto and Bahamondes (2011) studied 100 women, ages 18 to 50, over a 3-month period. The women were separated into three groups: (1) women without CPP, (2) women with CPP but without functional constipation, and (3) women with CPP with functional constipation as defined by Rome III criteria. It was discovered that the women in group 3 had more pregnancies, more cesarean sections, and more pelvic surgeries ($P < 0.0001$). In addition, the prevalence of other types of pain, stress, intense physical exercise, and sadness was higher in group 3 ($P < 0.0001$).

Women Who Are Perimenopausal

The demographics of women in the United States are undergoing considerable changes, largely due to aging of the baby boomer generation (born between 1946 and 1964)—the largest generational group in U.S. history. A woman born today will typically have a life span of 81 or more years, entering into menopause at the age of 51 or 52 years (Beckmann et al., 2014). Unlike their predecessors in previous generations, these women will spend more than one-third of their lives in menopause. The number of women older than 65 years is projected to rise steadily through 2060 (Colby & Ortman, 2015). These women will have the expectation of remaining healthy (physically, intellectually, and sexually) throughout their lifetime, including the "menopause years" (Beckmann et al., 2014). It is important that clinicians remain cognizant of the changing age demographics,

especially in their provision of primary and preventive care from a gynecologic perspective (Beckmann et al., 2014).

Learman et al. (2011) conducted a study with 557 women to determine whether age at first uterus-preserving treatment (UPT) predicts symptom resolution among women with common pelvic problems. The mean age of participants in this study was 43 years. The findings indicated that women who are 40 years or older when they undergo their first uterus-preserving treatment experience greater CPP symptom resolution than younger women. Promoting UPT as an alternative to hysterectomy may, in fact, be appropriate only for a subset of women who are 40 years or older (Learman et al., 2011). Based on the results of this study, the researchers concluded that age should be considered a risk factor when counseling younger women about treatment options for CPP.

Older Women

Taverner, Closs, and Briggs (2014) conducted a study aimed at development of grounded theory to describe and explain the experience of chronic pain and its impact on older adults. Eleven people, age 65 or older, participated in the study, and all experienced chronic pain due to a leg ulcer. All participants received treatment for their leg ulcers, but the pain became as chronic as the leg ulcers. According to the participants, the treatment to heal the leg ulcer actually exacerbated the pain. Once the participants developed a chronic pain condition, their quality of life was decreased; they suffered from depression, insomnia, social isolation, suicidal ideation, and desire for limb amputation. The most appropriate way to manage these individuals was to provide symptom management for chronic pain.

Influences of Culture

Increased susceptibility to pain is linked to factors such as English as a second language, race and ethnicity, income and education, gender, age, geographic location, veterans, cognitive disabilities, surgical history, cancer diagnosis, and end-of-life status (Institute of Medicine, 2011).

Knowing and appreciating the cultural background of a woman is a significant component of providing culturally competent health care. Cultural and social stratification influences decision making for both patient and clinician, as well as the treatment options that are offered and accepted. Should the clinician be shaking hands, making eye contact, or addressing the woman directly? If her husband is present, does the couple's culture dictate that the clinician include him in the conversation as well? How close should the clinician stand or sit when taking a history? These are all culturally significant questions to consider. In addition, women of different cultures express pain differently. Validating a woman's feelings and recognizing and appreciating her cultural and ethnic background are important not only in gaining her trust and establishing rapport, but also in understanding the scope of the problem the woman presents.

Culture can also affect symptom reporting and diagnosis. A retrospective review of charts of Mexican American women with IBS was performed to determine whether the symptoms reported met the Rome II criteria (Barakzai & Gregory, 2007). Only 63% of the participants in the study reported symptoms that met any of the Rome II criteria. These findings emphasize that the clinician must have a clear understanding of what the illness means to the woman to make an accurate diagnosis and create an appropriate treatment plan (Barakzai & Gregory, 2007).

Many women live in a culture where physical, sexual, and psychological abuse are commonplace. Women with histories of abuse report higher pain-related disability when compared to those reporting no abuse (As-Sanie et al., 2014). The clinician must remain cognizant of the possibility of abuse and incorporate related discussions into the conversation with each woman.

Pain and Gender

Pain is an intimate experience that only the person experiencing it can truly comprehend. Because pain is a subjective phenomenon, it should be reliably assessed from the woman's personal perspective. The emphasis on equality during the 1980s, however, downplayed gender differences; as a consequence, few studies assessed differences between men and women, including studies about pain. Pain research was based on the male response to pain, with the assumption that the findings could be generalized to women (Vallerand, 1995). Interestingly, as pain and gender studies became more prevalent, researchers observed that women were better able to verbalize the emotions they experienced with pain. Unfortunately, this finding caused women's responses to pain to be viewed as a psychologic issue and treated accordingly (Vallerand, 1995). As a consequence, women's responses to pain were often viewed with suspicion and the treatment for their pain was less aggressive.

In the late 1990s, the National Institutes of Health (NIH) Pain Research Consortium hosted a conference that focused on gender and pain. Also during this time, the International Association for the Study of Pain (IASP) formed a special-interest group—Sex, Gender, and Pain—that held its first meeting in 1999 in Vienna (Fillingim, King, Ribeiro-Dasilva, Rahim-Williams, & Riley, 2009). These two meetings served as springboards for the dramatic increase in research focusing on sex, gender, and pain.

In 2007, the IASP launched the Global Year Against Pain in Women, in recognition of the fact that a significant number of women worldwide have chronic pain conditions that negatively affect their lives, their families, and their communities. The current call to include more women in studies about pain also reflects the imperative that sex and gender differences be addressed by clinicians. Moreover, studying pain in women is important for driving attitudinal changes among clinicians who provide health care for women. Attitude can influence healthcare treatment, as can culture.

Also in 2007, a consensus report was published that was intended to serve as a guide to researchers studying sex and gender differences in pain and analgesia (Greenspan et al., 2007). This report underscored the point that there is no longer any debate about whether there are sex and gender differences in pain. The evidence reveals that they do, indeed, exist. What is needed now is to (1) develop a better understanding of which conditions lead to these differences, (2) determine which mechanisms underlie the differences, (3) learn how these differences inform pain management, and (4) explore differences in outcomes when similar treatments are used (Greenspan et al., 2007).

In 2008, the IASP published a Pain Clinical Update entitled *Gender, Pain, and the Brain*. This clinical update systematically reviewed findings from 30 research studies comparing gender differences in relation to pain management with opioid therapy and central nervous system responses as seen via positron-emission tomography (PET) or magnetic resonance imaging (MIR) (Derbyshire, 2008). The IASP Pain: Clinical Updates publishes information about pain management and therapy six times a year (IASP, 2016); to date, the updates have focused on various aspects of chronic pain, although none have been gender specific. In 2013, the IASP released a Pain Clinical Update focusing on the psychosocial aspects of chronic pelvic pain. However, the primary aim of this clinical update is to familiarize the reader with urologic chronic pelvic pain syndromes (UCPPS), specifically as they relate to pain and quality of life among men.

Pain is an individual experience that is shaped by a variety of biologic, psychological, and social factors (Tashani, Alabas, & Johnson, 2012). Over the last several years, a growing body of evidence has supported differences in pain experiences between genders. Ruau, Liu, Clark, Angst, and Butte (2012) reviewed 11,000 medical records and found the mean pain intensity rated on a 0 (pain free) to 10 (worst pain) scale was at least 1 point higher among women for a variety of painful conditions, including neck, back and joint pain. Similarly, in a study done by Etherton, Lawson, and Graham (2014), mean subjective pain ratings during cold pressor pain induction were higher among women than men. Also, in a study among individuals with chronic noncancer pain, women reported a greater number of tender points and a lower pain threshold than men (Ciaramella & Poli, 2015).

LeResche, Manel, Drangsholt, Saunders, and Korff (2005) found that gender differences in pain prevalence appear during adolescence. Rates of pain conditions increase as girls enter puberty, whereas rates for adolescent boys remain stable or rise notably less than for girls.

Safdar et al. (2009) studied analgesic administration in multiple emergency departments and found that this practice was not different between genders, although women presenting with complaints of severe pain were more likely than men to receive analgesics. In a systematic review of literature conducted by LeResche (2011), it was noted that clinicians' gender stereotypes, as well as the clinician's own gender, appear to influence diagnostic and treatment decisions for more chronic pain problems. The reasons for the differences in pain prevalence and the health care provided to different genders is not well understood (LeResche, 2011).

Individual differences in response to pain may significantly affect outcomes, including the development of chronic pain, overreliance on pain medication, and decreased psychosocial functioning. Psychosocial factors may be among the most important predictors in the development of chronic pain-related disability (Turk & Okifuji, 2002).

In fact, women who have multiple responsibilities as part of caring for their family view chronic pain as more of a threat because of its potential to affect their daily lives. For all these reasons, it is very important that the clinician carefully interview the woman who presents with chronic pelvic pain to assess the level of interference the pain may be having with her life and activities of daily living. Part of effective treatment may be working with her to identify how some of the activities can be accomplished.

References

Abercrombie, P. D., & Learman, L. A. (2012). Providing holistic care for women with chronic pelvic pain. *Journal of Obstetric, Gynecologic and Neonatal Nursing, 41*, 668–679.

Altman, G., & Lee, C. (2009). Chronic pelvic pain and associated disorders. *Kansas Nurse, 84*, 12–15.

American College of Obstetricians and Gynecologists. (2004, reaffirmed 2010). *Chronic pelvic pain: Clinical management guidelines for -obstetrician-gynecologists. Practice Bulletin No. 51.* Washington, DC: Author.

American College of Obstetricians and Gynecologists. (2008, reaffirmed 2014). *Medical management of ectopic pregnancy for obstetricians-gynecologists. Practice Bulletin No. 94.* Washington, DC: Author.

As-Sanie, S., Clevenger, L. A., Geisser M. E., Williams, D. A., & Roth, R. S. (2014). History of abuse and its relationship to pain experience and depression in women with chronic pelvic pain. *American Journal of Obstetrics & Gynecology, 210*, 317.e1–317.e8.

As-Sanie, S., Harris, R. E., Napadow, V., Kim, J., Neshewat, G., Kairys, A., . . . Schmidt-Wilcke T.. (2012). Changes in regional gray matter volume in women with chronic pelvic pain: A voxel based morphometry study. *Pain, 153*(5), 1006–1014.

Barakzai, M. D., & Gregory, J. (2007). The effect of culture on symptom reporting: Hispanics and irritable bowel syndrome. *American Academy of Nurse Practitioners, 19*, 261–267.

Beckmann, C. R. B., Ling, F. W., Herbert, W. N. P., Laube, D. W., Smith, R. P., & Casanova, R., . . . Weiss, P. M. (2014). *Obstetrics and gynecology* (7th ed.). Philadelphia, PA: Lippincott, Williams & Wilkins.

Bedaiwy, M. A., Patterson, B., & Mahajan, S. (2013). Prevalence of myofascial chronic pelvic pain and the effectiveness of pelvic floor physical therapy. *Journal of Reproductive Medicine, 58* (11–12), 504–510.

Berek, J. (2012). *Berek and Novak's gynecology* (15th ed.). Philadelphia, PA: Lippincott, Williams & Wilkins.

Bruckenthal, P. (2011). Chronic pelvic pain: Approaches to diagnosis. *Pain Management in Nursing, 12*(1), S4–S10.

Champaneria, R., Daniels, J. P., Raza, A., Pattison, H. M., & Khan, K. S. (2012). Psychological therapies for chronic pelvic pain: Systematic review of randomized controlled trials. *Nordic Federation of Societies of Obstetrics and Gynecology, 91*, 281–286.

Cheong, Y. C., Reading, I., Bailey, S., Sadek, K., Ledger, W., & Li, T. (2014). Should women with chronic pelvic pain have adhesiolysis? *BioMed Central Women's Health, 14*(36), 1–7.

Cho, S. H., & Hwang, E. W. (2010). Acupuncture for primary dysmenorrhea: A systematic review. *British Journal of Obstetrics & Gynaecology, 117*(5), 509–521.

Ciaramella, A., & Poli, P. (2015). Pathogenetic psychosomatic mechanisms in chronic pain: Gender differences among syndromes. *Journal of Psychosomatic Research, 78*(6), 597.

Colby, S. L., & Ortman, J. M. (2015). Projections of the size and composition of the U.S. population: 2014 to 2060 (Current Population Reports No. P25-1143). Retrieved from http://www.census.gov/content/dam/Census/library/publications/2015/demo/p25-1143.pdf

Demir, F., Ozcimen, E. E., & Oral, H. B. (2012). The role of gynecological, urological, and psychiatric factors in chronic pelvic pain. *Archives of Gynecology and Obstetrics, 286*(5), 1215–1220.

Derbyshire, S. W. G. (2008). Gender, pain, and the brain. *Pain Clinical Updates, 16*(3), 1–4. Retrieved from http://iasp.files.cms-plus.com/Content/ContentFolders/Publications2/PainClinicalUpdates/Archives/PCU08-3_1390262458261_5.pdf

Dunphy, L. M., Winland-Brown, J. E., Porter, B. O., & Thomas, D. J. (2015). *Primary care: The art and science of advanced practice nursing* (4th ed.). Philadelphia, PA: F.A. Davis Company.

Etherton, J., Lawson, M., & Graham, R. (2014). Individual and gender differences in subjective and objective indices of pain: Gender, fear of pain, pain catastrophizing and cardiovascular reactivity. *Applied Psychophysiology and Biofeedback, 39*, 89–97.

Fillingim, R. B., King, C. D., Ribeiro-Dasilva, M. C., Rahim-Williams, B., & Riley, J. L. (2009). Sex, gender, and pain: A review of recent clinical and experimental findings. *Journal of Pain, 10*(5), 447–485.

Ghosh, M., & Ojha, K. (2011). Medical and surgical management of chronic pelvic pain. *Obstetrics, Gynaecology and Reproductive Medicine, 21*(9), 249–253.

Greenspan, J. D., Craft, R. M., LeResche, L., Arendt-Nielsen, L., Berkley, K., Fillingim, R. B., & Pain SIG of the IASP. (2007). Studying sex and gender differences in pain and analgesia: A consensus report. *Pain, 132*, S26–S45.

Gyang, A. N., Feranee, J. B., Patel, R. C., & Lamvu, G. M. (2014). Managing chronic pelvic pain following reconstructive pelvic surgery with transvaginal mesh. *International Urogynecological Journal, 25*, 313–318.

Hart, D., & Lipsky, A. (2014). Acute pelvic pain in women. In J. Marks, R. Hockberger, & R. Walls (Eds.), *Rosen's emergency medicine: Concepts and practice* (8th ed., pp. 266–272). Philadelphia, PA: Elsevier Saunders.

Hoffman, B. L. (2012). Pelvic pain. In B. L. Hoffman, J. O. Schorge, J. I. Schaffer, L. M. Halvorson, K. D. Bradshaw, F. G. Cunningham, & L. E. Calver (Eds.), *Williams gynecology* (2nd ed., pp. 304–332). New York, NY: McGraw-Hill Medical.

Horwitz, J., Pundi, R. S., & Blankstein, J. (2011). Ovarian hyperstimulation syndrome treatment & management. *Medscape Reference*. Retrieved from http://emedicine.medscape.com/article/1343572-treatment

Howard, H. S. (2012). Sexual adjustment counseling for women with chronic pelvic pain. *Journal of Obstetric, Gynecologic and Neonatal Nursing, 41*(5), 692–702.

Ignatavicius, D., & Workman, M. (2002). *Medical–surgical nursing: Critical thinking for collaborative care*. Philadelphia, PA: W. B. Saunders.

Institute of Medicine. (2011). *Relieving pain in America: A blueprint for transforming prevention, care, education, and research*. Washington, DC: National Academies Press.

International Association for the Study of Pain (IASP). (2014). IASP taxonomy. Retrieved from http://www.iasp-pain.org/Taxonomy

International Association for the Study of Pain (IASP). (2016). Pain: Clinical updates. Retrieved from http://www.iasp-pain.org/Pain:ClinicalUpdates?navItemNumber=571

Johnson, J., Thomas, D. J., & Porter, B. O. (2015). Women's health problems. In L. M. Dunphy, J. E. Winland-Brown, B. O. Porter, & D. J. Thomas (Eds.), *Primary care: The art and science of advanced practice nursing* (4th ed., pp. 679–754). Philadelphia, PA: F. A. Davis.

Karnath, B., & Breitkopf, D. (2007). Acute and chronic pelvic pain in women. *Hospital Physician, 43*(7), 41–48.

Kassab, D., & Rollins, V. (2011). Should we screen patients with chronic pelvic pain for depression? *Evidence-Based Practice: Patient-Oriented Evidence That Matters, 14*(1), 13.

Kruszka, P. S., & Kruszka, S. J. (2010). Evaluation of acute pelvic pain in women. *American Family Physician, 82*(2), 141–147.

Lamvu, G. (2011). Role of hysterectomy in the treatment of chronic pelvic pain. *Obstetrics & Gynecology, 117*(5), 1175–1178.

Learman, L. A., Nakagawa, S., Gregorich, S. E., Jackson, R. A., Jacoby, A., & Kuppermann, M. (2011). Success of uterus-preserving treatments for abnormal uterine bleeding, chronic pelvic pain, and symptomatic fibroids: age and bridges to menopause. *American Journal of Obstetrics & Gynecology, 204*, 272.e1–272.e7.

Lentz, G., Lobo, R., Gershenson, D. M., & Katz, V. (2012). *Comprehensive gynecology* (6th ed.). Philadelphia, PA: Mosby Elsevier.

LeResche, L. (2011). Defining gender disparities in pain management. *Clinical Orthopaedics and Related Research, 469*, 1871–1877.

LeResche, L., Manel, L. A., Drangsholt, M. T., Saunders, K., & Korff, M. V. (2005). Relationship of pain and symptoms to pubertal development in adolescents. *Pain, 118*(1), 201–209.

Lindsay, L., & Farrell, C. (2015). Pharmacological management of neuropathic pain. *Prescriber, 26*(9), 13–18.

Mathias, S. D., Kuppermann, M., Libermann, R. F., Lipschutz, R. C., & Steege, J. F. (1996). Chronic pelvic pain: Prevalence, health-related quality of life, and economic correlates. *Obstetrics & Gynecology, 87*(3), 321–327.

Meltzer-Brody, S., & Leserman, J. (2011). Psychiatric comorbidity in women with chronic pelvic pain. *CNS Spectrums, 16*(2), 29–35.

Merlin, M. A., Shah, C. N., & Shiroff, A. M. (2010). Evidence-based appendicitis: The initial work-up. *Postgraduate Medicine, 122*(3), 189–195.

Modesto, W. O., & Bahamondes, L. (2011). Relationship between chronic pelvic pain and functional constipation in women of reproductive age. *Journal of Reproductive Medicine, 56*(9–10), 425–430.

Morelli, M., Rocca, M. L., Venturella, R., Mocciaro, R., & Zullo, F. (2013). Improvement in chronic pelvic pain after gonadotropin releasing hormone analogue (GnRH-a) administration in premenopausal women suffering from adenomyosis or endometriosis: a retrospective study. *Gynecological Endocrinology, 29*(4), 305–308.

Neis, K. J., & Neis, F. (2009). Chronic pelvic pain: Cause, diagnosis and therapy from a gynecologist's and an endoscopist's point of view. *Gynecological Endocrinology, 25*(11), 757–761.

Nelson, P., Apte, G., Justiz, R., Brismee, J. M., Dedrick, G., & Sizer, P. S. (2011). Chronic female pelvic pain: Part 2: Differential diagnosis and management. *Pain Practice, 12*(2), 111–141.

Olson, C., & Schnatz, P. F. (2007). Evaluation and management of chronic pelvic pain in women. *Journal of Clinical Outcomes Management, 14*(10), 563–573.

Potter, A. W., & Chandrasekhar, C. A. (2008). US and CT evaluation of acute pelvic pain of gynecologic origin in nonpregnant premenopausal patients. *Radiographics, 28*, 1645–1659.

Rapkin, A. J., & Nathan, L. (2012). Pelvic pain and dysmenorrhea. In J. Berek (Ed.), *Berek and Novak's gynecology* (15th ed., pp. 470–504). Philadelphia, PA: Lippincott Williams & Wilkins.

Rome Foundation, Inc. (2015). About the Rome Foundation. Retrieved from http://www.romecriteria.org/about

Ruau, D., Liu, L. Y., Clark, J. D., Angst, M. S., & Butte, A. J. (2012). Sex differences in reported pain across 11,000 patients captured in electronic medical records. *Journal of Pain, 13*(3), 228–234.

Safdar, B., Heins, A., Homel, P., Miner, J., Neighbor, M., DeSandre, P., & Todd, K. H. (2009). Impact of physician and patient gender on pain management in the emergency department: A multicenter study. *Pain Medicine, 10*(2), 364–372.

Shin, J. H., & Howard, F. M. (2011). Management of chronic pelvic pain. *Current Pain and Headache Reports, 15*, 377–385.

Silva, G. P., Nascimento, A. L., Michelazzo, D., Alves, F. F., Jr., Rocha, M. G., Rosa-e-Silva, J. C., . . . Poli-Neto, O. B. (2011). High prevalence of chronic pelvic pain in women in Ribeirão Preto, Brazil and direct association with abdominal surgery. *Clinics, 66*(8), 1307–1312.

Smith, C. A., Zhu, X., He, L., & Song, J. (2011). Acupuncture for primary dysmenorrhea. *Cochrane Database of Systemic Reviews, 1,* CD007854. doi:10.1002/14651858.CD007854.pub2

Solnik, M. J., & Munro, M. G. (2014). Indication and alternatives to hysterectomy. *Clinical Obstetrics and Gynecology, 57*(1), 14–42.

Stein, S. L. (2013). Chronic pelvic pain. *Gastroenterology Clinics of North America, 42*, 785–800.

Styer, A. K. (2013). Gynecologic etiologies of chronic pelvic pain. In A. Bailey & C. Bernstein (Eds.), *Pain in women: A clinical guide* (pp. 95–141). Boston, MA: Harvard Medical School.

Tachawiwat, K., & Cheewadhanaraks, S. (2012). Prevalence of irritable bowel syndrome among patients with mild–moderate and severe chronic pelvic pain. *Journal of the Medical Association of Thailand, 95*(10), 1257–1260.

Tashani, O. A., Alabas, O. A., & Johnson, M. I. (2012). Understanding the gender gap. *Pain Management, 2*(4), 315–317.

Taverner, T. (2014). Neuropathic pain: An overview. *British Journal of Neuroscience Nursing, 10*(3), 116–122.

Taverner, T., Closs, S. J., & Briggs, M. (2014). The journey to chronic pain: A grounded theory of older adults' experiences of pain associated with leg ulceration. *Pain Management Nursing, 15*(1), 186–198.

Trotman, G. E., & Gomez-Lobo, V. (2013). Pelvic pain in the adolescent. *North American Society for Pediatric and Adolescent Gynecology, 58*(1), 50–55.

Tu, F. F., Hahn, D., & Steege, J. F. (2010). Pelvic congestion syndrome–associated pelvic pain: A systematic review of diagnosis and management. *Obstetrical & Gynecological Survey, 65*(5), 332–340.

Turk, D. C., & Okifuji, A. (2002). Psychological factors in chronic pain: Evolution and revolution. *Clinical Psychology, 70,* 678–690.

Vallerand, A. (1995). Gender differences in pain. *Image: Journal of Nursing Scholarship, 27,* 235–237.

Whiteman, M. K., Hillis, S. D., Jamieson, D. J., Morrow, B., Podgornik, M. N., Brett, K. M., . . . Marchbanks, P. A. (2008). Inpatient hysterectomy surveillance in the United States, 2000–2004. *American Journal of Obstetrics & Gynecology, 198*(1), 34.e31–e37.

Williams, R., Hartmann, K., Sandler, R., Miller, W., & Steege, J. (2004). Prevalence and characteristics of irritable bowel syndrome among women with chronic pelvic pain. *Obstetrics & Gynecology, 104,* 452–458.

Yong, P. J., Sutton, C., Suen, M., & Williams, C. (2013). Endovaginal ultrasound-assisted pain mapping in endometriosis and chronic pelvic pain. *Journal of Obstetrics and Gynaecology, 33,* 715–719.

The International Pelvic Pain Society
Pelvic Pain Assessment Form

THE INTERNATIONAL
PELVIC PAIN
S O C I E T Y

| Pelvic Pain Assessment Form |

Physician: _____

Initial History and Physical Examination
Date: _____
This assessment form is intended to assist the clinician with the initial patient assessment and is not meant to be a diagnostic tool.

Contact Information
Name: _____ Birth Date: _____ Chart Number: _____
Phone: Work: _____ Home: _____ Cell: _____
Referring Provider's Name and Address: _____

Information About Your Pain
Please describe your pain problem (use a separate sheet of paper if needed) : _____
_____
_____
_____
_____

What do you think is causing your pain? _____
Is there an event that you associate with the onset of your pain? ☐ Yes ☐ No If so, what? _____
How long have you had this pain? _____ years _____ months

For each of the symptoms listed below, please "bubble in" your level of pain over the last month using a 10-point scale:
0 - no pain   10 – the worst pain imaginable

	0	1	2	3	4	5	6	7	8	9	10
How would you rate your pain?											
Pain at ovulation (mid-cycle)	O	O	O	O	O	O	O	O	O	O	O
Pain just before period	O	O	O	O	O	O	O	O	O	O	O
Pain (not cramps) before period	O	O	O	O	O	O	O	O	O	O	O
Deep pain with intercourse	O	O	O	O	O	O	O	O	O	O	O
Pain in groin when lifting	O	O	O	O	O	O	O	O	O	O	O
Pelvic pain lasting hours or days after intercourse	O	O	O	O	O	O	O	O	O	O	O
Pain when bladder is full	O	O	O	O	O	O	O	O	O	O	O
Muscle / joint pain	O	O	O	O	O	O	O	O	O	O	O
Level of cramps with period	O	O	O	O	O	O	O	O	O	O	O
Pain after period is over	O	O	O	O	O	O	O	O	O	O	O
Burning vaginal pain after sex	O	O	O	O	O	O	O	O	O	O	O
Pain with urination	O	O	O	O	O	O	O	O	O	O	O
Backache	O	O	O	O	O	O	O	O	O	O	O
Migraine headache	O	O	O	O	O	O	O	O	O	O	O
Pain with sitting	O	O	O	O	O	O	O	O	O	O	O

Provider Comments
_____
_____
_____
_____

Information About Your Pain
What types of treatments / providers have you tried in the past for your pain?   **Please check all that apply.**

☐ Acupuncture
☐ Anesthesiologist
☐ Anti-seizure medications
☐ Antidepressants
☐ Biofeedback
☐ Botox injection
☐ Contraceptive pills / patch / ring
☐ Danazol (Danocrine)
☐ Depo-provera
☐ Gastroenterologist
☐ Gynecologist

☐ Family practitioner
☐ Herbal medicine
☐ Homeopathic medicine
☐ Lupron, Synarel, Zoladex
☐ Massage
☐ Meditation
☐ Narcotics
☐ Naturopathic mediciation
☐ Nerve blocks
☐ Neurosurgeon
☐ Nonprescription medicine

☐ Nutrition / diet
☐ Physical therapy
☐ Psychotherapy
☐ Psychiatrist
☐ Rheumatologist
☐ Skin magnets
☐ Surgery
☐ TENS unit
☐ Trigger point injections
☐ Urologist
☐ Other _____

Pain Maps
Please shade areas of pain and write a number from 1 to 10 at the site(s) of pain. (10 = most severe pain imaginable)

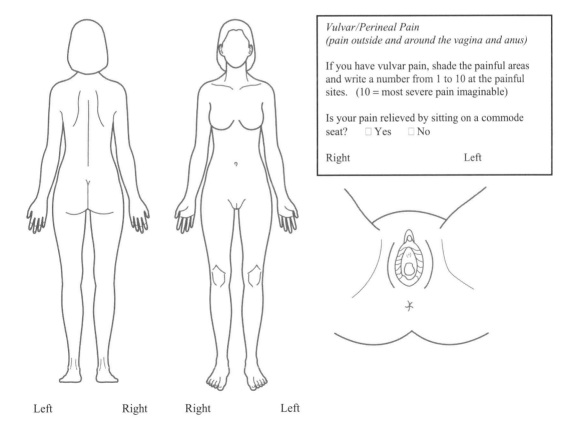

Vulvar/Perineal Pain
(pain outside and around the vagina and anus)

If you have vulvar pain, shade the painful areas and write a number from 1 to 10 at the painful sites.   (10 = most severe pain imaginable)

Is your pain relieved by sitting on a commode seat?   ☐ Yes   ☐ No

Right   Left

Left   Right   Right   Left

What physicians or health care providers have evaluated or treated you for **chronic pelvic pain**?

Physician / Provider	Specialty	City, State, Phone

Demographic Information
Are you (check all that apply):
    ☐ Married   ☐ Widowed   ☐ Separated   ☐ Committed Relationship
    ☐ Single   ☐ Remarried   ☐ Divorced
Who do you live with? _____

Education: ☐ Less than 12 years   ☐ High School graduate
               ☐ College degree   ☐ Postgraduate degree
What type of work are you trained for? _____
What type of work are you doing? _____

Surgical History
Please list all surgical procedures you have had **related to this pain**:

Year	Procedure	Surgeon	Findings

Please list all **other** surgical procedures:

Year	Procedure		Year	Procedure

Provider Comments
_____
_____
_____
_____

Medications

Please list **pain medication** you have taken for your pain condition in the past 6 months, and the providers who prescribed them (use a separate page if needed):

Medication / dose	Provider	Did it help?		
		☐ Yes	☐ No	☐ Currently taking
		☐ Yes	☐ No	☐ Currently taking
		☐ Yes	☐ No	☐ Currently taking
		☐ Yes	☐ No	☐ Currently taking
		☐ Yes	☐ No	☐ Currently taking
		☐ Yes	☐ No	☐ Currently taking
		☐ Yes	☐ No	☐ Currently taking
		☐ Yes	☐ No	☐ Currently taking

Please list all **other medications** you are presently taking, the condition, and the provider who prescribed them (use a separate page if needed):

Medication / dose	Provider	Medical Condition

Obstetrical History

How many pregnancies have you had? _____

Resulting in (#): _____ Full 9 months _____ Premature _____ Miscarriage / Abortion _____ Living children

Where there any complications during pregnancy, labor, delivery, or post partum?

☐ 4° Episiotomy ☐ C-Section ☐ Vacuum ☐ Post-partum hemorrhaging
☐ Vaginal laceration ☐ Forceps ☐ Medication for bleeding ☐ Other _____

Family History

Has anyone in your family had: ☐ Fibromyalgia ☐ Chronic pelvic pain ☐ Irritable bowel syndrome
☐ Depression ☐ Interstitial cystitis ☐ Other chronic condition _____
☐ Endometriosis ☐ Cancer, type(s) _____

Medical History

Please list any medical problems / diagnoses _____
_____
_____

Allergies (including latex allergy) _____

Who is your primary care provider? _____

Have you ever been hospitalized for anything besides childbirth? ☐ Yes ☐ No If yes, please explain _____
_____

Have you had major accidents such as falls or a back injury? ☐ Yes ☐ No

Have you ever been treated for depression? ☐ Yes ☐ No Treatments: ☐ Medication ☐ Hospitalization ☐ Psychotherapy

Birth control method: ☐ Nothing ☐ Pill ☐ Vasectomy ☐ Vaginal ring ☐ Depo provera
☐ Condom ☐ IUD ☐ Hysterectomy ☐ Diaphragm ☐ Tubal Sterilization
☐ Other _____

Menstrual History
How old were you when your menses started? _____
Are you still having menstrual periods? ☐ Yes   ☐ No

Answer the following only if you are still having menstrual periods.
Periods are: ☐ Light   ☐ Moderate   ☐ Heavy   ☐ Bleed through protection
How many days between your periods? _____
How many days of menstrual flow? _____
Date of first day of last menstrual period _____
Do you have any pain with your periods? ☐ Yes   ☐ No
    Does pain start the day flow starts? ☐ Yes   ☐ No   Pain starts _____ days before flow
    Are periods regular? ☐ Yes   ☐ No
    Do you pass clots in menstrual flow? ☐ Yes   ☐ No

Gastrointestinal / Eating
Do you have nausea?   ☐ No   ☐ With pain   ☐ Taking medications   ☐ With eating   ☐ Other
Do you have vomiting?   ☐ No   ☐ With pain   ☐ Taking medications   ☐ With eating   ☐ Other
Have you ever had an eating disorder such as anorexia or bulimia?   ☐ Yes   ☐ No
Are you experiencing rectal bleeding or blood in your stool?   ☐ Yes   ☐ No
Do you have increased pain with bowel movements?   ☐ Yes   ☐ No

The following questions help to diagnose irritable bowel syndrome, a gastrointestinal condition, which may be a cause of pelvic pain.
Do you have pain or discomfort that is associated with the following:

    Change in frequency of bowel movement   ☐ Yes   ☐ No
    Change in appearance of stool or bowel movement?   ☐ Yes   ☐ No
    Does your pain improve after completing a bowel movement?   ☐ Yes   ☐ No

---

Health Habits
How often do you exercise?   ☐ Rarely   ☐ 1–2 times weekly   ☐ 3–5 times weekly   ☐ Daily
What is your caffeine intake (number cups per day, include coffee, tea, soft drinks, etc)?   ☐ 0   ☐ 1–3   ☐ 4–6   ☐ > 6
How many cigarettes do you smoke per day? _____   For how many years? _____
Do you drink alcohol?   ☐ Yes   ☐ No
    Number of drinks per week _____
Have you ever received treatment for substance abuse?   ☐ Yes   ☐ No
What is your use of recreational drugs?   ☐ Never used   ☐ Used in the past, but not now   ☐ Presently using   ☐ No answer
    ☐ Heroin   ☐ Amphetamines   ☐ Marijuana   ☐ Barbiturates   ☐ Cocaine   ☐ Other _____
How would you describe your diet? (check all that apply)   ☐ Well balanced   ☐ Vegan   ☐ Vegetarian   ☐ Fried food
    ☐ Special diet _____   ☐ Other _____

Urinary Symptoms
Do you experience any of the following?

Loss of urine when coughing, sneezing, or laughing?	☐ Yes	☐ No
Difficulty passing urine?	☐ Yes	☐ No
Frequent bladder infections?	☐ Yes	☐ No
Blood in the urine?	☐ Yes	☐ No
Still feeling full after urination?	☐ Yes	☐ No
Having to void again within minutes of voiding?	☐ Yes	☐ No

The following questions help to diagnose painful bladder syndrome, which may cause pelvic pain
Please circle the answer that best describes your bladder function and symptoms.

	0	1	2	3	4
1. How many times do you go to the bathroom **DURING THE DAY** (to void or empty your bladder)?	3–6	7–10	11–14	15–19	20 or more
2. How many times do you go to the bathroom **AT NIGHT** (to void or empty your bladder)?	0	1	2	3	4 or more
3. If you get up at night to void or empty your bladder does it bother you?	Never	Mildly	Moderately	Severely	
4. Are you sexually active? ☐ Yes ☐ No					
5. If you are sexually active, do you now or have you ever had pain or symptoms during or after sexual intercourse?	Never	Occasionally	Usually	Always	
6. If you have pain with intercourse, does it make you avoid sexual intercourse?	Never	Occasionally	Usually	Always	
7. Do you have pain associated with your bladder or in your pelvis (lower abdomen, labia, vagina, urethra, perineum)?	Never	Occasionally	Usually	Always	
8. Do you have urgency after voiding?	Never	Occasionally	Usually	Always	
9. If you have pain, is it usually	Never	Mild	Moderate	Severe	
10. Does your pain bother you?	Never	Occasionally	Usually	Always	
11. If you have urgency, is it usually		Mild	Moderate	Severe	
12. Does your urgency bother you?	Never	Occasionally	Usually	Always	

© 2000 C. Lowell Parsons, MD Reprinted with permission.

KCl ____ *Not Indicated* ____ *Positive* ____ *Negative*

Coping Mechanisms

Who are the people you talk to concerning your pain, or during stressful times?

☐ Spouse / Partner   ☐ Relative   ☐ Support group   ☐ Clergy

☐ Doctor / Nurse   ☐ Friend   ☐ Mental   ☐ I take care of myself

How does your partner deal with your pain?

☐ Doesn't notice when I'm in pain   ☐ Takes care of me   ☐ Not applicable

☐ Withdraws   ☐ Feels helpless

☐ Distracts me with activities   ☐ Gets angry

What helps your pain?

☐ Meditation   ☐ Relaxation   ☐ Lying down   ☐ Music

☐ Massage   ☐ Ice   ☐ Heating pad   ☐ Hot bath

☐ Pain medication   ☐ Laxatives / Enema   ☐ Injection   ☐ TENS unit

☐ Bowel movement   ☐ Emptying bladder   ☐ Nothing

☐ Other _____

What makes your pain worse?

☐ Intercourse   ☐ Orgasm   ☐ Stress   ☐ Full meal

☐ Bowel movement   ☐ Full bladder   ☐ Urination   ☐ Standing

☐ Walking   ☐ Exercise   ☐ Time of day   ☐ Weather

☐ Contact with clothing   ☐ Coughing / sneezing   ☐ Not related to anything

☐ Other _____

Of all the problems or stresses or your life, how does your pain compare in importance?

☐ The most important problem   ☐ Just one of many problems

Sexual and Physical Abuse History

Have you ever been the victim of emotional abuse? This can include being humiliated or insulted. ☐ Yes   ☐ No ☐ No answer

Check an answer for <u>both</u> as a child and as an adult.

	As a child (13 and younger)	As an adult (14 and over)
1a. Has anyone ever exposed the sex organs of their body to you when you did not want it?	☐ Yes ☐ No	☐ Yes ☐ No
1b. Has anyone ever threatened to have sex with you when you did not want it?	☐ Yes ☐ No	☐ Yes ☐ No
1c. Has anyone ever touched the sex organs of your body when you did not want this?	☐ Yes ☐ No	☐ Yes ☐ No
1d. Has anyone ever made you touch the sex organs of their body when you did not want this?	☐ Yes ☐ No	☐ Yes ☐ No
1e. Has anyone forced you to have sex when you did not want this?	☐ Yes ☐ No	☐ Yes ☐ No
1f. Have you had any other unwanted sexual experiences not mentioned above?	☐ Yes ☐ No	☐ Yes ☐ No

If yes, please specify _____

2. When you were a child (13 or younger), did an older person do the following?

a. Hit, kick, or beat you?   ☐ Never   ☐ Seldom   ☐ Occasionally   ☐ Often

b. Seriously threaten your life?   ☐ Never   ☐ Seldom   ☐ Occasionally   ☐ Often

3. Now that you are an adult (14 or older), has any other adult done the following?

a. Hit, kick, or beat you?   ☐ Never   ☐ Seldom   ☐ Occasionally   ☐ Often

b. Seriously threaten your life?   ☐ Never   ☐ Seldom   ☐ Occasionally   ☐ Often

Leserman, J, Drossman D, Li Z. The reliability and validity of a sexual and physical abuse history questionnaire in female patients with gastrointestinal disorders. Behavioral Medicine 1995;21:141-148.

Short-Form McGill

The words below describe average pain. Place a check mark (√) in the column which represents the degree to which you feel that type of pain. Please limit yourself to a description of the pain in your pelvic area <u>only</u>.

What does your pain feel like?

Type	None (0)	Mild (1)	Moderate (2)	Severe (3)
Throbbing				
Shooting				
Stabbing				
Sharp				
Cramping				
Gnawing				
Hot-Burning				
Aching				
Heavy				
Tender				
Splitting				
Tiring-Exhausting				
Sickening				
Fearful				
Punishing-Cruel				

Melzak R. The Short-form McGill Pain Questionnaire. Pain 1987;30:191-197.

Pelvic Varicosity Pain Syndrome Questions

Is your pelvic pain aggravated by prolonged physical activity? ☐ Yes ☐ No
Does your pelvic pain improve when you lie down? ☐ Yes ☐ No
Do you have pain that is deep in the vagina or pelvis *during* sex? ☐ Yes ☐ No
Do you have pelvic throbbing or aching *after* sex? ☐ Yes ☐ No
Do you have pelvic pain that moves from side to side? ☐ Yes ☐ No
Do you have sudden episodes of severe pelvic pain that come and go? ☐ Yes ☐ No

Physical Examination – For Physician Use Only

Name:_____   Chart Number:_____

Date of Exam:_____   Height:_____ Weight:_____ BMI:_____

BP:_____ HR: _____ Temp:_____ Resp:_____ LMP:_____

ROS, PFSH Reviewed: ☐ Yes   ☐ No   Physician Signature:_____

General Appearance: ☐ Well-appearing   ☐ Ill-appearing   ☐ Tearful   ☐ Depressed
                       ☐ Normal weight   ☐ Underweight   ☐ Overweight   ☐ Abnormal Gait

_____
NOTE: Mark "Not Examined" as N/E

HEENT ☐ WNL   ***Lungs*** ☐ WNL   ***Heart*** ☐ WNL   ***Breasts*** ☐ WNL
    ☐ Other _____   ☐ Other _____   ☐ Other _____   ☐ Other _____

Right   Left

Abdomen
    ☐ Non-tender   ☐ Tender   ☐ Incisions   ☐ Trigger Points
    ☐ Inguinal Tenderness   ☐ Inguinal Bulge   ☐ Suprapubic Tenderness   ☐ Ovarian Point Tenderness
    ☐ Mass   ☐ Guarding   ☐ Rebound   ☐ Distention
    ☐ Other _____

Right   Left   Right   Left   Right   Left
   Trigger Points   **Surgical Scars**   **Other Findings**

Back
    ☐ Non-tender   ☐ Tender   ☐ Alteration in posture   ☐ SI joint rotation _____

Lower Extremities
    ☐ WNL   ☐ Edema   ☐ Varicosities   ☐ Neuropathy   ☐ Length discrepancy _____

Neuropathy
    ☐ Iliohypogastric   ☐ Ilioinguinal   ☐ Genitofemoral   ☐ Pudendal   ☐ Altered sensation

© April 2008, The International Pelvic Pain Society
This document may be freely reproduced and distributed as long as this copyright notice remains intact
(205) 877-2950   www.pelvicpain.org   (800) 624-9676 (if in the U.S.)

Fibromyalgia / Back / Buttock

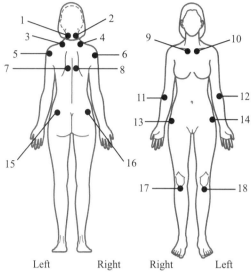

Left   Right   Right   Left

External Genitalia

☐ WNL   ☐ Erythema   ☐ Discharge   ☐ Q-tip test (show on diagram)   ☐ Tenderness (show on diagram)

Right   Left   Right   Left

Q-tip Test (score each circle 0-4) **Total Score** _____   **Other Findings**_____

Vagina

☐ WNL   ☐ Wet prep:_____ _____

☐ Local tenderness_____ ☐ Vaginal mucosa_____ ☐ Discharge_____

Cultures: ☐ GC   ☐ Chlamydia   ☐ Fungal   ☐ Herpes

☐Vaginal Apex Tenderness (post hysterectomy – show on diagram)

Right   Left   Right   Left

Transverse apex closure   **Vertical apex closure**

Unimanual Exam

- □ WNL
- □ Introitus
- □ Uterine-cervical unction
- □ Urethra
- □ Bladder
- □ R ureter
- □ R inguinal
- □ Muscle awareness

- □ Cervix
- □ Cervical motion
- □ Parametrium
- □ Vaginal cuff
- □ Cul-de-sac
- □ L ureter
- □ L inguinal
- □ Clitoral tenderness

Rank muscle tenderness on 0–4 scale

- □ R obturator_____
- □ R piriformis_____
- □ R pubococcygeus_____
- □ Total pelvic floor score_____

- □ L obturator_____
- □ L piriformis_____
- □ L pubococcygeus_____
- □ Anal Sphincter _____

Bimanual Exam

Uterus:	□ Tender	□ Non-tender	□ Absent
Position:	□ Anterior	□ Posterior	□ Midplane
Size:	□ Normal	□ Other_____	
Contour:	□ Regular	□ Irregular	□ Other
Consistency:	□ Firm	□ Soft	□ Hard
Mobility:	□ Mobile	□ Hypermobile	□ Fixed
Support:	□ Well supported	□ Prolapse	

Adnexal Exam

Right:

- □ Absent
- □ WNL
- □ Tender
- □ Fixed
- □ Enlarged _____ cm

Left:

- □ Absent
- □ WNL
- □ Tender
- □ Fixed
- □ Enlarged _____ cm

Rectovaginal Exam

- □ WNL
- □ Tenderness
- □ Nodules
- □ Mucosal pathology
- □ Guaiac positive
- □ Not examined

Assessment:_____

_____

_____

_____

_____

_____

Diagnostic Plan:_____

_____

_____

Therapeutic Plan:_____

_____

_____

The Institute for Women in Pain
Initial Female Pelvic Pain Questionnaire

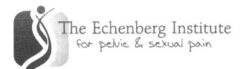

The Echenberg Institute
for pelvic & sexual pain

Phone: 610-868-0104 Fax: 610-868-0204

Please complete this questionnaire in its entirety, even if you feel some sections do not apply to you.

INITIAL FEMALE PELVIC PAIN QUESTIONNAIRE

Patient Information   Date: _____

Name: _____ DOB: _____ Age: _____

Race/Ethnic Identity: _____

Sexual Orientation: ___ Heterosexual ___ Homosexual ___ Bisexual ___ Asexual ___ Other: _____

Religious/Spiritual Affiliation (optional): _____

Medication Allergies: _____

(Office use: G P A VIP LC _____ Drive time: _____ Wgt _____ BP _____)

Demographic Information

1. **Are you (circle all that apply):**
   Single   Married (____ years)   Separated   Divorced
   Widowed   Committed Relationship (____ years)   Remarried

2. **Education:**
   Less than 12 years   High School graduate   Technical School
   College degree   Post-graduate degree

3. Who do you live with? _____

4. What type of work are you trained for? _____

5. What type of work are you doing? _____

6. What type of work does your partner do? _____

7. Has pain forced you to give up or change your type of work? ____ Yes ____ No

8. **If yes, how has pain changed your work?**
   a. Changed to a less strenuous, but full-time job? ____ Yes ____ No
   b. Changed to part-time work?   ____ Yes ____ No
   c. Unable to work?   ____ Yes ____ No
   d. If disabled, how long have you been unable to work? _____

Family History

9. **List anyone in your family,** *including relatives, (excluding yourself)* **who have had;**

❑ Fibromyalgia   ❑ Chronic pelvic pain   ❑ Irritable bowel syndrome
❑ Endometriosis   ❑ Migraine headaches   ❑ Interstitial Cystitis
❑ Depression/Anxiety   ❑ Cancer (type)   Other: _____

_____

10. **Please describe your pain problem**

_____

_____

_____

_____

_____

_____

_____

_____

_____

_____

_____

_____

_____

_____

_____

_____

_____

Groin pain? Yes ___ No ___
Abdominal Pain? Yes ___ No ___
Lower back pain? Yes ___ No ___
Pain with sitting? Yes ___ No ___

Dates (years only) of Ultrasound: _____

MRI: _____

CT Scan: _____

ANSWER ALL QUESTIONS AS IF YOU'RE HAVING YOUR MOST SEVERE DAY OF PAIN

On the diagrams below, shade in <u>all the areas of your body where you feel pain</u>.
If there is an area that hurts more than anywhere else, put an *X* on that area.

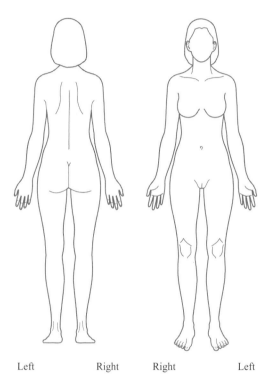

Left   Right   Right   Left

Vulvar/ Perineal Pain
(pain outside and around the vagina and rectum)

If you have vulvar pain, shade the painful areas.

Is your pain relieved by sitting on a commode seat?   ❑ Yes   ❑ No

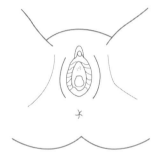

Then shade the inside view of the pelvis to show pain that is deep.

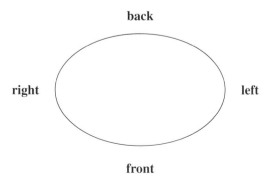

back

right   left

front

Medications

Please list <u>pain medication</u> you have taken for your pain condition in the past 6 months, and the providers who prescribed them (use a separate page if needed):

Medication/dose	Provider	Did it help?
		❑ Yes ❑ No ❑ Currently taking
		❑ Yes ❑ No ❑ Currently taking
		❑ Yes ❑ No ❑ Currently taking
		❑ Yes ❑ No ❑ Currently taking
		❑ Yes ❑ No ❑ Currently taking
		❑ Yes ❑ No ❑ Currently taking
		❑ Yes ❑ No ❑ Currently taking
		❑ Yes ❑ No ❑ Currently taking
		❑ Yes ❑ No ❑ Currently taking
		❑ Yes ❑ No ❑ Currently taking

Please list all <u>other medications</u> you are presently taking, the condition, and the provider who prescribed them (use a separate page if needed):

Medication/dose	Provider	Medical Condition

11. Your age when you first started having pain: _____
12. If your pain had gone away and now has returned, what age did it return? _____
13. What do you think is causing your pain? _____
14. Is there an event that you associate with the onset of your pain?   Yes   No
     If yes, what? _____
15. How long have you had this pain? _____ years _____ months

16. Please tell us how the pain started or the circumstances related to its onset:

     _____

     _____

17. How has the intensity of your pain changed over the past several months?
     ❑ Increased   ❑ Decreased   ❑ Stayed the same   ❑ Varied

18. **Which word or words would you use to describe the pattern of your pain?**
(Circle all that apply)

Continuous	Rhythmic	Brief
Steady	Periodic	Momentary
Constant	Intermittent	Transient

19. **Shade in the circle of the number that most appropriately rates your pain level:**

0 = No Pain   10 = Worst Possible Pain

0__1__2__3__4__5__6__7__8__9__10

a. Right now   O__O__O__O__O__O__O__O__O__O__O
b. At its <u>worst</u> in the past month   O__O__O__O__O__O__O__O__O__O__O
c. At its <u>least</u> in the past month   O__O__O__O__O__O__O__O__O__O__O
d. At its <u>average</u> in the past month   O__O__O__O__O__O__O__O__O__O__O
e. At <u>mid-cycle</u> (ovulation)   O__O__O__O__O__O__O__O__O__O__O
f. <u>Before</u> period or with menses   O__O__O__O__O__O__O__O__O__O__O
g. <u>With</u> period or menses   O__O__O__O__O__O__O__O__O__O__O
h. With <u>intercourse</u>   O__O__O__O__O__O__O__O__O__O__O
i. Entrance pain   O__O__O__O__O__O__O__O__O__O__O
j. Deep pain with intercourse   O__O__O__O__O__O__O__O__O__O__O
k. Pain or burning following intercourse   O__O__O__O__O__O__O__O__O__O__O
l. Pain with sitting   O__O__O__O__O__O__O__O__O__O__O
m. Pain in either groin   O__O__O__O__O__O__O__O__O__O__O
n. Worst <u>toothache</u> ever   O__O__O__O__O__O__O__O__O__O__O
o. Worst <u>headache</u> ever   O__O__O__O__O__O__O__O__O__O__O
p. Ideal <u>acceptable</u> level of pain?   O__O__O__O__O__O__O__O__O__O__O

20. **What does your pain feel like?**

(The words below describe average pain. **Please shade the circles in the correct column,** which represents the degree to which you feel that type of pain. Please limit yourself to a description of the pain in your *PELVIC AREA ONLY.*)

	None (O)	Mild (1)	Moderate (2)	Severe (3)
Throbbing	O	O	O	O
Shooting	O	O	O	O
Stabbing	O	O	O	O
Sharp	O	O	O	O
Cramping	O	O	O	O
Gnawing	O	O	O	O
Hot-Burning	O	O	O	O
Aching	O	O	O	O
Heavy	O	O	O	O
Tender	O	O	O	O
Splitting	O	O	O	O
Exhausting	O	O	O	O
Sickening	O	O	O	O
Fearful	O	O	O	O
Punishing/Cruel	O	O	O	O

PLEASE REMEMBER TO CONTINUE TO ANSWER ALL QUESTIONS AS IF YOU'RE HAVING YOUR MOST SEVERE DAY OF PAIN.

21. **Please shade the number that describes how, during the past month, pain has interfered with:**

    (0 = did not interfere   10 = completely interfered)

		0 1 2 3 4 5 6 7 8 9 10
a.	General Activity	O__O__O__O__O__O__O__O__O__O__O
b.	Housework	O__O__O__O__O__O__O__O__O__O__O
c.	Walking	O__O__O__O__O__O__O__O__O__O__O
d.	Sleeping	O__O__O__O__O__O__O__O__O__O__O
e.	Enjoyment of Life	O__O__O__O__O__O__O__O__O__O__O
f.	Mood	O__O__O__O__O__O__O__O__O__O__O
g.	Relations with Other People	O__O__O__O__O__O__O__O__O__O__O
h.	Sexual Relations	O__O__O__O__O__O__O__O__O__O__O

22. **Mark the number that summarizes your overall sense of well-being for the past month.**
    (When reflecting on your sense of well-being over the past month, you need to take into consideration your physical, mental, emotional, social and spiritual condition.)

    0 = <u>worst</u> you have ever been   10 = <u>best</u> you have ever been

    0   1   2   3   4   5   6   7   8   9   10

23. **Who are the people you talk to concerning your pain or during a stressful time?**

    ❑ Spouse/Partner   ❑ Doctor/Nurse   ❑ Support Group   ❑ Clergy
    ❑ Friend   ❑ Relative   ❑ Mental Health Provider   ❑ I take care of Myself

24. **How does your partner deal with your pain?**

    ❑ Doesn't notice when I'm in pain   ❑ Takes care of me
    ❑ Withdraws   ❑ Feels helpless   ❑ Not applicable
    ❑ Distracts me with activities   ❑ Gets angry

25. **What helps your pain?**

    ❑ Meditation   ❑ Relaxation   ❑ Lying down   ❑ Hot Bath
    ❑ Massage   ❑ Ice   ❑ Heating Pad   ❑ Nothing
    ❑ Injection   ❑ Pain Medication   ❑ TENS Unit   ❑ Prayer
    ❑ Laxatives   ❑ Emptying Bladder   ❑ Music   ❑ Other:_____

26. **What makes your pain worse?**

    ❑ Intercourse   ❑ Orgasm   ❑ Stress   ❑ Full Meal
    ❑ Bowel Movement   ❑ Full Bladder   ❑ Urination   ❑ Standing
    ❑ Walking   ❑ Exercise   ❑ Time of Day   ❑ Sitting
    ❑ Clothing Contact   ❑ Coughing/Sneezing   ❑ Weather   ❑ Not Related to Anything

27. **Of all the problems or stresses of your life, how does your pain compare?**

    ❑ The most important   ❑ Just one of many problems

28. **What types of treatment/providers have you tried in the past for your pain?**

❏ Acupuncture	❏ Family practitioner	❏ Nutrition/diet
❏ Anesthesiologist	❏ Herbal medicine	❏ Physical therapy
❏ Anti-seizure medications	❏ Homeopathic medicine	❏ Psychotherapy
❏ Antidepressants	❏ Lupron, Synarel, Zoladex	❏ Psychiatrist
❏ Biofeedback	❏ Massage therapy	❏ Rheumatologist
❏ Bladder instillations	❏ Meditation	❏ Skin magnets
❏ Botox injections	❏ Narcotics	❏ Surgery
❏ Contraceptive methods	❏ Naturopathic medication	❏ TENS unit
❏ Danazol (Danocrine)	❏ Nerve blocks	❏ Trigger point injections
❏ Depo-Provera	❏ Neurosurgeon	❏ Urologist
❏ Gastroenterologist	❏ Nonprescription medications	❏ Pain management
❏ Gynecologist	❏ Other _____	❏ Other _____

29. **Approximately how many healthcare practitioners have you seen up until this point for your pelvic pain symptoms?** _____

29a. **Have any of the following providers either told you or implied that your pain is "all in your head"?**

   i) **Healthcare Practitioner**   _____
   ii) **Family member**   _____
   iii) **Sexual partner**   _____
   iv) **Friend**   _____
   v) **Co-worker**   _____
   vi) **Classmate**   _____
   vii) **Yourself**   _____

29b. **What is the worst thing any doctor has told you about your pain?**

29c. **Indicate to us the top 3 people in your life who <u>believe</u> the level of pain you have been experiencing. (Eg: partner, family, friend, doctor)**

29d. **Who in your life helps you feel safe?**

What physicians or healthcare providers have evaluated you for chronic pelvic pain?

Physician/Provider	*Specialty*	*City, State*	*Phone Number*
a.			
b.			
c.			
d.			
e.			

GYN and Obstetrical History

30.   How many pregnancies have you had? _____

Resulting in #: ___ Full (9 months) ___ Premature ___ Miscarriage/Abortion ___ Living Children

Were there any complications during pregnancy, labor, delivery or post partum? ___ Yes ___ No

If yes, please check all that apply:

❑ 4° Episiotomy   ❑ C-section   ❑ Vacuum   ❑ Treatment for bleeding
❑ Vaginal laceration   ❑ Forceps   ❑ Post partum hemorrhaging   ❑ Other_____

31.   Birth control method:

❑ Nothing   ❑ Pill   ❑ Vasectomy   ❑ Vaginal ring   ❑ Depo Provera
❑ Condom   ❑ IUD   ❑ Hysterectomy   ❑ Diaphragm   ❑ Tubal Sterilization

Menstrual History

32.   How old were you when your menses started? _____

Are you still having menstrual periods? ___ Yes ___ No

If not, approximate date of your last menstrual period ?_____

If not, reason is: ❑ Hysterectomy ❑ Menopause ❑ Uterine ablation ❑ medical or hormonal suppression: _____

33.   Periods are/used to be:

❑ Light   ❑ Moderate   ❑ Heavy   ❑ Bleeding through protection

How many days between the start of each period? _____
How many days of menstrual flow? _____
Date of first day of last menstrual period? _____

Do you have pain with your periods?   ❑ Yes ❑ No
Does pain start the day flow starts?   ❑ Yes ❑ No   Pain starts _____ days before flow.
Are your periods regular?   ❑ Yes ❑ No
Do you pass clots in your menstrual flow? ❑ Yes ❑ No

Lower Bowel Symptoms

34.   Have you had a colonoscopy? _____ Yes _____ No   *If yes, when?* _____

35.   In general have you had?:

	Yes	No
a. Less than 3 bowel movements per week	O	O
b. More than 3 bowel movements per day	O	O
c. Hard or lumpy stools	O	O
d. Loose or watery stools	O	O
e. Straining during a bowel movement	O	O
f. Urgent need to have a bowel movement	O	O
g. Feeling of incomplete emptying with bowel movements	O	O
h. Passing mucous at the time of bowel movements	O	O
i. Abdominal fullness, bloating or swelling	O	O
j. Pain with bowel movement	O	O
k. Pain relieved with bowel movement	O	O

Gastrointestinal/Eating

36. **Do you have nausea?** ❑ No ❑ With pain ❑ Taking medications ❑ With eating
37. **Do you have vomiting?** ❑ No ❑ With pain ❑ Taking medications ❑ With eating

38. **How would you best describe your diet?**
    ❑ Well-balanced ❑ Vegan ❑ Vegetarian ❑ Fried food

39. **Have you ever had an eating disorder such as anorexia or bulimia?** ____ Yes ____ No
40. **Are you experiencing rectal bleeding or blood in your stool?** ____ Yes ____ No
41. **Do you have increased pain with bowel movements?** ____ Yes ____ No

The following questions help to diagnose irritable bowel syndrome, a gastrointestinal condition, which may be a cause of chronic pelvic pain.

42. **Do you have pain or discomfort that is associated with the following?**
    Change in frequency of bowel movement? ❑ Yes ❑ No
    Change in appearance of stool or bowel movement? ❑ Yes ❑ No
    Does your pain improve after completing a bowel movement? ❑ Yes ❑ No

---

Health Habits

43. **How often do you exercise?** ❑ Rarely ❑ 1-2x weekly ❑ 3-5x weekly ❑ Daily

44. **What is your caffeine intake?** ❑ 0 ❑ 1-3 ❑ 4-6 ❑ 6+
    (number of cups per day including coffee, tea, soft drinks, etc.)

45. **How many cigarettes do you smoke per day?** ____ For how many years? ____
46. **Do you drink alcohol?** ____ Yes ____ No Number of drinks per week? ____

47. **Have you ever received treatment for substance abuse?** ____ Yes ____ No
48. **What is your use of recreational drugs?**
    ❑ Never used ❑ Used in past, but not now ❑ Presently using
    ❑ Marijuana ❑ Cocaine ❑ Barbiturates ❑ Amphetamine ❑ Heroin ❑ Other

Vulvar Hygiene

49. **Do you use vaginal douches?** ____Yes ____ No ____ In the past, but not currently
    If yes, type and frequency: _____
    If in the past, type and frequency: _____

50. **Underwear (shade all that apply):**
    O Cotton O Silk O Synthetic O None O Unsure of fabric

**Urinary Symptoms**

51. **Have you had a cystoscopy?** ____ Yes ____ No   _If yes, when?_ _____
52. **Do you experience any of the following?**

Loss of urine when coughing, sneezing or laughing?	❑ Yes	❑ No
Difficulty passing urine?	❑ Yes	❑ No
Frequent bladder infections?	❑ Yes	❑ No
Blood in the urine?	❑ Yes	❑ No
Still feeling full after urination?	❑ Yes	❑ No
Having to void again within minutes of voiding?	❑ Yes	❑ No
If you took a long car ride (2–4 hours) would you have to make a stop to use the bathroom?	❑ Yes	❑ No

"Urinary urgency" is defined as a compelling desire to urinate, which is difficult to postpone because of pain, pressure or discomfort and a fear of worsening pain.

Please circle the answer that best describes your bladder function and symptoms, as if you are having a BAD day with your bladder.

	0	1	2	3	4
How many times do you go to the bathroom DURING THE DAY (to void or empty your bladder?)	3–6	7–10	11–14	15–19	20 or more
How many times do you go to the bathroom AT NIGHT (to void or empty your bladder?)	0	1	2	3	4 or more
If you get up at night to void or empty your bladder, does it bother you?	Never	Mildly	Moderately	Severely	
Do you have the urge to go again soon after voiding?	Never	Occasionally	Usually	Always	
If you have urgency (see definition above) is it usually:	Never	Mild	Moderate	Severe	
Does your urgency bother you?	Never	Occasionally	Usually	Always	
Do you have pain associated with your bladder OR in your pelvis (lower abdomen, labia, vagina, urethra or rectum?)	Never	Occasionally	Usually	Always	
If you have pelvic pain, is it usually:		Mild	Moderate	Severe	
Are you sexually active? \n ***If no, is it because of pain?**	Yes \n Yes	No* \n No			
If you are or have been sexually active do you now or have you ever had pain or symptoms during or after sexual intercourse?	Never	Occasionally	Usually	Always	
Does your pain bother you?	Never	Occasionally	Usually	Always	

Office use:

Sexual Pain History

53. Have you ever been sexually active? ____ Yes ____ No

If yes, please answering the following:

Have you been sexually active in the past 6 months? ____ Yes ____ No

Number of lifetime sexual partners (approximate): _____

Age at first intercourse: _____

Any pain during or after orgasm? ____ Yes ____ No

54. If pain or discomfort with sexual activity is part of your pelvic pain problem...:

a. Pain with first sexual experience?	❑ Yes	❑ No
b. Only with current partner?	❑ Yes	❑ No
c. Also with previous partner?	❑ Yes	❑ No
d. Is your current partner always aware of your pain or discomfort?	❑ Yes	❑ No
e. Is discomfort at vaginal opening, deeper, or both? *(please circle one!)*		
f. Were tampons ever a problem to insert?	❑ Yes	❑ No

Describe current sexual pain or discomfort and how it is affecting your relationship:

_____

_____

55. Does your partner have sexual difficulty? ____ Yes ____ No _____ Uncertain

If yes, please shade all that apply: O Erectile difficulties   O Rapid ejaculation

O Low sexual desire   O Fear of hurting   O Other

Sexual and Physical Abuse History

Have you ever been the victim of emotional abuse? This can include being humiliated or insulted.

____ Yes ____ No ____ No answer

56. Check an answer for both as a child and as an adult: As a child (13 and younger)   As an adult (14 and older)

	As a child (13 and younger)		As an adult (14 and older)	
a. Has anyone ever exposed the sex organs of their body to you when you did not want it?	❑ Yes	❑ No	❑ Yes	❑ No
b. Has anyone ever threatened to have sex with you when you did not want it?	❑ Yes	❑ No	❑ Yes	❑ No
c. Has anyone ever touched the sex organs of your body when you did not want this?	❑ Yes	❑ No	❑ Yes	❑ No
d. Has anyone ever made you touch the sex organs of their body when you did not want this?	❑ Yes	❑ No	❑ Yes	❑ No
e. Has anyone forced you to have sex when you did not want this?	❑ Yes	❑ No	❑ Yes	❑ No
f. Have you had any other unwanted sexual experiences not mentioned above?	❑ Yes	❑ No	❑ Yes	❑ No

57. When you were a child did an older person ever hit, kick, or beat you? Threaten your life?

____ *Yes* ____ *No*   O Never   O Seldom   O Occasionally   O Often

58. Now that you are an adult, has another adult ever hit, kick, or beat you? Threaten your life?

____ *Yes* ____ *No*   O Never   O Seldom   O Occasionally   O Often

Headache History

59. **Do you have a history of headaches?** ____ Yes ____ No

If yes, when did they begin? _____

What is the frequency of your headaches? _____

Are they associated with your menstrual cycles? ____ Yes ____ No

Do you suffer from migraine headaches? ____ Yes ____ No

What do you take for your headaches? _____

Sleep Problems

60. Do you have trouble falling asleep? ❑ Yes ❑ No

61. Do you have trouble staying asleep? ❑ Yes ❑ No

62. Do you take anything to help you sleep? ❑ Yes ❑ No

Seasonal Allergies

63. Do you have seasonal allergies? ❑ Yes ❑ No

If yes, allergic to:

_____

64. Do you take anything for your allergies? ❑ Yes ❑ No

If yes, what do you take:

_____

Surgical History

65. **Please list all surgical procedures you have had** _(related to your pain):_

Procedure	Surgeon	Year	Findings

66. **Please list all surgical procedures you have had** _(not related to your pain):_

Procedure	Surgeon	Year	Findings

Medical History

67. **Please list any other medical problems/diagnoses:**

   _____

   _____

   _____

   _____

68. **Have you ever been hospitalized for anything other than childbirth or surgeries?**
   ____ Yes ____ No   *If yes, please explain:*

   _____

   _____

   _____

69a. **Approximately how many times have you gone to an emergency room because of your pelvic pain symptoms?** _____

Physical Trauma History

69. **Through your entire life, have you had any painful injuries, torn ligaments, whiplash, straddle injuries, tailbone injuries, concussions, or broken bones, including ALL parts of your body?** If you can't remember, please ask a family member. ____ No ____ Yes
   If yes, please explain:

   _____

   _____

   _____

   Have you ever been in a car accident? ____ No ____ Yes. If yes, please explain:

   _____

   _____

   _____

70. **Please list all major physical activities and/or sports you have participated in competitively or recreationally and how many years of each.** *(This includes gymnastics, cheerleading, dance, horseback riding, soccer, softball, volleyball, track & field, running, etc)*

Activity or Sport	Years of Participation

<u>*Significant Emotional Stressors*</u>

71. In general, how would you describe your current relationship?	No tension Some tension A lot of tension
72. Do you and your current partner work out arguments with:	A lot of difficulty Some difficulty No difficulty
73. Do arguments ever result in you feeling down or bad about yourself?	Often Sometimes Never
74. Do you ever feel frightened by what your current partner says or does?	Often Sometimes Never
75. Has your current partner ever abused you emotionally?	Often Sometimes Never
76. Has your current partner ever abused you sexually?	Often Sometimes Never

Please clearly circle the answer that best suits your situation

77. **What other important stressors in your life should we know about? Please explain.**

78. **How does your pelvic pain problem affect your life?**

79. **What is the pain preventing you from doing?**

80. **What is your greatest fear regarding your pelvic pain symptoms?**

81. **Do your symptoms cause you more <u>pain</u> or <u>suffering</u>? Please explain**

VULVAR PAIN FUNCTIONAL QUESTIONNAIRE (V-Q)

These are statements about how your pelvic pain affects your everyday life. Please check one box for each item below, choosing the one that bst describes your situation. Some of the statements deal with personal subjects. These statements are included because they will help your healthcare provider design the best treatment for you and measure your progress during treatment. Your responses will be kept completely confidential at all times.

1. Because of my pelvic pain
    - ❑ I can't wear tight-fitting clothing like pantyhose that puts any pressure over my painful area.
    - ❑ I can wear closer fitting clothing as long as it only puts a little bit of pressure over my painful area.
    - ❑ I can wear whatever I like most of the time, but every now and then I feel pelvic pain caused by pressure from my clothing.
    - ❑ I can wear whatever I like; I never have pelvic pain because of clothing.

2. My pelvic pain
    - ❑ Gets worse when I walk, so I can only walk far enough to move around in my house, no further.
    - ❑ Gets worse when I walk. I can walk a short distance outside the house, but it is very painful to walk far enough to get a full load of groceries in a grocery store.
    - ❑ Gets a little worse when I walk. I can walk far enough to do my errands, like grocery shopping, but it would be very painful to walk longer distances for fun or exercise.
    - ❑ My pain does not get worse with walking; I can walk as far as I want to
    - ❑ I have a hard time walking because of another medical problem, but pelvic pain doesn't make it hard to walk.

3. My pelvic pain
    - ❑ Gets worse when I sit, so it hurts too much to sit any longer than 30 minutes at a time.
    - ❑ Gets worse when I sit. I can sit for longer than 30 minutes at a time, but it is so painful that it is difficult to do my job or sit long enough to watch a movie.
    - ❑ Occasionally gets worse when I sit, but most of the time sitting is uncomfortable.
    - ❑ My pain does not get worse with sitting. I can sit as long as I want to.
    - ❑ I have trouble sitting for very long because of another medical problem, but pelvic pain doesn't make it hard to sit.

4. Because of pain pills I take for my pelvic pain
   - ❑ I am sleepy and I have trouble concentrating at work or while I do housework.
   - ❑ I can concentrate just enough to do my work, but I can't do more, like go out in the evenings.
   - ❑ I can do all of my work, and go out in the evening if I want, but I feel out of sorts.
   - ❑ I don't have nay problems with the pills that I take for pelvic pain.
   - ❑ I don't take pain pills for my pelvic pain.

5. Because of my pelvic pain
   - ❑ I have very bad pain when I try to have a bowel movement, and it keeps hurting for at least 5 minutes after I am finished.
   - ❑ It hurts when I try to have a bowel movement, but the pain goes away when I am finished.
   - ❑ Most of the time it does not hurt when I have a bowel movement, but every now and then it does.
   - ❑ It never hurts from my pelvic pain when I have a bowel movement.

6. Because of my pelvic pain
   - ❑ I don't get together with my friends or go out to parties or events.
   - ❑ I only get together with my friends or go out to parties or events every now and then.
   - ❑ I usually will go out with friends or to events if I want to, but every now and then I don't because of the pain
   - ❑ I get together with friends or go to events whenever I want, pelvic pain does not get in the way.

7. Because of my pelvic pain
   - ❑ I can't stand for the doctor to insert the speculum when I go to the gynecologist.
   - ❑ I can stand it when the doctor inserts the speculum if they are very careful, but most of the time it really hurts.
   - ❑ It usually doesn't hurt when the doctor inserts the speculum, but every now and then it does hurt.
   - ❑ It never hurts for the doctor to insert the speculum when I go to the gynecologist.

8. Because of my pelvic pain
   - ❑ I cannot use tampons at all, because they make my pain much worse.
   - ❑ I can only use tampons if I put them in very carefully.
   - ❑ It usually doesn't hurt to use tampons, but occasionally it does hurt.
   - ❑ It never hurts to use tampons.
   - ❑ This question doesn't apply to me, because I don't need to use tampons, or I wouldn't choose to use them whether they hurt or not.

9. Because of my pelvic pain
   - ❑ I can't let my partner put a finger or penis in my vagina during sex at all.
   - ❑ My partner can put a finger or penis in my vagina very carefully, but it still hurts.
   - ❑ It usually doesn't hurt if my partner puts a finger or penis in my vagina, but every now and then it does hurt.
   - ❑ It doesn't hurt to have my partner put a finger or penis in my vagina at all.
   - ❑ This questions does not apply to me because I don't have a sexual partner.
   - ❑ Specifically, I won't get involved with a partner because I worry about pelvic pain during sex.

10. Because of my pelvic pain
    - ❏ It hurts too much for my partner to touch me sexually even if the touching doesn't go in my vagina.
    - ❏ My partner can touch me sexually outside the vagina if we are very careful.
    - ❏ It doesn't usually hurt for my partner to touch me sexually outside the vagina, but every now and then it does hurt.
    - ❏ It never hurts for my partner to touch me sexually outside the vagina.
    - ❏ This question does not apply to me because I don't have a sexual partner.
    - ❏ Specifically, I won't get involved with a partner because I worry about pelvic pain during sex.
11. Because of my pelvic pain
    - ❏ It is too painful to touch myself for sexual pleasure.
    - ❏ I can touch myself for sexual pleasure if I am very careful.
    - ❏ It usually doesn't hurt to touch myself for sexual pleasure, but every now and then it does hurt.
    - ❏ It never hurts to touch myself for sexual pleasure.
    - ❏ I don't touch myself for sexual pleasure, but that is by choice, not because of pelvic pain.

© 2005 Kathie Hummel-Berry, PT, PhD, Kathe Wallace, PT, Hollis Herman MS, PT, OCS
All providers of women's health services are hereby given permission to make unlimited copies for clinical use.

---

80. *Please feel free to share any more information about your pain that you feel we need to know.*

Questionnaire adapted from The International Pelvic Pain Society, Dr. Fred Howard, Dr. Hope Haefher and Dr. Robert Echenberg. Updated 12-2015. Retrieved from http://instituteforwomeninpain.com/assets/files/Initial%20Questionnaire.pdf.

The International Pelvic Pain Society
Chronic Pelvic Pain Patient Education Booklet

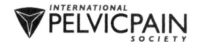

Chronic Pelvic Pain

What is Chronic Pelvic Pain (CPP)?

Chronic pelvic pain is one of the most common medical problems among women. Twenty-five percent of women with CPP may spend 2-3 days in bed each month. More than half of the women with CPP must cut down on their daily activities 1 or more days a month and 90% have pain with intercourse (sex). Almost half of the women with CPP feel sad or depressed some of the time.

Despite all the pain CPP causes, doctors are often not able to find a reason or cure to help these women.

CPP is any pelvic pain that lasts for more than six months. Usually the problem, which originally caused the pain, has lessened or even gone away completely, but the pain continues.

What is the difference between "acute" and "chronic" pain?

Acute pain is the pain that happens when the body is hurt, such as when you break your arm. There is an obvious cause for the pain. Chronic pain is very different. We may not know what the original cause of the pain was and it may be gone. The reason pain is still there might be because of changes in the muscles, nerves or other tissues in and near the pelvis. The pain itself has now become the disease.

What is "Chronic Pelvic Pain Syndrome"?

When constant, strong pain continues for a long period of time, it can become physically and mentally exhausting. To deal with the pain, the woman may make emotional and behavioral changes in her daily life. When pain has continued for so long and to such an extent that the person in pain is changing emotionally and behaving differently to cope with it, this is known as "Chronic Pelvic Pain Syndrome". Women with this condition will have the following:

- Pain present for 6 or more months
- Usual treatments have not relieved the pain or have given only little relief
- The pain is stronger than would be expected from the injury/surgery/condition which initially caused the pain
- Difficulty sleeping or sleeping too much, constipation, decreased appetite, "slow motion" body movements and reactions, and other symptoms of depression, including feeling blue or tearfulness.
- Less and less physical activity
- Changes in how she relates in her usual roles as wife, mother and employee.

Chronic pelvic pain has many parts. For example:
  1. Physical symptoms: pain, trouble sleeping, small appetite

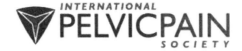

2. Emotional symptoms: depression, anxiety
3. Changes in behavior: spending time in bed, missing work, no longer enjoying usual activities

It is not "all in your head"!

Can CPP affect other parts of my body?

A woman who has CPP for a long time may notice that she starts to have problems in other parts of her body as well. It is common for pain to cause muscle tension. Tightness in the pelvic muscles can affect the bladder and the bowel causing problems with urinating or having a bowel movement. Patients also may notice pain in the back and legs due to problems with muscles and nerves. Once these problems have started, they may become more painful and troublesome than the pelvic pain, which started them. Doctors who specialize in treating chronic pelvic pain will examine all of your organ systems, including your bladder and bowel, not just your female organs.

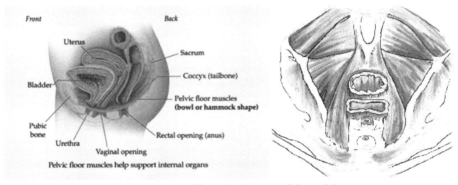

Pelvic floor muscles from the side and from the bottom of the pelvis

How do I feel pain?

Injured tissues in the body send signals through nerves to your spinal cord. The spinal cord acts like a gate. It can let the signals pass to the brain, stop the signals or change them, making them stronger or weaker. How the spinal cord acts depends on other nerve messages and signals from the brain. So, how you feel pain is affected by your mood, by your surroundings and by other things happening in your body at the same time.

When a person has chronic, long-lasting pain, the spinal cord gate may be damaged. This may cause the gate to remain open even after the injured tissue is healing. When this happens, the pain is still there even though the original cause of the pain was treated.

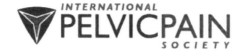

Sometimes women with chronic pain feel pain differently or more strongly than others. Something that does not cause pain for one person may cause pain in a person with chronic pain. We are not sure why this happens, but think it may be because of the way the nerves send pain information to the brain and how the brain processes this information.

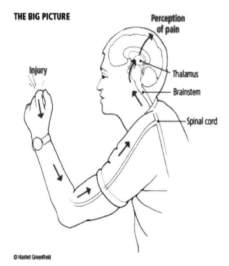

How the body sends pain messages to the brain

What are the characteristics of chronic pain?

There are four main factors:

1. Problem at the site of origin: There is or was an injury at the place where the pain first started. This injury can come from many things such as cysts on the ovaries, infections of the bowel or bladder, or scar tissue.
2. Referred Pain: Your body has two types of nerves. *Visceral* nerves carry information from the organs (stomach, intestines, lungs, heart, etc.). *Somatic* nerves bring messages from the skin and muscles. Both types of nerves travel to the same area on the spinal cord. When your *visceral* nerves are active for long periods of time with pain, it may activate the *somatic* nerves, which then carry the pain back to the muscles and skin. In CPP, the *somatic* nerves may carry the pain back to your pelvic and abdominal muscles and skin. That means that your pain may start in your bladder and spread to your skin and muscles, or the other way around.
3. Trigger points: These are specific areas of tenderness that happen in the muscle wall of the abdomen. Trigger points may start out as just one symptom of your pelvic pain or they may be the major source of pain for you. For this reason, treating the trigger points, for some women, can help make the pain much better. For other women, the original source of injury as well as the trigger points must be treated.
4. Action of the Brain: Your brain influences your emotions and behavior. It also works with your spinal cord to manage how you feel pain. For example, if you are depressed,

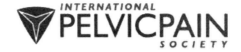

your brain will allow more pain signals to cross the gates of the spinal cord, and you will feel more pain. Treatment of how your brain processes pain can help manage chronic pain. Treatment can include psychological counseling, physical therapy and medications.

It is important to remember that all of these 4 levels of pain must be treated together for CPP therapy to be successful.

How will my doctor diagnose CPP?

Your doctor will take a history of your problem. It is very important to give your doctor a detailed and exact description of the problem. He/she will also do a physical examination. From this, the doctor will be able to decide what lab tests and procedures might be needed to find the reasons for your pain.

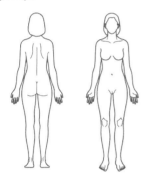

There are a number of things you can do to help your doctor diagnose and treat you:
- Get copies of your medical records, including doctor visits, lab tests, x-rays and surgical testing.
- If you have had surgeries, records of the surgical treatments including photos and videotapes are very helpful
- Carefully fill out the doctor's questionnaire. Take your time and try to remember all the details and the order in which they happened. Just filling out the questionnaire may help you remember details you had forgotten. Also, it may be easier to write out personal information that is difficult or embarrassing to talk about. Remember that the more information you give the doctor, the easier it will be for him/her to help you. Factors which may be very important in your care are:
  - How and when did your pain begin?
  - What makes the pain better or worse?
  - Does your pain change based on time of day, week or month?
  - How does your menstrual cycle or period affect the pain?
  - How does the pain affect your sleep?
  - Has the pain spread since it began?
  - Do you notice problems or pain with your skin (pain, itching, burning), muscles, joints or back?
  - Do you have pain with urination (peeing), constipation, diarrhea or other problems with your bowels?

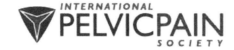

    o   Has the pain caused emotional changes like anxiety or depression?
    o   What have you done to help make the pain better? What has worked? What has not worked?
    o   What medical treatments have you had? Have they helped?
    o   What medications have you used in the past? What medicines are you taking now?
    o   What do you think is causing your pain?
    o   What concerns you most about your pain?

Your doctor will do a complete physical exam. The pelvis not only contains the female organs, but also contains bowel, bladder, blood vessels and nerves. It provides support for your upper body and connects the upper body to the lower body. For these reasons, not only will your female organs, vagina and rectum be examined, but also your posture, how you walk, your back, abdomen, legs and thighs. Special attention will be given to any changes in skin sensation, numbness or tenderness. A close examination of the vagina and also the labia (lips of the vagina) will be done. You may also have a rectal examination. During the exam, you may be asked at times to tense and relax specific muscles. Throughout all of this, your doctor will be looking for clues to damage or disease, which might have started the pain, and clues to which nerves are contributing to the pain.

What factors will my doctor consider when deciding how to help me?

Your doctor will consider a number of factors in deciding how best to treat your pain. Pain is in the nervous system, which includes the body <u>and</u> the mind. The pain is not all in your body but it is not all in your head either. For a treatment to be effective, it needs to treat the body and the mind. CPP is not caused by a single problem but by a number of problems interacting together. This means that you do not need a single "treatment". You will need several treatments for all the problems.

It is impossible to tell how much each pain factor adds to the whole problem. In fact, whatever caused your pain in the first place may become only a minor factor while the chronic pain is caused by secondary factors. Therefore, ALL factors must be treated, not just the ones that "seem" the most important.

How soon will I start to feel better?

It may take a long time before you start feeling better, even though your doctor is trying to provide you with relief as quickly as possible. It took a long time for your pain to become so bad, and it may take weeks or months for it to get better. Often the pain will not go away completely, but the goal is to make the pain manageable enough to do the things you normally like or want to do. During your treatment, as you are slowly improving, try to remain calm and patient and keep a positive attitude.

Will I receive pain medication?

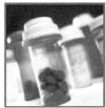

In the early stages of your treatment, you may be given pain medication. The treatment of CPP takes time to work and medication can keep you comfortable until they can take effect. Please remember that pain

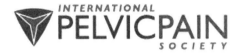

medication is just temporary treatment of the pain, but does not treat the problems that cause the pain. Pain medications may not take all of your pain away, but may make your symptoms more bearable.

All medications can have side effects, especially narcotic pain pills (like Norco or Percocet). Your doctor will probably try non-narcotic pain relievers first to avoid potential drug side effects.

You may be given a combination of medications instead of one. Some medications can work better when given together. You may get the most relief using some medications for pain and others for mood, such as antidepressants.

Taking medication every time you feel pain can make you hooked on medication. It is better to take your pain medication at scheduled times. Your doctor may give you a set number of pills to take at a certain time.

Your body may get used to the narcotic pills and the medication may help your pain less and less. Talk to your doctor about how well your medications are working at each visit. If in between visits, call your doctor to schedule an appointment. Changing pain medication is not something your physician can easily do based on a phone conversation.

It is your responsibility to use strong narcotic pain pills safely and correctly. Lost and stolen prescriptions will not be replaced. Your doctor may no longer provide care to you if you are getting narcotic pain pills from multiple doctors. Some doctors do not routinely prescribe narcotics and advise patients to obtain these medications from their primary care doctor only.

What about my muscle aches and pains?

Treating problems with your muscles are an important part of your care. A physical therapist may examine how you walk and how you stand. They will also look at the individual muscles of your abdomen, pelvis and legs. The therapist may do special tests for muscle strength, tenderness, length and flexibility. She/he will also decide if you have "trigger points" or areas where your muscles are especially tender or sore. Your physical therapist will give you different exercises to help you build healthier and stronger muscles. There are different treatments for this. You may learn special exercises. Some patients use special equipment such as ultrasound or muscle stimulators. You will also learn relaxation and breathing techniques. The physical therapist will work closely with your doctor to make a program of exercises and pain medications by mouth and/or injection as needed.

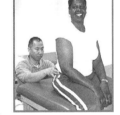

Will I be treated for emotional pain?

Chronic pain affects all aspects of your physical and emotional life. It may cause anxiety, depression, and problems with your work and home life. To give the best treatment, your doctor will treat the cause of the pain, but also all the other problems it has caused. A number of different therapies can be used to help you overcome these common problems in chronic pelvic pain syndrome. You can improve your anxiety and depression by learning to change the behaviors that contribute to your pain.

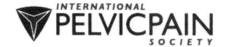

The pain you suffer also affects your family. They will receive education about how your pain affects them and how their reactions to your pain affect you. Teaching your support system about your pain, the causes and treatments will help them support you in your recovery.

What about surgical treatments?

Sometimes your doctor may decide to do surgery to look for other causes of pain or treat pain. This is decided based on a patient's history and exam.

So...what can I expect from treatment for CPP?

First off, you need to be realistic in your goals and hopes for treatment. Some CPP can never be completely cured. Some women are so uncomfortable with the evaluation and testing process that they are never able to get a significant amount of pain relief.

Do not expect instant results. Be patient with your treatment and follow all your doctor's instructions. Treatments may take up to 3-6 months to work, so continue to follow instructions even if you don't see results right away. During your treatment and therapies, you will have set appointments with your doctor and therapist rather than just coming in when the pain is particularly bad. You may start with weekly or monthly visits. You and your doctor will decide whether these should be more or less frequent based on your progress. Be sure not to miss an appointment as this can interfere with your treatment. If you miss an appointment and your pain becomes worse, it may take time to get it under control again.

Remember that the treatment of chronic pelvic pain is a slow process using many different kinds of therapy. It may not be possible to totally cure your pain. Successful treatment means decreasing your pain to a low level so that you are able to enjoy doing the things you want to do again.

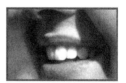

Introduction to Prenatal and Postpartum Care

CHAPTER 29

Anatomy and Physiologic Adaptations of Normal Pregnancy

Ellise D. Adams

INTRODUCTION

Anatomy and physiologic changes occur in a woman's body from the moment of conception. As signs and symptoms of pregnancy begin to occur, the woman suspects and seeks to confirm the pregnancy. Chapter 30 provides content on the signs and symptoms of pregnancy and methods for diagnosing pregnancy. Many signs of pregnancy are anatomic or physiologic adaptations of pregnancy (**Table 29-1**).

This chapter provides a body systems approach to the anatomic and physiologic adaptations of normal pregnancy. It should be explored along with Chapter 5 for a better understanding of gynecologic anatomy and physiology. Pregnancy represents a period in which changes are rapidly occurring in a woman's anatomic and physiologic processes. These changes support the increased metabolic demands of pregnancy, the increased demands of the developing fetus, and the physical demands of childbirth and lactation. An understanding of these processes provides the clinician with knowledge to make optimal clinical decisions related to the care of women during pregnancy.

BREAST CHANGES

During pregnancy, changing hormones levels contribute to breast changes and development in preparation for lactation. See Chapter 32 for more information about the process of lactation. Hormones contributing to breast changes during pregnancy include prolactin-inhibiting factor (PIF), estrogen, progesterone, and human placental lactogen (hPL). While prolactin levels rise in pregnancy, the corresponding rise in estrogen and PIF suppresses the effects of this increase, so that the woman does not produce breastmilk until after giving birth. Estrogen and progesterone cause the ducts and glandular tissue of the breast to proliferate (Wambach & Riordan, 2014)—a process aided by hPL and growth hormone. Many women experience the early, presumptive sign of pregnancy of heaviness, fullness, and tenderness in the breast. By term, the total breast weight has increased by 12 ounces (Blackburn, 2013). Later in pregnancy, heavier breasts can cause posture changes such as anterior flexion of the neck and slumping of the shoulders.

By the second trimester, the number of mammary alveoli and ducts increases and branching of the ducts takes place (Wambach & Riordan, 2014). Proliferation of the alveoli may be palpable, and these structures will feel nodular (Jarvis, 2016). Nipples become more erect, may lengthen, and widen with an increase in width of the areola (Thanaboonyawat, Chanprapaph, Lattalapkul, & Rongluen, 2013).

During pregnancy, the skin of the breast becomes thinner and striae develop on the breasts

TABLE 29-1	Presumptive, Probable, and Positive Signs of Pregnancy

Sign	Clinical Findings
Presumptive (subjective signs)	Amenorrhea, nausea, vomiting, increased urinary frequency, excessive fatigue, breast tenderness, quickening at 18–20 weeks
Probable (objective signs)	Goodell sign (softening of cervix) Chadwick sign (cervix is blue/purple) Hegar's sign (softening of lower uterine segment) Uterine enlargement Braxton Hicks contractions (may be palpated by 28 weeks) Uterine soufflé (soft blowing sound due to blood pulsating through the placenta) Integumentary pigment changes Ballottement, fetal outline definable, positive pregnancy test (could be hydatidiform mole, choriocarcinoma, increased pituitary gonadotropins at menopause)
Positive (diagnostic)	Fetal heart rate auscultated by fetoscope at 17–20 weeks or by Doppler at 10–12 weeks Palpable fetal outline and fetal movement after 20 weeks Visualization of fetus with cardiac activity by ultrasound (fetal parts visible by 8 weeks)

Data from Jarvis, C. (2016). *Physical examination and health assessment* (7th ed.). St. Louis, MO: Saunders Elsevier; King, T., Brucker, M., Kriebs, J., Fahey, J., Gegor, C., & Varney, H. (2015). *Varney's midwifery* (5th ed.). Burlington, MA: Jones & Bartlett Learning.

of many women. Darkening of the pigmentation of the areola may also occur. In the second trimester, colostrum begins to be excreted as the alveoli become progressively distended (Blackburn, 2013).

REPRODUCTIVE SYSTEM CHANGES

Uterine Changes

During pregnancy, the uterus changes from an almost solid organ to a thin-walled, hollow organ. The uterus holds, on average, 5 L of fluid during pregnancy (Blackburn, 2013). The uterine wall thickens from 10 to 25 mm by 16 weeks' gestation. It is hypothesized that the increased production of estrogen and progesterone initiates the process of uterine growth via hypertrophy of the uterine muscle cells. However, by term the uterine wall thins to 5 to 10 mm as a result of distention due to fetal growth (sometimes referred to as mechanical

distention) (Blackburn, 2013). The shape of the uterus also becomes more globular. Dextrorotation or rotation of the uterus to the right occurs early in pregnancy due to displacement of the uterus by the descending colon (Jarvis, 2016).

Hegar's sign—a probable sign of pregnancy—may be detectable by the fourth month of gestation. It occurs when the uterus bends in an anterior direction on the softened lower uterine segment or isthmus. As pregnancy progresses, the fundus rises out of the pelvis (**Figure 29-1**). At 12 weeks' gestation, the fundus is located at the level of the symphysis pubis. By week 16, it rises to midway between symphysis pubis and the umbilicus. By 20 weeks' gestation, the fundus is typically at the same height as the umbilicus. Until term, the fundus enlarges approximately 1 cm per week. As the time for birth approaches, the fundal height drops slightly. This process, which is commonly called lightening, occurs for a woman who is a primigravida around 38 weeks' gestation but may not occur

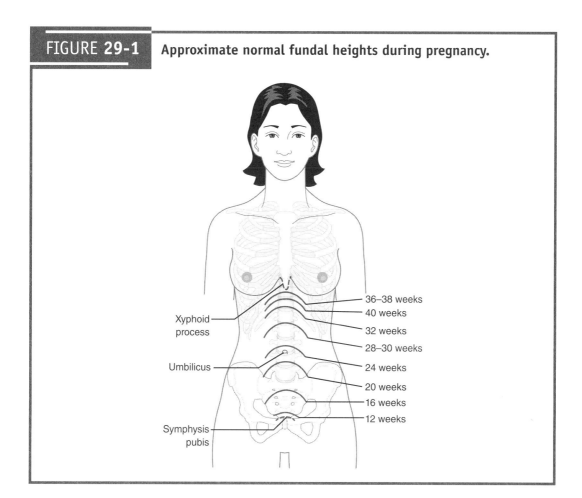

FIGURE 29-1 Approximate normal fundal heights during pregnancy.

for the woman who is a multigravida until she goes into labor (King et al., 2015).

The uterus is a muscular organ and contracts throughout pregnancy. Contractions that occur in early pregnancy are typically felt as mild and irregular in occurrence. These early contractions, commonly called Braxton Hicks contractions, may begin at 6 weeks' gestation but may not become noticeable until the second trimester for the woman experiencing her first pregnancy (primigravida). At 25 weeks' gestation, uterine contractility increases, with contractions occurring at a rate of 0.32 per hour. At term, contractions can occur at a rate of 2.33 per hour (Blackburn, 2013).

Uteroplacental blood flow also increases during pregnancy. Uterine soufflé—a quiet swishing sound—may be detectable during fetal heart rate auscultation. This sound is attributable to the maternal arterial blood arriving into the placenta (Jarvis, 2016). Uterine soufflé is one of the reasons it is suggested that the clinician check the maternal pulse when checking the fetal heart rate, thereby ensuring one is not confused with the other.

Cervical Changes

The nature and consistency of the cervix change during pregnancy. The woman's prepregnant cervix is firm to palpation. Conversely, a softened cervix, known as Goodell's sign, is considered a probable sign of pregnancy. At 4 weeks' gestation, the cervix becomes edematous and congested. Hypertrophy and hyperplasia of the cervical glands occur at this time as well, and the cervix takes on a bluish hue known as Chadwick's sign, a probable sign of pregnancy. A mucus plug develops in the os of the cervix to protect the growing fetus against intrauterine infection.

As the time for birth approaches, the cervix begins to soften and thin; this thinning of the cervix is called effacement. This is typically referred to as cervical ripening and is the result of increasing levels of estrogen and changes in the solubility of collagen. Near term, the cervix moves from a posterior position to an anterior position. Cervical ripening is one of the signs clinicians look for when determining the possibility of the onset of labor. The process of regular uterine contractions initially stimulates cervical stretching followed by cervical dilation (Blackburn, 2013).

Vaginal and Vulvar Changes

Increased vascularization of the vagina and pelvic viscera, softening of the connective tissue, and hypertrophy of the smooth muscle are also reproductive system changes noted during pregnancy. In the second trimester, these changes may increase a woman's libido and heighten her sexual response. There may also be generalized edema of the labia majora near term. These physiologic changes also represent preparatory steps for birth.

During pregnancy, the vaginal mucosa thickens and rugae (vaginal folds) become more pronounced, allowing for expansion of the vagina without trauma during the birthing process. Vaginal pH increases, which leads to an increased risk for candidiasis. Leukorrhea is common in pregnancy, manifesting as a thin or thick, white or yellow discharge without itching or irritation and most commonly occurring during the second trimester (Blackburn, 2013; King et al., 2015).

Increasing venous stasis due to mechanical pressure from the growing uterus and vasodilation may lead to vulvar varicosities. Obesity, poor muscle tone, sedentary lifestyle, and familiar tendencies may exacerbate the increased risk for varicosities.

Pelvic Floor Changes

Increasing levels of progesterone and relaxin during pregnancy soften the ligaments and muscles of the pelvic floor. These muscles and ligaments are further stretched by the gravid uterus and during vaginal birth. Anatomic changes of the pelvic floor during pregnancy and birth may predispose the woman to urinary and fecal incontinence, hemorrhoids, dyspareunia, uterine prolapse, and future perineal trauma, particularly when associated with overstretching and pelvic floor damage (Steen & Roberts, 2011).

INTEGUMENTARY SYSTEM CHANGES

During pregnancy, there is an increased production of sweat and sebaceous glands. Increased vascularity and pigmentation of the areola, genitalia, abdomen, and face (chloasma gravidarum) may occur. Linea nigra—a dark line beginning near the sternal notch and continuing downward to the symphysis pubis and genitalia—may appear due to increasing levels of melanocyte-stimulating hormone (Jarvis, 2016).

Striae gravidarum (stretch marks) may appear on the breasts, abdomen, hips, and thighs, due to the breakdown of connective tissue. These marks may appear deep red to purple in color during pregnancy but typically fade to light silver in the months following pregnancy. Despite advertisers' claims, there is no magic cream to prevent striae or to make them go away. Watching weight gain and eating nutritiously can help decrease their number and severity.

GASTROINTESTINAL CHANGES

Peristalsis slows during pregnancy, which may cause flatus, constipation, and diminished bowel sounds. Constipation may also stem from the displacement of the intestines by the gravid uterus, fluid reabsorption changes, and increased progesterone levels, all of which can result in decreased intestinal contractility.

The displacement of abdominal organs and altered esophageal sphincter and gastric tone related to increasing progesterone levels may cause dyspepsia in pregnancy. A woman who is pregnant may report taste changes and increased salivation. She is also predisposed to gallstone formation related to sluggish emptying of bile from the gallbladder combined with increased cholesterol saturation during pregnancy (Jarvis, 2016). See Chapters 30 and 31 for suggestions in how best to prevent or decrease the discomfort from these common complications.

CARDIOVASCULAR SYSTEM AND HEMATOLOGIC CHANGES

During pregnancy, the heart is displaced upward and to the left within the chest cavity by the gravid uterus's pressure on the diaphragm. As pregnancy progresses, the risk for inferior vena cava and aortic compression leading to supine hypotension increases when the woman lies in a supine position.

To avoid hypotension and potential syncope, the woman should be advised to lie in a left lateral position. Hemodynamic changes and anatomic changes also may alter vital signs in the pregnant woman (**Table 29-2**).

Cardiac output in pregnancy increases by 30% to 50% over that in women who are not pregnant (Blackburn, 2013; Ouziunian & Elkayam, 2012). This increase peaks in the early third trimester and is maintained until birth. Half of the total increase in cardiac output, however, occurs by the eighth week of pregnancy (Blackburn, 2013). Therefore, women with cardiac disease may become symptomatic during the first trimester. Stroke volume is also increased during pregnancy by 20% to 30%. These increases in cardiac output and stroke volume allow for the 30% increase in oxygen consumption observed during pregnancy.

TABLE 29-2	Vital Sign Changes in Pregnancy	
Vital Sign	**Changes in Pregnancy**	**Measurement Alterations in Pregnancy**
Heart rate and heart sounds	Volume of the first heart sound may be increased with splitting. Third heart sound may be detected. Systolic murmurs may be detected. Increases by 15–20 beats/min by 32 weeks' gestation.	Palpate the maternal pulse when auscultating the fetal heart rate to be able to distinguish between the two.
Respiratory rate	Increases by 1–2 breaths/min	None
BP	First trimester: same as prepregnancy values Second trimester: systolic BP decreases by 2–8 mm Hg and diastolic BP decreases by 5–15 mm Hg due to peripheral vascular resistance Third trimester: gradually returns to prepregnancy values	Use of an automated cuff may improve accuracy of measurement, as some pregnant women do not have a fifth Korotkoff sound. Systolic and diastolic BP may be 16 mm Hg higher when taken while the woman is sitting. BP readings may decrease in the maternal left lateral position.

Abbreviation: BP, blood pressure.
Data from Jarvis, C. (2016). *Physical examination and health assessment* (7th ed.). St. Louis, MO: Saunders Elsevier; Ouziunian, J., & Elkayam, U. (2012). Physiologic changes during normal pregnancy and delivery. *Cardiology Clinics, 30*, 317–329; Tan, E., & Tan, E. (2013). Alterations in physiology and anatomy during pregnancy. *Best Practice & Research Clinical Obstetrics & Gynaecology, 27*, 791–802.

During pregnancy, blood volume increases by 30% to 50%, or 1,100 to 1,600 mL (Ouziunian & Elkayam, 2012), and peaks at 30 to 34 weeks' gestation. The increase in blood volume improves blood flow to the vital organs and protects against excessive blood loss during birth. Fetal growth during pregnancy and newborn weight are correlated with the degree of blood volume expansion.

Of the blood volume expansion occurring during pregnancy, 75% is considered to be plasma (King et al., 2015). There is also a slight increase in red blood cell volume (RBC). The blood volume changes result in hemodilution, which leads to a state of physiologic anemia during pregnancy. As the RBC volume increases, iron demands also increase. Leukocytosis occurs in pregnancy, with white blood cell counts increasing to as much as 14,000 to 17,000 cells per mm^3 of blood (**Table 29-3**). Clotting factors increase as well, creating a risk for clotting events during pregnancy.

Systemic vascular resistance is reduced due to the effects of progesterone, prostaglandins, estrogen, and prolactin. This lowered systemic vascular resistance, in combination with inferior vena cava compression, is partly responsible for the dependent edema that occurs in pregnancy. Epulis of pregnancy, or hypertrophy of the gums accompanied by bleeding, may also occur and is due to decreased vascular resistance and increase in the growth of capillaries during pregnancy (Jarvis, 2016).

RESPIRATORY SYSTEM CHANGES

Increased edema of the pharynx and larynx during pregnancy may cause respiratory congestion in some women. Blood vessels in the nose vasodilate, resulting in engorgement of the capillaries, which may result in nose bleeds. The diaphragm is elevated because of the intra-abdominal pressure from the enlarging uterus and the effects of relaxin and progesterone. Chest wall circumference increases and chest compliance decreases. These anatomic findings reduce lung capacity in pregnancy by 5%. The risk for hyperventilation and dyspnea is heightened among pregnant women because of their increased respiratory rate and tidal volume; the latter may increase by 30% to 50% (Tan & Tan, 2013).

The 30% increase in oxygen consumption that occurs during pregnancy may further compromise respiration in women with conditions such as chronic asthma, obesity, or maternal smoking. However, higher PaO_2 levels and lower $PaCO_2$ levels create respiratory alkalosis. To compensate for these effects, the renal system excretes bicarbonate. A woman who is pregnant and who has insulin-dependent diabetes is at greater risk for diabetic ketoacidosis (Tan & Tan, 2013).

RENAL SYSTEM CHANGES

During pregnancy, the renal system is responsible for maintaining electrolyte and acid–base balance,

TABLE **29-3**	Laboratory Value Changes in Pregnancy			
Hematologic Measure	**Nonpregnant Women, Ages 19–65**	**First Trimester**	**Second Trimester**	**Third Trimester**
Hemoglobin	12–16 g/dL	11.6–13.9 g/dL	9.7–14.8 g/dL	9.5–15 g/dL
Hematocrit	37–47%	31–41%	30–39%	28–40%
Red blood cell count	3.5–5.5/mm^3	3.4–5.2/mm^3	2.8–4.5/mm^3	2.7–4.4/mm^3
White blood cell count	4.5–11/mm^3	4–13/mm^3	6–14/mm^3	6–17/mm^3

Data from Blackburn, S. T. (2013). *Maternal, fetal and neonatal physiology: A clinical perspective* (4th ed.). St. Louis, MO: Saunders Elsevier; King, T., Brucker, M., Kriebs, J., Fahey, J., Gegor, C., & Varney, H. (2015). *Varney's midwifery* (5th ed.). Burlington, MA: Jones & Bartlett Learning.

regulating increases in blood and extracellular fluid volume, excreting maternal and fetal waste products, and conserving essential nutrients. Anatomically, the kidneys are displaced and increase in size during pregnancy. The renal tubules dilate, leading to urinary stasis, which in turn increases the risk for urinary tract infections. Bladder tone is decreased due to the effects of progesterone, which can lead to urinary frequency and incontinence. Urinary frequency is more common in the first and third trimesters. Urinary incontinence is most common in women who have had more than one pregnancy (multiparas) (Tan & Tan, 2013).

Nutritional status and effectiveness of medications may be affected by the urinary changes that occur during pregnancy. Renal vascular dilation and the resulting increased renal plasma flow increase the glomerular filtration rate (GFR). GFR peaks at 180 mL/min by the end of the first trimester—a factor that may alter the clearance of medications that are excreted by the kidneys (Tan & Tan, 2013). Protein, albumin, and glucose excretion are also affected by changes in the GFR.

MUSCULOSKELETAL SYSTEM CHANGES

Several musculoskeletal changes occur during pregnancy related to the effects of progesterone, estrogen, and relaxin on ligaments and joints. Particularly notable is the relaxation of pelvic structures in the woman who is pregnant. As mentioned earlier, uterine enlargement causes the diaphragm to rise and the rib cage to increase in width at the base (Jarvis, 2016). The circumference of the neck enlarges. Noticeable alterations in posture manifest as lordosis and kyphosis; they are due to a shifting center of balance caused by the enlarging uterus. This change in posture can lead to carpal tunnel syndrome in some pregnant women (Jarvis, 2016). Gait changes also occur to accommodate these changes. Common discomforts such as sciatica, discomfort of the symphysis pubis, and stretching and pain of the round, broad, uterosacral, and cardinal ligaments accompany these anatomic changes.

ENDOCRINE SYSTEM CHANGES

A palpable, mild enlargement of the thyroid occurs early in the first trimester. Thyroid-stimulating hormone levels decrease initially, but return to normal by birth (Tan & Tan, 2013). The pituitary gland also increases in size by a factor of 3. The basal metabolic rate increases by 20% to 25% (King et al., 2015), and insulin secretion increases to meet the physiologic demands of pregnancy. Women with preexisting insulin resistance and women who are obese are at greater risk for developing gestational diabetes. In preparation for lactation and the birthing process, prolactin and oxytocin are released in increasing amounts throughout pregnancy.

NEUROLOGIC SYSTEM AND PSYCHOSOCIAL CHANGES

Pregnancy is a time of central nervous system changes accompanied by many psychosocial changes. Shifting levels of hormones throughout the trimesters of pregnancy may engender emotional lability and irritability. Changes in cognition such as decreased attention span, decreased ability to concentrate, and memory lapses are also often reported during pregnancy. Sleep alterations may reflect either the physical discomforts of pregnancy or hormonal shifts. Pregnant women with sleep alterations are at risk for depressive moods and stress, which are associated with poorer pregnancy outcomes (Okun et al., 2013).

Optic and otic changes may also occur during pregnancy. Fluid retention in pregnancy accompanied by corneal thickening may be expressed as corneal edema, hyposensitivity, and decreased intraocular pressure (Blackburn, 2013). The effects of estrogen may bring about a feeling of plugged ears. Transient minimal hearing loss and vertigo can also occur. Hoarseness and snoring may result from laryngeal edema.

CONCLUSION

Recognition of the normal anatomy and physiologic changes in pregnancy allows the clinician to provide appropriate anticipatory guidance to maintain the health of the mother and her fetus. When these changes are understood and appreciated, alterations in normal pregnancy may be recognized appropriately and managed in a timely and effective manner.

References

Blackburn, S. T. (2013). *Maternal, fetal and neonatal physiology: A clinical perspective* (4th ed.). St. Louis, MO: Saunders Elsevier.

Jarvis, C. (2016). *Physical examination and health assessment* (7th ed.). St. Louis, MO: Saunders Elsevier.

King, T., Brucker, M., Kriebs, J., Fahey, J., Gegor, C., & Varney, H. (2015). *Varney's midwifery* (5th ed.). Burlington, MA: Jones & Bartlett Learning.

Okun, M., Kline, C., Roberts, J., Wettlaufer, B., Glover, K., & Hall, M. (2013). Prevalence of sleep deficiency in early gestation and its associations with stress and depressive symptoms. *Journal of Women's Health, 22*(12), 1028–1037.

Ouziunian, J., & Elkayam, U. (2012). Physiologic changes during normal pregnancy and delivery. *Cardiology Clinics, 30,* 317–329.

Steen, M., & Roberts, T. (2011). The consequences of pregnancy and birth for the pelvic floor. *British Journal of Midwifery, 19*(11), 692–698.

Tan, E., & Tan, E. (2013). Alterations in physiology and anatomy during pregnancy. *Best Practice & Research Clinical Obstetrics & Gynaecology, 27,* 791–802.

Thanaboonyawat, I., Chanprapaph, P., Lattalapkul, J., & Rongluen, S. (2013). Pilot study of normal development of nipples during pregnancy. *Journal of Human Lactation, 29*(4), 480–483.

Wambach, K., & Riordan, J. (2014). *Breastfeeding and human lactation* (5th ed.). Burlington, MA: Jones & Bartlett Learning.

CHAPTER 30

Diagnosis of Pregnancy and Overview of Prenatal Care

Julia C. Phillippi

The editors acknowledge Robin G. Jordan, who was author of the previous edition of this chapter.

INTRODUCTION

There are an estimated 6.6 million pregnancies each year in the United States (Finer & Zolna, 2014), and clinicians often see women who are pregnant for initial diagnosis or primary care. Given that an estimated 51% of pregnancies are unplanned (Finer & Zolna, 2014), women may not have considered pregnancy as a reason for fatigue, nausea, or amenorrhea, and may seek care for these symptoms with a trusted clinician, regardless of specialization. This chapter focuses on the care of women who have a diagnosis of pregnancy at a gynecologic or episodic clinic visit. The purpose of the chapter is to assist clinicians who provide only primary or gynecologic care with basic information about the assessment and initial prenatal care needs of a woman who is diagnosed with a pregnancy. A diagnosis of pregnancy can be surprising, and beginning care immediately with a trusted clinician can provide stability and increase the likelihood the woman will receive early prenatal care.

For more in-depth information on antepartum care, consult midwifery and obstetric books such as *Varney's Midwifery* (King, Brucker, Kriebs, Fahey, & Varney, 2013), *Prenatal and Postnatal Care: A Woman-Centered Approach* (Jordan, Engstrom, Marfell, & Farley, 2014), and *Obstetrics: Normal and Problem Pregnancies* (Gabbe et al., 2012).

DIAGNOSIS OF PREGNANCY

Bodily changes related to alterations in hormone levels early in pregnancy include breast changes, fatigue, urinary frequency, and nausea and vomiting. These changes, known as presumptive signs of pregnancy, may cause women to suspect pregnancy or seek primary care. While amenorrhea is the most well-known sign of pregnancy, many women have irregular cycles or do not keep track of their menstrual periods. Any sexually active woman of childbearing age (approximately 11–44 years old) has the potential to be pregnant. Some women, especially teens, may be reluctant to disclose sexual activity or admit they are at risk for pregnancy. Clinicians should have a low threshold for requesting a pregnancy test at any gynecologic or primary care visit, especially if the woman has symptoms of pregnancy.

Urine pregnancy tests are inexpensive, noninvasive, reliable, and easy to perform in any clinic with the capability to handle urine. Pregnancy tests detect the presence of human chorionic gonadotropin (hCG), which is released from a fertilized egg (blastocyst) once it implants in the uterus. Urine pregnancy tests provide a positive or negative finding, known as a qualitative result, within minutes. Such tests are usually positive 14 days after fertilization or 4 weeks after the last menstrual period (LMP), which corresponds to the first missed menses (Demma & Grace, 2013). A positive urine test, either at home or in the office, provides near certainty that a woman is pregnant. False-positive results are unlikely in an otherwise healthy woman. If used correctly, home pregnancy tests are very accurate. A negative urine hCG test does not rule out pregnancy, as sperm can remain viable in the female reproductive tract for 3 days, and the fertilized ovum floats within the uterine cavity for up to 7 days prior to implantation (Blackburn, 2013).

Blood serum pregnancy tests can detect the presence of hCG 8 to 10 days after fertilization and can yield either qualitative or quantitative results (Gabbe et al., 2012). Serum pregnancy tests are more costly, and their results are not immediately available, so they are usually reserved for women with complications such as pain or bleeding. Quantitative serum tests provide a numeric measurement of the level of hCG. Repeated quantitative hCG tests are useful in determining viability of a pregnancy from implantation until 9 weeks, when hCG begins a physiologic decline (Gabbe et al., 2012).

Because urine tests are so effective and rarely have false-positive results, a single urine pregnancy test is all that is needed to diagnose pregnancy. This diagnosis can elicit a range of emotions among women. Some women may have been struggling with infertility and will be elated, while others may be blind-sided by the pregnancy or even devastated. Clinicians should approach this moment with compassion and without judgment, giving the woman time to absorb the news. It may be best to tell a teen of the diagnosis privately, away from her family or support person, to allow her a moment to process this information and provide an opportunity to assess her safety and desire to disclose the pregnancy to others. A woman's initial response to the diagnosis may also differ dramatically from her later feelings. While clinicians should use the woman's response to guide the visit, it is important to inform women of all their options and allow time for reflection. Chapter 17 explores women's options for unintended pregnancy in more detail.

After allowing the woman a moment to absorb the news, it is important to begin early pregnancy care. The estimated due date can be calculated from the woman's last period. In addition, an early ultrasound can provide valuable information about the pregnancy, including the estimated due date and the location of implantation. Other than establishment of the woman's safety and the estimated gestational age of the pregnancy, the content of the remainder of the visit can be adjusted to meet the woman's needs.

While establishment of prenatal care is important to ensure maternal safety and allow early fetal assessment, the woman may need a few days to adjust to the news. Women may wish to continue seeing a trusted clinician until they are ready and able to locate prenatal care. In addition, women without previous health insurance become eligible for Medicaid upon diagnosis of pregnancy and can qualify for free or reduced-cost prenatal care; if this is the case, they may need time to establish insurance coverage and find a compatible provider.

ASSESSMENT

Even if the woman plans to obtain care at another location, careful assessment and counseling is needed at the time of diagnosis to determine maternal and fetal safety and prevent complications. Careful assessment can detect potentially life-threatening conditions and prevent fetal abnormalities. Assessment should be holistic and include medical, social, and personal components to determine the need for immediate intervention or education. Subjective and objective information is used to determine the woman's risk for complications and form a plan to optimize pregnancy outcomes through appropriate education, testing, and services.

History

The health history is an essential component of the initial prenatal visit. See Chapter 6 for basic elements of a health history. Because pregnancy affects all components of the woman's medical care, the history should include an in-depth assessment of the woman's medical and obstetric history as well as information about her family, social support, and occupation. Key components of pregnancy assessment, beyond the normal history, are highlighted here for clarity.

Menstrual History

Data about a woman's last normal menses are needed to make a determination of gestational age and an estimated date of birth (EDB). To determine if the date of the LMP can be used to accurately date the pregnancy, the woman should be certain of the date of onset, it should be a normal flow and duration, and she should have a history of regular cycles (Phelan, 2008). Gestational age refers to the length of pregnancy after the first day of the LMP and is usually expressed in weeks and days; it is also known as menstrual age. Pregnancy is dated from the first day of the last menstrual period, because this is often a known date and pregnancy has historically been dated from this milestone.

The EDB for women with 28-day cycles can be determined by using Nägele's rule: Add 7 days to the first day of the LMP, then subtract 3 months (**Box 30-1**). If using a gestational wheel, software, or an app to calculate an estimated due date, be sure the version is accurate and accounts for the leap year when needed. If a woman has cycles that are longer or shorter than 28 days, the EDB will need to be adjusted. A woman with 30-day cycles would have 2 days added to the calculated EDB, while a woman with 26-day cycles would have 2 days subtracted.

If the woman is not certain of the date of her LMP, an ultrasound is needed to date the pregnancy (Whitworth, Bricker, Neilson, & Dowswell, 2010). If the top of the uterus, the uterine fundus, is below the pubic bone, a transvaginal ultrasound is most appropriate. Abdominal ultrasound is preferred when the uterine fundus is above the pubis. The accuracy of ultrasound dating declines as pregnancy progresses, so a quick referral is important (Gabbe et al., 2012).

Medical History

Birth Control Use at Conception Ask if the woman was using birth control at the time of conception. If she has an intrauterine device (IUD) in place, it needs to be removed as soon as possible (if the pregnancy is less than 12 weeks, the IUD can be removed immediately during the office visit),

---

BOX 30-1 Nägele's Rule

Here is an example of using Nägle's rule to calculate an estimated date of birth from the date of the last menstrual period.

```
 4/23 LMP of April 23
+    7 days
 4/30
– 3    months
 1/30 January 30 (of following year)
```

---

and she should receive an ultrasound to rule out ectopic pregnancy (Demma & Grace, 2013).

Prior Obstetric History In addition to recording the pregnancy history as outlined in Chapter 6, also ask about any pregnancy complications, gestational age at birth, length of labor, and pain relief used during vaginal births. Women with a previous cesarean birth will need further personalized counseling on the risks and benefits of vaginal versus cesarean birth.

Infectious Disease History A thorough history of prior infectious diseases and immunizations is needed to establish the woman's risk and need for testing and vaccination. Ask if the woman has ever known anyone with tuberculosis or traveled to areas where tuberculosis is common. If she is at risk, she should receive a tuberculin skin test when she can return in 48 to 72 hours. Past history of varicella is important, as well as the woman's vaccine history, to determine if she is at risk for chickenpox.

Women can receive vaccines in pregnancy (**Table 30-1**). The Centers for Disease Control and Prevention (CDC) updates the adult vaccine schedule often, and this information can be easily accessed on its website. The CDC website also includes detailed information about safety of vaccines for travel of local disease outbreaks during pregnancy (CDC, 2014). All women who are pregnant should be offered the influenza vaccine during flu season, though live attenuated influenza vaccine (LAIV [FluMist]) should not be given to pregnant women. All women should be encouraged to receive a tetanus, diphtheria, and acellular pertussis (Tdap) vaccination in the third trimester (CDC, 2016). Other vaccines, such as hepatitis B, can be administered if the woman is at risk (CDC, 2016).

During pregnancy, women have a decreased immune response to pathogens, making them more susceptible to infection. If a woman has cats, she should be careful to avoid contracting toxoplasmosis—an infection that is spread through cat feces. Someone else should change the cat litter box daily to prevent contact with the *Toxoplasma gondii* parasite. Wearing gloves while gardening, and careful hand washing are also essential. More information and patient handouts are available for free at the CDC website.

TABLE 30-1	Vaccines in Pregnancy

Recommended *Each* Pregnancy	Rationale	Timing
Influenza (flu)[a]	Women who are pregnant are at increased risk for flu-related complications.	Any gestation when the injection is available
Tetanus, diphtheria, pertussis (Tdap)	After maternal vaccination, antibodies cross the placenta and decrease the risk of pertussis infection in the newborn.	Third trimester (ideally 27–36 weeks' gestation)
Advised If at Risk	**Rationale**	**Timing**
Hepatitis B	If the woman is at risk for acquiring HBV, she should be vaccinated. Indications include risk of occupational exposure to blood, treatment for a sexually transmitted infection, more than 1 sex partner in the past 6 months, recent intravenous drug use, and HBsAg–positive sex partner.	3 injections beginning at any point in gestation
Contraindicated	**Rationale**	
Measles, mumps, rubella	This live virus vaccine has a (theoretical) risk to the fetus.	
Varicella	This live virus vaccine has a (theoretical) risk to the fetus.	

Abbreviations: HBsAg, HBV surface antigen; HBV, hepatitis B virus.
[a] Live attenuated influenza vaccine (LAIV [FluMist]) should not be given to pregnant women.

Women who are trying to conceive or who are pregnant should be warned to avoid ill children and adults and if working in occupations with bodily fluid exposure they should continue to use universal precautions and have a low threshold for using advanced personal protective equipment to avoid airborne pathogens. If exposed to infectious diseases, women who are pregnant should contact their clinician to determine if blood testing and immune globulin treatment are needed.

The woman's history of sexually transmitted infections (STIs) is also important. Ask if she has ever been diagnosed with an STI and inquire about treatment and follow-up. Also determine if she has undergone STI testing since having intercourse with her current partner. While a woman may not think she is at risk, all women who are pregnant have had bodily fluid exposure. A history of STIs is relevant because it is a risk factor for ectopic pregnancy, and genital herpes can affect the preferred route of birth. Current STIs need prompt diagnosis and treatment to prevent pregnancy and fetal complications. Treatment for STIs is often different in pregnancy, and the CDC is the source for up-to-date information on these practices (Workowski & Bolan, 2015). The current guidelines can be easily located on the CDC website with the keywords "sexually transmitted diseases" and "guidelines." In addition, the CDC has a free mobile app to expedite guideline use.

Genetic History

Clarify the woman's personal and family history, paying special attention to the items found in **Box 30-2**. If she is uncertain of her family history, she can report that information after she has a chance to disclose the pregnancy and speak with her relatives.

Paternal History

The medical and familial history of the genetic father of the baby is important to assess the risk for fetal abnormalities and determine the need for genetic or developmental screening. Relevant history items shown are shown in **Box 30-2**. The woman may not be able to state a full paternal history

---

BOX 30-2 Risk Factors for Fetal Genetic or Development Abnormalities in Maternal, Paternal, and Family History

- Maternal age > 35 years
- High-risk racial/ethnic group
- Mother and father related by blood
- Genetic conditions
- Congenital malformations of any body part
- Congenital blindness or deafness
- Stature disorders (very tall or very short family members)
- Developmental delays and mental retardation
- Maternal exposure to toxins
- Unexplained maternal or paternal infertility

Modified from Latendresse, G., & Deneris, A. (2015). An update on current prenatal testing options: First trimester and noninvasive prenatal testing. *Journal of Midwifery & Women's Health, 60*(1), 24–36. doi:10.1111/jmwh.12228.

and can bring this information to a later visit, if available.

Substance Exposure Including Medications, Illicit Drugs, and Chemicals

The first 12 weeks of pregnancy, as dated by the LMP, are a critical period for fetal development. Exposure to toxins during this period can permanently affect fetal development. Assessment of the woman's exposure to drugs and chemicals is crucial to assist her in avoiding toxins while continuing needed therapies.

Prescription Medications Prescription medications should be evaluated for safety in pregnancy (**Box 30-3**). Beginning in 2015, the U.S. Food and Drug Administration (FDA) requires manufacturers of all medications to provide detailed information about effects of their drugs in pregnancy (FDA, 2011). While high-quality data on many drugs and medications are limited, online resources can expedite obtaining current information. The drug prescribing information provides a brief summary about what is known about the drug in pregnancy. In addition, ToxNet is a free, online database maintained by the federal government that covers toxicology, hazardous chemicals, environmental health, and toxic releases. Reprotox is a database on the reproductive effects of medications and chemicals that is easy to use but requires a subscription.

For each prescribed medication, the drug information should be consulted and the risks and benefits of the medication considered in light of the woman's medical needs. Sometimes the risks of discontinuation of a drug for the woman outweigh minimal fetal risks. For instance, if a woman has a history of suicide attempts, discontinuation of

---

BOX 30-3 Sources of Information About Medications in Pregnancy

- FDA-approved drug prescribing information
- ToxNet: http://toxnet.nlm.nih.gov
- Reprotox: http://reprotox.org

her antidepressant may be dangerous. If a woman needs pharmacologic treatment for a medical condition, and her current drug has evidence of fetal toxicity, another class of drug with a different risk profile can be substituted during pregnancy. Changes in medication should be done with the woman as an active partner in the decision-making process, and specialists consulted as needed.

Nonprescription or Illicit Substance Use
Women should be counseled to avoid many nonprescription medications during pregnancy. It is difficult to provide women with a list of all "safe" medications, as research is often lacking to support this designation. However, acetaminophen and topical creams for itching and hemorrhoids have historically been recommended for symptom relief, even though conclusive safety information is not available (Thiele, Kessler, Arck, Erhardt, & Tiegs, 2013).

Women who are pregnant should be screened for alcohol use, especially binge drinking, using strategies defined in Chapter 7. Women who consumed greater than 7 drinks per week or more than 3 drinks on one occasion prior to pregnancy may benefit from additional support during pregnancy (American College of Obstetricians and Gynecologists, 2011). Alcohol use in pregnancy has been associated with spontaneous abortion, fetal death, and child developmental disorders (Andersen, Andersen, Olsen, Grønbæk, & Strandberg-Larsen, 2012). While there are few data on the harm associated with very small amounts of alcohol, guidelines advise complete cessation of consumption during pregnancy (American College of Obstetricians and Gynecologists, 2011).

Assess whether the woman is smoking or has smoked cigarettes or any substance, as this increases her risk of poor perinatal outcomes. Encourage her to quit as soon as possible or drastically cut back on the number of cigarettes she smokes each day, as smoking decreases placental perfusion. Research supports that psychological support during smoking cessation improves success rates and perinatal outcomes (Chamberlain et al., 2013). However, there is not sufficient evidence to determine if pharmacologic therapies for smoking cessation are safe in pregnancy (Coleman, Chamberlain, Davey, Cooper, & Leonardi-Bee, 2012).

In recent years, the use of narcotic pain relievers has increased in the United States. Use of these drugs often begins with medical use but may progress to dependence and illicit use. Women with opioid dependence need interprofessional care that includes medical treatment and support, as narcotics have effects on the developing fetus, and babies born to drug-using mothers have withdrawal symptoms (American College of Nurse-Midwives [ACNM], 2013). However, rapid cessation of use can have negative effects on maternal and fetal health as well (American College of Obstetricians and Gynecologists, 2012).

The history should also include the woman's current and past use of illicit substances such as marijuana, heroin, cocaine, and other street drugs. Women with recent use can benefit from referrals and support to assist them in recovery. While a drug screen can be performed, urine screens require the consent of the woman and have minimal value in detecting drug use, except for marijuana and opioids (American College of Obstetricians and Gynecologists, 2012). A main goal of the visit should be to develop trust with the woman so she returns for prenatal care, and the value of drug testing should be weighed against the importance of support (ACNM, 2013). If the woman states that she has been using drugs, a compassionate approach is essential in helping her access needed services (American College of Obstetricians and Gynecologists, 2012). Women with substance use in the distant past should be encouraged to use resources for support during pregnancy and parenting.

Chemical Exposure
Women can be exposed to chemicals and dangerous substances both at home and at work. Home exposure can take place while cleaning, gardening, or crafting. In addition, indoor and outdoor air quality may affect the woman's health and her baby (Ghosh, Wilhelm, & Ritz, 2013; Shah & Balkhair, 2011). **Table 30-2** summarizes specific substances to be included in initial data gathering and discussion, and women should be encouraged to avoid these toxic substances or mitigate their exposure to them.

Occupational exposure to chemicals is also important. Ask the woman to describe her current job and the work environment, and inquire if she is

TABLE 30-2	Potentially Toxic Environmental Exposures		
Substance	**Potential Exposure**	**Potential Problem**	**Recommendations**
Cigarette smoke	Second-hand smoke from being near lit cigarettes	Low birth weight, preterm birth	Leave the area Open a window
Lead	Older homes with lead pipes, lead paint, hobbies using lead (stained glass, furniture restoration, pottery making), pottery	Neurotoxin: learning deficits, developmental delays	Do not disturb pre-1970 paint Run water 30 seconds in lead pipes Drink bottled water
Mercury	Fish: swordfish, king mackerel, tilefish, shark, albacore tuna	Neurotoxin: learning deficits, developmental delays	Avoid fish with high mercury levels Check local freshwater fish safety advisories
Organic solvents	Occupations or hobbies involving adhesives, cleaning solvents, paints, resins, plastics, dyeing and printing materials	Birth defects	Eliminate contact Ensure adequate ventilation Wear personal protection, such as gloves and masks

exposed to chemicals/pesticides, solvents, metals, fumes, dust, noise, radiation, or other hazards. The Occupational Health and Safety Administration (OSHA) mandates that the names and health effects of all work-related chemicals be made available to employees in the workplace via Safety Data Sheets (SDSs). Asking the woman to obtain the relevant SDSs is a starting point for assessment of workplace chemical exposures.

Social History
Pregnancy is not only a physical event for a woman, but also a change in her family constellation requiring role readjustment. Ask the woman who she lives with and how they are related to her. Determine whether the household has adequate food, heat, and resources. If a woman lives in an insecure or dangerous environment, pregnancy can exacerbate tensions (Pallitto et al., 2013).

Women in abusive situations are more likely to have an unintended pregnancy (Pallitto et al.,

2013). A brief screening for intimate partner violence (see Chapter 13) is an essential component of the diagnostic visit. Adolescent girls who are pregnant should also be screened for parental, family, and sexual abuse and asked if they feel safe telling their family about the pregnancy. Lack of family and social support increases the risk of suicide in pregnancy (Hodgkinson, Beers, Southammakosane, & Lewin, 2014). Assessing the family structure and support allows for referral to social services for financial and family assistance programs as needed. While adult women have the option of accessing such resources, sexual or physical abuse of a minor must be reported.

Safety
Home Safety Women who are pregnant are more prone to musculoskeletal injuries. Moreover, if they become injured, the healing time may be prolonged due to the effect of some of the hormonal changes that occur during pregnancy. All normal

safety precautions are important to continue during the pregnancy to protect the mother and the fetus. For instance, seat belts should continue to be used throughout pregnancy. After diagnosis of pregnancy, women should decrease activities that involve extreme exertion or risk of injury; in particular, sports such as sky-diving, scuba diving, and rock climbing should be discontinued (Szymanski & Satin, 2012). Healthy women with a normal fitness level can continue to perform low-impact exercise throughout pregnancy.

Occupational Safety Occupational exposure to substances was discussed earlier, but clinicians should also ask women who are pregnant about the physical tasks involved in their job. During pregnancy, the joints of the body become more lax and prone to injury, and heavy physical work has been associated with poor birth outcomes (MacDonald et al., 2013). Proper body mechanics can prevent injury, but women should also adjust the amount and type of lifting as pregnancy progresses. Although women who are pregnant should not perform job tasks that involve lifting from the floor or lifting above the head, the exact acceptable weight for lifting depends on the frequency of lifting, the woman's gestation, and the height of the object (MacDonald et al., 2013). A woman who is pregnant should never lift more than 36 pounds in her job, but weight limits are much lower for repetitive or excisional lifting, especially after 20 weeks. The CDC and National Institute for Occupational Safety and Health have developed an easy-to-use graphic that identifies the recommended lifting limits in pregnancy (CDC, 2013). Some women will need a clinician's note to adjust their work tasks. However, many women, especially those in low-paid jobs, experience pregnancy-related discrimination and may not want to disclose their health status to their employer (Bornstein, 2012).

Physical Examination

All women who are newly pregnant should receive a complete physical examination. In addition to the routine elements of the physical examination described in Chapter 6, a brief oral-cavity assessment is warranted. Periodontal disease has been associated with an increased risk of preterm birth, and a referral can be beneficial to the woman (American College of Obstetricians and Gynecologists, 2013c). Some states even cover the cost of basic dental care in pregnancy for low-income women (Hwang, Smith, McCormick, & Barfield, 2012).

If the woman is due for a Papanicolaou test (also known as the Pap test [see Chapter 6]), it should be obtained using a speculum; light spotting is normal following the test. If this test is not needed, a speculum examination is not necessary, unless the woman is having symptoms of a vaginal infection. Prior to 12 weeks' gestation, a bimanual examination can be performed to estimate uterine size and assess the adnexa for tenderness. If the woman has anything more than mild tenderness during a gentle examination, she should be referred for ultrasound to rule out an ectopic pregnancy (Crochet, Bastian, & Chireau, 2013). (See the section on ectopic pregnancy for more information.)

After 12 weeks' gestation, the top of the uterus, known as the fundus, can be palpated abdominally. By 16 weeks' gestation, the fundus is midway between the symphysis and the umbilicus (**Figure 30-1**).If the uterus is larger or smaller than expected from the woman's LMP, an ultrasound can provide valuable information on the gestational age of the pregnancy and the number of fetuses.

Fetal heart tones can be heard with a handheld Doppler instrument (**Figure 30-2**) as early as 10 to 12 weeks after the LMP. The fetal heart tones are best heard by placing the probe on the uterus and slowly and systematically rotating the probe to pick up the fetal heartbeat. Normal range for fetal heart tones is 120 to 160 beats per minute.

Laboratory Testing

Specific laboratory tests are performed during the initial prenatal visit (**Box 30-4**). While some tests are based on the woman's risk factors or her preferences for testing, other tests are standard in pregnancy because they provide valuable information to improve maternal or newborn health. These essential tests should be performed at the diagnostic visit to maximize the opportunity to intervene with abnormalities. Present standard tests, including the test for infection with human immunodeficiency virus (HIV), to the woman as routine testing for all women. While women can "opt out" of any test, this approach maximizes consent for essential tests (CDC, 2010).

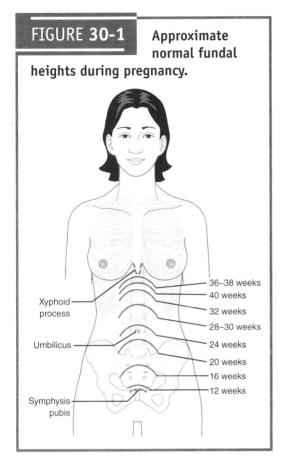

FIGURE **30-1** Approximate normal fundal heights during pregnancy.

Xyphoid process

Umbilicus

Symphysis pubis

36–38 weeks
40 weeks
32 weeks
28–30 weeks
24 weeks
20 weeks
16 weeks
12 weeks

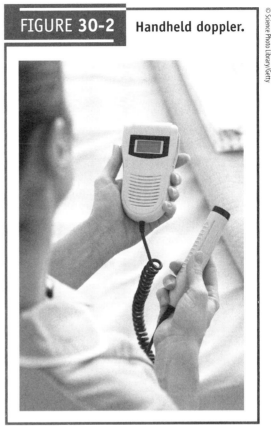

FIGURE **30-2** Handheld doppler.

MANAGEMENT

Patient Education

Education is an essential component of prenatal care. Priorities for the first-visit teaching include ensuring the woman has adequate resources and encouraging lifestyle modifications, if necessary. Beyond the medication, chemical exposure, and safety information previously discussed, the woman should be given a list of warning signs that include bleeding more than light spotting, severe abdominal pain, and extreme nausea and vomiting. An unrushed initial visit should include general information on topics such as sexuality during pregnancy, continuing exercise habits, wearing a seat belt, and avoidance of hot tubs and saunas; these topics can be covered at a later visit if needed.

Nutritional assessment and counseling are also components of comprehensive prenatal care. Appropriate weight gain is determined by the woman's body mass index (BMI) using guidelines established by the Institute of Medicine (2009), as presented in **Box 30-5**.

Women whose BMI is not within the normal range at the beginning of pregnancy can benefit from a consult with a dietician skilled in pregnancy nutrition (American College of Obstetricians and Gynecologists, 2013b). Detailed advice on the content and portion of food groups should be included in comprehensive prenatal care. This information may be best received after initial nausea and vomiting of early pregnancy has subsided. The government website http://www.ChooseMyPlate.gov is an excellent online resource for women and clinicians.

BOX 30-4 Laboratory Testing at the First Prenatal Visit

All Women and with Each Pregnancy

- Blood tests
  - Complete blood count including hemoglobin and hematocrit
  - Blood type and Rh factor
  - Antibody screen
  - Rubella titer
  - Hepatitis B surface antigen (HBsAg)
  - HIV
  - Syphilis test using Venereal Disease Research Laboratory (VDRL) or rapid plasma reagin (RPR) testing
- Urine tests
  - Culture
  - Chlamydia and gonorrhea
    - ▸ Gonorrhea testing may be optional for select women without risk factors

As Indicated by the Woman's History and Preferences

- Blood tests
  - Screening for diabetes (50-g glucose load and test venous blood glucose in 1 hour). Any value above 135–140 warrants further evaluation and/or testing.

  - ▸ For women with a history of impaired glucose metabolism or gestational diabetes, or with a current BMI ≥ 30
  - ▸ If the woman has current diabetes, screening is not needed
  - Varicella antibody screen
    - ▸ For women with no history of natural infection
  - Hepatitis C
    - ▸ For women with a history of blood transfusion before 1992 or any injected drug use
  - Thyroid-stimulating hormone
    - ▸ For women with a history of thyroid abnormalities
  - Maternal genetic testing
    - ▸ Cystic fibrosis testing (optional)
    - ▸ Hemoglobin electrophoresis for women of African descent
  - Fetal genetic and development screening
    - ▸ Maternal serum markers (optional)
      - □ For women 10–14 weeks' gestation
    - ▸ Noninvasive prenatal testing (NIPT)
      - □ For women at risk of fetal genetic disorders
    - ▸ Quad screening (optional)
      - □ For women 15–20 weeks' gestation
- Pap test

Data from Centers for Disease Control and Prevention (CDC). (2010). Sexually transmitted diseases: Treatment guidelines, 2010. *Morbidity and Mortality Weekly Report, 59*(RR-12), 1–110; Gabbe, S. G., Niebyl, J. R., Simpson, J. L., Landon, M. B., Galan, H. L., Jauniaux, E. R. M., & Driscoll, D. A. (2012). *Obstetrics: Normal and problem pregnancies* (6th ed.). Philadelphia, PA: Elsevier Saunders; National Institutes of Health (NIH) Consensus Panel. (2013). National Institutes of Health consensus development conference statement: Diagnosing gestational diabetes mellitus, March 4–6, 2013. *Obstetrics & Gynecology, 122*(2 pt 1), 358–369; American College of Obstetricians and Gynecologists. (2013a). ACOG Practice Bulletin No. 137: Clinical management guidelines for obstetrician-gynecologists. Gestational diabetes. *Obstetrics & Gynecology, 122*(2 pt 1), 406–416.

A federally operated assistance program—Special Supplemental Nutrition Program for Women, Infants and Children (WIC)—also offers dietary counseling and provides vouchers for healthy foods for women living at or below 185% of the federal poverty guidelines (U.S. Department of Agriculture, 2014).

A balanced diet with an increase of approximately 350 calories per day after the first trimester, spread over three meals and two snacks daily, is advised for most women. A generic prenatal vitamin supplement should be prescribed to ensure iron, folic acid, and vitamin needs are met.

BOX 30-5 **Prenatal Weight Gain Guidelines**

BMI < 18.5 (underweight): 28–40 lb

BMI 18.5–24.9 (normal): 25–35 lb

BMI 25–29.9 (overweight): 15–25 lb

BMI > 30 (obese): should gain 11–20 lb

Reprinted with permission from Institute of Medicine. (2009). *Weight gain during pregnancy: Reexamining the guidelines.* Washington, DC: National Academies Press. Courtesy of the National Academies Press, Washington, DC.

Foods to avoid during pregnancy related to their risk for infection are listed in **Table 30-3**.

While there are no conclusive data on safe doses, caffeine intake during pregnancy should be limited to approximately 200 mg daily, which is equivalent to two (8-oz) cups of coffee (Gabbe et al., 2012).

Tapering consumption over several days to a week can help prevent withdrawal headaches. High doses of caffeine (more than 6 cups of coffee per day) are associated with an increased risk of first-trimester miscarriage and pregnancy complications (Jahanfar & Jaafar, 2013). Nutritional supplements, beyond reputable prenatal vitamins, are not regulated by the FDA and may contain harmful substances and should be avoided in pregnancy.

Common Discomforts

Many women experience normal pregnancy-related discomforts. Often these common discomforts are the result of physiologic changes. An explanation for the physiologic basis of these common symptoms and information on relief measures should be provided as part of care. In addition, women should be informed of warning signs in pregnancy to assist them in differentiating between normal and abnormal symptoms.

TABLE 30-3 Foods to Avoid During Pregnancy

Food to Avoid	Increased Risk for . . .	To Reduce Risk. . .
Unpasteurized milk, soft cheeses (e.g., Camembert), gorgonzola, Mexican cheeses (e.g., queso fresco)	Listeriosis	Avoid
Prepackaged lunch meat, hot dogs, pâté and meat spreads	Listeriosis	Heat until steaming
Unpasteurized juices	*E. coli* infection, *Salmonella* enteritis	Avoid
Unwashed fruits and vegetables	Toxoplasmosis, *Salmonella* enteritis	Wash well prior to eating
Raw alfalfa sprouts	*E. coli* infection, *Salmonella* enteritis	Avoid
Raw eggs	*Salmonella* enteritis	Avoid
Rare meat	Toxoplasmosis	Cook meat to medium doneness
Raw fish and shellfish	Coliform bacteria and algae-related infection	Cook fish thoroughly

Data from March of Dimes. (2009). Food-borne risks in pregnancy. Retrieved from http://www.marchofdimes.com/professionals /14332_1152.asp.

As many as 91% of women who are pregnant experience some form of nausea and vomiting early in pregnancy (Castillo & Phillippi, 2015). Typically, pregnancy-related nausea and vomiting begins before 9 weeks, peaks at 12 weeks, and subsides by 20 weeks. Symptoms range from mild queasiness to overwhelming vomiting and can occur at any time of day. Most women have a mild to moderate nausea and vomiting and are able to hold down food and fluids at some point in the day. A variety of strategies can be used to lessen mild symptoms. Although a meta-analysis failed to find evidence that any one treatment is effective for a broad range of women (Matthews, Haas, O'Mathuna, Dowswell, & Doyle, 2014), little harm was demonstrated from lifestyle modifications and nondrug therapies, so women can experiment to find beneficial methods.

A common suggestion for obtaining relief or lessening of symptoms is to eat five to six small meals throughout the day. Bland, lukewarm or cold foods may better tolerated than spicy or hot foods. Protein or carbohydrates, especially if consumed 45 minutes before getting out of bed, may be helpful. Women should choose foods that smell and taste appealing (Castillo & Phillippi, 2015). Because the iron in multivitamins can exacerbate nausea, women can eliminate the full prenatal vitamin and take solely folic acid (at least 400 mcg/day) until their symptoms resolve. Women should also avoid anything that triggers symptoms, such as noxious odors or cooking. Other commonly recommended remedies include acupressure bands, marketed as Sea Bands, and ginger. Ginger can be consumed in candies, carbonated soda, or cookies or taken in capsules, with the maximum daily dose being 1,000 mg (Matthews et al., 2014).

Approximately 1 in 100 women experiences severe and persistent symptoms, known as hyperemesis gravidarum, that result in dehydration, ketonuria, and a 5% or greater weight loss (Castillo & Phillippi, 2015). Women with these symptoms need in-depth assessment and treatment and may benefit from pharmacologic therapies. Intravenous normal saline is appropriate to correct dehydration, but treatment should then focus on prevention. The only FDA-approved pharmacologic treatment for pregnancy-related nausea and vomiting is doxylamine succinate/pyridoxine hydrochloride (Diclegis).

Dosing starts with 2 (10 mg/10 mg) tablets at bedtime and can be increased up to 4 tablets per day. If this regimen fails to control symptoms, multidrug treatment is indicated (Castillo & Phillippi, 2015). Women who have struggled with hyperemesis with past pregnancies may benefit from Diclegis treatment early in pregnancy to avert severe symptoms.

Extreme fatigue is another common early pregnancy symptom and reaches a peak between 9 and 12 weeks' gestation (Demma & Grace, 2013). Women should be encouraged to rest as they are able, and many women feel improvement in this symptom in the second trimester. Nevertheless, fatigue often returns at the end of pregnancy.

Breast tenderness is a common pregnancy symptom that may occur as early as 2 weeks after fertilization. Increase in the breast size and darkening of the areola also begin early in the first trimester; these changes in the breast are caused by increased levels of progesterone and estrogen that prepare the breasts for lactation. Women experiencing breast discomfort should wear a properly fitted, supportive bra, which may mean obtaining a maternity or nursing bra in a larger size. Other common pregnancy discomforts, such as constipation and nasal stuffiness, can be treated with nonpharmacologic measures similar to those used in women who are not pregnant.

Genetic and Fetal Developmental Screening

A variety of genetic and developmental tests are available in pregnancy, and these tests should be offered equally to all women, regardless of their absolute risk for the condition (American College of Obstetricians and Gynecologists, 2007). If a woman or the genetic father of the baby has any risk factors for genetic or developmental disorders (**Box 30-2**), the woman can benefit from an early referral to a genetic counselor or maternal–fetal specialist. While in-depth discussion of genetic testing is beyond the scope of this chapter, common tests are discussed to facilitate access to screening and testing as desired by the woman.

Maternal Testing

All women should be offered testing for cystic fibrosis carrier status. Women need to be tested only once in their lifetime, as this status will not change. If the maternal test is positive, the father of the baby should be offered testing, because both parents must be carriers of the gene for the baby to be at risk of having cystic fibrosis, an autosomal recessive disease.

Women of African descent should be offered sickle cell carrier status using hemoglobin electrophoresis. Eight percent of African Americans in the United States are carriers of this trait (Taylor, Kavanagh, & Zuckerman, 2014). If a woman is a carrier, known as having sickle cell trait, she is at increased risk for bacteriuria and anemia in pregnancy (Jans, De Jonge, & Lagro-Janssen, 2010), and the father of the baby should be offered testing. If both parents are carriers of this autosomal recessive condition, the baby has a 25% risk of having sickle cell disease.

Fetal Testing

Fetal genetic screening should also be offered to each woman, regardless of her age. While Down syndrome is a commonly known genetic disorder, screening tests are available for a variety of aneuploidies, or abnormalities in chromosome number, as well as genetic variants that cause physical or cognitive disabilities (American College of Medical Genetics and Genomics et al., 2015). Although screening provides information on the likelihood of a fetus having a disorder, further testing is needed for diagnosis.

Fetal screening and diagnosis allow women to plan their location and provider for birth or decide about termination of pregnancy. Ideally, a woman should be given written information about genetic and developmental screening, including the risk of false positives, and given ample time with support people to decide whether she wants screening. Women with risk factors should be referred for consultation. Some of the tests are time sensitive, however. Thus, if pregnancy is advanced at the time of diagnosis, there may be limited opportunity for referral. Prior to ordering genetic screening tests, clinicians should consult current resources to determine if new treatments are available or if existing treatments have new applications. This area of clinical care for genetic diseases is rapidly expanding. In addition, the prices and indications for testing shift over time (American College of Medical Genetics and Genomics et al., 2015). While

screening can provide useful information, further testing will be needed for diagnosis.

First-trimester screening options include ultrasound and tests of maternal blood (**Table 30-4**). Maternal serum markers are chemicals and hormones that are affected if the fetus has aneuploidy. Ultrasound can be used to assess the fetal nuchal skin fold, which can be thickened with such an alteration in the number of chromosomes. The information from maternal serum markers can be combined with the maternal serum marker information to provide more information on the potential for fetal abnormalities.

Maternal blood can also be analyzed for pieces of cell-free fetal DNA. The amount of fetal DNA from various chromosomes can provide information about fetal genetics. This test, which is known as noninvasive prenatal testing (NIPT), is currently reserved for women at elevated risk for fetal aneuploidy due to maternal age related to the high cost of the test (Latendresse & Deneris, 2015). However, use may increase in the future, as NIPT has no risk to the fetus and has high sensitivity and specificity for chromosomal disorders (Latendresse & Deneris, 2015).

Some of the previously described tests can also be used in the second trimester (**Table 30-4**). In addition to these tests, the quad screen and ultrasound can be used to provide more information about the fetus. Whereas first-trimester tests focus on the risk of fetal genetic disorders, second-trimester tests can also provide information on fetal development, although they allow less time for parents to make decisions about the pregnancy.

The quad screen, performed in the second trimester, includes analysis of chemicals and hormones to assess risk of three types of trisomy. It also examines levels of alpha-fetoprotein, which can indicate whether the fetal neural tube has properly fused. False-positives are common with this test if the EDB is not accurate. Ultrasound is the most common form of developmental screening. An ultrasound by a trained sonographer can assess fetal anatomy after 18 weeks' gestation (Latendresse & Deneris, 2015).

Any abnormal finding on screening tests warrants referral for diagnostic testing, such as amniocentesis. The screening tests are good at pointing out when fetuses have abnormalities, known as

TABLE 30-4	Fetal Screening Tests

Screening Test	Components	Detects Increased Risk for . . .	Timing
Maternal serum screening	Determination of 2 hormone levels and comparison with norms	Trisomies 13, 18, and 21	10–14 weeks' gestation
Nuchal trans-lucency	Ultrasound evaluation of the thickness of the fetal nuchal fold	Aneuploidy, fetal anomalies	10–14 weeks' (ideally 11 weeks') gestation
Noninvasive prenatal testing	Examination of cell-free fetal DNA within maternal blood	Aneuploidy, limited fetal gene disorders	10 or more weeks' gestation
Quad screen	Serum screen of various markers from maternal blood	Neural tube defects, trisomies 13, 18, and 21	15–22 weeks' gestation
Anatomy ultrasound	Ultrasound of fetus, umbilical cord, and placenta and measurement of amniotic fluid levels	Fetal structural abnormalities in all body systems, aneuploidy	18+ weeks' gestation (difficult to see some structures late in gestation)

specificity, but they are associated with high rates of false-positive findings that can cause anxiety. Even if a low-risk woman has a positive screening test, the likelihood that her baby has an abnormality is small. Key points to consider when discussing genetic screening with women who are pregnant are presented in **Box 30-6**.

FIRST-TRIMESTER BLEEDING

Approximately 1 in 4 women who are pregnant will experience vaginal bleeding in the first trimester (Deutchman, Tubay, & Turok, 2009). Vaginal bleeding can originate from the vagina, cervix, or uterus. Bright red or pink blood means bleeding is actively ongoing, while dark red or brown blood signals the blood was expelled earlier. The timing, amount, and color of blood can be useful in determining the origin of the bleeding.

Light spotting around the expected menstrual period (4 weeks from the last menstrual period)

BOX 30-6　Key Points in Offering Fetal Screening

- All women should be offered screening tests for chromosomal abnormalities and neural tube defects (NTDs) up to 20 weeks' gestation.
- Nondirective counseling should be used when discussing testing options and obtaining informed consent.
- The risk for chromosomal disorders and NTDs is small for most women.
- Screening does not diagnose anomalies; it indicates increased risk. Further testing is needed for diagnosis.
- Women can freely decline genetic and developmental screening and diagnostic tests.

can be caused by implantation of the zygote in the uterine lining. This light spotting is not clinically significant and requires no additional assessment. Light spotting is also fairly common after intercourse. The bleeding may start out as pink or red and then taper to dark red or brown over hours or days. As long as the spotting is decreasing and the woman does not have any pain, she does not need further evaluation. If the blood is soaking through her underwear, or if she is in pain, an examination is needed.

Examination should include blood pressure, pulse, and a pelvic examination. A speculum should be used to visualize the vagina and cervix to determine the color, amount, and origin of the blood. Bleeding of the cervix is fairly common in pregnancy, but bleeding from the uterus can signal impending pregnancy loss. Cervical motion tenderness, adnexal pain, or an adnexal mass on bimanual exam can indicate ectopic pregnancy (Crochet et al., 2013). A quantitative hCG test provides valuable information, especially if the test can be repeated in 48 hours, because the quantitative level of hCG in maternal blood should double every 48 hours in viable pregnancies. If the hCG level is greater than 3,000 mIU/mL, a gestational sac should be visible in the uterus (Crochet et al., 2013). If a fetal heartbeat is seen on ultrasound, the risk of miscarriage is reduced (Gabbe et al., 2012). If a woman is having uterine bleeding after a confirmed pregnancy, check her blood type. Women with uterine bleeding who are Rh-negative will need Rho(D) immunoglobulin (RhoGam) to prevent them from developing antibodies to Rh-positive blood. Two doses of Rho(D) immunoglobulin are available in the United States, 50 mcg and 300 mcg, and either dose can be used in women with first-trimester bleeding, with the choice depending on cost and availability.

Early Pregnancy Loss

Approximately 30% of all implanted embryos and 15% of all clinically recognized pregnancies miscarry (Gabbe et al., 2012). Most miscarriages (also known as spontaneous abortions) occur in the first trimester and are related to embryo chromosomal abnormalities. Symptoms include uterine bleeding and cramping. A thorough evaluation, as described previously, is needed. If a woman's hCG level does not double or declines within 48 hours, miscarriage is a likely outcome. Transvaginal ultrasound can provide information about pregnancy viability 6 weeks after the LMP (Gabbe et al., 2012). At that point, a fetal heartbeat should be visible. If a fetus is not visible, the ultrasound can be repeated in 2 weeks in case the estimated due date was inaccurate.

If transvaginal ultrasound confirms fetal death with a single, first-trimester fetus, the woman can be given options to allow spontaneous miscarriage or to be referred for intervention. More than 60% of miscarriages will happen within 2 weeks of diagnosis (Demma & Grace, 2013). In an uncomplicated miscarriage, the woman experiences increasing cramping and bleeding that resolves rapidly after passage of a small mass of tissue, known as the products of conception. If she does not spontaneously miscarry within 2 weeks or if she has extensive bleeding (more than one pad per hour), feels faint, or has extreme pain, she will need additional assessment and care. If a qualified clinician is not easily available, emergency rooms are equipped to assist miscarriages. Options for intervention include oral medications and uterine evacuation through aspiration or dilation and curettage. Following a miscarriage, a clinical evaluation is needed to ensure physical and emotional healing and assess the need for contraception.

Ectopic Pregnancy

Ectopic pregnancy is a potentially life-threatening form of pregnancy complication resulting from implantation of the fertilized egg outside the uterus, usually in the fallopian tube. With a prevalence of approximately 2% of reported pregnancies (Marion & Meeks, 2012), ectopic pregnancy is a leading differential diagnosis when a woman has lower abdominal pain in the first trimester. Risk factors include a history of pelvic inflammatory disease or infertility. However, if a woman who is newly pregnant is experiencing lower quadrant pain, it is important to rule out ectopic pregnancy even if she does not have risk factors. Any women with cervical motion tenderness on bimanual examination should be evaluated for ectopic pregnancy, as should any woman early in pregnancy with pelvic or abdominal pain. Bleeding, ranging from spotting to the amount that occurs during a menstrual period, can also be a symptom (Crochet et al., 2013). If the woman's hCG level is more than 3,000 mIU/mL, a gestational sac should be visible within the uterus. Ectopic pregnancies tend to have slowly rising hCG levels that increase but do not double within 48 hours.

Women with ectopic pregnancies need treatment to avoid tubal rupture that could lead to maternal death. Management can include outpatient medication therapy or inpatient surgery; prompt referral can assist women in avoiding complications and preserving future fertility. Transfer of medical records can expedite treatment.

PLANNING FOR PREGNANCY CARE

A careful history and physical examination will provide information to determine if the woman with an unexpected pregnancy is at low risk and has adequate social support and resources, or if the woman has medical or social risk factors that require intensive follow-up. Women needing immediate medical assistance should receive a prompt referral to a specialist. Social services referrals can often take several days to coordinate. Low-risk women may need time to consider other aspects of their care as well.

All women who are pregnant should leave the initial visit with the items listed in **Box 30-7**. A follow-up call may allow the woman the opportunity to ask questions after she adjusts to the news of her pregnancy.

BOX 30-7 **Items to Provide to Women After Diagnosis of Pregnancy**

- Prenatal vitamin prescription
- Proof of pregnancy (for Women, Infants, and Children [WIC] and health insurance)
- Laboratory work order (if not drawn at clinic)
- Information about applying for health insurance
- Information about prenatal care
- Ultrasound order (if needed)

Referral for Routine Prenatal Care

Early and appropriate prenatal care can assist women in improving their health, connect them with needed resources, and provide education for birth and parenting. Optimal pregnancy care requires a holistic approach to a woman's physical, social, and emotional needs.

Many different types of prenatal care clinicians with different knowledge, skills, and philosophies of care can be consulted for ongoing care (ACNM & American College of Obstetricians and Gynecologists, 2011). Care led by midwives who are appropriately trained and educated has been shown to yield superior outcomes for low-risk women when compared with physician-led models (Sandall, Soltani, Gates, Shennan, & Devane, 2013). If women have substantial medical risk factors, they are best seen by an interprofessional team of providers that includes a physician and other specialized healthcare providers to provide a unified, multifaceted approach to a high-risk pregnancy (Zwarenstein, Goldman, & Reeves, 2013). Prenatal care can be provided individually or in a group setting, and a group form of care known as CenteringPregnancy has been shown to have superior outcomes when compared with traditional individual care (Ickovics et al., 2007).

Women may also want to consider their preferred location of birth as they choose a care provider. While the hospital is the dominant location of birth in the United States, out-of-hospital birth in birth centers and homes has been shown to be a safe option for low-risk women as long as a qualified attendant, emergency medications, and rapid transport to a higher level of care are available (American College of Obstetricians and Gynecologists & Society for Maternal–Fetal Medicine, 2015; National Collaborating Centre for Women's and Children's Health, 2014).

Pregnancy is not just a normal physiologic process; it is a transformative event, encompassing profound emotions and role change. Referrals and recommendations for prenatal care providers who will promote holistic pregnancy health should be made intentionally. Medical records from the initial diagnostic visit should be sent to the woman's chosen provider as soon as possible. Women should be supported in choosing a care provider that meets their personal needs.

References

American College of Medical Genetics and Genomics, American College of Obstetricians and Gynecologists, National Society of Genetic Counselors, Perinatal Quality Foundation, Society for Maternal–Fetal Medicine, Edwards, J. G., . . . Watson, M. S. (2015). Expanded carrier screening in reproductive medicine: Points to consider: A joint statement of the American College of Medical Genetics and Genomics, American College of Obstetricians and Gynecologists, National Society of Genetic Counselors, Perinatal Quality Foundation, and Society for Maternal–Fetal Medicine. *Obstetrics & Gynecology, 125*(3), 653–662.

American College of Nurse-Midwives (ACNM). (2013). *Position statement: Addiction in pregnancy.* Silver Spring, MD: Author.

American College of Nurse-Midwives (ACNM) & American College of Obstetricians and Gynecologists. (2011). *Joint statement of practice relations between obstetrician gynecologists and certified nurse-midwives/certified midwives.* Silver Spring, MD: Authors.

American College of Obstetricians and Gynecologists. (2007). ACOG Practice Bulletin No. 77: Screening for fetal chromosomal abnormalities. *Obstetrics & Gynecology, 109*(1), 217–227.

American College of Obstetricians and Gynecologists. (2011). At-risk drinking and alcohol dependence: Obstetric and gynecologic implications. Committee Opinion No. 496. *Obstetrics & Gynecology, 118*, 383-388.

American College of Obstetricians and Gynecologists. (2012). Opioid abuse, dependence, and addiction in pregnancy: Committee Opinion No. 524. *Obstetrics & Gynecology, 119*(5), 1070–1076.

American College of Obstetricians and Gynecologists. (2013a). ACOG Practice Bulletin No. 137: Clinical management guidelines for obstetrician-gynecologists. Gestational diabetes. *Obstetrics & Gynecology, 122*(2 pt 1), 406–416

American College of Obstetricians and Gynecologists. (2013b). ACOG Committee Opinion No. 549: Obesity in pregnancy. *Obstetrics & Gynecology, 121*(1), 213.

American College of Obstetricians and Gynecologists. (2013c). Committee Opinion No. 569: Oral health care during pregnancy and through the lifespan. *Obstetrics & Gynecology, 122*(2 pt 1), 417–422.

American College of Obstetricians and Gynecologists & Society for Maternal–Fetal Medicine. (2015). Obstetric Care Consensus No. 2: Levels of maternal care. *Obstetrics & Gynecology, 125*(2), 502–515. doi:510.1097/1001.AOG.0000460770.0000499574.0000460779f

Andersen, A.-M. N., Andersen, P. K., Olsen, J., Grønbæk, M., & Strandberg-Larsen, K. (2012). Moderate alcohol intake during pregnancy and risk of fetal death. *International Journal of Epidemiology,* 41, 405–413. doi:10.1093/ije/dyr189.

Blackburn, S. T. (2013). *Maternal, fetal, and neonatal physiology: A clinical perspective* (4th ed.). Maryland Heights, MO: Elsevier.

Bornstein, S. (2012). Work, family, and discrimination at the bottom of the ladder. *Georgetown Journal on Poverty Law Policy, 19.* Retrieved from http://scholarship.law.ufl.edu/facultypub/502

Castillo, M. J., & Phillippi, J. C. (2015). Hyperemesis gravidarum: A holistic overview and approach to clinical assessment and management. *Journal of Perinatal & Neonatal Nursing, 29*(1), 12–22. doi:10.1097/jpn.0000000000000075

Centers for Disease Control and Prevention (CDC). (2010). Sexually transmitted diseases: Treatment guidelines, 2010. *Morbidity and Mortality Weekly Report, 59*(RR-12), 1–110.

Centers for Disease Control and Prevention (CDC). (2013). Provisional recommended weight limits for lifting at work during pregnancy. Retrieved from http://blogs.cdc.gov/niosh-science-blog/files/2013/05/ClinicalGuidelinesImg-NewLogoFinal.jpg

Centers for Disease Control and Prevention (CDC). (2014, March 2014). Guidelines for vaccinating pregnant women. Retrieved from http://www.cdc.gov/vaccines/pubs/preg-guide.htm

Centers for Disease Control and Prevention (CDC). (2016). Recommended adult immunization schedule. Retrieved from http://www.cdc.gov/vaccines/schedules/downloads/adult/adult-combined-schedule.pdf

Chamberlain, C., O'Mara-Eves, A., Oliver, S., Caird, J. R., Perlen, S. M., Eades, S. J., & Thomas, J. (2013). Psychosocial interventions for supporting women to stop smoking in pregnancy. *Cochrane Library, 10,* CD001055. doi:10.1002/14651858.CD001055.pub4

Coleman, T., Chamberlain, C., Davey, M. A., Cooper, S. E., & Leonardi-Bee, J. (2012). Pharmacological interventions for promoting smoking cessation during pregnancy. *Cochrane Library, 9,* CD010078. doi:10.1002/14651858.CD010078

Crochet, J. R., Bastian, L. A., & Chireau, M. V. (2013). Does this woman have an ectopic pregnancy? The rational clinical examination systematic review. *Journal of the American Medical Association, 309*(16), 1722–1729.

Demma, J. M., & Grace, K. T. (2013). Prenatal care. In T. L. King, M. C. Brucker, J. M. Kriebs, J. O. Fahey, & H. Varney (Eds.), *Varney's midwifery* (5th ed., pp.657–721). Burlington, MA: Jones & Bartlett Learning.

Deutchman, M., Tubay, A.T., & Turok, D.K. (2009). First trimester bleeding. *American Family Physician,* 79(11), 985–994.

Finer, L. B., & Zolna, M. R. (2014). Shifts in intended and unintended pregnancies in the United States, 2001–2008. *American Journal of Public Health, 104*(S1), S43–S48.

Gabbe, S. G., Niebyl, J. R., Simpson, J. L., Landon, M. B., Galan, H. L., Jauniaux, E. R. M., & Driscoll, D. A. (2012). *Obstetrics: Normal and problem pregnancies* (6th ed.). Philadelphia, PA: Elsevier Saunders

Ghosh, J. K. C., Wilhelm, M., & Ritz, B. (2013). Effects of residential indoor air quality and household ventilation on preterm birth and term low birth weight in Los Angeles County, California. *American Journal of Public Health, 103*(4), 686–694.

Hodgkinson, S., Beers, L., Southammakosane, C., & Lewin, A. (2014). Addressing the mental health needs of pregnant and parenting adolescents. *Pediatrics, 133*(1), 114–122.

Hwang, S. S., Smith, V. C., McCormick, M. C., & Barfield, W. D. (2012). The association between maternal oral health experiences and risk of preterm birth in 10 states, pregnancy risk assessment monitoring system, 2004–2006. *Maternal and Child Health Journal, 16*(8), 1688–1695.

Ickovics, J. R., Kershaw, T. S., Westdahl, C., Magriples, U., Massey, Z., Reynolds, H., & Rising, S. S. (2007). Group prenatal care and perinatal outcomes: A randomized controlled trial. *Obstetrics & Gynecology, 110*(2 pt 1), 330–339.

Institute of Medicine. (2009). *Weight gain during pregnancy: Reexamining the guidelines.* Washington, DC: National Academies Press.

Jahanfar, S., & Jaafar, S. H. (2013). Effects of restricted caffeine intake by mother on fetal, neonatal and pregnancy outcome. *Cochrane Library, 2,* CD006965. doi:10.1002/14651858.CD006965.pub3

Jans, S. M., De Jonge, A., & Lagro-Janssen, A. (2010). Maternal and perinatal outcomes amongst haemoglobinopathy carriers: A systematic review. *International Journal of Clinical Practice, 64*(12), 1688–1698.

Jordan, R., Engstrom, J., Marfell, J., & Farley, C. L. (Eds.). (2014). *Prenatal and postnatal care: A women-centered approach.* Ames, IA: Wiley-Blackwell.

King, T. L., Brucker, M. C., Kriebs, J. M., Fahey, J. O., & Varney, H. (2013). *Varney's midwifery* (5th ed.). Burlington, MA: Jones & Bartlett Learning.

Latendresse, G., & Deneris, A. (2015). An update on current prenatal testing options: First trimester and noninvasive prenatal testing. *Journal of Midwifery & Women's Health, 60*(1), 24–36. doi:10.1111/jmwh.12228

MacDonald, L. A., Waters, T. R., Napolitano, P. G., Goddard, D. E., Ryan, M. A., Nielsen, P., & Hudock, S. D. (2013). Clinical guidelines for occupational lifting in pregnancy: Evidence summary and provisional recommendations. *American Journal of Obstetrics & Gynecology, 209*(2), 80–88.

Marion, L. L., & Meeks, G. R. (2012). Ectopic pregnancy: History, incidence, epidemiology, and risk factors. *Clinical Obstetrics and Gynecology, 55*(2), 376–386.

March of Dimes. (2009). Food-borne risks in pregnancy. Retrieved from http://www.marchofdimes.com/professionals/14332_1152.asp

Matthews, A., Haas, D. M., O'Mathuna, D. P., Dowswell, T., & Doyle, M. (2014). Interventions for nausea and vomiting in early pregnancy. *Cochrane Database of Systematic Reviews, 3,* CD007575. doi:10.1002/14651858.CD007575.pub3

National Collaborating Centre for Women's and Children's Health. (2014). *Intrapartum care: Care of healthy women and their babies during childbirth. Clinical Guideline 190: Methods, evidence and recommendations.* London, England: National Institute for Health and Care Excellence. Retrieved from http://www.ncbi.nlm.nih.gov/books/NBK328269/?report=reader

National Institutes of Health (NIH) Consensus Panel. (2013). National Institutes of Health consensus development conference statement: Diagnosing gestational diabetes mellitus, March 4–6, 2013. *Obstetrics & Gynecology, 122*(2 pt 1), 358–369.

Pallitto, C. C., García-Moreno, C., Jansen, H. A., Heise, L., Ellsberg, M., & Watts, C. (2013). Intimate partner violence, abortion, and unintended pregnancy: Results from the WHO Multi-country Study on Women's Health and Domestic Violence. *International Journal of Gynecology & Obstetrics, 120*(1), 3–9.

Phelan, S. (2008). Components and timing of prenatal care. *Obstetrics and Gynecology Clinics of North America, 35*(1), 339–353.

Sandall, J., Soltani, H., Gates, S., Shennan, A., & Devane, D. (2013). Midwife-led continuity models versus other models of care for childbearing women. *Cochrane Database of Systematic Reviews, 8,* CD004667. doi:10.1002/14651858.CD004667.pub3

Shah, P. S., & Balkhair, T. (2011). Air pollution and birth outcomes: A systematic review. *Environment International, 37*(2), 498–516.

Szymanski, L. M., & Satin, A. J. (2012). Exercise during pregnancy: Fetal responses to current public health guidelines. *Obstetrics & Gynecology, 119*(3), 603.

Taylor, C., Kavanagh, P., & Zuckerman, B. (2014). Sickle cell trait: Neglected opportunities in the era of genomic medicine. *Journal of the American Medical Association, 311*(15), 1495–1496.

Thiele, K., Kessler, T., Arck, P., Erhardt, A., & Tiegs, G. (2013). Acetaminophen and pregnancy: Short-and long-term consequences for mother and child. *Journal of Reproductive Immunology, 97*(1), 128–139.

U.S. Department of Agriculture. (2014). Women, Infants, and Children (WIC): WIC income eligibility guidelines. Retrieved from http://www.fns.usda.gov/wic/wic-income-eligibility-guidelines

U.S. Food and Drug Administration (FDA). (2011). FDA issues final rule on changes to pregnancy and lactation labeling information for prescription drug and biological products [Press release]. Retrieved from http://www.fda.gov/NewsEvents/Newsroom/PressAnnouncements/ucm425317.htm

Whitworth, M., Bricker, L., Neilson, J. P., & Dowswell, T. (2010). Ultrasound for fetal assessment in early pregnancy. *Cochrane Database of Systematic Reviews, 4,* CD007058. doi:10.1002/14651858.CD007058.pub2

Workowski, K. A., & Bolan, G. A. (2015). Sexually transmitted diseases treatment guidelines, 2015. *Morbidity and Mortality Weekly Report, 64,* 3.

Zwarenstein, M., Goldman, J., & Reeves, S. (2013). Interprofessional collaboration: Effects of practice-based interventions on professional practice and healthcare outcomes. *Cochrane Database of Systematic Reviews, 3,* CD002213. doi:10.1002/14651858.CD002213.pub3

CHAPTER 31

Common Complications of Pregnancy

Ellise D. Adams

During pregnancy, a host of anatomic and physiologic changes occur to support the pregnancy and maturation of the fetus in preparation for extrauterine life. An overview of the normal anatomic and physiologic changes that occur during pregnancy is provided elsewhere in this text (see Chapter 29). The focus of this chapter is on changes that may be associated with complications of pregnancy and the impact those complications can have on the mother and the fetus. Initial management of the complications, including referral to the appropriate clinician for continuation of care, is provided.

INFECTIONS COMMONLY DIAGNOSED DURING PREGNANCY

During pregnancy, the maternal immune system undergoes many changes. Cell-mediated response is not as active, the antigen–antibody response becomes more active, and the relationship between these two is altered (Blackburn, 2013). While these changes prevent fetal rejection by the maternal body, they also increase maternal risk of developing an infection. An important factor related to these changes is the passage of maternal antibodies across the placenta. Maternal immunoglobulin G (IgG) antibodies provide the fetus with passive immunity. In addition, the placenta provides protection in the form of macrophage cells, lymphocytes, phagocytes, and cytokines that defend against viruses and bacteria. Nevertheless, some viruses and bacteria are capable of crossing the placental barrier and can endanger the fetus.

Urinary Tract Infections

Urinary frequency due to bladder compression by the gravid uterus is a common discomfort of pregnancy. In some cases, however, urinary frequency may be a symptom of urinary tract infection (UTI). Pregnancy increases the risk of UTI and asymptomatic bacteriuria (ASB) due to decreased urinary tract peristalsis. The predominant causative agents of UTI and ASB in pregnancy are group B *Streptococcus* and *Escherichia coli* (Schneeberger, Kazemier, & Geerlings, 2014). Differential diagnoses to consider when assessing urinary symptoms in a woman who is pregnant include rupture of membranes and gestational diabetes.

To avoid bladder stasis, clinicians should encourage women who are pregnant to maintain adequate water intake and to rest in the left lateral position—this position shifts the enlarged uterus away from the vena cava and aorta, which in turn enhances cardiac output, kidney perfusion, and kidney function. To assist women who are pregnant in managing symptoms of urinary frequency, the clinician can also provide instruction in Kegel exercises (see Chapter 22).

Trimethoprim (a folate antagonist) should be avoided during the first trimester of pregnancy. Sulfonamides have an increased likelihood of causing hyperbilirubinemia in the neonate and should be avoided during the third trimester. Thus the combination of trimethoprim/sulfamethoxazole should not be prescribed during either the first or third trimesters (Briggs & Freeman, 2015; Brucker & King, 2015; Schneeberger et al., 2014). For further information on the treatment and management of urinary tract infections, see Chapter 21.

Pregnancy Complicated by Infections Caused by Cytomegalovirus, Parvovirus B19, Toxoplasmosis, Rubella, Varicella Zoster, and Group B *Streptococcus*

Despite the alterations that occur in the immune system during pregnancy, gestation is not considered to be an immunocompromised state. Alterations in the cell-mediated response do, however, increase maternal susceptibility to certain pathogens. Changes in maternal neutrophil function, for example, may result in lingering infections. This section discusses the implications of a pregnancy that is complicated by infections caused by cytomegalovirus, parvovirus B19, toxoplasmosis, rubella, varicella-zoster, and group B *Streptococcus*.

Cytomegalovirus

Cytomegalovirus (CMV) is a member of the large family of deoxyribonucleic acid (DNA) viruses known as herpesviridae; thus it is considered a herpesvirus. Women can acquire CMV through sexual contact, blood transfusions, and contact with urine or saliva of infected individuals. Most women who are pregnant acquire the infection as a result of contact with their own younger children or children in a daycare or preschool setting. Women who are immunocompromised are particularly susceptible to this viral infection.

CMV is transmitted transplacentally to the fetus following primary maternal infection or reactivation of a previous infection (Blackburn, 2013). It can also be transmitted through contact with maternal body fluids during birth or through breastfeeding. One-third to one-half of infants born to mothers with primary CMV infection will be affected to some degree (Stowell, Forlin-Passoni, & Cannon, 2010). Fetuses exposed in the first 20 weeks of pregnancy are at the greatest risk of developing congenital CMV. Congenital CMV can result in mental retardation, hearing loss, and cerebral palsy (Stowell et al., 2010). Newborn CMV infections are associated with hepatosplenomegaly, thrombocytopenia, hepatitis, and anemia. Maternal symptoms associated with CMV include flulike symptoms, although in many cases women remain asymptomatic.

Prenatal screening for CMV is not recommended (American College of Obstetricians & Gynecologists, 2015a), although risk screening is appropriate. Maternal diagnosis is typically made through serologic testing for IgG and IgM antibodies. When suspicion of congenital CMV arises, ultrasound is used to identify fetal complications such as abdominal and liver calcifications, hepatosplenomegaly, ascites, microcephaly, hydrops fetalis, and intrauterine growth retardation. The single best test for the diagnosis of congenital infection is detection of the virus in the amniotic fluid by culture or identification of a polymerase chain reactive (PCR) assays. Referral to a maternal–fetal specialist for management during the pregnancy is necessary.

All women who are pregnant should be taught how to prevent CMV transmission. Good hand washing and hygienic practices associated with shared items such as toys and hard surfaces are the best form of prevention.

Fifth Disease

Parvovirus B19 is a single-strand DNA virus that infects only humans and is the cause of fifth disease. Typically the infection is not a problem for a woman who is pregnant. Approximately half of all women who are pregnant are immune to parvovirus B19. Those who are not immune usually do not have serious complications if they develop an infection with this virus (Centers for Disease Control and Prevention [CDC], 2012a).

When a woman has a parvovirus B19 infection, she may develop a mild rash (although this is more commonly observed in children) and painful, swollen joints (polyarthropathy syndrome) (CDC, 2012a). The virus can cause the body to stop making red blood cells, which can lead to transient aplastic crisis, hydrops fetalis, congenital anemia, pure red cell aplasia, or persistent anemia (CDC, 2012a). Fewer than 5% of women with the infection will experience any of these outcomes, however, and most of the time the fetus is not affected (American College of Obstetricians and Gynecologists, 2015a). Transmission to the fetus occurs transplacentally (Blackburn, 2013). Women who are pregnant at greatest risk for contracting parvovirus B19 are those who are immunocompromised, who are exposed to school-age children, who are schoolteachers, and who are daycare workers.

Women who are pregnant should be screened for risk factors, and serologic testing should be performed in women who are pregnant who have been exposed to the virus. Women with negative IgM and positive IgG titers can be reassured that this status indicates immunity owing to a prior infection. Positive IgM and negative IgG titers indicate active infection, whereas individuals who are IgM and IgG negative are at risk for infection and should have serologic testing repeated in 2 to 4 weeks (American College of Obstetricians and Gynecologists, 2015a; Dijkmans et al., 2012). If infection is diagnosed, referral to a maternal–fetal specialist for management during the pregnancy is necessary. Ultrasound may detect hydrops fetalis, and amniocentesis can be used to detect PCR to aid in diagnosis.

All women who are pregnant should be taught methods to prevent parvovirus B19 transmission. Good hand washing and hygienic practices associated with shared items such as toys and hard surfaces are the best form of prevention.

Toxoplasmosis

Toxoplasmosis is caused by a parasite, *Toxoplasma gondii*. This infection is not passed from person to person except in pregnancy (congenital transmission), during blood transfusion, or by organ transplant. Transmission occurs through the following routes:

- Foodborne transmission (eating uncooked or contaminated meat, particularly pork, lamb, and venison), including poor hand hygiene following handling of contaminated raw meats or using utensils that were improperly washed after coming into contact with contaminated raw meat
- Animal-to-human transmission, which occurs most often from infected cats who shed the parasite in their feces and accidental ingestion of the parasite's oocytes occurs during cleaning of the litter box (American College of Obstetricians and Gynecologists, 2015a)

Transmission to the fetus occurs transplacentally (Blackburn, 2013) and the risk of transmission increases with advancing gestation. However, the most severe impacts to the fetus occur when exposure happens during the first trimester (American College of Obstetricians and Gynecologists, 2015a). Fetal effects may include vision or hearing loss, neurologic delays, and seizures. The infection is typically asymptomatic in adults who have an intact immune system. If symptoms develop, they may mimic the flu and hepatosplenomegaly may be present.

Prenatal screening for toxoplasmosis is not recommended (American College of Obstetricians and Gynecologists, 2015a), but risk screening is appropriate. Diagnosis is accomplished by serologic testing of IgM and IgG. Consistently high and rising maternal levels of IgM and IgG should lead to fetal surveillance. Ultrasound may detect microcephaly, hepatosplenomegaly, and intrauterine growth retardation, among other fetal complications. Amniocentesis can be used to detect PCR to aid in diagnosis. Referral to a maternal–fetal specialist for management during the pregnancy is necessary.

All women who are pregnant should be counseled about proper handling and cooking of raw meat; having someone else clean cat litter boxes or if that is not possible, wearing gloves and practicing good hand hygiene; using gloves if gardening; and thoroughly cleaning vegetables and fruits to avoid exposure to contaminated soil. Good hand washing and hygienic practices are the best forms of prevention.

Rubella (German Measles)

Rubella is caused by a virus that is transmitted by contact with an infected person who spreads the virus by airborne droplets when coughing or sneezing. Transmission to the fetus occurs transplacentally (Blackburn, 2013), with the greatest risk of congenital infection and birth defects occurring during the first 12 weeks of pregnancy (CDC, 2015a; U.S. National Library of Medicine [NLM], 2015). The most serious consequences of rubella infection that occur in early pregnancy include miscarriage, stillbirth, and an array of severe birth defects in the infant—deafness, eye defects such as cataracts or glaucoma, patent ductus arteriosus or other cardiac defects, microcephaly, intellectual development disorder (formally called mental retardation), bone lesions, and thrombocytopenia purpura.

Congenital rubella syndrome (CRS) is an illness that results from rubella infection during pregnancy (NLM, 2015). Infants with CRS usually present with more than one sign or symptom consistent with congenital rubella infection, although hearing impairment is the most common single defect (CDC, 2012b; NLM, 2015). Symptoms in children exposed during pregnancy may be delayed for 2 to 4 years. Many of the children who have CRS develop diabetes mellitus later in childhood. Maternal symptoms of infection include fever, malaise, and upper respiratory symptoms, followed by a maculopapular rash that usually begins on the face and proceeds downward.

All women who are pregnant should be screened at the first prenatal visit for immunity to rubella. Women who are pregnant and who have symptoms suggestive of rubella should have a viral culture, PCR, or IgM antibody testing. Fetal surveillance includes ultrasound to determine obvious defects. Referral to a maternal–fetal specialist for a woman who is pregnant and diagnosed with rubella, especially in the first half of pregnancy, is appropriate. Women without immunity to rubella should be counseled to avoid exposure to infected individuals. The rubella vaccine should not be given to women who are pregnant, as this vaccine consists of a live attenuated strain; in contrast, vaccination is recommended in the immediate postpartum period for those women with non-immune status. The clinician should explain the importance of avoiding pregnancy within 4 weeks of vaccination (CDC, 2015a).

Varicella-Zoster Virus (Chickenpox)

Varicella-zoster virus (VZV) is a DNA herpes-type virus that is highly contagious and easily transmissible by contact and droplets. The incidence of VZV infection is unknown, as it is not a reportable disease. While the incidence in the United States appears to be increasing, it is suspected that this increase is due to immigration of susceptible individuals and that the rate will decrease with implementation of vaccination programs (CDC, 2012b). Primary infection is known as chickenpox, whereas recurrent disease is known as herpes zoster (CDS, 2012b).

Primary varicella infection can present as a virulent course in adults, with greater risk for complications when compared with courses in children

(Blackburn, 2013). Pneumonia occurs in 14% of maternal cases and without antiviral therapy, mortality rates in pregnancy may reach 40% (American College of Obstetricians and Gynecologists, 2015a). Varicella can be transmitted transplacentally to the fetus. Fetal complications include congenital varicella syndrome in fetuses exposed prior to 20 weeks' gestation. Congenital varicella syndrome is associated with intrauterine growth restriction, low birth weight, skin lesions, microcephaly, paralysis, seizures, psychomotor retardation, limb hypoplasia, muscle atrophy, malformed digits, cataracts, gastrointestinal atresia or stenosis, and hydronephrosis (American College of Obstetricians and Gynecologists, 2015a; CDC, 2012b). Transmission that occurs late in pregnancy can result in congenital herpes zoster during infancy, prematurity, and fetal death.

Prenatal screening for varicella is not recommended (American College of Obstetricians and Gynecologists, 2015a), but risk screening is appropriate. Varicella can be diagnosed in women who are pregnant through clinical findings, although PCR assay of vesicle fluid is also available. For women who are pregnant without documented immunity to varicella, varicella-zoster immune globulin (VZIG) is indicated. The risk of a primary varicella infection is decreased if VZIG is administered within 96 hours of exposure, although this treatment may be effective up to 10 days following exposure (American College of Obstetricians and Gynecologists, 2015a). Fetal surveillance following maternal diagnosis includes assessment for anatomic abnormalities associated with congenital varicella syndrome. Referral to a maternal–fetal specialist for management during the pregnancy is necessary.

Prevention measures appropriate for all women who are pregnant, especially those without documented immunity, include avoiding infected individuals and instructions to contact the clinician as soon as possible following possible exposure. Immunization is not appropriate during pregnancy, but should be provided to postpartum women immediately following birth.

Group B Streptococcus

Group B *Streptococcus* (GBS) is a gram-positive bacteria that can cause infections of the blood (sepsis), lungs, brain, or spinal cord in newborns (American College of Obstetricians and

Gynecologists, 2011, reaffirmed 2013). Two types of GBS disease occur in newborns: (1) early-onset (occurring during the first week of life) and (2) late-onset disease (CDC, 2014a). GBS infection is the most common cause of neonatal sepsis and meningitis in the United States (CDC, 2014b).

The presence of GBS during pregnancy is typically asymptomatic and is associated with increased urinary tract infections and preterm labor and birth. This bacterium is transmitted to the newborn vertically through contact with a GBS-colonized vagina during vaginal birth. During the early newborn period, infants born to mothers who are GBS positive are at risk for developing pneumonia, septicemia, and meningitis. Newborn infections of GBS can occur up to 12 weeks of age and may be associated with speech and language delays, spastic quadriplegia, blindness, deafness, seizures, and hydrocephalus (CDC, 2010).

Women who are pregnant should be screened for GBS with cervical and vaginal cultures between 35 and 37 weeks' gestation. Women who are positive for GBS should receive care from a clinician equipped to provide intrapartum antibiotic prophylaxis during labor. Women whose GBS status is unknown at the time of labor should be provided with intrapartum antibiotic prophylaxis if they have high risk factors such as gestation less than 37 weeks, rupture of membranes for 18 hours or longer, maternal temperature of 100.4°F or higher, or a positive nucleic acid amplification test for GBS (CDC, 2010).

Sexually Transmitted Infections

Sexually transmitted infections (STIs) can create a serious risk to maternal and fetal health during pregnancy as well as to the newborn during the postpartum period. Chapter 20 provides detailed information about STIs and their treatment in women who are not pregnant. The identification of STIs early in pregnancy through appropriate screening and prompt treatment can minimize maternal, fetal, and neonatal complications.

Trichomoniasis

Trichomonas vaginalis is a flagellated, anaerobic protozoan that is transmitted primarily by sexual contact. The presence of trichomoniasis increases the risk for transmission of human immunodeficiency virus (HIV). Infection during pregnancy is associated with premature rupture of membranes, a two- to three-fold increase in preterm birth, and low birth weight in the newborn (CDC, 2015b).

There is no recommended routine screening for trichomoniasis in women who are pregnant, although screening should occur upon symptom recognition. Trichomoniasis is characterized by a vaginal discharge that is profuse, frothy, and green in color; this discharge may also have a foul odor. Vaginal pH may be less than 5.

Women who are pregnant may be treated at any stage during pregnancy with one dose of metronidazole 2 gm orally. For the mother who is lactating, an alternative treatment is metronidazole 400 mg, 3 times daily, for 7 days. Although several reported case series found no evidence of adverse effects in newborns exposed to metronidazole in breastmilk, some clinicians suggest suspending breastfeeding for 12 to 24 hours following treatment with the single-dose regimen (Briggs & Freeman, 2015; CDC, 2015b).

Human Immunodeficiency Virus

Human immunodeficiency virus (HIV) presents a danger to both the women who is pregnant and her newborn. There are three routes of transmission to the fetus and newborn: (1) maternal circulation during the first trimester of pregnancy; (2) maternal and fetal blood and fluid exchange at birth; and (3) lactation. Women who are pregnant and HIV positive must avoid procedures that increase the risk of the fetus's exposure to blood or body fluids, such as amniocentesis, fetal scalp electrode application, fetal blood sampling, and chorionic villi sampling. Newborns who contract HIV are at risk for failure to thrive, upper respiratory tract infections, chronic diarrhea, dermatitis, thrush, and other infections. Maternal treatment with antiretroviral agents, avoiding the aforementioned antepartum procedures, and avoiding breastfeeding can reduce the rate of transmission of the virus from 30% to less than 2% (CDC, 2015b).

All women who are pregnant should be screened for HIV at the first antepartum visit. Testing should occur in the third trimester for all women who are high risk. Refer women who test positive for HIV to a specialist for management and fetal surveillance. All women who are pregnant and HIV positive can benefit from patient teaching related to adequate rest, stress reduction, and consumption of a diet rich in fruits, vegetables, antioxidants, and omega-3 fatty acids to complement their pharmacologic treatment.

Hepatitis B

Hepatitis B may be transmitted to the fetus and newborn through secretions such as vaginal fluid, amniotic fluid, blood, saliva, and (most likely) breastmilk. Most newborns born with hepatitis B acquire it during the third trimester or during the birth process (Blackburn, 2013). Hepatitis B infections during pregnancy are associated with spontaneous abortion (SAB) and preterm birth.

All women who are pregnant should be screened for hepatitis B surface antigen (HBsAg) at the first antepartum visit. Those at high risk for infection can receive the vaccination during pregnancy (Briggs & Freeman, 2015). Women who are pregnant who test positive for hepatitis B should be referred to a specialist for treatment and management. Infants born to mothers who are HBsAg positive may continue to breastfeed (CDC, 2014a).

Syphilis

Syphilis is characterized by three stages, each of which has a unique set of symptoms. Syphilis is transmitted transplacentally to the fetus (Blackburn, 2013). If syphilis is contracted in pregnancy prior to 28 weeks' gestation, the newborn is at risk for developing congenital syphilis, which is characterized by snuffles or nasal discharge, rhagades (fissures, cracks, or linear scars in the skin, especially at the linear angles of the mouth or nose), hydrocephaly, saddle nose, saber shin, Hutchinson teeth or notched and tapered canines, diabetes, preterm birth, and fetal death (CDC, 2015b).

All women who are pregnant should be screened for syphilis at the first antepartum visit using nontreponemal antibody testing (CDC, 2015b). Testing for syphilis should be repeated after 28 weeks' gestation in women who report high-risk behaviors or live where there is documented high syphilis morbidity. Treatment for syphilis during pregnancy is the same regimen as for the woman who is not pregnant (see Chapter 20). Attentive

fetal surveillance is necessary, so referral to a maternal–fetal specialist is appropriate.

Gonorrhea

Gonorrhea is a sexually transmitted bacterial infection caused by *Neisseria gonorrhoeae*. In pregnancy, gonorrhea infections are associated with ectopic pregnancy, preterm birth, premature rupture of membranes, and intrauterine growth restriction. Transmission of the bacterium to the newborn occurs during exposure to the cervix of a woman who is pregnant and has the infection. Newborn illness usually occurs 2 to 5 days after birth and is manifested as ophthalmic neonatorium and sepsis (CDC, 2015b).

All women who are pregnant who are younger than 25 years and women who are older at increased risk should be screened at the first antepartum visit. If the risk for gonorrhea continues into the pregnancy, retesting should occur during the third trimester (CDC, 2015b). Treatment of gonorrhea during pregnancy is the same as for the women who is not pregnant (see Chapter 20). Because chlamydial infection is thought to coexist with gonorrhea, treatment includes agents to address both *N. gonorrhoeae* and *Chlamydia*. A test-of-cure is not needed for persons who receive a diagnosis of uncomplicated urogenital or rectal gonorrhea who are treated with any of the recommended or alternative regimens; however, any person with pharyngeal gonorrhea who is treated with an alternative regimen should return 14 days after treatment for a test-of-cure (CDC, 2015b).

Chlamydia

Chlamydia is the most common nationally notifiable STI in the United States (CDC, 2015b). This infection, which is caused by the bacterium *Chlamydia trachomatis*, can cause infertility after the first infection and often accompanies gonorrhea. Transmission to the newborn occurs during birth from exposure to the cervix of the infected women who is pregnant. Chlamydial infection during pregnancy is associated with SAB, ectopic pregnancy, premature rupture of membranes, postpartum endometritis, preterm birth, and stillbirth. The neonate who contracts chlamydia is 10 times more likely to die in the newborn period (CDC, 2015a). Neonatal conjunctivitis is likely 5 to 12 days after birth and subacute, afebrile pneumonia can occur 1 to 3 months after birth (CDC, 2015a).

All women who are pregnant who are younger than 25 years and women who are older at increased risk should be screened at the first antepartum visit. Retesting should occur during the third trimester. Women who are pregnant and test positive for chlamydia should be treated with azithromycin 1 gm orally, one dose, or amoxicillin 500 mg orally, 3 times daily, for 7 days. A test of cure should be done 3 to 4 weeks following treatment and again within 3 months (CDC, 2015b).

Herpes Simplex Virus

Herpes simplex virus (HSV) is differentiated into two types: type 1 (HSV-1) and type 2 (HSV-2). Most HSV genital infections occur as a result of exposure to HSV-2, although genital infections caused by HSV-1 are becoming increasingly more common (American College of Obstetricians and Gynecologists, 2007, reaffirmed 2014). Herpes infection during pregnancy is associated with SAB, preterm birth, and intrauterine growth retardation. Between 30% and 50% of newborns born to mothers who contract primary HSV late in the third trimester will acquire the disease (CDC, 2015b). There is a high mortality rate for these newborns prior to 4 weeks of age, yet fewer than 1% of newborns born to mothers with recurrent or contracted HSV in the first trimester will acquire the disease (Blackburn, 2013). Women who have active lesions at the time of birth should consider cesarean birth to decrease the newborn transmission rates of HSV.

Routine screening for HSV infection in pregnancy is not recommended, but women with a history of risky sexual practices or known exposure should be screened upon identification of risk. Type-specific serologic testing may be used to screen (CDC, 2015b). Acyclovir is compatible with pregnancy and may be administered for the initial episode (Briggs & Freeman, 2015). Immediate antiviral treatment reduces the severity of symptoms and reduces the duration of shedding (American College of Obstetricians and Gynecologists, 2007, reaffirmed 2014). Suppressive therapy, consisting of acyclovir 400 mg orally, 3 times daily, or valacyclovir 500 mg, 2 times daily, beginning at 36 weeks' gestation may prevent cesarean birth in women who are HSV positive (American College of Obstetricians and Gynecologists, 2007, reaffirmed 2014; CDC, 2015b). Women who are pregnant with symptoms of painful perineal lesions may benefit from cool compresses or perineal washes and loose-fitting undergarments and clothing.

Human Papillomavirus

Human papillomavirus (HPV) is characterized by the presence of precancerous, genital lesions, sometimes called warts (CDC, 2015b). During pregnancy, these lesions can grow, proliferate, and become friable. Some lesions may grow quite large, to the point that obstruction of the introitus is possible. The presence of large perineal lesions is not an indication for cesarean birth unless complete obstruction occurs or excessive bleeding is possible. In rare instances, the newborn may develop respiratory papillomatosis and subsequent obstruction of the pharynx.

Screening for HPV in conjunction with cervical cancer screening is recommended for women who are pregnant at the same screening intervals as for women who are not pregnant. Treatment for HPV with podofilox, podophyllin, and sinecatechin is not appropriate in pregnancy (CDC, 2015b). There are limited data to support the use of imiquimod during pregnancy, so its use should be avoided (Briggs & Freeman, 2015). Lesions during pregnancy can be observed closely and treatment delayed until after birth, as many resolve spontaneously at this time.

FIRST-TRIMESTER COMPLICATIONS

The first trimester of pregnancy is characterized by many discomforts, including nausea, vomiting, irregular menses, increased urination, and breast tenderness. The degree of expression of these symptoms varies among women. The wise clinician listens intently to the woman to discover when these symptoms move from common discomforts of pregnancy to complications. This section will assist the clinician in differentiating between what is often a common discomfort of early pregnancy such as nausea and vomiting and those symptoms that may indicate a complication of pregnancy, such as hyperemesis gravidarium.

Hyperemesis Gravidarium

Nausea and vomiting (also referred to as morning sickness, even though the symptoms can occur at any time) are discomforts commonly experienced during the first trimester of pregnancy. Hormonal shifts of estrogen, progesterone, and human chorionic gonadotropin (hCG) levels as well as a deficiency of vitamin B_6 are suggested as causes of commonly experienced nausea and vomiting (American College of Obstetricians and Gynecologists, 2015b). However, women who are pregnant and have uncontrolled nausea and vomiting that is associated with a weight loss of greater than 5% of their pre-pregnant weight must be evaluated for hyperemesis gravidarium. Hyperemesis gravidarium occurs in 0.5% to 2.0% of all pregnancies (American College of Obstetricians and Gynecologists, 2015b). Risk factors include history of hyperemesis gravidarium, multiple gestation, molar pregnancy, Caucasian ethnicity, primipara status, obesity, single relationship status, and younger age.

Women with hyperemesis gravidarium report uncontrolled nausea and vomiting, anorexia, fatigue, loss of work, and difficulty managing activities of daily living. Diagnosis of hyperemesis gravidarium requires assessment for ketonuria and dehydration, electrolyte imbalance, and weight loss. Differential diagnoses include gastroenteritis, cholecystitis, pancreatitis, hepatitis, and appendicitis. Care of the woman with hyperemesis gravidarium should be managed by a maternal–fetal specialist with the primary goal of correcting dehydration and electrolyte imbalance. Treatment may require hospitalization and include bed rest and fetal surveillance, intravenous fluids, parenteral nutrition, antiemetics, enteral feedings, and dietary counseling.

Vaginal Bleeding During Early Pregnancy

Bleeding during the first trimester of pregnancy must always signal to the clinician the possibility of pregnancy loss. Prompt identification of symptoms accompanying vaginal bleeding will assist the clinician to differentiate between simple spotting during pregnancy, SAB, ectopic pregnancy, and hydatidiform mole.

Spontaneous Abortion

SAB is considered to be loss of a pregnancy prior to 20 weeks' gestation. Risk factors that may be associated with SAB include advancing maternal age, endocrine disorders such as thyroid disease

and polycystic ovarian syndrome, history of SAB, viral and bacterial infections, anatomic reproductive disorders such as a malformed uterus, chronic diseases, and exposure to environmental hazards. Several types of SABs exist (**Table 31-1**), and the clinician must be able to differentiate between them.

Diagnosis of SAB requires assessing uterine size by either physical examination or ultrasound, identifying if fetal heart tones are present by either auscultation or ultrasound, examination of the cervical os to determine if it is dilated, and serial β-hCG measurements. Differential diagnoses include reproductive cancers, ectopic pregnancy, and hydatidiform mole. Upon identification of symptoms related to SAB, referral to a physician for management is appropriate. Rhogam administration following a SAB is indicated for women who have an Rh-negative blood type.

Ectopic Pregnancy

Ectopic pregnancy is the implantation of a fertilized ovum in locations other than the uterine cavity. It is the second leading cause of maternal mortality in the United States (Marion & Meeks, 2012). Approximately 95% of all ectopic pregnancies occur in the fallopian tube (American College of Obstetricians and Gynecologists, 2008, reaffirmed 2014). Growth of the fetus in the fallopian tube puts the woman who is pregnant at high risk for pregnancy loss, tubal rupture, excessive blood loss, and future infertility due to tubal scarring. **Box 31-1** summarizes risk factors associated with ectopic pregnancy.

Pelvic and abdominal pain and unexplained vaginal bleeding are the primary symptoms experienced by most women with ectopic pregnancy. The pain may be described as vague, sharp, diffuse, or unilateral. The woman may have had a time of amenorrhea, and pregnancy may or may not already be diagnosed. A ruptured ectopic pregnancy is characterized by a sudden onset of vaginal bleeding and sharp, severe, unilateral abdominal pain. Following rupture, symptoms of significant blood loss and resulting shock may include hypotension, shoulder pain, and breast tenderness.

Physical findings associated with ectopic pregnancy include cervical motion tenderness, a uterus that is not enlarged, adnexal mass, and adnexal

| TABLE 31-1 | Types of Spontaneous Abortion |

Type	Definition	Symptoms	Prognosis
Threatened	Symptoms of SAB present. Products of conception intact.	Minimal vaginal bleeding. Abdominal cramping. Uterine size is equal to dates. Cervical os is closed.	Possible pregnancy loss
Inevitable	Symptoms of SAB increased in severity, to include cervical dilation. Products of conception intact.	Moderate vaginal bleeding. Moderate to severe uterine cramping. Uterine size is equal to dates. Cervical os is dilated.	Poor
Incomplete	Symptoms of SAB present, to include cervical dilation. Partial products of conception expelled.	Heavy vaginal bleeding. Moderate to severe uterine cramping. Uterine size is equal to dates. Cervical os is dilated.	Poor
Complete	Products of conception expelled in entirety following symptoms of SAB.	Minimal vaginal bleeding. Prior uterine cramping has subsided. Uterus is pre-pregnancy size. Cervical os is either closed or dilated.	Pregnancy loss
Missed	Products of conception retained for up to 6 weeks following symptoms of SAB.	Vaginal bleeding has occurred, subsided, and reoccurs. No current uterine contractions, but there is a history of uterine cramping.	Pregnancy loss
Recurrent	Three or more SABs occurring consecutively.	See above.	Poor for maintaining future pregnancies without intervention; refer to assistive reproduction specialist

Abbreviation: SAB, spontaneous abortion.

tenderness. Diagnosis may take several steps and should be managed by a maternal–fetal specialist. Immediate data to collect to aid in the diagnosis include a transvaginal ultrasound to determine the contents of the uterus, pregnancy test, complete blood count, and β-hCG levels. Differential diagnoses include appendicitis, pelvic inflammatory disease, bowel irritability or obstruction, cholecystitis, pyelonephritis, and ovarian torsion.

Management prior to a confirmed diagnosis includes close observation to avoid the medical emergency of tubal rupture. Early diagnosis also may facilitate the use of methotrexate to dissolve the products of conception and avoid tubal rupture. The presence of signs and symptoms of rupture requires prompt medical attention in an institution that is equipped with surgical capabilities. Close follow-up of the woman who experiences an

BOX 31-1 **Risk Factors for Ectopic Pregnancy**

- Age 15–19 years
- Age > 35 years
- Racial minorities
- Previous ectopic pregnancy
- Any previous tubal surgery or tubal deformity
- History of pelvic inflammatory disease
- History of infertility
- Past or current use of intrauterine device
- Use of low-dose progestins or postcoital estrogens for contraception
- Assisted reproduction
- History of therapeutic abortion especially with complications

FIGURE 31-1 **Molar pregnancy.**

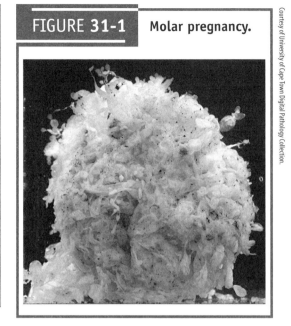

Courtesy of University of Cape Town Digital Pathology Collection.

ectopic pregnancy includes Rhogam administration when appropriate, monitoring β-hCG levels, emotional care due to pregnancy loss, and future fertility counseling.

Gestational Trophoblastic Disease (Hydatidiform Mole)

Hydatidiform mole, also called a molar pregnancy, is an abnormal proliferation of placental tissue that results in the development of a benign or malignant tumor. These abnormal growths appear as grapelike villae that fill the uterine cavity (**Figure 31-1**).

There are two types of molar pregnancies: (1) partial, in which nonviable fetal tissue may be present, and (2) complete, in which there is an absence of fetal tissue. In a partial molar pregnancy, the woman may present with symptoms of a missed SAB with uterine size as expected related to her last normal menstrual period (LNMP). Typically, women who present with a complete molar pregnancy have a uterine size greater than expected related to their LNMP and have experienced vaginal bleeding accompanied with passage of grapelike villae. Increased incidence of

complications is associated with a complete molar pregnancy. Risk factors associated with molar pregnancy include age younger than 20 years or older than 40 years, history of molar pregnancy, and living in Asia, South Pacific, or Mexico.

Women who have a molar pregnancy may experience the following symptoms: dark red or brown vaginal bleeding, abdominal tenderness especially over the ovaries, severe nausea and vomiting persisting beyond 12 weeks' gestation, extreme fatigue, pelvic pain, coughing and shortness of breath, hemoptysis, and weight loss. The woman may report passage of grapelike villae. Symptoms of preeclampsia may develop prior to 24 weeks. Gathering careful objective data assists with the diagnosis of a molar pregnancy. An ultrasound reveals a snowstorm pattern, lack of fetal parts, and lack of fetal movement. No fetal heart tones will be auscultated. Levels of β-hCG will be consistently high and rising.

Management requires a referral to a maternal–fetal specialist. If a malignancy is diagnosed, a referral to an oncologist is necessary. Evacuation of the molar tissue may be accomplished pharmacologically or surgically. Follow-up care will include monitoring β-hCG levels to determine if the levels are decreasing, contraception, consultation with a maternal–fetal specialist, avoidance of pregnancy for 6 to 12 months, and emotional care due to pregnancy loss.

SECOND-TRIMESTER COMPLICATIONS

The second trimester is typically a time when a woman who is pregnant has some resolution from the physical discomforts of the first trimester. The period of organogenesis has passed and the fetus is growing and developing at a rapid rate. Several of the complications discussed in this section can be identified during routine prenatal screening. The goal here is to provide a clinician with the ability to identify these complications and take appropriate action.

Cervical Insufficiency

Cervical insufficiency can be defined as the inability of the cervix to remain closed in the absence of uterine contractions in the second trimester (American College of Obstetricians and Gynecologists, 2014). This condition increases the risk for pregnancy loss. Women who are pregnant at risk for cervical insufficiency include those who have had cervical trauma due to cervical conization, loop electrosurgical excision procedures, or mechanical dilation during pregnancy termination. Additional suggested causes include birth trauma from cervical lacerations, a history of fetal loss at 14 weeks' gestation or later, and a history of multiple pregnancy terminations (American College of Obstetricians & Gynecologists, 2014; King et al., 2015).

Cervical insufficiency does not always present with clinical symptoms. If symptoms are present, they may include backache, uterine contractions, vaginal spotting, pelvic pressure, an increase in vaginal discharge, decrease in cervical length, and cervical dilation confirmed by speculum examination (American College of Obstetricians & Gynecologists, 2014). Referral to a maternal–fetal specialist is appropriate. In the past, the patient was told to restrict activity and was placed on bed rest; however, current evidence does not support this intervention. Prenatal surveillance for women at risk for cervical insufficiency, and therefore preterm labor and birth, may include serial transvaginal ultrasound beginning at 16 weeks' gestation and continuing until 24 weeks' gestation (American College of Obstetricians & Gynecologists, 2014).

Preterm Labor and Birth

Preterm birth (PTB) is defined as birth that occurs between 20 0/7 weeks' gestation and 36 6/7 weeks' gestation (American College of Obstetricians & Gynecologists, 2012). Preterm labor (PTL) is defined as the onset of regular contractions resulting in cervical change between 20 and 37 completed weeks of gestation (American College of Obstetricians & Gynecologists, 2012). Maternal infection and inflammation in the reproductive tract may be linked to 20% to 40% of all preterm births (Blackburn, 2013). Urinary tract infections and asymptomatic bacteriuria are associated with PTL. Common risk factors associated with PTL include maternal age younger than 15 years and older than 40 years; low socioeconomic status; African American ethnicity; low educational level; poor nutritional status; history of cervical or uterine anomalies or previous surgeries; history of low-birth-weight infants, preterm birth, or premature rupture of membranes; fewer than 18 months between pregnancies; multiple pregnancy terminations; multiple gestation; pregnancy-induced hypertension with current pregnancy; cervical insufficiency; polyhydramnios; and substance abuse (including smoking and alcohol). Women who are pregnant and have had a prior preterm birth and/or have a short cervix are at the highest risk for PTL and PTB in subsequent pregnancies (American College of Obstetricians & Gynecologists, 2015b). Despite all that is known about risk factors for preterm labor and birth, the majority of women with PTL and PTB have no identifiable risk factors.

Risk assessment and prompt management of potential PTL contribute to reduced incidence of preterm birth. Symptoms associated with PTL include menstrual-like uterine cramps; a low, dull backache and pelvic pressure prior to 36 weeks' gestation that may be due to fetal descent; diarrhea; increased vaginal discharge; leakage of clear fluid from the vagina; and vaginal bleeding. Women who are pregnant who exhibit any of these symptoms should be instructed to reduce physical and sexual activity, avoid breast stimulation, and increase hydration; they should also be followed closely to observe for cervical change, cervical shortening, and fetal well-being. Prompt recognition of these symptoms indicates referral to a maternal–fetal specialist and management in a facility equipped to care for preterm infants.

Gestational Diabetes Mellitus

Pregnancy is a time of metabolic changes that support the maternal anatomic and physiologic alterations and adequate fetal growth. Increases in maternal basal metabolism typically increase glucose utilization. Gestational diabetes mellitus (GDM) occurs when a woman who is pregnant develops a carbohydrate intolerance during pregnancy (American College of Obstetricians & Gynecologists, 2013a). As a result of the carbohydrate intolerance, between weeks 20 and 30, hyperglycemia occurs. A diagnosis of GDM occurs in 1% to 5% of pregnancies in the United States. Most (90%) of these cases will resolve in the postpartum period, but 50% of women whose GDM resolves during the postpartum period will develop type 2 diabetes mellitus 22 to 28 years later (American College of Obstetricians & Gynecologists, 2013a). The incidence is greatly influenced by body weight and can be reduced by 25% if normal body mass index is maintained through proper nutrition and exercise (American College of Obstetricians & Gynecologists, 2013a).

Women at risk for developing GDM include those with a previous history of GDM, obesity, history of diabetes mellitus in a first-degree relative, age greater than 25 years, and African American, Hispanic, Native American, or Asian ethnicity (**Table 31-2**).

Maternal complications associated with GDM include SAB, pyelonephritis, preterm labor and preterm birth, polyhydramnios, preeclampsia, and an increased rate of operative birth, particularly cesarean birth. Fetal and newborn complications associated with GDM include stillbirth; macrosomia leading to increased risk for operative birth, shoulder dystocia, or birth trauma; neonatal hypoglycemia; hyperbilirubinemia; hypocalcemia; polycythemia; and an increased risk for obesity and type 2 diabetes later in life (American College of Obstetricians & Gynecologists, 2013a).

All women who are pregnant should be screened for GDM between 24 and 28 weeks' gestation. Women whose BMI is equal to or greater than 30, who have a history of a first-degree relative with diabetes mellitus or a strong family history, and who have a history of GDM or other impairment of glucose metabolism should be screened during the first trimester. If this screen is negative, it should be repeated at 24 to 28 weeks' gestation (American College of Obstetricians & Gynecologists, 2013a). The most common approach to screening for GDM is to administer 50-gm oral

TABLE 31-2	Risk Factors for Gestational Diabetes	
Demographic Characteristics	**Medical and Family History**	**Previous Obstetric History**
Maternal age Member of an ethnic group at increased risk for type 2 diabetes mellitus • Hispanic • African American • Native American • South or East Asian • Pacific Islands for more than 25 years	Prepregnancy weight ≥ 110% of ideal body weight or BMI > 30 kg/m², significant weight gain in early adulthood or between pregnancies, or excessive gestational weight gain History of abnormal glucose tolerance Current use of glucocorticoids Polycystic ovary syndrome Essential hypertension First-degree relative with diabetes	History of adverse pregnancy outcomes associated with GDM • Infant more than 9 pounds at birth • Unexplained stillbirth • Infant with congenital anomalies History of GDM in prior pregnancy

Abbreviations: BMI, body mass index; GDM, gestational diabetes mellitus.

glucose, followed by a 1-hour venous blood glucose test. Women whose blood sugar is greater than 130 to 140 mg/dL should undergo a 3-hour glucose tolerance test with a 100-gm oral glucose dose. Diagnosis of GDM can be made with two elevated blood glucose values (**Table 31-3**).

Women with GDM are considered to have a higher-risk pregnancy, and should receive care either in collaboration with or through referral to a maternal–fetal specialist. The goal of care is to normalize the level of glycemic control to the level of a nondiabetic woman. Nutritional therapy and fetal surveillance are part of the standard of care, while pharmacologic management should be considered

for women who are unable to maintain their blood sugar with complementary care.

Blood Incompatibility

Blood types and Rh factors can have a significant impact on pregnancy and the newborn. During pregnancy, there is a potential for mixing of the maternal and fetal blood. In the Rh-negative woman who is pregnant with an Rh-positive fetus, this mixing of blood can cause the development of IgG antibodies to the Rh (D) antigen. Subsequent pregnancies with Rh-positive fetuses are then at risk when the IgG antibodies cross the placenta, attach to fetal cells, and create hemolysis; such

TABLE **31-3**	Screening and Diagnostic Criteria for Gestational Diabetes
Organization	**Plasma Glucose Diagnostic Values**

American College of Obstetricians and Gynecologists	1. *50-gram glucose screening test:*
	  a. GDM diagnosed if > 200 mg/dL
	  b. If > 130 mg/dL or > 140 mg/dL, move to 3-hour GTT
	2. *3-hour GTT at 24–28 weeks':*
	  GDM diagnosed if two values are over the following threshold values:
	  a. Carpenter/Coustan plasma or serum glucose level: fasting > 95 mg/dL; 1-hour > 180 mg/dL; 2-hour > 155 mg/dL; 3-hour > 140 mg/dL
	  b. National Diabetes Data Group plasma level: fasting > 105 mg/dL; 1-hour > 190 mg/dL; 2-hour > 165 mg/dL; 3-hour > 145 mg/dL

International Association of the Diabetes and Pregnancy Study Groups; American Diabetes Association	1. *Measure fasting plasma glucose, HbA1c, or random plasma glucose of all women or all high-risk women at initial prenatal visit:*
	  a. Overt diabetes diagnosed: fasting ≥ 126 mg/dL; HbA1c ≥ 6.5%; random plasma glucose ≥ 200 mg/dL that is subsequently confirmed via HbA1c or fasting blood glucose value
	  b. GDM diagnosed: fasting ≥ 92 mg/dL but < 126 mg/dL
	2. *If initial values do not detect overt diabetes or GDM, do 75-gram 2-hour GTT at 24–28 weeks':*
	  a. Overt diabetes diagnosed: fasting ≥ 126 mg/dL
	  b. GDM diagnosed if one value is over the following threshold values: fasting > 92 mg/dL; 1-hour plasma glucose > 180 mg/dL; 2-hour plasma glucose > 153 mg/dL

Abbreviations: GDM, gestational diabetes mellitus; GTT, glucose tolerance test; HbA1c, glycated hemoglobin.
Modified from American College of Obstetricians and Gynecologists. (2011). Gestational diabetes: Practice Bulletin No. 30. *Obstetrics & Gynecology, 98*, 525–538; International Association of Diabetes and Pregnancy Study Groups Consensus Panel, Metzger, B. E., Gabbe S. G., Persson B., Buchanan T. A., Catalano P. A., . . . Schmidt, M. I. (2010). International Association of Diabetes and Pregnancy Study Groups recommendations on the diagnosis and classification of hyperglycemia in pregnancy. *Diabetes Care, 33*, 676–682.

hemolysis may lead to erythroblastosis fetalis and stillbirth.

The risk associated with Rh factor isoimmunization has significantly decreased since the late 1960s due to the development of Rhogam, an anti-D immune globulin prophylaxis. Prophylaxis with Rhogam prevents development of the IgG antibodies. Women who are pregnant should be screened during the first trimester to determine their Rh status. An antibody titer should be ordered during the second trimester for those found to be Rh negative. Rhogam should be administered by the 28th week of gestation to women with a negative titer. A second dose of Rhogam is administered within 72 hours of birth for mothers who give birth to Rh-positive infants. When a potential for mixing of maternal and fetal blood occurs, the administration of Rhogam is indicated. Additional indications include placental abruption, prenatal procedures such as amniocentesis or chorionic villus sampling, spontaneous abortion, therapeutic abortion, ectopic pregnancy, hydatidiform mole, abdominal trauma, and external cephalic version.

Amniotic Fluid Complications

Amniotic fluid is essential for maintenance of a stable uterine temperature, fetal lung development, adequate movement by the fetus that encourages morphologic development, protection from trauma by providing a cushioned environment, and provision of a barrier to infectious agents (Blackburn, 2013). By 32 to 35 weeks' gestation, there is a mean of 780 mL of amniotic fluid. Although volumes vary, alterations in the amount of amniotic fluid may compromise fetal health.

Oligohydramnios

Oligohydramnios is defined as less than 500 mL of amniotic fluid at 40 weeks' gestation. It can be identified by an amniotic fluid index of less than 5 cm during the third trimester in a singleton pregnancy or less than 2-cm pocket in a twin gestation (King et al., 2015). This condition may occur at any time during pregnancy, but is generally considered to be rare. Oligohydramnios is associated with maternal hypertension, placental insufficiency, maternal dehydration or renal disorders, post-term pregnancies, and fetal renal or heart abnormalities. Later in pregnancy, oligohydramnios may be associated with post-term pregnancy, inhibition of fetal lung development, umbilical cord compression, fetal distress, and musculoskeletal anomalies. Care of women diagnosed with oligohydramnios is best managed by a maternal–fetal specialist.

Polyhydramnios (Hydramnios)

Polyhydramnios is defined as greater than 1.5 to 2 L of amniotic fluid, or greater than 24 cm as observed by ultrasound on an amniotic fluid index or the deepest vertical pocket of amniotic fluid measuring greater than 8 cm (King et al., 2015). The incidence of polyhydramnios is 0.93%, with 60% of cases considered to be idiopathic and 40% to 50% associated with no fetal difficulties (Blackburn, 2013). Polyhydramnios is most often associated with multiple gestation, maternal hyperglycemia, decreased fetal swallowing, and fetal cardiac abnormalities. It may complicate fetal descent and inhibit effective labor.

Premature Rupture of Membranes

Premature rupture of membranes (PROM) is defined as rupture of membranes prior to the onset of labor, whereas rupture of membranes prior to labor and before 37 weeks' gestation is called preterm premature rupture of membranes (PPROM) (American College of Obstetricians & Gynecologists, 2013b). PROM is a normal, physiologic phenomenon that occurs in 8% to 10% of all labors due to a weakened amniotic membrane. In most cases, the onset of contractions follows PROM within 24 hours (King et al., 2015). Rupture of membranes at any gestation increases the risk of infection, with this risk increasing with the duration of rupture. Women who are pregnant and at risk for PPROM include those with a history of PPROM, amniotic infection, and risks associated with preterm labor. Approximately 50% of women who experience PPROM will give birth within 1 week. Referral to a maternal–fetal specialist is required upon recognition of PPROM.

A sudden, spontaneous rupture of membranes (SROM) may be associated with umbilical cord prolapse. Umbilical cord prolapse is considered an obstetric emergency, and immediate transport to a healthcare facility is necessary. If the prolapse is diagnosed in the office setting, the woman should immediately be placed either in a knee-chest position or on her left side in lateral Sims position until she can be transported to the hospital (King et al., 2015). The clinician should never try to replace the cord.

The incidence of umbilical cord prolapse is between 1.4 and 6.2 cases per 1,000 pregnancies (Phelan & Holbrook, 2013). Risk factors related to umbilical cord prolapse may be classified as either spontaneous occurrences or iatrogenic factors. Spontaneous factors include fetal malpresentation, prematurity, cord and fetal anomalies, polyhydramnios, multiple gestation, SROM, PPROM, and grand multiparity. Iatrogenic factors associated with umbilical cord prolapse include amniotomy, amnioinfusion, attempted rotation of the fetal head or cephalic version, placement of internal fetal and uterine monitors, and placement of cervical ripening balloon catheters (Phelan & Holbrook, 2013). Steps to manage the prolapsed umbilical cord in the outpatient setting are as follows:

1. Position the mother in lateral or knee-chest position to relieve cord pressure.
2. Relieve pressure on the cord by inserting a gloved hand into the vagina, maintaining this position during transport.
3. Monitor the fetal heart rate.
4. Administer maternal oxygen.
5. Initiate intravenous access.

THIRD-TRIMESTER COMPLICATIONS

Complications late in pregnancy can compromise the health of the woman who is pregnant as well as the health of her fetus. Hypertensive disorders and bleeding disorders associated with the placenta are two common complications that require the clinician to carefully assess clinical findings and act promptly to provide care in an effort to improve and maintain the health of the mother and her newborn.

Hypertensive Disorders of Pregnancy

Preeclampsia

Preeclampsia occurs in 6% to 10% of pregnancies and is characterized by a systolic blood pressure of 140 mm Hg or higher, a diastolic blood pressure of 90 mm Hg or higher, and proteinuria of +1 on two occasions 4 hours apart or 300 mg or greater

in a 24-hour time frame or absent proteinuria but with the presence of thrombocytopenia, renal insufficiency, impaired liver function, pulmonary edema, or central nervous system or visual changes (American College of Obstetricians & Gynecologists, 2013b). Preeclampsia can be classified as severe with the addition of one or more of the following symptoms: a systolic blood pressure of 160 mm Hg or higher, a diastolic blood pressure of 110 mm Hg or higher on two occasions 4 hours apart in women who are pregnant and at least 20 weeks' gestation, new onset of central nervous system or visual changes, pulmonary edema, severe upper right quadrant or epigastric pain, impaired liver function, thrombocytopenia, or progressive renal insufficiency (American College of Obstetricians & Gynecologists, 2013b). Women at increased risk for developing hypertensive disorders in pregnancy include those with factors such as nulliparity, age greater than 35 years, African American ethnicity, family or personal history of preeclampsia, obesity, personal history of vascular disease, hydatidiform molar pregnancy, multiple gestation, and lower socioeconomic status.

Preeclampsia is associated with both maternal and fetal complications. Women are at risk for renal or liver failure, disseminated intravascular coagulopathy (DIC), abruptio placentae, emergent operative birth, and death. The fetus of a mother with preeclampsia may develop intrauterine growth restriction, oligohydramnios, or fetal distress during labor and may be born prematurely.

Women with symptoms of preeclampsia need to be cared for by a maternal–fetal specialist. Hospitalization, increased maternal and fetal surveillance, pharmaceutical administration, and emergency birth may be necessary. Patient teaching to complement surveillance includes self-monitoring of blood pressure and urine protein, daily fetal movement counts beginning at 28 weeks' gestation, activity restriction, and dietary counseling to reduce sodium and increase protein.

HELLP Syndrome

HELLP syndrome is considered to be a serious complication of preeclampsia, although it can also occur without being associated with preeclampsia. This syndrome is characterized by hypertension, elevated liver enzymes, and low platelets. Women with HELLP syndrome may complain of headache, epigastric or chest pain, and extreme fatigue, nausea, and vomiting. The serious risks associated with HELLP syndrome are hepatic rupture, DIC, and eclampsia.

Eclampsia

Eclampsia is a life-threatening complication of preeclampsia characterized by tonic–clonic seizure activity, which may be accompanied by loss of consciousness and intracranial hemorrhage. Women must receive prompt medical attention to include seizure precautions and immediate delivery of the fetus.

Late-Pregnancy Bleeding

The placenta is a vascular organ that forms during pregnancy to nourish the fetus and to assist in waste removal. For the fetus to grow appropriately, the placenta must function properly throughout pregnancy. Proper placement of the placenta, including proper attachment, is essential. Abnormalities such as placenta previa, abruptio placentae, and placenta accreta may compromise the fetus's well-being (**Figure 31-2**).

Placenta Previa

Placenta previa is implantation of the placenta in the lower segment of the uterus in a position that may obstruct the cervical os. Classification of placenta previa is explained in **Table 31-4**. Women at increased risk for placenta previa include those with a history of placenta previa, history of cesarean section and other uterine surgeries, history of SAB or therapeutic abortion, age 35 years or older, history of multiple pregnancies, and history of smoking and cocaine abuse. Complications associated with placenta previa include abruptio placentae, placenta accreta, fetal malpresentation, postpartum hemorrhage, disseminated intravascular coagulation, infertility, and increased perinatal mortality.

Painless vaginal bleeding is a hallmark symptom of placenta previa. Bleeding may occur after 24 weeks' gestation and is usually bright red but varies in amount. Women may experience fatigue and syncope. Symptoms of shock may occur with excessive bleeding. An ultrasound can determine the placement of the placenta. Cervical exams are contraindicated with active vaginal bleeding.

Management is dependent upon the classification of the placenta previa. No intervention is necessary if there is no bleeding, but education regarding vaginal bleeding and when to seek care related to volume of bleeding is necessary. Women diagnosed with complete or partial previa should be referred to a specialist and counseled regarding pelvic rest.

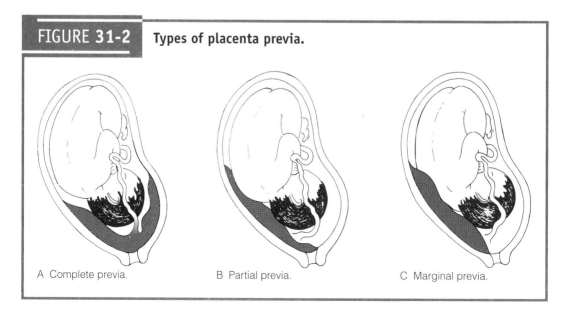

FIGURE 31-2 Types of placenta previa.

A Complete previa.

B Partial previa.

C Marginal previa.

TABLE 31-4	Classification of Placenta Previa

Classification	Description
Complete	Placenta totally covers the cervical os. Birth cannot be accomplished vaginally.
Partial	Placenta partially covers the cervical os. Birth is unlikely to be accomplished vaginally.
Marginal	Placenta lies within 2 cm of the cervical os but does not cover the cervical os. Birth may occur vaginally.
Low-lying	Placenta lies within 2–5 cm of the cervical os but does not cover the cervical os. This is the most common type of placenta previa. Vaginal birth is probable, as the placenta will most likely migrate as the pregnancy progresses.

Abruptio Placentae

Abruptio placentae is the premature separation of the placenta from the uterine wall. It can be classified as obvious or occult. With obvious abruptio placentae, there is external, obvious vaginal bleeding. With occult abruptio placentae, bleeding occurs along the central portion of the placenta and is concealed by a fetal head that is firmly applied to the cervical os. Maternal risk factors associated with abruptio placentae include hypertension, history of abruption, circumvallate placenta attachment, sudden uterine decompression as in sudden rupture of membranes, abdominal trauma, uterine cavity deformities, short umbilical cord, and smoking or cocaine use. The hemorrhage associated with abruptio placentae is a life-threatening complication. This condition is also associated with intrauterine growth retardation, fetal malformations, maternal anemia, disseminated intravascular coagulation, and postpartum endometritis.

Painful, bright red vaginal bleeding and the sudden onset of sharp, localized abdominal pain are characteristics of abruptio placentae. However, mild back or abdominal cramping and no vaginal bleeding may also be associated with abruptio placentae. Uterine tenderness may be both reported by the woman and elicited by the clinician. The maternal abdomen may be palpated as board-like and firm. Fetal heart tones may be diminished or absent, and fetal distress may be noted.

Suspicion of abruptio placentae requires referral to a maternal–fetal specialist, as this condition is considered an emergent situation. The woman needs to be cared for in a facility that can manage surgical intervention, manage a hypoxic newborn, and assist with maternal vascular support if necessary.

Placenta Accreta

Placenta accreta is a condition in which the villi adhere to the myometrium. Placenta increta extends into the myometrium, whereas placenta accreta extends through the myometrium. Implantation over a previous uterine scar seems to increase the risk of placenta accreta. The more cesarean sections a woman has had, the greater her risk for placenta accreta. In fact, as the incidence of cesarean has risen in the general population, the overall incidence of accreta has likewise increased (King et al., 2015).

Vaginal bleeding is a common symptom of placenta accreta. The amount of vaginal bleeding depends on the level of invasion into the myometrium and detachment. Referral to a specialist is important, as complete detachment from the uterine wall may not be possible and a hysterectomy may be indicated.

CONCLUSION

Effective care of the woman who is pregnant is provided through taking a holistic approach—caring for the maternal–fetal dyad physically and providing emotional care to the mother when necessary. Proactive risk screening will prevent some complications and allow for the prompt management

of others. Clinicians who encounter women who are pregnant can contribute significantly to positive outcomes by making appropriate referrals to maternal–fetal specialists when complications arise.

References

American College of Obstetricians and Gynecologists. (2007, reaffirmed 2014). Management of herpes in pregnancy: Practice Bulletin No. 82. *Obstetrics & Gynecology, 109,* 1489–1498.

American College of Obstetricians and Gynecologists. (2008, reaffirmed 2014). Medical management of ectopic pregnancy: Practice Bulletin No. 94. *Obstetrics & Gynecology, 111*(6), 1479–1485.

American College of Obstetricians and Gynecologists. (2011). Gestational diabetes: Practice Bulletin No. 30. *Obstetrics & Gynecology, 98,* 525–538.

American College of Obstetricians and Gynecologists. (2011, reaffirmed 2013). Prevention of early-onset group B streptococcal disease in newborns: Committee Opinion No. 485. Retrieved from https://www.acog.org/Resources-And-Publications/Committee-Opinions/Committee-on-Obstetric-Practice/Prevention-of-Early-Onset-Group-B-Streptococcal-Disease-in-Newborns

American College of Obstetricians and Gynecologists. (2012, reaffirmed 2014). Management of preterm labor: Practice Bulletin No. 127. *Obstetrics & Gynecology, 119,* 1308–1307.

American College of Obstetricians and Gynecologists. (2013a). Gestational diabetes mellitus: Practice Bulletin No. 137. *Obstetrics & Gynecology, 122*(2), 406–416.

American College of Obstetricians and Gynecologists. (2013b). Executive summary: Hypertension in pregnancy. *Obstetrics & Gynecology, 122*(5), 1122–1131.

American College of Obstetricians and Gynecologists. (2014). Cerclage for the management of cervical insufficiency: Practice Bulletin No. 142. *Obstetrics & Gynecology, 123*(2), 372–379.

American College of Obstetricians and Gynecologists. (2015a). Cytomegalovirus, parvovirus B19, varicella zoster and toxoplasmosis in pregnancy: Practice Bulletin No. 151. *Obstetrics & Gynecology, 125*(6), 1510–1525.

American College of Obstetricians and Gynecologists. (2015b). Preterm labor and birth. Retrieved from http://www.acog.org/Resources-And-Publications/Patient-Education-Pamphlets/Files/Preterm-Labor-and-Birth

Blackburn, S. T. (2013). *Maternal, fetal and neonatal physiology: A clinical perspective* (4th ed.). St. Louis, MO: Saunders Elsevier.

Briggs, G., & Freeman, R. (2015). *Drugs in pregnancy and lactation* (10th ed.). Philadelphia, PA: Wolters Kluwer.

Brucker, M., & King, T. (2015). Pharmacotherapeutics. In T. King, M. Brucker, J. Kriebs, J. Fahey, C. Gegor, & H. Varney (Eds.), *Varney's midwifery* (pp. 127–152). Burlington, MA: Jones & Bartlett Learning.

Centers for Disease Control and Prevention (CDC). (2010). Prevention of perinatal group B streptococcal disease. *Morbidity and Mortality Weekly Report, 59*(RR-10), 1–32.

Centers for Disease Control and Prevention (CDC). (2012a, February). Fifth disease. Retrieved from http://www.cdc.gov/parvovirusb19/index.html

Centers for Disease Control and Prevention (CDC). (2012b). Congenital rubella syndrome. In *Manual for the surveillance of vaccine-preventable diseases.* Retrieved from http://www.cdc.gov/vaccines/pubs/surv-manual/chpt15-crs.html

Centers for Disease Control and Prevention (CDC). (2014a). Group B strep infections in newborns. Retrieved from http://www.cdc.gov/groupbstrep/about/newborns-pregnant.html

Centers for Disease Control and Prevention (CDC). (2014b). Group B strep: What you need to know. Retrieved from http://www.cdc.gov/groupbstrep/about/transmission-risks.html

Centers for Disease Control and Prevention (CDC). (2015a). *Epidemiology and prevention of vaccine-preventable diseases* (13th ed.). Washington, DC: Public Health Foundation.

Centers for Disease Control and Prevention (CDC). (2015b). Sexually transmitted diseases treatment guidelines, 2015. *Morbidity and Mortality Weekly Report, 64*(3), 1–137.

Dijkmans, A. C., de Jong, E. P., Dijkmans, B. A., Lopriore, E., Vossen, A., Waltheer, F. J., & Oepkes, D. (2012). Parvovirus B19 in pregnancy: Prenatal diagnosis and management of fetal complications. *Current Opinions in Obstetrics & Gynecology, 24*(2), 95–101. doi:10.1097/GCO.0b013e3283505a9d

International Association of Diabetes and Pregnancy Study Groups Consensus Panel, Metzger, B. E., Gabbe S. G., Persson B., Buchanan T. A., Catalano P. A., . . . Schmidt, M. I. (2010). International Association of Diabetes and Pregnancy Study Groups recommendations on the diagnosis and classification of hyperglycemia in pregnancy. *Diabetes Care, 33,* 676–682.

King, T., Brucker, M., Kriebs, J., Fahey, J., Gegor, C., & Varney, H. (2015). *Varney's midwifery* (5th ed.). Burlington, MA: Jones & Bartlett Learning.

Marion, L., & Meeks, G. (2012). Ectopic pregnancy: History, incidence, epidemiology and risk factors. *Clinical Obstetrics and Gynecology, 55*(2), 376–386.

Phelan, S., & Holbrook, B. (2013). Umbilical cord prolapse: A plan for an OB emergency. *Contemporary OB/GYN, 58*(9), 28–36.

Schneeberger, C., Kazemier, B., & Geerlings, S. (2014). Asymptomatic bacteriuria and urinary tract infections in special patient groups: Women with diabetes mellitus and pregnant women. *Current Opinion in Infectious Diseases, 27*(1), 108–114.

Stowell, J., Forlin-Passoni, D., & Cannon, M. (2010, May). Congenital cytomegalovirus: An update. *Contemporary Pediatrics,* 38–51.

U.S. National Library of Medicine (NLM). (2015). Rubella. *MEDLINEPlus.* Retrieved from https://www.nlm.nih.gov/medlineplus/ency/article/001574.htm

CHAPTER 32

Postpartum Care

Deborah Karsnitz

The days and months following the birth of a newborn are defined as the postpartum period or puerperium. Traditionally, the puerperium begins after the birth of the fetal membranes and continues throughout 6 to 8 weeks postpartum. Designation of this particular time frame is attributed to the average time necessary for physiologic return to a pre-pregnant state. However, postpartum restoration, both physical and emotional, is influenced by various factors prompting individual differences in this time frame.

The days and months leading up to the birth of a newborn are filled with numerous appointments, planning, well wishes from friends and family, and a variety of physical and emotional changes. Once birth occurs, focus shifts to postpartum recovery, needs of the infant, and return to life after pregnancy.

This chapter briefly reviews the normal physiologic and psychologic changes that occur as the woman's body returns to a pre-pregnant state. Selected postpartum complications are also discussed. To obtain an in-depth understanding of these topics, resources are provided at the end of this chapter.

POSTPARTUM PHYSIOLOGY

Many physiologic changes occur during the postpartum period as organ systems, structures, and hormonal balances return to their pre-pregnant state. The puerperium begins immediately following the delivery of the placenta. Placental separation results in immediate physiologic events that promote maternal hemostasis and initiate restoration to a pre-pregnant state.

Hemostasis

Uterine contractions facilitate a shortening of myometrial fibers, which reduces uterine size and facilitates uterine compression to decrease bleeding. Increased blood volume, which was important during pregnancy, is no longer necessary. While some blood loss occurs during birth, 10% to 15% of blood volume is auto-transfused. In addition, extracellular fluid is mobilized and returned to circulation. Coagulation changes initially increase dramatically, then remain increased for 1 to 2 weeks postpartum. Total blood volume returns to a pre-pregnant state by 1 week postpartum. However, increased venous diameter and decreased blood flow may take as long as 6 weeks to return. For this reason, women have an elevated risk for thromboembolic events during the puerperium. Maternal heart rate remains increased for approximately 1 hour after a woman gives birth before returning to a pre-pregnant rate, while blood pressure can remain elevated for up to 4 days. Cardiac output is elevated after childbirth and remains somewhat elevated for approximately 1 week postpartum.

Uterus

Involution describes the process of the uterus returning to a pre-pregnant state (approximately 100 gm or less). Involution of the uterus occurs through contraction of uterine smooth muscles, autolysis of excess tissue, regeneration of endometrial tissue (resulting

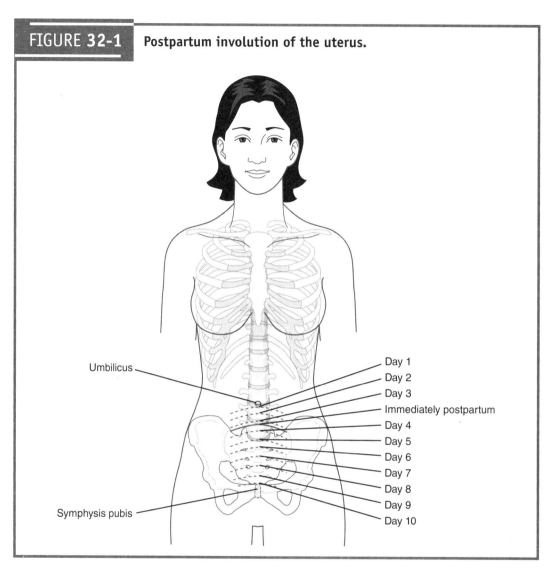

FIGURE 32-1 Postpartum involution of the uterus.

Umbilicus

Symphysis pubis

Day 1
Day 2
Day 3
Immediately postpartum
Day 4
Day 5
Day 6
Day 7
Day 8
Day 9
Day 10

in the shedding of decidual tissue), and regeneration of the placental site, leaving no scar behind. In most cases, the uterus becomes a pelvic organ by 10 to 14 days and is no longer palpable abdominally. The rate of uterine descent is typically 1 cm per day. The process for uterine restoration is usually completed by 6 weeks postpartum. See **Figure 32-1**.

Lochia

Lochia, the term used to denote vaginal discharge post birth, indicates the phases of restoration of the uterus and can vary in duration from 4 to 8 weeks. As the amount of bleeding differs among women, it is important to note that a continuous decrease in lochia amounts over time is an important consideration—stages of lochia do not always occur during specific time frames. Women may experience a transient increase in lochia discharge (7–14 days), referred to as the release of the eschar or sloughing of the placental site. **Table 32-1** identifies the postpartum stages of lochia.

TABLE 32-1	Ranges of Normal Postpartum Lochia		

Lochia Stage	Postpartum Days/Weeks	Lochia Color
Rubra	Days 2–5	Dark red
Serosa	Days 3–10	Lighter red
Alba	Weeks 2–8	White to yellow–white

Data from Azulay Chertok, I. R. (2013). The postpartum period and lactation physiology. In S. T. Blackburn (Ed.), *Maternal, fetal and neonatal physiology: A clinical perspective* (4th ed., pp. 142–162). St. Louis, MO: Saunders Elsevier; Fahey, J. O. (2015). Anatomy and physiology of postpartum. In T. L. King, M. C. Brucker, J. M. Kriebs, J. O. Fahey, C. L. Gegor, & H. Varney (Eds.), *Varney's midwifery* (5th ed., pg. 1101–1110). Burlington, MA: Jones & Bartlett Learning.

Cervix

Following childbirth, the cervix is often soft, edematous, and sometimes bruised. Within several days, however, it begins to return to an altered pre-pregnancy state. By 1 week postpartum, the cervix is further restored, with the external os being approximately 1 cm dilated. The cervical os no longer resembles the nulliparous os (dimple) and now has the appearance of a slit.

Vagina

Following the birth of a newborn, the vagina can appear bruised, edematous, and sometimes lacerated. The vaginal mucosa is smooth, rugae are absent, and tone is decreased. Within 3 to 4 weeks postpartum, the rugae are restored, although tone may remain decreased, improving over time but perhaps not to the same pre-pregnancy tone.

Endocrine System

Expulsion of the placenta signals dramatic hormonal changes as blood levels of estrogen, progesterone, human placental lactogen (hPL), and human chorionic gonadotropin (hCG) all decrease. These immediate changes initiate other systematic changes, including lactogenesis (Azulay Chertok, 2013). Estrogen returns to its pre-pregnant level within 1 to 2 weeks, and progesterone levels return to the pre-pregnant state within 48 hours.

Pituitary

Follicle-stimulating hormone (FSH) and luteinizing hormone (LH) levels remain low for 2 weeks postpartum, with a gradual rise to pre-pregnant levels. Lactation, however, can interfere with this return of LH and FSH to pre-pregnant levels. Subsequently, ovulation and return of menses vary in relation to frequency and duration of breastfeeding. Resumption of ovulation in women who are not breastfeeding usually occurs at some point between 45 and 94 days postpartum (Jackson & Glasier, 2011). Although few women regain fertility by 2 weeks postpartum, contraception counseling should include postpartum hormonal influences, whether a woman is solely breastfeeding and how often, and other influential factors related to return of ovulation and fertility.

Renal System

Postpartum return of bladder tone and reduced dilation of the renal track occur over a 6- to 8-week time frame or longer. Bladder displacement or trauma during labor and childbirth can predispose a woman to urinary tract infections.

Gastrointestinal System

Decrease in progesterone aids in the restoration of muscle tone, relieving reflux and constipation within 2 to 3 days postpartum. However, perineal trauma from childbirth, lack of fluids, or mobility can result in continued constipation.

POSTPARTUM CARE

The postpartum period signifies the end of a pregnancy and the beginning of a new journey. Despite significant physiologic and emotional transitions, following discharge from a hospital the woman is typically not evaluated until 6 weeks postpartum. Yet, during the 6 weeks prior to her first postpartum visit, she goes through physical restoration, role attainment, and formation of new relationships. Women in the United States are rarely given more than 6 weeks of maternity leave, and many do not have designated pay during this time frame. Many women are expected to resume regular activity within a few weeks. Except for selected complications, postpartum research in the United States is limited.

Culture

The postpartum period is rich with cultural influences, beliefs, and traditions that impact restoration, recovery, role transitions, and family dynamics. Cultural diversity should be included in all aspects of health care and should guide assessment, management, and education. Expectations of recovery can differ and should be assessed prior to educating women and their families. Most traditions during the postpartum period influence diet and rest, as well as lactation and newborn care. For example, a traditional Hispanic cultural practice, *la cuarentena*, nurtures a new mother for approximately 40 days (Waugh, 2011), while some Asian cultures observe "doing the month" (Liu, Petrini, & Maloni, 2014). Yet other cultures have expectations that regular activity will resume shortly after childbirth. In many cultures, the new mother is revered, yet considered vulnerable. Traditions are often intended to protect her from current as well as long-term illness. New mothers are encouraged to stay at home, avoid cold or spicy foods, and refrain from sexual activity for a specific period of time or until there is no further bleeding (Waugh, 2011). Family or female support is a central tenet in most cultural practices. As the new mother's needs are met, she is able in turn to focus solely on her newborn.

To improve health care and acknowledge cultural influences and traditions, clinicians should identify the family healthcare decision maker and include this individual in education and planning sessions. Understanding cultural diversity will facilitate a better relationship and a greater likelihood of addressing certain complications. It is important that cultural beliefs and practices be individually assessed. Because many subcultures exist within a larger culture, clinicians must avoid stereotypical assumptions. Women desire respect, attention to their individual needs, and provision of quality care (Small et al., 2014).

POSTPARTUM ASSESSMENT

Because the early postpartum period is exemplified by abrupt and dramatic changes, the woman must be reassured and educated regarding usual occurrences and their variances. Many factors can influence the duration of these changes, which vary depending on length of labor, type of birth, parity, and other circumstances. Once individual needs are met and reassurance provided, women can begin to fully focus on infant care, role adaptations, and eventual return to daily activity.

Adaptation

The process of adapting to a maternal role, whether or not it is the first time, differs for everyone. While some women immediately take on this new role, others find gradual transition more acceptable. Clinicians can help facilitate women's transitions by listening to the birth story, filling in gaps when possible, and helping the family acclimate to a new situation (Mercer, 1985). Many births are different than imagined. Subsequently, the *taking in* phase after childbirth helps the woman process her birth (Rubin, 1961), thereby, allowing the woman to gain an overall understanding of her birth experience. Eventually, a mother will move toward *taking hold* and begin self-recovery, care of the newborn, and attention to family (Rubin, 1961). Many family configurations are possible—single parent, biological parents, nonbiological parents, extended family, and more. For this reason, knowledge of family structure can facilitate meeting individual needs during the transition period.

Bonding, described by Klaus and Kennell (1976) as the early attachment formed during the first encounter between mother and infant, plays a significant role in the long-term emotional bond between mother and child. Nevertheless, studies indicate bonding continues to develop over time and can include other family members as well (Figueiredo, Costa, Pacheco, & Pais, 2009).

Many factors can influence bonding. Maternal bonding can be influenced by type of birth, medical problems, a lack of support, or emotional factors. Additionally, infant temperament or medical conditions can delay infant bonding (Bienfait et al., 2011; Pickler, 2009). Mothers experiencing difficult births, long labors, cesarean birth, or painful postpartum have been noted to delay bonding and subsequent care of the infant (Figueiredo et al., 2009). Furthermore, effects of anesthesia can interfere with infant reaction and subsequent maternal reaction (Figueiredo et al., 2009). In addition, infant cues such as crying, arm waving, and facial expressions impact the extent of bonding (Figueiredo et al., 2009).

Immediately after birth, the release of oxytocin facilitates a peaceful, loving feeling with the woman that can influence the mother's reaction (Galbally, Lewis, Ijzendoorn, & Permezel, 2011). Breastfeeding and various newborn sounds and behaviors also enable oxytocin release (Galbally et al., 2011). Oxytocin can increase euphoria, decrease stress and facilitate attachment (Feldman, Weller, Zagoory-Sharon, & Levine, 2007; Galbally et al., 2011).

Skin-to-Skin Contact (Kangaroo Care)

When possible, skin-to-skin contact (infant to parent or caregiver) should be encouraged and facilitated postpartum. Skin-to-skin contact has been shown to induce a physiologic response in the newborn and is known to promote stabilization of infant breathing, heart rate, and skin temperature (Feldman, 2004); it also influences the duration and frequency of breastfeeding (Moore, Anderson, Bergman, & Dowswell, 2012). Additionally, anxiety is decreased and women report greater confidence when returning home with a newborn when skin-to-skin contact was initiated following childbirth (Moore et al., 2012). Furthermore, newborns are reported to cry less and remain in an alert, calm, or drowsy state for a period of time after skin-to-skin contact is discontinued (Tallandini & Scalembra, 2006). The percentage of healthcare facilities promoting skin-to-skin contact continues to increase in the United States, with 54% (2011) reporting most newborns (90%) receive skin-to-skin contact

after a vaginal birth (Centers for Disease Control and Prevention [CDC], 2013a).

Family

Traditionally, the father's role has been that of the family caretaker, with little involvement in direct infant care. Today, however, fathers are taking a more active role in infant care and, in fact, are often the main caretaker for certain tasks.

Sibling adjustment to a newborn can be influenced by many factors, including family dynamics, culture, personality, gender, or interest. Age is not the significant factor as once reported, nor do first siblings experience behavior regressions or long adjustment periods (Volling, 2012). Familiar lifestyle is altered, however, and there can be periods of behavioral exhibitions such as mimicry of infant behaviors, toileting accidents, or even moments of aggression (Volling, 2012).

Helpful strategies involve family inclusion during prenatal visits, enrollment in sibling classes, sibling involvement during infant care, alone time with siblings, and encouragement of other family members to include siblings while visiting.

POSTPARTUM EXAMINATIONS

Early postpartum assessment focuses on physiological changes associated with return to the pre-pregnant state. Some changes occur immediately after childbirth (first few days to 1 week), whereas others emerge over a longer period of time. Subjective assessment of the postpartum woman includes her general overall feelings, orientation, comfort, sleep, nutrition, and emotions. Objective assessment includes examination of her general appearance, vital signs, neurologic system, heart and lungs, breasts, gastrointestinal system, urinary system, perineal area, anal area, and lower extremities, as well as laboratory analysis.

The initial postpartum examination should include a review of systems as well as teaching components of early postpartum considerations, what to expect, duration of these changes, and when to call a clinician. Postpartum teaching actually begins during prenatal care and continues throughout the puerperium. Postpartum teaching can also occur at various opportunities, such as with a systems review or during an examination. In addition, all women should receive a teaching booklet with clearly printed warning signs (when to call the clinician). **Table 32-2** illustrates common concerns in the early postpartum period.

Later postpartum examinations have similar components, but teaching will be different. Although both 2-week and 6-week examinations are preferable, the 2-week examination has become nonexistent in many practices. Most postpartum complications or concerns occur prior to 6 weeks, however, and delayed assessment can prevent early identification and treatment, thereby increasing the risk of severe illness. Additionally, breastfeeding assessment and support can increase

TABLE 32-2	Common Early Postpartum Concerns			
Condition	**Etiology**	**Duration**	**Management**	**Notes**
Afterbirth pains	Uterine contractions during involution	Immediate to several days	Empty bladder Prone position Breastfeeding Analgesics	Pain increased if second or more births, as well as over-distended uterus (multiple gestation) Breastfeeding may increase cramps initially NSAIDs
Diuresis/ diaphoresis	Physiologic elimination of excess retained water through voiding and perspiration	Usually days 2–5 but may begin as early as 12 hours and last up to 21 days	Keep bladder empty Reassurance Comfort measures	Approximately 3,000 cc/day Frequent showers Wear natural fibers Dress in layers Drink to thirst
Constipation	Slowed motility during labor and birth Decreased intake during labor Elimination during birth	Up to 1 week	Encourage mobility Increase fluids Increase high-fiber foods Mild laxatives/stool softeners	Fear can play a role if the woman experienced a laceration or episiotomy; provider reassurance is helpful Take as directed
Hemorrhoids	Venous distention, common during pregnancy and may be exacerbated during childbirth	Most painful 24–48 hours postpartum but often remain present at varying degrees	Tucks or witch hazel compresses Ice packs Ointments (Preparation H) Anesthetic sprays Warm sitz baths Stool softeners/ suppositories	Prevention by increasing fluids, fiber, mobility

Condition	Etiology	Duration	Management	Notes
Perineal discomfort	Secondary to laceration or episiotomy	Usually 1–3 weeks	Decrease edema Ice packs initially (24 hours) Topical anesthetics Warm sitz baths Kegel exercises Witch hazel compresses Analgesics	Varies according to degree of laceration/episiotomy or if sutures were required Improve circulation
Breast engorgement	Increased vascularity and congestion as milk supply increases	Usually occurs 2–3 days after childbirth and lasts 24–48 hours	Lactating women: Early initiation of breastfeeding Frequent feeding Warmth/heat Mild analgesics Nonlactating women: Support—supportive bra or breast binder Ice packs Analgesics	Encourage immediate breastfeeding Avoid supplementation or pumping if possible Avoid expressing milk Avoid standing in warm showers to increase let-down

Abbreviation: NSAIDs, nonsteroidal anti-inflammatory drugs.
Data from Andrighetti, T. P., & Karsnitz, D. B. (2014). Components of postnatal care. In R. G. Jordan, J. Engstrom, J. Margell, & C. L. Farley (Eds.), *Prenatal and postnatal care: a woman-centered approach* (pp. 423–440). Ames, IA: Wiley-Blackwell; Blackburn, S. T. (2013). *Maternal, fetal and neonatal physiology: A clinical perspective* (4th ed.). St Louis, MO: Saunders Elsevier; Kantrowitz-Gordon, I. (2015). Anatomy and physiology of postpartum. In T. L. King, M. C. Brucker, J. M. Kriebs, J. O. Fahey, C. L. Gegor, & H. Varney (Eds). *Varney's midwifery* (5th ed., pp. 1101–1110). Burlington, MA: Jones & Bartlett Learning.

duration of breastfeeding. **Table 32-3** highlights components of the 2- and 6-week examinations.

Activity

Women should ambulate soon after birth, even if it is simply to get out of bed to void. In fact, encouragement of increased fluid intake and the need to keep the bladder empty can facilitate early ambulation. Fatigue is common, is individualized, and can be increased after a long labor. The sooner activity increases, the sooner energy and strength will return and opportunities for thromboembolism will decrease. Women recovering from a cesarean section are encouraged to ambulate and can adjust activity as needed (American College of Obstetricians and Gynecologists, 2015a).

Clinicians should encourage postpartum exercise in a modified form soon after a vaginal birth. Walking is a great exercise that can improve mood as well as increase oxygen consumption and circulation. Women can gauge uterine healing by lochia flow and adapt exercise or return to activity as needed. Too much activity can increase bleeding, but with rest, this aspect of healing should quickly return to normal.

Abdominal exercises will aid the restoration of abdominal muscle tone and can begin immediately after a vaginal birth. Women are encouraged to begin slowly and increase exercising abdominal muscles according to their comfort level and healing. Initial abdominal exercise involves lying flat with knees bent while raising the head slowly. As healing progresses, repetitions can increase and abdominal crunches can be added (American College of Obstetricians and Gynecologists, 2015a).

Kegel exercises (strengthening vaginal musculature) can begin immediately after a vaginal birth.

TABLE 32-3   Postpartum Assessment

Initial Postpartum Examination	Subjective	Objective	Unusual Findings	Teaching
General	Well-being, emotions Ambulation Nutrition/fluids Rest Comfort Infant feeding Review birth story	Appearance weight	Discomfort, sadness Sadness Unable to ambulate No appetite Unable to rest	Ambulate often Drink when thirsty Sleep when infant sleeps Analgesics Infant feeding Formula: 2–3 hours Discuss birth experience
Vital signs	Breathing Shortness of breath	BP, temperature, pulse, respirations	BP > 140/90 mm Hg BP < 85/60 mm Hg Temperature > 38°C Pulse >100 bpm	Signs and symptoms of infection
Neurologic	Orientation to time and place	Alert, oriented	Excessive drowsiness Headaches	Headache Analgesic Report blurred or double vision
Cardiovascular	Chest pain or increased heart rate	Regular rate and rhythm	Noted chest pain Irregular rate and rhythm/ tachycardia	Report shortness of breath, chest pain
Pulmonary	Breathing	Lungs clear	Shortness of breath	Report shortness of breath

	Assessment	Normal	Abnormal	Intervention
Breasts	Pain, tenderness Milk production/colostrum, breastfeeding frequency and duration Nipple tenderness	Soft: days 1–2 Fullness: days 3–4 Nipples: intact, erect	Engorgement Nipples: cracked, bleeding Nipples: inverted/flat	Frequent breastfeeding Proper latch Binder or support if not breastfeeding Analgesia
Genitourinary	Voiding amounts Frequency Pain or inability to void	Bladder nondistended No CVAT	Pain with urination Frequency with inability to void Positive CVAT Bladder distention	Increased voiding noted for 3–5 days postpartum Inability to void can be due to perineal edema Increase fluids
Gastrointestinal	Abdominal pain or tenderness Bowel movement	Abdomen nontender Bowel sounds present	Abdominal tenderness Lack of bowel sounds Constipation/lack of flatulence Nausea or vomiting	Stool softeners Ambulation Increase fiber Increase fluids
Uterus	Cramping, pain Bleeding amount/color	Size: involution as expected Firm without tenderness Lochia	Size greater than expected Soft, boggy Lochia: amount increased, clots malodorous	Decreased activity Keep bladder empty Lie prone Heat pad
Perineum	Pain or tenderness	Intact	Erythema, edema	Ice or warm soaks, witch hazel Analgesics
Lower extremities	Able to ambulate Muscle soreness	Reflexes Some edema	Pain, erythema, or edema noted: generalized or local	Ambulate
Anus	Pain or tenderness, bleeding with bowel movement	Hemorrhoids	Hemorrhoids noted, edematous, bruised or bleeding	Hemorrhoid cream, tucks Stool softeners

(continues)

TABLE 32-3   Postpartum Assessment (continued)

2- or 6-Week Examination

Examination	Subjective	Objective	Unusual Findings	Teaching
General	Well-being Mood: EPDS Activity Nutrition/fluids Rest Family adaptation Infant feeding Lochia Voiding/stooling Sexuality	Appearance score < 10	Signs and symptoms of postpartum depression or anxiety EPDS score ≥ 10 Decreased activity Decreased appetite Unable to rest Breastfeeding concerns Increased bleeding Constipation	Discuss postpartum depression, anxiety Sleep when infant sleeps Family roles Infant feeding Stages of lochia Sexuality/contraception
Vital signs	Breathing	Weight BP, temperature, pulse, respirations	BP > 140/90 mm Hg BP < 85/60 mm Hg Temperature > 38°C Pulse > 100 bpm	Signs and symptoms of infection
Neurologic	Orientation to time and place	Alert, oriented	Headaches	Review tension headaches, analgesics
Cardiovascular	Palpitations	Regular rate and rhythm	Irregular rate and rhythm/tachycardia	
Pulmonary	Breathing	Lungs clear	Shortness of breath	
Breasts	Lactation Nipple tenderness Breast infection	Soft (depending on last breastfeed) Nipples: intact, erect	Nipples: cracked, redness, bleeding Nipple *Candida* Mastitis	Review breastfeeding schedule, signs and symptoms of mastitis or nipple *Candida*, pumping, and return to work

Abdomen/gastrointestinal	Pain or tenderness Nausea or vomiting Bowel movement	Soft Diastasis recti Bowel sounds	Herniation Abdominal tenderness No bowel sounds Constipation	Abdominal exercises Stool softeners Fiber Fluids
Genitourinary	Voiding amounts/frequency	Bladder nondistended No CVAT	Pain with urination Frequency with inability to void Positive CVAT Bladder distention	Signs and symptoms of urinary tract infection
Uterus	Lochia cessation Occurrence of menses since birth	Uterus not palpated	Palpation of uterus Lochia still present	Activity level Contraception
Perineum	No pain or tenderness at laceration/episiotomy site	Intact	Erythema, edema	
Vagina (6 weeks)	No discharge	Pink		
Cervix		Pink, firm		
Sexuality	Resumption of sexual intercourse			Sexuality
Lower extremities	Pain, tenderness, edema	No edema or redness	Pain, erythema, or edema noted: generalized or local	Ambulate Signs and symptoms of thrombophlebitis
Anus	Pain or tenderness, bleeding with bowel movement	Hemorrhoids	Hemorrhoids noted; edematous, bruised or bleeding	Hemorrhoid cream, tucks Stool softeners Fiber Fluids

Abbreviations: BP, blood pressure; CVAT, costovertebral angle tenderness; EPDS, Edinburgh Postnatal Depression Scale.
Republished with permission of Wiley from Andrighetti, T. P., & Karsnitz, D. B. (2014). Components of postnatal care. In R. G. Jordan, J. Engstrom, J. Margell, & C. L. Farley (Eds.), *Prenatal and postnatal care: A woman-centered approach* (pp. 423–440). Ames, IA: Wiley-Blackwell. Permission conveyed through Copyright Clearance Center, Inc.; Wambach, K., & Riordan, J. (Eds.). (2016). *Breastfeeding and human lactation* (5th ed.). Burlington, MA: Jones & Bartlett Learning.

This particular exercise not only strengthens and tightens vaginal tone, but also increases urinary tone and circulation to the perineal area, thereby promoting healing (Kocaoz, Eroglu, & Sivashoglu, 2013).

Exercise capability differs among individuals and can depend on the prior level of proficiency. However, all women should be encouraged to begin exercise shortly after giving birth. It is important to teach warning signs related to exercise, and to encourage women to report increased bleeding, change in color of lochia, pain, shortness of breath, leg pain, or dizziness that persists. If breastfeeding, women may choose to breastfeed prior to exercise for comfort measures. In addition, keeping hydrated is important.

Sexuality

Traditionally, women were told to not resume intercourse until the 6-week postpartum examination. However, there is no evidence to support this instruction, which is most likely based on uterine healing. Many couples resume sexual intercourse by 1 month and most by 2 months postpartum (Kennedy & Trussell, 2011). Resuming intimacy is a personal choice and associated with circumstances related to the birth, recovery, emotional readiness (both partners), and physiologic comfort. Additionally, numerous factors can interfere with or delay the resumption of intercourse, such as fatigue, vaginal bleeding, perineal discomfort, decreased lubrication, diminished desire, leaking breasts, body image, and fear of subsequent pregnancy. Furthermore, resumption of intimacy may be based on perception of partner's desire as well (Hipp, Kane Low, & van Anders, 2012). Clinicians can help alleviate anxiety by discussing comfort measures, birth control, and other forms of intimacy. Women should be supported in their choice and encouraged to resume intercourse when they are ready, and they should recognize that time frames will vary.

Contraception

Contraceptive choices for postpartum women require careful consideration and should be discussed at various times throughout pregnancy and postpartum. Discussion of different options will give women the opportunity to consider which choices best fit their lifestyle and circumstances.

Nonhormonal methods such as abstinence, withdrawal, condoms, or other barrier methods can be used earlier in the postpartum period in both women who are breastfeeding and not breastfeeding. Combined oral contraceptives and other combined methods are contraindicated until 21 days postpartum due to increased risk of venous thromboembolism (Hatcher et al., 2011). Women with risk factors for venous thromboembolism (VTE) should be further evaluated if they wish to use hormonal contraceptives. Copper intrauterine devices can be inserted immediately postpartum (within 10 minutes of birth) or after 4 weeks postpartum. Contraceptive options (type, efficacy, ease of use, lifestyle needs) will vary according to numerous factors, and are discussed in greater depth elsewhere in this text.

Women who are breastfeeding frequently, without supplementation and without occurrence of menses after childbirth, experience a natural form of contraception, known as lactation amenorrhea. The Lactation Amenorrhea Method (LAM) of contraception is 98% effective for the first 6 months postpartum (Kennedy & Trussell, 2011). Contraceptive options (type, efficacy, ease of use, lifestyle needs) will vary according to numerous factors. (See Chapter 11 for further discussion.)

Hormonal contraception while breastfeeding remains controversial. The World Health Organization (WHO, 2010) recommends that women who choose to breastfeed do not use hormonal methods containing estrogen during the first 6 weeks (contraindicated) and up to 6 months (relative contraindication) postpartum. Other sources disagree, suggesting that although there is some risk, not enough research has been conducted to support strong restrictions. The CDC (2010) recommends restriction of use of hormonal methods only during the first month postpartum. Although past recommendations suggested initiation of progestin-only contraceptives after 4 to 6 weeks postpartum, there have been no reports to indicate adverse effects on lactation or newborn health. The CDC (2010) supports initiation of such contraception during the first month postpartum, as the benefits outweigh the risks.

Breastfeeding

The means used to feed their infant can be a difficult decision for some women. Consideration of this issue should begin early during the prenatal period, with discussion continuing until the birth of the newborn and in the early postpartum period as needed. Evidence continues to showcase the benefits of breastfeeding for both mother and newborn. The U.S. Department of Health and Human Services (DHHS) has promoted breastfeeding as a *Healthy People* initiative, setting goals to improve health care. The *Healthy People* goals for 2020 include increased breastfeeding initiation and duration rates (DHHS, 2010). Furthermore, the American Academy of Pediatrics (AAP, 2012) supports breastfeeding as the newborn feeding method of choice and recommends exclusive breastfeeding for at least 6 months. The AAP further recommends continued breastfeeding with introduction of other foods for up to 1 year or more.

Breastfeeding initiation rates have increased dramatically over the past 30 years: from 26.5% (1970) to 77% (2009) (CDC, 2013b; DHHS, 2010). In addition, breastfeeding continuation at 6 months has increased from 35% (2000) to 49% (2010), and breastfeeding at 1 year has increased from 16% (2000) to 27% (2010) (CDC, 2013b). WHO and UNICEF (2009) recommend skin-to-skin contact for at least 1 hour after birth to facilitate initiation of breastfeeding.

The breast prepares for lactation throughout pregnancy, completing the task once the newborn begins to suckle. Hormones influence breast growth and development early in pregnancy (lactogenesis I), and women can begin secreting colostrum between 12 to 16 hours after childbirth. Lactogenesis II (milk production) begins following the delivery of the placenta, with subsequent decreases in progesterone and increases in prolactin being observed. Women usually experience fullness in their breasts during this time (2–3 days postpartum) and colostrum can be expressed. Arrival of milk usually occurs between 32 and 96 hours postpartum.

Breastfeeding should be initiated as soon as possible following the birth of a newborn. An earlier introduction of the newborn to breastfeeding will increase the likelihood of production of milk. Women report "feeling" a *let-down* reflex (flow of milk), which occurs when the woman breastfeeds, holds, cuddles, or sometimes just thinks about the newborn. The let-down or milk ejection reflex occurs when oxytocin is released from the posterior pituitary gland, causing contraction of the myoepithelial cells and transport of the milk to the nipple. Prolactin levels increase with suckling and maintain lactation.

Correct latch and suck are very important for nipple integrity as well as continued nutritional intake. Newborns should be assessed for proper latch and swallowing to ensure they are getting milk. Women (especially during the early postpartum) find supporting the breast assists with latch. The "C" hold (the woman's thumb placed above the areola and her index finger below the areola) assists the mother during attempts at latch and is helpful while learning to breastfeed. It is important to remind the mother to take precautions to not compress the nipple.

Positioning

Comfort and proper positioning of the newborn and the mother contribute to successful breastfeeding. Encourage the mother to choose a comfortable position using pillows or rolled blankets for support. Many different positions can facilitate effective breastfeeding (**Table 32-4**). Teaching all positions allows the mother to choose which works best in different situations.

The *cradle* position (the most common position) involves the mother holding the infant in her arms with the baby facing the mother (stomach to stomach). The infant's head is higher than the hips and the infant's nose is aligned with the mother's nipple, with chin placement below the nipple.

The *cross-cradle* position is similar to the cradle position, but the infant is held in the mother's opposite arm, with her hand holding the infant's head. This position is ideal for early breastfeeding when a newborn needs better head control.

The *clutch* or "football" position allows the mother to use a pillow at her side to support the infant. The infant is placed on the pillow lying somewhat on the side, facing the mother's breast and tilted toward the breast. This position is excellent for a woman post-cesarean section and also allows for infant better head control.

The *lying down* position allows the mother to lie on her side and also place the infant on her side, facing the mother. A rolled blanket can help support the infant's back. This position is also helpful if a woman has experienced a cesarean section.

TABLE 32-4 Common Body Positions for Breastfeeding

Position	Description	Advantages	Illustration
Cradle or Madonna position	The infant is side-lying, facing the mother, with the side of the head and body resting on the mother's forearm of the arm next to the breast to be used.	This is the most commonly used nursing position and tends to feel most natural for the mother. However, it offers the least amount of control over the infant's head.	
Cross-cradle posture	The infant is side-lying, facing the mother, with the side resting on the mother's forearm of the arm on the opposite side of the breast being used.	This posture is considered especially useful for the mother of a newborn or preterm infant. It offers greater control over the infant's head	
Football or clutch	A sitting position in which the infant lies on her or his back, curled between the side of the mother's chest and her arm. The infant's upper body is supported by the mother's forearm. The mother's hand supports the infant's neck and shoulders. The infant's hips are flexed up along the chair back or other surface that the mother is leaning against.	This position is helpful for women post cesarean section and those who have large pendulous breasts or are nursing multiple infants.	

Semi-reclining	The mother leans back and the infant lies against her body, in chest-to-chest contact, usually prone.	This is the most comfortable position for women recovering from a cesarean section, those who have large pendulous breasts, and those who choose to co-sleep with their infants.
Side-lying	The mother lies on her side. The infant is side-lying, chest to chest with the mother. The mother's arm closest to the mattress supports the infant's back.	This position is helpful for women who have had a cesarean section or have large or pendulous breasts.
Australian	The mother is "down-under," lying on her back, with the infant supported on her chest.	This posture allows the infant to be in maximal control of the feeding and is especially valuable when the milk flow is faster than the infant can handle.

Modified from International Lactation Consultant Association; Mannel, R., Martens, P. J., Walker, M. (Eds.). (2013). *Core curriculum for lactation consultant practice* (3rd ed.). Burlington, MA: Jones & Bartlett Learning.

Latch

Once the mother is comfortable and has chosen a position, encourage her to bring the infant to her breast rather than bring her breast to the infant. The infant's nose should be aligned with her nipple as she supports the breast and allows the infant to latch. Proper latch is demonstrated by the infant securing a large part of the areola, rather than just nipple, as well as visualizing and hearing the infant swallow. The infant's lips should flare outward and a seal should be formed around the breast. If smacking or clicking sounds are heard, reposition the latch. To break the seal (if repositioning is needed), the mother should place her index finger in the corner of the infant's mouth and apply mild downward pressure.

Table 32-5 identifies some items to be assessed regarding the infant's breastfeeding behavior.

Milk Supply

Women choosing breastfeeding need education and support. Breast assessment is crucial to determine if a woman will need further assistance if she chooses to breastfeed. Whether the nipples are erect, flat, or inverted can impact the type of breastfeeding support needed. Additionally, common misconceptions must be addressed. Breast size has no impact on breastfeeding, but some other factors can delay milk production (lactogenesis II). Specifically, lactogenesis can be affected by delayed initiation of breastfeeding, ineffective suckling, cesarean birth, increased stress, medical conditions, and obesity (Nommsen-Rivers, Chantry, Peerson, Cohen, & Dewey, 2010), which in turn can impact successful continuation of breastfeeding (Brownell, Howard, Lawrence, & Dozier, 2012).

Whereas some women experience decreased milk production, other women have an overabundance of milk, which can lead to inadequate emptying or milk stasis. The let-down reflex in such a case can overwhelm the infant's ability to swallow or take in breastmilk effectively. The infant will often make choking sounds, attempt to turn away, or detach from the breast. Also, the mother will have increased leaking, which can interfere with other activities. Evaluation includes newborn assessment for problems associated with swallowing (gastroesophageal reflux). Teaching includes position change, pumping or expression of milk to eliminate milk stasis, and use of one breast only for several feedings. If problems continue after a few weeks, consideration of pharmacologic assistance can be considered.

Galactagogues

There is a lack of evidence promoting effectiveness of specific pharmacologic or herbal remedies

---

TABLE 32-5   **Breastfeeding Assessment of the Newborn**

Assessment	Expected Findings	Provider Notes
Rooting	Infant turns face toward breast	Cue that infant is ready to feed Do not wait until infant cries
Latch	Jaw angled at 120–160°	Allows for better grasp of areola
	Tongue extends past lower gum	Better milk flow
	Audible or visible swallow	Indicates infant getting milk (should not hear smacking or clicking sound)
	Tight seal (tongue under breast, lips flanged)	Seal needs to be broken by placement of mother's index finger

as treatments for decreased milk supply, although some common galactagogues have been used with some success. Pharmaceuticals such as metoclopramide (Reglan) and domperidone (Motilium) have been used to increase milk supply. However, side effects include elevation of the QT segment on EKG with domperidone use (Osadchy, Moretti, & Koren, 2012) and tardive dyskinesia with metoclopramide (Betzold, 2004), prompting addition of a "black box" warning to this drug's label. Additionally, herbal remedies, such as fenugreek, may be used to increase milk supply and can be taken as capsules or tea (Betzold, 2004).

BREASTFEEDING COMPLICATIONS

Mastitis

Lactation mastitis—inflammation in an area of the breast—most commonly occurs during breastfeeding within several weeks to 6 months (Amir, Forster, Lumley, & McLachlan, 2007). Women report unilateral localized erythema, breast tenderness, and warmth at the site, and can present with accompanying fever and flu-like symptoms. Mastitis is usually short-lived and should not interfere with breastfeeding. Breastfeeding continuation is encouraged and will usually aid recovery.

Mastitis can be infective or noninfective depending on the mode of occurrence. Plugged ducts or milk stasis is most often related to noninfective mastitis. Infective mastitis can occur secondary to entry of bacteria from nipple trauma/cracking, stress and fatigue, milk stasis, or sometimes without explanation. Bacteria causing this condition include *Staphylococcus aureus* (coagulase-negative *Staphylococcus* is most common), *Escherichia coli*, *Enterobacteriaceae*, *Mycobacterium tuberculosis*, and *Candida albicans*. Infective mastitis can occasionally occur in both breasts.

The incidence of mastitis ranges from 4% to 27% (Amir et al., 2007). Risk factors include stress and fatigue, cracked or fissured nipples, plugged ducts, milk stasis/engorgement, over-supply of milk, breast trauma or restriction (too-tight bra), poor nutrition, and vigorous exercise. Risk increases with a prior history of mastitis (Wambach, 2016). Recent studies have shown that milk cultures identify bacteria normally present on the skin

as causative agents. Symptoms between groups comparing normal bacteria and potential pathogenic bacteria did not result in major differences in symptoms or duration. Pathogenic bacteria have been found to be related to sore nipples prior to mastitis (Osterman & Rahm, 2000).

Treatment includes continuation of breastfeeding, increased rest, fluids, nutrition, application of moist heat, anti-inflammatory medications, and possible use of antibiotics. Standard treatment for lactation mastitis includes a penicillinase-resistant penicillin or cephalosporin (which eradicates *S. aureus*) for 10 to 14 days. Symptoms should resolve by 48 hours; if they do not, consider the possibility of methicillin-resistant *S. aureus* (MRSA) infection and obtain a milk culture (Amir, Trupin, & Kvist, 2014).

Women with mastitis should be encouraged to empty the breasts and maintain frequency of feedings. Altering the feeding schedule can increase the risk of milk stasis and subsequent mastitis. Likewise, proper latch will ensure nipple integrity.

Breast Abscess

Untreated mastitis or infection that does not respond to antibiotic therapy can result in a breast abscess. An abscess is a collection of pus (boil-like) that will most likely need to be incised and drained. Culture will determine the appropriate antibiotic treatment.

When abscess is present, breastfeeding is encouraged, albeit usually on the unaffected breast. If treatment with drains or position of the abscess does not interfere with latch, infants can breastfeed on the affected breast. Additionally, expression or pumping of milk may be necessary (Wright, 2015).

Nipple Candidiasis

Candidiasis, commonly referred to as thrush, is caused by *Candida albicans*, a fungus that thrives in a warm, moist environment such as the infant's mouth or within the mother's nipples. Infant exposure can occur during vaginal birth and be subsequently transmitted to the mother's nipples while breastfeeding. Nipple candidiasis occurs bilaterally and usually presents with sudden onset. Women describe deep red coloration, burning, and shooting or stabbing pain in both nipples that occurs during and after breastfeeding (Barrett, Heller, Stone, & Murase, 2013). Women or infants receiving antibiotic treatment are at risk for acquiring a yeast infection. As the infection can pass between mother and infant, both should be treated to eradicate the fungal infection (Wright, 2015).

The most common treatment for nipple candidiasis is application of Nystatin (painted on the infant's tongue and in the oral cavity) after each breastfeeding. Fluconazole (Diflucan) is prescribed for both mother and infant if infection persists (Wright, 2015). Infants should receive treatment regardless of visualized thrush. Mothers should also be assessed for a vaginal yeast infection and subsequently treated (Wambach, 2016). For a more in-depth discussion of breastfeeding, see the resources at the end of this chapter.

SELECTED POSTPARTUM COMPLICATIONS

Postpartum recovery is typically uneventful. Indeed, with proper nutrition, rest, and support, most women can return to daily activity without complication. However, occasionally complications do occur, for which recovery necessitates medical management.

Puerperal Infection

The Joint Committee on Maternal Welfare defines puerperal morbidity as a temperature greater than 38° C (100.4°F) that occurs on any 2 days (after the first 24 hours) within the first 10 days postpartum (The Joint Commission, 2010). Although commonly defined as an infection of the genital tract following childbirth, miscarriage, or termination, puerperal infections can occur secondary to dehydration, urinary or respiratory infections, and mastitis. Additionally, puerperal morbidity may be caused by cardiovascular or thromboembolic events, mood and anxiety disorders, or other medical conditions.

Historically, the "lethal triad"—hemorrhage, infection, and blood pressure—was the major cause of morbidity and mortality in postpartum women (King, 2012). Infection after childbirth had significant consequences prior to the introduction of hand washing and eventually antibiotics (Carr, 2000). Despite a generally decreased trend in puerperal genital tract infection in the 20th century, infection remains a significant cause (11%) of pregnancy-related morbidity and mortality (Berg, Callaghan, Syverson, & Henderson, 2010). Recent trends indicate an increase in puerperal morbidity and mortality from complications related to medical conditions within the first year after childbirth (King, 2012). In the past decade, the incidence of puerperal sepsis has increased in the United States while decreasing in many other countries (Bick, Beake, & Pellowe, 2011). Although the reason for this increase might potentially be better data recording, it may also be related to increased obesity, surgical birth, chronic health problems, or access to care (Hankins et al., 2012; King, 2012).

Most infections following a vaginal birth are polymicrobial and occur at the placental site, laceration, or episiotomy. Abdominal wound infections occur after rupture of membranes and secondary to ascent of colonized bacteria. Common pathogens include those existing normally in the genital tract or bowel and others found on the skin surface, nasopharynx, or environment. Bacteria most often associated with puerperal infection include the following:

- Aerobes:
  - Gram-positive cocci—group A, B, and D streptococci; *Enterococcus, Staphylococcus aureus, Staphylococcus epidermis*
  - Gram-negative bacteria: *Escherichia coli, Klebsiella, Proteus* species
  - Gram-variable species: *Gardnerella vaginalis*
- Anaerobes:
  - Cocci: *Peptostreptococcus* and *Peptococcus* species
  - Others: *Clostridium, Bacteroides,* and *Fusobacterium* species, as well as *Mobiluncus* species
- Others: *Mycoplasma* and *Chlamydia* species and *Neisseria gonorrhoeae* (Cunningham et al., 2014)

Cesarean section is the most common risk factor for puerperal infection (Baxter, Berghella, Mackeen, Ohly, & Weed, 2011). Most postpartum infections occur within the first few weeks following childbirth, though women are often not scheduled to return for a follow-up visit until 6 to 8 weeks. For this reason, some infections go unreported or women present to an emergency room for diagnosis and treatment (Maharaj, 2007). A study in Denmark (n = 1,871 women) revealed that only 66% of women reported postpartum symptoms to their clinician and 9% to a healthcare facility (Ahnfeldt-Mollerup, Petersen, Kragstrup, Christensen, & Sorensen, 2012).

Puerperal Fever

Puerperal fever is defined as a temperature greater than 38°C (100.4°F) that occurs on any 2 days (after the first 24 hours) within the first 10 days postpartum (The Joint Commission, 2010). Fever can occur from factors such as dehydration, engorgement, thrombophlebitis, or other infections unrelated to the genital tract. A fever spiking to 39°C (102.2° F), abruptly occurring within 24 hours after cesarean birth, may indicate group B *Streptococcus* infection (Cunningham et al., 2014).

Uterine Infection

Uterine infection (metritis) can occur in the endometrium (endometritis), myometrium (myometritis), and parametrium (endoparametritis) and is one of the more common infections diagnosed postpartum. Metritis occurs in 1% to 2% of women following vaginal birth, but this incidence rises dramatically (27%) following cesarean birth (Sweet & Gibbs, 2009). The American College of Obstetricians and Gynecologists recommends a single dose of prophylactic antibiotics within 60 minutes prior to a cesarean birth (American College of Obstetricians and Gynecologists, 2011, reaffirmed 2014). Single-dose therapy has dramatically decreased the risk for uterine infection—by as much as 75% (Smaill & Gyte, 2010). Risk factors for uterine infection include cesarean birth, long labor, frequent vaginal examinations, prolonged rupture of membranes, internal uterine or fetal monitoring, instrumental birth, tissue trauma, traumatic birth, uterine exploration, postpartum hemorrhage, retained placental fragments, common medical conditions, obesity, and low socioeconomic status.

Symptoms include persistent elevated temperature of 38°C to 39°C (100.4–102.2°F) or higher depending on the type of infection, along with chills, malaise, tachycardia, uterine tenderness, pelvic pain on examination, scanty, odorless or malodorous, seropurulent lochia, and uterine subinvolution. Onset and severity can occur in the early postpartum period (24 hours) to 2 to 3 weeks postpartum or longer depending on the type of causative organism.

Management, in addition to physical examination, includes laboratory analysis consisting of urine and blood cultures, urinalysis, and a complete blood count. The white blood cell count can exceed 20,000 cells/mm^3. If lung infection is suspected, a chest x-ray should be included in the diagnostic process.

Broad-spectrum antimicrobial therapy is the treatment of choice for a uterine infection. Mild uterine infection following a vaginal birth *only* can be treated with oral antibiotics, such as ampicillin (Principen) and gentamycin (Garamycin). Women with moderate to severe uterine infections will be hospitalized for intravenous therapy. Nearly 90% of women respond to treatment within 48 to 72 hours and may be discharged home after being afebrile for at least 24 hours (Cunningham et al., 2014). If left untreated, uterine infection can result in salpingitis, peritonitis, septic pelvic thrombophlebitis, or necrotizing fasciitis.

The incidence of uterine infection would decrease dramatically with a reduction in the number of cesarean births, in addition to improved obstetric management (prenatal infection surveillance and treatment), limiting the number of vaginal examinations during labor, and appropriate use of procedures such as internal monitoring, induction, episiotomy, rupture of membranes, and uterine manipulation.

Wound Infection

Puerperal wound infections can occur at either the site of a laceration or episiotomy (vaginal birth) or abdominal incision (post cesarean birth). Women often report increased pain at the wound site with or without accompanying fever. Wound infections increase the likelihood of hospitalization and, like other puerperal infections, can interrupt or cause discontinuation of breastfeeding (Ahnfeldt-Mollerup et al., 2012).

Incidence of wound infection varies widely, from 0.8% to 10% for perineal infections (Maharaj, 2007) and from 2% to 16% for abdominal infections. These variations in estimates are attributed to lack of definition, underreporting, change of clinician or healthcare facility, and poor data collection (Ahnfeldt-Mollerup et al., 2012). Organisms frequently associated with wound infection include *S. aureus*, *Streptococcus*, and both aerobic and anaerobic bacilli.

Risk factors for wound infection are similar to those for uterine infection. Women present with localized pain and erythema and edema present at the wound edges. At times, exudate and wound dehiscence may occur. Fever is often low grade, approximately 38.3°C (101°F). Dysuria can ensue secondary to perineal infection.

Wound infection management depends on location and severity. Management for an infection occurring in a laceration or episiotomy can include suture removal, opening, debridement, and cleansing. Administration of a broad-spectrum antibiotic is indicated. Most perineal wounds do not need further repair unless third- or fourth-degree extension occurs. Abdominal wound infections require similar management with inclusion of antibiotics and occasionally drainage. If dehiscence occurs in an abdominal wound, repair may be necessary. Abdominal wound management can include daily debridement and packing depending on the severity of infection (Cunningham et al., 2014).

Urinary Tract Infection

Urinary tract infection (UTI) is a common cause of puerperal morbidity (Maharaj, 2007). Urinary stasis, which may result from multiple factors (e.g., decreased bladder tone, increased bladder volume, use of epidural anesthesia, inability to empty completely, pain or edema from perineal trauma), increases the likelihood of infection. Women receiving catheterization are also at increased risk for UTI. Common pathogens include *Escherichia coli* (early postpartum, 90%), *Proteus mirabilis*, and *Klebsiella pneumoniae* (Cunningham et al., 2014). Bacteria that ascend into the kidney will result in pyelonephritis.

Symptoms of UTI include frequency, urgency, low abdominal pain, and dysuria, whereas symptoms of pyelonephritis include a low-grade fever with spikes, flank pain, costovertebral angle tenderness (CVAT), nausea, and vomiting. Diagnosis is made by urine culture.

Uterine Subinvolution

Subinvolution occurs when uterine restoration is interrupted and unable to return (involute) to pre-pregnant size during the standard postpartum time frame. Typically, by 2 weeks postpartum the uterus should not be able to be palpated abdominally and should be located below the symphysis pubis. Subinvolution can be the result of inhibition of the myometrial fibers to contract effectively. Other causative factors may include retained placental fragments, infection, or myomata. Additionally, increased activity can slow uterine restoration. Placental site subinvolution occurs when the uteroplacental arteries do not close properly, filling with thrombi and delaying regeneration of the placental site. This condition has been identified as later causing hemorrhage, usually around 2 weeks postpartum (Petrovitch, Jeffrey, & Heerema-McKenney, 2009).

Symptoms often include reports of increased, continued bleeding as well as cessation and then return of bleeding. Subinvolution is noted on examination with presentation of a boggy, larger-than-expected uterus for that time period. If subinvolution occurs secondary to infection, along with increased size, uterine tenderness and malodorous lochia are usually present.

Management depends on the presenting symptoms. Increased or persistent bleeding requires ultrasound to assess for retained placental fragments. Ultrasound may not always show fragments, however, so occasionally uterine exploration is performed. If infection is suspected, treatment with broad-spectrum antibiotics is indicated. When there are no signs of placental fragments or infection, treatment with methyl-ergonovine (Methergine) or ergonovine (Ergotrate) 0.2 mg orally, every 6 hours for 24 to 48 hours, is indicated. Women are encouraged to rest, increase fluids and nutrients, and return for follow-up in 2 weeks.

Secondary (Delayed) Postpartum Hemorrhage

Postpartum hemorrhage remains a leading cause of maternal morbidity and mortality despite advances in its management and reductions in its incidence during the 20th century (Berg et al., 2010; Kramer et al., 2013). Secondary postpartum hemorrhage is defined by increased bleeding occurring after the first 24 hours following childbirth and until 12 weeks postpartum (American College of Obstetricians and Gynecologists, 2006, reaffirmed 2013). Secondary postpartum hemorrhage occurs in approximately 1% of women, usually within the first 2 weeks (80%) postpartum (American College of Obstetricians and Gynecologists, 2006, reaffirmed 2013).

Risk factors for secondary postpartum hemorrhage are similar to those for immediate postpartum hemorrhage, including uterine atony, retained placental fragments, and infection. However, most cases occur secondary to subinvolution of the placental site (Cunningham et al., 2014). Additionally, women who present with increased bleeding during the first week postpartum (days 2–5) should be evaluated for von Willebrand's disease (vWD) (Pacheco et al., 2010). This disease, which occurs when there is a deficiency of von Willebrand's factor (a protein necessary for platelet adherence), affects 1% to 2% of women. Levels of von Willebrand's factor increase during pregnancy, but then decrease postpartum, usually by 48 hours after childbirth (Pacheco et al., 2010).

Signs and symptoms of secondary postpartum hemorrhage include increased or persistent heavy bleeding, cessation of bleeding followed by its sudden return, and possibly signs and symptoms of hypovolemia or shock. A sudden, transient episode of increased bleeding, usually 7 to 10 days postpartum, is related to sloughing of the eschar (placental site) and not considered a postpartum hemorrhage.

Management of secondary postpartum hemorrhage includes ultrasound for detection of placental fragments (suction and evacuation if needed) and treatment with uterotonics or curettage. Uterotonics such as ergonovine, methylergonovine, oxytocin, or a prostaglandin analogue are usually sufficient. Curettage is less likely to be performed due to the increased risk for perforation attributable to the soft nature of the puerperal uterine wall.

Puerperal Hematoma

Genital tract hematoma occurs when extravasated blood accumulates as a result of vascular trauma during birth or the birth procedure. Hematoma formation can also occur spontaneously. Puerperal hematoma occurs in approximately 1 in 300 to 1,500 births, usually presenting immediately or within several hours after birth (Cunningham et al., 2014). Vulvar hematomas usually stem from ruptured blood vessels, especially in the vulva, vagina, or broad ligament.

Risk factors for puerperal hematoma include instrumental or surgical birth, as well as failure to discern or repair a torn vessel. Other risk factors include vulvovaginal varicosities, medical conditions, coagulopathies, preeclampsia, primiparity, multiple gestation, and prolonged labor.

Signs and symptoms include persistent bleeding despite a firm uterus; increased vulvar, vaginal, or rectal pain and pressure; and presentation of a fluctuant edema with bluish coloration. Increased lateral uterine or flank pain or signs and symptoms of shock necessitate assessment for broad ligament or subperitoneal hematoma.

Small hematoma formation can be expectantly managed by marking the affected area and observing for size increase. Moderate to large hematomas will usually need surgical incision and drainage.

Postpartum Venous Thrombophlebitis and Venous Thromboembolism

The advent of early and frequent ambulation after birth dramatically decreased the incidence of puerperal thromboembolism. However, the incidence of puerperal morbidity and mortality from thromboembolism remains significant, and pulmonary embolism is responsible for 9.3% of pregnancy-related deaths (2006–2010)—a rate that has remained consistent (Creanga et al., 2014).

A variety of risk factors contribute to thromboembolic events, including surgical birth, obesity, comorbid illnesses, and advanced maternal age. Despite increased risk after cesarean section, recent data from the Nationwide Inpatient Sample (2006–2009) indicated that nearly 47% of VTE cases occur subsequent to vaginal birth (Ghaji, Boulet, Tepper, & Hooper, 2013). Women are at increased risk for thromboembolic events during postpartum due to hypercoagulability, stasis, and vascular trauma (Virchow's triad). Notably, hormonal effects from progesterone and venous pressure from the growing uterus increase the possibility of venous stasis. Birth-related risk factors include cesarean section, operative vaginal birth, infection, vascular trauma, immobilization, and postpartum hemorrhage. Other risk factors include maternal history of varicosities, inherited thrombophilias, obesity, smoking, age greater than 35 years, antiphospholipid antibody syndrome, sickle cell disease, heart disease, diabetes, and other medical conditions.

Signs and symptoms depend on the thromboembolic event. During the postpartum period, women with superficial thrombophlebitis (SVT) present with localized extremity pain, a firm cord-like structure, edema, erythema, and warmth at the site. Ultrasound is indicated to rule out underlying deep vein thrombosis (DVT). DVT often occurs with abrupt onset of severe leg pain, which worsens when ambulating or standing. Generalized edema of the entire leg is present, and the woman may present with a slight temperature and mild tachycardia. There may or may not be localized tenderness and warmth at the site of the thrombosis. Positive Homan's sign is no longer considered diagnostic of DVT, as it could also indicate muscular strain.

Laboratory analysis can include D-dimer studies. However, D-dimer levels can increase in pregnancy for a number of reasons, so they are not considered diagnostic. Nevertheless, a negative D-dimer result can be encouraging. Compression ultrasound of the proximal veins is considered the initial diagnostic study (Cunningham et al., 2014).

Management for DVT includes anticoagulation therapy (at least 6 months' duration) and rest until symptoms resolve. Once leg pain diminishes and most symptoms resolve, gradual ambulation can begin. Women should be fitted and taught proper use of compression stockings. Warfarin (Coumadin) can be used while breastfeeding. Other management includes nonsteroidal anti-inflammatory agents.

Postpartum Preeclampsia/Eclampsia and Late Preeclampsia

Preeclampsia is a hypertensive disorder that most commonly presents prenatally. It is typically characterized by hypertension and proteinuria, and can range from mild to severe in presentation. Although less common, puerperal preeclampsia usually presents within 24 to 48 hours after birth, and late preeclampsia presents after 48 hours and before 4 months postpartum (Sibai & Stella, 2009).

Risk factors include current diagnosis of gestational hypertension or preeclampsia (the disease can worsen postpartum). Additionally, there is an increased risk of pulmonary edema from postpartum extravascular fluid shift, use of intravenous fluids during labor and birth, and renal dysfunction secondary to severe preeclampsia. Puerperal preeclampsia also increases the risk for eclampsia (seizures), thromboembolism, and stroke.

The presentation of preeclampsia is more subtle during the postpartum period than in its prenatal form. Women typically present with headaches, visual changes, nausea and vomiting, and epigastric pain. Hypertension and proteinuria are not necessarily the primary signs of developing preeclampsia. Neurologic symptoms are more common during postpartum.

Management includes treatment with intravenous magnesium sulfate, other antihypertensive therapy, and hospitalization for at least 24 hours (Cunningham et al., 2014).

Postpartum Thyroiditis

Postpartum thyroiditis—that is, inflammation of the thyroid gland—can present anytime during the first postpartum year (usually 1–4 months) as either hypothyroiditis or hyperthyroiditis or both, alternating from one to the other (Neville, 2011). Overabundant release of thyroid hormones occurs initially (3 months postpartum), lasting 2 to 3 months, followed by insufficient release; thus hyperthyroidism usually presents first. In contrast, hypothyroiditis usually occurs 4 to 8 months postpartum. Incidence varies from 5% to 10%, although some cases may be unreported. Signs and symptoms are subtle and may not be readily recognized, as manifestation of thyroiditis can mimic common postpartum occurrences.

Risk factors include women with autoimmune disorders, diabetes, or history of thyroid dysfunction. The risk of this complication increases 25% in women with type 1 diabetes (Neville, 2011). A positive thyroid antibody test during the first trimester is correlated with a nearly 50% risk of postpartum thyroiditis (Stagnaro-Green & Pearce, 2012).

Signs and symptoms of hyperthyroiditis include fatigue, anxiety, palpitations, insomnia, irritability/nervousness, weight loss, and goiter. Signs and symptoms of hypothyroiditis include fatigue, inability to concentrate, depression, dry skin, constipation, weight gain, and goiter. Women can experience dysphoria, which sometimes may lead to misdiagnosis of postpartum psychosis. Because some signs and symptoms of hyperthyroiditis and hypothyroiditis are similar to some mental health disorders, thyroid function studies are indicated when assessing women for perinatal mood and anxiety disorders.

Laboratory analysis for hyperthyroiditis include thyroid-stimulating hormone (TSH; low levels), presence of thyroid peroxidase antibodies, and decreased TSH receptor antibodies. Diagnosis of hypothyroiditis includes TSH (elevated) and a positive test for anti-thyroid peroxidase antibodies.

Management depends on the phase and severity of symptoms. Beta blockers are the treatment of choice for hyperthyroiditis, whereas thyroid supplementation is prescribed for hypothyroiditis. Breastfeeding need not be interrupted or discontinued during treatment.

Thyrotoxicosis (thyroid storm), a potentially life-threatening condition, can occur during the first month postpartum. Its onset is abrupt, short-lived, and characterized by fever, nausea, vomiting, diarrhea, tachycardia, and tremor. Treatment is imperative and includes hydration and decrease of excessive circulating thyroid hormones (Neville, 2011).

Postpartum Mood and Anxiety Disorders

Postpartum mood and anxiety disorders (PMAD) are common complications of childbearing whose incidence varies from 7% to 20%, depending on the study (Gaynes et al., 2005; Zender & Olshansky, 2009). Anxiety disorders, including generalized anxiety disorder (GAD), panic disorder (PD), obsessive–compulsive disorder (OCD), and post-traumatic stress disorder (PTSD), often accompany depression (58%) (Zender & Olshansky, 2009). Women have nearly a 30% lifetime prevalence of anxiety disorders. Mood and anxiety disorders are most often reported around 2

months postpartum, but their signs and symptoms can occur at various times throughout the first year after childbirth or at even more distant times (Zender & Olshansky, 2009).

The etiology of PMAD has not been settled, despite ongoing research in this area, but a combination of genetics and environmental factors is thought to influence its development (Alder, Fink, Bitzer, Hosli, & Holzgreve, 2007). The hypothalamus–pituitary–adrenal (HPA) axis and noradrenergic and serotonergic systems should work in harmony. When dysfunction occurs, postpartum mood and anxiety disorders can develop.

Risk factors for PMAD, along with physiologic changes after childbirth (hormonal, HPA), include stressors such as social and economic influences, lack of sleep, demands of a new infant, role adaptation, and family needs (Karsnitz & Ward, 2011). Additional factors include substance use, preterm birth, young maternal age, single-parent status, and comorbid illnesses. In particular, a personal or family history of mental illness or a personal history of postpartum mood or anxiety disorders increases risk.

Signs and symptoms vary according to severity and type of illness. Women describe symptoms that range from mild to severe (an inability to perform daily activities or thoughts of harming self). Mental health stigma often inhibits women from reporting these symptoms, however, so clinicians must be particularly aware of screening all women. **Table 32-6** describes clinical presentations for postpartum mood and anxiety disorders.

Management depends on severity and/or comorbid illness. Diagnosis and treatment of PMAD can be complex. A team approach with a mental health specialist provides the best opportunity for appropriate care.

Screening

Assessment for PMAD should begin at the first prenatal visit and be ongoing throughout pregnancy and postpartum as indicated. The American College of Nurse-Midwives (ACNM, 2003) supports universal screening of women. Recently, other professional organizations have changed prior recommendations and now fully support screening for depression (American College of Obstetricians and Gynecologists, 2015b), for example,

TABLE 32-6	Postpartum Mood and Anxiety Disorders: Clinical Presentations and Symptoms

Postpartum Mood Disorders

Blues (Symptoms < 14 Days)	Depression	Psychosis
Tearful	Tearful	Hallucinations
Irritability	Irritability or anger	Delusions
Mood swings	Mood swings	Inability to communicate
Fatigue	Fatigue	Rapid mood change
Appetite changes	Lack of interest in the baby	Paranoia
	Sleep disturbances	Inability to sleep
	Appetite disturbances	Hyperactivity
	Guilt or shame	Disorganized thoughts
	Feelings of isolation	
	Hopelessness	
	Loss of pleasure	
	Feelings of harming the baby or self	

Postpartum Anxiety Disorders

Generalized Anxiety Disorder	Obsessive–Compulsive Disorder	Panic Disorder	Post-traumatic Stress Disorder
Excessive worry	Intrusive thoughts	Fear of dying	Flashbacks or nightmares
Sleep disturbances/fatigue	Checking	Dizziness, shortness of breath	Anxiety
Appetite changes	Cleaning	Heart palpitations	Panic attack
Feelings of dread	Hypervigilance of infant	Feeling impending doom	Powerlessness
Physical symptoms		Extreme anxiety	Increased arousal
Restlessness		Irritable bowel	Avoidance of situations
Lack of concentration			Detachment

Reproduced from Karsnitz, D. B., & Ward, S. (2011). Spectrum of anxiety disorders: Diagnosis and pharmacologic treatment. *Journal of Midwifery & Women's Health, 56*(3), 266–281. Reprinted with permission from John Wiley & Sons.

has identified a need for screening at least once during the perinatal period. The U.S. Preventive Services Task Force (USPSTF, 2016) recommends screening for all adults, including pregnant and postpartum women. The American Association of Family Physicians follows the USPSTF recommendations.

The Edinburgh Postnatal Depression Scale (EPDS), the most commonly used self-report screening tool, has been validated in numerous studies, is available in many languages, and is accessible without cost. The EPDS has a sensitivity of 86% and specificity of 78% with a positive predictive value of 73% (Cox, Holden, & Sagovsky,

1987). Other screening tools include the Postpartum Depression Screening Scale (PDSS), the Patient Health Questionnaire (PHQ-9), the Beck Depression Inventory (BDI). and the Center for Epidemiological Studies' Depression Scale (CED-D). Despite their ease of use and widespread availability, such self-report screening tools are generally underutilized.

Postpartum Blues

Many believe postpartum blues to be a mild form of postpartum depression. Postpartum blues affects nearly 80% of all postpartum women, is transient, and is short-lived, occurring most often in the first 7 to 10 days postpartum. To counteract this condition, women should be encouraged to rest when possible, increase nutrition and fluids, get fresh air, and ask for family support.

Postpartum Depression

Postpartum depression can occur at any time within the first year postpartum but often presents around 2 months. Because signs and symptoms of depression may mimic common prenatal occurrences (fatigue or sleep disturbance), depression can begin prenatally, only to become exacerbated in the early postpartum period. Signs and symptoms lasting longer than 2 weeks should be considered postpartum depression. Assessment should always include suicidal ideation or consideration of a plan to commit suicide.

Management includes treatment with antidepressants. First-line treatment consists of selective serotonin reuptake inhibitors (SSRIs). Additionally, cognitive-behavioral therapy or group support therapy can be helpful. Of note, treatment with antidepressants could trigger a manic episode and subsequent psychosis in a woman with undiagnosed bipolar disorder (King, Johnson, & Gamblian, 2011). For this reason, it is important to collaborate with a mental health clinician when caring for patient woman with postpartum depression.

Postpartum Psychosis

Postpartum psychosis often presents early in the postpartum period (the first few days to 1 week after childbirth) and is usually abrupt in onset.

Incidence is 1 to 2 per 1,000 women. Women with bipolar disorder or previous diagnosis of a mental health disorder are at increased risk for postpartum psychosis. Other risk factors include sleep deprivation for an extended period (Posmontier, 2010). Postpartum psychosis can have devastating consequences, and suspicion of this condition warrants immediate referral for inpatient mental health treatment.

Generalized Anxiety Disorder

Generalized anxiety disorder (GAD) can be difficult to diagnose during the postpartum period, as extreme anxiety or worry (impacting daily activity) must occur for at least 6 months to warrant this diagnosis. Prevalence during postpartum is 4.4% to 8.2% (Ross & McLean, 2006). Risk factors include past or present history of GAD, family history of GAD, life stressors, and the hormonal fluctuations associated with the postpartum.

Pharmacologic treatment, as in depression, consists of SSRIs. Cognitive-behavioral therapy is often indicated to help women identify triggers and subsequent coping mechanisms (Vythilingum, 2008).

Panic Disorder

Panic disorder is characterized by recurrent panic attacks, occurring at any time with or without necessary triggers. The prevalence of this condition during pregnancy is 1.3% to 2% (Ross & McLean, 2006). Panic disorder impacts the woman's quality of life, affecting both work and social events. Women experiencing panic disorder will often avoid an environment that can potentially trigger an attack.

Risk factors include hormonal influences, substance abuse, and stressful circumstances. Panic disorder is also a risk factor for postpartum depression (Rambelli et al., 2010). Treatment includes psychotherapy and psychotropic agents.

Post-traumatic Stress Disorder

Post-traumatic stress disorder (PTSD) occurs when the individual experiences a real or perceived threat of death to self or another, then is exposed to the same or a similar environment in which the trauma first occurred (Beck & Watson, 2010). Individuals experiencing PTSD report feelings of extreme fear and helplessness. Estimates of the prevalence of postpartum PTSD range from 1.5% to 6.6% (Beck, 2006).

Birth experiences and perceptions vary among women and can have long-term consequences. PTSD related to childbirth can result in attachment or relationship issues, and has been indicated in development of postpartum depression. Debriefing or discussion of events surrounding childbirth can be helpful and further assist with understanding specifics of the experience. Furthermore, examining aspects of the birth that are unclear can correct misinformation and give the woman an opportunity to express any concerns or fears. Management includes treatment with SSRIs and psychotherapy (Meades, Pond, Ayers, & Warren, 2011).

Complementary Therapy

Complementary therapies can be used for postpartum mood and anxiety disorders. In particular, omega-3 fatty acid supplements, St. John's wort, and kava root can be helpful in women with PMAD (King et al., 2011). Nevertheless, it is important to recognize that most complementary treatments are not evidence based. Furthermore, women should be assessed for current use of any complementary therapies before beginning treatment. Teaching

should include variations in strength, use of active ingredients, or ways in which substances are derived.

CONCLUSION

The postpartum period encompasses numerous physiological and psychological changes as women return to a pre-pregnant state and transition to a new or additional role. The plans for interactions between new mothers and members of the healthcare community in the United States do not fit well with this time frame, as healthcare providers often do not communicate with women until 6 weeks postpartum. Postpartum complications usually occur before this 6-week visit, however, and breastfeeding is frequently discontinued prior to this visit. Clinicians have an opportunity to facilitate an uneventful recovery while employing judicious assessment for recognition of complications. Consideration of cultural influences, education, and team approach will impact treatment and promote long-term health care.

For additional resources on postpartum care, refer to **Box 32-1**.

BOX 32-1   Additional Resources About Postpartum Care

Postpartum Web Resources

Academy of Pediatrics, information on breastfeeding: http://search.aap.org/?source=aap.org&k
    =breastfeeding
Baby-Friendly USA: http://www.babyfriendlyusa.org
Edinburgh Postnatal Depression Scale: http://www.fresno.ucsf.edu/pediatrics/downloads/edinburghscale.pdf
La Leche League International: http://www.lalecheleague.org
MEDLINE Plus (Internet). Bethesda, MD: National Library of Medicine. Herbs and Supplements:
    http://www.nlm.nih.gov/medlineplus/druginformation.html
Postpartum Support International: http://www.postpartum.net

Postpartum/Breastfeeding Textbook Resources

King, T. L., Brucker, M. C., Kriebs, J. M., Fahey, J. O., Gegor, C. L., & Varney, H. (Eds.). (2015). *Varney's
    midwifery* (5th ed.). Burlington, MA: Jones & Bartlett Learning.
Jordan, R. G., Engstrom, J., Marfell, J., & Farley, C. L. (Eds.). (2014). *Prenatal and postnatal care:
    A woman-centered approach*. Ames, IA: Wiley Blackwell.
Wambach, K., & Riordan, J. (Eds). (2016). *Breastfeeding and human lactation* (5th ed.). Burlington, MA:
    Jones & Bartlett Learning.

References

Ahnfeldt-Mollerup, P., Petersen, L. K., Kragstrup, J., Christensen, R. D., & Sorensen, B. (2012). Postpartum infections: Occurrence, health care contacts and association with breastfeeding. *Acta Obstetricia et Gynecologica Scandinavica, 91*(12), 1440–1444.

Alder, J., Fink, N., Bitzer, J., Hosli, I., & Holzgreve, W. (2007). Depression and anxiety during pregnancy: A risk factor for obstetric, fetal and neonatal outcome? A critical review of the literature. *Journal of Maternal–Fetal and Neonatal Medicine, 20*(3), 189–209.

American Academy of Pediatrics (AAP). (2012). Breastfeeding and the use of human milk. *Pediatrics, 129*(3), 827–841.

American College of Nurse-Midwives (ACNM). (2003). Position Statement: Depression in women. Retrieved from http://www .midwife.org/ACNM/files/ACNMLibraryData/UPLOADFILENAME /000000000061/Depression%20in%20Women%20May%20 2013.pdf

American College of Obstetricians and Gynecologists. (2006, reaffirmed 2013). Postpartum hemorrhage: Practice Bulletin 76. *Obstetrics & Gynecology, 108*, 1039–1047.

American College of Obstetricians and Gynecologists. (2010). Committee on Obstetric Practice. Committee Opinion No. 453: Screening for depression during and after pregnancy. *Obstetrics & Gynecology, 115*, 394–395.

American College of Obstetricians and Gynecologists. (2011, reaffirmed 2014). Use of prophylactic antibiotics in labor and delivery: Practice Bulletin No. 120. *Obstetrics & Gynecology, 117*, 1472–1483.

American College of Obstetrician and Gynecologists. (2015a). *Committee opinion: Screening for perinatal depression.* Retrieved from http://www.acog.org/Resources-And-Publications /Committee-Opinions/Committee-on-Obstetric-Practice /Screening-for-Perinatal-Depression

American College of Obstetricians and Gynecologists. (2015b). Physical activity and exercise during pregnancy and the postpartum period. Committee on Obstetric Practice: Committee Opinion No. 650. *Obstetrics & Gynecology, 126*, 135–142.

Amir, L. H., Forster, D., Lumley, J., & McLachlan, H. (2007). A descriptive study of mastitis in Australian breastfeeding women: Incidence and determinants. *BMC Public Health, 7*, 62–71.

Amir, L. H., Trupin, S., & Kvist, L. J. (2014). Diagnosis and treatment of mastitis in breastfeeding women. *Journal of Human Lactation, 30*, 10–13.

Andrighetti, T. P., & Karsnitz, D. B. (2014). Components of postnatal care. In R. G. Jordan, J. Engstrom, J. Margell, & C. L. Farley (Eds.), *Prenatal and postnatal care: A woman-centered approach* (pp. 423–440). Ames, IA: Wiley-Blackwell.

Azulay Chertok, I. R. (2013). The postpartum period and lactation physiology. In S. T. Blackburn (Ed.), *Maternal, fetal and neonatal physiology: A clinical perspective* (4th ed., pp. 142–162). St. Louis, MO: Saunders Elsevier.

Barrett, M., Heller, M. M., Stone, H. F., & Murase, J. E. (2013). Dermatoses of the breast in lactation. *Dermatologic Therapy, 26*(4), 331–336.

Baxter, J. K., Berghella, V., Mackeen, A. D., Ohly, N. T., & Weed, S. (2011). Timing of prophylactic antibiotics for preventing postpartum infectious morbidity in women undergoing cesarean delivery. *Cochrane Database Systematic Reviews, 12*. doi:10.1002/14651858.CD009516

Beck, C. T. (2006). The anniversary of birth trauma: Failure to rescue. *Nursing Research, 55*(6), 381–390.

Beck, C. T., & Watson, S. (2010). Subsequent childbirth after a previous traumatic birth. *Nursing Research, 59*(4), 241–249.

Berg, C., Callaghan, W. M., Syverson, C., & Henderson, Z. (2010). Pregnancy-related mortality in the United States, 1998–2005. *Obstetrics & Gynecology, 116*, 1302–1309.

Betzold, C. M. (2004). Galactagogues. *Journal of Midwifery & Women's Health, 49*, 151–154.

Bick, D., Beake, S., & Pellowe, C. (2011). Vigilance must be a priority: Maternal genital tract sepsis. *Practicing Midwife, 14*(4), 16–18.

Bienfait, M., Maury, M., Haquet, A., Faillie, J., Franc, N., & Combes, C. (2011). Pertinence of the self-report mother-to-infant bondig scale in the neonatal unit of a maternity ward. *Early Human Development, 87*(4), 281–287.

Blackburn, S. T. (2013). *Maternal, fetal and neonatal physiology: A clinical perspective* (4th ed.). St Louis, MO: Saunders Elsevier.

Brownwell, E., Howard, C. R., Lawrence, R. A., & Dozier, A. M. (2012). Delayed onset lactogenesis II predicts the cessation of any or exclusive breastfeeding. *Journal of Pediatrics, 161*(4), 608–614.

Carr, L. (2000). *Dying to have a baby: The history of childbirth.* Department of Obstetrics, Gynecology and Reproductive Sciences. Manitoba: University of Manitoba. Retrieved from http://www .neonatology.org/pdf/dyingtohaveababy.pdf

Centers for Disease Control and Prevention (CDC). (2010). U.S. medical eligibility criteria for contraceptive use, 2010. *Morbidity and Mortality Weekly Report, 59*, 1–85.

Centers for Disease Control and Prevention (CDC). (2013a). Breastfeeding report card: United States/2013. Retrieved from http://www .cdc.gov/breastfeeding/pdf/2013BreastfeedingReportCard.pdf

Centers for Disease Control and Prevention (CDC). (2013b). Progress in increasing breastfeeding and reducing racial/ethnic differences—United States, 2000–2008 births. *Morbidity and Mortality Weekly Report, 62*(5), 77–80.

Cox, J. L., Holden, J. M., & Sagovsky, R. (1987). Detection of postnatal depression: Development of the 10-item Edinburgh Postnatal Depression Scale. *British Journal of Psychiatry, 150*, 782–786.

Creanga, A. A., Berg, C. J., Syverson, C., Seed, K., Bruce, F. C., & Callaghan, W. M. (2014). Pregnancy-related mortality in the United States, 2006–2010. *Obstetrics & Gynecology, 125*, 5–12.

Cunningham, F. G., Leveno, K. J., Bloom, S. L., Spong, C. Y., Dashe, J. S., Hoffman, B. L., . . . Sheffield, J. S. (2014). *Williams obstetrics* (24th ed.). New York, NY: McGraw-Hill Education.

Fahey, J. O. (2015). Anatomy and physiology of postpartum. In T. L. King, M. C. Brucker, J. M. Kriebs, J. O. Fahey, C. L. Gegor, & H. Varney (Eds.), *Varney's midwifery* (5th ed., pg. 1101–1110). Burlington, MA: Jones & Bartlett Learning.

Feldman, R. (2004). Mother–infant skin-to-skin contact (Kangaroo Care): Theoretical, clinical, and empirical aspects. *Infants & Young Children: An Interdisciplinary Journal of Special Care Practices, 17*(2), 145–161.

Feldman, R., Weller, A., Zagoory-Sharon, O., & Levine, A. (2007). Evidence for a neuroendocrinological foundation of human affiliation: Plasma oxytocin levels across pregnancy and the postpartum period predict mother–infant bonding. *Psychological Science, 18*(11), 965–970.

Figueiredo, B., Costa, R., Pacheco, A., & Pais, A. (2009). Mother-to-infant emotional involvement at birth. *Maternal & Child Health Journal, 13*(4), 539–549.

Galbally, M., Lewis, A., Ijzendoorn, M., & Permezel, M. (2011). The role of oxytocin in mother–infant relations: A systematic review of human studies. *Harvard Review of Psychiatry, 19*(1), 1–14.

Gaynes, B. N., Gavin, N., Meltzer-Brody, S., Lohr, K. N., Swinson, T., Gartlehner, G., . . . Miller, W. C. (2005). *Perinatal depression: Prevelance, screening accuracy and screening outcomes evidence report/technology assessment (Summary) No. 119.* AHRQ Publications No. 05-E006-2. Rockville, MD: Agency for Healthcare Research and Quality. Retrieved from http://archive.ahrq.gov/downloads/pub/evidence/pdf/peridepr/peridep.pdf

Ghaji, N., Boulet, S. L., Tepper, N., & Hooper, W. C. (2013). Trends in venous thromboembolism among pregnancy-related hospitalizations, United States, 1994–2009. *American Journal of Obstetrics and Gynecology, 209*(5), 1–8.

Hankins, G., Clark, S. L., Pacheco, L. D., O'Keefe, D., D'Alton, M., & Saade, G. R. (2012). Maternal mortality, near misses, and severe morbidity: Lowering rates through designated levels of maternity care. *Obstetrics & Gynecology, 120*, 929–934.

Hatcher, R. A., Trussell, J., Nelson, A. L., Cates W. Jr., Kowal, D., & Policar, M. S. (2011). *Contraceptive technology* (20th ed.). New York, NY: Ardent Media.

Hipp, L. E., Kane Low, L., & van Anders, S. M. (2012). Exploring women's postpartum sexuality: Social, psychological, relational, and birth-related contextual factors. *Journal of Sexual Medicine, 9*(9), 2330–2341.

International Lactation Consultant Association; Mannel, R., Martens, P. J., Walker, M. (Eds.). (2013). *Core curriculum for lactation consultant practice* (3rd ed.). Burlington, MA: Jones & Bartlett Learning.

Jackson, E., & Glasier, A. (2011). Return of ovulation and menses in postpartum nonlactating women: a systematic review. *Obstetrics & Gynecology, 117*(3), 657-662. doi:10.1097/AOG.0b013e31820ce18c

Kantrowitz-Gordon, I. (2015). Anatomy and physiology of postpartum. In T. L. King, M. C. Brucker, J. M. Kriebs, J. O. Fahey, C. L. Gegor, & H. Varney (Eds). *Varney's midwifery* (5th ed., pp. 1101–1110). Burlington, MA: Jones & Bartlett Learning.

Karsnitz, D. B., & Ward, S. (2011). Spectrum of anxiety disorders: Diagnosis and pharmacologic treatment. *Journal of Midwifery & Women's Health, 56*(3), 266–281.

Kennedy, K. I., & Trussell, J. (2011). Postpartum contraception and lactation. In R. A. Hatcher, J. Trussell, A. L. Nelson, W. Cates Jr., D. Kowal, & M. S. Policar, *Contraceptive technology* (20th ed., pp. 483–502). New York, NY: Ardent Media.

King, J. C. (2012). Maternal mortality in the United States: Why is it important and what are we doing about it? *Seminars in Perinatology, 36*, 14–18.

King, T. L., Johnson, R., & Gamblian, V. (2011). Mental health. In T. L. King & M. C. Brucker (Eds.), *Pharmacology for women's health* (pp. 750–791) Sudbury, MA: Jones and Bartlett.

Klaus, M. H., & Kennell, J. H. (1976). *Maternal–infant bonding: The impact of early separation or loss on family development.* St. Louis, MO: Mosby.

Kocaoz, S., Eroglu, K., & Sivashoglu, A. A. (2013). Role of pelvic floor muscle exercises in the prevention of stress urinary incontinence during pregnancy and the postpartum period. *Gynecologic and Obstetric Investigation, 75*(1), 34–40.

Kramer, M. S., Berg, C., Abenhaim, H., Dahhou, M., Rouleau, J., Mehrabadi, A., & Joseph, K. S. (2013). Incidence, risk factors, and temporal trends in severe postpartum hemorrhage. *American Journal of Obstetrics and Gynecology, 209*(5), 449.e1–449.e7.

Liu, Y. Q., Petrini, M., & Maloni, J. A. (2014). "Doing the month": Postpartum paractice in Chinese women. *Nursing & Health Sciences.* doi:10.1111/nhs.12146

Maharaj, D. (2007). Puerperal pyrexia: A review. Part II. *Obstetrical & Gynecological Survey, 62*(6), 400–406.

Meades, R., Pond, C., Ayers, S., & Warren, F. (2011). Postnatal debriefing: Have we thrown the baby out with the bath water? *Behaviour Research and Therapy, 49*(5), 367–372.

Mercer, R. T. (1985). The process of maternal role attainment over the first year. *Nursing Research, 34*(4), 198–204.

Moore, E. R., Anderson, G. C., Bergman, N., & Dowswell, T. (2012). Early skin-to-skin contact for mothers and their healtyh newborn infants. *Cochrane Database Systematic Review, 3,* CD003519. doi:10.1002/14651858

Neville, M. W. (2011). Thyroid disorders. In T. L. King & M. C. Brucker (Eds.), *Pharmacology for women's health* (pp. 539–559). Sudbury, MA: Jones & Bartlett.

Nommsen-Rivers, L., Chantry, C. J., Peerson, J. M., Cohen, R. J., & Dewey, K. G. (2010). Delayed onset of lactogenesis among first-time mothers is related to maternal obesity and factors associated with ineffective breastfeeding. *American Journal of Clinical Nutrition, 92*(3), 574–584.

Osadchy, A., Moretti, M. E., & Koren, G. (2012). Effect of domperidone on insufficient lactation in puerperal women: A systematic review and meta-analysis of randomized controlled trials. *Obstetrics and Gynecology International, 2012* (2012), Article ID 642893. http://dx.doi.org/10.1155/2012/642893

Osterman, K. L., & Rahm, V. (2000). Lactation mastitis: Bacterial cultivation of breast milk, symptoms, treatment and outcome. *Journal of Human Lactation, 16,* 297–302.

Pacheco, L. D., Costantine, M. M., Saade, G. R., Mucowski, S., Hankins, G. D., & Sciscione, A. C. (2010). vonWillebrand disease and pregnancy: a practical approach for the diagnosis and treatment. *American Journal of Obstetrics and Gynecology, 203*(3), 194–200.

Petrovitch, I., Jeffrey, R. B., & Heerema-McKenney, A. (2009). Subinvolution of the placental site. *Journal of Ultrasound Medicine, 28*(8), 1115–1119.

Pickler, R. (2009). Understanding, promoting, and measuring the effects of mother-infant attachment during infant feeding. *Journal of Obstetric, Gynecologic & Neonatal Nursing, 38*(4), 468–469.

Posmontier, B. (2010). The role of midwives in facilitating recovery in postpartum psychosis. *Journal of Midwifery & Women's Health, 55,* 430–437.

Rambelli, C., Montagnani, M. S., Oppo, A., Banti, S., Borri, C., Cortopassi, C. . . . Mauri, M. (2010). Panic disorder as a risk factor for postpartum depression: Results from the Perinatal Depression Research & Screening Unit (PND-ReScU). *Journal of Affective Disorders, 122,* 138–143.

Ross, L. E., & McLean, L. M. (2006). Anxiety disorders during pregnancy and the postpartum period: A systematic review. *Journal of Clinical Psychiatry, 67,* 1285–1298.

Rubin, R. (1961). Basic maternal behavior. *Nursing Outlook, 9*(11), 683–686.

Sibai, B. M., & Stella, C. L. (2009). Diagnosis and management of atypical preeclampsia–elampsia. *American Journal of Obstetrics and Gynecology, 200,* 481.e1–481.e7.

Smaill, F. M., & Gyte, G. M. (2010). Antibiotic prophylaxis versus no prophylaxis for preventing infection after cesarean section. *Cochrane Database Systematic Reviews, 1.* CD007482. doi:10.1002/14651858.CD007482.pub2

Small, R., Roth, C., Raval, M., Shafiei, T., Korfker, D., Heaman, M., . . . Gagnon, A. (2014). Immigrant and non-immigrant women's experiences of maternity care: A systematic and comparative review of studies in five countries. *BMC Pregnancy and Childbirth, 14*(152). doi:10.1186/1471-2393-14-152

Stagnaro-Green, A., & Pearce, E. (2012). Thyroid disorders in pregnancy. *Nature Reviews: Endocrinology, 8*(11), 650–658.

Sweet, R. L., & Gibbs, R. S. (2009). *Infectious diseases of the female genital tract* (5th ed.). Baltimore, MD: Lippincott Williams & Wilkins.

Tallandini, M., & Scalembra, C. (2006). Kangaroo mother care and mother–premature infant dyadic interaction. *Infant Mental Health Journal, 27*(3), 251–275.

The Joint Commission. (2010). Preventing maternal death. Retrieved from http://www.jointcommission.org/sentinel_event_alert_issue _44_preventing_maternal_death

U.S. Department of Health and Human Services (DHHS). (2010). *Healthy people 2020. Maternal, infant, and child health objectives (MICH)21: Increase the proportion of infants who are breastfed.* Retrieved from https://www.healthypeople.gov/2020/topics -objectives/topic/maternal-infant-and-child-health/objectives

U. S. Preventive Services Task Force (USPSTF). (2016). Screening for depression in adults: U. S. Preventive Services Task Force recommendation statement. *Journal of the American Medical Association, 315*(4), 380–387. doi:10.1001/jama.2015.18392

Volling, B. (2012). Family transitions following the birth of a sibling: An empirical review of changes in the firstborn's adjustment. *Psychological Bulletin, 138*(3), 497–528.

Vythilingum, B. (2008). Anxiety disorders in pregnancy. *Current Psychiatry Reports, 01,* 331–335.

Wambach, K. (2016). Breast-related problems. In K. Wambach & J. Riordan (Eds.), *Breastfeeding and human lactation* (5th ed., pp. 291–324). Burlington, MA: Jones & Bartlett Learning.

Wambach, K., & Riordan, J. (Eds.). (2016). *Breastfeeding and human lactation* (5th ed.). Burlington, MA: Jones & Bartlett Learning.

Waugh, L. J. (2011). Beliefs associated with Mexican immigrant families' practice of la cuarentena during postpartum recovery. *Journal of Obstetric, Gynecologic and Neonatal Nursing, 40*(6), 732–741.

World Health Organization (WHO). (2010). *Medical eligibility criteria for contraceptive use* (4th ed.). Geneva, Switzerland: WHO, Reproductive Health and Research Division.

World Health Organization (WHO), UNICEF. (2009). *Baby-Friendly Hospital Initiative 2009: Revised, updated, and expanded for integrated care.* Geneva, Switzerland: Author.

Wright, E. M. (2015). Breastfeeding and the mother–newborn dyad. In T. L. King, M. C. Brucker, J. M. Kriebs, J. O. Fahey, C. L. Gegor, & H. Varney (Eds.), *Varney's midwifery* (5th ed., pp. 1157–1184.). Burlington, MA: Jones & Bartlett Learning.

Zender, R., & Olshansky, E. (2009). Women's mental health: Depression and anxiety. *Nursing Clinics of North America, 44,* 355–364.

INDEX

Note: Boxes, figures, and tables are indicated with *b*, *f*, and *t* following the page numbers.

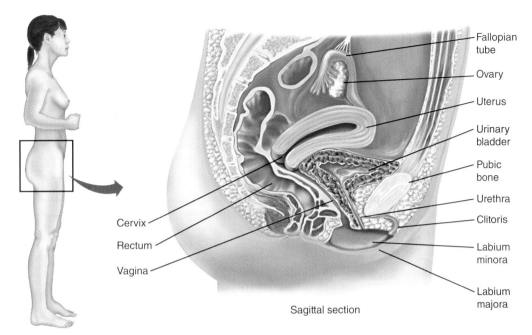

Fallopian tube

Ovary

Uterus

Urinary bladder

Pubic bone

Urethra

Clitoris

Labium minora

Labium majora

Cervix

Rectum

Vagina

Sagittal section

COLOR PLATE 1 Midsagittal view of a woman's pelvic organs.

COLOR PLATE 2 Female external genitalia.

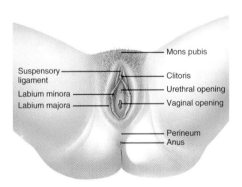

Mons pubis

Suspensory ligament

Clitoris

Urethral opening

Labium minora

Vaginal opening

Labium majora

Perineum

Anus

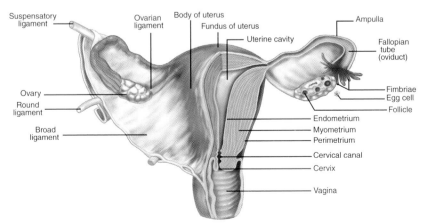

Suspensatory ligament

Ovarian ligament

Body of uterus

Fundus of uterus

Uterine cavity

Ampulla

Fallopian tube (oviduct)

Fimbriae

Egg cell

Follicle

Ovary

Round ligament

Broad ligament

Endometrium

Myometrium

Perimetrium

Cervical canal

Cervix

Vagina

COLOR PLATE 3 An anterior view of the female internal genital anatomy showing the relationships of the ovaries, fallopian tubes, uterus, cervix, and vagina.

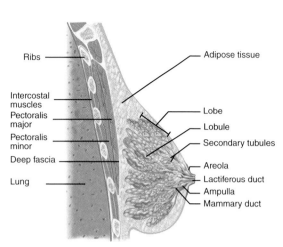

Ribs

Intercostal muscles

Pectoralis major

Pectoralis minor

Deep fascia

Lung

Adipose tissue

Lobe

Lobule

Secondary tubules

Areola

Lactiferous duct

Ampulla

Mammary duct

COLOR PLATE 4 The structure of a woman's breast and mammary glands: sagittal section.

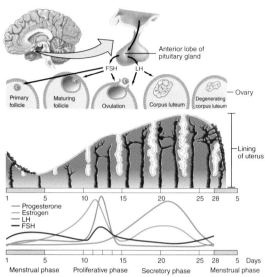

Anterior lobe of pituitary gland

FSH   LH

Primary follicle   Maturing follicle   Ovulation   Corpus luteum   Degenerating corpus luteum   Ovary

Lining of uterus

— Progesterone
— Estrogen
— LH
— FSH

1   5   10   15   20   25   28   5   Days

Menstrual phase   Proliferative phase   Secretory phase   Menstrual phase

COLOR PLATE 5 Influence of steroid hormones on the ovaries and endometrium.

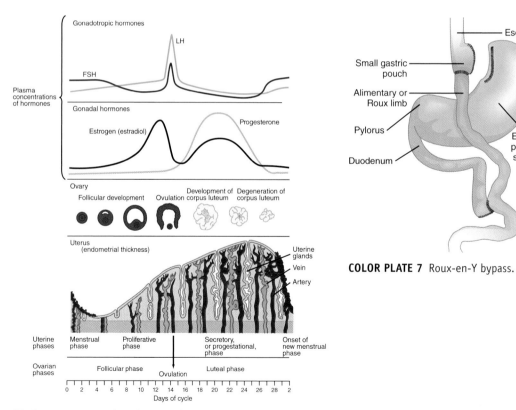

Gonadotropic hormones

LH

FSH

Plasma concentrations of hormones

Gonadal hormones

Progesterone

Estrogen (estradiol)

Ovary

Follicular development   Ovulation   Development of corpus luteum   Degeneration of corpus luteum

Uterus (endometrial thickness)

Uterine glands

Vein

Artery

Uterine phases: Menstrual phase   Proliferative phase   Secretory, or progestational, phase   Onset of new menstrual phase

Ovarian phases: Follicular phase   Ovulation   Luteal phase

0   2   4   6   8   10   12   14   16   18   20   22   24   26   28   2

Days of cycle

COLOR PLATE 6 Ovarian phases and endometrial development.

Esophagus

Small gastric pouch

Alimentary or Roux limb

Pylorus

Duodenum

Excluded portion of stomach

COLOR PLATE 7 Roux-en-Y bypass.

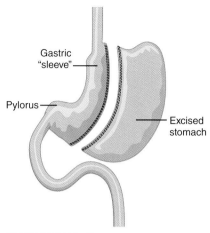

COLOR PLATE 8 Sleeve gastrectomy.

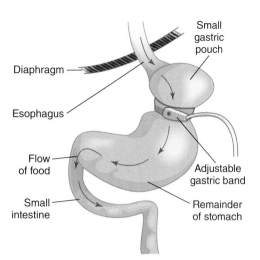

COLOR PLATE 9 Gastric banding.

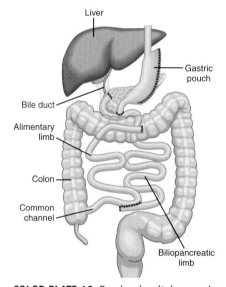

COLOR PLATE 10 Duodenal switch procedure.

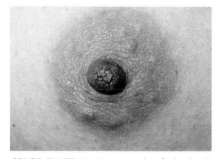

COLOR PLATE 11 An example of nipple discharge.
© Dr. H. C. Robinson/Science Source

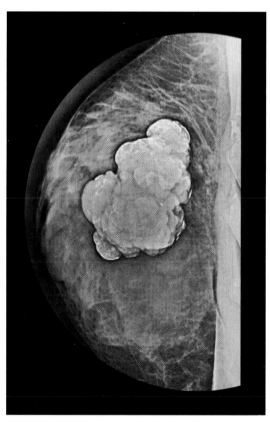

COLOR PLATE 12 An example of a breast mass.
© CNRI/Science Source

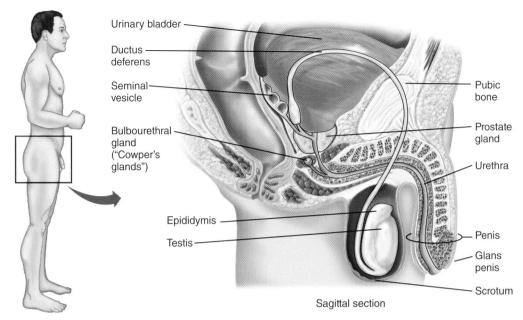

Urinary bladder

Ductus deferens

Seminal vesicle

Bulbourethral gland ("Cowper's glands")

Epididymis

Testis

Pubic bone

Prostate gland

Urethra

Penis

Glans penis

Scrotum

Sagittal section

COLOR PLATE 13 Midsagittal view of the male reproductive organs.

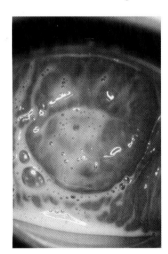

COLOR PLATE 14 An example of vaginal discharge from trichomoniasis.
© ISM/Phototake

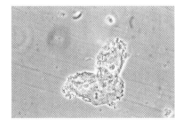

COLOR PLATE 15 A micrograph of bacterial vaginosis.
Courtesy of CDC/M. Rein.

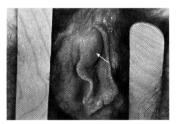

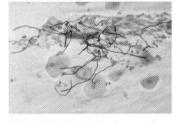

COLOR PLATE 16 A micrograph of vulvovaginal candidiasis.
Courtesy of CDC.

COLOR PLATE 17 Bartholin's cyst.
Courtesy of CDC/Susan Lindsley.

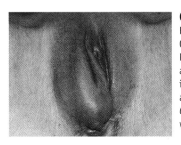

COLOR PLATE 18 Bartholin's abscess.
Reproduced from Ozdegirmenci, O., Kayikcioglu, F., & Haberal, A. (2009). Prospective randomized study of marsupialization versus silver nitrate application in the management of Bartholin gland cysts and abscesses. *Journal of Minimally Invasive Gynecology, 16*(2), 149–152. Copyright 2009, with permission from Elsevier.

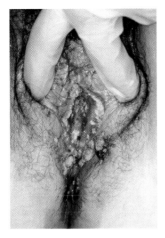

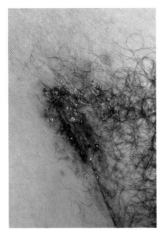

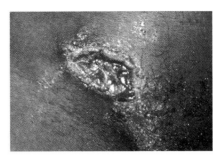

COLOR PLATE 21 Chancroid lesion.
Courtesy of CDC/J. Pledger.

COLOR PLATE 19 Genital warts.
Courtesy of CDC/Joe Millar.

COLOR PLATE 20 Genital herpes lesions.
© Dr. P. Marazzi/Science Source

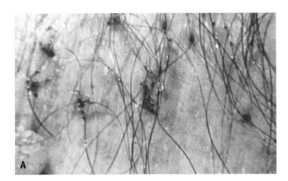

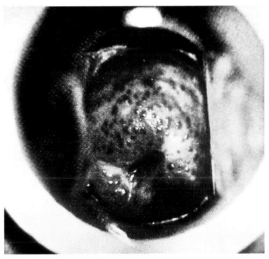

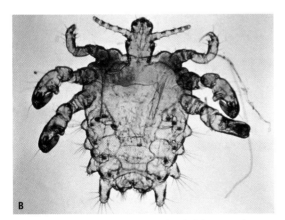

COLOR PLATE 23 Cervical petechiae with trichomoniasis.
Courtesy of CDC.

COLOR PLATE 22 Pediculosis pubis (A) is caused by *Phthirus pubis* (B).
A. Courtesy of CDC/Joe Miller. B. Courtesy of CDC/WHO.

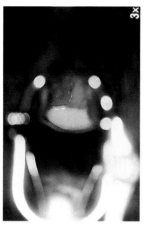

COLOR PLATE 24 Chlamydial mucopurulent cervical discharge.
Courtesy of CDC.

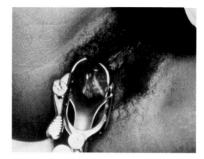

COLOR PLATE 25 Gonorrheal mucopurulent cervical discharge.
Courtesy of CDC.

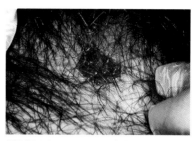

COLOR PLATE 26A Syphilitic chancre (primary syphilis).
Courtesy of CDC/Joe Miller/Dr. N.J. Fiumara.

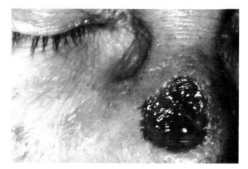

COLOR PLATE 26C A gumma, which is a soft noncancerous growth resulting from the tertiary stage of syphilis.
Courtesy of CDC/J. Pledger.

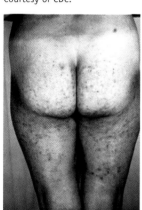

COLOR PLATE 26B Syphilitic rash (secondary syphilis).
Courtesy of CDC/J. Pledger, BSS, VD.

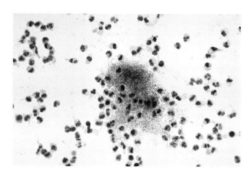

COLOR PLATE 27 Urine microscopy for a urinary tract infection.
© Dr. Frederick Skvara/Visuals Unlimited, Inc.

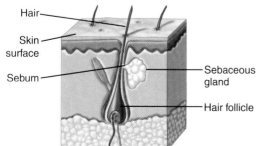

Hair
Skin surface
Sebum
Sebaceous gland
Hair follicle

COLOR PLATE 28 Normal pilosebaceous unit.
Modified from National Institute of Arthritis and Musculoskeletal and Skin Diseases. (2015). Questions and answers about acne. NIH Publication No. 15-4998. Retrieved from http://www.niams.nih.gov/Health_Info/Acne/default.asp.

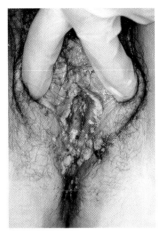

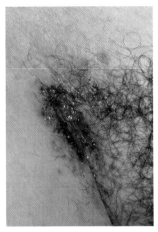

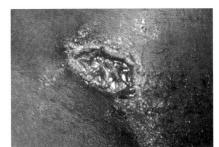

COLOR PLATE 21 Chancroid lesion.
Courtesy of CDC/J. Pledger.

COLOR PLATE 19 Genital warts.
Courtesy of CDC/Joe Millar.

COLOR PLATE 20 Genital herpes lesions.
© Dr. P. Marazzi/Science Source

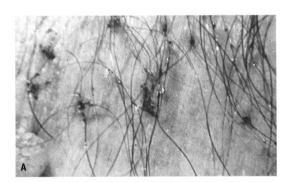

A

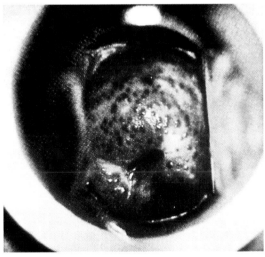

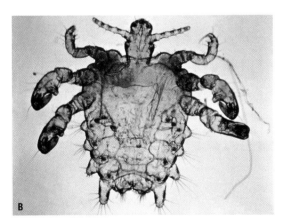

B

COLOR PLATE 23 Cervical petechiae with trichomoniasis.
Courtesy of CDC.

COLOR PLATE 22 Pediculosis pubis (A) is caused by *Phthirus pubis* (B).
A. Courtesy of CDC/Joe Miller. B. Courtesy of CDC/WHO.

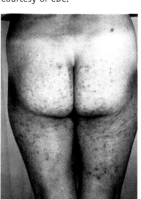

COLOR PLATE 24 Chlamydial mucopurulent cervical discharge.
Courtesy of CDC.

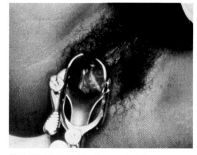

COLOR PLATE 25 Gonorrheal mucopurulent cervical discharge.
Courtesy of CDC.

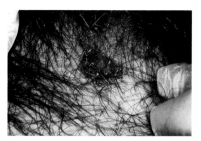

COLOR PLATE 26A Syphilitic chancre (primary syphilis).
Courtesy of CDC/Joe Miller/Dr. N.J. Fiumara.

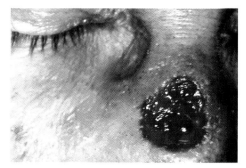

COLOR PLATE 26C A gumma, which is a soft noncancerous growth resulting from the tertiary stage of syphilis.
Courtesy of CDC/J. Pledger.

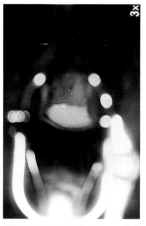

COLOR PLATE 26B Syphilitic rash (secondary syphilis).
Courtesy of CDC/J. Pledger, BSS, VD.

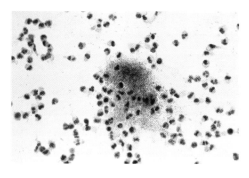

COLOR PLATE 27 Urine microscopy for a urinary tract infection.
© Dr. Frederick Skvara/Visuals Unlimited, Inc.

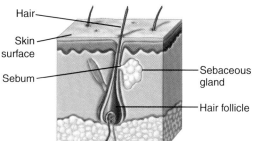

Hair
Skin surface
Sebum
Sebaceous gland
Hair follicle

COLOR PLATE 28 Normal pilosebaceous unit.
Modified from National Institute of Arthritis and Musculoskeletal and Skin Diseases. (2015). Questions and answers about acne. NIH Publication No. 15-4998. Retrieved from http://www.niams.nih.gov/Health_Info/Acne/default.asp.

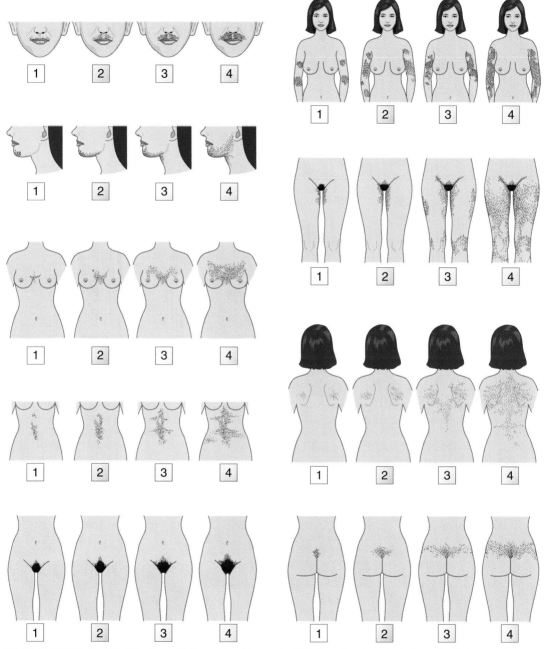

COLOR PLATE 29 Modified Ferriman–Gallwey hirsutism scale. This is a visual method of scoring hair growth in women, modified from the original scale reported by Ferriman and Gallwey in 1961. Each of the nine areas is given a score ranging from 0 (no hair) to 4 (extensive terminal hair). The scores for each of the nine areas are totaled, and a score of 8 or greater indicates hirsutism.

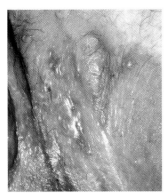

COLOR PLATE 30
Genital hidradenitis
suppurativa.
© Mediscan/Visuals
Unlimited, Inc.

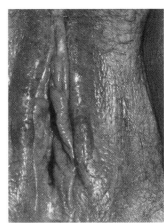

COLOR PLATE 31
Irritant contact
dermatitis.
Reproduced from
Stewart, K.M. (2010).
Clinical care of vulvar
pruritis, with emphasis
on one common
cause, lichen simplex
chronicus. *Dermatologic
Clinics, 28*(4),
669–680. Copyright
2010, with permission
from Elsevier.

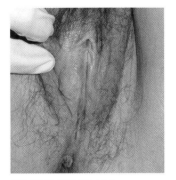

COLOR PLATE 32 Lichen
sclerosus.
Courtesy of Rylander, E. (2007).
Lichen sclerosis. Retrieved from
www.issvd.org.

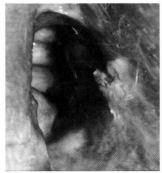

COLOR PLATE 33 Lichen planus.
Courtesy of Rylander, E. (2007).
Lichen planus: Type 3 (erosive).
Retrieved from www.issvd.org.

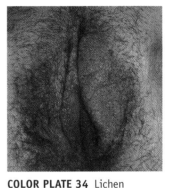

COLOR PLATE 34 Lichen
simplex chronicus.
Reproduced from Stewart, K.M.
(2010). Clinical care of vulvar
pruritis, with emphasis on one
common cause, lichen simplex
chronicus. *Dermatologic Clinics,
28*(4), 669-680. Copyright 2010,
with permission from Elsevier.

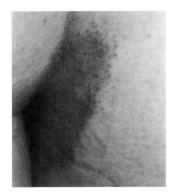

COLOR PLATE 35 Genital
psoriasis.
Reproduced from Stewart, K.M.
(2010). Clinical care of vulvar
pruritis, with emphasis on one
common cause, lichen simplex
chronicus. *Dermatologic Clinics,
28*(4), 669–680. Copyright 2010,
with permission from Elsevier.

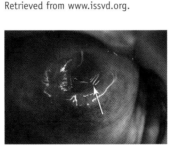

COLOR PLATE 36 Cervical polyp.
© Dr. P. Marazzi/Science Source

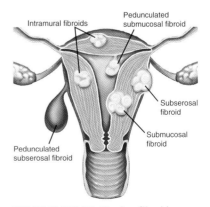

Intramural fibroids

Pedunculated
submucosal fibroid

Subserosal
fibroid

Submucosal
fibroid

Pedunculated
subserosal fibroid

COLOR PLATE 37 Uterine fibroids,
classification by location.